M

Palliative Care Nursing

Quality Care to the **End of Life**

Marianne Matzo, PhD, GNP-BC, FPCN, FAAN, is Professor and Frances E. and A. Earl Ziegler Chair in Palliative Care Nursing at the University of Oklahoma Health Sciences Center College of Nursing in Oklahoma City. She also is an Adjunct Professor in the Department of Geriatric Medicine, the University of Oklahoma College of Medicine; a member of the Doctoral Faculty at the Union Institute and University, Cincinnati, Ohio; and a Soros Scholar for the Project on Death in America. She was awarded a doctorate in Gerontology from the University of Massachusetts–Boston and a master's degree in nursing from the Gerontological Nurse Practitioner program at the University of Massachusetts–Lowell. Her funded research explores issues of sexual health promotion and assessment in patients receiving hospice and palliative care. Dr. Matzo has presented educational programs regionally, nationally, and internationally on many topics related to care of the dying person, gerontological nursing, and curriculum development. She has authored four books, including two published by Springer Publishing, 23 book chapters, and 42 peer-reviewed publications.

Deborah Witt Sherman, PhD, APRN, ANP-BC, ACHPN, FAAN, is Professor and Assistant Dean of Research at the University of Maryland School of Nursing and Assistant Director of the Developing Center for Excellence in Palliative Care Research. Dr. Sherman is also a member of the Palliative Care Consultation Service at the University of Maryland Medical Center. In 2009, Dr. Sherman received the Hospice and Palliative Care Nurses Association's "Leading the Way Award," which recognizes her implementation of the first Palliative Care Nurse Practitioner Program in the United States. Dr. Sherman also serves as faculty of Tenshi College in Hakkaido, Japan, where she implemented Japan's first Palliative Care Masters Program in Nursing.

Dr. Sherman's education includes a BSN from Mount Saint Mary's College, Newburgh, New York; a master's degree from Pace University, Tarrytown, New York; a doctoral degree in nursing from New York University, and a post-master's certificate in adult health from New York University. She was awarded the Prestigious Project on Death in America Faculty Scholars Fellowship, funded by the Soros Foundation. Dr. Sherman served for seven years as the co-director of the Bronx VA Medical Center Interprofessional Palliative Care Fellowship Program. Dr. Sherman received a Post-Doctoral AIDS Research Fellowship Award from the Aaron Diamond Foundation and has had two studies funded by the National Institutes of Health. Dr. Sherman has been faculty for the End of Life Nursing Education Consortium (ELNEC), and served as a member of the steering committee in developing the National Consensus Guidelines for Quality Palliative Care. She is a member of several nursing and palliative care editorial boards and has published numerous data-based and other scholarly articles and books related to palliative care.

Palliative Care Nursing

Quality Care to the **End of Life**

EDITORS

Marianne Matzo, PhD, GNP-BC, FPCN, FAAN
Deborah Witt Sherman, PhD, APRN, ANP-BC, ACHPN, FAAN

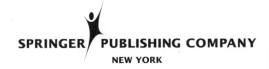

SPRINGER PUBLISHING COMPANY
NEW YORK

Springer Publishing Company, LLC.
11 West 42nd Street
New York, NY 10036
www.springerpub.com

Acquistions Editor: Margaret Zuccarini
Cover design: Bill Smith Group
Composition: Six Red Marbles

E-book ISBN: 978-0-8261-5792-8

10 11 12 13 / 5 4 3 2 1

The author and the publisher of this Work have made every effort to use sources believed to be reliable to provide information that is accurate and compatible with the standards generally accepted at the time of publication. Because medical science is continually advancing, our knowledge base continues to expand. Therefore, as new information becomes available, changes in procedures become necessary. We recommend that the reader always consult current research and specific institutional policies before performing any clinical procedure. The author and publisher shall not be liable for any special, consequential, or exemplary damages resulting in whole or in part, from the readers' use of, or reliance on, the information contained in this book. The publisher has no responsibility for the persistence or accuracy of URLs for external or third-party Internet Web sites referred to in this publication and does not guarantee that any content on such Web sites is, or will remain, accurate or appropriate.

Library of Congress Cataloging-in-Publication Data

Palliative care nursing: quality care to the end of life/Marianne LaPorte Matzo, Deborah Witt Sherman [editors].—3rd ed.

    p.; cm.

Includes bibliographical references and index. ISBN 0-8261-5794-7 (hc)

  1. Terminal care. 2. Palliative treatment.
  [DNLM: 1. Terminal Care. 2. Hospice Care—psychology. 3. Palliative Care. WY 152 P1677 2005] I. Matzo, Marianne. II. Sherman, Deborah Witt.

RT87.T45P343 2005
616.02[H11032]9—dc22   2005051706

Printed in the United States by Bang Printing

Contents

SECTION I

CARING FOR THE WHOLE PERSON IN PALLIATIVE CARE

SECTION II

SOCIAL AND PROFESSIONAL ISSUES IN PALLIATIVE CARE

SECTION III

PSYCHOSOCIAL CONSIDERATIONS

SECTION IV

PHYSICAL ASPECTS OF DYING

Contributors

Elizabeth A. Ayello, PhD, RN, ACNS-BC, ETN, FAPWCA, FAAN
Faculty
Excelsior College School of Nursing
Albany, NY

Cindy R. Balkstra, MS, RN, CNS-BC
President
Georgia Nurses Association
Atlanta, GA

Marilyn Bookbinder PhD, RN
Director of Nursing
Beth Israel Medical Center
New York, NY

Mary Brennan, M.S., ACNP-BC
Clinical Assistant Professor
New York University
New York

Nessa Coyle, NP, PhD
Pain and Palliative Care Service
Memorial Sloan-Kettering Cancer Center
New York, NY

Constance M. Dahlin, MS, APRN, BC, ACHPN, FAAN
Advanced Practice Nurse – Palliative Care Services
Massachusetts General Hospital
Boston, MA

Robert B. Davis, RN, FNP
University of Virginia Health System
Charlottesville, VA

Judith B. Dyne, MS, RN, APRN, BC
Assistant Professor of Nursing
Utica College
Utica, NY

Amy E. Guthrie, MSN, APRN, CNP/CNS, ACHPN
OHSU Palliative Medicine/Comfort Care Team
Portland, OR

Jane A. Hill, MS, RN
Associate Professor
The University of Oklahoma Health Sciences Center
Oklahoma City, OK

Christine Kovach, PhD, RN
Professor
University of Wisconsin
Milwaukee, WI

Lisa M. Krammer, RN, MSN, ANP, AOCN, ACHPN
Palliative Care Nurse Practitioner
Northwestern Memorial Hospital
Chicago, IL

Mary Layman-Goldstein, RN, MS, ANP-BC, ACHPN
Nurse Practitioner
Pain and Palliative Care Service
Memorial Sloan-Kettering Cancer Center
New York, NY

Pamala D. Larson, RN, PhD, CRRN, FNGNA
Associate Dean and Professor
University of Wyoming
Laramie, WY

Judy Lentz, RN, MSN, NHA
CEO
Hospice and Palliative Nurses Association
Pittsburgh, PA

Carla Mariano, EdD, RN, AHN-C, FAAIM
Professor
New York University
New York, NY

Jeanne Martinez, RN, MPH, CRNH
Quality Specialist
Palliative Care & Home Hospice Program
Northwestern Memorial Hospital
Chicago, IL

Polly Mazanec, PhD, APRN, BC, AOCN
Palliative Care Advanced Care Practice Nurse
Hospice of the Western Reserve
Cleveland, OH

Marlene McHugh, DNP-C, FNP-BC, RN
Associate Director of Palliative Care Service
Montefiore Medical Center
New York, NY

Kathleen Ouimet Perrin, PhD, RN, CCRN
Professor
Department of Nurshing
St. Anselm College
Manchester, NH

Lynn R. Noland, PhD, FNP
Assistant Professor
School of Nursing
University of Virginia
Charlottesville, VA

Mertie L. Potter, ND, APRN, DC
Associate Professor
Department of Nursing
St. Anselm College
Manchester, NH

Sheila Reynolds, MS, GCNS, BC
University of Wisconsin
Milwaukee, WI

Eileen A. Ring-Hurn, RN, MS, CMT
Nurse Educator
Seven Rivers Regional Medical Center
Crystal River, FL

Judith Schwartz, PhD, RN
Nurse Ethicist, Consultant – End of Life
New York, NY

R. Gary Sibbald, BSc, MD, FRCPC (Med Derm) MACP DABD, Med FAPWCA
Director of Medical Education & Wound Clinic
Women's College Hospital
Toronto, Ontario
Canada

Patsy R. Smith, PhD, RN
Assistant Professor
The University of Oklahoma Health Sciences Center
Oklahoma City, OK

Anita J. Tarzian, PhD, RN
Ethics and Research Consultant
Baltimore, MD

Mary Beth Williams, RN, MN
Vice President, Operations
Access Community Health Network
Chicago, IL

Kevin Y. Woo, PhD, MSc, RN, ACNP, GNC(C)
Lecturer
Department of Public Health Sciences
University of Toronto
Toronto, Ontario
Canada

Foreword:
Extending the Embrace of Palliative Nursing

The field of palliative nursing began relatively recently, yet the demands of society have resulted in rapid advancement to maturity in this dimension of health care. Nurses led the introduction of hospice in America and similarly have pioneered palliative care programs, working with interdisciplinary teams to transform systems of care which are unprepared to care for the seriously ill.

Palliative nursing continues to evolve and extend its embrace to all ages, disease groups, and settings of care. Nurses have known since the introduction of hospice in America in the 1970s that the philosophy of comfort-focused care should be extended to many vulnerable populations at a time of life often characterized by its suffering rather than as a time that honors a life and the sacred nature of life's end.

This textbook has mirrored the advancement of palliative nursing. It acknowledges that palliative care nursing cures what can be cured, relieves suffering through effective pain and symptom management as well as spiritual support, and continuously offers comfort. The previous editions introduced concepts and methods of education which helped to move palliative nursing forward as an evidenced-based practice of whole person care. This edition is an important advance and Matzo and Sherman have extended the embrace of palliative nursing by addressing the life span needs of people facing illness and eventual death, and have focused on the palliative care needs of patients with various life–threatening illnesses. The contributors have strengthened this embrace through clinically insightful discussions of the most important concerns expressed by patients and families experiencing life–threatening illness. You, the readers of this book, are a part of the history of this evolving profession. Through this text, we collectively celebrate the embrace of palliative care nursing.

Betty Ferrell, PhD, FAAN
Research Scientist

Palliative care is a philosophy of care that provides a combination of disease-modifying and supportive, compassionate therapies intended to alleviate pain and other symptoms while addressing the emotional, social, cultural, and spiritual needs of patients and families who are experiencing life-threatening progressive illness (National Consensus Project, 2009). The current trend is toward the integration of hospice and palliative care and the inclusion not only of individuals with cancer or AIDS, but also of patients with end-stage organ diseases, neurodegenerative diseases, and dementia. Palliative care is offered from the time of diagnosis with advanced disease until death, and continues for families during the bereavement period.

As Project on Death in America Faculty Scholars, the editors have assumed the responsibility in their roles as nurse practitioners, educators, and researchers to work collaboratively with nursing colleagues in developing, implementing, and evaluating nursing initiatives in palliative care within the United States, as well as internationally.

Palliative Care Nursing: Quality Care to the End of Life, in the first, second, and third editions, has been written as a contribution to the initiatives of the nursing profession regarding palliative care. This third edition of *Palliative Care Nursing* addresses content, knowledge, attitudes, and skills, which address the undergraduate and graduate AACN End-of-Life nursing competencies. This text is applicable to students, to educators, and to practicing nurses. Nursing students enrolled in advanced practice palliative care master's programs, including nurse practitioner, post-master's certificate, and clinical nurse specialist programs will find this book an asset in providing care to patients with complex physical, emotional, social, and spiritual needs across health care settings. With knowledge of advanced pathophysiology, pharmacology, and physical assessment, advanced practice palliative care nurses can prescribe a vast array of pharmacological and nonpharmacological interventions that are discussed in this book. Throughout the illness and dying trajectory, graduate nurses also assume leadership roles as members of interdisciplinary palliative-care teams and develop standards of care, clinical guidelines, and health care policies, and they serve as consultants in the development of clinical practice, education, and research initiatives. Advanced practice palliative care nurses also educate and mentor undergraduate-prepared nursing colleagues and participate in or develop research proposals to support evidence-based practice. The information presented in this text therefore will serve as a foundation to advanced palliative care competencies.

This text is organized to emphasize the importance of a holistic perspective and an understanding of the patient and family—as individuals with diverse spiritual and cultural needs and expectations. Section I addresses these more abstract needs of patients, families, and health care providers, with an emphasis on culture and spirituality and the value of complementary holistic modalities in promoting health, wholeness, and sexual health throughout the course of a serious illness and even as death approaches. In Section II, societal aspects of palliative and end-of-life care are discussed, including societal perspectives, the evolution of palliative care nursing, and ethical and legal issues. The psychological aspects of palliative care are addressed in Section III, including communication, the needs of family caregivers, and the experience of loss, grief, death, and bereavement. The four chapters in Section IV cover the physical aspects of living with a life-threatening illness, specifically information related to various disease states such as cancer, end-stage organ diseases, neurological disorders, and HIV/AIDS, as well as pain and symptom management and the needs and experiences of individuals who are seriously ill and dying. The authors believe that decisions regarding physical interventions at the end of life must be addressed on the basis of knowledge of the spiritual, social, and psychological beliefs, values, expectations, and wishes of the patient and family.

Comprising the largest number of health care professionals in the country, nurses have a tremendous potential to change the care of the dying and their families. Nursing professionals can capitalize on the individual's desire for autonomy and control of his or her life by reinforcing the importance and value of actively participating in the decisions at the end of life through advanced care planning. As nurses frame the discussion of illness, dying, and death within the context of hope and meaning and as an opportunity for choices and continued achievement of goals, uncertainty is replaced with certainty, hopelessness with faith, and despair with empowerment. The possibility exists that dying and death then will become one of the most meaningful and significant acts of life.

Palliative care nursing therefore offers an exquisite blend of holistic, humanistic caring coupled with aggressive management of pain and symptoms associated with advanced disease. Educational and research initiatives will transform the care offered to patients and families and improve their quality of life until death.

Through collaborative interdisciplinary care, patients and families can regain a sense of trust and security in knowing that their holistic needs are being addressed, and that a peaceful, respectful death is their right. Palliative care nursing promotes quality of life for patients and families who are experiencing life-threatening illness throughout the illness/dying trajectory and thereby has changed the experience of dying in America. The envisioned possibilities are that life-threatening illness and dying are recognized as opportunities for continued growth and transcendence., and for healing on emotional and spiritual levels.

Deborah Witt Sherman
Marianne Matzo

Caring for the Whole Person in Palliative Care

April 12

Today, I admitted Candy Harris to our home-care agency. Candy is a 42-year-old woman who until a month ago worked as a nurse with developmentally delayed children. She has been married to Ron for the last 20 years; a picture taken of them at their Senior Prom sits on a bookshelf. They have two children aged 5 and 8 years and live in a new neighborhood development. She seemed so sad when I arrived, but I would be, too, if I were in her situation. I find admissions like this so difficult; she is close to my age and we are so similar in other ways.

She tells me the history of her disease in a very matter-of-fact way. For the 9 months prior to her diagnosis, Candy had noticed increased flatus that had not gotten better, despite alterations in her diet. For the 2 months prior she said that she had little appetite, but still had gained 5 pounds. She felt bloated all the time and the waistbands of her clothes were tight. Her mother started menopause in her early 40's and died at age 56 of breast/ovarian cancer. Candy thought that her symptoms were related to the early start of menopause and so decided to visit her nurse practitioner for a physical exam and pap smear.

Given Candy's symptoms and her positive family history of cancer, the nurse practitioner ordered an abdominal CT scan in addition to a complete physical work-up. An ovarian mass was detected and Candy was scheduled for a laparotomy. Stage III ovarian cancer was diagnosed. The surgeon was able to use cytoreduction to decrease the tumor volume to <2 cm in diameter, and the oncologist suggested platinum-based combination chemotherapy. She was in shock that all this was happening to her so fast. The children were really too young to completely understand what was going on and her husband insisted that they were going to "fight this."

Candy had just finished her third cycle of chemotherapy. She is very weak and in need of home healthcare support. Candy was sitting in a chair in the living room when I arrived. Her hair had all fallen out and her eyes were red, as though she had been crying, and she was holding a rosary in her hand. One section of the wall was covered with get-well cards; she referred to this area as her "prayer wall." As I was assessing her, she burst into tears and told me that she thinks "God is punishing her for something" and that this is why she

has cancer. This was not the first time that I have heard this from a patient. Believing in the importance of atoning for her sins, Candy has been attending mass whenever she has the strength, praying the rosary regularly, and asking the church congregation to pray for her. She has gone to confession and received the "Sacrament of the Sick." She also admitted that she wanted to "cover all of her bases" and that she has turned to holistic interventions in addition to her chemotherapy so that her body, mind, and soul will also heal. After her initial diagnosis, she researched complementary interventions for cancer and started on a macrobiotic diet with additional B12 and D vitamins.

Candy receives Reiki twice a week and is seeing a therapist weekly. She said that she and her husband use mental imagery and relaxation techniques to imagine her body defenses as a powerful source to annihilate the cancer cells. Candy said that she has so much to live for, that she has a lot of good friends, a loving husband, and great kids. She really doesn't know what she has "done wrong" but she asks for God's forgiveness and hopes to get on with her life.

As a nurse, I marvel at her will to live and her determination to beat this disease. She seems to draw her strength from her religion and her relationships. Her strength is an inspiration to all who care for her.

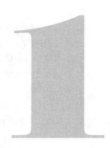

Culture and Spirituality as Domains of Quality Palliative Care

Deborah Witt Sherman

Key Points

- Culture and spirituality structure human experience, values, and behaviors.
- Spirituality provides a sense of connection to self, others, nature, and God and is important in crisis and illness.
- Cultural competence involves knowledge of your own and other cultural groups.
- Cultural assessment has several areas to be addressed.
- Palliative care addresses the cultural and spiritual needs of patients and families.
- Spirituality and religiosity help individuals to cope with serious illness and play a role in the dying process.
- Suffering is a part of the human condition and is experienced in physical, emotional, and spiritual ways.
- Suffering is reciprocal involving not only the patient but also his/her family.
- Hope plays a role in promoting spiritual well-being.
- Health professionals must learn how to conduct a spiritual assessment and have conversations about spiritual and religious issues.
- Spiritual care discovers, reverences, and tends to the human spirit.
- Knowledge of spiritual and religious perspectives on death informs spiritual care.
- Spiritually and culturally competent care requires self-reflection and self-care of health professionals.

Case Study: Mrs. Martinez is an 84-year-old Latino woman, who has progressive pain and weakness due to sensory neuropathy, secondary to diabetes and arthritis. During the course of her illness, she has maintained her independence and good spirits. Mrs. M. believes that her faith in God has enabled her to endure her chronic pain. She states "Sometimes I pray when I am in deep, serious pain. I pray and all at once the pain gets easy. I feel it has helped me more than the medication. I believe in God. He is my guide and protector." Mrs. Martinez lives with her daughter, son-in-law, and grandchildren.

They are a source of comfort and support and are very concerned about her well-being. Unfortunately, Mrs. Martinez recently had a stroke, which resulted in left hemiplegia. After an initial hospital stay, her family insisted that they care for her at home. On a visit to their home, the healthcare professional observes a shrine of Mary in the front yard, as well as crucifixes and pictures of Jesus in every room. In addition to traditional medications prescribed by her physician, Mrs. Martinez takes herbal remedies in an attempt to restore her health. The healthcare professional acknowledges the cultural and spiritual values and beliefs of Mrs. Martinez as considerations in providing quality palliative care.

Introduction

Culture and spirituality are among the most important factors that structure human experience, values, behaviors, and illness patterns. As a system of shared symbols and beliefs, culture supports a person's sense of security, integrity, and belonging and provides a prescription for how to conduct life and approach death (End of Life Nursing Education Consortium (ELNEC), 2001). Every culture has a worldview or construct of reality that defines the individual within that reality. Patients' cultural backgrounds are therefore fundamental in defining and creating their reality and determining their purpose in life (Ersek, Kagawa-Singer, Barnes, Blackhall, & Koenig, 1998). A transformation of identity begins when an individual is diagnosed with a terminal illness. Cultural rituals provide the sacred elements that support patients and families during times of illness and transition. Specific rituals assist individuals and families in coping with death, which is the final transition in life. The rituals of death change the identity of the patient from the living to the dead, and also the identity of the family member, for example, from spouse to widow or widower (Kagawa-Singer, 1998). Culture provides a framework of expectations about communication with others including health professionals and the role of family, and influences the dynamics of decision making regarding health issues and the dying process itself (Barclay, Blackhall, & Tulksy, 2007).

Spirituality plays a vital role in times of crisis and illness, as it provides a sense of connection to self, others, nature, and God, and is a means to cope with loss, grief, and death (Weaver, Flannelly, & Flannelly, 2001). Life-threatening illness is a crisis on many levels-physical, psychological, familial, social, and spiritual (Doka & Morgan, 1993). Given the uniqueness and individuality of each person, even people of the same culture and spirituality may have different backgrounds, experiences, needs, concerns, and interpretation of illness. In addition to the individuality of the person, the nature of the life-threatening illness may be different and the person may be at different points in adapting to the reality of the disease. Spiritual and cultural concerns may permeate the illness experience or may arise at any point across the illness/dying trajectory. For patients and families who are experiencing life-threatening illness, the concerns may be of suffering that may take multiple forms relative to the mind-body-spirit. It is now recognized that the uncertain and long-term nature of many life-threatening illnesses pose the potential for pain, alterations in body image, and confrontation with death, which may lead to spiritual distress. The renewed focus on incorporating spiritual care into nursing practice is congruent with nursing's commitment to holistic practice and the renewed valuing of human experiences that defy scientific description and explanation (O'Neill & Kenny, 1998). Within the past few years, research has shown that religious beliefs and spiritual practices affect the meaning of illness, physical and emotional well-being, coping with illness, and healthcare decisions, particularly for individuals facing life-threatening illness.

Spiritual and cultural competences are central tenets of palliative care. As a philosophy of care, palliative care combines active and compassionate therapies to support and comfort individuals and families who are living with life-threatening illness. Palliative care strives to meet the physical, psychological, social, and spiritual expectations and needs, while remaining sensitive to personal, cultural, and religious beliefs and practices (National Consensus Project, 200 9). Undergraduate-prepared nurses and advanced-practice nurses must become spiritually and culturally competent in the care they offer across the illness/dying trajectory. Such care is critical to enhancing the quality of life and quality of dying and to supporting the intrinsic dignity of patients and their families.

Understanding Culture

Culture is defined as a way of life, which provides a worldview, fundamental in defining and creating a person's reality, determining his/her meaning and purpose in life, and providing guidelines for living (Ersek et al., 1998). As cultural perspectives evolve, changes are evident in the beliefs, values, and attitudes of a cultural group or its members. Cultures are not monolithic, but rather there is a range of potential responses to each issue in every cultural group. Thus, there may be within-group variations, such as those attributed to acculturation differences, as well as to differences related to age, education, geographic location, and social context (Kagawa-Singer & Blackhall, 2001; Barclay et al., 2007). It is important to inquire whether an individual patient adheres to the beliefs and practices of his/her cultural group, rather than assuming that he/she holds the same values and beliefs (Crawley, Marshall, Lo, & Koenig, 2002).

Although culture is often identified with ethnicity, it is a far broader concept, which encompasses the components of gender, age, sexual orientation, differing abilities, educational level, employment, and place of residency (ELNEC, 2001). As examples, cultures may value male children more than female; the young more than the old, heterosexuals rather than homosexuals, the educated and employed more than the uneducated or unemployed; individuals with stable domiciles more than the homeless; and the healthy more than the physically, emotionally, or intellectually challenged. The diversity of the population with regard to many of these factors may increase their vulnerability in terms of perceived cultural status. Concepts of culture and ethnicity may be useful for making generalizations about populations; however, if they limit appreciation of the unique differences of people and are used to predict individual behavior, they may lead to stereotyping (Koenig, 2002).

Cultural background also relates to issues of power, decision making, language and communication, sources of support within the community, degree of fatalism or activism in accepting or controlling death, maintaining hope, and even views of the patient and family about death (Sherman, 2001). Cultural differences are further evident in terms of the relationship between the older adult and his/her family. In certain cultures, the older person is viewed as the patriarch or matriarch of the family who has the final word in personal and family matters. In other cultures, the older person defers decision making to members of the family, as interdependence among the family and community members is more valued than individual autonomy (Ersek et al., 1998). Dependent on cultural expectations, families may believe that it is their duty to protect the patient from bad news, which is believed to burden the individual or cause emotional distress or harm. Full disclosure of diagnosis and prognosis to the patient may therefore be considered harmful by families (Barclay et al., 2007). As the cultural diversity of patients and practitioners in the United States continues to increase, there is a risk for cross-cultural misunderstanding surrounding care at the end of life. Cross-cultural understanding and communication techniques increase the likelihood that both the process and outcome of healthcare are satisfactory for all involved (Kagawa-Singer & Blackhall, 2001).

CULTURAL PERSPECTIVES IN HEALTHCARE

Understanding the cultural backgrounds of patients is fundamental to the development of a trusting and supportive relationship between patient, family, and healthcare professionals, and essential in developing a plan for healthcare that is consistent with their cultural expectations and health beliefs. Andrews and Boyle (1995) discussed three types of health belief systems: magico-religious, biomedical, and holistic. In the magico-religious paradigm, a person believes that God or supernatural forces control health and illness. In the biomedical paradigm, to which most Americans subscribe, illness is believed to be caused by a disruption in physical or biochemical processes that can be manipulated by healthcare. In the holistic paradigm, health results from a balance or harmony among the elements of nature and illness is produced by disharmony. Examples of the magico-religious system is a Haitian patient who believes that his symptoms are caused by spirits, or the Mexican American who uses herbs, oils, incense, or religious figurines to drive away evil spirits or to relieve gastric pains. In the biomedical system, Americans or Europeans seek cure of illness through advanced medical technology and pharmacologic management. Based on the holistic belief system, a Chinese woman may attribute her headache to a stagnation of Qi, believing in the need for balance between Yin and Yang, while a Native American patient may wear a bag of herbs around his neck blessed by the medicine man to maintain his strength (Grossman, 1996).

Recognition of these health beliefs systems is evident in the healthcare practices of many cultures. The health beliefs of the African American, Chinese, Asian Indian, Latino and Hispanic, and Native American will be discussed on the basis of recent studies or cultural inquiries and provide a framework for offering culturally competent Hospice and palliative care to members of these cultural groups. The only truly accurate way to know what individuals believe in or the effect that their culture or religion plays in their life is to ask them. The following information will guide the nurse regarding areas to be assessed.

Cultural Perspectives of African-Americans

Within the African-American culture, there is a strong sense of community and of the importance of family, friends, and the church community as sources of support. The extended African-American family consists of mother, father, children, grandparents, aunts, uncles, nieces, nephews, and cousins with a willingness to accept all relatives regardless of their circumstances (McDavis, Parker, & Parker, 1995). Older adults are prized in the African-American family and they play key roles in the family, church, and community. Many grandparents accept the responsibility for rearing their grandchildren, while the parents of those children work or receive higher education. Children are taught to take care of their parents and to be devoted to them. In addition, older African-American family members play a significant role in passing on cultural values, customs, and traditions to the children (McDavis et al., 1995).

With respect to healthcare, African–Americans are often distrustful of the healthcare system, given a history of oppression from slavery and racism. Common themes of justice and respect have reinforced the importance of self-determination. In a study of attitudes, values, and questions of African Americans regarding participation in Hospice Programs, Taxis (2005) identified three main barriers: 1) a lack of information about Hospice and inaccurate assumptions regarding Hospice care; 2) cultural barriers resulting from an avoidance of discussions regarding end-of-life planning; and 3) institutional barrier resulting from a mistrust of the healthcare system. Bullock (2006) reported that even using a faith-based promotion model of advanced care planning, 75% of the 102 African–American participants refused to complete advance directives. The participant's decisions were based on such factors as spirituality, view of suffering, dying, and death, social support networks, and mistrust of the healthcare system. For African Americans, advance care planning conflicts with their beliefs and attitudes about fighting to the end, not giving up hope, and enduring suffering. In a study of 473 adults (220 blacks and 253 whites), Ludke and Smucker (2007) found that relative to whites, blacks were significantly less likely to consider Hospice if they were near the end of life even if their doctor recommended its use. However, blacks who had a prior exposure to Hospice and who trusted their doctor were more willing to consider Hospice.

Since family is central to the care of the dying, and with the assistance and supportive relationships established with church members and neighbors, there is a decreased need for outside support (Sherman, 2001). Given strong family loyalty, there is reluctance to hospitalize family members. As a measure of respect and devotion, elder African-Americans are placed in nursing homes only as a last resort (McDavis et al., 1995).

In the African–American culture, death is integrated into the totality of life. Ancestor worship involves the communion with the living dead through memories, and the deceased are remembered by name. When the deceased are no longer remembered by people alive, they become part of the anonymous dead, but by this time their spirit has been reborn in a new child (Sherman, 2001)

To explore the meaning of death and the experience of grieving, Abrums (2000) conducted life history interviews of nine church-going women, ranging in age from 19 to 82 years, from a small black storefront Baptist church in the Pacific Northwest. The findings indicated that the women in the church had been taught to be strong in the face of death and to handle their grief "head on." The women believed that they would one day be reunited with their loved ones. The terminology of dying was through use of the words "passed on," "passed away," or "died." Participants described many spirit visits for the purpose of offering warnings or as direct messages. Belief in an afterlife was sustained by day-to-day experiences of visions or messages from another world. It was believed that God spoke to them in many ways through premonitions, perceived as the voice of God. There was strong perception of the journey of life in which there was a job to do on earth and a purpose to one's life. No life was in vain. Time was needed to prepare for death and to make peace with God as dying individuals. Participants also described the importance of hope, acceptance, and responsibility to comfort the dying and the bereaved. Abrums (2000) concluded that health professionals should learn to value the spiritual beliefs and grieving behaviors of members of other cultures, rather than viewing them as maladaptive. Supporting the dying and their family in their beliefs is important in providing spiritual care. Verbal recognition of specific actions taken by family to support the dying provided a sense of comfort and support to the family in their grief. The people in this storefront church were often comforted by the recognition that God sustained them in times of adversity and God would protect their loved ones. This acknowledgement of the family's belief system by health professionals can augment the healing process during times of loss and grief.

Cultural Perspectives of the Chinese

In the Chinese culture, the primary theme related to social structure is the centrality of the family. From the centrality of the family arise cultural expectations, such as: 1) duty to family manifested by respect and reverence for parents; 2) conformance to family and societal norms and especially not bringing shame to the family; 3) family recognition through achievement; 4) emotional self-control manifested through reserved and formal public verbal and nonverbal communications; 5) family disagreement, or demands, kept to a minimum; 6) collectivism evidenced by people keeping a focus on the family and community over self; and 7) humility manifested by a lack of striving for individual achievement but achievement that is related to the family (Kemp & Chang, 2002).

Given the traditionally hierarchical and patriarchal family structure of the Chinese, the oldest adult male is the primary decision maker. In family matters, there is significant influence of elders. Health decisions may be made by the family, and are based on what is best not only for the elder patient but also for the family. In general, yes and no questions should be avoided as yes is considered to be the polite answer and is nearly always given.

In China, the primary religion is Buddhism. The essence of Buddhism is the Four Noble Truths, specifically that: 1) all sentient beings suffer; 2) the cause of suffering is desire manifested by attachment to life, security, and to others; 3) the way to end suffering is to cease to desire; and 4) the way to cease desire is to follow the Eightfold path of: knowledge of the Four Noble Truths, right intent, right speech, right action, right endeavor, right mindfulness, and right meditation. It is believed that following the Eightfold Path leads to emancipation from rebirth (Kemp & Chang, 2002).

In the Chinese culture, it is also important to understand the importance of balance of the Yin and Yang, which are complementary forces. A second important concept is that of traditional Chinese medicine (TCM), which is based on channel (meridian) systems, in which various body channels carry vital or life energy called chi. Imbalance or disruption of channels leads to illness and the treatment goal of TCM is to restore balance. A third important concept in understanding Chinese approaches to health and illness is the use of allopathic medicine, as well as TCM.

Issues central to the care of the Chinese at the end of life center around family and communications (Kemp & Chang, 2002). Symptom management may be complicated by patient's and family's reluctance to complain because of respect for others in position of authority. Concerns also center around fears of addiction, desire to be a good patient, and fear of distracting the physician from treating the disease. In some cases, elders may even deny symptoms when asked directly; however, the use of the visual analog scale and numeric rating scale can be used to assess pain. For example, patients may want to keep warm during illness by wearing sweaters or socks in bed and drinking warm liquids and avoiding cold drinks. As death nears, the family may wish to call monks or nuns for ritual prayers (Kemp & Chang, 2002).

Communications at the end of life are also complicated by reluctance to discuss prognosis and diagnosis. Chinese families often withhold information from patients and may pretend that he/she does not know what is happening. Families believe that discussing end-of-life issues is like wishing death upon the elder, or may lead to hopelessness, especially since terminal illness is not socially accepted. As death approaches, it is believed that a person's final days should be characterized by calm and the patient should not be involved in decision making. The best way to handle the conspiracy of silence is to ask the patient to whom the information should be given and who should make decisions. Families often feel it is their cultural obligation to care for the person who is dying, and, therefore, Hospice services are often refused (Kemp & Chang, 2002).

The best way to handle the conspiracy of silence is to ask the patient to whom the information should be given and who should make decisions. Families often feel it is their cultural obligation to care for the person who is dying, and, therefore, Hospice services are often refused (Kemp & Chang, 2002).

Cultural Perspectives of (Asian) Indians

Among (Asian) Indians, extended families are prevalent and elders are highly respected. The husband's parents often move in with family after retirement, when the family decides to have children, or if there is illness. Elders are highly valued, as is their role as grandparents in raising children. Value is placed on independence and privacy in Indian culture, and family issues are discussed within the immediate family before outside help is sought (Bhungalia & Kemp, 2002). Healthcare decisions usually require family input.

Many Indians are of the Hindu faith. The goal of Hinduism is to free the soul from endless incarnation and suffering inherent in existence. The endless reincarnations of the soul are the result of karma or actions of the individual in this present life and the accumulation of actions from past lives.

The caste system is part of Hinduism. In this system, society is divided into four social classes: the highest class is the priest class, or Brahmans, and the lowest class is the laborer class, or Sudras. A person's class is inherited at birth based on his/her karma. Hindu beliefs that may affect patient care include the following:

- Karma or the consequences of one's actions or behaviors, which influences the circumstances of life and may have caused an illness;
- The importance of meditation and prayer; and
- The practice of vegetarianism in which Hindus pray a specific prayer before eating to ask forgiveness for eating a plant or vegetable in which a soul may dwell.

The Indian system of medicine is known as Ayurveda, which means knowledge of life. Indian medicine mixes religion and secular medicine, with more than

80% of people in India relying on herbal remedies to cure or prevent illness. In this system, the root of disease is not always inside the body, but may be related to the environment or other factors. In the Ayurveda system, the body comprises three primary forces, called dosha, specifically the Vata, Pitta, and Kapha. Each represents characteristics derived from the five elements of space, air, fire, water, and earth; the balance between these forces is essential to health. Once there is imbalance between the forces, balance is sought using different therapies, which includes approximately 1400 plants used in Ayurvedic medicine. Most Indians eat two to three meals a day, eating with the fingers of their right hand, and avoiding distractions while eating, such as watching television or excessive talking. Some foods are considered hot and others cold and should not be eaten in combination, as it is believed to affect bodily functions.

With respect to end-of-life care, it is important for the ill individual to complete unfinished business and resolve relationships. Home is the preferred place of death, with many family members present. Symptoms may not be reported, as it is believed that suffering is inevitable and the result of karma. Many seek a conscious dying process without mental clouding from medications. As death approaches, the following rituals are valued:

- A lamp may be placed near the patient's head; turn the body to face east, towards Mecca; sacred ash may be applied to the forehead.
- A few drops of water from the sacred Ganges River may be placed in the dying person's mouth, while a mantra is softly chanted in the patient's right ear.
- Prayer and incense are part of the rituals of the dying process.

After death, family members should be the only ones to touch the body, and ideally a family member of the same sex should clean the body. After the body is cleansed, a cloth is tied under the chin and over the top of the head, and the body is wrapped in red cloth. Embalming and organ donation are prohibited, and there is a preference for cremation. Following the death, religious pictures at home are turned toward the wall and mirrors may be covered. It is believed that for 12 days the soul wanders in the home, trying to let go of life and the material world. During this time, the family prays and chants, and on the 12th day, the soul is reincarnated (Bhungalia & Kemp, 2002).

Cultural Perspectives of Latinos and Hispanics

The cultural group referred to as Latinos refers to individuals of Hispanic background. By conducting 10 focus groups and interviews with 17 gatekeepers in Latino communities, Sullivan (2001) identified Latino views regarding end-of-life care. The results indicated that many Latinos felt that they could not communicate effectively with healthcare providers due to language barriers, and were not able to understand informed consent even when interpreters were used. None of the Latino participants wanted to die in a nursing home, believing that it is the families' responsibility to care for their relative. Most participants were also not aware of Hospice services or had false information. Although participants expressed diverse views, one third of participants were against the use of life support, particularly if it prolonged the suffering of the patient. Participants also believed that their religious beliefs, especially fatalism and reliance on God, were central to their decision making regarding end-of-life care. There was division among the participants regarding the extent to which they wanted to be informed about a fatal diagnosis, citing that being informed may accelerate the illness. Many Latinos also perceived racial discrimination and cultural insensitivity as barriers to quality care and healing (Sullivan, 2001).

In the Hispanic culture, there are several considerations that relate to quality care at the end of life (Sherman, 2001). It is recognized that in Hispanic culture, there is strong family support and a belief that the dying person should be protected from his/her prognosis. Women show extreme grief or hysteria, while men show little or no grief. Death is often confronted with a humorous sarcasm and is viewed as an equalizer (DeSpelder & Strickland, 1999). Mexican Americans, as well as other Hispanics, are likely to call the priest for the sacrament of the sick, and the bereaved may take shifts being with the deceased person. There is strong support of family as a unit. The funeral is the single most important family ceremony and goes on for several days, as there is the belief that it takes time to grieve. Individuals are prohibited from speaking ill of the person who has died, and the bereaved visit the grave frequently. The day of the dead is celebrated in November and coincides with All Saints' Day, the feast of the commemoration of the dead. Although death is viewed as an adversity, references to dying and death are common in the culture as children play with toys symbolizing death, and the funeral is an important family ceremony. It is a time of celebration with special foods, music, and the decoration of graves. It is believed that the dead return to the world of the living for this special celebration, and families are scorned if they neglect their responsibilities. The bereaved are discouraged from crying too many tears, as excessive grief may make the pathway traveled on by the dead slippery and burden them in the journey (DeSpelder & Strickland, 1999).

Given that cultural values profoundly influence the experience of health and illness for individuals, Martinez (1995) conducted a qualitative study of 14 Hispanic participants, ranging in age from 60 to 89, along with 6 health professionals and 2 clergy who practice in the community. They perceived health as creating balance in life and as faith that one will be cared for by God, family, and community. Participants held holistic views of self and emphasized the spiritual aspects of life in relation to health. Mental health was described as knowing what is right, living a life consistent with one's beliefs and values, trusting that life will work out, and maintaining faith in God. Caring for self was through caring for others for whom one had responsibility. In dealing with illness, there was a blending of modern medicine and traditional healing remedies. It was also appropriate to include family members in making health decisions.

Cultural Perspectives of Native Americans

For Native Americans, the focus of identity is on the tribe, rather than having simply Native American ancestry. This is important because values and beliefs vary among tribes and the different bands among the "First Nations." There may be similarities in nations originating in the same region, but there are also tribal distinctions (Brokenleg & Middleton, 1993). For many Native Americans, however, life and death are viewed as a natural part of the life cycle and as a part of human existence. Time is considered as a recurring cycle, rather than a linear process. Native Americans are concerned with how this cycle affects people in this life, and death is viewed as a motivation to treat people kindly and lead a good life (Brokenleg & Middleton, 1993; Sherman, 2001).

From a cultural perspective, Native Americans avoid eye contact and are stoic regarding the expression pain and suffering, and traditional tribal medicines are used (Sherman, 2001). Prayer is a medium through which one might accept the outcome of a situation, and it is not appropriate to question "why" something is happening, as there is an acceptance of the natural order of things (Brokenleg & Middleton, 1993). Death may be forecast by unusual spiritual or physical events. As examples, the sign of an owl may signify that someone close will soon die, and a blue light seen coming from the direction of a dead relative's home or room indicates death (Brokenleg & Middleton, 1993).

Given their reverence for the body in life and death, autopsies and cremation are not acceptable (Sherman, 2004a). Funerals are usually at home, with members of the community expected to stay with the mourners. A death song is sung that represents the summary of a person's life and acknowledgment of death. The dead are considered guardian spirits. After death, the spirit lingers near the site of the death for several days. Native Americans use a funeral pyre and adorn the corpse with flowers, feathers, and skins. For 6 months to 1 year, the name of the deceased is not called, in order to confirm their separation from the living. All material possessions of the deceased are given away so that the family can begin its new life without the presence of that person (Brokenleg & Middleton, 1993). In the Cocopa tribe, violent grief is expressed until cremation, when they invite the spirits to join them in celebration. In the Hopi tribe, death is kept at a distance because it threatens order and control. The expression of grief remains limited and funerals are attended by few and held privately. For Native Americans, hallucinations in which they see and converse with the dead are regarded as a part of mourning (DeSpelder & Strickland, 1999).

Based on focus groups representing many Native American tribes and conducted by Native American nurses, Lowe and Struthers (2001) identified seven themes representing core principles relevant to healthcare. These themes include: 1) caring, which embodies characteristics of health, relationships, holism, and knowledge, and is characterized as a "partnership in healing"; 2) traditions, which refers to: valuing and connection with heritage; respect, which includes characteristics of honor, identity, and strength and refers to the components of presence and compassion; connection, which honors all people, the past, present, and future, harmony with nature, and explores differences and similarities; holism, which includes balance and culture; trust, which is characterized through relationship, presence and respect; and spirituality which includes unity, honor, balance, and healing and includes components of touching, learning, and utilizing traditions to recognize oneness and unity.

DEVELOPING CULTURAL COMPETENCE

A culturally competent healthcare system "acknowledges and incorporates at all levels the importance of culture, the assessment of cross-cultural relations, vigilance toward the dynamics that result from cultural differences, and the expansion of cultural knowledge, and adaptation of services to meet culturally unique needs" (Cort, 2004, p. 68). Achieving cultural competence is a dynamic state in which health professionals gain knowledge of their own cultural and social backgrounds and become aware of the history, traditions, and values of other groups, including understanding the history, food, and lifestyles of people from other countries (Cort, 2004). According to the Schim and Miller, cultural competence model, there are four components of cultural competence:

1) Cultural diversity, which is reflected in every aspect of the healthcare system in the United States and recognizes diverse populations with unique values, beliefs, and customs;

2) Cultural awareness, which implies knowledge and information exchange regarding health, beliefs,

and practices specific to various communities, and cultural variations within groups;

3) Cultural sensitivity, which requires the recognition of individual attitudes and beliefs and a refinement of communication skills related to active listening, use of silence and touch, conversational distance, language patterns, and the effective use of translators; and

4) Cultural competence, which is the ultimate goal and incorporates diversity (fact), awareness (knowledge), and sensitivity (attitude) into everyday practice and behaviors (Doorenbos & Schim, 2004).

Cultural diversity refers to differences between people based on treasured beliefs, shared teachings, norms, customs, language, and meaning that influence the individual's and families' response to illness, treatment, death, and bereavement (Showalter, 1998). Cultural diversity is evident in the perception of pain, ways of coping with life-threatening illness, and the behavioral manifestations of grief, mourning, and funeral customs (DeSpelder & Strickland, 1999). The acknowledgement of such concepts and their relationships may provide a framework for cultural assessment and an opportunity to provide quality care respectful of differences with regard to cultural expectations and needs. Failure to take culture seriously means that health professionals elevate their values above the values of others, which is culturally destructive rather than culturally skilled (Kagawa-Singer & Blackhall, 2001). Therefore, it is important to support trusting and effective patient and provider interactions through respect, and acknowledgement of cultural diversity and avoidance of misperceptions.

For those experiencing life-threatening illness, several issues are relevant with respect to culture. One such issue is patient autonomy, which emphasizes the rights of patients to be informed about their condition, its treatments, and the right to choose or refuse life-prolonging care. However, this reflects the American beliefs regarding independence and individual rights, which may not be shared by patients and families from other cultures (Kagawa-Singer & Blackhall, 2001). For example, those from Asian cultures may believe that the family as a whole should make decisions regarding the aged individual. This is an example of "family-centered" rather than "patient-centered" decision-making styles (Barclay et al., 2007).

Another issue influenced by culture is responses to inequities in care. When not addressed, this issue may lead to feelings of mistrust regarding the intentions of healthcare providers and a lack of cooperation and collaboration between the patient, family, and healthcare provider. Discussions of the cost of technology and the ineffectiveness of treatment may be perceived by the patient as a devaluation of his/her life (Crawley et al., 2002). As a result, there may be an increased desire for futile aggressive care at the end of life, and

dissatisfaction with care. This issue is relevant to the care of African-American patients and families who are more likely to want aggressive medical care at the end of life and less likely to have Do-Not-Resuscitate (DNR) orders. To address this issue, practitioners can ask directly if the individual trusts someone who is not from his/her same background. Practitioners can work toward addressing inequities in care, or can attempt to understand and accommodate desires for more aggressive care (Kagawa-Singer & Blackhall, 2001).

Furthermore, communication or language barriers may lead to bidirectional misunderstanding and unnecessary physical, emotional, social, or spiritual suffering. It is therefore important to avoid medical jargon, make language simple, check for understanding or hire a trained interpreter. The use of family or untrained interpreters should be avoided, as they may misinterpret phases, censor sensitive or taboo topics, or filter and summarize discussions rather than translating them completely (Crawleyet al., 2002; Flores, 2005).

There may also be differences in religion and spirituality, which may create a lack of trust between the patient and professional from different backgrounds. To create a sense of connection, healthcare professionals need to ask about religious or spiritual beliefs and practices and how the patient could be supported in addressing religious or spiritual needs.

Another issue, which may need to be negotiated, is truth-telling. Individuals from certain cultures may develop mistrust or anger if the healthcare team insists on informing patients about their diagnosis or prognosis against the wishes of their family. Families often believe that such knowledge will result in a sense of hopelessness for the patient, which contributes to their suffering. In this situation, it would be appropriate for the healthcare provider to ask whether the patient would want to know everything about his/her illness, and be cognizant of nonverbal communication when discussing serious information (Kagawa-Singer & Blackhall, 2001).

Consideration should also be given to the issue of family involvement in decision making. Disagreement and conflict between family and healthcare professionals may occur when the family insists on making decisions for patients who have decisional capacity. As healthcare professionals, it is important to identify the key members of the family and involve them in the discussions as desired by the patient. If the patient is capable of making decisions for himself/herself, yet the family requests that information be withheld from the patient and that they make the decisions, it is helpful to conduct a family meeting in which the patient, family members, and healthcare professionals are present. This may provide an opportunity to clarify issues, address conflicts, and provide clarity about the decisions and preferences of the patient.

At the end of life, cultural differences may also exist regarding the desire to enroll in Hospice care. Health professionals need to understand the feelings and perceptions of patients and families from varying cultural perspectives, and emphasize that Hospice is not a replacement for the family, but as a way of providing resources to support the quality of life for patients and families (Kagawa-Singer & Blackhall, 2001).

Although there may be diversity in terms of desires, preferences, and expectations across cultures, there are also similarities. In a study of the needs and experiences of non-English-speaking Hospice patients and families in an English-speaking country, McGrath, Vun, and McLeod (2001) found, based on focus groups which included Indian, Filipino, Chinese, and Italian cultural groups and their caregivers, that participants from all groups expressed the same issues. These included the importance of support from families; the pressures on family members to care for relatives at the end of life; lack of knowledge about Hospice and palliative care services; lack of choice in how they wished to care for their family member; difficulty in talking about dying; and desire to care for a family member at home.

In providing quality palliative care for patients and their families, consideration should also be given to the following principles of culturally sensitive care (CSWE Faculty Development Institute, 2001). The first principle is to *be knowledgeable about cultural values and attitudes.* Healthcare professionals should attend to a patient's needs in a sensitive, understanding, and non-judgmental way, and respond with flexibility as much as possible. The second principle is for healthcare practitioners *to attend to diverse communication styles,* including spending time listening to the person's needs, views, and concerns. The third principle is to *ask the patient for his or her preferences for decision making* early in their care. As a fourth principle, it is important to *recognize cultural differences and varying comfort levels* with regard to personal space, eye contact, touch, time orientation, learning styles, and conversation styles.

The fifth principle is to *use a cultural guide from the patient's ethnic or religious background* to clarify cultural problems or concerns if communication with the patient or family is unclear. If necessary, ask the older adult to identify a family spokesperson and respect the appointment made by patient, even if the person is not a family member or does not live nearby. If the elder's preference is for family involvement, family meetings are opportunities to identify family's needs and concerns, and an opportunity for the family to understand the patient's goals of care and end-of-life wishes.

A sixth principle is to *get to know the community, its people, and resources* to identify the availability of social support and needed resources. Healthcare professionals may establish relationships with key community resources to assist the seriously ill older adult and his or her family. As a seventh principle, health practitioners should *create a culturally friendly physical environment* by designing facilities with artwork or pictures valued by the cultural groups to whom care is most commonly provided. Written materials should be available in the language of patients to enhance their understanding of their disease and treatment options and provide their sense of partnership in making healthcare decisions.

As an eighth principle, it is appropriate for the health professionals to *determine the acceptability of patients being physically examined by a practitioner of a different gender.* Patients should also be asked if they would want to have a family member present during the physical examination. Recognize that symptom recognition, as well as its reporting and meaning, may vary based on the patient's cultural background. A ninth principle is for health professionals to advocate *for availability of services, accessibility in terms of cost and location, and acceptability of services* that are compatible with cultural values, and practices of the person.

Lastly, the tenth principle is for health professionals to *conduct a self-assessment of their own beliefs* about illness and death and how they influence one's attitudes; how significant are culture and religion in health professionals' personal attitudes toward death; what kind of death would they prefer; what efforts should be made to keep a seriously ill person alive and the disposition of their bodies; and what is their experience of participating in rituals to remember the dead.

Having considered the importance of a comprehensive cultural assessment, it is also valuable for health professionals to have knowledge of the principles of culturally sensitive care. With this knowledge and understanding, health professionals are able to develop a culturally appropriate plan of care that addresses the cultural needs and expectations of patients and their families and supports their trust of health professionals and satisfaction with healthcare.

In providing culturally sensitive care, DeSpelder (1998) also suggests that health professionals listen for and mirror the language patterns based on an individual's culture. Small differences in language, such as saying "passed away" or "passed on", can indicate much about the speaker's experience. For example, "passed away" may describe the deceased from the survivor's perspective, whereas "passed on" may imply a belief in life after death. Nurses also can attend to the cultural needs of their patients by gathering information about distinctive rituals, practices, and beliefs, particularly an understanding of what is meaningful to the individual person. This assessment involves listening, observing, and asking about practices of patients and families that may be unfamiliar to the nurse. Furthermore, nurses can determine the strengths an individual draws on when encountering death, dying, or bereavement, such as internal resources provided by the individual's belief system or past experiences; and external resources, such as the comfort provided by cultural customs (DeSpelder & Strickland, 1999). As nurses interact with patients and families from diverse cultures, they have the experiential opportunity to learn about cultural values, expectations, and needs regarding illness, dying, and death. In caring for patients and families at the end of life, nurses can enhance the quality of life and quality of dying by promoting a respectful and peaceful death through the recognition of their spiritual and cultural needs.

Cultural mistrust is a dynamic that has implications not only for individual healthcare providers but also for administrators of healthcare systems (Cort, 2004). Measures carried out by Hospices to overcome cultural mistrust may include 1) hiring competent African-American staff and minority volunteers; 2) respecting differences in cultural preferences; 3) conducting public education campaigns, by television or community and local organizations, newsletters, and church presentations; 4) involving African-American pastors in capacities that permit them to serve as bridges of trust between their communities and the healthcare system; and 5) avoiding perceptions of injustice and inequality by promising only the services that can be delivered (Cort, 2004).

Cultural competency is a set of academic and personal skills that allow practitioners to increase understanding and appreciation of cultural differences between groups (American Medical Student Association, 2001). Practitioners need to appreciate and accept cultural differences, to learn to culturally assess a patient to avoid stereotyping, and to explain an issue from another's cultural perspective. Areas of dissonance between patients and healthcare providers include historical distrust, varying interpretations regarding disability, the influence of family structure on decision making, and differences in willingness to treat diseases without symptoms, such as high cholesterol, or appreciating illness even when there are no observable manifestations.

Cultural competence entails listening with sympathy and understanding, acknowledging and discussing differences and similarities between perceptions of illness and its treatment, recommending treatments while remembering the patient's cultural perspectives, and negotiating and compromising when worldviews are in conflict (American Medical Student Association, 2001; Crawley et al., 2002). In improving the relationship between the health professional and the patient across cultures, it is important to maintain non-judgmental attitudes towards unfamiliar beliefs and practices, and to determine what is appropriate and polite caring behavior. It is respectful to begin by being more formal with patients, addressing them by their surname, rather than by first name. Recognize that it may be a sign of disrespect to look directly into another's eye or to ask questions regarding treatment. Shaking of the hands as a form of introduction, although valued in American culture, may be inappropriate by a female when

introducing herself to an Orthodox Jewish or Muslin male (Grossman, 1996). Furthermore, a firm handshake may be interpreted by members of Native American tribes as aggressive or rude.

Asian–Americans may tend to have subtle and indirect communication styles that rely heavily on nonverbal cues, such as facial expression, body movements, use of physical space, and tone of voice. For example, a patient may bow his head or may disengage from you if he is in disagreement with the plan of care (Grossman, 1996). Nodding of the head in Asian or Hispanic populations may be merely a social custom, showing politeness and respect for a person in authority rather than a sign of agreement. Given this possibility, the healthcare provider may then ask specific questions that require the patient to express his/her feelings and wishes (Crawley et al., 2002).

It is important to ask questions to explore the patients' beliefs about health, illness, and prevention. Accept the fact that many patients use complementary therapies as well as Western medicine, and not discount the possible effects of the supernatural on health. As health professionals, it is important to have knowledge of the patient's family and kinship structure to help ascertain the values, differing gender roles, issues concerning authority and decision making within a household, and the value of involving the family in the treatment (Grossman, 1996). Discussion with patients and their families may also involve the importance of food and eating as potentially enhancing a sense of community and as a way of supporting customs and heritage. Such information can assist the healthcare team in providing appropriate dietary instructions. For examples, Islamic law forbids Muslim patients to ingest alcohol, or pork or meat from animals that are not appropriately slaughtered. Jewish patients may observe the laws of kashrut, which prescribe specific ways of food preparation and prohibit the eating of pork, shellfish, and wild birds. Individuals from Cuban backgrounds may prefer a diet that is high in calories, starches, and saturated fats, and modification of such a diet may mean just adhering to a modest serving size (Grossman, 1996).

Nurses' Cultural Self-Awareness and Development of Cultural Competency

By being aware of their own feelings, attitudes, preferences, and biases, nurses can be more in touch with themselves, acknowledging their right to their own beliefs, but not allowing those values and beliefs to take precedence over those expressed by patients and families. In order for nurses to care effectively for patients from diverse cultural groups, they also must be willing to learn about the cultures of their patients and presuppositions. The first step is to find educational sources that provide information about the various cultures, while recognizing that there are individual differences even within the same culture because of differences in social stratum, personal experiences with illness and death, and individual preferences and values. By asking someone of a particular culture to help them understand the taboos and meanings of experiences and events, nurses can actively learn about other cultures. Nurses must also recognize that losses have different meanings from person to person and culture to culture and may be viewed as major or minor.

The key to accommodating cultural diversity is for nurses to understand their own values, beliefs, and customs related to the celebration of life, and coping with illness and death. Irish, Lundquist, and Nelsen (1993) suggest that health professionals assess the degree in which they are proactive in their attitudes and activities toward diversity by asking themselves the following questions:

- Have I actively sought information to enhance my own awareness and understanding of multicultural diversity?
- Have I consciously pondered my own attitudes and behaviors as they either enhance or hinder my relationships with others?
- Have I evaluated my use of terms or phrases that may be perceived by others as degrading or hurtful?
- Have I suggested or initiated workshops or discussions about multicultural diversity?
- Have I openly disagreed with racial, cultural, or religious jokes, comments, or slurs?
- Have I utilized in my work setting appropriate occasions to discuss the multicultural climate in the organizations with my colleagues and with institutional administration?
- Have I complained to the author when I see a broadcast, advertisement, or newspaper article that is racially, culturally, or religiously biased? (p. 45)

Furthermore, DeSpelder (1998) suggests that healthcare professionals develop end-of-life cultural competence when they reflect on their own attitudes, beliefs, and practices toward dying and death. Nurses may explore for themselves:

- their own beliefs about death and what influenced these attitudes;
- how significant religion is in their attitudes toward death;
- what kind of death they would prefer;
- if diagnosed with a terminal illness, whom they would want to tell;
- what efforts should be made to keep a seriously ill person alive;
- how they would want their bodies to be disposed; and

- what their experience is of participating in rituals to remember the dead.

Cultural Assessment

Developing cultural competency requires that nurses listen carefully and gather cultural information. The patient's background may provide clues about a person's beliefs; however, these are only assumptions unless validated by asking patients about their beliefs, needs, expectations, and wishes. Knowledge about a person's cultural group should serve only as a starting point or guideline in assessing individual beliefs and behaviors (Kagawa-Singer, 1998; Lipson, Dibble, & Minarik, 1996).

In conducting a cultural assessment, there are several areas to be addressed:

- Identify the birthplace of the patient.
- Ask a patient about his/her immigration experience.
- Determine his/her level of ethnic identity.
- Evaluate the degree of acculturation as evidenced by his/her use of the English language, the length of time in the United States, and his/her adaptation.
- Determine his/her family structure.
- Identify the use of informal networks and sources of support within the community.
- Identify who makes decisions, such as the individual patient, the family, or another social unit.
- Assess his/her primary and secondary language.
- Determine the person's verbal and nonverbal communication patterns.
- Consider gender and power issues within relationships.
- Evaluate the patient's sense of self-esteem.
- Identify the influence of religion or spirituality on patients' and families' expectations and behaviors.
- Ascertain the patient's perceptions regarding discrimination or racism.
- Identify cooking and dining traditions and the meaning of food.
- Determine the patient's educational level and socioeconomic status.
- Assess attitudes, beliefs, and practices related to health, illness, suffering, and death.
- Determine patients' and families' preferences regarding location of death.
- Discuss expectations regarding healthcare.
- Determine the degree of fatalism or activism in accepting or controlling care and death.
- Evaluate the patient's knowledge and trust regarding the healthcare system.
- Assess the value and use of pharmacologic, nonpharmacologic, and complementary therapies.
- Discuss how hope is maintained (American Medical Student Association, 2001; ELNEC, 2001; Ersek et al., 1998).

UNDERSTANDING SPIRITUALITY

Spirituality and religiosity are often fundamental to the way patients face chronic illness, suffering, loss, dying, and death. Spirituality and religiosity are integral to holistic care and are important considerations, particularly since spirituality may be a dynamic in the patient's understanding of his/her disease and way of coping. Religious convictions may also affect healthcare decision making (Puchalski, 2001a). Spiritual ideas are fundamental to palliative care since both are concerned with non-abandonment, the value of interpersonal relationships, and recognize the value of transcendent support (Purdy, 2002).

Although spirituality and religion are often used interchangeably in common conversations, spirituality is a broader concept than religiosity. Spirituality comes from the Latin word *spiritus,* which refers to breath, air, and wind. Spirituality refers to the energy in the deepest core of the individual. It is the integrating life force that allows us to transcend our physical being and gives us ultimate meaning and purpose in life (Conrad, 1985). Spirituality represents the harmonious interconnectedness with self, others, nature, and God, and can also be communicated through, art, music, and relationships with family or the community (Puchalski & Romer, 2000). Spirituality further involves a melding of the individual's past, present, and future (Hicks, 1999). Even individuals who have no specific religion or faith background are spiritual beings and can have spiritual needs.

Spirituality, as a concept, also includes references to the soul, as well as spiritual needs, perspectives, and spiritual well-being. Moberg (1984) conceptualized spiritual well-being as encompassing a horizontal dimension that refers to a sense of purpose and mission in life and life satisfaction, and a vertical dimension that refers to a sense of well-being in relation to God. Downey (1997) describes spirituality as the awareness that there are levels of reality not immediately apparent and that there is a quest for personal integration in the face of forces of fragmentation and depersonalization. Therefore, spirituality is that aspect of human beings that seeks to heal or be whole (Puchalski, 2001b).

Moore (1992) has discussed the individual's spiritual quest, which is a process of "re-sacralization" of the self and the world in which we live. Individuals are embarking on spiritual journeys to discover the transcendent in daily life and in interpersonal relationships. The spiritual need is one of finding the mystery and sacredness of daily existence. Wink (1999) believes that individuals are searching for meaning outside of the confines of their religion. This is particularly important for individuals who are aging and who may be experiencing a chronic, debilitating, or life-threatening illness and who are questioning the meaning of not only their life but also their suffering. Within this context, the spirit of the person seeks to transcend suffering through the virtues of love, hope, faith, courage, acceptance, and a sense of meaning in the encounter with death (Arnold, 1989).

Throughout a person's lifetime, and particularly as people age, religion and spirituality assist them to confront their finitude and vulnerability; to uncover meaning, value, and dignity in illness and death; to establish connection with others and a higher life force; and to find hope, love, and forgiveness in the midst of fear and despair. As such, spirituality engenders serenity and transcendence, thereby buffering stress (Doka, 1993).

As a chaplain, Ryan (1997) emphasizes the five fundamental spiritual needs of all people, which include: 1) finding meaning in life, particularly during adverse circumstances; 2) the need for a relationship with a higher life force or transcendent being; 3) the need to transcend the sources of suffering; 4) the need for hope no matter how difficult life can be; and 5) the need to have others who share our life journey and care for us. As one example, a 68-year-old woman with advanced breast cancer revealed her spiritual need when she stated "I only wish there was one person in this world who could tell me that they love me."

Religiosity is one means of expressing spirituality as are prayer and meditation (Puchalski, 1998a). Religiosity refers to beliefs and practices of different faiths and an acceptance of their traditions, such as Catholicism, Eastern perspectives, Islam, Judaism, and Protestantism. For many people, religion forms a basis for meaning and purpose in life, and provides the moral codes by which to live. As illness can call into question the person's purpose in life and work, spiritual and religious issues often arise. Seventy-eight percent of Americans indicate that they receive comfort and support through religious beliefs and have greater trust in health professionals who ask them about their spiritual or religious needs (Koenig, 2002; Ehman, Ott, Short, Ciampa, & Hanson-Flaschen, 1999).

Spirituality and Palliative Care

Even as the physical body declines, healing, which means to make whole, can occur as spiritual needs are identified and spiritual care is given to restore a person to wholeness. Healing can be accomplished through the spiritual journey of remembering, assessing, searching for meaning, forgiving, reconciling, loving, and maintaining hope (Puchalski, 1998a). Holistic care, including care of the soul or spirit, is important to quality palliative care, whose goal is to enhance a person's quality of life across the illness trajectory. People do want their spiritual needs addressed at the end of life and feel that health professionals should speak to patients about their spiritual concerns (Gallop, 1997). Furthermore, elder individuals who are dying express the need for companionship and spiritual support, particularly human contact, and to have the opportunity to pray alone or with others (Nathan Cummings Foundation, 1999).

When providing palliative care for patients and their families, it is important to remember the following principles (Doka & Morgan, 1993):

■ Each person has a spiritual dimension.
■ Illness and death can be opportunities for spiritual growth.
■ Spiritual care may be different for each individual dependent on his/her religious or cultural background.
■ Spirituality is supported through formal and informal ways, such as religious practices, secular practices, symbols, rituals, art forms, prayer and meditation.
■ Care should be offered in settings that accommodate the needs of religious or spiritual practices and rituals, and promote spiritual work.

Spirituality and Health

Physicians, psychologists, and other professionals are researching the role of spirituality in healthcare. Research indicates that spirituality is related to mortality, coping, and recovery, since people with regular spiritual practices tend to live longer, utilize health beliefs in coping with illness, pain, and life stress, and have enhanced recovery from illness and surgery (Puchalski, 2001a). A systematic review of the literature during the 20th century revealed, based on 724 quantitative studies, a significant relationship between religious involvement and better mental health, greater social support, and less substance abuse (Koenig et al., 1992). In a study of religious coping in 850 hospitalized patients, a significant inverse correlation ($p < .001$) was found between religious coping and depressive symptoms (Koenig et al., 1992). In another study examining the speed of recovery from depression of 87 medical inpatients, Koenig (1998) reported that of nearly 30 baseline characteristics, intrinsic religiosity was 1 of only 5 independent predictors of the speed of recovery.

In a study of religiosity, Bergan and McConatha (2000) reported that religious affiliation and private religious devotion increased with age across the lifespan. Based on a sample of 2025 community-dwelling elder residents, it was found that religious attendance provided a persistent protective effect against mortality, even after controlling for the most potential confounders, such as social support, health status, and physical functioning.

Studies also indicate that those who are religious or spiritual have lower blood pressure, fewer cardiac events, better result following heart surgery, and longer survival in general (Koenig, 2002). Furthermore, spirituality counteracts stress-related physiologic states that impair healing and facilitates coping with chronic

pain, disability, and serious illness by enhancing a sense of control that interrupts the cycle of anxiety and depression (Koenig, 2002). Those who participate in religious services express less loneliness and isolation as they receive support from others and believe that God is with them.

Religion or spirituality also facilitates coping with chronic pain, disability, and serious illness by providing an indirect form of control that helps to interrupt the cycle of anxiety and depression. For some individuals, prayer provides a form of control by believing that through prayer they can influence their medical outcome, while, in contrast, others deliberately turn over to God their health situation (Koenig, 2002). The belief that God is with them provides relief from loneliness and isolation. Individuals who attend religious services also have an opportunity for socialization and support from others, while praying for others in need often provides a distraction from one's own pain (Koenig, 2002). These findings are supported by more recent reviews of the literature by Okon (2005) who conducted a review of the spiritual, religious, and existential aspects of palliative care, and by Sinclair, Pereira, and Raffin (2006) who provide a thematic review of the spirituality literature regarding palliative care. Both articles provide comprehensive discussions related to differences between religion and spirituality, spiritual assessment, instruments to measure spirituality, correlates to health, and spiritual interventions.

In terms of health consequences, religious involvement has been associated with improved attendance at medical appointments, greater adherence to medical regimens, and improved medical outcomes. Studies indicate that those who are religious or spiritual have lower blood pressure, fewer cardiac events, better results following heart surgery, and longer survival in general (Koenig, 2002). Furthermore, religious or spiritual practices are believed to influence sympathetic and parasympathetic nerve pathways connecting thoughts and emotions to circulatory and immune system changes, and counteracting stress-related physiologic states that impair healing (Koenig, 2002).

Interested in religiosity and spirituality, Heintz and Baruss (2001) conducted a study based on a sample of 30 people whose mean age was 72.6 years. While some religious behaviors, such as frequent religious practice, prayer, and church attendance were correlated with some dimensions of spirituality, many of the scores on the Expressions of Spirituality Inventory were independent of self-reported religious behaviors. These results reinforced the differences between the concepts of religiosity and spirituality.

In a qualitative study of 41 male and female residents aged 66–92 years, most of the older adults believed that a higher power was present in their lives, which supported them constantly, and was perceived as protecting, guiding, helping, teaching, and healing them (Mackenzie, Rajogopal, Meibohm, & Lavizzo-Mourey, 2000). God was perceived to work through the mundane world, such as through the work of physicians, loving friends, and helpful strangers. Many felt that their relationship with God formed the foundation of their psychological well-being. The authors concluded that the subjective experience of spiritual support may form the core of the spirituality-health connection for older adults.

The Role of Religiosity and Spirituality in Coping with Serious Illness

As patients are faced with chronic or serious illness and eventually near death, they may experience despair, with spiritual and religious concerns intensified or awakened (Lo et al., 2002). The patient may struggle with the physical aspects of the disease, as well as the pain related to mental and spiritual suffering. They may ask "Why did this happen to me?" "Why is God allowing me to suffer?" "What will happen after I die?" "Will I be remembered or missed?" or "Will I be able to finish my life's work? (Puchalski, 2002). True healing requires an answer to these questions as healing can be experienced as acceptance of illness and peace with one's life (Puchalski, 2001a).

It is through spirituality that people find meaning in illness and suffering and are liberated from their despair. Spiritual care changes chaos to order, and seeks to discern what if any blessings might be revealed in spite of and even through tragedy (Purdy, 2002). As people are dying, they want to be listened to, to have someone share their fears, to be forgiven by God or by others, and believe that they will live on in the hearts of others or through their good works (Puchalski, 2002).

In a study of 19 individuals with advanced cancer, Thomas and Retsas (1999) learned through in-depth interviews that people with cancer developed a spiritual perspective that strengthened their approach to life and death. As cancer progressed, participants described the transaction of self-preservation by discovering deeper levels of understanding self, which incorporates a higher level of spiritual growth, spiritual awareness, and spiritual experiences.

Individuals at the end of life also express spiritual needs. Based on a qualitative study of nine Hospice patients, Hermann (2000) reported their need for religion, companionship, involvement, and control to finish business, experience nature, and the need for a positive outlook. Participants perceived spirituality as a broad concept that may or may not involve religion and that spiritual needs were closely linked to the purpose and meaning in life. In studying older patients approaching the end of life from advanced heart disease, it was

found that 24% of the variance in their global quality of life was predicted by their spirituality (Beery, Baas, Fowler, & Allen, 2002).

Taylor and Outlaw (2002) conducted a qualitative study to understand the use of prayer among persons with cancer ($n = 30$) and recognized that individuals with cancer use prayer to cope with their illness. Participants viewed prayer as personal communication involving or allowing transcendence. The communication or prayer was initiative and receptive. The initiative aspect of praying was to talk to God, get in touch with God, or beseech God, while the receptive aspect of prayer was characterized by phrases like being quiet, being accessible, and listening to God. For these individuals, prayer meant being constantly conscious of God and coming into that higher intention in life. Participants' illness increased their awareness of the inadequacy of relying on self and the need to rely on a greater power. They described prayer as an active cognitive process, while others described prayer as a more passive process or as "prayer of the heart." Assistive strategies for praying included constructing a prayer, writing a prayer, relaxing, reading religious material, and how one prayed depended on the purpose of the prayer. Some individuals prayed about healing, or that "God's will be done." Many prayed for forgiveness or to be a better person. Most prayed for family and friends who needed peace and support, and also included thanks and praise in their prayers that they were given another day to live. Through the process of prayer, many individuals believed that they benefited, whether their prayer was answered or not. From prayer, they expected that the "best will happen," or that they will receive comfort, forgiveness, or salvation. As health professionals, the implications for prayer are that clinicians can help by fostering a condition and environment conducive to prayer and can facilitate patient's use of prayer, which is unique to individuals.

In a phenomenological study of spirituality and life-threatening illness, Albuagh (2003) interviewed seven participants who had either cancer or heart or lung disease for at least 1 month. Participants described a sense of comfort from aspects of spiritual life, such as belief in support from God, feelings of not being alone, and the power of prayer. The participants expressed a trust in God, believing that God would provide the means to get through the experience either by restoring their health or through death. The strength of their spiritual beliefs, feelings of being blessed despite or through the illness, and a deeper meaning to life after facing life-threatening illness were described. The study supports the need to acknowledge patients' spirituality and assist them in meeting their spiritual needs.

Through a qualitative study involving 28 African-American and European-American adult patients with cancer and their caregivers, Taylor (2003) examined participants' expectations of nurses in meeting their spiritual needs. Participants identified six approaches of nurses in addressing spiritual needs: 1) showing kindness and respect; 2) talking and listening; 3) prayer, such as offering verbal prayer or saying, "You are in my thoughts and prayers"; 4) connecting with authenticity and genuineness; 5) quality temporal nursing care, such as coming back to check on the patient; and 6) mobilizing religious or spiritual resources. The authors concluded that nurses need to consider their role in spiritual care and educate the public about their role as holistic healthcare providers.

The effects of spirituality on well-being of people with lung cancer were studied by Meraviglia (2004). Based on a sample of 60 adults who were predominately Caucasian and women, it was found that higher meaning-in-life scores were associated with higher psychological well-being and lower symptom distress. Prayer was positively related to psychological well-being, explaining 10% of its variance. Regression analysis indicated that meaning in life mediated the relationship between functional status and physical responses to lung cancer and explained 9% of the variance in symptom distress. The author concluded that this study supported the importance of providing spiritual care for patients with cancer.

Lorenz, Shapiro, Cleay, Asch, and Wenger (2005) examined religiousness and spirituality among HIV-infected Americans. Based on a sample of 2266 patients receiving care for HIV infection, 80% reported a religious affiliation and the majority indicated that they rely on religious or spiritual means when making a decision or confront problems. Women, older patients, and non-whites were more spiritual, but the clinical stage of the disease was not associated to religiosity or spirituality. It was concluded that religious or spiritual organizations should be used to support patients diagnosed with HIV infection.

Mako, Galek, and Poppito (2006) reported that of the 57 patient with advanced-stage cancer in a palliative care hospital, 96% reported spiritual pain due to intrapsychic conflict, interpersonal loss, or conflict in relation to the diying. Depression was correlated with the intensity of spiritual pain but not with physical pain or severity of illness. The authors conclude that unaddressed spiritual pain contributes to overall suffering.

Based on a study of 50 adult Hospice patients, Prince-Paul (2008) also reported strong positive correlations among spiritual well-being, communicative acts, and quality of life at the end of life (QOLEOL), when controlling for physical symptoms, explaining 53.5% of the variance.

Spirituality or Religiosity During the Dying Process

The attitudes an individual holds regarding the dying process and death are embedded in his/her cultural and religious values. Values affect the way individuals conceptualize death and behave in relation to death (Meagher & Bell, 1993). Many people return to the religious legacies of their childhood during the dying process since it may have been the first time that they heard about death and learned about Christian resurrection (Satterly, 2001).

At this time, it would be important to explore guilt as central to a person's religious pain, as well as the concept of forgiveness from his/her religious perspective. Religious rituals for cleansing or religious doctrine may allay feelings of remorse and guilt, providing for renewal of the soul and redemption. In supporting elders in spiritual pain, it may also be helpful to consider the concept of love. Most religious traditions provide a hopeful belief in the unconditional love of God, as well as reinforcing how unconditional love can be allowed to self, especially when an individual may have previously engaged in self-criticism or self-hatred (Satterly, 2001).

As individuals approach death, Doka (1993) identified the spiritual need of individuals to die in a way that is consistent with their self-identity. For example, if a person's approach to life has also been to remain in control and "not give up the fight," then it would be expected that they may not want to forego aggressive therapies, even if the chances of cure, or remission are low. Their spiritual need may be to continue to fight the disease. For those who are dying, Doka (1993) also emphasizes the spiritual task of finding hope that extends beyond the grave, as one seeks a sense of symbolic immortality. Individuals often need to feel that they are leaving a legacy, whether through having children or being remembered through their contributions to community, or through artwork, music, or their writings.

Suffering and Spirituality

Suffering is a part of life and the human condition, with suffering either personally experienced in a physical, emotional, social, or spiritual way, or experienced as witnesses to another's suffering. Cassell (1982) defines suffering as "the state of severe distress associated with events that threaten the intactness of a person" (p. 639). Suffering can be defined as the endurance of, or submission to, affliction, pain, or loss. Suffering is usually psychological, as a result of distressing circumstances that arise in the process of living, but can also be the effects of physical pain. Cassell (1982) believes that many aspects of a person can be sources of, or be affected by, suffering, such as personality, character, the past, relationships, life experiences, roles, one's rights and responsibilities, family, and cultural background.

According to Kahn and Steeves (1996), suffering is a private-lived experience of a whole person, unique to each individual. As such, suffering cannot be assumed present or absent in any given clinical condition or situation because suffering is dependent on the meaning of the event or loss. The experience of suffering is also both intrapersonal and interpersonal because it involves the person's own coping with suffering and the caring of others (Kahn & Steeves, 1996). Although we may not find answers about why we suffer, as a part of the human family we build relationships, communities, and society to reach out to one another to relieve suffering and sustain us in our struggle (McGann, 1997).

Suffering varies with the type of disease, type of personality, and the relationship between these factors. "The loss of physical integrity and the impending destruction of the unity of one's person can cause profound suffering" (DeBellis et al., 1986, p. 6). Within the context of illness, suffering can occur because of unfavorable prognoses, loss of function, disability, the complexity of treatment, failure to achieve relief of symptoms, the expense of treatment, and the effects of disease on all social relationships and economic security (DeBellis et al., 1986).

Millspaugh (2000a), as a chaplain, describes suffering as spiritual pain which involves an awareness of death, loss of relationships, loss of self, loss of purpose, and loss of control, which can be lessened by life affirming and transcending purpose and internal sense of control. The loss of self involves fears about death, loss of independence, loss of body image, loss of a God who can be bribed, and loss of relationships to others. It also involves loss of the established self. As spiritual pain is often marked by a sense of being alone, the task of the practitioner is to earn the person's trust and to walk with him or her by being present with the belief that a greater Spirit is at work-a joining of spirits which provides the sufferer with a sense of being understood, and feeling a sense of control in the situation (Millspaugh, 2005b).

Although, suffering and pain often are referred to interchangeably, they are not identical. In some cases, they are both present; at times, one exists without the other. The transition from pain to suffering can occur when pain is unrelieved and out of control or when the source of pain is unknown. The persistence of pain and uncertainty therefore can increase suffering exponentially. Yet, suffering can continue even when pain is controlled. Based on a sample of 177 end-stage cancer patients who had an expected life expectancy of less than 1 month to live in a Hospice, Adunsky, Aminoff, Arad, and Bercovitch (2008) found, using the Mini-suffering State Examination, that there was a low level of suffering, despite maintaining a constant rate (68%) of the use of opioids at admission and the last week of life. The reduction of the level of suffering in end-of-life cancer patients, in the face of pain needs, may be attributed to the medical and nursing care offered through Hospice care.

At the end of life, suffering may also be exacerbated because of protracted or chronic illness, multiple simultaneous diseases and comorbid conditions, recurrent disease, and awareness of mortality. Because suffering has to do with a personal understanding of the physical, emotional, and spiritual self and their interrelationships, we learn about suffering only by the ways in which an individual expresses an awareness of the threats to his/her personal wholeness (Smith, 1996). Chochinov, Jack, Hassard, McClement, and Harlos (2006) in validating the Dignity model, reported on the basis of 211 patients receiving palliative care that "not being treated with respect or understanding" and "feeling a burden to others" were the issues most identified as having an influence on dignity. In a logistic regression model, "feeling life no longer had meaning or purpose" was the only variable which predicted overall sense of dignity. Addressing these issues is believed to be the cornerstone of dignity-conserving care.

Using heuristic research, Wayman and Gaydos (2005) explored the question, "what is the experience of self-transcending through suffering?" Four people were interviewed who self-identified themselves as self-transcending. The themes were presented linearly but participants were able to move freely between themes. Participants identified a *turning point* in their suffering when they turned from self-identification with their suffering, as it became a part of their lives but not who they were. This was a wake-up call and invitation to change. Then there was a *pause,* in which there was a forced pause in all activity due to treatment. This pause was followed by *confrontation* with their experience of suffering and their response, accepting their suffering for what it was. Participants *surrendered* to a new truth, which led to *extraordinary experiences* of peace and interconnectedness. These experiences became the *touchstones of* change as they reminded themselves of the lessons of suffering and the changes they had made. Participants were changed after transcending their suffering, valuing their lives more, and became more truly who they really were. Their transcending encouraged an unfolding of the hidden, with their inner selves becoming more congruent with their outer selves. This led to the desire for meaningful work and a sense of gratitude for the experience. Their humility grew as they honestly assessed themselves. The experience of self-transcending is the patient's struggle and life journey, which can be supported when nurses facilitate opportunities for pause and reflection, and give reassurance and compassion which facilitate a patient's sense of wholeness and well-being.

In a study of terminally ill patients ($n = 96$) on palliative care units and Hospice, Schroepfer (2007) identified four critical events as motivating individuals to consider hastening their death: specifically perceived insensitive and uncaring communication of a terminal diagnosis, experiencing unbearable physical pain, unacknowledged feelings regarding treatment, and dying in a distressing environment. In order to address these issues, the authors recommend changes in policies and practices that promote time for communication by health professionals coupled with appropriate training in communication skills. It is further recommended that support be offered by members of the interdisciplinary team to reduce suffering and take a proactive rather than reactive approach to end-of-life care.

Reciprocal Suffering of Patients and Family

Within the context of life-threatening illness, suffering, in the form of physical, emotional, social, and spiritual distress, often becomes an experience not only of the patient but also of the family caregivers, as the suffering of one amplifies the distress of the other (Foley, 1995). Family members, like patients themselves, are in transition from living with the disease to anticipating the death of their loved one from the disease (Davies, Reimer, & Marten, 1994). They fear that death will occur in their absence, and may therefore refuse to leave the patient's side for even a moment. There is also a strong compulsion to attend to the patient's every need with disregard for their own needs (Klein, 1998). As the patient's illness progresses, the needs of the family also intensify and change, with both the patient and family caregivers potentially experiencing a significant compromise in the quality of their lives (Sherman, 1998).

Although family members may express the rewards of caring for terminally ill relatives, such care can have major psychosocial and physical effects, including heightened symptoms of depression, anxiety, psychosomatic symptoms, restrictions of roles and activities, strain in relationships, and poor physical health (Higginson, 1998). As witnesses to the patient's pain and suffering, family caregivers may also experience a sense of powerlessness, and are often frightened and confused by the dramatic physical and emotional changes they perceive in their loved one as the disease progresses (Loscalzo & Zabora, 1998).

Coyle (1995) gives examples of suffering, such as when patients experience despair, loneliness, and vulnerability; feel trapped by fear and bewilderment; experience loss and worry about treatment decisions; worry about being a burden; have financial concerns; experience abandonment; or fear dying yet are weary of life, and experience pain or the loss of hope. Families suffer as they assume the responsibilities of caregiving, watch the patient's deterioration, become exhausted, neglect their own needs, experience uncertainty about goals of care, and become anxious about the place of care. The suffering of family members also occurs because of fear of the dying process and the experience of the loss of life as it was, the person they knew, and of hope, as well as guilt in wanting death to come soon.

There are also many conflicting emotions and adjustment tasks, including conflict among feelings of loss, sadness, guilt, difficulty in knowing how to talk with the person who is dying, and worry about dying and death (Beeney, Butow, & Dunn, 1997). Furthermore, the family caregiver must adapt to changes in family roles and responsibilities, while attempting to meet the increased emotional needs of other family members and performing standard family functions (Doyle, 1994). Given that 25% of caregivers lose their job due to caregiver responsibilities and nearly one third of families lose their major source of income or their savings, families also experience significant financial burdens (Lederberg, 1998). This may lead to feelings of anger, jealousy, and an increase in the family caregiver's own needs because of heightened psychological distress. In addition, there is often a loss of social mobility, as well as social abandonment by friends, which negatively impact on the quality of life of family caregivers (Lederberg, 1998).

From a spiritual perspective, family members may question the meaning of the illness and suffering. They often spend considerable time reviewing painful aspects of the past with feelings of regret for disagreements, conflicts, or failures and a wish that relationships with the patient and with each other were somehow different. Buck and McMillan's (2008) study of the unmet spiritual needs of caregivers of patients with advanced cancer, emphasizes that, based on a sample of 110 caregivers of Hospice home care patients, the highest spiritual needs of caregivers related to outlook such as seeing smiles, thinking happy thoughts, laughing, and being with family. Caregivers' unmet total needs were predicted by caregivers' outlook, caregivers' religion, and the patient's distress score. To reduce caregiver suffering, it was concluded that healthcare providers must be aware of the needs for positive thinking, reminiscing of happier times through story telling or the use of pictures, and that chaplains may offer comfort through the reading of religious texts and speaking with caregivers about spiritual issues.

With each family member's unique experience of the stress, families may find it difficult to come together to effectively cope with the imposed life changes (Sherman, 1998). In their search for meaning, patients and families affirm spiritual values, change life priorities, and examine how the experience of illness has contributed to their personal growth. Like their dying loved one, they live day to day to make the most of the present as they prepare for death on practical, cognitive, emotional, and spiritual levels (Davies et al., 1994). The hope is that through palliative nursing care, both patients and family members can transcend their reciprocal suffering and experience growth as they face the challenges of life-threatening or terminal illness (Sherman, 1998).

THE CARE OF THOSE WHO ARE SUFFERING

Cassell (1982) believes that the ways to relieve suffering are, first, through the assignment of meaning to the injurious condition or event and, second, through transcendence, which is the most powerful way of restoring an individual's personhood to wholeness. Watson (1986) proposes four generic meanings of suffering, which include *correction* in which an individual is being corrected of his/her wrongdoing; *affirmation* in which a person is affirmed of his/her "rightdoing" and the ability to be a role model for others; *naturalism* in which the individual is experiencing general human destiny; and altruism in which an individual's suffering will have benefit to others. In caring for those who are suffering, health professionals may help individuals come to a healthy, maintainable higher meaning to their suffering. From a theological perspective, Smith (1996) discusses the religious response to suffering and the possibility of transcendence of suffering through intellectual, ethical, and experiential dimensions of religion. The intellectual dimension involves the realization of some transcendent meaning, which connects the suffering person with some greater reality and delivers the individual from the threat of meaninglessness that is raised by illness and pain. The ethical dimension of religious life provides a perspective regarding how to interpret and respond to suffering. Suffering may be seen as a test of one's virtue or fidelity to God, a test of the worth of religious commitment, or as an opportunity of personal transformation. Within the experiential dimension of religion, the life of oneself and others and of the relationship of these lives to each other and to God are contemplated. The religious experience of suffering may therefore enable an individual to provide redemptive relationships with others, including God, and experience transcendence.

In caring for the suffering, Spross (1996) believes that the role of the nurse is one of coaching. "Coaching is an interpersonal intervention that requires the therapeutic use of the self, involving one's mind, past experience, words, heart, and hand-to comfort those who suffer" (Spross, 1996, p. 201). In coaching, the nurse

■ establishes a trusting partnership;
■ assesses those who are at risk for suffering or who are vulnerable;
■ reassures patients that although their suffering may not disappear, they will not be abandoned;
■ identifies factors that may be eliminated or modified to alleviate suffering; and
■ intervenes to facilitate expression of feelings, find meaning in suffering, and help patients and families redefine the quality of life.

Spross (1996) states that the ability to alleviate suffering or find meaning in the experiences of suffering depends on the intrapersonal and interpersonal qualities of the nurse. The nurse must be self-accepting, be secure in his or her own self-concept, and feel confident in strengthening others. As coach, the nurse values others and communicates that the individual's feelings, goals, and opinions are respected, while conveying that the person is trustworthy, responsible, capable of self-direction, and able to identify relevant goals and find meaning in life.

Watson (1986) believes that nurses and other health professionals can relieve suffering in six ways: first, by being a companion to sufferers by identifying the pain of their losses, and exploring the circumstance and extent of the loss; second, by listening for statements of meaning from sufferers and allowing the person's natural instincts and energy to surface the issue of higher meaning; third, by valuing any self-disclosure on meaning that a sufferer offers, by analyzing the meaning of the statements and learning what the statement reveals about the sufferer's view of him- or herself; fourth, by encouraging the sufferer's interpretation of their own experience; fifth, by validating the sufferer's interpretation of his/her own experience while clarifying the meaning, seeking further definition of the meaning, and offering alternatives for reframing the meaning; and last, by identifying supportive resources and hoping for the sufferer to extend his or her identity and meaning in the future.

In alleviating the suffering of others, Bird (1986) offers seven principles to be considered within the context of nursing practice:

1) Remember that institutions do not dehumanize patients; staff members do.
2) Assume responsibility for morale whenever you are in the chain of command.
3) Be a whole person yourself, with a healthy sense of humor and attitude.
4) Do not add clinical ineptitude to the further suffering of patients.
5) Be empathetic rather than sympathetic to patient's needs; otherwise, human suffering can emotionally devastate one.
6) Offer holistic care and well-chosen words to allay suffering.
7) Determine to touch the life of at least one patient daily with some depth.

Halifax (1999) believes that healthcare providers, patients, and families can go to the root of their own suffering and transform the suffering into inherent wisdom. As a Buddhist, she reminds health professionals to come to the caregiving relationship with loving kindness, compassion by being in touch with one's own and others' suffering, joy in the well-being of others, and equanimity.

The Role of Hope in Spiritual Well-Being

Cousin (1979) reminds us that death is not the ultimate tragedy of life, but rather being separated from our connection with others, and separated from a desire to experience the things that make life worth living, separated from hope. Spirituality may help people to cope with their dying as it may offer hope. In early illness, the hope may be for the cure of the disease and treatment, and later on for the hope of prolongation of life. When cure is not possible, hope may be to see a loved one, to have a day without pain, to celebrate a certain life event, or have the time to travel or complete unfinished business. Eventually, hope may be for a peaceful death. It may be hope that allows seriously ill individuals to find courage and strength to transcend their suffering, and teach others how to die with dignity.

In redefining hope for the seriously ill or the dying, Corr (1991) distinguishes between hope and a "wish," stating that hope is grounded in reality, while wish is not. Mitchell (1997) offers a definition that hope is not a belief that something is going to go well, but rather that it is a belief that whatever happens will make sense, no matter how it turns out. For patients who are dying, hope may be defined as "an inner life force that helps each dying person to live life until the moment of death" (Parker-Oliver, 2002). Indeed, hope may be defined as the positive expectation for meaning attached to an event, recognizing that individuals shape their hopes by finding new meanings for living (Parker-Oliver, 2002). Hope allows for a sense of control and promotes an active rather than passive participation in life's events. Even in dying, people have the hope to discover new meanings.

The challenge for healthcare professionals is therefore to help individuals find hope as they search for meaning in their illness, suffering, and death. This can happen as professionals assist individuals to identify key relationships, facilitate caring relationships, and encourage the opportunity to heal relationships and complete unfinished business. Byock (1997) encourages the completion of relationships by saying "I forgive you," "Forgive me," "I love you," "Thank you," and "Goodbye." Through the encouragement of short-term, attainable goals, hope can also be promoted as well as by recognizing and encouraging a sense of determination and courage in the face of adversity. Gum and Snyder (2002) conclude that hope can me maintained when providers provide clear information, control symptoms, and maintain functionality.

Hope can also found within the context of spirituality as spiritual beliefs systems hold hope for happiness, and a promise of an afterlife. Spirituality offers hope for living on in the world through a connection with others, traditions, and rituals and through establishing legacies. Hope can also be easily discovered by just asking the patient what is meaningful to them and what they want to do with the remainder of their lives. Based on a study of 69 participants, age 65 or older, Theris (2001) reported a significant difference in hope based on the religion of participants. Based on a one-way ANOVA and Scheffe tests, Catholic participants expressed greater hope than those of the Jewish faith, and another significant difference existed between participants of the Protestant and Jewish faiths. There was also a significant, positive correlation between spirituality and level of hope ($r = .73$, $p = .000$). In a multiple regression analysis, which was used to test for the combined contribution of spirituality and connectedness with others to levels of hope, only spirituality emerged as a significant predictor of hope. The authors concluded that connection with oneself and connection with a higher being was especially important in the maintenance of hope in nursing home residents. Such results are consistent with the findings of Buchanan (1993), who reported, based on a sample of 160 older adults who were depressed and nondepressed, that higher levels of spirituality, hope, health, and social support were positively correlated with meaning in life, and that there was an inverse relationship between meaning in life and depression.

Based on qualitative studies of elder Hospice patients, Herth (1992) found that hope facilitated the transcendence of the present situation and movement toward new awareness and enrichment of being, while Duggleby (2000) found that hope was a process of enduring suffering through a trust in a higher power and making meaning of their lives. Despite the stage of illness and a situation of poor prognosis, practitioners can provide hope and a positive outlook by discussing goals of care, offering symptom control, providing supportive resources, and promising the patient that they will not abandon them (Barclay et al., 2007).

For those who are dying, the focus of hope changes from a hope in the future or a redefinition of the future, to a hope on living day to day. The focus of hope for those with advanced disease is also hope for no more suffering, life after death, and hope their families will not suffer when they are gone (Duggleby, 2001). At times, the most important way to provide hope is by listening attentively and being physically present, which convey a sense of value and affirmation of worth. Hope is then gained that they will not be abandoned and isolated (Duggleby, 2000). Hutchings (2007) conducted a qualitative study of eight people who were dying, guided by Parse's Theory of Human Becoming. The interviews illustrated that persons at the end of life still envision hopes and possibilities despite declining function and decreased energy. Such findings help health professionals understand that dying patients co-create meaning day by day while emphasizing the importance of bearing witness to the struggles, joys, and hope of dying persons.

The concept of hope in palliative care was also examined by Fanos and colleagues (2008), based on 16 patients diagnosed with amyotrophic lateral sclerosis (AML). Although there was no significant relationship found between hope and functional status, qualitative interviews revealed that patients with AML have hope related to cure, social support, spiritual beliefs, adapting to changing capacities, and the possibility of living in the moment as well as self-transcendence. It was concluded that there was a range of themes from narcissism to altruism with a heightened concern for others and that the palliative care team can play an important role by promoting discussions regarding hope in its many forms.

Learning about Spiritual Assessment and Caregiving

Health professionals need to be attuned not only to their own cultural beliefs but also to their own spirituality before participating in spiritual care. Personal preparation for spiritual caregiving includes the professional's self-evaluation of personal spirituality; reviewing personal beliefs, opinions and biases; understanding the meaning of spirituality; becoming aware of how one's own religious beliefs influence caregiving; and establishing a trusting patient-provider relationship (Hermann, 2000).

As in the care of all patients and families, health professionals caring for patients and their families must learn the specific techniques for addressing spirituality in clinical practice, including how to conduct a spiritual assessment. This also requires that the health professional be totally present and open by listening actively to spiritual issues (Hermann, 2000). Learning spiritual assessment and caregiving can also occur through a combination of teaching/learning strategies, including small group discussions, reflective writing, storytelling, use of poetry, case presentation and discussion, panel discussions with chaplains, patients, and healthcare practitioners, role playing with standardized patients, and attending lectures on the role of spirituality in healthcare (Puchalski, 2001b).

In providing spiritual care, healthcare professionals must remember that religion is only one way of enhancing spiritual well-being. Conversations about life, love, hope, trust, and forgiveness may renew the spirit of both patients and healthcare providers. Although the perspectives of health professionals is of personal value in one's role as a health practitioner, it is important to be non-judgmental, never imposing one's own beliefs and values on the patient or family, always remembering that it is the spiritual or religious perspective of the patient or family that is important. Indeed, the therapeutic value of the self will be recognized through listening, presence, and non-abandonment.

Millspaugh (2005b) suggests that in providing spiritual care for individuals who are suffering, practitioners must be able to maintain boundries, emphathize, contain their own suffering, focus and attend to the suffer's agenda, use theology, as well as the social and behavioral sciences to inform assessments and interventions, and engender a sense of security and comfort.

Conversations about Spiritual or Religious Issues

Conversations regarding spiritual needs often begins with the use of open-ended questions, such as "Do you have any thoughts about why this is happening to you?" Practitioners can also encourage the patient to say more by such statements as "Tell me more about that?" When exploring spiritual concerns, practitioner should acknowledge and normalize patient's concerns by comments, such as "Many patients ask the same question," and responding with emphatic comments, such as "That sounds like a painful situation" (Lo et al., 2002).

Pitfalls in discussions about spiritual or religious issues near the end of life often occur by trying to solve the patient's problems or resolve unanswerable questions; going beyond the practitioner's expertise or role in providing spiritual care; imposing one's beliefs on the patient; or providing premature reassurance, which may appear superficial or deter the disclosure of other important issues or emotions (Lo et al., 2002). When patients inquire about the religious background of the practitioner, they may be inquiring to determine whether it is safe to talk about spiritual or religious issues, or they may prefer to talk to someone who shares the same religious faith. However, practitioners may answer the question regarding their religious background, but need not explicate on their religious or spiritual beliefs (Lo et al., 2002). If the patient asks for details, it is appropriate to refocus the conversation back to the patient.

In addition to clarifying the patient's spiritual concerns and needs by following spiritual cues, and exploring emotions with emphatic support, healthcare professionals may also do the following:

- Make wish statements, such as "I also wish you were not ill."
- Identify common goals for care and reach agreement on clinical decisions.
- Mobilize support for the patient and family from family, church members, or the community (Lo et al., 2002).

In situations when the patient or his/her family is praying for a miracle even in medically futile situations, the role of health professionals is to respect their beliefs and remain supportive by trying to understand their worldview and the role their beliefs have in coping. Criticism or confrontation will lead to distrust and close the dialogue between healthcare professionals and the patient. When older patients and their families feel that they can talk to health professionals about their religious or spiritual beliefs, there is greater chance that they will accept what the professional is saying. A response may be that "Sometimes God answers our prayers for healing in interpersonal ways that may ultimately be more important than physical healing" (Koenig, 2002, p. 492.)

Conducting a Spiritual Assessment

Holistic care involves not only assessment of physical, emotional, and social needs, but also of spiritual needs and expectations. A spiritual history is a history about a person's values or beliefs that explicitly opens the door to conversations about the role of spirituality and religion in the person's life (Puchalski & Romer, 2000). Although it is not the health professional's responsibility to solve spiritual problems or provide answers, health practitioners need to conduct a spiritual assessment to identify when a patient or family member is experiencing spiritual distress. It is important to create an environment that nurtures the patient's exploration of spiritual needs and concerns and supports them in their search for answers. A spiritual history or assessment should be completed with each new patient visit and on annual examinations, as a part of taking routine history taking (Puchalski, 2001b). A spiritual history inquires about the role religion or spirituality plays in the patient's ability to cope with illness. Affiliation with a religious or spiritual community is important for many individuals and serves often as an extended family for many adults, especially those who live alone or have limited family support (Koenig, 2002). In taking a spiritual history, Puchalski (1998b) suggests that the acronym FICA be used:

- "F" refers to faith as identified by the question "What is your faith or beliefs and do you consider yourself religious or spiritual?"
- "I" refers to influence which is assessed by the question "How does your faith or spirituality influence your medical decisions?"
- "C" refers to community and is related to the question "Are you a part of a spiritual or religious community?" and
- "A" refers to addressing spiritual concerns as exemplified by the question "Would you like someone to address your spiritual needs or concerns?"

A spiritual history is important not only in identifying ways individuals may cope with adverse life circumstances, but also to examine potential negative effects in which religious beliefs are a source of distress and emotional turmoil (Koenig, 2002). Religious pain is a condition in which the patient feels guilty over the violation of the moral codes or values of his/her religious tradition. This may arise due to major transgressions such as abortion, adultery, overt cruelty, or from minor transgressions such as not seeking a second opinion or failing to take better care of one's self. As a result, the patient may feel that that God is disappointed in his/her past or present behaviors, actions, or thoughts (Satterly, 2001). Feelings of guilt are often accompanied by a fear of punishment from God, that God does not love them, or has abandoned them in their time of need.

Individuals may believe that future punishment from God can be avoided if enough self-pain is endured here and now (Satterly, 2001). Such may be the case for individuals who refuse pain medications, and may warrant spiritual exploration by members of the palliative care team. Chaplains have the knowledge and skills to discuss spiritual issues related to a patient's perceived need for pain and suffering and they may provide an alternative perspective concerning the patient's perception of either a punishing or forgiving God. In some cases, a patient may refuse to speak with the chaplain or clergy because he/she is angry with God, thereby rejecting religion or spirituality as a source of comfort. It is important for healthcare professionals to recognize that religious or spiritual pain is highly personal and deeply subjective, and does not have to make "sense" to the professional in order for a patient to experience it (Satterly, 2001).

Religious beliefs may also influence an individual's decisions about medical treatments, particularly if they become seriously ill, such as decisions related to cardiopulmonary resuscitation or withholding or withdrawal of life-prolonging treatments. Medical therapies may also be refused if a patient is a Jehovah's Witness or Christian Scientist; in such situations, health professionals need to understand the patient's viewpoint and show respect for his/her beliefs (Koenig, 2002).

As another approach, Highfield (2000) uses the letters from the word "SPIRIT" to remember question appropriate to a spiritual interview, specifically:

S Spiritual belief system (religious affiliation);
P Personal spirituality (beliefs and practices of affiliation that the patient and family accepts);
I Integration with a spiritual community (role of the religious/spiritual group; individual's role in the group);
R Ritualized practices and restrictions (beliefs that healthcare providers should remember during care);
I Implications for medical care;
T Terminal events planning (impact of beliefs on advance directives; contacting the clergy).

Spiritual assessment further includes assessment of personal beliefs, sources of meaning and hope, values, belief in an afterlife, and sense of connection to self, others, nature, and God. Health practitioners begin to address spirituality by asking such questions as "How are your spirits? "How do you define your spirit?" "What nourishes your spirit?" or "How have you relieved your spiritual pain in the past?" (O'Connor, 1993). For adults with life-limiting or threatening illness, valuable questions to explore include the following:

- Are you suffering in physical, emotional, social, or spiritual ways?
- What is the meaning of illness and suffering?
- Do you see purpose in your suffering?
- Are you able to transcend your suffering?
- Are you at peace, or feeling hope and despair?
- Do your personal beliefs help you to cope with anxiety about pain, and death and provide a way for achieving peace? (Puchalski & Larson, 1998)

Hermann (2000) further asks in a spiritual assessment such questions as "What gives your life meaning and purpose?" "Do you have goals you would still like to achieve?" "How has your diagnosis changed the meaning of your life?" "What kinds of things do you hope for?" and "To whom do you turn for help?" Practitioners should also observe for objective data such as signs of depression, flat affect or refusal of treatment, presence of religious, spiritual or inspirational books or other literature, or jewelry (Hermann, 2000).

Health professionals may recognize spiritual pain as the person expresses sorrow or grief, verbalizes a sense of meaninglessness or emptiness to life, fear and avoidance of the future, sense of hopelessness and despair, anger towards God, as well as isolation of self and others (Matthews, 1999). It is important to realize that indications of spiritual pain can be both verbal and nonverbal, and that just as physical pain may change in nature and intensity over time, so too can spiritual pain change over time. As death approaches, new spiritual issues may arise, which may or may not be accompanied by spiritual pain (O'Connor, 1993). Furthermore, although health professionals may wish to alleviate spiritual pain, it is important to recognize the meaning and value of experiencing pain from the patient's perspective. Some individuals may believe that pain will lead to salvation or as a way of coming closer to God.

Instruments to Measure Spirituality

In the past several years, there has been a focus on the role of spirituality, as distinct from religion, in coping with illness. However, there remains a dearth of well-validated, psychometrically sound instruments

to measure aspects of spirituality (Peterman, Fitchett, Brady, Hernandez, & Cella 2002). One instrument that is a psychometrically sound measure of spiritual well-being is the Functional Assessment of Chronic Illness Therapy—Spiritual Well-Being (FACIT—Sp). This instrument comprises two subscales, one measuring a sense of meaning and peace and the other assessing the role of faith in illness. The FACIT-Sp has convergent validity with five other measures of spirituality and religion in samples of early state and metastatic cancer diagnoses, as well as documented reliability. A total score can be obtained.

A second spirituality assessment instrument with clinical utility is the Paloutzian and Ellison's Spiritual Well-Being Scale, which has also been administered to 70 family members caring for a relative with life-limiting illness. This 20-item instrument yields three scores: a total score of spiritual well-being (overall score); an existential well-being score, which relates to feelings about meaning and purpose in life, feelings about the future, and sense of well-being; and a religious well-being score which represents a sense of support and connection with God (Kirschling & Pittman, 1989).

Such instruments are of value in conducting research studies that explore the relationships of spirituality and quality of life for patients on palliative care. By identifying a patient's or family member's sense of spiritual well-being or spiritual distress, spiritual interventions may be provided to maintain or improve spiritual well-being and, hopefully, the quality of life and quality of dying as perceived by patients and family members.

Spiritual Caregiving

"Spiritual care is so much more than religious care. Spiritual care discovers, reverences, and tends the spirit-that is the energy or place of meaning and values—of another human being" (Driscoll, 2001, p. 334). In providing spiritual care, health professionals express the capacity to enter the world of others, to respond to fears, concerns, and feelings with compassion, and bear witness to the physical, emotional, social and spiritual dimensions of their suffering. As adults age, healthcare professionals can provide an opportunity to find intrinsic dignity, which is the dignity that comes from being a human being with inherent value and worth. By reviewing past life experiences, health professionals can assist the individual to reflect on their life accomplishments, the value of their relationships with others, and to forgive or be forgiven by others, and to say goodbye. Support can be given to patients to complete unfinished tasks or goals, and make peace with themselves or with God.

During hospitalizations, health professionals may ask if the person would like to speak with the clergy or chaplain or have the opportunity to attend a hospital worship service. Patients may also be asked if they would like someone to pray with or for them or have spiritual reading materials. Prayer has been identified as the most frequently reported alternative treatment modality of elders, with women and blacks using prayer as a coping strategy significantly more than men and whites (Dunn & Horgas, 2000). At times, if the patient is of the same faith background as the health professional, the patient may request prayer. However, prayer is appropriate only when the patient wants it and will be comforted by it (Koenig, 2002). Prayer should not be prescribed because the risk is that the intention is not patient-centered, but provider-centered, and in that context prayers offered by health professionals may be viewed as coercive (Koenig, 2002). The existing religious or spiritual beliefs of the patient should be supported and encouraged, yet the end of life is not the appropriate time to introduce new or unfamiliar spiritual beliefs or practices (Koenig, 2002). In a study of 30 individuals with cancer, Taylor, Outlaw, Bernardo, and Roy (1999) reported that several individuals described hesitancies about petitionary prayers for particular things, cure, or for themselves, and described inner conflicts about releasing control to God.

If a person is not religious or does not want a health professional to address religious issues, spiritual conversations around hope, love, courage, and forgiveness can occur in the provider–patient relationship (Koenig, 2002). Patients and health professionals of different faith backgrounds can appreciate the commonalties of basic human needs, such as love and hope, and explore issues of coping and what it means to live with an illness. Although health professionals can assess spiritual needs and address uncomplicated spiritual issues, caring and listening is the intervention, not giving advice or trying to address spiritual problems (Koenig, 2002).

Addressing spiritual problems is the role of the chaplain or clergy, as a member of the interdisciplinary team. The chaplain is a healthcare professional who has been trained to offer spiritual care to all people of any or no religious tradition and whose primary focus is the spiritual needs of patients, families, and staff (Driscoll, 2001). Like other members of the palliative care team, chaplains are alert to the expressed needs of the patient. As counselors, they take time to listen, discern the significance of the words spoken, intuit what is the importance of what is unspoken, and affirm the value of shared silence (Purdy, 2002). Often, spiritual support is listening to rhetorical questions, wanting an honest hearing of the question, rather than an answer. Patients may want to explore with chaplains whether God exists, the meaning of mortality, what Heaven is like, who goes to Hell, the integrity of doubt, the possibility of a miracle, the need to forgive, or the loneliness of suffering (Purdy, 2002). Patients and their families experience spiritual support when interdisciplinary team members

actively listen to their anxiety and allow discussion of the question, "Are we doing the right thing here?" (Purdy, 2002). Health professionals can also provide support by silent witnessing, and presencing, as well as serving as a liaison with other health professionals in addressing physical, emotional, and spiritual needs (Hicks, 1999).

Humor also has an effect on the spiritual aspect of healing, as many patients find humor "spiritually uplifting." As an element of spirituality and a coping method for spiritual growth and healing, humor can be transcendent, momentarily removing one from an isolated state to join in surprise at ludicrous human situations (Johnson, 2002). In a study of nine women with breast cancer, participants stated that they looked for meaning in their lives through spirituality and humor, as humor helped them to laugh at themselves and life. For some, it appeared that God had a sense of humor and that finding humorous moments was a step to recovery as humor heals and gives hope to survive the moment (Johnson, 2002).

Health professionals can also encourage patients to socialize with friends, family, and children, as well as encouraging them to help others, even if only by active listening. Supporting others often preserves a person's meaning in life and sense of usefulness. Adults can also pass on their legacy to others by recording personal histories, telling stories, and reminiscing about the past. Conducting a life review by asking questions, such as tell me about tranquil times in your life, chaotic time, what was your childhood like, what obstacle you overcame, what have you achieved, what are your fondest memories, help individuals to recontextualize and reframe mistakes and failure, allow forgiveness of self and others, reclaim an unlived life, and take advantage of current opportunities to participate in enjoyed activities (Jenko, Gonzalez, & Seymour, 2007). If the person is isolated, the health practitioner can suggest his/her watching spiritual or religious television programs or provide an opportunity to enjoy his/her favorite sacred or secular music, or other forms of art (Hermann, 2000). Practitioners may encourage opportunities for patients to experience nature in whatever ways they can, such as a walk or wheelchair ride in the garden or courtyard, or as they sit outside feeling the air and warmth of the sun.

Spiritual uplifting in the present moment can also occur as the practitioner attempts to create meaning and a source of pleasure in the present moment. As one example, a bed-bound patient with Parkinsonism found a moment of meaning and pleasure in the day by retelling to the nurse practitioner a story from his childhood, while anticipating a favorite meal to be brought in by his family the following day. Spiritual care can also involve "making meaning" through other forms of life review, such as looking at old photographs or personal memorabilia, reading old letters, or diary entries. By such efforts, healthcare professionals can acknowledge the individuality of a person and promote his/her sense of connection to self, others, and nature, thereby supporting his/her spirits and sense of well-being.

Chochinov and Cann (2005) reinforce not only general approaches to spiritual care, such as those offered by palliative care and psychotherapeutic approaches, but also specific approaches, such as relief of symptoms, as well as exploring guilt, encouraging forgiveness of self and others, and complementary practices that promote healing. Other supportive interventions include music and art and supportive-affective programs that focus on the spirit, emotions, and relationships.

Spiritual support may also be available through Parish nursing, which expands home health and public health provider roles. Parish nursing uses the faith community as a cooperative means of successful health promotion and maintenance for the older adult (Boland, 2000). In a survey of parish, oncology, and Hospice nurses, the most frequently identified spiritual interventions were referral, prayer, active listening, facilitation and validation of patient's thoughts and feelings, conveying acceptance, and instilling hope (Sellers & Haag, 1998).

SPIRITUAL AND RELIGIOUS PERSPECTIVES ON DEATH

Losses in life often challenge our faith and philosophical systems. Those who experience loss and grief may differ regarding religious and spiritual perspectives from which they seek answers, search for meaning, and to which they turn for ritual, comfort, and support (Doka & Davidson, 1998). Understanding the ways that spirituality or religiosity facilitates or complicates the adjustment to loss and grief is a critical task to those involved in palliative care.

Death from a Jewish Perspective

Judaism began when the descendants of Abraham's grandson Israel were enslaved in Egypt. Moses led them to Palestine. During this time, Jewish law, known as the Torah, was divinely revealed to Moses. The Sabbath is celebrated from sunset on Friday to sunset on Saturday evening. The Sabbath is the day of rest. The degree to which a Jew observes the Sabbath and other rituals depends on whether he or she is Orthodox, Conservative, or Reformed. (Sherman, 2004a). The focus of those of the Jewish faith is on life and its preservation and in fostering and establishing religion in the life of people on earth, rather than focusing on the world beyond. The Jewish faith offers consolation in death by affirmation of life. Sickness and death are viewed as neither punishment nor reward. Death is not considered evil but rather inevitable and natural, as it comes from God

and should not be feared. Jewish teachings are that the soul exists before the body comes into existence and continues to live on after the body is dead. Although the Orthodox believe in resurrection, this belief may be figurative rather than literal (Grollman, 1993).

Jewish death practices help the bereaved to realize that the loved one is dead and to gradually fill the void in a constructive way. The memory of the deceased must be perpetuated. Although Jews are usually buried, cremations are also done. A religious rite is the rending of mourners' clothes, signified by the cutting of a black ribbon that is pinned to the mourners' clothing in the funeral chapel or cemetery. This signifies the loss of a loved one. The Jewish funeral is a rite of separation, in which the casket actualizes the experience. The rabbi recites prayers expressive of the spirit of Judaism and the memory of the deceased. Shiva refers to the 7 days of intensive mourning beginning right after the funeral. The bereaved remain at home and condolence calls are made to pay respects to the family. The shiva candle burns for 7 days and the family prepares the meal of consolation, known as seudat havra'ah. Following shiva comes the 30 days of sloshim. During this time normal activities are resumed but entertainment is avoided. If a parent dies, the mourning continues for an entire year. The mourner's prayer is called the Kaddish, which is recited during the weekly Sabbath as a pledge to dedicate one's life to God, acknowledge the reality of death, and affirm life. The anniversary of the death is called yahrzeit. The Kaddish prayer is recited and yahrzeit candles are again kindled (Grollman, 1993).

Death from the Roman Catholic Perspective

In Catholicism, it is believed that Jesus experienced suffering, grief, and death. Jesus's death and the death of all others are viewed as a part of God's divine providence. As sinners, human beings experience the tragedy of death, yet are beneficiaries of its forgiveness and liberation. In Catholicism, resurrection is integral to death. Catholics believe that Christ died and rose from the dead, and that faith will allow them to see death as an entry into life with God. Confession and communion are important rituals conducted by priests. The sacrament of the anointing of the sick provides bodily and spiritual renewal and has replaced the term "the last rites," which was viewed as a harbinger of death.

Since the second Vatican Council, the Catholic contemporary view places emphasis on risen life. There is a move from a preoccupation with sin and death toward an orientation of blessing for a Christian life. Christians follow Jesus into the mystery of death in order to find a life like his own (Miller, 1993). The funeral becomes one of thanksgiving and consolation; the funeral mass is offered on behalf of the deceased, aiding them to the other side of death and giving the bereaved the consolation of hope. It is believed that Christ accompanies the dying person to heaven and that dying is an act of faith in God (Miller, 1993).

Death from the Protestant Perspective

In Protestantism, spirituality is viewed as a dimension of humanness, a process of interaction, and an awareness of relationship. Spirituality cannot be lived in the abstract but rather is lived through one's religion, which is regarded as a cultural institution (Klass, 1993). God is viewed as a single being, who spoke to his people through the Bible; God protects but also judges. Each Protestant has a direct and personal relationship with God, unmediated by priest or sacrament. The church is viewed as a voluntary association of believers. The Protestant community is the local congregation or particular denomination supporting interpersonal relationships, yet is often split along racial, ethnic, and social class lines (Klass, 1993). Anointing the sick is accepted by some groups. Although there are no last rites, prayers are given to offer support.

Death is a challenge because it raises the problem of evil and the problem of the meaningfulness of suffering. Suffering and overcoming evil are the core of Protestant teaching. For Protestants, the focus is salvation, which depends on the moral quality of life on earth. Heaven is known in hope, but not as a guarantee. The belief in an afterlife is through experiences of memory and sense of presence and shared community. Although Jesus is a model for physical, emotional, social, and spiritual suffering, the individual faces the cosmos alone. The issue is not how the individual can participate in Jesus's suffering, but rather the individual's accepting the gift of God's grace in Jesus's death (Klass, 1993).

Death from the Islamic Perspective

Islam means submission. Muslim means one who submits. A Muslim is one who submits to Allah, the Arabic word for God. Muslims, Jews, and Christians worship the same God. The founder of Islam is Mohammad, who received a vision while meditating, which later became the Koran. The five pillars of Islam are confession of faith daily in front of witnesses, prayer five times a day, fasting during the month of Ramadan, almsgiving, and a pilgrimage to Mecca. Fasting during Ramadan is not required of the sick. Second-degree male relatives (e.g., cousins or uncles) should be contacted when a person is sick. They determine if a person or family should be told the diagnosis or prognosis. The Islamic teachings encourage Muslims to seek treatment when they are sick including modern medicine, spiritual healing, and traditional healing practices such as recitation of verses of the Noble Qur`an. They believe in divine predestination and perceive suffering as atonement for one's sins. When asking about the life expectancy of a patient, they are more likely to be comfortable with less definitive answers such as "it is in the hands of God" as Allah determines the time of death (Zafir al-Shahri and al-Khenaizan (2005).

Death is viewed as the beginning of a different form of life in which there are blessing from Allah. Some families may ask to have the patient face Mecca (East) and his/her head should be elevated above the body. Discussions about death are not usually welcomed. Grief may be expressed by slapping or hitting the body. Same-sex Muslims should handle the body after death; otherwise the individual should wear gloves so as not to touch the body. Islam forbids cremation, and burial should happen as soon as possible (Zafir al-Shahri & al-Khenaizan (2005)).

Death from Eastern Perspectives

Hinduism originated in India, with belief in the cycles of being born and dying in an infinite series of lives or successive creations. Hinduism teaches the belief in karma, which is that every act of a human being, even an internal act, such as desire, has an effect on who that person becomes. One becomes virtuous by good actions and bad by bad actions (Ryan, 1993). A Supreme Being exists in the individual's soul and is the ultimate all.

Originating in India, Buddhism does not include a belief in a God or a soul. Buddism teaches that suffering is a part of life and that in death there is a transference of consciousness out of the body (Smith-Stoner, 2006). Buddhists believe in karma and rebirth. Karma is the principle of cause and effect. Buddhists train their minds to remain calm and peaceful as death approaches. Buddha taught that a way to overcome ignorance and attain truth is through the path to enlightenment or changed state of awareness called Nirvana. Buddhists believe that the way to Nirvana is through meditation, while others believe it can be attained through faith.

Yet another Eastern tradition is that of Confucianism, which has its origins in China and stresses the importance of improving human relationships. The proper relationship between the living and dead is one of continuous remembrance and affection, through which one attains social immortality. The value of rituals is that they relate the living with the dead. Memories of parents and ancestors are kept through regular remembrance rituals, which also provide a vehicle for the expression of the human emotions of grief and affection.

Taoism has its origins in China. In Taoism, the focus is on nature and remedying society's disorder and lack of harmony. One looks toward nature to discover the principles of life. Life is viewed as the companion of death, and death is viewed as the beginning of life and part of the living-dying process. Taoism offers a way of transcending the limits of the world, as there are ceaseless transformations where the person is not lost. The yin and yang are the basic principles for all natural change. The yang is the light half, which is characterized as masculine, active, hot, bright, dry, and hard. The yin is the dark half, which is characterized as feminine, passive, cold, dark, wet, and soft. They are viewed as complementary forces that transform into the other. There is no light without dark, evil without good, or life without death (Ryan, 1993).

Many Asian patients—Chinese, Japanese, Koreans-have an Eastern perspective in which formal behaviors are valued. It is believed that to rebel against death reveals a fundamental lack of understanding about life. Therefore, sadness and grief are kept private. Such behavior sets a good example and contributes to one's good reputation (Ryan, 1993). Patients may seek comfort in images, such as Buddha, Krishna, or the Divine Mother, or in repeating holy mantras. Those from an Eastern perspective believe that a person's final dying thoughts may determine one's rebirth.

Spiritual Issues in Death and Dying for Those Who Have No Conventional Religious Beliefs

Religion traditionally has provided a context for understanding and interpreting death. However, individuals who are not religious can still find comfort and meaning through spirituality and by stepping back from the material world (Orion, 1993). Individuals with no conventional religious beliefs often interpret life on the basis of a sense of being a part of a larger whole and from a scientific worldview. There is belief that an individual's life has a beginning and an ending, but the life process is indefinite. Whether the process is defined in terms of social or biological continuity, the brevity of life does not suggest insignificance. A particular life is short and seemingly inconsequential but assumes value and importance as a significant element in the entire ongoing process. Even brief life is viewed as a contribution to the life process.

Those without conventional religious beliefs often consider the present as the real world and take full responsibility for their decisions. There is the belief that immortality occurs by biological immortality such as living on in the genetic pool of one's descendants, or living on in the memories of others or one's contributions to the world (Orion, 1993). The focus is on actualizing human potential. From the naturalistic perspective, death is not avoided or denied. Death is viewed as real, final, and inevitable and a mark of humans' solidarity with nature and the evolutionary process.

Naturalism leads an effort to place the death of an individual in a framework of the process of living and dying, emergence, and extinction. In this framework, death is:

- a working out of the natural law by which all living things die;
- the absorption of the differentiated person in the natural process;
- a contribution to the evolutionary process;
- cessation of life's potential for negative and positive contributions; and
- re-absorption into new ways in nature (Orion, 1993).

Fear of death can be overcome by remembering that everything dies, but existence goes on. When death is seen as part of the natural order or part of the universal condition, it can be tolerated more easily. Life and death are continuous parts of the whole (Orion, 1993).

Given the dearth of studies regarding the perspectives of atheists in palliative medicine, Smith-Stoner (2007) conducted a study of 88 individuals who self-identified as atheists, which is defined as someone who does not accept that there are any Gods, heaven, hell, devils, souls, miracles, an afterlife, or anything else supernatural. Based on an analysis of open- and closed-ended survey questions, the results of end-of-life preferences indicate that participants' view of a good death included respect for nonbelief and the withholding of prayer or any other references to God. However, consistent with a definition of spirituality which includes intrapersonal, interpersonal, and a natural focus, atheists expressed a deep desire to find meaning in their own lives (intrapersonal), to maintain connection with family and friends (interpersonal), and to continue to experience and appreciate the natural world.

Based on a qualitative study, it was also reported that patients with cancer use prayer to cope with their illness. Participants described prayer as an active cognitive process involving talking to God, or beseeching God, while others described a passive process involving listening to God and accepting that "God's will be done" (Taylor & Outlaw, 2002).

NURSES' NEED FOR SELF-REFLECTION AND SELF-HEALING IN PALLIATIVE CARE

Doka and Morgan (1993) describe the caregivers' assumptions and principles of spiritual care. First, nurses represent diverse spiritual or cultural backgrounds and, like patients, have the right to expect respect for their belief systems. Second, nurses should be offered opportunities to explore their own values and attitudes about life and death and their meaning and purpose in life. Third, nurses should be aware that they have the potential for providing spiritual care, and should be encouraged to offer spiritual care to dying patients and their families, as needed. Fourth, just as all caregivers, nurses should be flexible and realistic in setting spiritual goals. Fifth, ongoing care of the dying and bereaved may cause a severe drain of energy and uncover old and new spiritual issues for the caregiver. Spiritual growth and renewal is, therefore, a necessary part of staff support and a personal priority for each caregiver.

Indeed, in caring for dying patients and bereaved families, nurses may have experiences that create a grief response of their own because they have lost someone in whom they have invested themselves emotionally. Nurses' grief response, like that of their patients, will be influenced by their spiritual and cultural values and beliefs. If accumulated grief is not worked through, the nurse is vulnerable to the same manifestations of unresolved grief as any other individual who has had a loss but failed to complete the grief work (Rando, 1984; Sherman, 2004b). Nurses, therefore, need to resolve their own feelings of loss, with their spiritual convictions supported, sense of failure alleviated, and emotional strength replenished (Rando, 1984; Sherman, 2004b).

In coping with the stress of caring for the dying, Rando (1984) believes that nurses progress through five stages: 1) focusing on professional knowledge and factual information; 2) experiencing the trauma of the patient's illness, often accompanied by guilt and frustration as the nurse confronts the patient's impending death; 3) moving through the pain and coming to an acceptance of the reality of death; 4) identifying the pain and suffering with sensitivity, but freeing themselves from the incapacitating effects; and 5) relating compassionately with the dying person in full acceptance of impending death. In caring for patients in palliative care, nurses must develop an awareness of their own emotional, physical, or spiritual limits, and develop an awareness of their own energy levels. By realizing the need for self-care, acknowledging their own feelings about dying and death and the stresses in caring for the dying that are most troublesome to them individually, nurses can prevent caregiver burnout (Rando, 1984).

In developing awareness and supporting nurses' spiritual well-being, nurse educators may ask their students or nursing colleagues the following questions:

- What expectations do you have about yourself in caring for the dying and bereaved?
- What would define success in your work?
- What are the three most difficult aspects of your work in caring for patients with life-threatening illness?
- What are you doing to help yourself cope with stress and replenish yourself to avoid becoming overstressed?

"Nurses must recognize their stress reactions and symptoms and employ self-care strategies to replenish themselves in physical, emotional, mental, and spiritual ways to overcome the various sources of stress" (Sherman, 2004b, p. 53). In reducing burnout in palliative-care nursing, *physical health* is promoted as nurses care for their bodies by eating well, engaging in restful and relaxing activities, and counterbalancing fatigue by making improvements in lifestyle. *Emotional* health is bolstered by developing a calm mind with peaceful thoughts through such activities as meditation or listening to quiet music, as well as consciously letting go of negative thoughts and emotions. *Mental health* is strengthened by making choices, setting priorities, letting go of conflict, and saying no, while keeping open to new opportunities and possibilities. And *intuitional health* is nurtured by listening to the soul's wisdom and recognizing the need for balance and wholeness.

In overcoming interpersonal stressors, particularly when relations with others are difficult, nurses may find it helpful to reflect on the rewards of their work and the moments in which they have made the greatest difference in the lives of their patients and families. To cope with feelings of grief and loss, nurses can take time to reflect on what happened at the time of the patient's death and lessons learned and speak to colleagues or journal about feelings, perceptions, and experiences (Sherman, 2004b).

Within the context of end-of-life care, and given that spirituality has emerged as a vital component of health, it becomes necessary for nurses to acknowledge their own spiritual beliefs and values and to deal with their own spiritual and cultural issues. Based on a sample of 155 Israeli oncology nurses, Musgrave and McFarlane (2004) reported that nurses' attitudes toward spiritual care are influenced by their spiritual well-being, intrinsic and extrinsic religiosity, and education. In a descriptive, qualitative study of the spiritual care perspectives and practices of 204 Hospice nurses, Belcher and Griffiths (2005) recognized that the majority of the sample stated that they personally expressed their spirituality by attending church and related activities, that there was an openness and level of comfort in being a spiritual caregivers, and that there was no role conflict in spiritual expression. The majority of Hospice nurses learned of the spiritual needs of their patients and families through personal interactions and the support of pastoral counselors or learning from their own personal life experiences. As Hospice nurses, most indicated that they conducted spiritual assessment and recognized the importance of addressing spiritual needs, although their basic educational programs did little to prepare them. It was clear that Hospice nurses value education regarding spirituality, which they believe enhances the quality of care. Clark and colleagues (2007) examined the spirituality of members of a Hospice interdisciplinary team (n = 215). Based on the Jarel Spiritual Well-Being

Scale, the Chameic-Case Spirituality Integration Scale, and the Job Satisfaction Scale, respondents reported high levels of spiritual well-being, self-actualization, and job satisfaction. Structural path analyses revealed that job satisfaction is more likely realized by a model that transforms one`s spirituality into processes of integrating spirituality at work and self-actualization.

According to Hunnibell, Reed, Quinn-Griffin and Fitzpatrick (2008), nurses in Hospice and palliative care, as well as oncology nurses, manifest self-transcendence, which is characterized by awareness of the spiritual self, one's relationship to others, a higher being, and find meaning and purpose in life. Based on a sample of 563 nurses (244 Hospice nurses and 319 oncology nurses), both groups of nurses scored high on the Self-transcendence Scale, though Hospice nurses had higher scores. For both groups of nurses, the greater the level of self-transcendence, the lower the nurses scores of burnout, measured by the Maslach Burnout Inventory, as emotional exhaustion, depersonalization, and personal accomplishment. Oncology nurses manifested higher levels of burnout than Hospice nurses, particularly with respect to depersonalization. It was suggested that nurses should be encouraged to connect with other nurses and form support groups to share their experiences. Strategies such as keeping a journal, sharing one's stories, and recognizing positive individual contributions to care may increase sense of worth and reduce professional burnout.

The importance of spiritual care was emphasized in a position statement published by the Hospice and Palliative Care Nurses Association (2007). The statement emphasized the commitment of Hospice and palliative care nursing to compassionate care at the end of life, acknowledging the importance of spiritual care, encouraging support of The National Consensus Project Guidelines for Quality Palliative Care on spirituality, encouraging organizational support in the provision of spiritual care, commitment to education and resources to promote spiritual care, and recognition of the right of individuals to decline spiritual care.

In caring for people with life-threatening and progressive illness, nurses must remain in tune with their own spiritual needs, healing themselves as well as others. To do so, Halifax (1999) suggests a contemplative exercise for nurses to remain centered, renewed, and whole as they care for others. Sitting in a relaxed position, with eyes closed and aware of the rhythm of the breath, the nurse focuses one at a time on each of the following five phrases, which are repeated slowly twice. The nurse then allows the phrase to pass into the background of her or his awareness, moving attention to the breath and to the next phrase. The phrases are as follows:

- May I offer my care and presence unconditionally, knowing that it may be met with gratitude, indifference, anger, or anguish.

- May I offer love, knowing that I cannot control the course of life's suffering or death.
- May I remain in ease and let go of my expectations.
- May I view my own suffering with compassion just as I do the suffering of others.
- May I be aware that my suffering does not limit my good heart.
- May I forgive myself for things left undone.
- May I forgive all who have hurt me.
- May those whom I have hurt forgive me.
- May all beings and I live and die in peace.

Coulehan and Clary (2005) suggest that poetry can play a role in healing, as the written word becomes an instrument of healing, and an opportunity for practitioners to reframe negativity, learn to function in the face of uncertainty, and supports a compassionate presence in the care of the seriously ill and dying. Writing and reading poetry assists practitioners in understanding their own beliefs, feelings, attitudes, and response patterns, and in the process fosters empathic connection and a relationship that heals both patients and practitioners.

Spiritually and culturally competent care, therefore, requires self-reflection and self-care of nurses. Replenishing one's own vessel in spiritually and culturally renewing ways is important in supporting nurses' caregiving potential. For, it is only by doing so that nurses will come to the bedside with the strong healing presence and true compassion needed to alleviate the suffering of patients and their families.

Case Study conclusion: Mrs. Martinez's weakness and fatigue progressed, with only a slight improvement in her left sided weakness. She spent the last 6 months of her life in the loving care of her family with the support of Hospice. The nurse continued to address Mrs. Martinez's physical needs, which were increasing pain, constipation, and nausea, while recognizing the multidimensional aspects of her suffering. Mrs. Martinez enjoyed her visits with the Hospice chaplain, who was a Catholic priest. He prayed with her at her request, administered weekly Holy Communion, and anointed her with the Sacrament of the Sick. Like Mrs. Martinez, the family expressed their appreciation for the chaplain's spiritual sensitivity and care. Spiritual support was further offered by the nurse practitioner who recognized the value of life review and sat with Mrs. Martinez and the family as they watched family videotapes and reminisced about special occasions. With help from the nurse, the daughter would take her mother in the wheelchair to sit for short periods in the yard. Mrs. Martinez's face relaxed as she listened to the birds and enjoyed her watching grandchildren.

Till the very last days of her life, Mrs. Martinez experienced the love and support of her family. Sips of herbal teas were encouraged to give her strength or relieve the nausea. Latino music was played, reminding her of her cultural connection. Members of her church visited and prayer novenas were conducted. Mrs. Martinez died in her own room with her family and the Hospice nurse at her side. The nurse and family discussed the cultural and spiritual practices of the family in preparing for Mrs. Martinez's funeral and plans to celebrate her life.

During a follow-up bereavement visit, Mrs. Martinez's family acknowledged their appreciation for the culturally and spiritually sensitive care received by the Hospice team. Mrs. Martinez's daughter told the nurse that they considered her as a member of their family. This comment reveals the depth of connection that can be established with older patients and their family, and the importance of cultural and spiritual sensitivity in providing quality palliative care.

CONCLUSION

Illness and dying are occurrences that take us to the very core of our being. Although they are intensely personal experiences, they occur within the context of our spiritual and cultural traditions. Culture and spirituality can therefore not be separated from who we are, as they are often the very source of our nourishment and physical, emotional, social, and spiritual well-being. Through sensitive and competent cultural and spiritual care, nurses can protect patients and families from the ultimate tragedy of depersonalization. They will be able to sustain them in a personalized environment that recognizes their individual needs, reduces their fears, and offers them hope and dignity. Sulmasy (1997) believes that "when patients collapse spiritually in the face of illness, a clinician with the right perspective will understand much more acutely how desperate their plight really is and will treat the wounds of such patients with even more liberal applications of the wine of fervent zeal and the oil of compassion" (p. 52). Frankl (1988) reminds us that man is not destroyed by suffering, but by suffering without meaning.

Cultural and spiritual values, beliefs, and practices profoundly influence life and living and death and dying. Identifying cultural and spiritual factors pertinent to a patient's health are critical to the development of a successful plan of care that supports a person's sense of worth, integrity, and the continued actualization of their

potentials. Within the context of culturally and spiritually diverse beliefs and practices, health professionals should preserve beliefs and practices of individuals that have beneficial effects on health, encourage the adaptation or adjustment of practices that are neutral or indifferent, and suggest the re-patterning of those practices that are potentially harmful to health (Leininger, 1995).

Culturally and spiritually competent care requires self-reflection and self-care if healthcare professionals are to be therapeutic. As such, healthcare professionals need to replenish their own vessels in culturally and spiritually renewing ways to actualize their caregiving potential. In doing so, healthcare practitioners can offer a strong healing presence, true compassion, and sensitivity to the cultural and spiritual needs of older patients and their families (Sherman, 2001).

Consideration of the cultural and spiritual backgrounds of patients and attention to their cultural and spiritual needs often enable older patients to live as fully as possible until death, and to maintain or restore quality to their lives. Byock (1997) reminds us that through competent and compassionate end-of-life care, older adults and all other patients can achieve a sense of inner well-being even as death approaches, and that "when the human dimension of dying is nurtured, for many the transition from life can be as profound, intimate, and precious as the miracle of death"(p. 57).

EVIDENCE-BASED PRACTICE

Level IV Evidence: Descriptive, Correlational, Qualitative

Mako, C., Galek, K., & Poppito, S. (2006). Spiritual pain among patients with advanced cancer in palliative care. *Journal of Palliative Medicine, 9*(5), 1106–1113.

Background. Empirical research indicates that the spiritual pain of patients influences the disease process and further understanding of the complexity of spiritual pain is warranted.

Purpose. To explore the multidimensional nature of spiritual pain as it relates to physical pain, symptom severity, and emotional distress in patients with end stage cancer.

Design. Quantitative evaluation of the intensity of spiritual pain, physical pain, depression, and intensity of illness, as well as a qualitative exploration by chaplains of the nature of spiritual pain and interventions identified by patients to relieve spiritual pain.

1.1 | Plan for Achieving Competencies: Spiritually and Culturally Competent Palliative Care

KNOWLEDGE NEEDED	ATTITUDE	SKILLS	UNDERGRADUATE BEHAVIORAL OUTCOMES	GRADUATE BEHAVIORAL OUTCOMES	TEACHING/LEARNING STRATEGIES
Cultural perspectives regarding illness and death: —Native American; —African and African-American; —Hispanic; —Asian; —Cultural values underlying advanced directives and medical decision making; —Research regarding culture and end-of-life issues.	■ Appreciate varying cultural perspectives of death. ■ Value research in informing cultural care.	■ Demonstrate sensitivity to cultural beliefs and customs.	■ Develop a plan of care with the patient and family that addresses their cultural perspectives on death and cultural needs. ■ Critique and utilize research in guiding culturally competent care.	■ Address conflicts that result from differences in cultural perspectives on death of patients, families, and healthcare providers. ■ Participate in conducting research regarding culture and health-related outcomes.	■ Have students interview two individuals of diverse cultural backgrounds and compare beliefs, values, expectations, and traditions related to illness and death. Compare the information obtained from information written in textbooks or journal articles. Share findings in class. ■ Critique five research articles related to cultural beliefs and healthcare issues. Synthesize the findings and discuss the implications for nursing practice.
Quality nursing care: Addressing cultural needs of patients and their families—nurses' cultural self-awareness and development of cultural competency—cultural assessment and interventions.	■ Recognize students'/nurses' own cultural beliefs and values.	■ Convey unconditional acceptance of patients and families of various cultural backgrounds. ■ Demonstrate the completion of a cultural assessment.	■ Create an environment which supports cultural beliefs, values, traditions, and rituals.	■ Develop a comprehensive plan of care which takes into account cultural values, needs, and expectation. ■ Educate other healthcare providers in providing culturally competent care.	■ In post-conference or seminar, encourage students to express feelings of appreciation regarding their own cultural heritage while introducing the topic of ethnocentrism in connection with the value of cultural diversity. ■ Have students identify who was significant in teaching or transmitting to them their cultural identity and discuss the impact of their identity on their present life. ■ Have students identify how members of their cultural group approach personal or emotional problems. ■ In the clinical setting, conduct a cultural assessment of a patient/family and report findings in post-conference or seminar. ■ In post-conference or seminar, create and discuss a list of behaviors or comments which may be viewed as culturally insensitive based on past, personal, or professional experiences. Role-play compassionate and effective communication regarding cultural issues relevant to palliative care.
Spirituality and culture as factors that structure responses to	■ Affirm nurses' commitment to holistic practice.	■ Act in accordance with the patients' and families'	■ Incorporate spiritual and cultural care in nursing practice.	■ Role-model and expect of others spiritually and culturally	■ Write a position paper about the role of spirituality and culture in providing nursing care.

KNOWLEDGE NEEDED	ATTITUDE	SKILLS	UNDERGRADUATE BEHAVIORAL OUTCOMES	GRADUATE BEHAVIORAL OUTCOMES	TEACHING/LEARNING STRATEGIES
life-threatening illness.	■ Emphasize the value of spirituality and culture in providing end of life care.	spiritual and cultural values and wishes.		competent care for patients and families.	
The spiritual nature of the person	■ Value and support the spirituality of human beings. ■ Appreciate the needs of the dying to make peace with life and death.		■ Provide spiritually competent care to patients and families experiencing life threatening illness by considering spiritual well-being.	■ Create an environment in which the spiritual nature of people is recognized, valued, and supported. ■ Assist patients and families to find a source of spiritual energy or reaffirm students'/ nurses'/spiritual focus.	■ Based on the spiritual assessment of a particular patient and family, develop a spiritual plan of care. Review the plan of care with clergy/chaplain.
Suffering as a human condition —reciprocal suffering of patients and family—care of those who are suffering.	■ Acknowledge suffering as a multidimensional experience. ■ Recognize that suffering may be personal or experienced as witness to another's suffering. ■ Appreciate that suffering and pain are not identical. ■ Consider the effect of suffering on health and quality of life of patients, families, and healthcare providers.	■ Demonstrate therapeutic use of self in alleviating suffering.	■ Assist patients and family to identify the meaning of suffering and refer to members of other disciplines as appropriate.	■ Assess the impact of suffering on patient, family, healthcare providers, and community. ■ Implement the role of nurse as a coach in caring for those who are suffering. ■ Support patients and family in achieving some transcendent meaning to their suffering.	■ Based on a case study, identify the dimensions of suffering and nursing strategies to alleviate suffering.
Spiritual and religious perspectives of death: —Jewish —Roman —Catholic —Protestant —Islam —Eastern perspectives	■ Appreciate varying spiritual and religious perspectives of death. ■ Value research in informing spiritual care.	■ Demonstrate sensitivity to spiritual and religious beliefs and customs.	■ Develop a plan of care with the patient and family that addresses their spiritual and religious perspectives on death and associated needs.	■ Address conflicts that result from differences in spiritual and religious perspectives on death of patients, families, and	■ Role-play as a way of learning about different spiritual/ religious beliefs and values in a nonjudgmental way. Self-critique attitudes and interaction followed by feedback from faculty and peers. ■ Critique five research articles related to spiritual or religious beliefs and

(Continued)

Table 1.1 *(Continued)*

KNOWLEDGE NEEDED	ATTITUDE	SKILLS	UNDERGRADUATE BEHAVIORAL OUTCOMES	GRADUATE BEHAVIORAL OUTCOMES	TEACHING/LEARNING STRATEGIES
—No conventional religious beliefs —Research regarding spirituality			■ Critique and utilize research in guiding spiritual caregiving.	healthcare providers. ■ Participate in conducting research regarding spirituality and health-related outcomes.	healthcare issues. Synthesize the findings and discuss the implications for nursing practice. ■ Distribute 3×5 cards and ask the students what happens at the time of death on side one and how that belief serves them on side two of the card. Ask the students to pass the card to another student. They are to take on the belief of the other student as their own. They are now asked how this new belief may benefit them.
Quality nursing care: Addressing spiritual needs of patients and families: —spiritual caregiving —spiritual assessment —spiritual interventions and care —educating nurses and physicians regarding spirituality.	■ Recognize students'/nurses' own spiritual and religious beliefs and values. ■ Value nurses' presence, compassion, and hopefulness in providing quality spiritual care. ■ Appreciate the role of chaplains and clergy in offering spiritual care.	■ Convey unconditional acceptance of patients and families of diverse spiritual and religious beliefs and backgrounds. ■ Demonstrate the completion of a spiritual history/assessment.	■ Create an environment that nurtures the the patient's exploration of spiritual needs and concerns. ■ Address patients' and families' spiritual and religious needs through presencing, active listening, unconditional regard, and support of meaningful rituals.	■ Identify patients and family who are at risk for spiritual distress. ■ Develop a comprehensive plan of care to alleviate spiritual suffering. ■ Educate other healthcare in providing spiritually competent care.	■ Write a position statement identifying students'/nurses' personal beliefs and assumptions as it relates to spirituality or religiosity. ■ Conduct a values clarification exercise for students/nurses to identify their own spiritual values. ■ Discuss the role of clergy as members of the interdisciplinary team in post-conference or seminar. ■ Discuss illustrative cases where patient's spirituality or religiosity negatively affected their health outcomes and potential spiritual interventions.
Nurses' needs for self-reflection and self-healing in palliative care.	■ Affirm nurses' right to be respected for their belief systems. ■ Acknowledge students'/nurses' personal potential for providing spiritual and and cultural care. ■ Appreciate the potential drain of energy and resurfacing of personal spiritual issues related to care giving.		■ Develop an awareness of students'/nurses' own spiritual, emotional, and physical limits. ■ Establish a personal plan of care for maintaining health and promoting personal and professional growth.	■ Assess colleagues at risk for caregiving burnout. ■ Advocate for systems that support students'/nurses' self-care and personal and professional growth.	■ Write a personal plan of care to address the students'/nurses' physical, emotional, social, and spiritual needs, and strategies to promote personal and professional growth within the next 6 months. ■ Create a suggestion box and contribute one recommended change, which would support the nurses' caregiving potential within the educational setting. ■ Discuss in the classroom, post-conference, or seminar ways in which students/nurses have been able to provide spiritual care and the responses of the individual and family. ■ Beginning with a 5-min relaxation exercise, have students/nurses write a poem asking a transcendent life force for support. Have each student/nurse read their poem, twice slowly.

Sample. 57 patients with advanced cancer in a palliative-care hospital.

Results. 96% reported spiritual pain which was described as intrapsychic (anxiety , loss, regret, interpersonal feeling unwanted and disconnected from others), and in relation to the divine (abandoned by God, being without faith or a religious community). Intensity of spiritual pain was correlated with depression, but not with physical pain or severity of illness. However, a third of participants describe their pain in somewhat physical terms. Those receiving morphine for physical pain were more likely to express spiritual pain. The intensity of spiritual pain was not associated with age, gender, disease course or religious affiliation. The most frequently requested intervention is listening and presence.

Conclusion. Spiritual pain is universal and multidimensional. Alleviation of physical pain by morphine may allow access to underlying spiritual issues. Spiritual pain is communicated through an emotional realm. Though there is overlap between spiritual pain and depression, there is differentiation requiring different interventions. More attention needs to be given to exploring the complexity of pain and of spiritual pain as a factor.

Commentary. This study is of significance to palliative-care practitioners in recognizing that spiritual pain can occur in the absence of physical pain and that dignity conserving interventions are of benefit. This study discussed in the review of the literature Melzack and Wall's theory of pain as a multidimensional construct but did present as conceptual framework or theory which guided the study. There was no discussion of the inclusion criteria, data collection procedures, or protection of human subjects. The variables were not measured with instruments with reliability or validity. The methods for qualitative data analysis were not described. Paragment et al.s three dimensions of spiritual pain was used to classify the qualitative data regarding spirituality, which may have limited reporting of other findings that did not fit the three dimensions. The authors conclude that unaddressed spiritual pain may impede recovery and contribute to overall suffering. It is recognized that spiritual pain is associated with anxiety, but the concepts of recovery and suffering were not directly measured. The findings support the need for assessment of spiritual distress and the need for future research, which will inform the identification and implementation of appropriate spiritual interventions.

To identify the knowledge, attitudes, and skills of undergraduate and graduate nurses' behavioral outcomes and teaching/learning strategies, please refer to the Education Plan (Table 1.1).

REFERENCES

Abrums, M. (2000). Death and meaning in a storefront church. *Public Health Nursing, 17*(2), 132–142.

Adunsky, A., Aiminoff, B., Arad, M., & Bercovitch, M. (2008). Mini-suffering state examination: Suffering and survival of end of life cancer patients in a Hospice setting. *American Journal of Hospice and Palliative Medicine, 24*(6), 493–498.

Albuagh, J. (2003). Spirituality and life-threatening illness: A phenomenologic study. *Oncology Nursing Forum, 30,* 593–598.

American Medical Student Association. (2001). Cultural competency in medicine. Retrieved from http://www.amsa.org/programs/gpit/cultural

Andrews, M., & Boyle J. (1995). *Transcultural concepts in nursing care.* Philadelphia, PA: J. B. Lippincott.

Arnold, E. (1989). Burnout as a spiritual issue: Rediscovering meaning in nursing practice. In V. Carson (Ed.), *Spiritual dimensions of nursing practice* (pp. 320–353). Philadelphia, PA: Saunders.

Barclay, J., Blackhall, L., & Tulsky, J. (2007). Communication strategies and cultural issues in the delivery of bad news. *Journal of Palliative Medicine, 10*(4), 958–977.

Beeney, L., Butow, P., & Dunn, S. (1997). Normal adjustment to cancer: Characteristics and assessment. In R. K. Portenoy & E. Bruera (Eds.), *Topics in palliative care: Vol. 1* (pp. 213–244). New York: Oxford University Press.

Belcher, A., & Griffiths, M. (2005). The spiritual care perspectives and practices of Hospice nurses. *Journal of Hospice and Palliative Nursing, 7*(5), 271–279.

Bergan, A., & McConatha, J. (2000). Religiosity and life satisfaction. *Activities Adapt Aging, 24*(3), 23–24.

Beery, T., Baas, L., Fowler, C., & Allen, G. (2002). Spirituality in persons with heart failure. *Journal of Holistic Nursing, 20*(1), 5–25.

Bhungalia, S., & Kemp, C. (2002). (Asian) Indian health beliefs and practices related to end of life. *Journal of Hospice and Palliative Nursing, 4*(1), 54–58.

Bird, L. (1986). Suffering, thanatology, and whole-person medicine. In R. DeBellis, E. Marcus, A. Kutscher, C. Smith Torres, V. Barrett, & M. Siegel (Eds.), *Suffering: Psychological and social aspects in loss, grief, and care* (pp. 31–39). New York: Haworth Press.

Boland, C. (2000). Parish nursing: Addressing the significance of social support and spirituality for sustained health-promoting behaviors in the elderly. *Journal of Holistic Nursing, 16*(3), 355–368.

Brennan, M. R. (1994). *Spirituality in the homebound elderly.* Unpublished doctoral dissertation, Catholic University of America, Washington, DC.

Brokenleg, M., & Middleton, D. (1993). Native Americans: Adapting, yet retaining. In D. Irish, K. Lundquist, & V. Nelsen (Eds.) *Ethnic variations in dying, death, and grief* (pp. 101–112). Philadelphia, PA: Taylor & Francis.

Buchanan, D. (1993). *Meaning in life, depression, suicide in older adults: A comparative survey study.* Unpublished doctoral dissertation, Rush University, Chicago, IL.

Buck, H., & McMillan, S. (2008). The unmet spiritual needs of caregivers of patients with advanced cancer. *Journal of Hospice and Palliative Nursing, 10*(2), 91–105.

Bullock, K. (2006). Promoting advance directives among African Americans: A faith -based model. *Journal of Palliative Medicine, 9*(1), 183–194.

Byock, I. (1997). *Dying well: The prospect for growth at the end of life.* New York: Riverhead Books.

Cassell, E. (1982). The nature of suffering and the goals of medicine. *New England Journal of Medicine, 306,* 639–645.

Chochinov, H., & Cann, B. (2005). Interventions to enhance the spiritual aspects of dying. *Journal of Palliative Medicine, 8*(1), S-103- S-115.

Chochinov, H. Krisjanson. L., Jack, T., Hassard, T., McClement, S., & Harlos, M. (2006). Dignity in terminally ill: Revisited. *Journal of Palliative Medicine, 9*(3), 666–672.

Clark, L., Leedy, S., McDonald, L., Muller, B., Lamb, C., & Mendez, T.,et al. (2007). Spirituality and job satisfaction among Hospice interdisciplinary team members. *Journal of Palliative Medicine, 10*(6), 1321–1328.

Coulehan, J., & Clary, P. (2005). Healing the healer: Poetry in palliative care. *Journal of Palliative Medicine, 8*(2), 382–387.

Conrad, N. L. (1985). Spiritual support for the dying. *Nursing Clinics of North America, 20,* 415–425.

Corr, C. (1991). A task-based approach to coping with dying. *Omega-Journal of Death and Dying, 24*(2), 81–94.

Cort, M. (2004). Cultural mistrust and use of Hospice care: Challenges and remedies. *Journal of Palliative Medicine, 7*(1), 63–71.

Cousins, N. (1979). *Anatomy of an illness.* New York: Norton.

Coyle, N. (1995). Suffering in the first person. In B. R. Ferrell (Ed.), *Suffering* (pp.21–32). Sudbury, MA: Jones and Bartlett.

Crawley, L., Marshall, P., Lo, B., & Koenig, B. (2002). Strategies for culturally effective end of life care. *Annals of Internal Medicine, 136,* 673–679.

Davies, B., Reimer, J., & Marten, N. (1994). Family functioning and its implications for palliative care. *Journal of Palliative Care, 10,* 35–36.

DeBellis, R., Marcus, E., Kutscher, A., Smith Torres, C., Barrett, V., & Siegel, M. (1986). *Suffering: Psychological and social aspects in loss, grief, and care.* New York: Haworth Press.

DeSpelder, L. (1998). Developing cultural competency. In K. Doka & J. Davidson (Eds.), *Living with grief* (pp. 97–106). Washington, DC: Hospice Foundation of America.

DeSpelder, L., & Strickland, A. (1999). *The last dance: Encountering death and dying.* Mountain View, CA: Mayfield.

Doka, K., & Davidson, J. (1998). *Living with grief.* Philadelphia, PA: Hospice Foundation of America.

Doka, K., & Morgan, J. (1993). *Death and spirituality.* Amityville, NY: Baywood.

Doorenbos, A., & Schim, S. (2004). Cultural competence in Hospice. *American Journal of Hospice and Palliative Care, 21*(1), 28–32.

Downey, M. (1997). *Understanding Christian spirituality.* Mahwah, New Jersey: Paulist Press.

Doyle, D. (1994). *Caring for a dying relative: A guide for families.* New York: Oxford University Press.

Driscoll, J. (2001). Spirituality and religion in end of life care. *Journal of Palliative Medicine, 4,* 333–335.

Duggleby, W. (2000). Enduring suffering: A grounded theory analysis of the pain experience of elderly hospice patients with cancer. *Oncology Nursing Forum, 27,* 825–830.

Duggleby, W. (2001). Hope at the end of life. *Journal of Hospice and Palliative Nursing, 3*(2), 51–57.

Dunn, K., & Horgas, A. (2000). The prevalence of prayer as a spiritual self-care modality of elders. *Journal of Holistic Nursing, 18*(4), 337–351.

Ehman, J. W., Ott, B. B. Short, T. H., Ciampa, R. C., & Hansen-Flaschen, J. (1999). Do patients want physicians to inquire about their spiritual or religious beliefs when they become gravely ill? *Archives in Internal Medicine, 159,* 1803–1806.

End of Life Nursing Education Consortium (ELNEC). (2001). *Module 5: Cultural considerations.* City of Hope Medical Center and American Association of Colleges of Nursing. Available from the American Association of Colleges of Nursing: www.aacn.nche.edu/elnec.

Ersek, M., Kagawa-Singer, M., Barnes, D., Blackhall, L., & Koenig, B. (1998). Multi-cultural considerations in the use of advance directives. *Oncology Nursing Forum, 25,* 1683–1689.

Flores, G. (2005). The impact of medical interpreter services on the quality of healthcare: A systematic review. *Medical Care Research Review, 62,* 255–299.

Foley, K. (1995). Pain, physician-assisted suicide, and euthanasia. *Pain Forum, 4,* 163–176.

Gallop, G. (1997). *Spiritual beliefs and the dying process. A national survey conducted for the Nathan Cummings Foundation and the Fetzer Institute.* New York: Nathan Cummings Foundation.

Grollman, E. (1993). Death in Jewish thought. In K. Doka & J. Morgan (Eds.), *Death and spirituality* (pp. 21–32). Amityville, NY: Baywood.

Grossman, D. (1996). Cultural dimensions in home health nursing. *American Journal of Nursing, 96*(7), 33–36.

Gum, A., & Synder, C. (2002). Coping with terminal illness: The role of hopeful thinking. *Journal of Palliative Medicine, 5,* 883–894.

Halifax, J. (1999, October). *Being with dying: Contemplations on death and dying.* Presentation at the Art of Dying III Conference: Spiritual, Scientific and Practical Approaches to Living and Dying by the New York Open Center and Tibet House, New York, NY.

Heintz, L., & Baruss. L. (2001). Spirituality in late adulthood. *Psychological Reports, 88*(3), 651–654.

Hermann, C. (2000). A guide to the spiritual needs of elderly cancer patients. *Geriatric Nursing, 21,* 324–325.

Herth, K. (1992). Fostering hope in terminally ill people. *Journal of Advanced Nursing, 15,* 1250–1259.

Hicks, T. (1999). Spirituality and the elderly: Nursing implications with nursing home residents. *Geriatric Nursing, 20*(3), 144–146.

Highfield, M. (2000). Providing spiritual care to patients with cancer. *Clinical Journal of Oncology Nursing. 4*(3), 115–120.

Higginson, I. J. (1998). Introduction: Defining the unit of care: Who are we supporting and how? In E. Bruera & R. K. Portenoy (Eds.), *Topics in palliative care: Vol. 2* (pp. 205–207). New York: Oxford University Press.

Hospice and Palliative Care Nurses Association. (2007). HPNA position paper: Spiritual care. *Journal of Hospice and Palliative Care Nursing, 9*(1), 15–16.

Hunnibell, L., Reed, P., Quinn-Griffin, M., & Fitzpatrick, J. (2008). Self-transcendence and burnout in Hospice and Oncology nurses. *Journal of Hospice and Palliative Nursing, 10*(3), 172–179.

Hutchings, D. (2007). Struggling in change at the end of life: A nursing inquiry. *Palliative and Supportive Care, 5,* 31–39.

Hyland, K. (1996). *The influence of religiosity on an older person's adjustment to the nursing home environment.* Unpublished doctoral dissertation, Long Island University, Brookville, New York.

Irish, D., Lundquist, K., & Nelsen, V. (1993). *Ethnic variations in dying, death, and grief.* Philadelphia, PA: Taylor & Francis.

Jenko, M., Gonzalez, L., & Seymour, M. (2007). Life review with the terminally ill. *Journal of Hospice and Palliative Nursing, 9*(3), 159–167.

Johnson, P. (2002). The use of humor and its influences on spirituality and coping in breast cancer survivors. *Oncology Nursing Forum, 29,* 691–695.

Kagawa-Singer, M. (1998). The cultural context of death rituals and mourning practices. *Oncology Nursing Forum, 25,* 1752–1756.

Kagawa-Singer, M., & Blackhall, L. (2001). Negotiating cross-cultural issues at the end of life. *Journal of the American Medical Association, 286,* 2993–3001.

Kahn, D. L., & Steeves, R. (1996). An understanding of suffering grounded in clinical practice and research. In B. R. Ferrell (Ed.), *Suffering* (pp. 3–27). Sudbury, MA: Jones and Bartlett.

Kaldjian, L. C. (1998). End of life decisions in HIV-positive patients: The role of spiritual beliefs. *AIDS, 12*(1), 103–107.

Kemp, C., & Chang, B. (2002). Culture and the end of life: Chinese. *Journal of Hospice and Palliative Nursing, 4,* 173–177.

Kirschling, J., & Pittman, J. (1989). Measurement of spiritual well-being: A Hospice caregiver sample. *Hospice Journal, 5*(2), 1–11.

Klass, D. (1993). Spirituality, Protestantism, and death. In K. Doka & J. Morgan (Eds.), *Death and spirituality* (pp. 51–73). Amityville, NY: Baywood.

Koenig, H. G. (1998). Religious coping and health status in medically ill hospitalized older adults. *Journal of Nervous Mental Disease, 186,* 513–518.

Koenig, H. G. (1999, March). *The healing power of faith: When serious illness strikes.* Paper presented at the Harvard University Spirituality and Healing Conference, Denver, CO.

Koenig, H. G. (2002). An 83-year old woman with chronic illness and strong religious beliefs. *Journal of the American Medical Association, 288,* 487–493.

Koenig, H. G., Cohen, H. J., Blazer, D., Pieper, C., Meador, K., Shelp, G., et al. (1992). Religious coping and depression among hospitalized elderly medically ill men. *American Journal of Psychiatry, 149,* 1693–1700.

Lederberg, M. (1998). The family of the cancer patient. In J. Holland (Ed.), *Psychooncology* (pp. 981–993). New York: Oxford University Press.

Leininger, M. (1995). *Transcultural nursing: Concepts, theories, research, and practice.* New York, NY: McGraw-Hill Inc.

Lipson, J., Dibble, S., & Minarik, P. A. (1996). *Culture and nursing care: A pocket guide.* St. Louis, MO: Mosby.

Lo, B., Uston, D., Kates, L., Arnold, R., Cohen, C., Faber-Langendoen, K., et al. (2002). Discussing religious and spiritual issues at the end of life: A practical guide for physicians. *Journal of the American Medical Association, 287,* 749–754.

Lorenz, K. Hays, R., Shapiro, M., Cleay, P., Asch, S., & Wenger, N. (2005). Religiousness and spirituality among HIV-infected individuals. *Journal of Palliative Medicine, 8*(4), 774–780.

Loscalzo, M., & Zabora, J. (1998). Care of the cancer patient: Response of family and staff. In E. Bruera & R. K. Portenoy (Eds.), *Topics in palliative care: Vol. 2* (pp. 209–246). New York: Oxford University Press.

Lowe, J. & Struthers, R. (2001). A conceptual framework of nursing in native American culture. *Journal of Nursing Scholarship, 33,* 279–283.

Ludke, R., & Smucker, D. (2007). Racial differences in the willingness to use Hospice services. *Journal of Palliative Medicine, 10*(6), 1329–1336.

Mackenzie, E., Rajogopal, D., Meibohm, M., & Lavizzo-Mourey, R. (2000). Spiritual support and psychological well-being: Older adults' perceptions of the religion and health connection. *Alternative Therapies in Health & Medicine, 6*(6), 37–45.

Mako, C., Galek, K., & Poppito, S. (2006). Spiritual pain among patients with advanced cancer in palliative care. *Journal of Palliative Medicine, 9*(5), 1106–1113.

Matthews, D. (1999, March). *The faith factor: Is religion good for your health.* Paper presented at the Harvard University Spirituality and Healing Conference, Denver, CO.

McDavis, R., Parker, W., & Parker, W. (1995). Counseling African Americans. In N. Vace, S. DeVaney, & J. Wittmer (Eds). *Experiencing and counseling multicultural and diverse populations* (pp. 217–248.). Bristol, PA: Accelerated Development.

McGann, J. (1997). *Comfort my people: Finding peace as life ends.* Rockville Center, New York: Long Island Catholic.

McGrath, P., Vun, M., & McLeod, L. (2001). Needs and experiences of non-english speaking Hospice patients and families in an english speaking country. *American Journal of Hospice and Palliative Care, 18*(5), 305–312.

Meagher, D., & Bell, C. (1993). Perspectives on death in the African American community. In K. Doka, & J. D. Morgan (Eds.). *Death and spirituality* (pp. 113–130). Amityville, New York: Baywood Publishing Company, Inc.

Meraviglia, M. (2004). The effects of spirituality on well-being of people with lung cancer. *Oncology Nursing Forum, 31*(1), 89–94.

Miller, E. (1993). A Roman catholic view of death. In K. Doka & J. Morgan (Eds.), *Death and spirituality* (pp. 33–49). Amityville, NY: Baywood.

Millspaugh, D. (2005a). Assessment and response to spiritual pain: Part I. *Journal of Palliative Medicine, 8*(5), 919–923.

Millspaugh, D. (2005b). Assessment and response to spiritual pain: Part II. *Journal of Palliative Medicine, 8*(6), 1110–1117.

Mitchell, D. (1997). The good death: Three promises to make at the bedside. *Geriatrics, 52*(8), 91–92.

Moore, T. (1992). *Care of the soul: A guide for cultivating depth and sacredness in everyday life.* New York: Harper-Collins.

Mull, C., Cox, C., & Sullivan, J. (1987). Religion's role in the health and well-being of well elders. *Public Health Nursing, 4*(3), 151–159.

Musgrave, C.& McFarlane, E. (2004). Israeli oncology nurses' religiosity, spiritual well-being, and attitudes toward spiritual care: A path analysis. *Oncology Nursing Forum, 31,* 321–327.

Nathan Cummings Foundation. (1999 February 12). Spiritual beliefs and the dying process: Key findings. Retrieved from http://www.ncf.org/ncf/publications/reports/fetzer/fetzer_keyfindings.html.

O'Connor, P. (1993). A clinical paradigm for exploring spiritual concerns. In K. Doka & J. Morgan (Eds.), *Death and spirituality* (pp. 133–150). Amityville, NY: Baywood.

O'Neill, D., & Kenny, E. (1998). Spirituality and chronic illness. *Image: Journal of Nursing Scholarship, 30,* 275–279.

Orion, P. (1993). Spiritual issues in death and dying for those who do not have conventional religious beliefs. In K. Doka & J. Morgan (Eds.), *Death and spirituality* (pp. 93–112). Amityville, NY: Baywood.

Parker-Oliver, D. (2002). Redefining hope for the terminally ill. *American Journal of Hospice and Palliative Care, 19*(2), 115–120.

Peterman, A., Fitchett, G., Brady, M., Hernandez, L., & Cella, D. (2002). Measuring spiritual well-being in people with cancer: The functional assessment of chronic illness therapy-Spiritual well-being Scale (FACIT-Sp). *Annals of Behavioral Medicine, 24*(1), 49–58.

Prince-Paul, M. (2008). Relationships among communicative acts, social well-being, and spiritual well-being on the quality of life at the end of life in patients with cancer enrolled in Hospice. *Journal of Palliative Medicine, 11*(1), 20–25.

Puchalski, C. (1998a). Facing death with dignity. *The World and I, 3,* 34–39.

Puchalski, C. (1998b). FICA: A spiritual assessment. Unpublished manuscript.

Puchalski, C., & Romer, A. (2000). Taking a spiritual history allows clinicians to understand patients more fully. *Journal of Palliative Medicine, 3*(1), 129–137.

Puchalski, C. (2001a). Spirituality and health: The art of compassionate medicine. *Hospital Physician, 37*(3), 30–36.

Puchalski, C. (2001b). Spirituality and health: The art of compassionate medicine. *Hospital Physician, 37*(3), 30–36.

Puchalski, C. (2002). Spirituality and end of life care: A time for listening and caring. *Journal of Palliative Medicine, 5,* 289–294.

Puchalski, C., & Larson, D. (1998). Developing curricula in spirituality and medicine. *Academic Medicine, 73,* 970–974.

Purdy, W. (2002). Spiritual discernment in palliative care. *Journal of Palliative Medicine, 5,* 139–141.

Rando, T. (1984). *Grief, dying, and death: Clinical interventions for caregivers.* Champaign, IL: Research Press.

Roberts, J. A. (1997). Coping with gyneco-logic cancer. *American Journal of Obstetrics and Gynecology, 176,* 166–172.

Ryan, D. (1993). Death: Eastern perspectives. In K. Doka & J. Morgan (Eds.), *Death and spirituality* (pp. 75–92). Amityville, NY: Baywood.

Ryan, S. (1997). Chaplains are more than what chaplains do. *Visions, 7*(3), 8–9.

Satterly, L. (2001). Guilt, shame, and religious and spiritual pain. *Holistic Nursing Practice, 15*(2), 30–39.

Schroepfer, T. (2007). Critical events in the dying process: The potential for physical and psychosocial suffering. *Journal of Palliative Medicine, 10*(1), 136–146.

Sherman, D. W. (1998). Reciprocal suffering: The need to improve family caregiver's quality of life through palliative care. *Journal of Palliative Medicine, 1,* 357–366.

Sherman, D. W. (2001). Spiritual and cultural competence in palliative care. In M. Matzo, & D. W. Sherman (Eds.). *Palliative care nursing: Quality care to the end of life* (pp. 3–47). New York: Springer Publishers.

Sherman, D. W. (2004a). Cultural and spiritual backgrounds of older adults: Considerations for quality palliative care. In M. L. Matzo & D. W. Sherman (Eds.), *Gerontological palliative care nursing* (pp. 3–30). St. Louis, MO: Mosby.

Sherman, D. W. (2004b). Nurses' stress and burnout: How to care for yourself when caring for patients and their families experiencing life-threatening illness. *American Journal of Nursing, 104*(5), 48–57.

Sinclair, S. Pereira, J., & Raffin, S. (2006). A thematic review of the spirituality literature within palliative care. *Journal of Palliative Medicine, 9*(2), 464–479.

Smith, R. (1996). Theological perspectives. In B. R. Ferrell (Ed.), *Suffering* (pp. 159–171). Sudbury, MA: Jones and Bartlett.

Smith-Stoner, M. (2006). Caring for Buddhists at end of life. *American Academy of Hospice and Palliative Medicine Bulletin,* Summer, 6–7.

Smith-Stoner, M. (2007). End of life preferences for atheists. *Journal of Palliative Medicine, 10*(4), 923–928.

Spross, J. (1996). Coaching and suffering: The role of the nurse in helping people face illness. In B. R. Ferrell (Ed.), *Suffering* (pp. 173–208). Sudbury, MA: Jones and Bartlett.

Sulmasy, D. (1997). *The healer's calling: A spirituality for physicians and other healthcare professionals.* New York: Paulist Press.

Sullivan, M. (2001). Lost in translation: How Latinos view end of life care. Retrieved from [http:// www.lastacts.org].

Taylor, E. J. (2003). Nurses caring for the spirit: Patients with cancer and family caregiver expectations. *Oncology Nursing Forum, 30,* 585–590.

Taylor, E. J., Outlaw, F. H., Bernardo, T. T., & Roy, A. (1999). Spiritual conflicts associated with praying about cancer. *Psychooncology, 8*(5), 386–394.

Taylor, E., & Outlaw, F. (2002). Use of prayer among persons with cancer. *Holistic Nursing Practice, 16*(3), 46–60.

Taxis, J. (2005). Attitudes, values, and questions of African Americans regarding participation in Hospice programs. *Journal of Hospice and Palliative Nursing, 8*(2), 77–85.

Theris, T. (2001). Nurturing hope and spirituality in the nursing home. *Holistic Nursing Practice, 15*(4), 45–56.

Thomas, J., & Retsas, A. (1999). Transacting self-preservation: A grounded theory of the spiritual dimensions of people with terminal cancer. *International Journal of Nursing Studies, 36*(3), 191–201.

Watson, J. (1986). Suffering and the quest for meaning. In R. DeBellis, E. Marcus, A. Kutscher, C. Smith Torres, V. Barrett, & M. Siegel (Eds.), *Suffering: Psychological and social aspects in loss, grief, and care* (pp. 175–187). New York: Haworth Press.

Wayman, L., & Gaydos, H. (2005). Self-transcending through suffering. *Journal of Hospice and Palliative Nursing, 7*(5), 263–270.

Weaver, J. Flannelly, L., & Flannelly, K. (2001). A review of research on religious and spiritual values in two primary gerontological journals. *Journal of Gerontological Nursing, 27*(9), 47–54.

Wink, P. (1999). Addressing end of life issues: Spirituality and inner life. *Generations, 23*(1), 75–80.

Zafir al-Shahri, M., & al-Khenaizan, A. (2005). Palliative care for Muslim Patients. *Supportive Oncology, 3*(6), 432–436.

Holistic Integrative Therapies in Palliative Care

Carla Mariano

Key Points

- Holism focuses on unity, mutuality, meaning, and the interrelationship of all beings, events, and things.
- People can grow and learn from illness and dying. Individuals can die healed.
- Holism is the theoretical and philosophical foundation for all alternative/complementary integrative healing modalities.
- Holistic integrative therapies can be used by the nurse, client, and family. They are therapies of healing and empowerment.
- Relaxation is the basis for most holistic modalities.
- Imagination can play a powerful role in healing.
- Although there are many forms of meditation, all attempt to quiet the mind and focus one's attention inward.
- Sense therapies such as music (sound), aromas (smell), and touch (kinesthetics) have very potent natural healing properties that can adjust chemical or other imbalances with the body.
- Reminiscence and life review allow one to reintegrate past issues and experiences in the present to achieve a sense of meaning and ego integrity.
- Journal writing often helps those who cannot express verbally how they feel or what they are experiencing.
- Touch is essential to the quality of one's existence. It needs to be reintroduced as a significant modality in nursing practice.
- Herbs have many healing qualities but should be used knowledgeably.
- Homeopathy is a longstanding method of holistic medicine in which "like cures like" and remedies are tailored to the individual.
- Prayer is unique to each individual both in form and in content.
- There is a consciousness in dying where individuals become aware of their own deaths in phases.
- Self-care for health professionals who care for dying persons is imperative. Self-care areas include spiritual, emotional, physical, mental, and relationships.

Case Study: J.A., a 40-year-old male in the terminal stages of AIDS, was admitted to the hospital 1 week ago. This was his third hospitalization in 6 months. He was experiencing difficulty breathing, dehydration, extreme weakness, and fatigue. Because J.A. had lost so much weight, he was uncomfortable much of the time with muscle and joint aches. Additionally, J.A. was very anxious and found it difficult to sleep at night or rest during the day, increasing his discomfort and fatigue. He was fearful that any physical treatments or manipulation would exaggerate his pain, and he often became angry when the nurses administered morning and evening care.

J.A. was offered therapeutic touch (TT) treatments to see if it might be helpful in relaxing him. At first he refused, stating that he did not want to be touched. The nurse clarified that TT would not cause him any physical pain and that it did not in fact involve touching his body. She explained that it might be relaxing for him and might also help him to rest and sleep. The nurse suggested that if J.A. was willing, she do a 10-minute "trial" session to see if TT helped. After putting a sign on the door "Do not disturb for 15 minutes," the nurse encouraged J.A. to breathe slowly and deeply and close his eyes. She then centered herself, breathing slowly and deeply, and set the intention for the wholeness and wellbeing of J.A. Working about 7–10 inches away from his body, she began to assess J.A.'s energy field to ascertain his energy flow and any blockages. She then passed her hands repeatedly through his field from head to toe to get the energy flowing and balance J.A.'s field. The nurse continued for about 5 minutes, noticing that J.A.'s muscles were becoming relaxed, his expression becoming softened, and he becoming quiet.

Introduction

This chapter introduces the reader to a variety of holistic modalities that are used in nursing practice today and can be used in palliative care. The modalities are defined and shown where they are most useful. In addition, this chapter includes a section on exercises that can be used readily by nurses and incorporated into their practice. It also includes resources where more information on each of these modalities can be obtained. In the education of nurses, it is particularly important for nursing faculty to incorporate these healing modalities into the curriculum for both undergraduate and graduate-level students.

Holism focuses on unity, mutuality, meaning, and the interrelationship of all beings, events, and things. The words "heal" and "health" come from *haelan*, which means to be or become whole. Holism emphasizes the basic wholeness and integrity of the individual. It views the body, mind, emotion, and spirit as inseparable and interdependent. All behaviors, including health, illness, and dying are manifestations of the life process of the whole person (Quinn, 1995).

Holistic nursing care draws on nursing knowledge, theories, expertise, and intuition, as nurses and clients become therapeutic partners in a shared evolving process toward healing. Holistic care

■ believes that people can grow and learn from health, illness, and dying;
■ promotes clients' active participation in their own healthcare, wellness, and healing;
■ uses appropriate interventions in the context of the client's total needs;
■ works to alleviate clients' physical signs and symptoms; and
■ concentrates on the underlying meanings of symptoms and illness events, and changes in the clients' life patterns and perceptions (Mariano, 2007a,1998).

Numerous modalities (Micozzi, 2006) are used in the provision of holistic care. Some of these that are particularly useful in end-of-life care are discussed in this chapter. Nurses can practice holistic care in any setting where healing occurs.

HEALTHCARE AND USE OF COMPLEMENTARY/ALTERNATIVE MODALITIES IN THE UNITED STATES

The American public is increasingly demanding healthcare that is compassionate and respectful, provides options, is economically feasible, and is grounded in holistic ideals. A shift is occurring in healthcare where people desire to be more actively involved in health decision making. They have expressed their dissatisfaction with conventional (Western allopathic) medicine and are calling for a care system that encompasses health, quality of life, and relationship with their providers. An issue of Center for Disease Control's (CDC) Advanced Data from Vital and Health Statistics on complementary and alternative medicine (CAM) use in the United States noted characteristics commonly associated with CAM therapies:

"Individualized diagnosis and treatment of patients; an emphasis on maximizing the body's inherent healing ability; and treatment of the 'whole' person by addressing their physical, mental, and spiritual attributes rather than focusing on a specific pathogenic process as emphasized in conventional medicine" (Barnes, Powell-Griner, McFann, & Nahin, 2004).

Western medicine is proving wholly or partially ineffective for a significant proportion of the common chronic diseases. Furthermore, highly technological healthcare is too expensive to be universally affordable. Holistic care that promotes health is more cost effective and culturally acceptable to diverse and disparate populations whose belief systems are more congruent with whole system and holistic approaches to treatment. The use of alternative methods for economic and cultural reasons by these populations often outweighs their use of conventional treatments (Mariano, 2009).

Barnes et al. (2004) found that those who had been hospitalized in the past year were more likely to use CAM than those who had not been in the hospital in the past year. Most people use CAM to treat and/or prevent musculoskeletal conditions or other conditions associated with chronic or recurring pain. Adult CAM users were most likely to utilize CAM because they believed that CAM combined with conventional medical treatments would help (54.9%). Twenty-eight percent of adult CAM users believed that conventional medical treatments would not help them. And 13% of adult CAM users used CAM because they felt that conventional medicine was too expensive.

A Survey of Consumer Use of CAM by American Association for Retired Persons and National Center for Complementary and Alternative Medicine (AARP and NCCAM) (2007) found that people 50 years and older tend to be high users of CAM. Nearly two thirds of the respondents (63%) have used one or more CAM therapies. A significant aspect of this study was that among all respondents who saw a physician, only one in five (25%) had discussed CAM with a physician and 77% did not discuss CAM with their doctor because of the following:

- The physician never asked them (42%).
- The respondents did not know they should (30%).
- There was not enough time during the office visit (19%).
- They do not think the doctor knows the topic (17%).
- The doctor would have been dismissive or told them not to do it (12%).

Nearly three fourths of respondents (74%) in this study said that they take one or more prescription medications. Twenty percent of respondents reported currently taking more than five prescription medications. Three fourths (75%) of those currently taking one or more prescription medicines also take one or more over-the-counter medicines. Three fourths (75%) of the respondents who had used herbal products or dietary supplements reported that they currently take one or more prescription medicines.

It is clear that people aged 50 years and older are likely to be using CAM. It is also clear that this population is frequently using prescription medications. Common use of CAM as a complement to conventional medicine—and the high use of multiple prescription drugs—further underscores the need for healthcare providers and clients/patients/families to have an open dialogue to ensure safe and appropriate integrated healthcare. The lack of this dialogue points to a need to educate both consumers and healthcare providers about the importance of discussing the use of CAM, how to begin that dialogue, and the implications of not doing so.

The chronically and terminally ill consume more healthcare resources than the rest of the population. Approximately 75% of all healthcare spending in the United States currently is for the treatment of chronic disease and 25% of Medicare spending is for costs incurred during the last year of life. The great interest in CAM practices among the chronically ill, those with life-threatening conditions, and those at the end of their lives suggests that increased access to some services among these groups could have significant implications for the health care system (White House Commission on Complementary and Alternative Medicine Policy (WHCCAMP) 2002).

With the number of older Americans expected to increase dramatically over the next 20 years, alternative strategies for dealing with the elderly population and end-of-life processes will be increasingly important in public policy. If evaluations show that some uses of CAM can lessen the need for more expensive conventional care in these populations, the economic implications for Medicare and Medicaid could be significant. If safe and effective CAM practices become more available to the general population, special and vulnerable populations should also have access to these services, along with conventional healthcare. CAM would not be a replacement for conventional healthcare, but would be part of the options available for treatment. In some cases, CAM practices may be an equal or superior option. CAM offers the possibility of a new paradigm of integrated healthcare that could affect the affordability, accessibility, and delivery of healthcare services for millions of Americans (Institute of Medicine (IOM), 2005; WHCCAMP, 2002).

HEALING AND DYING

"Healing the dying sounds like an oxy-moron. . . . But to heal is not necessarily to cure. . . . To heal is to bring various levels of oneself—cellular, physical, intrapersonal, interpersonal, societal, spiritual, perhaps even cosmic—into new relationship with each other" (Olson, 2001, p. 3). The nurse must assess the relationship of the individual who is dying with self, others, and a higher power, and provide appropriate interventions to assist in the development or maintenance of new or right relationships.

"Dying healed means that a person has finished the business of life, said goodbyes, and reached life's goals. An individual knows who he is, and has a sense of integration of self and life" (Olson, 2001, p. 3). She or he realizes that one's life was unique and one's death matters to someone. One looks inward and realizes that life's difficulties have created a certain wisdom. Significant others have had time to grieve and plan for changes, and comfort and peace are attained. Control of the dying process is maintained as long as possible by the individual and as much as possible as the person is willing. Dying is seen as a stage of life. It is part of a larger philosophy and perception in which both life and death have meaning.

As mentioned previously, healing the dying necessitates regard for relationships and connectedness. We speak of transcendence when implying a sense of connectedness between self and a greater reality. Transcendence "integrates self with past and future, giving meaning to life. It is a set of introspective activities that reflect concern for others or for meaning" (Olson, 1997, p. 128). Many of the integrative modalities described in this chapter facilitate self-transcendence. As noted by Olson and Dossey (2009), positive outcomes for the self-transcendent person, even when nearing death, include less depression, neglect, and hopelessness; a greater sense of well-being and ability to cope with grief and death; and the ability to live and find meaning in the present and connect with a higher power.

This caring relationship emphasizes quality rather than length of life. Healing the dying includes palliative care, and focuses on relationships of all kinds. There is the provision for opportunities and choices where the dying person can live life to its fullest, and at some point comfortably forgive, let go, release, and experience a peaceful death.

The nurse is in a partnership with the dying client, sharing rather than denying the experience. The focus of nursing care is on providing sacred space and the milieu for a calm and peaceful death. The nurse works with the client to foster hope and cultivate an appreciation of the seemingly irrelevant things in life. Learning to appreciate simple occurrences such as a sunset or the joys of life can cultivate a more positive view of life and one's present experience. Enhancing avenues of support, whether professional, social (family and friends), or support groups, can often facilitate grieving and increase a sense of meaning in illness. Developing unrecognized inner strengths and resources is of great importance to the person who is dying or grieving.

The Chinese symbol for crisis indicates that crisis can be a challenge but simultaneously offers an opportunity for growth and a different perspective. The Greek word for crisis (krisis) signifies a "turning point." Grief can serve as a building block for personal growth and healing. Asking the dying person about spiritual needs gives the client an occasion to verbalize unmet needs. All of this requires skill, knowledge, compassion, caring, anticipation, and organization on the part of the nurse, as well as a willingness to face one's own impermanence and mortality. It also necessitates caring for oneself.

SPECIFIC HOLISTIC HEALING MODALITIES

Holism is the theoretical and philosophical foundation for alternative/complementary integrative healing modalities. Numerous kinds of these modalities are used in healthcare today. This chapter will cover only a few of those that are most useful in end-of-life care. Many of these modalities can be used effectively by the nurse as well as the client, for example, centering, relaxation, imagery, meditation, prayer, herbology, and homeopathy. Others are described in use with clients, such as sense therapies, reminiscence and life review, touch, and Reiki. In addition to their calming influence and physiological benefits, these techniques also may alter the perception of pain. Another valuable aspect of these modalities is that their use can empower clients and families. When clients learn to heal themselves, they are empowered. When they learn these techniques, they can do it themselves, which oftentimes gives them a sense of control (Mariano, 2004, 2007a). And when families are taught to use these modalities, they feel as if they are contributing something positive to the care of their loved one.

Centering

Centering is a process by which one quiets the mind and focuses one's thoughts. It calms the mind and allows the practitioner to access inmost resources that are powerful forces in healing. Krieger (1997) notes that

> "Being on-center does not mean being still, immobile, rigid. . . . In centering, we are quiet and 'listen' to another language. Our attention goes to the heart region, where we find our own center of peace and know it as an attribute of our true self. We find that this sense of deep serenity is reminiscent to the truer peace we find in untrammeled nature and, with a thrill of personal discovery, realize that it is through such profound natural experiences that we can be at-one with the universe" (p. 22).

Centering is a shift in consciousness, an integrated sense of being. Bodily movements become quieted, and yet one is in an actively conscious state. One feels a unique stillness and peace. There is a sense of inner equilibrium and well-being. Perception deepens, and one is less aware of the chaos of the moment, the day, and the mind's chatter. Practice in the act of centering (closing eyes, quieting one's mind and activities, focusing on one's center or inner peace) leads to intuition and inner wisdom (Krieger, 1997, 2002).

By remaining "on-center," the nurse is able to convey to the client an awareness, a sensitivity, an empathy, and a deep sense of peace and regard that often creates a relaxation response in the client. One must give oneself permission to center, as the environment is always calling us to be present for *it* rather than for ourselves.

But when one is centered and personally present, compassion becomes real, and this state is needed for those who would facilitate healing. One important exercise that the nurse can practice is to center before entering into each client encounter— detaching from any prior encounter, and to approach each client with awareness and with, as Carl Rogers says, "unconditional positive regard" (Laurant & Shlien, 1984).

Creating Intention

Creating intention affects the mental, emotional, and physical realms. It is a powerful way to establish an optimal milieu for a caring-healing interaction.

> "Examine the following intention: 'I am here for the greater good of this person. I set aside my own concerns and worries and am fully present to the person here and now.' With this intention the nurse is consciously setting aside his or her own concerns and focusing on the patient; s/he has set into motion the dynamic that this interaction will be 'for the greater good of this person'; and s/he is making a conscious decision to be fully present. The nurse, through this intention, creates an environment that promotes and sustains a caring-healing interaction" (Thornton & Mariano, 2009).

Relaxation

Relaxation is a state in which there is an absence of physical, mental, and emotional tension. A pleasant sensation and the lack of stressful or uncomfortable thoughts also accompany relaxation. It is often referred to as the opposite of the fight-or-flight or freeze response.

Relaxation allows the body/mind to quieten and focus inward. One can retreat mentally from one's surroundings, still thoughts, relax muscles, and maintain a state of relaxation, attaining the benefits of decreased tension, anxiety, and pain. Regardless of the approach (use of meditation, yoga, muscle and breathing exercises, hypnosis, prayer, and other forms of stress management), the end result of the relaxation response is a movement of the person toward calmness, balance, and healing. The guidelines for relaxation are found in Exhibit 2.1.

Relaxation techniques are the basis of many holistic modalities. Relaxation has three aims: 1) as a prevention to protect body organs from unnecessary stress and wear; 2) as a treatment to alleviate stress in numerous conditions, for example, hypertension, tension headache, insomnia, asthma, immune deficiency, panic, pain; and 3) as a coping skill to calm the mind and to help thinking to become clearer and more effective (Benson, 1995; Payne, 2005). Positive information in memory also becomes more accessible when a person is relaxed.

There are numerous benefits to the relaxed state, including lowered blood pressure, decreased heat rate, increased body temperature, decreased anxiety associated with painful situations, easing of muscle tension pain such as in contractures, a general sense of intense calm, decreased symptoms of depression and stress, decreasing fatigue. Other benefits include helping the client to sleep, increasing the effects of medications, improvements in side effects of cancer therapy (decreased nausea, vomiting, and anxiety) and AIDS therapy, assisting in preparation for surgery or other treatments, and helping to dissociate from pain (Freeman, 2004; Payne, 2005). In addition to the therapeutic benefits, relaxation techniques also give clients a sense of control by enabling them to bring about certain psychological and mental responses by themselves.

Anselmo (2009), Lawson and Horneffer (2002), and Payne (2005), provide excellent guidelines for the nurse in preparing the client for relaxation and actual scripts to guide one through various relaxation exercises. Exhibit 2.1 includes guidelines or key points for relaxation.

EXHIBIT 2.1: GUIDELINES FOR RELAXATION

- Be familiar with the relaxation exercise before introducing it to the client.
- Encourage use of familiar relaxation techniques that the client knows.
- Assess the client's level of tension, level of readiness to learn to relax, pain, anxiety, fear, and perception of reality or history of depersonalization.
- Ask the client what it means for him/her to be relaxed.
- Assess the client's ability to remain comfortably in one position for 10–20 minutes. Decrease as much environmental stimuli as possible.
- Assist the client to develop a positive expectation of what is to occur. Describe the potential benefits of relaxation and enlist cooperation.
- Reduce the opportunity for self-blame if the session does not go as expected.
- Have the client close his or her eyes
- Use a tone of voice that is quiet and calm, conversational at first, and decreasing in volume as the session goes on.
- Use either tapes or a live voice. Music can provide background if desired.
- Guide the client through a basic breathing exercise (see "Exercises" section).
- Phrase all suggestions in a positive form, e.g., "*Let go* of your tension," "Feel the tightness *melting* away," "*Loosen and soften* your muscles," "Allow the tension to *drift* away."
- Clients may experience a release of emotion as they relax, such as tears, vomiting, or faster and more shallow breathing. Gently ask if the client can put words to those feelings. Allow time for expression before continuing.
- At the completion of the session, bring the client gradually back to reality by having the client take deep breaths, move the hands and feet, and stretch if able.
- Have the client evaluate the experience.
- Engage the client's cooperation in continuing practice until the next session.

A basic breathing exercise and relaxation exercise that can be used with the client or by the nurse is found in the "Exercises" section at the end of this chapter.

Imagery

Imagining is a powerful technique of focusing and directing the imagination. One uses all the senses—vision, sound, smell, taste, movement, position, and touch. Imagery influences an individual's attitudes, feelings, behaviors, and anxiety, which can either lead to a sense of hopelessness or promote a perception of well-being that assists in changing opinions about disease, treatment, and healing potential. "Imagery [is the] internal experience of memories, dreams, fantasies, and visions—sometimes involving one, several, or all the senses that serve as the bridge for connecting body, mind, and spirit" (Schaub & Dossey, 2009, p. 295). Imagery can affect people physically, emotionally, mentally, and biochemically, and the body and mind respond as if the event is actually occurring.

Guided imagery and interactive guided imagery (having the client directly interact with the image) are techniques to access the imagination through a guide. There are numerous types of imagery:

- Receptive imagery (inner knowing or "bubble-up" images).
- Active imagery (a focus on the conscious formation of an image).
- Correct biological imagery (recognizing the impact of negative images on physiology and creating positive correct biological images).
- Symbolic imagery (images emerging from both the unconscious and conscious that shape attitudes, belief systems, and cultural experiences, often mythic symbols).
- Process imagery (a step-by-step rehearsal of any procedure, treatment, surgery, or other event prior to its occurrence).
- End-state imagery (rehearsal of an image of being in a final, healed state).
- General healing imagery (images that have a personal healing significance such as a wise person, an animal, the sun, etc.).
- Packaged imagery (another person's images such as commercial tapes).
- Customized imagery (images specific to an individual).

Guided imagery has many applications in end-of-life care, including relaxation, stress reduction, pain relief, symptom management, grief work, and assisting clients to comprehend meaning in their illness experience (Rossman, 1999; Van Kuiken, 2004). It is useful not only in mobilizing latent, innate healing abilities of the client by intensifying the impact of healing messages

that the autonomic nervous system sends to the immune system and other bodily functions, but also in the self-care of the nurse. It has been found helpful in relieving chronic pain and headaches, stimulating healing, tolerating medical procedures, exploring emotions that may have caused illness, solving difficult problems, envisioning and planning for the future, and listening to one's inner advisor.

It is usually helpful for the nurse to have training in the use of interactive guided imagery because of possibly overwhelming effects with this type of imagery (Rossman, 1999). Otherwise, as Schaub and Dossey (2009) note, imagery scripts are more effective when one learns the speaking skills of voice modulation, specific word emphasis, and the use of pauses. Guidelines for the nurse to use in teaching the client the imagery process are presented in Exhibit 2.2.

Basic imagery exercises that nurses can use with clients are under the "Exercises" section at the end of this chapter.

Meditation

Meditation is a quiet turning inward. It is the practice of focusing one's attention internally to achieve clearer consciousness and inner stillness. There are numerous methods and schools of meditation, all having an individual interpretation of the practice. However, all methods believe in emptying the mind and letting go of the mind's chatter that preoccupies us.

Meditation, which originated in the Eastern tradition and is integral to Hinduism, Taoism, and Buddhism, is both a state of mind and a method. The state is one where the mind is quiet and listening to itself. The practitioner is relaxed but alert. The method involves the focusing of attention on something such as the breath, an image, a word, or action such as tai chi or qigong. There is a sustained concentration but it should be effortless.

The objective of meditation is to detach from external events as well as one's own mental activity. Rather than examining thoughts that may enter the mind, the person disregards them and allows them to drift away.

EXHIBIT 2.2: GUIDELINES TO IMAGERY

- Have the client relax. Help the client to identify the problem or goal of imagery.
- Develop a basic understanding of the physiology involved in the healing process. Begin with a few minutes of relaxation, meditation, or paying attention to the breath exercise.
- Assist the client to develop images of:
  —the problem
  —inner healing resources (beliefs, coping strategies, etc.)
  —external healing resources (medications, treatments, family, etc.)
  □ End with images of the desired state of well-being.

There is no criticism or judgment, but an attitude of a beginner's mind: a mind that is open and receptive, clear of attachment to any thoughts. The body is relaxed and the mind is emptied of all thought except awareness of the image, word, or breath. "Passive concentration" keeps the meditator in a state of awareness and alertness rather than drowsiness, and intently focused on the present moment. There should be no blame, guilt, or recrimination if the meditator loses focus or if the mind wanders; one is instructed simply to return the mind to its original focus. Reentry into the normal waking state should be gentle and relaxed. Meditation requires practice on a regular schedule, usually once or twice daily to achieve maximal results.

There are various reasons for practicing meditation: to find peace, achieve awareness and enlightenment, find oneself, experience true reality, and enhance a sense of well-being. Research has demonstrated that relaxed forms of meditation decrease heart rate and blood pressure, increase breathing volume while decreasing the number of breaths per minute, increase peripheral blood flow, improve immune function, and decrease skeletal muscle tension, epinephrine level, gastric acidity, motility, anxiety, depression, traumatic stress, and alcohol and drug consumption (Anselmo, 2009; Bonadonna, 2003; Freeman, 2004; Gauding, 2005; Gross et al., 2004). It is believed that meditation activates the right cerebral hemisphere and the parasympathetic nervous system, thereby quieting the nerves and allowing intuitive, wordless thinking to occur. In addition to physiological benefits, the advantages of meditation cited by Payne (2005) are listed in Exhibit 2.3.

A simple meditation that can be practiced by the nurse or with a client is in the "Exercises" section at the end of this chapter.

Sense Therapies

Sense therapies use the senses to treat physical and psychological problems and to adjust chemical or other imbalances within the body. These can include behavioral vision therapy, eye movement, desensitization, flower remedies, hydrotherapy, and light therapy. Two therapies will be explored under sense therapies: music therapy and music thanatology, and aromatherapy.

Music Therapy. Morris (2009) defines music therapy as the "behavioral science concerned with the systematic application of music to produce relaxation and desired changes in emotions, behavior, and physiology" (p. 327). The elements of music, sound, rhythm, hearing, melody, harmony, and movement are part of people's primary experiences. Listening to, creating, or moving to music assists people in improving, changing, or better integrating aspects of themselves. Music has a power that cannot be expressed in verbal language.

There are references to the therapeutic powers of music in philosophy, art, and literature throughout the ages. Music is used in healing ceremonies throughout the world. Our own experiences demonstrate the psychological effect that music has on us. Despite varying musical tastes, certain types of music create specific moods: for example, a march, ominous music, lively music at sports events, quiet, relaxing music in waiting rooms, or a mother's singing and rocking her baby in times of distress (McCraty, Barrios-Chaplin, Atkinson, & Tomasino, 1998).

Music therapy can reduce biopsychological stress, pain, anxiety, and isolation. It assists clients in reaching a deep state of relaxation, developing self-awareness and creativity, improving learning, clarifying personal values, and coping with a variety of psychophysiological problems. It also provides clients with integrated body/mind episodes and encourages them to become active participants in their own healing. Appropriate music produces the relaxation response, often removing a client's inner restlessness and quieting ceaseless thinking. It is used as a healing technique to quiet the mind and bring about inner relaxation (LeRoux, 2006; Morris, 2009). Research has demonstrated that music reduces acute and chronic pain (Freeman, 2004), is beneficial in treating or managing dementia symptoms (Koger & Brotons, 2000), reduces agitated behaviors in elderly individuals (Remington, 2002), and reduces pain and nausea (Sahler, Hunter, & Liesveld, 2003).

Because music therapy focuses on process and not on outcome, one need not have any musical skills or talents to derive benefits. Frank-Schwebel (1999) recommends that clients be induced to a relaxed state through breathing, suggestive imagery, or a relaxation exercise. Music selected by the client or the nurse is played, and the client is invited to explore images, sensations, emotions, memories, and visions brought on by the music. No one type of music works well for all individuals in all situations. A variety of soothing selections (popular, New Age, classical, country, opera, folk, jazz, choral hymns, etc.) should be available because one

---

EXHIBIT 2.3: ADVANTAGES OF MEDITATION

- A better understanding of the self and increased receptivity to insights arising from one's deeper being. Practicing meditation can bring the experience of self for the dying, where the individual may attain calm and often a sense of purpose.
- A new sense of relaxation and inner peace.
- A clearer mind and improved concentration.
- More harmony with and within the self.
- As a result of the detachment, an acceptance that many unpleasant emotional responses are short-lived sensations created by one's thoughts.
- An emphasis on living in the present and valuing the here and now.

cannot always predict a client's particular preference or response to the music. Often the client experiences an altered state of consciousness, which is usually very relaxing. After the listening, the client is brought back to reality to discuss the experience. In some instances, the client chooses the music and moves or paints to the music. The nurse should assess the factors described in Exhibit 2.4 in preparing to use music therapy (Morris, 2009).

Music has the greatest effect when the client is appropriately prepared. Find a quiet environment and have the client assume a comfortable position. Suggest that the client maintain a passive attitude, neither forcing nor resisting the experience, and remind the client to focus all concentration on the music.

Music Thanatology. Music thanatology, developed by Schroeder-Sheker (1994, 2005) and Freeman et al. (2006), is a relatively new field that addresses the needs of the dying by assisting the client in completing the transition between life and death. Specially trained therapists, using harp, voice, and chanting, assist the client in leave-taking during the last hours of life by reinforcing peace, acceptance, and a calm anticipation of death. Schroeder-Sheker (1994) describes music thanatology as a "palliative medical modality employing prescriptive music to tend the complex physical and spiritual needs of the dying . . . music thanatology is concerned with the possibility of a blessed death and the gift that conscious dying can bring to the fullness of life" (p. 83). This music is live (not taped), dynamic, and prescriptive. It is individual to each patient and each death, much like childbirth. According to Schroeder-Sheker, music thanatology has been found to be most effective in deaths from cancer, AIDS, burns, and slowly degenerative diseases.

Schroeder-Sheker (1994) identifies six foundational assumptions of music thanatology:

1) It recognizes dying as a spiritual process and as an opportunity for growth.

EXHIBIT 2.4: ASSESSMENT FOR MUSIC THERAPY

- The client's music history and music preferences.
- The client's identification of music that make the client happy, excited, sad, or relaxed.
- The client's identification of music that is distasteful and that makes the client tense.
- Assessment of the importance of music in the client's life.
- The frequency of music playing in the client's life.
- Previous participation in relaxation/imagery techniques combined with music; the client's mood—this will determine the type of music to be played.

2) The musical deathbed vigil, often called "musical-sacramental-midwifery," is a contemplative practice requiring serious inner work and integration of the physical, emotional, mental, and spiritual aspects of the caregiver.
3) Death is not an enemy and it is not a failure. It is a critical chapter of human biography.
4) The way in which each person dies is equally important as the way in which that person lived. Beauty, reverence, dignity, and intimacy are central to life and especially so for death. The infirmary music can bring things to the surface in a nonthreatening way or serve the role of meditation. Music is a flow, weaving body, soul, and spirit together.
5) This work is a vocation, not merely a career. It requires clear intention and attention at each deathbed vigil.
6) Death and dying should be returned to the human, personal realm rather than denying or ignoring loss and leave-taking and thus reducing them to legal or corporate medical matters.

Music thanatology focuses on music for the dying versus music for the living. The dying person should not spend energy, only receive energy.

> "The entire surface of the skin can become an extension of the ear, thus enabling the patient to absorb infirmary music, creating the possibility for even deeper emotional, mental, and spiritual reception. . . . The sole focus is to help the person move toward completion and to unbind from anything that prevents, impedes, or clouds a tranquil passage" (Schroeder-Sheker, 1994, pp. 93–94).

Aromatherapy. Aromatherapy is an offshoot of herbal medicine in which aromatic plant extracts are inhaled or applied to the skin as a means of treating illness and promoting physical, psychological, and spiritual benefits as well as positive changes in mood and outlook (Buckle, 2009). Though aromatherapy and herbal medicine use many of the same plants, in aromatherapy the plants are distilled into oils of exceptional potency (Allison, 1999, p. 86).

The advantage of these oils comes from their influence on the limbic system, which coordinates mind and body activity. This system is very sensitive to odors and encodes them into associations and memories, which when awakened alter basic physical functions such as heart rate, blood pressure, breathing, and hormone level. When these oils are rubbed into the skin or inhaled, they set off a reaction leading to rapid and significant alterations in memory, heart rate, and other bodily mechanisms. Some boost energy, some promote relaxation, and others have pharmaceutical effects. However, no treatment should ever involve more than a few drops of oil.

There are hundreds of plants used for aromatherapy (Davis, 2005; Price & Price, 2006). Some of the more common ones that are useful in the care of the dying include chamomile, which is used to overcome anxiety, anger, tension, stress, and insomnia; lavender, for exhaustion, depression, and stress; marjoram, used for those who are physically debilitated; neroli, for countering depression, anxiety, nervous tension, and fearfulness; peppermint and rosewood for treating nausea; and chamomile, camphor, fennel, lavender, peppermint, and rose for relieving vomiting (Buckle, 2009; Eaton-Kelley, 2006; Piotrowski, 2005). Aromatherapy also is used in the relief of pain (lavender, capsicum, bergamot, chamomile, rose, ginger, rosemary, lemongrass, sage, and camphor) (Buckle, 2004, 2009; Huebscher & Schuler, 2004; Kim, 2006). It is most useful in the enhancement of mood, increasing vitality, and relaxation (Buckle, 2009; Brownlee, 2005). These plants and oils can be found in natural or health food stores.

Reminiscence and Life Review

Life review or reminiscence therapy is the remembering of significant past events that enable one to reintegrate past issues and experiences in the present for the purpose of achieving a sense of meaning and ego integrity. The concept has been most frequently used with elderly individuals but is just as effective with those nearing the end of life. Reminiscence is a natural phenomenon. It is the process of recounting past events to someone else, or it can be a more complex process of transpersonal focusing and inward reflection. The level of complexity depends on the wish of the client and the training of the nurse. Life review can be oral, including audio and video recordings, or written. Journal and letter writing can also be useful techniques in life review. Photographs and personal items often provide the opportunity for reminiscence and give information about the client that assists the nurse in providing personal and meaningful care.

Life review is a process of unfolding and emerging and therefore cannot be hurried. A life review can be one or many sessions. Olson (2001) provides a guide for a structured life review that usually includes six to eight sessions:

- Use open-ended questions. Ask about childhood and earliest memories and be sure to be supportive if the client recalls sad events.
- Again using open-ended questions, proceed through their life history by asking about adolescence, family and home, adulthood, and later life.
- Have a summary session inquiring about the following: "Generally, what kind of life do you think you have had? What would you do over again?"

To promote the process, the nurse should encourage the client to express himself or herself, involve significant others, assure confidentiality of the information, be sure the client has sufficient physical strength and a desire for sharing, listen carefully, use touch as appropriate, and allow the client periods of silence to reflect. Life review provides integration, a feeling that this life was individual and unique. The client may verbalize sadness as well as achievement, but the objective is to allow a person to see the meaning in his/her life.

Journal Writing

Keeping a log or journal is a very effective healing technique to use for individuals who are experiencing life-threatening illness and during the grieving process. It allows the person to express innermost feelings and thoughts without fear of criticism. It is often helpful for those who are uncomfortable or unable to articulate how they feel or what they are going through. Writing can also assist the person to make new connections and reframe past experiences. The healing emanates from the actual writing and expression, and not from an analysis of the content of the journal. The writing may be totally private or shared with others. Many clients do not think of this technique, and the nurse may suggest it. Roach and Nieto (1997) and Rew (2009) offer some suggested topics for journal writing:

- special thoughts of the dying person or about the deceased
- feelings that were never expressed
- saying good-bye
- ways that grief or dying has helped one grow
- lessons learned from life that one wants to share
- positive aspects of the past, present, and future.

There are numerous topics for journal writing, or the client can just write thoughts and feelings as they occur. The individual may find comfort in writing when difficult times occur, for example, unanticipated news about diagnosis or prognosis, dealing with family members, or writing to God, a loved one, or one's disease. Often the journal becomes one's own record of grieving. It often serves as a chronicle of personal growth, insights, and wisdom gleaned from the experience of dying or loss.

Touch

In the later stages of life, individuals are often deprived of tender and nurturing physical contact such as being touched in a way that is healing, nourishing, relaxing, and pleasurable. Touch is essential to one's quality of existence. It provides comfort, warmth, and renewed vitality—a sense of security and assurance that we are not alone. Reasons for the lack of touch of the dying include fear, discomfort, stereotypes about dying people, and a sense of one's own vulnerability. However, the benefits of touch on individuals are many. There is an increase of circulation and mobility (e.g., range of motion or hand grasp); a decrease in pain, increase in vitality, increase in physical functioning (Cook, Guerrerio, & Slater, 2004; Wardell, Rintala, & Tan, 2008), the experience of being nurtured and cared for; a boost in self-esteem; increased motivation to receive and give attention to self and others; energy and emotional release; a sense memory triggering relaxation response; relief from loneliness and isolation; decreased feelings of abandonment and deprivation; verbal interaction; and calming reassurance and support (MacInytre et al., 2008; Maville, Bowen, & Beham, 2008). It often induces much-needed sleep. In this day of technological care, touch may be the one caring tool to help a client feel better.

There are many forms of touch considered to be holistic/integrative modalities (Allison, 1999; Aspen Reference Group, 2003; Dossey & Keegan, 2009; Fontaine, 2004; Micozzi, 2006; Walker & Walker, 2003). These include, but are not limited to, the following:

Acupressure—the application of pressure, using fingers, thumbs, palms, or elbows to specific sites along the body's energy meridians to stimulate, disperse, and regulate the body's healing energy for the purpose of relieving tension and reestablishing the flow of energy along the meridian lines.

Body therapy—a general term used for approaches (e.g., Alexander technique, chiropractic, Rolfing, shiatsu, Feldenkrais) that use hands-on techniques to manipulate and balance the musculoskeletal system to facilitate healing, increase energy, relieve pain, and promote relaxation and well-being.

Reflexology—the application of pressure to specific reflex areas on the feet or hands that correspond to other parts of the body in order to locate and correct problems in the body.

Massage—the practice of kneading or otherwise manipulating a person's muscles and other soft tissue with the intent of inducing physical and psychological relaxation, improving circulation, relieving pain and sore muscles, and improving the individual's well-being. Procedural massage is done to diagnose, monitor, or treat the illness itself, focusing on the end result of curing the illness or preventing further complications. In the past, massage has been one of nurses' most important interventions for pain reduction, comfort, tension release, prevention of atrophy of muscles and stiffness of joints, and inducing sleep. A back massage has left many a patient refreshed and feeling cared for. It would behoove us in nursing to reintroduce massage into our practice armamentarium.

Therapeutic touch (TT)—developed by Dolores Krieger and Dora Kunz. This is a specific modality of centering intention while the practitioner moves the hands through the client's energy field for the purpose of assessment and treatment. It is based on the philosophy that universal life energy flows through and around us, and any interruption in this free flow of energy leads to illness. The goal is to balance and repattern the body's energy so that it flows most efficiently to promote health and prevent disease. The TT practitioner scans the client's energy flow, replenishing it where necessary, releasing congestion, removing obstructions, and restoring order and balance in the ill system. This approach is also an effective complementary care approach for facilitation of the body's natural restorative processes, thereby accelerating healing, promoting relaxation, reducing pain and anxiety, and treating chronic conditions (Denison, 2004; Krieger, 1997, 2002; Newshan, 2003).

According to Macrae (1987), a well-known TT practitioner:

"Since therapeutic touch is an interaction, it has the potential to heal the practitioner as well as the patient. . . You can also use the principles of TT to assist in healing yourself . . . the use of mental imagery can facilitate both the energy transfer and the rebalancing of the [practitioner's] field. If you have pain or discomfort somewhere: (1) Sit quietly and center yourself; (2) Visualize the healing energy (as light, if you wish) coming down from above and flowing through you; (3) Visualize the energy clearing away the pain or discomfort (as light shines through a dark area)" (pp. 79–80).

Compassionate touch, developed by Nelson (1994) specifically for hands-on care given to those who are elderly, ill, or dying, is described as

"a gentle, sensitive, and non-intrusive program of massage, attentive touch, and supportive comfort care for those individuals who are temporarily or permanently less active. . . . It also includes individuals of any age who are actively beginning the mysterious life transition that we call death" (p. 1).

Compassionate touch is a hands-on technique stemming not from the hands but from the heart. It combines massage and attentive touch with active listening, reflective communication, relaxation, imagery, and breathing awareness exercises. It focuses on not only the physical condition of the client, but also on the psychosocial, emotional, and spiritual needs as well.

According to Nelson (1994),

"compassion for another implies a feeling of unconditional regard for that other; it also implies a genuine, sincere interest in that person's well-being. The compassionate heart shares in, and is affected by the suffering of another. . . The compassionate individual is able to put aside his or her own concerns for a time in order to give attention to someone else. Some say compassion is love in action" (p. 1).

Compassionate touch is not something we give; it is a way of being. It is a way of providing contact, reassurance, relief, and comfort for those who may be frightened, depressed, out of control, abandoned, overwhelmed, confused, or in despair. It is a means of relating to others rather than a prescribed set of techniques to be practiced on others. It is a spontaneous event of relationship that unfolds moment to moment. Compassionate touch can be administered by anyone who feels inspired to reach out toward a fellow human being in need.

Reiki is based on Buddhist teachings, using hands-on touch to support and intensify energy in the physical, emotional, intellectual, and spiritual areas. "Universal and individual energy are aligned and balanced through the application of gentle hands-on touch to energy pathways of the body" (Abrahms, 1999, p. 133). Those who use Reiki attribute it with reducing stress and stress-related illnesses, including acute and chronic conditions; helping in debilitating disease because it bolsters the immune system by increasing energy; and contributing to an overall sense of well-being in the client.

The philosophy of Reiki contends that a person is vitalized by an essential energy that comes from the universal life force. Everyone has access to this life force, and one becomes ill when the energy flow is interrupted or stopped. Opening pathways for energy flow is the prime objective of Reiki. Learners of Reiki must themselves receive an attunement by an expert Reiki master in an initiation ceremony so that they are attuned to the energy transfer process.

Reiki bodywork is not massage. The touch is gentle and aims not to manipulate tissue, but rather to transmit universal life force to the client. The practitioner uses both hands, palms down, fingers held together, and proceeds in a pattern over the client's body. Each positioning of the hands is maintained for 3–5 minutes without any movement of the fingers or change in the initial gentle touch. During these hand placements, the universal life force flows through the practitioner to the client to balance the client's energy where necessary (Micozzi, 2006; Miles & True, 2003).

Reiki bodywork is very individualized, and the client's perception of the energy transfer is unique to each person. Most find it rejuvenating and relaxing. The effects may be felt immediately or several days later. Following attunement/initiation of the caregiver, Reiki can be used as a method of self-healing as well as caring for others.

As can be seen, numerous holistic healing modalities can be used during end-of-life care.

Herbology

Herbology is also known as *phytotherapy* or *phytomedicine*. Herbal remedies have been used in various cultures for centuries and are increasingly popular in the United States as health products and medicines. In fact, herbal use is the fastest growing category of alternative/complementary therapy in the United States. McCaleb, Leigh, and Morien (2000) define herbs as plants or plant parts (bark, fruit, stem, root, or seed) that are used in fresh, dried, or extracted form for promoting, maintaining, or restoring health. Herbs are prepared in many forms: tinctures, extracts, capsules, tablets, lozenges, teas, juices, vapor treatments, poultices, compresses, salves, liniments, and bath products (Bascom, 2002; Springhouse Corporation, 2005).

Herbs are classified for their effects as follows (Skidmore-Roth, 2009; Springhouse- Corporation, 2005):

- Adaptogenic herbs (which increase the body's resistance to illness)
- Anti-inflammatory herbs
- Antimicrobial herbs
- Antispasmodic herbs
- Astringent herbs (which are applied externally)
- Bitter herbs to increase the secretion of digestive juices, stimulate appetite, and promote liver detoxification
- Carminative herbs (aromatic oils) to soothe the lining of the gastrointestinal (GI) tract and reduce gas, inflammation, and pain
- Demulcent herbs to soothe and protect inflamed and irritated tissue and mucous membranes
- Diuretic herbs
- Expectorant herbs
- Hepatic herbs to tone the liver and increase the production of hepatocytes
- Hypotensive herbs
- Laxative herbs
- Nervine herbs to (a) strengthen and restore, (b) ease anxiety and tension; and (c) stimulate nerve activity
- Stimulating herbs to stimulate physiologic and metabolic activities
- Tonic herbs, which enliven and invigorate by promoting the "vital force," the key to health and longevity
- Pain-relieving herbs.

Although herbs are natural substances and overall risk seems to be low, they cannot be used indiscriminately. Herbs are medicinal and may have serious side effects and interactions with prescription drugs. Additionally, there is a lack of regulation of commercial herbal products in the United States and lack of standardized dosage ranges and preparations. Yet, so many Americans choose to take herbal remedies because they are much less costly than prescription drugs, their access is virtually unlimited and unrestricted, they are effective, and many people are becoming disenchanted with traditional healthcare. However, before taking any herbal remedy, one must know what it does, how to use it, and the possible adverse effects.

Many clients may hesitate to inform their health-care provider that they are using herbs. It is therefore important for the nurse to assess clients' use of herbs and advise them accordingly. Several researchers offer the following guidelines (Bascom, 2002; Skidmore-Roth, 2009; Springhouse Corporation, 2005):

1) In a nonjudgmental manner, encourage the client to disclose use of herbal treatments and obtain a history of herb use as complete as possible, including all products taken, amounts, and brand names. If the client is seeing a herbalist, report any prescription drugs.
2) Determine if the client is using herbal remedies instead of, or as an adjunct to, conventional treatment. Is the herb being used to treat a specific condition or for general health?
3) Inform the client of various benefits, risks, and side effects of the herbal remedy, and any potentially serious adverse reactions that may occur when herbs are used with other drugs or substances the client is using. Labels on the products should contain information about product ingredients and use. Recommend standardized herbs.
4) Warn elderly clients, pregnant women, children, and those with known adverse drug reactions, allergies, chronic skin rashes, or preexisting liver disease that they have an increased risk of adverse effects from herbal medicines.
5) Advise the client to notice any unusual symptoms and to report these to the health provider immediately.
6) Advise the client not to take herbal products for serious medical conditions unless they are used under the care of a well-trained healthcare provider. Urge clients to take only the recommended dosages of herbal remedies.
7) Advise the client to be informed of reputable herbal companies and careful about products sold through magazines, brochures, and the Internet.
8) Tell the client to see a health provider well-trained in herbology when using herbal remedies. Health food store clerks are salespersons, not trained practitioners.
9) Keep a referral list of knowledgeable herbologists.

The field of herbology is expanding at an enormous rate and many books are now available for the nurse to refer to in the care of clients. It is important that the nurse become informed about herbs because increasingly our clients will be coming to us while concurrently using herbal remedies.

Homeopathy

"Homeopathy" comes from the Greek words *homeo*, which means similar, and *pathos*, which means disease or suffering (Boiron Group, 2009). It is based on the law of similars, or like cures like, where stimulating the natural healing properties in the body cures a disease or alleviates a symptom (Freeman, 2004). In other words, when a substance identical to what would produce the symptoms of the disease is introduced into the body in very small or minute doses, it stimulates the person's healing energy. This is very different from what Hahnemann (the father of homeopathy) called allopathy, from the Greek words *allos*, meaning different, and *pathein* or *pathos*, meaning disease or suffering (Weiner, 1998).

The philosophy of homeopathy strongly contends that health and disease are a holistic phenomenon and the individual must be considered from a body, mind, and spirit perspective; that there is an inherent capacity in all living things to respond to illness in a self-curative way; that there is an "unknowability" about certain disease processes; and that rather than focusing on the disease, treatment may begin with the symptom but the client is treated as a whole and as an individual rather than as a diagnosis with common symptoms. Treatment is individualized and tailored to the uniqueness of each person.

Homeopathic remedies are prepared from natural substances—plant, animal, and mineral. The use of micro doses, that is, highly diluted doses, ensures the minimization of toxicity and side effects. Homeopathic medicines are available in various dosage forms: pellets, tablets, liquids, suppositories, and ointments. The U.S. Food and Drug Administration (FDA) recognizes homeopathic remedies as official drugs and regulates the manufacturing, labeling, and dispensing of homeopathic remedies. Simple homeopathic medications of low potencies are available over the counter; however, dilutions for more complicated and chronic conditions are available only from a homeopathic practitioner. Homeopathic remedies are safe, economical, simple to administer, mild in action, and have very few serious or prolonged adverse effects (Micozzi, 2006).

Homeopathic remedies are valuable for a number of symptoms: arnica (marked muscle soreness and acute pain); hypericum (nerve pain, shooting pain); bryonia (trauma, pain on movement); bellis perennis (muscle injury from surgery); ipecacuanha (nausea and vomiting); aconite (fear and shock); calendula (bleeding, preventing infection, increasing granulation); chamomilla (irritability, sensitivity); belladonna (fever); and nux vomica (insomnia) (Wauters, 2007).

Prayer

Whatever holistic/complementary therapy we use may not be as important as how we use it. Our providing safe space where healing can occur is what is most important—and that means using ourselves as an instrument of healing. Clients with life-threatening illness often question "Why?" and may need support in their desire to connect with something larger and outside of themselves. Focusing on them as spiritual beings allows them to explore the meaning and purpose of their illness and can bring comfort, often alleviating pain (Dossey, 1996, 1998; Wright, 2005). Burkhardt and Nagai-Jacobson (2009) offer a number of useful guides and instruments to facilitate spiritual assessment.

As O'Brien (2003a) notes, "Prayer is as unique as the individual who prays. Whether one's prayer is of petition, adoration, reparation, or thanksgiving, both the form and the content may vary greatly" (p. 105). Prayer is a simple act of turning our attention to the sacred. Depending on one's beliefs, this can be the God of whatever religion or culture, a higher power, or the ultimate reality. Prayer can be active or passive, involve words, or be wordless. It can involve asking something for oneself or another, expressing repentance for wrong-doing and asking for forgiveness, giving praise and honor, summoning the presence of the Almighty, or offering gratitude (Ameling, 2000; O'Brien, 2003b). Many forms of prayer are meditative in nature, e.g., centering prayer, mantra, prayer beads, and have the benefits of meditation previously discussed in the section on "Meditation." Others are inter-cessory, an active form of prayer that seeks an outcome through intentionality where we ask for healing for another or ourselves. This also can be done at a distance which is referred to as nonlocal healing (Dossey, 1998). Clients also can benefit from prayerful listening to sacred music or sounds, writing or art, or expressing their intent toward the sacred through some body movement or posture (Taylor, 2003).

Prayer is often an important solace to clients who are ill; however, illness may create a barrier to prayer. In those instances, nurse's prayer for and with the client can be a meaningful spiritual intervention as long as permission is obtained when possible. The nurse should assess the client to ascertain if prayer is desired and then follow the client's expressed wish. Taylor (2003) suggests some assessment questions that the nurse can use:

- "How important or helpful is prayer to you?"
- "Would praying together now be comforting?"
- "What type of prayer would be helpful or comforting to you now?"
- "What helps or hinders you as you pray?"
- "How has your illness affected the way you pray or think about prayer?"
- "Have your prayers changed since you became sick?"
- "Do you find it harder to pray sometimes? How do you deal with that?"
- "Have your beliefs about prayer been challenged or changed by illness?" (p. 182)
- "At times like this, some start thinking about if and how their prayers 'get answered.' Have you thought about this?"

A few minutes spent on assessing and possibly praying with a client can often lower a client's anxiety or assist the nurse's understanding of how prayer facilitates the client's coping.

THE HEALING JOURNEY AT THE END OF LIFE

Individuals become aware of their own deaths in phases, and this awareness can lead to consciousness in dying. Olson and Dossey (2009) and Olson (1997) identify some tasks for dying consciously, specifically:

1) *Live fully* until death comes. Direct or participate in treatment decisions, determinations about the kinds of care, and other decisions until you are comfortable with accepting the assistance of others.

2) *Plan* to say good-bye to family and friends, finish things you wanted to do, make final decisions, regarding the last will and testament, the estate, organ donation, and so forth. Consider what an ideal death would be like. Who do you want with you, or do you want to be alone? Who are the important people in your life and have you told them? Are there certain rituals you want at your death, for example, a memorial service, cremation? What kind of ceremony do you want? Are there certain treasures that you want particular people to have? Are there particular prayers, poems, or music you want read or played?

3) *Participate* in emotional and spiritual tasks such as forgiving yourself and others, feeling that life mattered and the world is different because you were here, and knowing and accepting love as one changes. Forgiving yourself and others necessitates recognizing that we are responsible for what we are holding onto; confessing one's story to self and others, looking for the good points in ourselves and others; making amends where possible; looking to a higher power for help; and considering what we have learned (Borysenko, 1990). Forgiving others and ourselves helps one recognize unconditional love and connect more with the source of our joy instead of focusing on loss, sadness, and pain. Unconditional love helps release one from fear and anxiety.

4) *Rehearse* the dying process. Through an awareness of dying, learn to diminish the fear of death and to "let go of this life" when it is time to do so. Imagery, relaxation, meditation, and prayer scripts on learning forgiveness, becoming peaceful, letting go, opening the heart, forgiving self and others, releasing pain and grief, conscious dying, moving into the light, and closure can facilitate the detachment from pain and grief, the establishment of comfort and peace, and the achievement of closure. Olson and Dossey (2009) is an excellent source for some of these scripts. However, the nurse should have some practice experience prior to their use with clients.

BENEFITS OF HOLISTIC INTEGRATIVE THERAPIES

Nurses can make a critical difference in ensuring that clients receiving palliative care obtain maximum benefit at minimum risk when they integrate complementary/alternative modalities and conventional therapies. Clients benefit because of the following:

- Holistic therapies build on the body's capabilities and are aimed toward strengthening the body's own defenses and healing abilities so that it can do for itself. Strengthened and healthy defenses offer relief that exceed symptom management.
  - □ Holistic integrative therapies view people holistically, realizing that they are complex combinations of unique bodies, minds, emotion, and spirits. CAM considers this interconnectedness, as it assesses and addresses the physical, mental, emotional, environmental, and spiritual aspects of the person. Healing practices are tailored to the individual. This is especially important for palliative care where each person is experiencing a unique dying process. As a result, questions, emotional problems, socioeconomic concerns, and spiritual issues that affect health can be shared. Learning about the total person facilitates addressing needs holistically. Whole-person practices offer attentive and customized healing measures.
- Holistic therapies empower clients and families. People are taught about self-care practices, guided in using them, and assisted in exploring obstacles that could stand in the way of doing so. Also, family members and caregivers can be taught simple holistic techniques to use with their loved ones and themselves, thereby empowering the caregivers/family to participate in their loved one's care and reduce their own stress.
- Most holistic therapies are safer and gentler than conventional therapies. A variety of physical and mental changes, combined with the high volume and nature of medications used in terminal phases of illness, carry many risks for dying clients. Although there are conditions for which drugs provide remarkable benefit, there are other conditions that can be managed and improved through lower risk CAM approaches.

With the many benefits that can be derived from using complementary/alternative therapies and a holistic approach, nurses can best assist those in the dying process by integrating CAM with conventional therapies. This requires that nurses understand the intended and safe use of various CAM therapies, educate clients/families in appropriate CAM use, and prepare themselves to offer selected CAM therapies as part of their practice.

SELF-CARE FOR THE HEALER

Working with the dying and their families can create much stress for the nurse. It is sometimes referred to as "death overload." Olson (1997) notes that caregivers of dying persons often re-examine their own belief systems and may suffer an existential crisis of faith. Health professionals grieve the loss of their clients, and when the losses come too quickly, they may not complete the grieving process before the next death. This may lead to feelings of guilt, anger, irritability, frustration, helplessness, inadequacy, sleeplessness, and depression. Problems may arise in interaction with clients, family members, and other staff. Olson (1997) further notes the consequences when staff are not dealing well with the deaths of clients (p. 207):

- avoiding patients/families;
- poor clinical judgment;
- unrealistic expectations;
- staff absences;
- outbursts of anger;
- lack of anticipatory planning;
- staff conflict;
- scapegoating;
- interdisciplinary power struggles;
- staff fatigue;
- ambivalence toward patients/families.

These problems can affect an individual or an entire team. Therefore, it is imperative that health professionals learn self-care techniques. In discussing bereavement care and the role of nurse healers, Roach and Nieto (1997) identify five self-care areas and questions that need to be explored when working with the dying and their families:

1) Spiritual self-care—Is spirituality important in my life? What is my relationship with God or a higher power? Why am I here and what is my purpose? What is my relationship to the universe?
2) Emotional self-care—Can I identify my emotions? How do I deal with them? Am I usually in control? Can I discuss my emotions? Am I open to others and do I respect the feelings of others or do I jump to conclusions? When do my emotions get out of control?
3) Physical self-care—What areas of my lifestyle are unhealthy or do I have a healthy lifestyle? What can I do to improve my lifestyle?
4) Mental self-care—Am I knowledgeable and do I continually increase my knowledge? Am I satisfied with the status quo or am I open to new ideas? What am I doing to stimulate my mind?
5) Relationships self-care—Am I open and honest with myself and others? Do I have satisfying relationships with others? Am I willing to accept the thoughts and

feelings of others even though they are different from my own or am I judgmental? Must I have all the control or can I share it? Do I have a balance between work, home, and leisure? (pp. 171–175).

Worden (1982) identified four tasks of mourning that are equally applicable to staff. Accepting the reality of the loss, although painful, is necessary for healing to occur. It may sometimes feel as if the nurse in end-of-life care is in chronic grieving because of the number of dying clients. But denying the emotional pain, especially of a favored patient, only slows or inhibits the healing process from occurring.

Although more obvious in the significant others, experiencing the pain of the loss also occurs in the staff, including anger, depression, and guilt. Healing support of each other involves encouraging the expression of feelings and emotions such as sadness, anger, guilt, resentment, and pain. Validating the normalcy of the feelings and emotions is also important. One should identify coping strategies that might work or are not working; forgive oneself and others; and remember shared experiences with the deceased client.

Rediscovering meaning is a period of yearning, searching, and discovery. One yearns for the lost person(s) or assumed state of ordinariness, searches for some type of normalcy to reenter the everyday living or working situation, and then discovers the meaning of the loss or losses. Meaning to each of us is individual, unique, and personal. But if one can find meaning, one seems to adjust more easily. Some find meaning in religion, some in support or supportive groups, and some in going inward. Some may never find the answer to the questions "Why did they have to die?" or "Why am I surrounded by so much death?" However, even if these questions are not answered, one may find a new meaning to life—to the present and to the future.

Reinvesting in life or work is somewhat like hope (Roach & Nieto, 1997). One realizes that there is a purpose to this type of work, that the future can be full and good. There is a letting go of remorse and fear of the future, a sense of empowerment, and a sense of one's place in the world. With letting go, the nurse is free to remember the meaningful times with clients and the lessons learned. Although many techniques described above help in reinvesting in work, it also is useful for one to engage in an area of interest outside of work: enroll in a class, take a trip, do special things for oneself, or review one's job goals and setting. Reinvesting in work does not necessarily mean that everything is solved; however, it can be the motivation for growth. This growth can be expressed as feeling more intensely, empathizing more completely, caring more fully, and developing more sensitivity to and compassion for others.

As noted earlier, those who care for the terminally ill are at risk for stress associated with many losses. There is also opportunity for a career leading to joy, a sense of personal and professional proficiency, and a capability of living life to the fullest. Olson (1997) identifies three aspects of developing growth when working with the dying. Identifying one's motivation for practicing end-of-life care is important. Is it unresolved personal issues; a professional challenge beyond the physical that involves a search for meaning and peace; a desire to witness the growth of each individual as one comes to terms with mortality and the nature of life; a spiritual calling; a joy in physical care that involves a variety of techniques including complementary modalities such as breathing, TT, and relaxation? Whatever the motivation, exploring this question leads the nurse in end-of-life care to a certain insight and wisdom.

Coping techniques include those strategies used to change the negative effects of stress (Mariano, 2007b). It can be forgiving self and others, and maintaining health through good nutrition, weight control, regular exercise, adequate sleep, and sufficient resources to maintain oneself in a healthy state. Other kinds of physical activities include massage, diaphragmatic breathing, and distraction. Time needs to be scheduled so that the staff can focus on themselves. An example of diaphragmatic breathing is found in the "Exercises" section of this chapter. Those who use this technique regularly can do so on cue, even at the bedside of a dying patient. Distraction includes humor, a massage break, having lunch out, a day off, or just a break. One needs these distractions to rest and refresh one's spirit. Scheduling things that are not reminders of patients, death, or dying are important aspects in addition to grieving and remembering.

Developing the spiritual self includes knowing that one's life has meaning and confronting one's mortality. These are key aspects in caring for the dying and their significant others. "*Healing the Dying* means healing oneself by forming connections with the Universe and all that it is. It means a path one can count on, a way one travels with confidence" (Olson, 2001, p. 252). Searching for meaning necessitates learning to listen, quieting the mind's chatter, hearing the whisper of the inner self, and connecting to one's spirituality. A sense of connection with meaningfulness and purpose can be with an organized religion, with a group, or the path of an inner process. There are many ways to develop an ability to listen to the inner self: meditation, creating an environment that supports peace, for example, nature or sound; reading literature about the development of a spiritual path; setting a regular time to practice; keeping a journal; sharing one's spiritual journey with like-minded people; and enjoying life. Whatever the technique, there is a growing sense of unity and purpose in being. One belongs here, one has a mission and a purpose.

This chapter has presented some of the more common alternative/complementary/ integrative healing modalities that are and can be used by nurses and by students of nursing. It should be noted that centering, relaxation, imagery, meditation, reminiscence and life review, and journal writing are basic and can be practiced by nurses and students with little or no experience. The sense therapies, touch therapies, and Reiki bodywork necessitate further study, which are offered through a few master's degree programs and workshops. Whenever one learns these therapies, it is imperative that nurses practicing end-of-life care be familiar with healing modalities and their beneficial effects for clients during the dying process.

A COMMENTARY ON EVIDENCE-BASED PRACTICE RESEARCH AND HOLISTIC INTEGRATIVE THERAPIES

There is a great need for an evidence base to establish the effectiveness and efficacy of holistic/integrative therapies, and research in this area will become increasingly important in the future. However, according to Hyman (2006), there are two fundamental problems with using randomized control clinical trials (RCT) to study holistic healing modalities. The first is that holistic healing modalities are often part of a system, a philosophical approach that is centered on facilitating and promoting balance and health in the body, rather than ameliorating a particular symptom. In an RCT, the holistic/healing modality often is examined out of context, and, consequently, the results often do not indicate the accurate effectiveness of these treatments. Secondly, most outcome measures used in the scientific community today are based on tangible physical/mental or disease symptomatology. One of the formidable tasks for nurses will be to identify and describe outcomes of holistic/integrative therapies such as healing, well-being, and harmony to develop instruments to measure these outcomes. In addition, methodologies need to be expanded to capture the wholeness of the individual's experience because the philosophy of these therapies rests on a paradigm of wholeness.

There is presently much discussion about what method is most appropriate for the study of holistic phenomena. Van Weel and Knotterneus (1999) note that evidence-based medicine (EBM) falls short in the clinical context of patients with chronic complex illnesses. EBM tends to concentrate on research methodology and reduces clinical practice to the technical implementation of research findings. Clinical practice most often employs multiple interventions that do not add up to an evidence-based approach based on a single intervention. Clinical research fails to focus on the combined outcome of multiple interventions because of the complexity, cost, and absence of effective tools for studying such approaches.

Researchers are being challenged to look at alternative philosophies of science and research methods that are compatible with investigations of humanistic and holistic occurrences. We need to study phenomena by exploring the context in which they occur and the meaning of patterns that evolve. Also needed are approaches to interventions studies which are more holistic, taking into consideration the interactive nature of the body-mind-emotion-spirit-environment. Rather than isolating the effects of one part of an intervention, we need more comprehensive interventions and more sensitive instruments that measure the interactive nature of each client's biological, psychological, emotional, spiritual, sociological, and environmental patterns. Researchers must begin to look at whole practices and whole systems which typify whole person treatment. Comprehensive comparative outcome studies are needed to ascertain the usefulness, indications, and contraindications of integrative therapies. And researchers must also evaluate these interventions for their usefulness in promoting wellness as well as preventing illness.

The IOM report titled *Complementary and Alternative Medicine in the United States* (IOM, 2005) and participants at the recent "IOM Summit on Integrative Medicine and the Health of the Public" (Feb. 25–27, 2009) strongly emphasize that investigations of CAM (holistic/healing) practices entails a moral commitment of openness to diverse interpretations of health and healing, a commitment to finding innovative ways of obtaining evidence, and an expansion of the knowledge base, relevant and appropriate to practice. One way to honor social pluralism is in the recognition of medical pluralism, meaning the broad differences in preferences and values expressed through the public's prevalent use of CAM modalities. The proper attitude is one of skepticism about any claim that conventional biomedical research and practice exhaustively account for the human experiences of health and healing.

Dossey (2003) discusses a conundrum that researchers in this area face.

> "In healing research, we face a paradox. Most healers acknowledge that healing cannot be forced to happen. At some point the healer must relax into a state in which he or she permits the healing process to proceed in its own way. This strategy of stepping aside has been called 'doing through non-doing,' 'purposeful purposelessness,' a 'controlled accident.' Although irrational, the accounts of actual healers worldwide abound with descriptions of this sort. Perhaps there is a lesson here as we attempt to craft definitions of the terms involved in healing. Maybe we need to preserve a certain level of imprecision, irrationality, and illogic in how we talk about this field. This does not mean that we should jettison discipline and skills in favor of an 'anything goes' approach, but that we recognize that the discipline of healing requires a level of freedom or play within certain limits. This level of freedom is [what] engineers build into bridges and skyscrapers - what they call tolerance - that allows the structure to sway without buckling....a strictly rigid bridge or building that has no sway, that cannot drift off

center a bit, can be a disaster. Just so, ...if a term is to serve us, it must be permitted to move within certain boundaries, to manifest nuances when evidence and circumstances change" (p. A12).

The nature of many holistic phenomena presents a challenge to their "scientific" exploration and understanding. Because of the nonempirical effects of some healing therapies, how do we ascertain the effectiveness of some therapies when we presently can only measure the physical, emotional or psychological parameters? How do we know something is useful to the client when there is no biophysical change and yet the client reports positive evaluations of these interventions? How do we know something works? How do we measure existential peace, or well-being, or openheartedness, or spiritual truth and connection, or psychic power? How do we measure transcendence or the universal life force? Do we need to measure there things? Are practice, theory, and research partly based on faith and mystery? Answers to these questions are beyond the scope of this discussion; however, other ways of knowing such as intuition, esthetic and personal knowing, and unknowing as a way of knowing must be given credibility in the research world focusing on healing and holistic/integrative therapies (Mariano, 2005; Mariano, 2008).

EXERCISES

Passive Relaxation[1]

Procedure for participants who are lying down:

- With your eyes closed, let your attention focus on your breathing . . . notice how gentle, slow, and regular it is becoming . . . imagine each breath out carrying your tensions away, leaving you more relaxed than you were before . . . if you want to, take one deep breath . . . then allow your breathing to settle into its own rhythm . . . easy, calm, and even . . . and forget about it.
- I'm going to ask you to take a trip around the body, checking that all the muscle groups are as relaxed as possible and letting go any tension that might still remain. If outside thoughts creep in, hold them in a bubble and let them flow away. I'll begin with the feet.
- Bring your attention to your toes . . . are they lying still? If they are curled or stretched out in some way not entirely comfortable, wiggle them gently. As they come to rest, feel all the tension leaving them . . . feel them sinking down, heavy and motionless.

- Let your feet roll out at the ankles. This is the most relaxed position for them. Let all the tension flow out of them . . . enjoy the sensation of just letting them go.
- Moving on to the lower legs: Feel the tension leaving the calf muscles and the shins. As the tension goes, so they feel heavier . . . so they feel warm and pleasantly tingling.
- The thighs next: to be fully relaxed they need to be slightly rolling outwards . . . feel the relaxing effect of this position. . . make sure you have released all tension, and feel your thighs resting heavily on the surface you are resting on.
- Focus for a moment on the sensation of sagging heaviness throughout your legs . . . let the muscles shed their last remaining hint of tension and settle into a deep relaxation. And now, think of your hips. Let them settle into the surface you are lying on. . . recognize any tension that lingers in the muscles . . . then relax it away . . . let it go on relaxing a bit further than you thought possible.
- Settle your spine into the rug or mattress . . . become aware of how it is resting on a surface. Let it sink down, making contact whenever it wants to . . . all tension draining out of it.
- Let your abdominal muscles lose their tension. Let them go soft and loose. Feel them spreading as they give their last vestige of tension . . . notice how your relaxed abdomen rises and falls with your breathing . . . rises as the air is drawn in and falls as the air is expelled . . . abdominal breathing is relaxed breathing.
- Move up to your chest and shoulders, to muscles that are prone to carry tension . . . feel them letting go . . . feel them spreading . . . feel them easing into the surface, limp and heavy . . . feel them drooping down towards your feet . . . imagine them shedding their burdens . . . and as the space between your shoulders and your neck opens out, imagine your neck a bit longer than it was before.
- Now, direct your thoughts to the muscles of your left arm. Check that it lies limply on a surface. Notice the feeling of relaxation and allow this feeling to sweep down to your wrist and hand. Think of the fingers, are they curved and still? . . . neither drawn up nor stretched out . . . neither opened nor closed, but gently resting . . . totally relaxed. As you breathe out, let the arm relax a little bit more . . . let it lie heavy and loose . . . so heavy and loose that if someone were to pick it up, then let it go, it would flop down again like the arm of a rag doll.
- Repeat the last paragraph with the muscles of the right arm.
- Your neck muscles have no need to work with your head supported, so let them go . . . enjoy the

feeling of letting go in muscles that work so hard the rest of the time to keep your head upright. If you find any tension in the neck, release it and let this process of releasing continue, even below the surface . . . feel how pleasant it is when you let go the tension in these muscles.

- Bring your attention now to your face, to the many small muscles whose job it is to manage your expressions. At the moment there's no need to have any expression at all on your face, so allow your muscles to feel relaxed . . . imagine how your face is when you are asleep . . . calm and motionless.
- Now, think about the jaw . . . and as you do, allow it to drop slightly so that your teeth are separated . . . feel it relaxing with your lips gently touching. Check that your tongue is still, and lying in the middle of your mouth, soft and shapeless. Relax your throat so that all tension leaves it and the muscles feel smooth and resting.
- With no expression on your face, your cheeks are relaxed and soft. If you think of your nose, it is just to register the passage of cool air traveling up your nostrils while the warmer air passes down. . . breathe tension out with the warm air . . . breathe stillness in with cool air.
- Check that your forehead is smooth . . . not furrowed in any direction . . . and as you release its remaining tension, imagine it being a little higher and a little wider than it was before . . . continue this feeling into your scalp and behind your ears . . . feel a sense of calm as you do this.
- Let your thoughts focus on your eyes as they lie behind gently closed lids. Think of them resting in their sockets, floating, rather than fixed . . . and as they come to rest, so do your thoughts.
- Spend a few minutes continuing to relax, deepening the effect of the above sequences . . .
- You now have relaxed all the major muscle groups in your body. Think about them now as a whole . . . a totally relaxed whole . . . soothed by your gentle breathing rhythm, feel the peacefulness of this idea . . .
- Images may drift in and out of your mind . . . see them as thoughts passing through. Feel yourself letting go of them. Say to yourself: "I am feeling calm, I am feeling peaceful." Let your mind conjure up a sense of contentment.

Imagery

The instructor picks one of the following: a sunny beach, a river bank, or a scented garden. If trainees suffer from hay fever, the first item is the best choice. Imagery is best used after a short relaxation exercise.

A Sunny Beach

- See yourself lying on the hot sand of a sunny beach within an enclosed bay. It is sheltered from storms and protected from ocean currents. It is safe. You watch the light dancing on the water; you smell the sea air as it fills your nostrils; you hear the gulls calling above the sound of waves; you feel the warm sun on your skin. The grains of dry sand run through your fingers, forming little bumps and hollows beneath your hand.

A River Bank

- Imagine you are lying in the soft, juicy long grass of early summer. You are in a green meadow that rolls down to the river. Scents rise up from the wildflowers, sweeping over you in waves. The sun is warm, but a gentle breeze softens its intensity. Closing your eyes, you become aware of the sound of water flowing, of birds calling, and of leaves rustling.

A Scented Garden

- Picture yourself lying on a newly mown lawn with the sun beating down on the moist cuttings, drawing out their fragrance. Reach out and feel the coolness of the damp grass. Through your half-closed eyelids you can see the tops of the trees swaying against the sky. Light breezes carry the scent of honeysuckle.

Following one of these short passages of visualization, trainees can relax for a few minutes, before the session is brought to an end.

Relaxation[1]

I would like you to be as comfortable as you possibly can. Take a couple of deep breaths. Inhale deeply. Exhale very slowly and very completely. Focus on your breathing. Again, inhale very deeply and exhale very slowly. Become aware of your ability to relax your muscles. Allow every muscle in your body to be as relaxed as possible, starting with the feet. Allow the feet to become very, very comfortable. Relax the feet completely. As the muscles relax, you may notice a tingling sensation in the soles and toes of the feet. This simply indicates that the muscles are relaxing.

Be aware as this sensation of relaxation begins to move upward from the feet to the ankles. This sensation of relaxation flows from the ankles to the calves of the legs. The muscles of the calves release the tension and relax. The calves become very comfortable as the tension is released.

[1] *From:* S. Roach & B. Nieto, 1997, *Healing and the Grief Process.* Copyright 1997 by Delmar Publications.

This comfortable, relaxed sensation moves from the calves to the upper legs and thighs. These muscles also relax and become very comfortable. Feel the muscles on the sides of the legs, the outside of the legs, the inner legs, and on the top of the legs as they become very comfortable and relaxed.

The sensation of relaxation moves up towards the buttocks and toward the pelvic area. Occasionally you may feel a muscle twitch. This is just another sign that relaxation is occurring. The tension of the muscles of the buttocks, pelvic area, and the lower abdomen is released. The internal organs relax and the muscles that surround them feel completely tension free.

The sensation of relaxation moves up the body to the upper abdomen, to the chest, and from the lower back toward the upper back. The muscles are relaxing from the chest and the upper back to the shoulders.

This relaxation extends to the neck and the throat. Feel the tension draining from the back of the neck. Tension is draining away from the back of the neck and the back of the head. As tension drains away, a sense of relaxation settles in. These feelings are so comfortable and so pleasant. Feel the muscles of the throat, the jaw, and across the bridge of the nose relaxing.

The tension in the arms is released, and these muscles feel relaxed. Relaxation spreads to the hands and the fingers as the tension is released.

From the feet, to the head, to the arms, to the fingertips, the whole body is completely and totally relaxed. Take a few moments to savor this comfortable state of total relaxation of body and mind.

Closure. Allow time for the client to appreciate this restful state of complete relaxation. After a few minutes, instruct the client to bring his/her attention back to the present. At times, the nurse may want to count slowly from 1 to 10 as the client progressively returns to a more wakeful state.

Meditation[1]

Using a Mantra

1) Select a word to focus on. It can be a neutral word, such as "one," or a Sanskrit mantra such as "Om Shanti," "Sri Ram," "So-Hum." It could also be a word or phrase that has some special significance within your personal belief system. In his recent book, *Beyond the Relaxation Response*, Benson (1985) describes how a word or phrase of special personal significance (such as "I am at peace" or "Let go, let God") deepens the effects of meditation.
2) Repeat this word or phrase, ideally on each exhalation.
3) As any thoughts come to mind, just let them pass over and through you, and gently bring your attention back to the repetitive word or phrase.

Continuing Breaths

1) As you sit quietly, focus on the inflow and outflow of your breath. Each time you breathe out, count the breath. You can count up to 10 and start over again, or keep counting as high as you like, or you can use Benson's method of repeating "one" on each exhalation.
2) Each time your focus wanders, bring it back to your breathing and counting. If you get caught in an internal monologue or fantasy, don't worry about it or judge yourself. Just relax and return to the count again.
3) If you lose track of the count, start over at 1 or at a round number like 50 or 100.
4) After practicing breath-counting meditation for a while, you may want to let go of the counting and just focus on the inflow and outflow of your breathing.

Whichever form of meditation you try, you might want to start out with short periods of 5 to 10 minutes and gradually lengthen them to 20 to 30 minutes over a period of 2 to 3 weeks. Most people find that it takes persistent and disciplined effort over a period of several months to become proficient at meditating. Even though meditation is the most demanding of relaxation techniques to learn, it is for many people the most rewarding. Research has found that among all relaxation techniques, meditation is the one that people are most likely to persist in doing regularly.

If you are truly interested in establishing a meditation practice, you may want to find a class, group, or teacher to study with. This will make it easier for you to continue your practice.

Script for Breathing for Relaxation and Health[2]

■ Close your eyes . . . Focus your mind on your breath . . . Just follow the air as it goes in . . . and as it goes out.

---

[1]*From:* Edmund J. Bourne, 1995, *The Anxiety and Phobia Workbook* (2nd Ed.), Copyright 1995 by New Harbinger Publications, Inc. All rights reserved.

[2]*From:* Julie T. Lusk, *30 Scripts for Relaxation, Imagery and Inner Healing,* Vol. 1. Copyright 1992 by Julie T. Lusk. Vols. 1 and 2 are available from Whole Persons Associates, 210 W. Michigan, Duluth, Minnesota 55802, 800-247-6789. Julie T. Lusk is also the author of *Refreshing Journeys,* a relaxation audiotape available from Whole Persons Associates, and *Desktop Yoga,* available from Perigee Books, 800-631-8751.

- Feel it as it comes in . . . and as it goes out . . . If your mind begins to wander, just bring it back to your breath.
- Feel your stomach rise . . . your ribs expand . . . and your collarbone rise . . . Breathe in naturally and slowly.
- On your next exhalation, release all the air from your lungs without straining . . . Let it all go . . . Let it all out . . . Prepare your lungs to receive fresh oxygen.
- Now take in a full, deep breath and let the air go to the bottom of your lungs. . . Feel your stomach rise . . . your chest expand, and the collarbone area fill.
- Now empty your lungs from top to bottom . . . Let all the air out . . . Compress your stomach to squeeze out all the stale air and carbon dioxide. Squeeze out every bit of air . . . Let it all go.
- Take in another deep breath . . . As you breathe in, your diaphragm expands and massages all the internal organs in the abdominal region . . . aiding your digestion.
- Breathe out . . . Relax . . . Feel the knots in your stomach untie . . . Let go.
- Breath in . . . Your diaphragm is stimulating your vagus nerve, slowing down the beating of your heart . . . relaxing you.
- Breath out . . . Let it all go . . . Relax . . . Relax more and more . . . Breathing heals you . . . calms you . . . soothes you.
- Breathe in again, fully and completely. Oxygen is entering your bloodstream, nourishing all your organs and cells . . . protecting you.
- Breath out . . . Release all the poisons and toxins with your breath . . . Your breathing is cleansing you . . . healing you.
- Breathe in.
- Now imagine exhaling confusion . . . and inhaling clarity.
- Imagine exhaling darkness . . . and inhaling light.
- Imagine exhaling hatred . . . and inhaling love.
- Exhaling anxiety . . . and inhaling peace.
- Exhaling selfishness . . . and inhaling generosity.
- Exhaling guilt . . . and inhaling forgiveness.
- Exhaling weakness . . . and inhaling courage.
- Breathe in through your nose and sigh out through your mouth. Let the air stay out of your lungs as long as it is comfortable, and then take another breath.
- Let your breath return to its normal and natural pace. Continue to breathe in slowly, smoothly, and deeply . . . Your breathing is steady, easy, silent.
- Each time you exhale . . . allow yourself to feel peaceful . . . calm . . . and completely relaxed . . . If your mind wanders, bring your attention back to your breath.

- Stretch and open your eyes, feeling refreshed and rejuvenated, alert, and fully alive.

Repeat the above instructions until everyone is alert.

White Light of Healing Energy Imagery[1]

Begin to imagine that there is a sphere of white light of healing energy about 4 inches above your head. The white light is now touching the top of your head. Begin to feel this light as it flows from the top of your head and allow it to flow down through the entire inside of the body.

The healing light has filled the inside of your head . . . and it now flows down your shoulders, back, down your arms, and into your fingertips. The white light is now flowing into your chest . . . around your sides . . . into your middle and lower back . . . below your waist . . . around your sides flowing into your abdomen . . . into your buttocks . . . and into your pelvis. The light now flows down your thighs . . . to your lower legs . . . and to your feet.

The white light has now completely filled the inside of your body. There is now a wonderful abundance of this healing light . . . and it begins to bubble up and flow back out through the top of your head . . . down the outside of your body . . . coating the entire outside of your body. The more you allow it to flow throughout your body . . . the more abundant it is. Send the healing white light to specific areas that need extra attention, such as places of discomfort or disease.

Inner Guide Imagery[2]

As you begin to feel even more relaxed now. . . going to a greater depth of inner being . . . more relaxed . . . more secure and safe . . . let yourself become aware of the presence of not being alone. With you right now is a guide . . . who is wise and concerned with your well-being. Let yourself begin to see this wise being with whom you can share your fears or your joys. You have trust in this wise guide.

If you do not see anyone, let yourself be aware of hearing or feeling this wise being, noticing the presence of care and concern. In whatever way seems best for you . . . proceed to make contact with the wise inner guide. Let yourself establish contact with your guide now . . . in any way that comes. Your guide may appear to you in any form, such as a person, an animal, or inner presence/peace . . . or as an image of the very wisest part of you.

[1] *From:* Barbara Montgomery Dossey, "Imagery," in *Holistic Nursing: A Handbook for Practice* (5th Ed.), edited by Barbara Montgomery Dossey & Lynn Keegan. Copyright 2009 by Jones and Bartlett Publishers.
[2] Ibid.

Notice the love and wisdom with which you are surrounded. This wisdom and love are present for you now . . . Let yourself ask for advice . . . about anything that is important for you just now. Be receptive to what emerges . . . Let yourself receive some new information. This inner guide may have a special message to share with you . . . Listen with openness and pure intention to receive.

Allow yourself to look at any issue in your life. It may be a symptom, a choice, or decision . . . Tell your wise guide anything that you wish . . . Listen to the answers that emerge. Imagine yourself acting on the answers and directions that you received . . . Imagine yourself calling upon the wisdom and love of this wise guide to help you in the days to come. Now in whatever way is best for you . . . bring closure to the visit with this inner guide. You can come back here any time you wish. All you have to do is take the time.

Imagery: Finding One's Special Place[1]

Begin by placing your body in a comfortable position, arms and legs uncrossed, your back well supported. Now take three deep breaths, and during each breath relax even more. Let the exhalation be a letting-go kind of breath, letting go of tension. With each breath, take in what you need and with each exhalation, release anything you don't need. Bring your attention to the top of your head. Feel your scalp relax and let your brow soften and smooth out. Allow the muscles around your eyes to relax. And let any tension flow out through your cheeks as you exhale. Suggest that your jaw relax. Imagine a wave of relaxation flowing down your shoulders, into your arms, elbows, and forearms, all the way into your hands and fingers. Now focus on your chest, releasing any tension around your heart or lungs, relax the muscles around your ribs. Wrap that relaxation around your back and let a wave of relaxation travel down the spine. Allow the muscles along the spine to lengthen and release. Soften and relax the buttocks and pelvis. Let the belly be very soft so that the breath moves easily down into the abdomen. Invite the legs to join in the relaxation now, as it moves through the thighs, knees, calves, ankles, and feet. Let any last bit of tension or tightness drain out through your feet or toes. When you feel relaxed and comfortable, let me know with a nod of your head. As your body remains relaxed and comfortable, imagine yourself in a very special place, somewhere that is full of natural beauty, safety, and peace. It may be a place you have been to before or it may be a place you want to create in your imagination. Take some

time and let yourself be drawn to one place that is just right for you today. Let me know when you are present there (wait for response). Describe what it is like there. What do you see? Are there any smells? Are there any sounds? What is the temperature like? Where are you in this special place? How do you feel here? Take some time to do whatever you would like to do here, to relax or do some activity. Feel free to do whatever you want. This is your place. (Pause 3 to 4 minutes).

In a few moments, it will be time to come back into a waking state. Know that you can return to this place again anytime you want. Now gently bring yourself back, letting the images fade but keeping with you this relaxed and peaceful feeling. Remember what has been important about this experience. Become aware of the current time and place. Begin to move your body, take a deep breath, open your eyes, and feel relaxed and awake.

At this point, the guide can take a few minutes to allow the person to share his/her experience.

Imagery in Oncology[2]

Cancer might well be the most feared disease of our time. Many people live their lives in dread and fear of cancer. The traditional medical treatments are terrifying and excruciating. Many nurses find it beneficial to work with the client's negative images and beliefs.

Some nurses have reported making tapes (there are also some available commercially) in which the client is encouraged to imagine chemotherapy or radiation therapy as something positive. Some clients prefer to view it as beams of energy or light.

The practitioner might ask "How do you imagine the chemotherapy?" Despite the response, the nurse can be helpful in supporting the transformation of the images into something beneficial and positive. "Imagine the medicine going into exactly the cells that most need it. The side effects will be minimal." There are a great variety of techniques and applications that enhance the healing journey through the experience of cancer.

Quick Uses of Imagery in the Clinical Setting

IVs. When a patient is receiving intravenous fluids, he/she can envision fluid flowing to every part of the body, removing toxins and flushing them out. The patient can see nutrients providing nourishment to every cell.

[1]From: K. Shames, 1996. *Creative Imagery in Nursing.* Copyright 1996 by Delmar Publications.

[2]Ibid.

Pain medications. Similarly, the patient can enhance the benefits of pain medication by envisioning its soothing effects as it travels through the bloodstream, sedating any irritated areas and bringing a deep sense of relief throughout. It is suggested that relaxation be used at the first sign of discomfort; focus the patient on the breath. Imagine the body releasing its natural medicine to all areas that are tense or uncomfortable. If pain begins to interfere with activity or rest, ask for medication before becoming so uncomfortable that it would be difficult to work with relaxation and the following imagery:

Imagine the pain medication to be exactly the strength it needs to be. See, feel, or sense the muscles around the painful area softening and relaxing as you breathe into the discomfort. See or feel the pain medication moving to that area, numbing the pain as if it had deposited a layer of frost.

Imagine a dial registering a number from 1 to 10 that represents your pain now. See the number come down to your tolerance level. Allow an image to form of a special, quiet, restful place and allow yourself to be there as you rest.

Antibiotics. Some patients like to imagine their antibiotic medication in the bloodstream as hunters stalking their prey. They can envision that the medication stays where the most protection is needed, particularly around burns or incisions, ready to pounce. If more medication is needed, there is an endless supply in the imagination.

Anticoagulants. Likewise, clients using anticoagulants can envision their blood becoming thinner, flowing to exactly the right places to prevent clotting. They can see the medication as extraordinarily efficient and relish watching as it does its magic.

Oxygen. As you take a deep breath, send nourishing healing oxygen into every cell of your lungs, expanding each cell like a balloon. As you exhale, imagine letting the balloons completely deflate and blow any tension or toxins that remain in the body out into the air. Continue doing this slowly for a few minutes, watching the balloons expand and contract.

Healing Image. Imagine little workers repairing the muscles and bones while they are resting, allowing the healing process to begin. See the bone rich in calcium, and see little bone cells growing like coral, increasing in number and density.

Ideal Images. Many clients continue to envision their healing process long after the crises have passed. One way to do this is to imagine themselves in 3 or 6 months. They can imagine themselves exactly as they would wish to be. They can observe how they look, how they walk, their facial expressions. They might imagine themselves running or swimming, looking healthy and happy.

It is also a good practice for nurses to see themselves as they want to be. Focus on the image; how does it feel to be whole? Many nurses find that using imagery supports their patients totally and empowers them in their work. According to one nurse, after incorporating imagery frequently, "I finally felt as if I were making a difference, despite the disempowering aspect of the environment."

Diaphragmatic Breathing

Diaphragmatic breathing is a useful technique for relaxing and beginning the centering process. Consciously realizing the path each inhalation takes through the respiratory passages, and inhaling so that the abdomen and lungs expand, allowing each breath to move to the bottom of the respiratory tree by moving the diaphragm downward and outward moves the whole person toward feeling more relaxed. As the slow, long exhalation occurs, a person feels shoulders moving downward and tensions slowly leaving the body. To help with stress at work, a nurse should practice diaphragmatic breathing at home, in either a supine or sitting position. Putting one's hand on the abdomen is an easy way to know if the abdomen is involved in the breath, or if shallow, tense breaths are a pattern. Once a pattern of abdominal breathing is the norm, the nurse can think of phrases such as, "I can feel this way whenever I take a deep breath and cross my fingers." Connecting the relaxed feeling to the physical act of crossing fingers (or another physical cue) helps the body remember how it feels to relax. A nurse who regularly practices this technique will have the ability to break the cycle of stress and muscle tension in just a few seconds, even at the bedside of a dying patient. The pattern is as follows:

- Recognize the feeling of tension.
- Take an abdominal breath—on inhalation the stomach expands.
- On exhalation the stomach contracts— allow the shoulders to sag and experience the relaxation during the exhalation.
- Use a physical cue that has been practiced.

This technique, or pattern, is useful by itself to help relax for a few minutes or to lead to more profound states of relaxation.

Case Study conclusion: Following the TT treatment, J.A. fell asleep. He told the nurse later that this was the most rested he felt since coming to the hospital and with rest that maybe he could deal better with his pain. The staff decided that J.A. would receive a TT treatment each morning and evening, during his hospitalization.

RESOURCES

Academy for Guided Imagery
P.O. Box 2070
Mill Valley, CA 94942
(800)726–2070; fax (415)389–9342
www.healthy.net/agi/index_explorer.html

American Association for Music Therapy (AAMT)
P.O. Box 27177
Philadelphia, PA 19918
(215)265–4006

American Herbalist Guild
1931 Gaddis Road
Canton, GA 30115
(770)751–6021
www.americanherbalist.com

American Holistic Nurses Association
323 N. San Francisco St. Suite 201
Flagstaff, AZ 86001
(800)526–2462
www.ahna.org

American Massage Therapy Association
820 Davis Street, Suite 100
Evanston, IL 60201–4444
(847)864–0123
www.amtamassage.org

American Psychological Association
750 First Street NE
Washington, DC 20002–4242
(800)374–2721

Association for Applied Psychophysiology and Biofeedback
Biofeedback Certification Institute of America
10200 W. 44th Avenue, Suite 304
Wheat Ridge, CO 80003
(303)420–2902
www.bcia.org

Center for Mindfulness in Medicine, Health Care and Society
University of Massachusetts Medical Center
419 Belmond Avenue Worcester, MA 01604
www.mindfulnesstapes.com

Compassionate Touch
20 Swan Court
Walnut Creek, CA 94596 (510)935–3906

Contemplative Outreach, Ltd.
[centering prayer] P.O. Box 737
10 Park Place, Suite 2B
Butler, NJ 07405
(973)838–3384;
e-mail: office@coutreach.org
www.centeringprayer.com/cntrgpryr.htm

International Center for Reiki Training
29209 Northwestern Highway, #592
Southfield, MI 48034
(800)332–8112
Maharishi Vedic School
[TM program] 636 Michigan Avenue
Chicago, IL 60605
(312)431–0110
www.maharishi.org

National Association for Holistic Aromatherapy
836 Hanley Industrial Court St. Louis, MO 63144
(888)ASK-NAHA; (888)275–6242

National Association of Music Therapy (NAMT)
8455 Colesville Road, Suite 930
Silver Spring, MD 20910
(301) 589–3300

National Association of Nurse Massage Therapists
(800)262–4017
http://members.aol.com/naumtl

National Center for Complementary and Alternative Medicine (NCCAM)
P.O. Box 7923
Gaithersburg, MD 20898
(888)644–6226; e-mail: info@nccam.nih.gov/

National Center for Homeopathy
801 N. Fairfax Street, Suite 306 Alexandria, VA 22314
(703)548–7790
www.homeopathic.org

National Certification for Acupuncture and Oriental Medicine (NCCAOM)
11 Canal Center Plaza, Suite 300 Alexandria, VA 22314
(703)548–9004
www.nccaom.org

Nurse Healers — Professional Associates
International [therapeutic touch]
3760 South Highland Drive, Suite 429
Salt Lake City, UT 84106
(801)942–5900 (801)273–3399;
e-mail: rmgood@worldnet.att.net
www.therapeutictouch.org

Transcendental Meditation (888)532–7686
Transcendental Meditation Program (888)LEARN TM
www.tm.org

REFERENCES

AARP/NCCAM (National Center for Complementary and Alternative Medicine). (2007). *Complementary and alternative medicine: What people 50 and older are using and discussing with their physicians.* Washington, DC: AARP.

Abrahms, E. (1999). Reiki. In N. Allison (Ed.), *The illustrated encyclopedia of body-mind disciplines* (pp. 133–136). New York: Rosen.

Allison, N. (1999). Guided imagery. In N. Allison (Ed.), *The illustrated encyclopedia of body-mind* disciplines (pp. 71–73). New York: Rosen.

Ameling, A. (2000). Prayer: An ancient healing practice becomes new age again. *Holistic Nursing Practice, 14*(3), 40–48.

Anselmo, J. (2009). Relaxation. In B. Dossey, & L. Keegan, (Eds.), *Holistic nursing a handbook for practice* (5th ed., pp. 259–293). Sudbury, MA: Jones and Bartlett.

Aspen Reference Group. (2003). *Holistic health promotion and complementary therapies: A resource for integrated practice.* Gaithersburg, MD: Aspen.

Barnes, P., Powell-Griner, E., McFann, K., & Nahin, R. (2004). *Complementary and alternative medicine use among adults: United States, advance data from vital and health statistics, No.343.* Hyattsville, MD: U.S. Department of Health and Human Services, Center for Disease Control and Prevention, and National Center for Alternative and Complementary Medicine. (Available online: http://www.mbcrc.med. ucla.edu/PDFs/camsurvey2.pfd).

Bascom, A. (2002). *Incorporating herbal medicine into clinical practice.* Philadelphia, PA: Davis.

Benson, H. (1995). *Beyond the relaxation process.* New York: Berkley Books.

Boiron Group. (2009). *The smart guide to homeopathy.* Newtown Square, PA: Author.

Bonadonna, R. (2003). Meditation's impact on chronic illness. *Holistic Nursing Practice, 17,* 309–319.

Borysenko, J. (1990). *Guilt is the teacher, love is the lesson.* New York: Warner Books.

Brownlee, C. (2005). Mapping aroma: Smells light up distinct brain parts. *Science News, 167*(22), 340–341.

Buckle, J. (2004). Aromatherapy. In L. Freeman (Ed.), *Mosby's complementary and alternative medicine: A research-based approach* (2nd ed.). St. Louis, MO: Mosby.

Buckle, J. (2009). Aromatherapy. In B. Dossey & L. Keegan (Eds.), *Holistic nursing a handbook for practice* (5th ed., pp. 483–498). Sudbury, MA: Jones and Bartlett.

Burkhardt, M., & Nagai-Jacobson, M. (2009). Spirituality and health. In B. Dossey & L. Keegan (Eds.), *Holistic nursing a handbook for practice* (5th ed., pp. 617–645). Sudbury, MA: Jones and Bartlett.

Cook, C., Guerrerio, J., & Slater, U. (2004). Healing touch and quality of life in women receiving radiation treatment for cancer. *Alternative Therapies in Health and Medicine, 10*(3), 34–41.

Davis, P. (2005). *Aromatherapy: An a-z: The most comprehensive guide to aromatherapy ever published.* London: Random House.

Denison, B. (2004). Touch the pain away: New research on therapeutic touch and persons with fibromyalgia syndrome. *Holistic Nursing Practice, 18,*142–150.

Dossey, L. (1996). *Prayer is good medicine.* San Francisco, CA: Harper Collins.

Dossey, L. (1998). *Reinventing medicine: Beyond mind-body to a new era of healing.* San Francisco, CA: Harper.

Dossey, L. (2003). Samueli conference on definitions and standards in healing research:

Working definitions and terms. In *Definifions and Standards in Healing Research. Alternative Therapies in Health and Medicine Supplement, 9*(3), A10-A12.

Dossey, B., & Keegan, L. (2009). *Holistic nursing: A handbook for practice* (5th ed.). Sudbury, MA: Jones and Bartlett.

Eaton-Kelley, K. (2006). Frankincense and the terminally ill patient. (R. J. Buckle Associates Certification no.303).

Frank-Schwebel, A. (1999). Music therapy. In N. Allison (Ed.), *The illustrated encyclopedia of body-mind disciplines* (pp. 366–369). New York: Rosen.

Fontaine, K. (2004). *Complementary and alternative therapies for nursing practice.* Upper Saddle River, NJ: Prentice-Hall.

Freeman, L. (2004). *Complementary and alternative medicine: A research-based approach* (2nd ed.). St. Louis, MO: Mosby.

Freeman, L., Caserta, D., Lund, S., Rossa, S., Dowdy, A., & Partenheimer, A. (2006). Music thantalogy: Prescriptive harp music as palliative care for the dying patient. *American Journal of Hospital Palliative Care, 23*(2), 100–104.

Gauding, M. (2005). *The meditation bible: The definitive guide to meditations for every purpose.* New York: Sterling Publications.

Gross, C., Kritzer, M. J., Russas, V., Treesak, C., Frazier, P., & Hertz, M., et al. (2004). Mindfulness meditation to reduce symptoms after organ transplant. *Alternative Therapies in Health and Medicine, 10*(3), 58–66.

Huebscher, R., & Schuler, P. (2004). *Natural, alternative and complementary health care practices.* St. Louis, MO: Mosby.

Hyman, M. (2006). The evolution of research: Meeting the needs of systems medicine, part 1. *Alternative Therapies in Health and Medicine, 12*(3), 10–13.

Institute of Medicine. (IOM). (2005). *Complementary and alternative medicine in the United States.* Washington, DC: The National Academies Press.

Kim, H. (2006). Evaluation of aromatherapy in treating postoperative pain: Pilot study. *Pain Practice, 6*(4), 273–276.

Koger, S. M., & Brotons, M. (2000). *Music therapy for dementia symptoms.* Cochrane Database Systematic Review. CD001121.

Krieger, D. (1997). *Therapeutic touch inner workbook.* Santa Fe, NM: Bear.

Krieger, D. (2002). *Therapeutic touch: A transpersonal healing.* New York: Lantern Books.

Laurant, R., & Shlien, J. (1984). *Client centered therapy and the person centered approach.* New York: Praeger.

Lawson, K., & Horneffer, K. (2002). Roots and viewing a pilot of a mind-body-spirit program. *Journal of Holistic Nursing, 20,* 250–263.

LeRoux, F. (2006). *Music is healing.* Charleston, SC: Book-Surge.

Macrae, J. (1987). *Therapeutic touch: A practical guide.* New York: Knopf.

Mariano, C. (1998). Preparing nurses to deliver holistic care. *Spectrum, 10*(22), 14–15.

Mariano, C. (2004). Holistic nursing today. *Creative Nursing, 10*(1), 4–8.

Mariano, C. (2005). *Nursing ethics and research within the holistic paradigm.* Unpublished paper presented at the Erickson Annual Lecture, University of Texas, Austin Texas.

Mariano, C. (2007a). Holistic nursing as a specialty: Holistic nursing: Scope and standards of practice. *Nursing Clinics of North America, 42*(2), 165–188.

Mariano, C. (2007b). The nursing shortage: Is stress management the answer? *Beginnings, 27*(1), 3.

Mariano, C. (2008). Contributions to holism through critique of theory development and research. *Beginnings, 28*(2), 12–13.

Mariano, C. (2009). Current trends and issues in holistic nursing. In B. Dossey & L. Keegan, (Eds.), *Holistic nursing a handbook for practice* (5th ed., pp.75–89). Sudbury, MA: Jones and Bartlett.

MacInytre, B., Hamilton, J., Fricke, T., Ma, W., Hehle, S., & Michel, M. (2008). The efficacy of healing touch in coronary artery bypass surgery recovery. A randomized clinical trial. *Alternative Therapies in Health and Medicine, 14*(4), 24–32.

Maville, J., Bowen, J., & Benham, G. (2008). Effect of healing touch on stress perception and biological correlates. *Holistic Nursing Practice, 22*(2), 103–110.

McCaleb, R., Leigh, E., & Morien, K. (2000). *The encyclopedia of popular herbs.* Roseville, CA: Prima.

McCraty, R., Barrios-Chaplin, B., Atkinson, M., & Tomasino, D. (1998). The effects of different types of music on mood, tension and mental clarity. *Alternative Therapies, 4*(1), 75–84.

Micozzi, M. (2006). *Fundamentals of complementary and alternative medicine* (3rd ed.). New York: Churchill Livingston.

Miles, P., & True, G. (2003). Reiki: Review of a biofield therapy history, theory, practice, and research. *Alternative Therapies, 9*(2), 62–72.

Morris, D. (2009). Music therapy. In B. Dossey & L. Keegan (Eds.), *Holistic nursing a handbook for practice* (5th ed., pp. 327–346). Sudbury, MA: Jones and Bartlett.

Nelson, D. (1994). *Compassionate touch: Hands-on care giving for the elderly, the ill and the dying.* Barrytown, NY: Station Hill Press.

Newshan, G. (2003). Large clinical study shows value of therapeutic touch program. *Holistic Nursing Practice, 17,* 189–192.

O'Brien, M. (2003a). *Spirituality in nursing standing on holy ground.* Sudbury, MA: Jones and Bartlett.

O'Brien, M. (2003b). *Prayer in nursing the spirituality of compassionate caregiving.* Sudbury, MA: Jones and Bartlett.

Olson, M. (1997). Death and grief. In B. Dossey (Ed.), *Core curriculum for holistic nursing* (pp. 126–133). Gaithersburg, MD: Aspen.

Olson, M. (2001). *Healing the dying* (2nd ed.). New York: Delmar Thompson Learning.

Olson, M., & Dossey, B. (2009). Dying in peace. In B. Dossey & L. Keegan (Eds.), *Holistic nursing, a handbook for practice* (5th ed., pp. 393–414). Sudbury, MA: Jones and Bartlett.

Payne, R. (2005). *Relaxation techniques: A practical handbook for the health care professional.* (3rd ed.). Edinburgh: Elsevier.

Piotrowski, A. (2005). Inhale peppermint to relieve postoperative nausea. (R. J. Buckle Associates Certification no. 293).

Price, L., & Price, S. (2006). *Aromatherapy for health professionals* (3rd ed.). New York: Churchill Livingston.

Quinn, J. (1995). The healing arts in modern health care. In D. Kunz (Ed.), *Spiritual aspects of the healing arts* (pp. 176–192). Wheaton, IL: Quest Books.

Remington, R. (2002). Calming music and hand massage with agitated elderly. *Nursing Research, 51,* 317.

Rew, L. (2009). Self-reflection. In B. Dossey & L. Keegan (Eds.), *Holistic nursing: A handbook for practice* (5th ed., pp. 195–207). Sudbury, MA: Jones and Bartlett.

Roach, S., & Nieto, B. (1997). *Healing and the grief process.* New York: Delmar.

Rossman, M. (1999). Interactive guided imagery. In N. Allison (Ed.), *The illustrated encyclopedia of body-mind disciplines* (pp. 77–78). New York: Rosen.

Sahler, J., Hunter, B., & Liesveld, J. (2003). The effects of using music therapy with relaxation imagery in the management of patients undergoing bone transplantation. *Alternative Therapies in Health and Medicine, 9*(6), 70–74.

Schaub, B., & Dossey, B. (2009). Imagery. In B. Dossey & L. Keegan (Eds.), *Holistic nursing: A handbook for practice* (5th ed., pp. 295–326). Sudbury, MA: Jones and Bartlett.

Schroeder-Sheker, T. (1994). Music for the dying. *Journal of Holistic Nursing, 12*(1), 83–99.

Schroeder-Sheker, T. (2005). Prescriptive music: Sounding our transitions. *Explore: The Journal of Science and Healing, 1*(1), 57–58.

Skidmore-Roth, L. (2009). *Mosby's handbook of herbs and natural supplements* (4th ed.). St. Louis, MO: Mosby.

Springhouse Corporation. (2005). *Nursing herbal medicine handbook* (3rd ed.). Springhouse, PA: Springhouse.

Taylor, E. (2003). Prayer's clinical issues and implications. *Holistic Nursing Practice, 17,* 179–188.

Thornton, L., & Mariano, C. (2009). Evolving from therapeutic to holistic communication. In B. Dossey & L. Keegan (Eds.), *Holistic nursing: A handbook for practice* (5th ed., pp. 533–545). Sudbury, MA: Jones and Bartlett.

Van Kuiken, D. (2004). A meta-analysis of the effect of guided imagery on practice outcomes. *Journal of Holistic Nursing, 22,* 164–179.

Van Weel, C., & Knotterneus, J. (1999). Evidence-based interventions and comprehensive treatment. *Lancett, 13* (353), 916–918.

Walker, M., & Walker, J. (2003). *Healing massage.* Scarborough, Ontario: Thompson Delmar Learning.

Wardell, D., Rintala, D., & Tan, G. (2008). Study descriptions of healing touch with veterans experiencing chronic neuropathic pain from spinal cord injury. *Explore, 4*(3), 187–195.

Wauters, A. (2007). *The homeopathic bible: The definitive guide to remedies.* NY: Sterling Publishers.

Weiner, M. (1998). *The complete book of homeopathy.* Arden City Park, NY: Avery.

White House Commission on Complementary and Alternative Medicine Policy

WHCCAMP *Final Report* (2002). Washington, DC: U.S. Government Printing Office.

Worden, J. (1982). *Grief counseling and grief therapy: A handbook for the mental health practitioner.* New York: Springer.

Wright, L. (2005). *Spirituality, suffering, and illness: Ideas for healing.* Philadelphia, PA: F. A. Davis Co.

Sexual Health and Intimacy

Marianne Matzo

Key Points

- Sexual health concerns exist even in late stage disease.
- Sexual health concerns for seriously ill patients are extremely diverse.
- There is very little documentation concerning seriously ill patients' wishes and expectations regarding their sexual health throughout the course of their illness trajectory.

Case Study: Sally is a 37-year-old woman who was one of my hospice patients; she has had a brain tumor for 3 years. During one of my visits Sally was talking about her partner and their loss of intimacy since about a year after her diagnosis. Regarding her relationship with her significant other she said, "we've grown apart, it's very sad." They thought about counseling when their relationship had begun to change, but "didn't think we were ready for that big a step, we were wrong." She said she is dissatisfied with her sex life, "I think about it sometimes, I miss it, I don't know where it went." When I asked her where she would rank her sexual needs at this point in her life, she said "toward the top." I asked her, if she could, be more specific, and she said "my favorite foods, then sex."

Introduction

Quality-of-life (QOL) issues are of the utmost importance with respect to the provision of palliative care. While assessment and intervention to address an individuals' ability to complete activities of daily living and basic needs are an integral part of palliative care, sexuality and intimacy are not discussed openly, if at all. Sexual health within the context of palliative care may be directly impacted by the disease on anatomical structures. However, direct anatomical effect is not the only concern; changes in a person's sexual interest or desire may also be affected by direct or indirect consequences of medical treatment or in association with being terminally ill.

For many people, when one talks about sexuality the immediate reference is to intercourse. Different approaches can be taken to the study of sexuality and intimacy, but the focus of this chapter is on *sexual health* which is broader than either of these terms alone. One definition of sexual health is the integration of somatic, intellectual, and social aspects of being sexual (Penson et al., 2000). The somatic aspect includes the physical ability to be intimate with a partner, be sexually functional (i.e. to have desire, become aroused, and obtain sexual fulfillment) (Robinson, Bockting, Rosser, Miner, & Coleman, 2002). The intellectual aspect is the ability to communicate about sexual needs and desires, to act intentionally and responsibly, and to set appropriate sexual boundaries. Sexual health affirms sexuality as a positive force that can enhance other aspects of a person's life (Robinson et al., 2002). Social aspects include the ability to be intimate with a partner, sexual desire, self acceptance and respect, and feeling of belonging to and involvement in one's culture.

The sexual healthcare needs of the seriously ill patient facing the end of their life has received some recognition in the professional literature (Anderson & Wof, 1875; Ashby, Kissane, Beadle, & Rodger, 2007; Caruso-Herman, 1989; Cort, Monroe, & Oliviere, 2004; Farkas, 1992; Freyer, 2004; Gideon & Taylor, 1981; Gilley, 1988; Grigg, 2002; Hordern, 1999; Katzin, 1990; Kutner, Kassner, & Nowels, 2001; Laury, 1987; Moynihan, 2007; Rice, 2000a, 2000b; Smith, 1989; Stausmire, 2004; Wells, 2002; Wickett, 1986) but limited research studies to support the assertions made in these publications. However, there is a growing recognition of the importance of public health concerns related to sexuality and their implications for health, well-being and quality of life (WHO, 2004). There is a need for data regarding patient needs to inform a sexual health plan of care. In response to this, the WHO department of reproductive health and research has begun to recognize sexual health as a separate dimension of QOL warranting clinical investigation (WHO, 2004).

An IOM (IOM, 2007) report addresses the importance of cancer care for the whole patient. The right concludes that in order to ensure appropriate psychosocial health, healthcare practitioners (HCPs) should facilitate effective communication between patients and care providers. In reality, one study of an oncology population documented that 28% of the patients indicate that their physicians do not pay attention to anything other than their medical needs (Young, 2007). Psychologic distress that the patient or her partner experiences during diagnosis and treatment of malignancy can impair a healthy sexual response cycle (Krychman, Pereira, Carter, & Amsterdam, 2006).

The theoretical framework that is holistic and that has applicability in palliative care is the Sexual Health Model (Robinson et al., 2002) (Fig. 1). The model reflects the complexity of human sexuality by identifying ten broad components posited to be essential aspects of healthy human sexuality:

1) Talking about sex: This is a cornerstone of the model and includes the ability to talk comfortably and explicitly about sexuality, especially one's own sexual values, preferences, attractions, history, and behaviors.
2) Culture and sexual identity: Culture influences one's sexuality and sense of sexual self, understanding how one's cultural heritage impacts sexual identities, attitudes, and behaviors will influence sexual health.
3) Sexual anatomy and functioning: Sexual health assumes a basic knowledge, understanding, and acceptance of one's sexual anatomy, sexual response, and sexual functioning, as well as freedom from sexual dysfunction and other sexual problems.

4) Sexual health care: This encompasses knowing one's body, obtaining regular exams for sexually transmitted diseases and cancer, and responding to physical changes with appropriate medical intervention.

5) Overcoming challenges to sexual health: Challenges to sexual health such as sexual abuse, substance abuse, compulsive sexual behavior, sex work, harassment, and discrimination are critical in any discussion of sexual health.

6) Body image: Body image is an important aspect of sexual health, challenging the notion of one, narrow standard of beauty and encouraging self-acceptance is relevant to all populations.

7) Masturbation/fantasy: This includes a realistic appreciation of the important role of masturbation and fantasy. Encouraging masturbation as a normal adjunct to partnered sex can decrease the pressures on women to engage in penetrative sex with their partners more frequently than they desire.

8) Positive sexuality: This is the eighth component which includes a developmental approach to sexual health over the lifespan, recognizing the reality that all human beings need to explore their sexuality in order to develop and nurture who they are. The importance of exploring and celebrating sexuality from a positive and self-affirming perspective is an essential feature of this model, the assumption being that when people are comfortable with their sexuality they will know and be able to ask for what is sexually pleasurable for them.

9) Intimacy and relationships: Intimacy is a universal need that people try to meet through their relationships.

10) Spirituality and values: This is the assumption of congruence between one's ethical, spiritual, and moral beliefs and one's sexual behaviors and values. In this context, spirituality may or may not include identification with formal religions, but the need to address moral and ethical concerns (Robinson et al., 2002).

TALKING ABOUT SEX

Many studies regarding sexual health document some seemingly universal themes related to communication about sexuality and intimacy between patients and their HCPs. These tend to fall into two categories: needs and communication. Regarding need, patients do have questions and concerns about their sexual health that they would like to discuss with their HCP (Ananth, Jones, King, & Tookman, 2003; Grigg, 2002; Smith, 1989; Stead et al., 1999). A survey of HCPs (n = 1,946) (Bachmann, 2006) documented that 60% of the respondents estimated at least three fourths of their patients had sexual dysfunction, but 58% indicated they initiated assessment of sexual health concerns in less

than one quarter of their patients. Second, concerning communication, patients indicate they do not initiate these conversations because they think HCPs are too busy, they do not want to "bother" them, they think that they should just be "grateful to be alive," that it is a private matter (Kralik, Koch, & Telford, 2001), or they think if something could be done about the situation, the HCP would raise the issue (Smith, 1989).

HCPs have indicated the reason sexual health is not routinely assessed is they believe the patient will bring it up if it is a concern; the perception that people are "too sick" to be sexual (Caruso-Herman, 1989) lack of their own comfort with the topic (Caruso-Herman, 1989; Dunn, 2004; Epstein & Street, 2007; Grigg, 2002; Wilmoth, 2006) preconceived ideas, attitudes, and values regarding sexuality (Grigg, 2002; Wilmoth, 2006) perceived lack of time for this conversation (Dunn, 2004) and the feeling that there are "more important" issues to be addressed (Ananth et al., 2003; Smith, 1989). Additionally, lack of communication about sexual health may be the result of the lack of evidence to support raising the issue (Stead, 2004). Sexual health is also not emphasized in HCP professional education (Caruso-Herman, 1989; Dunn, 2004; Grigg, 2002; IOM, 2007; Penson et al., 2000) which can result in this lack of communication, a conspiracy of silence, and a dominant communication pattern of evasiveness (Grigg, 2002).

The most effective communication is that which addresses the needs of the patient at each stage of their illness when they will have differing unmet needs. Communication with cancer patients is a dichotomous situation in that the disease is both life threatening while potentially treatable or curable (Epstein & Street, 2007), which creates much uncertainty and stress on the patient. Little is known about patient preferences for information, particularly the timing of communicating certain types of information (Tulsky, 2005).

SEXUAL ANATOMY AND FUNCTIONING

Any aspect of a terminal/life threatening disease (either from the disease itself or from the treatment) can impact sexual health. For example, women with advanced ovarian cancer (OVCA) have an overall survival rate of 15–30% (Armstrong, Burdy, & Wenzel, 2006) and approximately 70% will recur at some point (American Cancer Society (ACS)Facts and Figures, 2006). This translated into approximately 21,650 new cases of OVCA in 2008 and 15,520 women dying from the disease (Karlan, 2008).

Risk factors for poorer sexual functioning after being diagnosed with gynecological cancer are age, treatment, time since treatment, poor self esteem/body image, physical symptoms, poor performance status, depression, and anxiety (Stead & Stead, 2004). Ovarian cancer is usually treated with a hysterectomy, oophorectomy, and chemotherapy, which can all affect sexual functioning, through a decrease in estrogen production (resulting in vaginal atrophy, loss of vaginal lubrication, and hot flashes) and loss of sexual interest resulting from changes in body, fatigue, and nausea (Carmack-Taylor, 2005; Stead, 2004).

Even women with OVCA over the age of 55 have reported distress over the loss of reproductive potential (Stewart, Wong, & Duff, 2001). In one study, over 50% of the women with ovarian cancer reported moderate to severely worsened sexual function (Stewart et al., 2001). Carmack Taylor et al. (2004) compared the sexual health of women with breast cancer, ovarian cancer, and postmenopausal women and concluded that low desire, vaginal dryness, and dyspareunia are more common and severe in women with ovarian cancer (Carmack Taylor et al., 2004). Another study documented that, for women with ovarian cancer, their satisfaction with care for sexual problems was lower than with their overall cancer care (Lindau et al., 2007).

Treatments for cervical cancer result in numerous issues that can impact sexual health. Surgery shortens the proximal vagina by one third and radiation therapy causes stenosis, drying, and dyspareunia, which typically results in the need for the use of dilator and estrogen creams in order to help prevent vaginal atrophy (Suhatno, 2000). Hormonal changes result from surgical removal of the ovary or irradiation without protecting the ovary (Suhatno, 2000). Psychological issues related to the diagnosis that can have a negative impact on sexual health are fear of the disease and metastasis, vaginal odor, and the perception of some women that they "deserve" the disease because of their previous sexual behavior (Suhatno, 2000).

Alterations in sexual health for men primarily focus on erectile function. Cancer treatments can interfere with erection by damaging a man's pelvic nerves, pelvic blood vessels, or hormone balance. Prostate, bladder, and colon cancer are often treated with radiation to the pelvis. The higher the total dose of radiation and the wider the section of the pelvis irradiated, the greater the chance of an erection problem later (ACS, 2009). Erectile dysfunction (ED) is a common complication of diabetes (secondary to autonomic neuropathy, vascular insufficiency, or psychological factors) in at least half of men over age 50 (Kaye & Jick, 2003). ED can also occur as a result of cardiovascular disease, hypertension, hypercholesterolemia, smoking, and the abuse of drugs including alcohol.

After standard radical prostatectomy, between 65% and 90% of men will become impotent, depending on their age. If the surgeon does not remove or damage the nerves on either side of the prostate, the impotence rate drops to between 25% and 30% for men under 60. The impotence rate is higher for men over 70, even if nerves on both sides are not damaged or removed (Zippe & Pahlajani, 2008). After surgery, there is no ejaculation of semen although even with a dry orgasm, the sensation should still be pleasurable (ACS, 2009).

One observational study of erectile dysfunction after chemotherapy for non-small-cell lung cancer documented that erectile dysfunction was present for 8 months before the cancer was diagnosed (Hejna, Fiebiger, Reiter, & Raderer, 2001). Hedestig, Sandman, and Widmark (2003) conducted in-depth interviews with seven men (ages 62–69) with localized prostate cancer (Hedestig et al., 2003). These men reported that they were not as sexually active as before diagnosis, experienced reduced potency and diminished pleasure in ejaculation, felt their manhood was restricted and that they had difficulty discussing sexual problems. Men will sometimes report pain in the genitals during sex, or if the prostate gland or urethra has been irritated from cancer treatment, ejaculation may be painful (ACS, 2009).

Sexual health can be impacted by almost any life-threatening illness and should be assessed in every patient. Asking if there are concerns regarding sexual health may be a good first question in determining how a person's diagnosis, subsequent treatment, or current health has affected them. Not all patients will report concern regarding their sexual health function, in these cases, no further intervention is needed except to encourage the patient to let the HCP know if his situation changes. Not asking about sexual health may be more comfortable to the HCP, but will not impact the sexual health care of the patient.

Information to help patients with these concerns primarily focuses on preventing pain (genital and nongenital) during sex and interventions to help men get and keep an erection. In 1998 the Food and Drug Administration (FDA) approved sildenafil citrate (Viagra) to treat impotence. Oral phosphodiesterase-5 inhibitors (PDE-5) help achieve an erection by increasing blood flow to the penis. About half of men with impotence due to medical (rather than psychological) problems are helped to some extent by these drugs (ACS, 2009). Nerve damage from prostate cancer treatment may not respond as well to these drugs as some other physical causes of impotence.

Other treatments for ED include intracavernosal injection therapy and surgically implanted penile prostheses. Noninvasive drug-free solutions such as vacuum erection devices (VED) remain popular despite the availability of PDE-5 inhibitors. The VED is easy to use and a man can produce an erection in 2–3 minutes (which can increase spontaneity and patient compliance). Vacuum therapy is a tube, or cylinder, that is placed over the penis. A vacuum is then applied to increase penile blood flow (due to negative pressure). The use of the VED has expanded and is now used in combination with PDE-5 inhibitors in penile rehabilitation following radical prostatectomy and radiation therapy (Zippe & Pahlajani, 2008).

Pain during intercourse is one of the most common sexual problems for women (genital or nongenital) and can interfere with the feeling of pleasure during sex. Nongenital pain may be secondary to soreness in one arm after a radical mastectomy or tingling and numbness the hands and feet after chemotherapy. The ACS (2009) makes the following recommendations for patients regarding overcoming nongenital pain. First, plan sexual activity for the time of day they feel the least pain. If using pain medicine, take it an hour before planned sexual activity so it will be in full effect during sex. Second, find a position for touching or intercourse that puts as little pressure as possible on the sore areas, support the sore area and limit its movement with pillows. If a certain motion is painful, choose a position that does not require it or ask your partner to take over the hip movements during intercourse. Encourage patients to talk to their partner regarding what brings the most pleasure. Third, encourage the patient to focus on their feelings of pleasure and excitement; with this focus, the pain may fade into the background (ACS, 2009).

Genital-related pain results from a loss of vaginal lubrication and vaginal muscle scarring and shortening. Cancer treatments and menopause typically decrease the amount of vagina lubrication. Common brands of lubricants include K-Y Jelly and Astroglide. Some products include herbal extracts (such as aloe or lavender) that can cause irritation or allergic reactions and warming gels can cause a burning sensation in some people. Replens and K-Y Liquibeads are vaginal moisturizers that can be used 2 or 3 times a week to help keep the vagina moist and at a more normal acid balance (pH). The effects of these products last longer than those of lubricants, and can be purchased without a prescription. Lubrin and Astroglide Silken Secret are other moisturizers that are marketed as longer lasting than typical lubricants (ACS, 2009).

Vaginal dilators are often used after radiation to the pelvis, cervix, or vagina. It is recommended that vaginal dilators are offered to patients undergoing radical radiotherapy to the pelvis as part of their cancer treatment, together with support and education. A vaginal dilator is a tube of plastic or rubber used to dilate the vagina and to help women learn to relax the vaginal muscles (ACS, 2009). Regular intercourse and/or the use of vaginal dilators may minimize stenosis. Vaginal changes develop over time, even up to 5 years post treatment, and may impact sexual function, sexual health, and well-being in addition to considerable distress for a woman and her partner (Denton, 2000). Dilators work best when used early after radiation or surgery to prevent vaginal shrinkage prior to the vagina tightening. If a woman goes for many months without a sexual relationship, it is very important that the dilator be used to keep the vagina in shape (ACS, 2009). Instructions for use are found in Table 3.1.

3.1 | Using a Vaginal Dilator

- Minimum use is three times weekly for an indefinite time period. Dilators can be used in conjunction with sexual intercourse to achieve a combined frequency of vaginal dilation.
- Find a private and comfortable place where you can relax and use the dilator. Dilators can be used in the shower or bath if this provides privacy, and/or allows you to relax your pelvic floor muscles. If you wish, your significant other can also be encouraged to be involved.
- A water-soluble lubricant should be placed on the dilator and around the entrance to the vagina prior to insertion. Some doctors will prescribe Premarin cream to be used for this purpose.
- There are various positions in which to use the dilator: you can either lie down on your back with knees slightly apart and bent, or stand with a leg raised on the side of the bed or bath to insert the dilator.
- Inserting the dilator into the vagina requires a firm, gentle pressure. Insert it as deeply as is comfortable, without forcing the dilator. Do pelvic floor exercises during insertion.
- Once the dilator is inside the vagina it should be moved in a forward and backward motion, then a left to right motion. If possible gently rotating the dilator using the handle.
- Your doctor will fit you for the dilator. It is usual to start with the smallest size and progress to the largest (size 4) in the days/weeks following treatment, as it is comfortable.
- When the dilator is in as far as possible, leave it in your vagina for about 15 minutes. You can pass the time by reading, watching TV, listening to music, or even talking on the phone. If the dilator slips out, gently push it more deeply into your vagina.
- The dilator should be removed slowly rotating in clockwise/anticlockwise movements.
- Vibrators may also be used in conjunction with the use of dilators.
- Slight vaginal loss and blood staining is not uncommon when using dilators. If you experience heavy vaginal bleeding or pain contact your doctor.
- When you remove it, wash it with a mild soap and water. Be sure to rinse all the soap off so no film is left to irritate your vagina the next time you use it.

Overcoming Challenges to Sexual Health and Body Image

A urostomy, colostomy, or ileostomy presents challenges to maintaining sexual health. Patients should be reminded to empty the bag and check the seal to reduce the risk of the bag leaking during intercourse. A special small-sized ostomy pouch could be worn during sexual activity, or if a two-piece system is used, the pouch can be turned around on the faceplate so that the emptying valve is to the side. If an elastic support belt is worn on the faceplate, it can be tucked into the belt during sex or the bag can be taped to their body. Some people may be more comfortable wearing a T-shirt to cover the appliance. To reduce rubbing against the appliance, encourage patients to choose positions that will keep their partner's weight off the ostomy. If the patient prefers to be on the bottom during intercourse they can put a small pillow above the ostomy faceplate so that their partner can lie on the pillow rather than on the appliance. Those with a colostomy may be able to plan sexual activity for a time of day when the colostomy is not usually active. The colostomy can be irrigated and a stoma cover or a small safety pouch during sex (ACS, 2009).

Some cancers of the head and neck are treated by surgery to remove part of the bone structure of the face. These are public scars that can be devastating to self-image. Surgery on the jaw, palate, or tongue can also change the way people are able to talk. Advances in facial replacement devices and plastic surgery include ears and noses made out of plastic, tinted to match the skin, and attached to the face (ACS, 2009). These interventions can have a tremendous impact on body image and self esteem.

Treatment for primary tumors of the bone typically includes amputation of the limb which can result in the need to make some changes during intercourse. Wearing a prosthesis during sex may help with positioning and ease of movement, but the straps that attach it can get in the way. Without a prosthesis the partner with an amputation may have trouble staying level during intercourse; pillows can be used to support the body. Phantom limb pain can interfere with sexual desire and distract a person during sex; the patient should be encouraged to take pain medications prior to intercourse.

Masturbation

Another component of the Sexual Health Model is masturbation. A stratified probability sample survey of the British general population, aged 16–44 years, was conducted from 1999 to 2001 ($n = 11,161$) using face-to-face interviewing and computer-assisted self-interviewing (Gerressu et al., 2008). These data were used to estimate the population prevalence of masturbation, and to identify sociodemographic, sexual behavioral, and attitudinal factors associated with reporting this behavior. Seventy-three percent of men and 36.8% of women reported masturbating in the 4 weeks prior to interview. Among both men and women, reporting masturbation increased with higher levels of education and social class and was more common among those reporting sexual function problems.

For women, masturbation was more likely among those who reported more frequent vaginal sex in the last 4 weeks, a greater repertoire of sexual activity (such as reporting oral and anal sex), and more sexual partners in the last year. In contrast, the prevalence of masturbation was lower among men reporting more frequent vaginal sex. Both men and women reporting same-sex partner(s) were significantly more likely to report masturbation (Gerressu et al., 2008). Terminally ill people are likely no different than the general population regarding their masturbation habits. Palliative care practitioners should routinely ask their patients if anything interferes in their ability to masturbate and then work with the patient to correct the problem if it is identified.

Sexuality, Intimacy, and Relationships

Lemieux, Kaiser, Pereira, and Meadows (2004) conducted a qualitative study which assessed patient perspectives regarding sexuality in palliative care. Overall, it was found that emotional connections took precedence over the physical expressions of love, although sexuality was considered to be very important even during the final stages of life. Barriers to sexual expression included lack of privacy, shared rooms, staff interruptions, and single beds. The patients generally agreed that holistic palliative care should include the impact of illness on sexuality, and these patients would prefer to be asked about these issues in a sensitive manner (Lemieux et al., 2004).

Cort et al. (2004) discussed that sexuality is an integral aspect of palliative care, and couples are often seeking assistance and support in their relationship. Often, palliative care patients will feel a decreased self-control and a decreased sense of self (Cort et al., 2004). Despite age or physical health, people remain sexual beings and sexual health needs do not end when a person is diagnosed with a terminal illness. With respect to relationships, partners often fear causing pain to their significant other. In addition, other problems can occur, such as concerns about body image, altered sexual function, relationship issues, feelings of loss and grief, and bereaved partners (Cort et al., 2004).

Case Study conclusion: At the end of my visit to Sally I asked her what she wanted from her health care practitioners regarding sexual health promotion. She said "Don't just focus on my body, but help with the relationship." Sally died four days later.

CONCLUSION

There is a significant lack of literature addressing issues of sexuality in palliative care that can guide evidence-based practice. Sexual health is a broader concept than sexuality alone and moves past sexual intercourse to include a combination of intimacy, closeness, communication, and emotional support. Qualitative data obtained from patients reveals that they would prefer to be asked about these topics and given the opportunity to discuss them if so desired.

However, it appears that practitioners in palliative care settings often feel uncomfortable or unqualified to discuss these issues with their patients. Some suggestions provided for these practitioners include role-playing, increasing their knowledge base regarding these issues, and practicing their ability to discuss these issues in order to reduce discomfort. The practitioner can include general questions sexual health (e.g. "do you have any concerns about your sexual health?") and proceed to more specific questions about opportunities for kissing, holding hands, "snuggling," massage, oral sex, masturbation (e.g., "are you able to pleasure yourself sexually" or "are you able stimulate yourself to release sexual tension?") as examples of physical intimacy that promotes feelings of love and connectedness. In this way, palliative care clinicians can further enhance the quality of life for their patients throughout the trajectory of their illness.

EVIDENCE-BASED PRACTICE

Lindau, S. T., Schumm, L. P., Laumann, E. O., Levinson, W., O'Muircheartaigh, C. A., & Waite, L. J. (2007). A study of sexuality and health among older adults in the United States. *New England Journal of Medicine*, 357, pp. 762–74.

Purpose. This study aimed to increase understanding regarding the sexual behaviors and sexual function of older adults. A National probability sample of 3005 adults living in the United States (1550 women and 1455 men) ages 57–85 were interviewed in their homes and anthropometric measurements were performed for data regarding sexual function; blood, salivary, and vaginal mucosal specimens were collected; and physical function and sensory function were assessed.

Findings. Women were significantly less likely than men at all ages to report sexual activity. Sexual activity was lower among people age 75–85 years than in younger responders, but even in this oldest age group 54% reported having sex at least 2–3 times a month and 23% reported having sex once a week or more. Among those who reported that they were sexually active, half reported that they were bothered by at least one sexual problem. For women, these included low desire (43%), vaginal dryness (39%), and inability to climax (34%). Men reported erectile difficulties (37%) and 14% of all men reported using medication or supplements to improve sexual function. Both genders who rated their general health as poor were less likely to be sexually active. Only 38% of the men and 22% of the women reported discussing sex with their physician since the age of 50 years.

Conclusions. Sexual activity continues into old age, although women are less likely than men to have a spouse or other intimate partner and to be sexually active. There are a large proportion of elders who have sexual problems, but these are rarely discussed with physicians.

Implications for Practice. Assessment of sexual activity should be a part of a holistic health assessment regardless of age, health status, or gender. The findings from this study indicated that patients are not likely to raise concerns regarding sexual health with their health care provider (HCP), so assessment of these health concerns rests with the HCP.

REFERENCES

ACS. (2009). *Ways of dealing with sexual problems*. Retrieved 5/1/2009, 2009, from http://www.cancer.org/docroot/MIT/content/MIT_7_2X_Ways_of_Dealing_With_Specific_Sexual_Problems.asp.

American Cancer Society Facts and Figures. (2008). Atlanta: ACS.

Ananth, H., Jones, L., King, M., & Tookman, A. (2003). The impact of cancer on sexual function: A controlled study. *Palliative Medicine, 17*, 202–205.

Anderson, B., & Wof, F. (1875). Chronic physical illness and sexual behavior: Psychological issues. *Journal of Consulting and Clinical Pyschology, 54*(2), 168–175.

Armstrong, D., Burdy, B., & Wenzel, L. (2006). Intraperitoneal cisplatin and paclitaxel in ovarian cancer. *New England Journal of Medicine, 354*, 34–43.

Ashby, M. A., Kissane, D. W., Beadle, G. F., & Rodger, A. (2007). Psychosocial support, treatment of metastatic disease and palliative care. *The Medical Journal of Australia, 164*, 43–49.

Bachmann, G. (2006). Female sexuality and sexual dysfunction: Are we stuck on the learning curve? *Journal of Sexual Medicine, 3*(4), 639–645.

Best Practice guidelines on the use of vaginal dilators in women receiving pelvic radiotherapy. (2005). Edgbaston: Birmingham Women's Hospital.

Carmack-Taylor, C. L. (2005). Spousal intimacy after cancer. *Gynecologic Oncology, 99*(3, Suppl. 1), S217–S218.

Carmack Taylor, C. L., Basen-Engquist, K., Shinn, E. H., Bodurka, D. C., Carmack Taylor, C. L., Basen-Engquist, K., et al. (2004). Predictors of sexual functioning in ovarian cancer patients. [Comparative Study Research Support, Non-U.S. Gov't Research Support, U.S. Gov't, P.H.S.]. *Journal of Clinical Oncology, 22*(5), 881–889.

Caruso-Herman, D. (1989). Concern for the dying patient and family. *Seminars in Oncology Nursing, 5*(2), 120–123.

Cort, E., Monroe, B., & Oliviere, D. (2004). Couples in palliative care. *Sexual and Relationship Therapy, 19*(3), 337–354.

Denton, A. (2000). National audit of the management and outcome of carcinoma of the cervix treated with radiotherapy in 1993. *Clinical Oncology, 12*(1), 347–353.

Dunn, M. E. (2004). *Restoration of couple's intimacy and relationship vital to reestablishing erectile function* (Vol. 104, pp. 6S–10S).

Epstein, R. M., & Street, R. L. (2007). *Patient-Centered Communication in Cancer Care: Promoting Healing and Reducing Suffering.* Bethesda, MD: National Cancer Institute.

Farkas, C. G. (1992). Neglected issues in the care of dying patients: Nonverbal communication and sexuality. *Loss, Grief and Care, 6*(2–3), 125–129.

Freyer, D. R. (2004). Care of the dying adolescent: Special considerations. *Pediatrics, 113*(2), 381–388.

Gerressu, M., Mercer, C. H., Graham, C. A., Wellings, K., Johnson, A. M., Gerressu, M., et al. (2008). Prevalence of masturbation and associated factors in a British national probability survey. [Research Support, Non-U.S. Gov't]. *Archives of Sexual Behavior, 37*(2), 266–278.

Gideon, M. D., & Taylor, P. B. (1981). A sexual bill of rights for dying persons. *Death Education, 4*(4), 303–314.

Gilley, J. (1988). Intimacy and terminal care. *Journal of the Royal college of General Practitioners, 38,* 121–122.

Grigg, E. (2002). The issues of sexuality and intimacy in palliative care. In *Palliative care for people with cancer* (pp. 202–218). London: Arnold.

Hedestig, O., Sandman, P. O., & Widmark, A. (2003). Living with untreated localized prostate cancer: A qualitative analysis of patient narratives. [Research Support, Non-U.S. Gov't]. *Cancer Nursing, 26*(1), 55–60.

Hejna, M., Fiebiger, W. C., Reiter, W. J., & Raderer, M. (2001). Spontaneous erections in a patient with erectile dysfunction after palliative chemotherapy for non-small cell lung cancer. [Case Reports]. *Urologia Internationalis, 67*(2), 163–164.

Hordern, A. (1999). Sexuality in palliative care: Addressing the taboo subject. In S. Aranda & M. O'Connor (Eds.), *Palliative care nursing: A guide to practice* (pp. 197–211). Melbourne: Ausmed.

IOM. (2007). *Institute of Medicine. Cancer Care for the Whole Patient: Meeting Psychosocial Health Needs.* Washington, DC: The National Academies Press.

Karlan, B. Y. (2008). AMG 386, an investigational antiangiopoietin peptibody, combine with paclitaxel in advanced recurrent ovarian cancer. *Community Oncology, December,* 1–4.

Katzin, L. (1990). Chronic illness and sexuality. *American Journal of Nursing, 90*(1), 54–59.

Kaye, J. A., & Jick, H. (2003). Incidence of erectile dysfunction and characteristics of patients before and after the introduction of sildenafil l in the United Kingdom: Cross sectional study with comparison patients. *BMJ, 326,* 424–425.

Kralik, D., Koch, T., & Telford, K. (2001). Constructions of sexuality for midlife women living with chronic illness. *Journal of Advanced Nursing, 35*(2), 180–187.

Krychman, M. L., Pereira, L., Carter, J., & Amsterdam, A. (2006). Sexual oncology: Sexual health issues in women with cancer. *Oncology, 71*(1–2), 18–25.

Kutner, J. S., Kassner, C. T., & Nowels, D. E. (2001). Symptom burden at the end of life: Hospice providers' perceptions. *Journal of Pain and Symptom Management, 21*(6), 473–480.

Laury, G. V. (1987). Sexuality of the dying patient. *Medical Aspects of Human Sexuality, 21*(6), 102–109.

Lemieux, L., Kaiser, S., Pereira, J., & Meadows, L. M. (2004). Sexuality in palliative care: Patient perspectives. *Palliative Medicine, 18*(7), 630–637.

Lindau, S. T., Schumm, L. P., Laumann, E. O., Levinson, W., O'Muircheartaigh, C. A., & Waite, L. J. (2007). *A study of sexuality and health among older adults in the United States. New England Journal of Medicine* (Vol. 357, pp. 762–774).

Moynihan, T. (2007). Sexuality in palliative care. *Journal,* 1–8. Retrieved from http://www.utdol.com/utd/content/topic.do?topicKey = endoflif/7006&view = print

Penson, R. T., Gallagher, J., Gioiella, M. E., Wallace, M., Borden, K., Duska, L. A., et al. (2000). Sexuality and Cancer: Conversation Comfort Zone,*5,* 336–344.

Rice, A. (2000a). Sexuality in cancer and palliative care 1: Effects of disease and treatment. *International Journal of Palliative Nursing, 6*(8), 392–397.

Rice, A. (2000b). Sexuality in cancer and palliative care 2: Exploring the issues. [Review]. *International Journal of Palliative Nursing, 6*(9), 448–453.

Robinson, B. B. E., Bockting, W. O., Simon Rosser, B. R., Miner, M., & Coleman, E. (2002). The sexual health model: Application of a sexological approach to HIV prevention. *Health Education Research, 17*(1), 43–57.

Smith, D. B. (1989). Sexual rehabilitation of the cancer patient. *Cancer Nursing, 12*(1), 10–15.

Stausmire, J. M. (2004). Sexuality at the end of life. *American Journal of Hospice and Palliative Medicine, 21*(1), 33–39.

Stead, M. L. (2004). Sexual function after treatment for gynecological malignancy. *Current Opinion in Oncology, 16,* 492–495.

Stead, M. L., Crocombe, W. D., Fallowfield, L. J., Selby, P., Perren, T. J., Garry, R., et al. (1999). Sexual activity questionnaires in clinical trials: Acceptability to patients with gynaecological disorders,*106,* 50–54.

Stead, M. L., & Stead, M. L. (2004). Sexual function after treatment for gynecological malignancy. [Review]. *Current Opinion in Oncology, 16* (5), 492–495.

Stewart, D. E., Wong, F., & Duff, S. (2001). What doesn't kill you makes you stronger: An ovarian cancer survivor survey. *Gynecologic Oncology, 83,* 537–542.

Suhatno, N. (2000). Palliative care in cervical cancer. *Japanese Journal of Cancer Chemotherapy, 27*(2), 440–448.

Tulsky, J. A. (2005). Interventions to enhance communication among patients, providers, and families. *Journal of Palliative Medicine, 8* (Suppl.1), S–95–S–102.

Wells, P. (2002). No sex please, I'm dying. A common myth explored. *European Journal of Palliative Care, 9*(3), 119–122.

WHO. (2004). Sexual health-a new focus for WHO. *Journal,* (67) 8. Retrieved from http://www.who.int/reproductive-health/hrp/progress/67.pdf

Wickett, A. (1986). Sex and the terminally ill patient. *Euthanasia Review, 1*(2), 79–84.

Wilmoth, M. C. (2006). Life after cancer: What does sexuality have to do with it? *Oncology Nursing Forum, 33*(5), 905–910.

Young, P. (2007). Caring for the whole patient: The institute of medicine proposes a new standard of care. *Community Oncology, 4*(12), 748–751.

Zippe, C. D., & Pahlajani, G. (2008). Vacuum erection devices to treat erectile dysfunction and early penile rehabilitation following radical prostatectomy. *Current Urology Reports, 9*(6), 506–513.

Societal and Professional Issues in Palliative Care

Societal Perspectives Regarding Palliative Care

Marilyn Bookbinder
Marlene McHugh

Key Points

- Historical perspectives on death and dying in America.
- Emergence of chronic disease trajectories and palliative care for adults and pediatric patients.
- Emerging topics in palliative care important to nurses' practices.
- Evidence of the need for nursing science to build quality palliative care and end-of-life care models.
- Need for generalist and specialist level education for nurses.
- Future of health care and advances in science in health care delivery of palliative care.

Case Study: Mr. Wong is a 60-year-old Chinese American man, diagnosed a year ago with non-small cell lung cancer. The patient has been told he has "lung disease" but his son insists that he not be told of his diagnosis or prognosis. He has lost 20 lbs in the previous 2 months, and is having pain, shortness of breath and difficulty in swallowing. Mr. Wong is concerned about the hospital bills and his limited financial resources. He and his wife live in a four-story walk-up. Mr. Wong does not belong to a religious community and feels abandoned by God. The home health care team is increasingly frustrated with the fact that Mr. Li is not able to fully participate in decisions about his "care." He is becoming more withdrawn and his wife is increasingly tearful and distressed regarding her ability to care for her husband.

At the turn of the 20th century, Americans died from diseases such as yellow fever, small pox, diphtheria, and cholera. Death was often rapid, with little time to say goodbye to loved ones. In 1900, life expectancy was less than 50 years of age for both men and women, while in the year 2000, the median age of death was 77 years. Currently, Americans are struggling to develop a healthcare system that is both cost-effective and can ensure a "good life" and a "good death." This chapter addresses the changes and issues surrounding death in society in the 21st century, their impact on quality patient care, and the role of educators in preparing nurses to care for patients and families experiencing life-threatening illness. Two landmark studies from the 1990s—specifically, the "Study to Understand Prognosis and Preferences for Outcomes and Risks of Treatments" (SUPPORT, 1995) and the Institute of Medicine's (IOM) report "Approaching Death: Improving Care at the End of Life" (Field & Cassel, 1997)—provide evidence of the need to improve the care of the dying in America. This is the challenge for nurses and all health professionals in the 21st century.

CHANGES IN THE DEFINITION OF DEATH IN SOCIETY

Over the last few decades, the concept of death has raised many moral and ethical dilemmas for society. The *Encyclopedia Britannica* (2008) defines death as "the total cessation of life processes that eventually occurs in all living organisms." It goes on to say that "human death has always been obscured by mystery and superstition, and its precise definition remains controversial, differing according to culture and legal systems." Indeed, the experience of death has changed: Death in the first half of the 20th century usually occurred from an acute or unexpected event; today, many deaths occur following degenerative diseases that entail a long and declining course. In Kübler-Ross's (1967) seminal research and interviews with dying patients raised awareness about the dual concept of death: death, the event, and dying, the process. Though questioned today, her psychological stages of dying, specifically, denial, anger, bargaining, depression, and acceptance, revolutionized our thinking about death. Although no consensus currently exists about when dying or end of life begins, the American Geriatrics Society (AGS) (2007) Position Statement on "Caring for Dying Patients" offers clinicians guidelines for making this determination with the following statement: "People are considered to be dying when they have a progressive illness that is expected to end in death and for which there is no treatment that can substantially alter the outcome."

Although the precise determination of death is not a focus of this chapter, nurses need to be aware of this issue, as they may care for patients whose families fear that their loved ones will be declared dead prematurely, for example, when the determination of death is extended to assure viability of organs for transplantation. The ability to prolong and sustain life with artificial means necessitates the need for additional definitions of death. For legal purposes, brain death is considered to be the irreversible cessation of circulatory and respiratory function or the irreversible cessation of all functions of the entire brain, including the brain stem. Bioethicists and sociologists recommend the notion of "social death," referring to individuals who have lost their personhood by losing function of their cortex (Brody, 1988). Botkin and Post (1992) proposed that death be viewed as a syndrome, requiring that a cluster of related attributes be present before a diagnosis of brain death can be made.

The different views of death reflect the multidimensional nature of the concept. Professionals need to be cognizant of the varying definitions and the issues raised by each perspective, such as follows:

■ When should we remove life support and how should we support families?
■ What are the risks and benefits of feeding versus not feeding patients at the end of life?
■ When and from whom should we remove organs for transplantation?

- What skills and training do nurses need to serve as advocates to dying patients and families?
- What evidence is available to help nurses provide best practices in caring for patients and families experiencing life-threatening and terminal illness?
- What cultural and societal norms need to be addressed with patients and families facing advanced chronic illness?
- What system barriers need to be identified to support patients and families through the continuum of palliative care? For example, a patient with an advanced illness such as chronic pulmonary disease may not have a skilled nursing need that allows them to receive home care.
- What special needs are emerging within chronic illness populations throughout the lifespan? Just a generation ago, most children with severe disabilities died before reaching maturity. Today, with improvements in medical science and technology, more than 90% survive to adulthood. Nurses need to be aware of survivorship issues for various populations.
- What specific knowledge will nurses need to address the issues and consequences of genetic testing?

In palliative care, death is also viewed as an outcome or endpoint measure for improving end-of-life care. A "good death" is defined as one free from avoidable stress and suffering for patients, families and caregivers, in general accord with patients' and families' wishes, and reasonably consistent with clinical, cultural, and ethical standards. In contrast, a "bad death" is one in which there is needless suffering, disregard for patients' or families' wishes or values, and a sense among participants or observers that the norms of decency have been offended (Field & Cassel, 1997).

MORBIDITY AND MORTALITY STATISTICS FOR THE UNITED STATES: LEADING CAUSES OF DEATH

Life expectancy in the United States was the highest ever in 2006, and infant mortality was 6.7 infant deaths per 1,000 live births, a 2.3% decline from the 2005 rate of 6.9. The latest report prepared by the Centers for Disease Control and Prevention's (CDC) National Center for Health Statistics (NCHS), entitled "Deaths: Preliminary Data for 2006," finds that in 2006, life expectancy in the United States reached a new high of 78.1 years, a 0.3% increase from 2005 and up from 77.2 years in 2001. Life expectancy increased for both men and women, and for African Americans and Caucasians. Statistics from 2006 show a record high for both white and black males (76 and 70 years, respectively), as well as for white and black females (81 and 76.9 years, respectively). These data reflect an increase of over 25 years in life expectancy in the United States since 1900, which can be

attributed in part to advances in sanitation, nutrition, and immunization, advances that have eradicated or greatly reduced diseases.

Overall, death rates for the total U.S. population dropped in 2006. The national age-adjusted death rate decreased significantly, from 799 deaths per 100,000 in 2005 to 776.4 deaths per 100,000 in 2006. In addition, death rates for 8 of the 10 leading causes of death in the United States all dropped significantly in 2006, including a very sharp drop in mortality from influenza and pneumonia. The four leading causes of death in the United States in 2006 continued to be heart disease, cancer, cerebrovascular disease, and chronic obstructive pulmonary disease (COPD). Age-adjusted death rates decreased significantly between 2005 and 2006 for 11 of the 15 leading causes of death: Diseases of the heart, malignant neoplasms, cerebrovascular diseases, chronic lower respiratory diseases, accidents (unintentional injuries), diabetes mellitus, influenza and pneumonia, septicemia, intentional self-harm (suicide), chronic liver disease and cirrhosis, and essential hypertension and hypertensive renal disease.

Between 2005 and 2006, the largest decline in age-adjusted death rates occurred for influenza and pneumonia, with a 12.8% decline. Other declines were observed for chronic lower respiratory diseases (6.5%), stroke (6.4%), heart disease (5.5%), diabetes (5.3%), hypertension (5%), chronic liver disease and cirrhosis (3.3%), suicide (2.8%), septicemia or blood poisoning (2.7%), cancer (1.6%) and accidents (1.5%). Age-adjusted death rates for Alzheimer's disease, nephritis, nephrotic syndrome and nephrosis, Parkinson's disease, and assault (homicide) did not change significantly between 2005 and 2006.

BEYOND TABOOS IN ACKNOWLEDGING DEATH

Discussions about death make most people uncomfortable, including healthcare providers, and can trigger people's feelings about their own demise. How individuals and their families approach death is entwined with their cultural, ethnic, religious, and nonreligious backgrounds. Some individuals are inspired to search for meaning, peace, or transcendence, which can replace fear and despair with hope and serenity (Byock, 2007). For others, grief, shame, guilt, and anger become overwhelming emotions, which prolong the period of grief or surface later in other areas of the mourner's life. In many households, it is taboo to speak of death, especially in the presence of children. Parents often consider death as morbid and too much for children to handle. Children may even be sent off to a relative and told a lie, such as "Mommy has gone on a long trip," to avoid the topic.

America is a country of many races and cultures, and with each passing year, more healthcare providers are recognizing the challenge of caring for patients from diverse linguistic and cultural backgrounds. In addition to providing quality care to an aging and diverse population, clinicians need to integrate patients' and families' racial, ethnic, cultural, religious, and nonreligious rituals and beliefs into care planning. Nurses must assess patients' perceptions, preferences, and behaviors and individualize communication and care strategies so as to respect these differences in the context of their organizational systems. Consumers of all cultures are becoming more educated and vocal about their needs and options, especially those having Internet access to sophisticated medical information.

All cultures have developed ways to cope with death. Understanding these different responses to death can help professionals recognize the grieving process in patients and families of other cultures. Interfering with these practices may hinder necessary grieving processes. Helping families cope with the death of a loved one includes showing respect for the family's cultural heritage and encouraging them to decide how to honor the death. Important questions that should be asked of people who are dealing with the loss of a loved one include the following:

1) What are the cultural rituals for coping with dying, the deceased person's body, the final arrangements for the body, and honoring death?
2) What are the family's beliefs about what happens after death?
3) What does the family feel is a normal expression of grief and acceptance of the loss?
4) What does the family consider to be the roles of each family member in handling death?
5) Are certain types of death less acceptable (for example, suicide), or are certain types of death especially hard to handle for that culture (for example, the death of a child)?

In a cross-cultural patient/provider relationship, both parties may be called upon to acknowledge and respect health concepts and practices different from their own. Although this is an opportunity for growth and enrichment, it can also cause discomfort. Tension arises when different health belief systems confront one another. Common responses to the unknown or unfamiliar are anxiety, wariness, and even anger or fear. Nurses need to examine their own thoughts and feelings about these differences to become objective professionals advocating for the preferences of cultures different from their own.

To address the need for culturally and linguistically appropriate services (CLAS) in healthcare, the Office of Minority Health of the Department of Health and Human Services (DHHS) published national standards in 2000, and cultural competence has become a requirement for academic curricula and national certifications. For example, Georgetown University's National Center for Cultural Competence (2007) offers clinicians a tool to assess their level of competence. The Health Resources and Services Administration (HRSA) (2002), an agency of the DHHS, also offers specific guidelines for assessing cultural competence.

All healthcare personnel should learn to regard the patient and his or her family as unique and aim to develop skills to assess the role of culture in any given situation. It is important that clinicians develop consensus about how they will determine patient and family education regarding end-of-life issues, and provide culturally relevant resources and other sources of support.

WHERE PEOPLE DIE

Although surveys have shown that most cancer patients in the U.S. express a preference to die at home (Hays, 2003; Tang, 2003), about 75% of Americans with chronic illnesses die in a hospital or nursing home setting, with large regional differences (Grunier & Mor, 2007). According to the Center for Gerontology and Health Care Research (2004), between 1989 and 2001, the overall rate of home deaths increased (from 16% to 23%), hospital deaths decreased (from 62% to nearly 50%), and the likelihood of dying in nursing homes rose from 19% to 23%.

A systematic review of 66 observational studies found that being white, native-born, married, of higher socioeconomic status, and living farther away from a university health center are all factors associated with home death, whereas being black, Latino or other non-white increased the likelihood of hospital death (Grunier & Mor, 2007). About 55% to 60% of persons older than age 65 die in the hospital (Brunnhuber, Nash, Meier, Weissman, & Woodcock, 2008).

In previous centuries, the majority of people died at home. By mid 1970s, more than 70% of deaths were occurring in hospitals and other institutional settings (National Hospice Organization (NHO), 1997a). The shift in the location of dying has had a dramatic impact on the nature of dying. Patients dying at home were usually cared for by family members, with little or no high-technology equipment. The institutionalization of death raised a new set of challenges and problems for caregivers. Challenges included increased decision making about the extent of aggressive treatments; how to support and provide proper care for the dying; how to deal with the isolation and depersonalization of institutions; and how best to meet the nonphysical but critically important sociological, spiritual, and emotional needs of patients and family members. Additional regulations placed on institutions from managed care organizations often resulted in earlier discharges, shortened lengths of stay, and follow-up home care needs far greater than previously experienced. This is validated in data from 1988 through 1994, in which program payments for Medicare-covered home care services grew more than 500%, from $1.7 billion to $12.7 billion, and the number of certified home-health agencies grew from approximately 5,700 to 7,800 (Health Care Financing Administration (HCFA), 1996; Field & Cassel, 1997).

The literature describes an often fragmented approach to the care of the dying in institutions that resulted in undermining the patient's identity, wishes, and sense of self-worth. Institutionalization often served to isolate the family and to rob them of the opportunity to confront their own impending loss and adapt to the new roles and responsibilities ahead. Given proper support, most experts agree that families are able to resolve issues and become a strong source of support and caregiving for the patient. Byock's (1997) book, entitled *Dying Well,* illustrates through stories the prospect for growth and ability to achieve death-with-dignity at the end of life for patients and families. The hospice movement grew in response to this fragmentation of healthcare; the strongest proponents for change were the community and healthcare professionals who recognized inadequacies in end-of-life care.

Recent data from the National Hospice and Palliative Care Organization (NHPCO) show that most hospice patients (70.3%) die in the place they call "home" (National Hospice and Palliative Care Organization (NHPCO), 2008). In addition to private residences, this includes nursing homes and residential facilities. The percentage of hospice patients receiving care in an inpatient facility increased from 17.0% to 19.2%. Only 10.5% of patients died in a hospital setting that was not operated by a hospice team.

Nurses must be able to provide palliative care in all settings and to know where patients and families can access good end-of-life care. People are living longer and spending more time in various healthcare settings, making it common for nurses to coordinate care plans across settings as well, e.g., the home care nurse communicates with the acute hospital nurse and the acute care hospital case manager with long-term care facility or community-based home care nurse. Patient care plans need to transcend settings and providers and include the domains of good palliative care, e.g., advanced directives, symptom management, and psychosocial and spiritual care.

ILLNESS TRAJECTORIES

Americans are living longer with chronic or terminal illnesses, resulting in the need for increased assistance, symptom management, and hospice care services. The paths leading toward death are varied. Patients who understand that they have a progressive disease from which they will likely die may not see themselves, or

be seen by their families and friends, as dying. This group is differentiated from those thought to be imminently dying (i.e., likely to die within minutes to days), and those who are terminally ill but not thought to be actively dying (i.e., having a life expectancy of days to months and sometimes years). The latter group may have a period of prolonged "chronic living-dying" between the diagnosis of incurable illness and imminent death (McCormick & Conley, 1995). Patients in this group may be able to carry out their daily activities while coping with the prospect of death. Pediatric patients, for example, can live years to decades with illnesses such as cystic fibrosis. In the case of chronically ill older adults, premature death may occur suddenly from a superimposed viral illness, such as pneumonia.

The aging population is at increased risk for developing multiple chronic or life-threatening diseases, including heart disease, cancer, stroke, respiratory diseases, and other terminal illnesses, such as Alzheimer's disease. Healthcare costs can increase and quality of life and independence may be compromised for older adults and the terminally ill by weakness, falls, delirium, urinary incontinence, sleep disturbances, and serious depression. Living months or years with disease presents patients, families, and clinicians with social, moral, ethical, and medical dilemmas.

The National Institute on Aging's agenda (NIA, 2000) targeted three areas for research: (1) Preventing or reducing age-related diseases, disorders, and disability; (2) Maintaining physical health and function; and (3) Enhancing older adults' societal roles and interpersonal support and reducing social isolation. In 2008, the National Institutes of Health (NIH) added complementary and alternative medicine (CAM) information to their NIH Senior Health web site, as seniors (41% of adults aged 60–69) are frequent users of CAM, including products such as vitamins and herbal supplements, and practices such as chiropractic manipulation, acupuncture, meditation and massage.

Most recently, Brunnhuber et al. (2008) disseminated a synthesis of the evidence supporting key elements of palliative care: the control of common symptoms such as pain, dyspnea, and fatigue, communication and goal setting, and effective, efficient transition management. The report also depicts three disease trajectories for people with advanced chronic illness and progressive illness (Figure 4.1):

1) Progressive disability and eventual death over a period of weeks or a few months, most often seen in patients with the most common solid malignances: accounting for about 20% of deaths over the age of 65 years.
2) Slow decline with acute exacerbations and often a sudden death, most often due to chronic organ failure (e.g., lung, kidney, or heart failure): About 25% of deaths are over the age of 65 years.

3) Long period of slow decline with worsening self-care ability; death often from an unpredictable intercurrent illness; the underlying condition is typically a chronic neurodegenerative disease.

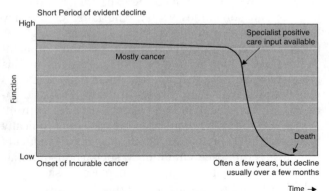

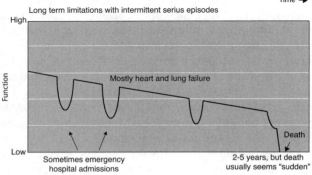

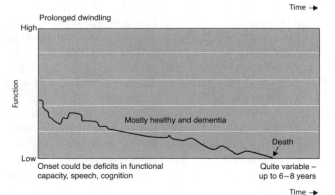

Figure 4.1   Typical illness trajectories for people with progressive chronic illness.
Source: © BMJ Publishing Group 2008. Reprinted with permission.

ETHICAL ISSUES

Technologies that sustain life by artificial means have increased our ability to prolong life, yet they have raised many moral, ethical, and legal dilemmas. Nurses are an essential voice in these discussions in their roles as patient and family advocates, clinicians, leaders, healthcare policy-makers, educators, and researchers. Education in the legal, moral and ethical principles, and decision-making models is essential if nurses are to have an impact in determining the quality of care offered to individuals at the end of life and if they are to empower patients to take an active role in achieving quality outcomes.

The American Nurses Association (ANA) *Code of Ethics for Nurses* addresses nurses' ethical obligations to relieve suffering associated with the dying process. Nurses caring for a dying patient should not hesitate to respond to a patient's pain level with full and effective pain medication and are reminded of the nurses' central role in assessing the presence of pain in the dying patient and assuring that the patient at the end of life has pain controlled to a level that is acceptable to the patient. The ANA's position statement, *Promotion of Comfort and Relief of Pain in Dying Patients, 1991,* directs nurses to use full and effective doses of pain medication to achieve adequate symptom control even if death is hastened as a result. In this situation, relief of pain and promotion of comfort is the intended effect, and the hastening of death may result secondarily from the drug's side effects on consciousness and respiration. For the dying patient, relief of pain and promotion of comfort is a primary goal and administering increasing doses of medication to achieve this goal is ethical even when the risks of death are increased (President's Commission for the Study of Ethical Problems in Medicine, 1983).

Nurses need to be clear regarding the moral differences between the actions of providing effective pain relief to a dying patient and participating in euthanasia or assisted suicide. The ANA *Code of Ethics for Nurses* and several position papers not only define the differences between euthanasia and assisted suicide, terms often used interchangeably, but also discuss acceptable actions nurses may take to ease suffering at the end of life. The *Code* clearly states that nurses have a moral obligation to prevent and relieve suffering of dying patients but that they must never act deliberately to terminate the life of any person. To administer an overdose of intravenous morphine, for example, with the intent of speeding the dying process, is contrary to the values and moral obligations of the profession.

Patient-Requested Euthanasia and Assisted Suicide

Euthanasia and assisted suicide have distinct definitions. Euthanasia, or "mercy killing,' is an intentional act that involves putting to death someone who is experiencing suffering or prolonged dying (ANA Position Statement, 1994). Patient-requested euthanasia refers to a practice by which the means of hastening death are administered directly by the healthcare provider (Matzo & Emanuel, 1997), for example, by injecting the patient with a lethal dose of medication.

Brody (1992), a nationally known physician/ethicist, originated the term "assistance in dying" and claimed that patients capable of decision making could request assistance to achieve a "good death." Assisted suicide is described as a practice by which healthcare providers supply, but do not directly administer, the means for a patient to voluntarily hasten his or her own death. This is usually done by prescribing lethal doses of medication that the patient then ingests (Field & Cassell, 1997; ANA Position Statement 1994).

Since the 1970s, notable events have shaped a new conceptualization and new legislation related to the end of life and causing or assisting death (Exhibit 4.1). The activities of Dr. Jack Kevorkian, a nonlicensed pathologist, who admitted to assisting more than 130 people to commit suicide, fueled the media and heightened public awareness about euthanasia and assisted suicide. Although he was found guilty in 1999 of second-degree murder and sentenced to 10 to 25 years of imprisonment, many Americans still view assisted dying as a "responsible alternative" to their fear of dying a lonely, undignified, prolonged, painful, or institutionalized death (Annas, 1995).

Oregon became the first state to legalize PAS, but not euthanasia, in 1997 via the Death with Dignity Act, which allows physicians to prescribe lethal dosages of medication to competent, terminally ill patients who request them. More recently, the state of Washington legalized PAS in 2008. This is a health policy issue that will continue to be closely examined by local and federal governments, academic institutions, and legal, nursing, and medical scholars.

Two surveys since the enactment of the Oregon law have provided some evidence about actual practices. Ganzini et al. (2000) found that physicians granted approximately one in six requests for a prescription for a lethal dose of medication, and one in ten requests actually resulted in suicide. The authors reported that effective palliative care interventions led most patients to change their minds about committing suicide. In a second study, undertaken to understand physicians' reactions to requests for assisted suicide, 35 Oregon physicians who had received requests from patients were interviewed (Dobscha, Heintz, Press, & Ganzini, 2004). Requests for assisted suicide had a powerful impact on physicians and their practices. Physicians reported feeling unprepared, and experienced apprehension and discomfort before and after receiving requests. Frequent sources of discomfort included concerns about adequately managing symptoms and suffering, not wanting to abandon patients, and incomplete understanding of patients' preferences, especially when physicians did not know the patients well. Participation in assisted suicide required a large investment of time and was emotionally intense. Physicians did not express major regrets about their decisions to assist or not. Many physicians felt that the process and discussions increased their confidence and assertiveness in discussing end-of-life issues with other patients. Physicians rarely sought support from their spouses about the emotional aspects of their experiences. The data also confirm other results that suggest patients who receive good symptom control at the end of life choose life over death (Coyle, 1992; Foley, 1995).

Although public debates about assisted dying have focused almost exclusively on physician practices (Bachman et al., 1996), nurses' reports of their experiences with assisted dying are increasing. Schwarz's (1999) integrated review of bioethics and nursing literature (from 1990 to 1999) reveals the dilemmas faced by many nurses in discriminating between "hastening" and "assisting" death when caring for patients with severe symptom distress at the end of life. When 80 nurses were interviewed about the circumstances under which they felt justified in performing patient-requested euthanasia, 21% of the nurses were ethically able to justify active euthanasia and 16% indicated that they viewed patient autonomy and the presence of severe suffering as justifications (Davis et al., 1995). In Asch's (1996) study of 1,139 critical care nurses' self-reported clinical experiences with assisted dying, 16% ($n = 129$) reported participating in assisted suicide or patient-requested euthanasia. Recurring themes in their comments included concerns about overuse of life-sustaining technology, a profound sense

EXHIBIT 4.1: EVENTS RAISING PUBLIC AWARENESS ABOUT ASSISTED DYING

1985: The first "right to die" case of Karen Ann Quinlan, NJ. Parents request permission to withdraw use of a respirator on their comatose young daughter. Respirator removed in 1976 and patient dies in 1985.

1990: Patient Self-Determination Act: Hospital patients are informed of their right to make treatment decisions. 1995 Americans continue to view assisted dying as a reasonable alternative to the fear of dying a lonely, undignified, prolonged, and painful, institutionalized death.

1995: Study to Understand Prognosis and Preferences for Outcomes and Risks of Treatments (SUPPORT). Five-year study results include inadequate pain management of end-of-life care.

1997: United States Supreme Court rules to maintain support for aggressive palliative care.

1997: Death with Dignity Act legalizes physician-assisted suicide in Oregon.

1998: Dr. Kevorkian's activities criticized by physicians and ethicists for assisting more than 130 people to commit suicide.

1999: Dr. Kevorkian found guilty of second-degree murder and sentenced to 10 to 25 years in prison.

2000: California "Natural Death Act" empowers patients to specify end-of-life wishes in a living will.

2005: Terry Schiavo, an American woman who suffered brain damage, was in a persistent vegetative state, and dependent on a feeding tube; the case attracted widespread media and public attention because of conflict between caregivers (spouse and parents).

2008: Washington State passes physician-assisted suicide legislation.

of responsibility for the patient's welfare, and a desire to relieve patient suffering to overcome the perceived unresponsiveness of physicians toward that suffering. Matzo and Emanuel's (1997) survey of 441 oncology nurses (71% response rate) revealed that 131 nurses (30%) received up to 20 requests for lethal drugs in the previous year. Of this group, 1% (n = 6) acknowledged helping a patient to commit suicide and 4.5% (n = 20) reported performing patient-requested euthanasia.

Ferrell, Virani, Grant, Coyne, and Uman (2000) surveyed 2,333 nurses for their perspectives on end-of-life care; the results support the need for closer examination of nurses' participation in assisted dying. Although fewer than 1% of the nurses reported participation, these findings are troubling in light of the prohibition of such practices by the ANA Code for Nurses, and indicate the need to better understand nurses' conduct. There is much support for the argument that if good symptom management were provided to dying patients, requests for assisted dying could be virtually eliminated (Coyle, 1992; Hall, 1996; Kazanowski, 1997; Kowalski, 1997; Murphy, 1992). This is especially important because skilled palliative care and hospice clinicians report being capable of making the dying process tolerable, if not completely comfortable, for almost 95% of their patients (Coyle, 1992; Foley, 1996; Quill, 1993).

Understanding why a terminally ill patient wishes to die has become a focus for improving end-of-life care and a key component of the physician-assisted suicide debate. In identifying the factors that contribute to a patient's desire for hastened death, the psychological factors of depression and hopelessness have been discovered to be as, if not more, important than physical pain in influencing a patient's wish to die (Breitbart et al., 2000).

Coyle and Sculco (2004) conducted a qualitative study of seven patients living with advanced cancer, revealing the many meanings of the expression "desire for hastened death." These include (a) a manifestation of the will to live; (b) a dying process so difficult that an early death was preferred; c) an intolerable immediate situation; (d) to extract themselves from an unendurable situation; (e) a last control effort; (f) a way to draw attention to one's uniqueness; (g) a gesture of altruism; (h) an attempt to manipulate a family situation; and (i) a despairing cry depicting the misery of the situation. The investigators recommend that nurses assess the context of the patient's situation, life history, and experiences and use the expression "desire for hastened death" as a communication tool, not necessarily as a literal request.

Sedation

The following definitions by the American Academy of Hospice and Palliative Medicine (AAHPM) (2006) provide clarification for nurses about various forms of sedation:

- Ordinary sedation.
  The ordinary use of sedative medications for the treatment of anxiety, agitated depression, insomnia, or related disorders, in which the goal of treatment is the relief of the symptom without reducing the patient's level of consciousness.
- Palliative sedation.
  The use of sedative medication at least in part to reduce patient awareness of distressing symptoms that are insufficiently controlled by symptom-specific therapies. The level of sedation is proportionate to the patient's level of distress, and alertness is preserved as much as possible.
- Palliative sedation to unconsciousness.
  The administration of sedatives to the point of unconsciousness, when less extreme sedation has not achieved sufficient relief of distressing symptoms. This practice is used only for the most severe, intractable suffering at the very end of life.

Position papers by the ANA and the Hospice and Palliative Care Nurses Association (HPNA) focus on the relief of intractable pain and suffering and support the use of palliative sedation to manage refractory and unendurable symptoms in imminently dying patients (Bruce, Hendrix, & Gentry, 2006). Policies and procedures vary for the implementation of palliative sedation. It is important that nurses review the literature, understand the ANA Code of Ethics, their state practice acts, and institutional policies and procedures governing their clinical practice.

Additional targeted research is needed regarding the barriers nurses encounter when trying to provide the best end-of-life care and access to palliative or hospice care for dying patients. Nurse educators, in particular, are challenged to help their students who are caring for highly symptomatic dying patients to distinguish between those acts presumed to be morally and professionally permissible and illegal acts of "assisted" dying (Schwarz, 1999).

EVIDENCE OF THE NEED TO IMPROVE END-OF-LIFE CARE

Two major studies have identified priority areas for end-of-life care that provide some conceptual benchmarks from which quality indicators can be measured: SUPPORT (1995) and the IOM report (Field & Cassel, 1997). Few clinical research projects have generated as much public interest or as many published articles as the SUPPORT study. This $29 million multiyear research project (funded by the Robert Wood Johnson Foundation) was the first to reveal the failure of the American healthcare system to provide effective and compassionate care to seriously ill and dying patients. The study began with a two-year prospective observational study (Phase 1) of 4,301 patients, followed by a two-year controlled clinical trial (Phase 2) in which 4,804 patients and their physicians were randomized by specialty group to an intervention group (n = 2,652) or control group (n = 2,152). The "intervention" took the form of a specially trained nurse who had multiple contacts with patient, family, physician, and hospital staff to elicit preferences, encourage attention to pain control, and facilitate advance care planning and physician/patient communication.

Results from Phase 1 documented the lack of communication between patients and physicians and provided characteristics about hospital deaths. Specifically, the results indicated that 46% of Do Not Resuscitate (DNR) orders were written within two days of death; 47% of physicians knew when their patients wanted to avoid CPR; 38% of patients who died spent at least 10 days in the ICU; 50% of patients who died in the hospital had moderate to severe pain (reported by families) at least half the time; and there was a high use of hospital resources. No improvements were found in the above outcomes following the Phase 2 nurse intervention. The findings from the SUPPORT study have provided the impetus for leaders in all health disciplines to develop and implement initiatives in research, education, and practice to improve end-of-life care for patients and their families.

The IOM produced the second series of landmark reports. The first report, "Approaching Death: Improving Care at the End of Life" (Field & Cassell, 1997), is based on the collaborative efforts of a committee of 12 experts in medicine and nursing who cared for chronically ill and severely ill patients. The IOM report summarized issues that needed to be addressed regarding end-of-life care: (1) A review of the state of the knowledge in end-of-life care; (2) Evaluation methods for measuring outcomes; (3) Factors impeding high-quality care; (4) Steps toward agreement on what constitutes "appropriate care" at the end of life. The committee's four major findings, listed below, suggest starting points for quality improvement (QI) work in terms of patient care, organizations, education, and research:

1) Too many people suffer endlessly at the end of life both from errors of omission (when caregivers fail to provide palliative and supportive care known to be effective) and from errors of commission (when caregivers do what is known to be ineffective and even harmful).
2) Legal, organizational, and economic obstacles conspire to obstruct reliably excellent care at the end of life.
3) The education and training of physicians and other healthcare professionals fail to provide them with knowledge, skills, and attitudes required to care for the dying patient.

4) Current knowledge and understanding are inadequate to guide and support consistent practice of evidence-based medicine at the end of life.

Two reports that followed – "Improving Palliative Care for Cancer" (Foley & Gelband, 2001) and "When Children Die: Improving Palliative and End-of-Life Care for Children and Their Families" (Field & Behrman, 2002) –continued the argument that medical and other support for people with fatal or potentially fatal conditions often fall short of what is reasonably, if not simply, attainable. The IOM reports highlight the inadequacy of current knowledge to guide the practice of clinicians in end-of-life care and the need for support from policy makers. Federal and private sources of funding to improve care at the end of life have increased. Examples include support from private foundations such as the Open Society Institute's Project on Death in America, the Commonwealth Fund, and the United Hospital Fund of New York, and the Robert Wood Johnson Foundation. Requests for research applications are available from federal and professional organizations in targeted areas such as reducing barriers to symptom management in palliative care and improving end-of-life care in the underserved elderly.

Nurses led several major efforts that focused on improvement in end-of-life care. The National Institute of Nursing Research (NINR) and Agency for Healthcare Research and Quality (AHRQ) commissioned an evidence report as the basis for a State-of-the Science Conference held in Washington in 2004. Five broad questions were asked: (1) What defines the transition to end-of-life care? (2) What outcome variables are valid indicators of the quality of the end-of-life experience of the dying person and for the surviving loved one? (3) What patient, family, and healthcare system factors are associated with better or worse outcomes at end of life? (4) What processes and interventions are associated with improved or worsened outcomes? and (5) What are future research directions for improving end-of-life care?

In 2007, 12% of the U.S. population was older than 65 years of age. In the next 30 years, that number is expected to double, as baby boomers successively reach age 65. Considering the discussions taking place in the media, online, and in other arenas, these boomers will place importance on dying well, just as they have emphasized living well. Hospice provides the quality care that allows people to live well at the end of life (NHPCO, 2003).

Just one generation ago, most children with severe disabilities died before reaching maturity. Today, more than 90% survive to adulthood. In 2000, an estimated 18 million U.S. children under 18 years of age had special healthcare needs. The lifespans of these children have been extended because of improved technology and medical advances (Rearick, 2007). Studies indicate that 31% of families lose significant portions of or all of their savings caring for these children (Brunnhuber et al., 2008; Plonk & Arnold, 2005). Despite these statistics, there is currently a dearth of organized palliative care services for children in the United States.

A recent study (Twaddle et al., 2007) examining the quality of palliative care services in 35 academic hospitals provides the beginning of the benchmark data. This multidisciplinary team used a multicenter, cross-sectional, retrospective design, and reviewed 1596 patient records against 11 key performance measures (KPM) (Exhibit 4.2), which were derived from evidence-based practice standards. Results suggest wide variability in adherence among hospitals, ranging from 0 to100% (with 0 meaning no adherence and 100% meaning complete adherence). Greater values in KPM indicated greater improvement in quality outcomes, cost, and length of stay. Institutions that benchmarked above 90% did so by incorporating KPM into care processes and using systematized triggers, forms, and default pathways. These results suggest that a "palliative care bundle" (i.e., selected KPMs) leads to improvement in areas of deficiency when all components of care are given to patients. For example, patients who had pain and other symptoms and who were assessed within 48 hours of admission were more likely to report relief of the symptom within the same time frame than those patients who were not assessed.

A nurse-led multidisciplinary palliative care team in one urban institution developed and tested a Palliative Care for Advanced Disease Pathway (PCAD). The

pathway provided a systematic approach to the care of dying patients. The research team selected three hospital floors (oncology, geriatrics and an inpatient palliative care / hospice unit) on which to develop and test the PCAD. Two general medical units received usual care. Four indices from a chart audit tool evaluated change over time in the mean number of (1) symptoms assessed, (2) problematic symptoms addressed, (3) interventions consistent with PCAD, and (4) consultations requested. Results showed that patients on PCAD were more likely to have DNR orders than the comparison units, more symptoms assessed, problematic symptoms addressed, and interventions consistent with state-of-the-science end-of-life care (Luhrs et al., 2005). The pathway has been downloaded by thousands of clinicians (see www.StopPain.org) and adapted for the electronic medical record of the Veterans Affairs Medical Centers (Bookbinder et al., 2005) and intensive care units in an urban trauma center (Mosenthal, 2004). These results suggest that a clinical pathway may serve as an important treatment and educational tool to improve the care of the imminently dying inpatient.

THE EVOLUTION OF HOSPICE AND PALLIATIVE CARE

The hospice concept originated in the Middle Ages when pilgrims traveling to the Holy Land found their minds and bodies restored when they stopped at way stations attended by religious orders. Hospices, originally opened by the Irish Sisters of Charity in Dublin, Ireland, in 1879, moved to London by 1905. Dame Cicely Saunders, a nurse who later became a social worker and physician, is credited with opening Saint Christopher's Hospice in London, where she championed the need for a multidisciplinary approach and round-the-clock administration of opioids when caring for dying patients. Saunder's approach to care focused on comfort, skilled nursing, family counseling, physical therapy, and addressing spiritual needs (Storey, 1996). These fundamental elements of care characterize quality palliative care.

Florence Wald, another nurse recognized for her pioneer work in the hospice movement in the United States, envisioned the need to maximize quality of life for the terminally ill. Following a trip to Saint Christopher's in the 1960s, she returned home to conduct a feasibility study of the need for a hospice in Connecticut. The United States subsequently opened its first hospice in Branford, Connecticut, in 1974 (Friedrich, 1999). Inducted into the Women's Hall of Fame in 1998, Florence Wald was known for her exemplary work in influencing hospices throughout the country, promoting holistic and humanistic care for the dying, and advocating nurses' education regarding care at the end of life. Until her passing away on November 8, 2008,

---

EXHIBIT 4.2: SUGGESTED KEY PERFORMANCE MEASURES IN A PALLIATIVE CARE "BUNDLE"

1) Pain assessment within 48 hours of admission.
2) Use of a quantitative pain rating scale.
3) Reduction or relief of pain within 48 hours of admission.
4) Bowel regimen ordered with opioid administration.
5) Dyspnea assessment within 48 hours of admission.
6) Reduction or relief of dyspnea within 48 hours of admission
7) Documentation of patient status (prognosis, psychosocial symptoms, functional status, overall symptom distress within 48 hours of admission.
8) Psychosocial assessment within last year or 4 days after admission.
9) Patient / family meeting to discuss patient treatment preferences or plans for discharge disposition within 4 days of admission.
10) Documentation of discharge plan within 4 days of admission
11) Discharge planner arranged services required for discharge.

Source: Twaddle, M.L., Maxwell, T.L., Cassel, J.B., Liao, S., Coyne, P.J., Usher, B.M., et al. (2007). Palliative care benchmarks from academic medical centers. *Journal of Palliative Medicine, 10,* 86–98.

she continued to promote the hospice model as the gold standard for offering the best end-of-life care to patients and their families.

Access to hospice traditionally has been limited to patients who have a life expectancy of less than six months and are no longer pursuing active treatment. Medicare Hospice Data from 1998-2005 showed that the number of patients receiving hospice care nationally increased 27% from 1998 to 2000 and 63% from 2000 to 2005. The average length of stay has been steadily increasing. For example, in 2005, Mississippi, Alabama, and Oklahoma had average lengths of stay of 122, 113, and 108, respectively, while the national average was 67 days. Overall, these data indicate that the use of the benefit has grown considerably (Center for Medicare and Medicaid Services, 2005). Palliative care, however, can begin at the time a patient is diagnosed with a life-threatening illness. With the increase in emphasis on national education in palliative care for physicians and nurses, more providers are referring patients with life-limiting advanced or chronic illnesses to a palliative care team because this referral does not carry the absolute association with death that hospice care does. Patients with COPD or congestive heart failure are prime examples of persons whose life expectancy is unknown. Hospice programs typically require a DNR order, and insurers may not allow high-tech life-prolonging therapies or may limit access to medical specialists. Palliative care programs also strive to relieve the pain and suffering associated with any life-threatening illness, but they do not mandate forgoing life-prolonging therapies. The goal of treatment remains the achievement of the optimal quality of life for patients and families.

The medicare hospice benefit is based on a probability prediction that an individual with a terminal or incurable illness will not survive longer than six months. Palliative care experts, however, have long recognized the need to provide access to comprehensive services earlier in the disease trajectory. Newer models of palliative care address both disease-specific therapies as well as supportive-comfort therapies that promote the optimal function and well-being of patients and their family caregivers. The Canadian Palliative Care Association's model (Ferris & Cummings, 1995) documents how palliative care needs to intensify at the end of life. The core issues of palliation, comfort, and function are salient throughout the course of the disease. A palliative care model recognizes the need to address symptom distress, physical impairments, and psychosocial disturbance even during the period of aggressive primary therapy with goals of cure or the prolongation of life (Portenoy, 1998).

The World Health Organization (WHO) (2002) defines palliative care as an approach that improves the quality of life of patients and families who face life-threatening illness by providing pain and symptom relief, and spiritual and psychosocial support from diagnosis to the end of life and bereavement. Palliative care:

1) provides relief from pain and other distressing symptoms;
2) affirms life and regards dying as a normal process;
3) intends neither to hasten nor postpone death;
4) integrates the psychological and spiritual aspects of patient care;
5) offers a support system to help patients live as actively as possible until death;
6) offers a support system to help the family cope during the patient's illness and in their own bereavement;
7) uses a team approach to address the needs of patients and their families, including bereavement counseling, if indicated;
8) will enhance quality of life, and may also positively influence the course of illness;
9) is applicable early in the course of illness, in conjunction with other therapies that are intended to prolong life, such as chemotherapy or radiation therapy, and includes those investigations needed to better understand and manage distressing clinical complications.

Palliative care and hospice programs have grown in the United States in response to a population living with chronic, debilitating, and life-threatening illness and to clinician interest in effective approaches to providing care. Most recently, five major palliative care organizations led a National Consensus Project (NCP) for Quality Palliative Care to improve the quality of palliative care in the U.S. This effort resulted in "Clinical Practice Guidelines for Quality Palliative Care" (2004). The guidelines are organized into eight domains of care (see Exhibit 4.3) and aim to promote quality and reduce variation in new and existing programs, develop and encourage continuity of care across settings, and facilitate collaborative partnerships among palliative care programs, community hospices, and other healthcare

EXHIBIT 4.3: DOMAINS OF QUALITY PALLIATIVE CARE

1) Structure and Processes of Care.
2) Physical Aspects of Care.
3) Psychological and Psychiatric Aspects of Care.
4) Social Aspects of Care.
5) Spiritual, Religious, and Existential Aspects of Care.
6) Cultural Aspects of Care.
7) Care of the Imminently Dying Patient.
8) Ethical and Legal Aspects of Care.

Source: National Consensus Project for Quality Palliative Care. (2004). *Clinical practice guidelines for quality palliative care.* Pittsburgh, PA: Author.

settings. Fundamental processes that cross all domains include assessment, information sharing, decision making, care planning, and care delivery.

Developers incorporated established standards of care from Australia, New Zealand, Canadian, Children's Hospital International, and the NHPCO . Studies will be needed to evaluate the usefulness of the guidelines to foster access to care; continuity across settings, such as home, residential, hospital, and hospice; development of national benchmarks for care; uniform definitions that assure reliable quality care; and encourage performance measurement and quality improvement initiatives for palliative care services. To review the consensus guidelines online, go to www.nationalconsensusproject.org.

Factors that also have contributed to the palliative care movement in the United States include the growing aging population, assisted suicide debate, reduced patient autonomy, and inappropriate end-of-life care (i.e., overtreatment of medical conditions and undertreatment of pain and depression). Quality outcomes of good palliative care ensure that patients' values and decisions are respected; comfort is a priority; psychosocial, spiritual, and practical needs will be addressed; and opportunities will be encouraged for growth and completion of unfinished business (NCP, 2004).

The nation's major public-private partnership organization charged with advancing the quality of healthcare, the National Quality Forum (NQF) (2006), developed *A Framework for Preferred Practices for Palliative and Hospice Care Quality: A Consensus Report*. The framework launches a set of 38 preferred practices associated with quality palliative care. In an effort to guide hospitals starting new or strengthening existing palliative care and hospice care programs, The Center to Advance Palliative Care (CAPC) (2008), convened a consensus panel to develop recommendations for key operational features for hospital programs. Twenty-two recommendations are grouped into 12 domains and include "must-have" and "should-have" features (www.capc.org/tools-for-palliative-care-programs/guidelines/nqf-brochure.pdf). The recommendations address the Institute of Medicine's six dimensions of quality: safe, effective, timely, patient-centered, efficient, and equitable. The preferred practices document marked a key step in the standardization of palliative care and hospice.

Nurses can help patients and their families with life-threatening illnesses and advanced disease to identify their preferences for care and decision making, including where to die and when to limit or withdraw interventions. By identifying and continually assessing these preferences for care, nurses have a pivotal role in guiding patient care across settings.

Hospitals are increasingly investing in palliative care services to improve patient care, enhance patient satisfaction, and reduce ICU and total bed days

and costs. According to a CAPC analysis of the latest data released in the 2007 American Hospital Association (AHA) Annual Survey of Hospitals, 1240 hospitals nationwide provide palliative care programs compared to 632 programs in 2000-a five-year increase of 96% (CAPC, 2008). Overall, these programs have been found to be effective in facilitating patient transitions from acute, high-cost hospitals to more suitable settings, such as the home.

CHANGES IN HEALTH CARE DELIVERY MODELS

Prognostication. Physicians and nurses struggle with decisions about appropriate care for patients who are near death. Predicting how long someone will live with an incurable illness is a difficult and complex task. Lynn, Teno, and Harrell (1995) describe the construction of a model for more accurate prognostications of death. It includes a risk of death estimate plus 14 patient characteristics: diagnosis, serum sodium level, temperature, respiratory rate, heart rate, oxygenation, creatinine level, mean blood pressure, bilirubin and albumin levels, Glasgow coma score, age, days in hospital, and having cancer as a comorbidity. These authors assert that their statistical model coupled with the physician's estimates is better than either one alone.

Weeks et al. (1998) examined data from 917 adults with stage III or IV non–small-cell lung and metastatic colon cancer in Phases 1 and 2 of the SUPPORT study across five U.S. teaching sites. Results indicated that patients were substantially more optimistic about their prognosis than their physicians were. In 82% of the physician–patient pairs, the patients' estimates of their chance of living 6 months were higher than the physicians' estimates; in 59% of the pairs, the patient estimate exceeded the physician estimate by two prognostic categories. Patients who were more optimistic about their prognosis lived longer than patients who were less optimistic. Patients who believed that they would survive at least six months favored life-extending therapy over comfort care at more than double the rate of those who believed they had less than six months to live. Patients greatly overestimated their chances of surviving six months while physicians' prognostic estimates were more precise: physicians (estimating 90% survival) accurately predicted 71% of the deaths.

These studies indicate two important findings. First is the need for better communication between physicians and their patients about prognosis. This discussion could help patients make more informed treatment decisions consistent with their values and could facilitate earlier access to palliative or hospice care. The second relates to the need to better understand the source of patients' beliefs, preferences, and the ways in which they arrive at decisions about their care. This may be critical in designing interventions that are effective in changing end-of-life patterns of communication and care.

Prognostication in nonmalignant disease is proving to be even more difficult. A systematic review (Glare et al., 2003) of 11 primarily prospective cohort and longitudinal studies suggested the lack of reliable prognostic models for this nonmalignant group contributed to the unfilled need for palliative care services for older patients with life-threatening illness (Coventry, Grande, Richards, & Todd, 2005). The review identified common predictors of survival for this population: increased dependency in activities of daily living, comorbidities, nutritional status and weight loss, and abnormal vital signs and laboratory tests.

Studies have begun to identify cultural differences in expectation around conditions of prognostic information (Barclay, Blackhall, & Tulsky, 2007). Investigators found that while most white and African American patients expect to be provided with full information to make informed decisions, in some other cultures (e.g., Asian, Navajo, African, Central and South American, and Eastern European cultures), nondisclosure of bad news or use of nonverbal means is expected. Authors advise clinicians that preferences vary and assumptions based on ethnic background can be misleading, indicating the need for prior discussions about appropriate levels of information.

The need for palliative care in non-cancer patients with chronic illnesses is often not recognized (Rodriguez, Barnato, & Arnold, 2007). In patients with heart failure, prognostication is especially difficult and physicians may not integrate preferences into goals of care.

In the SUPPORT study, only 25% of patients hospitalized with heart failure recalled a discussion with physicians about resuscitation and 20% changed preferences after discharge (Rodriguez, Barnato, & Arnold, 2007).

The sensitivity and specificity of tools estimating survival are being perfected. According to Brunnhuber et al. (2008), the PaP, a palliative prognostic indicator, is known to be the best validated tool with advanced cancer patients. The PaP is commonly used by clinicians and includes symptoms, performance status, and lab values (Pirovano et al., 1999). Prognostication of non-cancer disease can be more difficult.

Optimism. Another factor that is consistently associated with aspects of mental and physical health is optimism. Optimism has been shown to shape one's own assessment of a stressor as well as coping resources and subsequent coping efforts. Dispositional optimism, defined as generalized expectations that good things will happen , and situational optimism, which can be thought of as expectations that good things will happen in a given situation, have both been found to be positively associated with mental and physical health and quality of life (De Moor et al., 2006). These findings suggest

that in addition to physical assessment of individuals, nurses need to assess patients' psychosocial aspects of coping.

Financial Aspects. Between 2004 and 2006, U.S. hospital costs rose by nearly 20%, primarily because of the larger numbers of patients seeking care in hospitals, and the increase in availability of costly life-sustaining interventions. Hospitals now receive 75 cents of every medicare dollar. The medical costs incurred during the last years of life are high; over 50% of lifetime medical expenses occur after the age of 65, and 33% after 85 years of age. In the last year of life, an individual incurs about 30% of his or her lifetime medicare expenditures. However, spending on palliative and hospice interventions accounts for a small percentage of this (Brunnhuber et al., 2008).

Recent survey results indicate the cost savings that accrue from interdisciplinary palliative care teams. One survey (Morrison et al., 2008), showed that hospitals saved from $279 to $374 per day per palliative care patient and savings reached $1700–$4900 on each admission of palliative care patients. Savings included significant reduction in pharmacy, laboratory, and intensive care costs. This can mean a savings of more than 1.3 million for a 300-bed hospital and more than 2.5 million for the average academic medical center. These data indicate that "better care can go hand in hand with a better bottom line."

Nurses caring for patients with advanced and chronic illness, need to develop care plans with patients and families that clarify palliative issues regarding goals of care. It is important that primary nurses take the lead in advocating for patient and family preferences by communicating at goals of care conferences and with the palliative care team directly. Nurses need further educational opportunities, such as case presentations and clinical rounds and mentors, that improve the skill set needed to care for patients with advanced and chronic illnesses.

GENERALIST AND SPECIALIST PALLIATIVE CARE

The need for various levels of palliative care for both adults and children is likely to continue rising, with the increased incidence of cancer and other chronic diseases, as the population ages, and with improved survival from chronic illness. It is important that we plan to meet the increased need with specialized education of providers across the continuum of care, using cost- effective measures. Palliative care should be at the core of the work of every health professional. The term "general palliative care" refers to the provision of palliative care, in the community or in hospitals, by healthcare professionals who are not specialists in palliative care. General practitioners, nurses, and other members of the primary care team are recognized to be central to its provision. Pain and symptom assessment and advance care planning are core domains for all generalist level clinicians. Home care nurses have an important role in coordination and the maintenance of continuity for the chronically ill palliative care patient at home. New information technologies, using telemedicine in the home, are accelerating communication and identification of need and access to specialty-level services, such as palliative care.

Palliative care specialists (advance practice nurses and physicians) address diverse quality-of-life concerns and promote interdisciplinary care emphasizing distinction of life and of dying, promotion of comfort and relief of suffering, and respect for autonomy and family involvement. As specialists, they serve as role models and educators in clinical practice. They work to develop the theoretical and empirical body of knowledge in palliative care through research, develop and implement institution-based models of palliative care, and institute quality improvement programs. Palliative care specialists focus on complex patients, such as those with multiple or difficult symptom-control problems, who require comprehensive care for multiple needs (e.g., needing family support or nursing-home-based management for monitoring and titration of medication), and comprehensive care of the imminently dying. Although palliative care is now recognized as a specialty, palliative care as a model of care is a therapeutic approach ideally integrated into the care of all patients with life-threatening diseases across the illness or dying trajectory (NCP, 2004).

IMPROVING THE EDUCATION OF PROFESSIONALS

The SUPPORT study (1995) documented nurses' opinions that improved communication, time, and repeated information about end-of-life issues were necessary for families to make decisions regarding interventions for life-threatening illnesses (Hiltunen et al., 1995). These findings highlight the role of the nurse as companion and confidante to patients and families and support a shared decision-making model in end-of-life treatment discussions. This is especially relevant given that only 15% of patients nationally have an advance directive.

Efforts are increasing to educate professionals in the United States. The American Medical Association's "Education for Physicians on End-of-Life Care" (EPEC) curriculum (Emanuel, von Gunten, & Ferris, 1999), supported by a grant from the Robert Wood Johnson Foundation, is designed to educate physicians across the country on essential clinical competencies in end-of-life care. The American Society of Clinical Oncology, in collaboration with the National Cancer Institute and

the EPEC Project, offers workshops to help optimize care for patients throughout the course of their illness. A complementary program for nurses entitled the "End of Life Nursing Education Consortium" (ELNEC), also

EXHIBIT 4.4: COMPETENCIES NECESSARY FOR NURSES TO PROVIDE HIGH-QUALITY CARE TO PATIENTS AND FAMILIES DURING THE TRANSITION AT THE END OF LIFE

1) Recognize dynamic changes in population demographics, health-care economics, and service delivery that necessitate improved professional preparation for end-of-life care.
2) Promote the provision of comfort care to the dying as an active, desirable, and important skill, and an integral component of nursing care.
3) Communicate effectively and compassionately with the patient, family, and healthcare team members about end-of-life issues.
4) Recognize one's own attitudes, feelings, values, and expectations about death and the individual, cultural, and spiritual diversity existing in these beliefs and customs.
5) Demonstrate respect for the patient's views and wishes during end-of-life care.
6) Collaborate with interdisciplinary team members while implementing the nursing role in end-of-life care.
7) Use scientifically based standardized tools to assess symptoms (e.g., pain, dyspnea [breathlessness] constipation, anxiety, fatigue, nausea/vomiting, and altered cognition) experienced by patients at the end of life.
8) Use data from symptom assessment to plan and intervene in symptom management using state-of-the-art traditional and complementary approaches.
9) Evaluate the impact of traditional, complementary, and technological therapies on patient- centered outcomes.
10) Assess and treat multiple dimensions, including physical, psychological, social and spiritual needs, to improve quality at the end of life.
11) Assist the patient, family, colleagues, and one's self to cope with suffering, grief, loss, and bereavement in end-of-life care.
12) Apply legal and ethical principles in the analysis of complex issues in end-of-life care, recognizing the influence of personal values, professional codes, and patient preferences.
13) Identify barriers and facilitators to patients' and caregivers' effective use of resources.
14) Demonstrate skill at implementing a plan for improved end-of-life care within a dynamic and complex healthcare delivery system.
15) Apply knowledge gained from palliative care research to end-of-life education and care.

Source: American Association of Colleges of Nursing. (2005). *Peaceful death: Recommended competencies and curricula guidelines for end-of-life nursing care* [Electronic version]. Retrieved December 28, 2004 from http:/www.aacn.niche.edu/publications/deathfin.htm

funded by the Robert Wood Johnson Foundation, is a partnership of the American Association of Colleges of Nursing (AACN) and the City of Hope National Medical Center (COH). As of 2008, courses have been tailored to oncology, pediatrics, critical care, and geriatrics. Exhibit 4.4 outlines the AACN's recommended competencies and curricula for nurses to provide high-quality care to patients and families during the transition at the end of life. Exhibit 4.5 lists the content areas for modules in the ELNEC training curriculum. These content areas have been integrated into many clinical rotations in various practice settings. Palliative care competencies are now an essential part of generalist-level nursing and medical curricula. An ELNEC Super Core curriculum now includes separate tracks for undergraduate and graduate programs. For more information about these programs, visit www.aacn.nche.edu/ELNEC. Nursing faculty and clinicians trained in the ELNEC program are being called upon to disseminate this education to all healthcare providers throughout the world.

In addition to obtaining competency in palliative care, specialist level nurses will need to have knowledge in genomic information (Exhibit 4.6). Since the onset of the Human Genome Research Project in 1990, the pace has accelerated in genetic science. The objective of the project was to understand the genetic makeup of the human species, According to the International Society of Nurses in Genetics, these scientific advances have transformed the way patients, healthcare providers, and healthcare insurers define health and well-being. With a new paradigm for health and well-being comes a new conceptualization of healthcare services that includes consideration for the impact of genetics on disease etiology, predisposition, incidence, treatment and treatment outcomes. As a result of rapid technological advances, evolving healthcare needs and a growing interest among the public, there is and will continue to be an increasing number of people requiring genetic healthcare services (ISONG, 2003).

The rapid advancement of genetic and genomic science and technology has already had a significant impact on nursing's role and responsibilities in the 21st century, bringing new questions and ethical challenges.

EXHIBIT 4.5: MODULES INCLUDED IN ELNEC TRAINING

1) Nursing Care at the End of Life.
2) Pain Assessment & Management.
3) Symptom Management.
4) Ethical/Legal Issues.
5) Cultural Considerations in End-of-Life Care.
6) Communication.
7) Loss, Grief, Bereavement.
8) Achieving Quality Care at the End of Life.
9) Preparation for and Care at the Time of Death.

The ANA's *Code of Ethics for Nurses* (2001) provides a framework for nurses that is responsive to these challenges. The *Code* is a comprehensive statement of nurses' duties and obligations and specifically addresses ethical issues. Each of the nine provisions in the code need to be included in nursing curricula. The following

EXHIBIT 4.6: SOURCES OF INFORMATION ABOUT GENOMIC-BASED RESEARCH, GENOMIC-BASED CLINICAL TRIALS, AND RESOURCES RELATED TO GENETIC TESTING

Web Address & Description

1) grants.nih.gov/grants/guide0/index.html
   ☐ The archive can be browsed, or searched by keywords.
2) ninr.nih.gov/ninr/
   ☐ The National Institute of Nursing Research's Web site contains information about extramural research opportunities as well as research training opportunities such as the Summer Genetics Institute.
3) www.genome.gov
   ☐ The National Human Genome Research Institute's Web site contains information about policy and ethics, research opportunities, and educational opportunities.
4) www.who.int/genomics/en
   ☐ The World Health Organization's Web site provides helpful links for clinicians, educators and researchers in regard to global genomic issues.
5) www.gemcris.od.nih.gov/
   ☐ GeMCRIS allows users to access an array of information about human gene transfer trials registered with the NIH, including medical conditions under study, institutions where trials are being conducted, investigators carrying out these trials, gene products being used, route of gene product delivery, and summaries of study protocols.
6) www.cdc.gov/genomics/hugenet/
   ☐ Human Genome Epidemiology Network, or HuGENetTM is a global collaboration of individuals and organizations committed to the assessment of the effect of human genome variation on population health and how genetic information can be used to improve health and prevent disease.
7) www.genetests.org
   ☐ A publicly funded medical genetics information resource developed for healthcare providers and researchers. Contains up to date information on what genetic tests are currently available and what laboratories are conducting them.
8) www.intgen.org
   ☐ The International Genomics Consortium's Web site that contains information about genomics research extending from the Human Genome Project.
9) www.isong.org
   ☐ The International Society of Nurses in Genetics Web site contains information about this society that supports nurse scientists conducting genetic and genomic research as well as many other aspects related to the genetic health of the global society.

examples illustrate the application of the ethical concepts to current genetic and genomic issues and challenges. The first provision states that nurses take into account the values of every individual. These values, which differ from person to person, become evident when decisions are made regarding tests, treatments, reproduction, or participation in research. Considerations might include the hereditary risks for developing disease and the benefits and risks of genetic testing. Nursing responsibilities include advocacy and maintaining privacy and confidentiality (described in provision three). Throughout the *Code,* but explicitly in provision five, there is guidance on acquiring the knowledge and skills necessary for professional practice. Nurses need ongoing education in these areas to effectively use their competencies on a daily basis. Increasingly, diseases are being recognized as having a genetic component, and tests are being developed to identify susceptibility genes. As a result of these advancements, nurses have a responsibility to participate in the education of the public, including education on disease risk based on genomic information (Badzek, Turner, & Jenkins, 2008).

PROMOTING QUALITY PALLIATIVE CARE

Research results indicate that there is an overwhelming need for improved symptom management at the end of life for both adults and children with serious life-threatening illness. Patients at the end-of-life experience many of the same symptoms and syndromes regardless of their underlying condition. To decrease patient and family suffering at the end of life and improve symptom control, in-hospital programs are adopting a palliative care model that offers comprehensive care for seriously ill patients and their families. Nine case studies of pioneer palliative care programs are described in a Milbank Memorial Fund Report (2000), sponsored by the Robert Wood Johnson Foundation. More nurses with specialized palliative and hospice care expertise are being trained to provide patient care, serve as role models for staff, assure that standards are evidence based, and develop monitoring and evaluation programs to meet benchmarks set by professional organizations for quality care at the end of life. This work is especially important because nearly 35 years after the start of the hospice movement in the United States, only half of adults who die of cancer receive hospice care. Nurses have an important role in identifying patients eligible for hospice and palliative care and facilitating access to specialty services for patients and families.

Palliative care services are lacking for children. According to an Institute of Medicine Report in 2002, 53,000 children in the United States die each year, and another 400,000 have life-threatening illnesses In a Boston study of 165 children with cancer, 49% died in the hospital, and half of these were in the ICU. According to parents, 89% of the children suffered "a lot" or a "great deal" from at least one symptom in the last month of life, mostly pain, fatigue, and dyspnea (Wolfe et al., 2000). Currently, only a handful of organized palliative care services for children exist in the United States. Palliative care programs designed for adults are inappropriate and ineffective for children (Stevens, Dalla Poza, Caelletto, Cooper, & Kilham, 1994; Whitman, 1993). One reason cited was the unwillingness of providers and parents to relinquish curative, invasive therapies even when there was little or no realistic hope for favorable outcomes. Often, aggressive therapy is not abandoned until shortly before death so families and providers have little or no time to address their emotions or begin to grieve.

Pediatric nurses will need to understand the needs of patients and the impact of the child's illness on family members. Nurses must be prepared to address the psychological, emotional, physical, and spiritual needs of patients and families. They also will need to be able to advocate for the care of the pediatric patient, given that the legal power to make care decisions rests solely with parents, who may be reluctant to involve their children, even adolescents, in discussions and decisions about their care. Also, unlike elderly adults, there are children who lack health insurance entirely. All clinicians who care for pediatric patients should have a basic level of training in palliative bereavement, and end-of-life care (Field & Behrman, 2002).

The number of children living with life-threatening disease and chronic illness will increase. Programs to improve quality palliative and end-of-life care will continue to grow. For more information about education in palliative care for pediatrics, go to the End-of-Life Nursing Education Consortium for Pediatric Palliative Care (EL-NEC-PPC) (www.aacn.nche.edu/ELNEC/factsheet.htm).

Removing Barriers to Providing Excellent End-of-Life Care

Several structures, processes, and outcome measures are needed in organizations to identify and remove barriers to providing effective end-of-life care. A "top-down, bottom-up" approach is necessary. This means a mandate is needed from top administration that includes support and resources, coupled with a multidisciplinary team of experts, masterful in using a systematic process for creating change (Bookbinder et al., 2005). Structures geared toward reducing variation in practice and optimizing the achievement of best practices and outcomes can serve as a benchmark against which we can measure and constantly improve. In addition to hospital-required policies and procedures, structures include standards of care, guidelines, and tools that direct patient care management such as protocols, algorithms, care paths, flow charts, and standardized orders.

Quality structures can be internally initiated or externally imposed. By 2001, the Joint Commission on Accreditation of Healthcare Organizations (JCAHO, 2004) required hospitals to implement new pain management standards, including routine assessment and reassessment of pain and care at the end of life. This national initiative requiring relief of pain and suffering occurred within 15 years of the American Pain Society's Quality Assurance Standards for Relief of Acute and Cancer Pain (American Pain Society, 1995; WHO, 2002). This dramatic change in healthcare culture regarding the need for pain relief offers hope to palliative care initiatives aimed at good end-of-life care.

Protocols and algorithms have become popular clinical tools in a managed care era of "doing more with less time and resources." These tools aim to streamline processes of care, deliver consistent and timely interventions, and improve quality of life, particularly at the end of life. Tools such as the *Palliative Care Clinical Practice Protocol for Dyspnea* (Hospice Nurses Association, 1996), *Symptom Management Algorithms for Palliative Care* (Wrede-Seaman, 2008), and the *Pocket Guide to Hospice / Palliative Medicine* (AAHPM, 2003) offer clinicians a methodology for assessing symptoms, etiology, directions for treatment options, and guidelines for pharmacological and nonpharmacological interventions.

Pathways (care paths), flow sheets, and standardized orders also are products of the managed care era and are intended to "reduce variation" in services and practices, and thereby reduce costs Although the many needs of dying patients have been identified (SUPPORT, 1995), few end-of-life clinical pathways have been developed and tested (Panella, Marchisio, Barbieri, & De Stanislao, 2008; Ellershaw & Murphy, 2005; Bookbinder et al., 2005); NHO, 1997b; Gordon, 1996). Goals for these pathways include (1) respecting patient autonomy, values, decisions; (2) continually clarifying goals of care; (3) minimizing symptom distress at the end of life; (4) optimizing appropriate supportive interventions and consultations; (5) reducing unnecessary interventions; (6) supporting families by coordinating services; (7) eliminating unnecessary regulations; (8) providing bereavement services for families and staff; and (9) facilitating the transition to alternate care settings, such as hospice, when appropriate (Bookbinder et al., 2005).

Family perception of end-of-life care is increasingly being used to measure outcomes of care. Teno et al. (2004) conducted a mortality follow-back survey of family members or other knowledgeable informants representing 1,578 decedents. They found that family perceptions of patients who were involved in end-of-life decision making indicate positive end-of-life outcomes, for example, peaceful death, patient preferences were met, goals of care were agreed upon, and grief resolution.

Building Evidence-Based Practice

There are varying terms used to describe the process of bringing research into practice. Terms include "evidence-based practice," "evidence-based healthcare (EBHC)," "evidence-based nursing," and "evidence-based medicine." All four terms refer to the process of searching for the best level of evidence available to provide the basis for clinical protocols, policies, procedures, and decision-making (Wysocki & Bookbinder, 2005). Nurses need a knowledge base for understanding how evidence plays a critical role in their day-to-day practice. Using evidence is especially important for nursing as we continue to provide leadership in building palliative care programs (NQF, 2006) and continue the research needed to advance the science of nursing and palliative care (Coyle & Bookbinder, 2008).

Although few end-of-life care practices are currently based upon strong scientific evidence (Field & Cassell, 1997), research is available to help nurses shape their role in providing state-of-the-art care to patients and their families at the end of life. Research results indicate the need for healthcare settings to: (a) systematically identify and remove obstacles to excellent care of the seriously ill and dying patient; (b) identify end-of-life and palliative care issues in vulnerable populations such as children, older adults, and those who are chemically dependent; (d) test models and tools (algorithms and care paths) aimed to improve symptom control and end-of-life outcomes such as comfort and relief from physical, emotional, social, and spiritual distress; (e) develop programs to educate professionals in end-of-life care and evaluate the various formats for education; and (f) continue to develop professional competencies that demonstrate "best practices" at the bedside. Also important is the need for professionals to: (a) improve communication and understanding about treatment goals and outcomes among physicians, nurses, patients, and families; (b) understand the contributing factors to nurses' reported behaviors in assisted suicide; and (c) determine patient prognosis and earlier preparation for end-of-life care planning, especially in the "chronic-living-dying" population.

Nurses need to be familiar with frameworks for assessing the level of evidence of a study finding. Professional organizations, such as the Oncology Nursing Society (ONS), provide resources to help nurses evaluate the quality, quantity, and consistency of evidence (www.ons.org/research). In the ONS evidence-based model, evidence is ranked from Levels I to III with subcategories (see www.onsopcontent.ons.org/toolkits/evidence). ONS Level I is evidence from a meta-analysis of multiple, well-designed controlled studies; experimental studies; and well-designed nonrandomized studies. ONS Level II evidence is obtained from systematic reviews of non-experimental studies, and ONS

Level III is evidence derived from qualitative studies, case reports, and expert opinion. The strength of the evidence is strongest for Level I studies and weakest for Level III studies.

Brunnhuber et al. (2008) recently summarized the current state of research in palliative care. Reviewers identified the challenges in conducting research and using the evidence, including the difficulties in recruitment and retention in clinical trials of participants and families facing the end of life, and lack of funding for research. The authors also report that systematic reviews gave insufficient information regarding methods, limiting the findings' reproducibility. Despite a slow-moving evidence base, nurses will continue to be a collective national voice for nursing science. Partnerships among clinicians and researchers to conduct multisite trials are necessary to build a palliative care database specific to nursing practice. To build a research warehouse for palliative care, nurses will need to ask critical clinical questions and participate in research or quality improvement projects that generate new knowledge and evaluate and test standards of care and clinical practice. Knowledge will need to be generated by researchers, practitioners, educators, nursing administrators, health policy makers, and state and federal regulators to ensure quality care for patients and families along the illness continuum.

Case Study conclusion: The case of Mr. Wong and his family offers examples of domains of palliative care which should be addressed as per the National Consensus Project Guidelines for Quality Palliative Care. As Mr. Wong's disease progresses, he becomes weaker and unable to move from the bed. When asked how he is feeling, he always whispers "fine" and denies any symptoms. His wife believes he will be cured if only he will "eat" and that he must "try harder." Mr. Wong is actively dying. A nurse who visits Mr. Wong discusses the options of Hospice care or admission to an in-patient palliative care unit. She offers culturally sensitive care (Cultural Aspects of Care). The home health nurse contacts the nurse at hospice and he is admitted to Home Hospice Care. The Hospice team works with the family regarding symptom management and intake of food and fluids (Structure and Process of Care). The goals of care are discussed and the family wishes to move forward with a palliative care plan (Ethical and Legal Aspects of Care). The patient is successfully managed at home with twice weekly RN visits, and weekly social work visits. The patient becomes more SOB and tells his wife that he knows he is dying. He is becoming increasing restless and depressed and his symptoms are managed successfully (Physical and Psychological Aspects of Care). Mr. Wong dies peacefully two weeks after admission, with the family at his bedside. The Hospice nurse is present and manages his symptoms of pulmonary congestion and dyspnea (Care of the Imminently Dying). The family is offered bereavement services by the hospice and palliative care team (Psychological Care of Family).

CONCLUSIONS

Views toward death and dying in American culture continue to change at a relatively consistent pace as evidence is compiled documenting the need to improve the care of the dying and their families. This challenge to nurse educators and their students is a formidable one in the decades ahead, as the population ages, the need for management of chronic illness increases, and the impact of improved technology and genomic science influences patient and family decision making. Nurses leading the field need advanced education and training in palliative care. All nurses will need generalist-level palliative care education and will need to know when the services of an interdisciplinary specialist-level palliative care team are indicated and how to access those services. Curriculum designers will need to supplement didactic education with clinical rotations that span settings so that students gain an operational skill-set that provides coordination and continuity. Nurses need to be aware of evidence-based clinical practice guidelines in palliative care, and how to implement and evaluate them to achieve desirable patient and family outcomes. Nurse educators need to encourage students to participate in collaborative research efforts that will improve nursing science and patient and family outcomes. A new agenda for healthcare reform is imminent, the outcome of which may include changes in patients' access to services. Nurses will have opportunities to influence decision making and policies that effect optimal palliative and end-of-life care. They will be critical coordinators of care and advocates for patients as our nation moves to provide access to healthcare for all.

The Case Study that follows illustrates the nurses need to be knowledgeable of the domains of palliative care and evidence-base practice and how to apply these to daily professional nursing practice across settings.

EVIDENCE-BASED PRACTICE

Kerchoff, K., Palzkill, J., Kowalkowski, J., Mork, A., & Grelarsdottir, E. (2008). Preparing families of intensive care patients for withdrawal of life support. *American Journal of Critical Care Nursing*, 17(2), 113–122.

Background. Most deaths in intensive care occur after withdrawal of life support. Although preparation of patients' families is recommended, the specific information required has not been theoretically developed or tested.

Objective. To assess the feasibility of testing four tailored messages to prepare families of patients having a planned withdrawal of life support, to assess barriers to conducting such a study, and to obtain preliminary data on measurable effects that could be used to compare such preparation with usual care. Self-regulation theory was used to structure the messages.

Methods. Families were randomly assigned to usual care ($n = 10$) or to an intervention group ($n = 10$) that received 1 of 4 tailored messages to prepare them for withdrawal of life support.

They were contacted 2 to 4 weeks later to complete the Profile of Mood States and to give their evaluation of the experience, inclusive of the information received.

Results. Compared with the usual-care group, the intervention group was significantly more satisfied with the information they received and understood better what was to happen. The intervention group had lower negative mood scores and higher positive mood scores than did the usual-care group, although the difference was not significant. Unsolicited comments by the usual-care participants were requests for the specific information that had been received by the intervention group.

Conclusions. The information provided was considered helpful. A larger sample might yield more significant differences. Further work is needed on other aspects of preparation such as healthcare support, spiritual issues, and preparation for funeral arrangements.

REFERENCES

American Academy of Hospice and Palliative Medicine. (AAHPM). (2006). *Statement on palliative sedation.* Retrieved September 1, 2008 from http://www.aahpm.org/positions/sedation.html

American Academy of Hospice and Palliative Medicine. (2003). *Pocket guide to hospice/ palliative medicine.* Glenview, IL: Author.

American Association of Colleges of Nursing. (2005). *Peaceful death. Recommended competencies and curricula guidelines for end-of-life nursing care* [Electronic version]. Retrieved December 28, 2004 from http://www.aacn.niche.edu/Publications/deathfin.htm

American Association of Colleges of Nursing. (2001). *End-of-life nursing education consortium for pediatric palliative care (EL-NEC-PPC).* Retrieved February 5, 2009 from http://www.aacn.nche.edu/ELNEC/factsheet.htm

American Geriatrics Society. (AGS). (2007). *Position statement on the care of dying patients.* [Electronic version]. Retrieved November 14, 2008 from http://www.americangeriatrics.org/products/positionpapers/careofd.shtml

American Nurses Association. (2001). *Code of ethics for nurses.* Silver Spring, MD: Author. Retrieved November 14, 2008 from http://allnurses.com/nursing-activism-healthcare/code-ethics-nurses-118268.html

American Nurses Association. (1994). *ANA position statement: Assisted suicide.* Silver Spring, MD: Author.

American Nurses Association. (1991). *ANA position statement: Promotion of comfort and relief of pain in dying patients.* Silver Spring, MD: Author.

American Pain Society Quality of Care Committee. (1995). Quality improvement guidelines for the treatment of acute pain and cancer pain. *Journal of the American Medical Association, 274*(23), 1874–1880.

Annas, G. J. (1995). How we die. *Hastings Center Report, 25,* 512–514.

Asch, D. A. (1996). The role of critical care nurses in euthanasia and assisted suicide. *New England Journal of Medicine, 334,* 1374–1401.

Bachman, J., Alcser, K., Doukis, D., Lichtenstein, R., Corning, A., & Brody, H. (1996). Attitudes of Michigan physicians and the public towards legalizing physician-assisted suicide and voluntary euthanasia. *New England Journal of Medicine, 334,* 303–309.

Badzek, L., Turner, M., & Jenkins, J. F. (2008). Genomics and advancing nursing. Genomics and nursing practice: Advancing the nursing profession. *On-line Journal of Issues in Nursing. A Scholarly Journal of the American Nurses Association, 13, January 31,* 2008.

Barclay, J., Blackhall, L., & Tulsky, J. (2007). Communication strategies and cultural
issues in the delivery of bad news. *Journal of Palliative Medicine, 10,* 958–977.

Bookbinder, M., Blank, A. E., Arney, E., Wollner, D., Lesage, P., McHugh, M., et al. (2005). Improving end-of-life care: Development and pilot-test of a clinical pathway. *Journal of Pain and Symptom Management, 29*(6), 529–543.

Botkin, J. R., & Post, S. G. (1992). Confusion in the determination of death. *Perspective in Biology and Medicine, 36*(1), 129–138.

Breitbart, W., Rosenfeld, B., Pessin, H., et al. (2000). Depression, hopelessness, and desire for hastened death in terminally ill patients with cancer. *Journal of the American Medical Association, 284,* 2907–2911.

Brody, H. (1988). Brain death and personal existence: A reply to Green and Wikler. *Journal of Medicine and Philosophy, 4,* 8.

Brody, H. (1992). Assisted dying: A compassionate response to a medical failure. *New England Journal of Medicine, 327,* 1384–1388.

Bruce, S. D., Hendrix, C. C., & Gentry, J. H. (2006). Palliative sedation in end-of-life care. *Journal of Hospice and Palliative Nursing, 8*(6), 320–327.

Brunnhuber, K., Nash, S., Meier, D. E., Weissman, D. E., & Woodcock, J. (2008). *Putting evidence into practice: Palliative care.* London: BMJ Publishing Group.

Byock, I. R. (2007). To Life! Reflections on spirituality, palliative practice, and politics. *American Journal of Hospice and Palliative Medicine, 23*(6), 436–438.

Byock, I. R. (1997). *Dying well.* New York: Riverhead Books.

Center for Gerontology and Health Care Research. (2004). *Policy relevant data on care at the end of life.* Retrieved January 31, 2009 from http://www.chcr.brown.edu/dying/usastatistics.htm

Center to Advance Palliative Care. (CAPC). (2008). *Better care of sickest patients can save hospitals money, says largest study of its kind.* Retrieved January 31, 2009 from http://www.capc.org/news-and-events/releases/news-release-9-08-08

Center for Medicare and Medicaid Services. (2005). *Medicare hospice expenditures and units of care*. Retrieved February 14, 2009 from http://www.cms.hhs.gov/ProspMedicareFeeSvcPmtGen/ downloads/ FY05update_hospice_expenditures_and_units_of_ care.pdf

Centers for Disease Control and National Center for Health Statistics . *U.S. mortality drops sharply in 2006, latest data show*. [Electronic version]. Retrieved November 2, 2008 from http://www.cdc.gov/nchs/pressroom/08newsreleases/mortality2006.htm

Coventry, P. A., Grande, G. E., Richards, D. A., & Todd, C. J. (2005). Prediction of appropriate timing of palliative care for older adults with nonmalignant life-threatening disease: A systematic review. *Age and Aging, 34,* 218–227.

Coyle, N. (1992). The euthanasia and physician suicide debate: Issues for nursing. *Oncology Nursing Forum, 19*(Suppl. 7), 41–46.

Coyle, N., & Bookbinder, M. (2008). Nursing science in palliative care and end-of-life care. In J. Phillips & C. King (Eds.), *Advancing oncology nursing science* (pp. 75–91). Pittsburgh, PA: Oncology Nursing Society.

Coyle, N., & Sculco, L. (2004). Expressed desire for hastened death in seven patients living with advanced cancer: A phenomenologic inquiry. *Oncology Nursing Forum, 31*(4), 1–8.

Davis, A. J., Phillips, L., Drought, T. S., Sellin, S., Ronsman, K., & Hershberger, A. K. (1995). Nurses' attitudes toward active euthanasia. *Nursing Outlook, 43,* 174–179.

Death. (2008). In *Encyclopedia Britannica online*. Retrieved February 14, 2009 from http://www.britannica.com/EBchecked/ topic/154412/death

De Moor, J. S., De Moor, C. A., Basen-Engquist, K., Kudelka, A., Bevers, M. W., Cohen, L., et al. (2006). Optimism, distress, health-related quality of life, and change in cancer antigen 125 among patients with ovarian cancer undergoing chemotherapy. *Psychosomatic Medicine, 68,* 555–562.

Dobscha, S. K., Heintz, R. T., Press, N., & Ganzini, L. (2004). Oregon physicians' responses to requests for assisted suicide: A qualitative study. *Journal of Palliative Medicine, 7,* 469–471.

Ellershaw, J. E., & Murphy, D. (2005). The Liverpool care pathway (LCP): Influencing the UK national agenda on care of the dying. *International Journal of Palliative Nursing, 11*(3), 132–134.

Emanuel, L. L., von Gunten, C. F., & Ferris, F. D. (1999). *The education for physicians on end-of-life care (EPEC) curriculum*. From the EPEC Project, Feinberg School of Medicine, Northwestern University, Chicago.

Ferrell, B., Virani, R., Grant, M., Coyne, P., & Uman, G. (2000). Beyond the supreme court decision: Nursing perspectives on end-of-life care. *Oncology Nursing Forum, 27,* 445–455.

Ferris, F. D., & Cummings, I. (Eds.). (1995). *Palliative care: Towards a consensus in standardized principles of practice*. Ottawa: Canadian Palliative Care Association.

Field, M. J., & Behrman, R. E. (Eds.). (2002). *When children die: Improving palliative and end-of-life care for children and their families*. Washington, DC: National Academies Press.

Field, M. J., & Cassel, C. K. (Eds.). (1997). *Approaching death: Improving care at the end-of-life*. Washington, DC: National Academies Press.

Foley, K. M. (1995). Pain, physician-assisted suicide, and euthanasia. *Pain Forum, 4,* 163–178.

Foley, K. M. (1996). Controlling the pain of cancer. *Scientific American, 164* -165.

Foley, K. M., & Gelband, H. (Eds.). (2001). *Improving palliative care for cancer*. Washington, DC: National Academies Press.

Friedrich, M. J. (1999). Hospice care in the U.S.: A conversation with Florence S. Wald. *Journal of the American Medical Association, 281,* 1683–1685.

Ganzini, L., Nelson, H. D., Schmidt, T. A., Kraemer, D. F., Delorit, M. A., & Lee, M. A., et al. (2000). Physicians' experiences with the Oregon Death with Dignity Act. *New England Journal of Medicine, 342,* 557–563.

Glare, P., Virik, K., Jones, M., Hudson, M., Eychmuller. S., Simes, J., et al. (2003). A systematic
review of physicians' survival predictions in terminally ill cancer patients. *British Medical Journal, 327,* 195–198.

Gordon, D. B. (1996). Critical pathways: A road to institutionalizing pain management. *Journal of Pain and Symptom Management, 11,* 252–259.

Grunier, A., & Mor, V. (2007). Where people die: A multilevel approach to understanding influences on site of death in America. *Medical Care Research and Review, 64,* 351–378.

Hall, J. (1996). Assisted suicide: Nurse practitioners as providers? *Nurse Practitioner, 21,* 63–71.

Haward, R. A. (1998). Review of evidence-based cancer medline. *Annals of Oncology, 9,* 1073- 1078 .

Hays, J. C., Galanos, A. N., Palmer, T. A., McQuoid, D. R., & Flint, E. P. (2001). Preference for place of death in a continuing care retirement community. *Gerontologist, 41,* 123–128.

Health Care Financing Administration. (HCFA). (1996). Trends in medicare home health agency utilization and payment: CYs 1974–1994. *Health Care Financing Review 1996* (Statistical Suppl.), 76–77.

Health Resources and Services Administration. (HRSA). (2002). *U.S. Department of Health and Human Services*. Retrieved February 5, 2009 from http://www.hrsa.gov/culturalcompetence/curriculumguide

Hiltunen, E. F., Puopolo, A. L., Marks, G. K., Marsden, C., Kennard, M. J., Follen, M. A., et al. (1995). The nurse's role in end-of-life treatment discussions: Preliminary report from the SUPPORT project. *Journal of Cardiovascular Nursing, 9*(3), 68–77.

Hospice Nurses Association. (1996). *Hospice and palliative care clinical practice protocol: Dyspnea*. Pittsburgh, PA: Author.

International Society of Nurses in Genetics. (2003). *Position statement: Access to genomic healthcare: The role of the nurse*. Retrieved February 5, 2009 from http://www.isong.org/about/ ps_genomic.cfm

Joint Commission on Accreditation of Hospitals Organization. (2004). *Pain management standards*. Retrieved December 28, 2004 from http://www.jcaho.org

Kazanowski, M. (1997). A commitment to palliative care: Could it impact assisted suicide? *Journal of Gerontological Nursing, 23*(3), 36–42.

Kowalski, S. (1997). Assisted suicide: Where do nurses draw the line? *Nursing and Health Care, 14,* 70–76.

Kübler-Ross, E. (1967). *On death and dying*. New York: Touchstone.

Luhrs, C.A., Meghani, S., Homel, P., Drayton, M., O'Toole, E., Paccione, M., et al. (2005). Pilot of a pathway to improve the care of imminently dying oncology inpatients in a Veterans Affairs (VA) medical center. *Journal of Pain and Symptom Management, 29*(6), 544–551.

Lynn, J., Teno, J. M., & Harrell, F. E. (1995). Accurate prognostications of death: Opportunities and challenges from clinicians. *Western Journal of Medicine, 163,* 250–257.

Matzo, L. M., & Emanuel, E. J. (1997). Oncology nurses practices of assisted suicide and patient-requested euthanasia. *Oncology Nursing Forum, 24,* 1725–1732.

McCormick, T. R., & Conley, B. J. (1995). Patients' perspectives on dying and on the care of dying patients. *Western Journal of Medicine, 163*, 236–243.

Milbank Memorial Fund Report. (2000). *Pioneer programs in palliative care: Nine case studies.* New York: Milbank Memorial Fund.

Morrison, R. S., Penrod, J. D., Cassel, J. B., Caust-Ellenbogen, M., Litke A., Spragens, L., et al. (2008). Cost savings associated with US hospital palliative care consultation programs. *Archives of Internal Medicine, 168*, 1783–1790 .

Mosenthal, A. C. (2004). Bringing palliative care to the critically injured. *UMDNJ Research Bulletin, 5*(2). Retrieved December 3, 2008 from http://www.umdnj.edu/research/publications/fall04/05_palliative_care.htm

Murphy, P. A. (1992). Perspective: Nursing-the real issue. *Trends in Health Care, Law, and Ethics, 10*, 124–127.

National Center for Cultural Competence. (2007). [Electronic version]. Retrieved on October 1, 2008 from http://www11.georgetown.edu/research/gucchd/nccc.

National Consensus Project for Quality Palliative Care. (2004). *Clinical practice guidelines for quality palliative care.* Pittsburgh, PA: Author. Retrieved February 1, 2009 from http://www.nationalconsensusproject.org

National Hospice and Palliative Care Organization. (NHPCO). (2003). *Hospice facts and figures.* Retrieved December 28, 2004 from http://www.nhpco.org/files/public/Hospice_Facts_110104.pdf

National Hospice and Palliative Care Organization. (NHPCO). (2008). *Facts and figures on hospice.* Retrieved November 1, 2008 from http://www.nhpco.org/files/public/Statistics_Research/ NHPCO_facts-and-figures_2008.pdf

National Hospice Organization. (1997a). Working party on clinical guidelines in end-of-life care. *Changing gears: Guidelines for managing care in the last days of life in adults.* Arlington, VA: Author.

National Hospice Organization. (1997b). *A pathway for patients and families facing terminal illness.* Arlington, VA: Author .

National Institutes of Health. (2000). National Institute on Aging. Research agenda for 2001–2005 [Electronic version]. Retrieved February 3, 2000 from http://www.nia.nih.gov/AboutNIA/StrategicPlan/

National Institutes of Health. National Institute of Aging. Complementary & alternative medicine information added to NIHSeniorHealth web site. Retrieved February 22, 2009 from http://www.nia.nih.gov/NewsAndEvents/PressReleases/PR-20081212CAM.htm

National Quality Forum. (NQF). (2006). *Framework and preferred practices for palliative and Hospice care quality: A consensus report.* Washington, DC: Author. Also available at www.qualityforum.org/publications/reports.

Office of Minority Health, Department of Health and Human Services. (2000). *National standards on culturally and linguistically appropriate services (CLAS) in health care.* Federal Register 65, 247 (*December 22*, 2000). Retrieved December 8, 2008 from http://www.ahrq.gov/fund/fr/fr122200.htm

Oncology Nursing Society . (2009). *Putting evidence into practice. Improving oncology patient outcomes.* Retrieved February 14, 2009 from http://www.ons.org/outcomes/pep.shtml

Panella, M., Marchisio, S., Barbieri, A., & Di Stanislao, F. (2008). A cluster randomized trial to assess the impact of clinical pathways for patients with stroke: Rationale and design of the Clinical Pathways for Effective and Appropriate Care Study [NCT00673491]. BMC Health Services Research, 8, 223. Retrieved February 5, 2009 from http://www.biomedcentral.com/1472–6963/8/223/abstract

Pirovano, M., Maltoni, M., Nanni, O., Marinari, M., Indelli, M., Zaninetta, G., et al. (1999). A new palliative prognostic score: A first step for the staging of terminally ill cancer patients. Italian multicenter and study group on palliative care. *Journal of Pain and Symptom Management, 17*, 231–239.

Plonk, W. M. Jr., & Arnold, R. M. (2005). Terminal care: The last weeks of life. *Journal of Palliative Medicine, 8*(5), 1042–1054.

Portenoy, R. K. (1998). Defining palliative care. Retrieved from http://www.stoppain.org

President's Commission for the Study of Ethical Problems in Medicine and Biomedical and Behavioral Research. (1994). *Deciding to forego life-sustaining treatment.* Washington, DC: U.S. Government Printing Office. Available from http://content.nejm.org/cgi/content/extract/330/21/1524

Quill, T. E. (1993). Doctor, I want to die. Will you help me? *Journal of the American Medical Association, 270*, 870–873.

Rearick, E. (2007). Enhancing success in transition service coordinators: Use of transformational leadership. *Professional Case Management, 12*(5), 283–287.

Rodriguez, K. L., Barnato, A. E., & Arnold, R. M. (2007). Perceptions and utilization of palliative care services in acute care hospitals. *Journal of Palliative Medicine, 10*(1), 99–110.

Schwarz, J. K. (1999). Assisted dying and nursing practice. *Image: Journal of Nursing Scholarship, 31*, 367–373.

Stevens, M. M., Dalla Pozza, L., Caelletto, B., Cooper, M. G., & Kilham, H. A. (1994). Pain and symptom control in pediatric palliative care. *Cancer Survey, 21*, 211–231.

Storey, P. (1996). *Primer of palliative care* (2nd ed.). Dubuque, IA: Kendall/Hunt.

SUPPORT Principal Investigators. (1995). A controlled trial to improve care for seriously ill hospitalized patients: The Study to Understand Prognoses and Preferences for Outcomes and Risks of Treatments (SUPPORT). *Journal of the American Medical Association, 274*, 1591–1598.

Tang, S. T. (2003). When death is imminent: Where terminally ill patients with cancer prefer to die and why. *Cancer Nursing, 26*, 245–251.

Teno, J. M., Clarridge, B. R., Casey V., Welch L. C., Wetle T., Shield, R., et al. (2004). Family perspectives on end-of-life care at the last place of care. *Journal of the American Medical Association, 291*(1), 88–93.

Twaddle, M. L., Maxwell, T. L., Cassel, J. B., Liao, S., Coyne, P. J., Usher, B. M., et al. (2007). Palliative care benchmarks from academic medical centers. *Journal of Palliative Medicine, 10*, 86–98.

Weeks, J., Cook, F., O'Day, S. J., Peterson, L., Wenger, N., Reding, D., et al. (1998). Relationship between cancer patients' predictions of prognosis and their treatment preferences. *Journal of the American Medical Association, 278*, 1709–1714.

Whitman, E. H. (1993). Terminal care of the dying child: Psychosocial implications of care. *Cancer, 71*, 3450–3462.

Wolfe, J., Holcombe, G. E., Klar, N., Levin, S., Ellenbogen, J. M., Salen-Schatz, S., et al. (2000). Symptoms and suffering at the end of life in children with cancer. *New England Journal of Medicine, 342*, 326–333.

World Health Organization. (WHO). (2002). *Palliative care.* Retrieved December 28, 2004 from http://www.who.int/cancer/palliative/en/

Wrede-Seaman, L. (2008). *Symptom management algorithms: A handbook for palliative care.* Yakima, WA: Intellicard.

Wysocki, A., & Bookbinder, M. (2005). Implementing clinical practice changes: A practical approach. *Home Health Care Management and Practice, 17*(6), 502–507.

The Nurse's Role in Interdisciplinary and Palliative Care

Lisa M. Krammer
Jeanne Martinez
Eileen A. Ring-Hurn
Mary Beth Williams

Key Points

- Palliative-care nursing utilizes the conceptual framework of "whole-person" suffering, which includes the physical, psychological, spiritual, and social dimensions.
- In order to deliver quality, comprehensive, whole-person care, the goals of curative and palliative care are woven together concurrently and delivered throughout the disease continuum.
- The foundation for the palliative care philosophy and palliative care nursing is family-centered care, where the patient and family rather than the disease are the primary focus.
- Excellent palliative care embraces cultural, ethnic, and faith differences and preferences while interweaving the principles of ethics, humanities, and human values into every patient and family care experience.
- A core value of palliative care is the commitment to collaborate through an interdisciplinary process. Understanding the distinction between interdisciplinary and multidisciplinary practice is imperative for successful delivery of palliative care.
- A dynamic and outcomes-orientated interdisciplinary team requires collaboration, leadership, coordinated decision making, and conflict resolution.
- The palliative-care nurse and advanced-practice nurse combine the science of nursing with ethics, philosophy, the humanities, diverse worldviews, and individual and family life experiences in order to provide exceptional palliative care to families who are coping with a life-threatening illness.

Case Study: Ms. K. is a divorced 58-year-old woman with metastatic ovarian cancer with malignant bowel obstruction transitioning out of the hospital to home. One year ago, she was diagnosed with stage III ovarian cancer, and completed aggressive radiation and chemotherapy treatment. After treatment, Ms. K. had some fatigue and weight loss, but was otherwise symptom-free for most of the past 6 months. Five days ago, she was admitted to the hospital with nausea, projectile vomiting, and severe abdominal pain. She was diagnosed with a partial bowel obstruction, secondary to recurrence of her cancer. She was initially treated with a nasogastric (NG) tube, intravenous octreotide, and opioids for pain. On day 4, Ms. K. requested removal of the NG tube, because "the tube hurts worse than my stomach pain did." After much discussion, the nurse practitioner (NP) caring for Ms. K. advocated for NG removal, with continuation of the palliative medication, but expressed her concern to Ms. K. that she could begin frequent vomiting again after the tube removal. Ms. K. said she understood, but wanted to continue only the medication. Subsequent nursing reports focused on monitoring and reducing Ms. K.'s episodes of vomiting after removal of the NG tube. Ms. K continued to experience 1–2 episodes of vomiting every 24 hours.

On her next assessment, the NP asked Ms. K what else she needed. Ms. K. said, "I need to get home as soon as possible." The NP asked about her sense of urgency, as the vomiting was still not under control. Ms. K replied, "I feel so much better having the tube out, and just vomiting one time per day or so. I also don't have much time left. I want to label all of my things at home to give away, so there is no fighting among my family. And I need to list out important prayers and songs for my funeral. My son is in the Army, and I don't want to burden him with these decisions." She added tearfully, "I'm not sure I will even see him again."

Introduction

In assessing a patient with advanced illness and acute, severe symptoms, it is important that goals of care, which encompass physical, spiritual, and psychosocial issues, are addressed. Once immediate physical symptoms are managed or improved, nursing and the rest of the interdisciplinary team (IDT) needs to elicit the patient's goals of care, in order to most efficiently implement a care plan that reflects the patient's priorities. This chapter will describe the significance of the IDT process and the fundamental elements of effective IDT process. Also, the complex dimensions within nursing roles involved in successful family care at the end of life are presented.

PALLIATIVE CARE FAMEWORKS

Conceptual Model of Care

In order to relieve suffering, palliative care nursing utilizes a conceptual framework for end-of-life care practice. An effective model of care for the delivery of palliative nursing, adapted from hospice nursing, is Dame Cicely Saunder's conceptual model of "whole person" suffering. Saunders espouses that whole-person suffering has four dimensions: physical, psychological, spiritual, and social (Krammer, Muir, Gooding-Kellar, Williams, & von Gunten, 1999; Mount, Hanks, & McGoldrick, 2006). Under this concept, suffering affects each domain of the bio-psycho–social–spiritual aspects of care. This conceptual model forms the basis for the description of palliative care nursing practice in this chapter.

Delivery Model of Care

Within the traditional medical model of care lies a perceived dichotomy between curative/death-defying care and palliative care. It is almost as though the goal of care is *first* and *only* cure, then only if unable to cure, to relieve suffering. Often, this perceived dichotomy prevents or delays the introduction of palliative care measures for patients and their families. In order to provide quality, comprehensive, whole-person care, should not the goals of curative and palliative care be woven together concurrently? It would seem to be generally appropriate to relieve suffering *at the same time* as pursuing curative life-prolonging therapies (Ferrell et al., 2007; Von Gunten & Muir, 2000).

An effective framework for the delivery of palliative care throughout the disease continuum can be most readily visualized as an "umbrella of care." Debate exists as to the beginning and end of the umbrella's arch. For some healthcare clinicians, palliative care starts with the initial diagnosis of an illness, at which time the management of symptoms and the psychosocial stressors of the disease upon the patient and family are vigorously addressed with active curative-focused therapy. Although this scope may be considered ideal, the majority of palliative care providers emphasize the maximization of function and quality of life in those with far-advanced disease. For all providers, palliative care culminates in the management of complex physical, psychological, social, and spiritual issues that patients and members of their families will experience during the final phase of life and will include bereavement care for the family (Krammer et al., 1999; Twycross, 2003).

With the emergence of palliative care as a distinct medical specialty (Cairms & Yates, 2003; Leslie, Adams, & Canter, 2002; Von Gunten & Lupu, 2004), an ever growing number of hospitals have begun to develop comprehensive, academic palliative care progra1ms (El Sayem et al., 2004; Ferrell et al., 2007; Morrison, Maroney-Galin, Kralovec & Meier, 2005), consisting of one or all of the following program elements: acute palliative care inpatient units (Ferrell et al., 2007; Santa-Emma, Roach, Gill, Spayde & Taylor, 2002); palliative consultation teams (Ferrell et al., 2007; Virik & Glare, 2002); outpatient palliative care clinics (Strasser et al., 2004) and home hospice programs. This programmatic approach allows patients with advanced progressive disease and their families to have access to palliative care expertise in all settings, including the acute care hospital, out-patient clinic, home, or nursing home. With a comprehensive palliative care program, the IDT will utilize the same philosophy and model of care as they work throughout the continuum with the patient and family in a coordinated and collaborative manner to achieve mutually established goals.

PRINCIPLES OF PALLIATIVE CARE

A core principle of palliative care across the entire disease spectrum and in all settings is the concept that the patient and family constitute the unit of care. The patient and family, rather than the disease, are the primary focus of care. The constructs of family-centered care form the foundation of the palliative care philosophy. Palliative care addresses the meaning of disease, suffering, life, and death within the context of each family unit (National Consensus Project, 2009). Palliative care recognizes that each family member will experience the disease process and all of its implications within the context of his or her particular worldview, and individual care plans are developed to reflect these world-views.

Another core palliative care principle is the commitment to collaborate through an IDT process (Cairms & Yates, 2003; Leslie et al., 2002; Meier & Beresford, 2008; National Consensus Project, 2009). In order to facilitate a family in crisis to establish and then achieve mutually agreed upon goals, the palliative care team integrates and coordinates the assessment and interventions of each team member and creates a comprehensive plan of care. Good palliative care is significant in the manner in which it embraces cultural, ethnic, and faith differences and preferences, while interweaving the principles of ethics, humanities, and human values into every patient- and family-care experience (Loscalzo & Zabora, 1998; Morrison & Meier, 2004; Rosen, 1998).

Further, clinical ethics is an essential footprint for the provision of end-of-life care. Whereas clinicians often learn the *theoretical* principles behind ethics (Beauchamp, 2003; Beauchamp & Childress, 1994; Morrison & Meier, 2004), palliative care necessitates that these principles be incorporated into the practice or "put into motion" 24 hours a day, 7 days a week (Block, 2007; Roy & MacDonald, 1998). Palliative care embodies this concept of "ethics in motion" (C. Muir, personal communication, September 12, 2008), as each IDT member, including patient and families, contemplate the ethical questions in advanced disease and in end-of-life decision making. Ethical challenges present themselves to the palliative care IDT on an hourly basis. The following vignettes are a sampling of the ethical issues faced by the IDT in routine daily practice.

Professional Boundaries

Ms. D. is a 35-year-old patient, admitted to the palliative care unit for the third time in the past 2 months. Ms. D. was diagnosed with breast cancer 3 years ago. She is now admitted for terminal delirium. She is expected to die this admission. One staff nurse who has cared for her on the three previous admissions has become very close to the patient and family. She tells the staff that she will be visiting the patient on her day off, and she is to be called at any time if the patient's status changes. She has given her home phone number to the family, promising to be there at the time of the patient's death. Are the nurse's actions appropriate? How should other members of the palliative care team respond to the nurse's request to be called? Should the patient's and family's desires about the nurse's presence be considered in deciding the appropriate boundaries of professional staff?

Physician-Assisted Suicide

Mr. S., diagnosed with head and neck cancer, was admitted to the palliative care unit 3 weeks ago. Upon admission, he was found to have increased somnolence, dyspnea, fever, tachycardia, and low blood pressure. The tumor on his right neck recurred about 2 months ago. At that time, the patient received radiation for palliation. However, since then the tumor has continued to grow through the skin and is now visible, about 12 cm in diameter, with a strong odor. The patient's wife of 47 years has been managing her husband's care at home, but now finds it difficult to move him, and distressing to do his dressing changes. Upon admission, the staff prepared the family that the patient may be imminently dying. However, Mr. S.'s condition became relatively stable after completing a short course of IV antibiotics. He remains somnolent and bedridden, but is arousable when spoken to. The nurses have begun to have difficulty caring for him; for example, the odor has increased and pieces of the patient's neck flesh and ear have been coming off with each dressing change. The nurses have begun to express feelings of helplessness, wondering why this patient "is taking so long to die". They feel particularly bad for his elderly wife who takes two buses to the hospital to see her husband every day. One nurse expressed that "if there is any patient who needed physician-assisted suicide, it is Mr. S." In retrospect, should Mr. S. have been treated with antibiotics? What is the best way for the nurses to manage their feelings about caring for Mr. S.? And who is suffering the most in this situation-Mr. S., his wife, or the nursing staff?

Autonomy in Decision Making

Mr. L. is a 60-year-old widower diagnosed with recurrent colon cancer. He is in the final stages of dying and unable to communicate. Mr. L. has been in hospice care, and was admitted to a hospice bed in the hospital 2 days ago. A few months after his diagnosis, Mr. L. had previously completed a living will indicating that he did not want any heroic measures at the end of life. He also completed and signed documents appointing a close friend to be his power of attorney for health affairs. At that time, Mr. L. informed this friend that he and his attending physician had agreed to a Do-Not-Resuscitate (DNR) status when his disease no longer responded to treatment. Mr. L.'s 31-year-old son has now arrived from out of state to visit his father in the hospital. He is very upset that his father is in a hospice bed and is a DNR status. He is requesting that the DNR order be rescinded, and his father transferred to another unit in the hospital where he will be "actively treated." What rights does the patient's son have in making decisions for his father? Is the healthcare team obligated to follow the patient's living will when the patient can no longer make his own decisions? What is the role of this power of attorney? Each member of the IDT has a unique relationship with, and view of, the patient and family. These varied perspectives reveal vital information that is invaluable when identifying and clarifying potential conflicts and facilitating resolution. It is through the use of an IDT process that each ethical issue in palliative care is collaboratively and interdependently addressed and evaluated.

THE INTERDISCIPLINARY TEAM

Palliative care's reliance upon the IDT as a key factor for successful outcomes requires an understanding of the distinction between interdisciplinary and multidisciplinary practice. In the traditional multidisciplinary team, the physician primarily directs care of the patient, and the family needs may or may not be considered (see Table 5.1). Multiple disciplines of the health care

team may be involved in the individual assessments and in the delivery of care, although efforts by these team members are often uncoordinated and independent. The primary mode of communication between disciplines is the medical chart. The result is often incomplete communication between professions, lack of accountability, and a tendency for each discipline to develop its own patient care goals. Family needs are often unidentified and most often are not incorporated into the overall plan of care.

In contrast, in an interdisciplinary model, communication and decision making between team members is collaborative, with leadership shared and based upon primary patient and family needs and goals (Crawford & Price, 2003). The identity of the IDT supersedes personal identities and agendas (Cummings, 1998; Porchet, 2006), and the concept of the "sum of the whole is greater than its parts" is valued and respected. The interdisciplinary model facilitates team members to 1) directly interact with the patient and family, 2) share information among team members, 3) provide consultation to one another, and 4) work interdependently together in order to achieve the goals identified by the patient and family.

Table 5.1 lists the most common members of the palliative care IDT, explains their functions within the team, and discusses their interrelationships with the palliative care nurse. As a coordinator of care and a core member of the IDT, the nurse has the responsibility to spearhead the development of therapeutic relationships, not just between herself and the patient and family, but also with all pertinent members of the team, which in turn ensures effective and goal-driven supportive communication and patient outcomes. The palliative care nurse needs to continually reassess the goals of the patient and family, their treatment preferences, and support. A hallmark of quality palliative care is the collaborative role that the nurse develops with the physician and other IDT members. Often, the physician has had a long-term relationship with the patient and family, and as the needs for traditional medical-model "curative" care lessen and palliative care measures increase, this may represent a "loss" for the physician. As the nurse develops a relationship with the patient and family, the collaborative relationship with the physician may also be a source of support for the physician personally as well as professionally for decision making. The nurse is a primary conduit for information, critical assessments, and evaluation of the patient and family goals within the IDT. A critical aspect of palliative care involves the identification and subsequent resolution of often divergent goals of the patient, family, or the healthcare team. The palliative care nurse is often in the ideal position to be instrumental in coordinating and effecting a comprehensive family-focused plan of care.

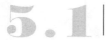

| | The Interdisciplinary Team (IDT) Member's Role, Function, and Interrelationship with the Palliative Care (PC) Nurse |

ADVANCED PRACTICE NURSE

Function: Incorporates the role of advanced clinician, educator, researcher, and consultant to families, staff, colleagues, and communities. *Interrelationship:* Acts as a consultant, educator, role model, and mentor to the PC nurse to synergistically achieve quality outcomes for patients and families.

BEREAVEMENT COUNSELOR

Function: Identifies through IDT assessment high-risk family members for bereavement and provides anticipatory grief counseling. Coordinates bereavement services for families including counseling sessions, grief support groups, memorial services, and community outreach programs. *Interrelationship:* Relies on the PC nurse assessment of the family upon a patient's death in order to begin bereavement care. Values the PC nurse's role in identifying high-risk family members for grief and bereavement.

PATIENT/FAMILY

Function: The focus of care of the IDT. The goals identified by the patient/family direct the participation of other members of the team. *Interrelationship:* The patient/family understands that the PC nurse is the coordinator of interdisciplinary care and continuously confers with the PC nurse regarding patient/family needs.

PALLIATIVE CARE PHYSICIAN

Function: Consults with primary care physician and collaborates with IDT to provide expertise in pain management, communication, and treatment decisions at the end of life for patients and families. *Interrelationship:* Understands that the PC nurse has the greatest prolonged contact with the patient and family and relies upon the holistic assessment and interventions of the nurse in order to develop a comprehensive medical care plan in collaboration with the IDT.

PASTORAL CARE COUNSELOR

Function: Provides in-depth assessment of the spiritual needs of patient/family including search for meaning and purpose of life. Acts as a liaison with community clergy and a resource for the IDT regarding ethical questions, faith traditions, and world religions. *Interrelationship:* Respects the spiritual assessment of the PC nurse and is consulted when family issues require advanced assessment and intervention. Acts as a resource for PC nurse when needing to debrief after a difficult death or experience.

PRIMARY CARE PHYSICIAN

Function: Initiates a relationship with the palliative care team with referral of a new patient/family. Provides a medical history of the patient's illness and any other pertinent medical and psychosocial information; continues to be the primary physician or transfers the role to the PC physician. *Interrelationship:* Assessments and interventions of the PC nurse and those of the IDT are coordinated with the primary physician to establish a comprehensive plan of care for the patient and family.

SOCIAL WORKER

Function: Provides history (via genogram) regarding the strengths, resources, and realities of patient/family system. Interventions include emotional support through individual, family, high-risk, and bereavement counseling. Provides referrals for families to the community as needed for social services. *Interrelationship:* Delivery of care involves ongoing collaboration with PC nurse who is continuously identifying psychosocial needs and outcomes of the patient and family.

THE RAPIES (PHARMACY, OCCUPATIONAL, PHYSICAL, DIETARY, SPEECH, ART, MUSIC, TOUCH, MASSAGE)

Function: Provide education and/or "hands-on" therapy of specialized discipline to maximize independence and quality of life of patient and family. *Interrelationship:* Participates in plan of care when consulted by PC nurse and reports outcomes of interventions through collaboration with the PC nurse.

(Continued)

Table 5.1 *(Continued)*

VOLUNTEER
Function: Gives of time freely to contribute to patient and family needs by direct service, administrative support of the palliative care program, public relations, and community education. *Interrelationship:* Reports observed family dynamics to PC nurse in order to revise plan of care if needed.

VOLUNTEER COORDINATOR
Function: Recruits, screens, educates, supervises, and retains volunteer staff to provide supportive services to patients and families. *Interrelationship:* Plans assignments of volunteers based upon identified needs of family by PC nurse; Involves PC nurse in volunteer training.

Characteristics of an Effective Interdisciplinary Team

A dynamic and outcomes-oriented IDT requires collaboration, leadership, coordinated decision making, and conflict resolution. Collaboration is defined as the ability to work with others, especially on intellectual endeavors (Merriam-Webster, 2008). It is the process of collaboration that empowers team members to act as decision makers within the group. For example, if a question on nausea and vomiting arises, various members of the team may provide observations and opinions in an effort to maximize the relief of all components of nausea and vomiting. Using a true collaborative process, the ultimate decision maker regarding this aspect of care would not come to a conclusion solely benefiting one member or one member's own perspective, but rather would make a decision reflecting the team's total input. Through collaboration, effective patient- and family-driven quality outcomes are achieved (Porter-O'Grady, Alexander, & Minkara, 2006).

The principles and tenets of palliative care are applicable throughout one's lifespan. From the very young to the elderly, each group faces unique circumstances as they endure a life-limiting illness (Bolmsjo 2008; Browning & Solomon, 2005; Himelstein, Hilden, Morstad Boldt & Weissman, 2004; Kapo, Morrison, & Liao 2007; Malloy, Sumner, Virani & Ferrell, 2007). An effective IDT will attend to these particular needs and will include specialists as warranted by the distinctive characteristics of the patient and family. For example, in the setting of a pediatric patient, in addition to the core IDT members, the IDT may consist of pediatric specialists such as child life specialists, pediatric advanced practice nurses, and chaplains trained in pediatrics; whereas an elderly patient's IDT may include, among others, physical and occupational therapists trained in the aging population, a geriatrician, and a geriatric nurse practitioner. It is the responsibility of the IDT to continually assess and make changes in the IDT members as appropriate.

Palliative care differs from the traditional medical model in which the physician is the sole leader of the multidisciplinary team. In the palliative care model, leadership is filled by the member of the IDT who is best educated and qualified to address and focus upon specific patient or family goals. In addition to achieving patient and family outcomes, leadership is essential to facilitate and optimize the professional potential of each team member's contribution (National Consensus Project, 2009).

Also, in the traditional multidisciplinary team, the physician, as team leader, is the primary decision maker for the care team. In contrast, in a true IDT process, coordinated decision making among team members is necessary to achieve quality patient and family outcomes. In order to sort out which member or members of the team would be the most appropriate in contributing to the decision-making process, the following questions, should be considered: "Who has the information necessary to make the decision?" "Who needs to be consulted before the decision is made?" "Who needs to be informed of a decision after it is made?" (Cummings, 1998; Porchet, 2006). Certain levels of decision making may be made by individual members of the team (e.g., titrating a pain medication based on patient needs), whereas other levels will require the input from the entire team as a whole (e.g., developing a care plan). Poor, fragmented decision making results from failure to include appropriate team members in the decision-making process (Cummings, 1998; Porchet, 2006).

Due to the interdependency among IDT members, professional conflict will inevitably arise, which may be beneficial and stimulating to an IDT. Respect and trust in each team member's skills, knowledge, expertise, and motivation are imperative. Lack of respectful conflict will result in group uniformity, which may stifle the creativity and the professional advancement and development of team members. Diverse ideas and opinions are often the impetus for innovative solutions for patient care problems, and in the process may deepen the professional dialogue within the team. However, conflict becomes destructive when it is personalized or viewed as a threat to a member's role. Thus, the art in managing conflict is not to avoid it, but to manage it effectively so that team members, patients, and families can receive its full benefits.

THE DEVELOPING ROLE IN NURSING IN PALLIATIVE CARE

In the book *Intimate Death,* de Hennezel writes:

"When death comes so close, and sadness and suffering rule, there is still room for life, and joy, and surges of feeling deeper and more intense than anything known before . . . to witness the preciousness of these last moments of life and to the extraordinary privilege of being able to share them has some value . . . to deepen our respect for the value of life itself" (de Hennezel, 1997).

In order to identify the essence of palliative care nursing, the values and beliefs of the role of the palliative care nurse and the qualities and themes inherent to the person that provides end-of-life care are to be delineated. As deHennezel describes it, working with patients at the end of their lives and with the families who are adjusting to illness and eventual loss enables those who work with these families not only to learn about the value of life but also to transform themselves continuously in the process.

The palliative care nurse combines the science of nursing with ethics, philosophy, the humanities, diverse worldviews, and individual and family life experiences in order to provide holistic care to families who are coping with a life-limiting illness.

THE NURSE'S ROLE IN INTERDISCIPLINARY CARE

The following case example is that of an advanced-practice nurse (APN) bringing a specific and well-defined set of qualities, knowledge, and judgments to caring for individuals and families at the end of life. This includes advanced scientific and biophysical knowledge, analytical skills, and mastery of a broad repertoire of communication and interpersonal skills. Specialized knowledge and proficiency in the ability to incorporate ethics, humanities, cultural diversity, family, spiritual, and psychological issues into care is also demanded (Coyne, 2003; Kuebler, 2003; Meier & Beresford, 2006).

The Calkin model of advanced nursing practice (Bryant-Lukosius, 2004; Spross & Baggerly, 1989) serves as an excellent model on which to base palliative care advanced practice nursing. Calkin defines the clinical judgment abilities of three nursing practice levels as novice, expert by experience, and the master's-prepared nurse. The following case study illustrates Saunder's four dimensions of human suffering within the context of Calkin's model. The case study also will demonstrate the APN sub-roles of expert clinician, educator, consultant, researcher, and collaborator (Chulk, 2008; Spross & Baggerly, 1989).

Clinical Case Study: A Woman with Neuropathic Pain Secondary to Metastatic Breast Cancer: Mrs. S. is a 52-year-old woman who is suffering from the sequelae of stage 4 metastatic breast cancer for the past 3 years. All curative interventions including surgical resection, chemotherapy, radiotherapy, hormone therapy, and experimental therapy have failed to halt the progression of her disease, which now affects her lung, liver, and bones, most notably her spine. Mrs. S.'s major distressing physical symptom is severe neuropathic pain, which radiates around her back to her abdomen. This pain has limited her ability to bathe, cook, eat, get dressed, and walk. Essentially all activities of daily living have been stripped from her and she is now confined to bed under the care of her husband. Prior to her cancer, she prided herself in being extremely independent. Currently, her neuropathic pain is being managed by steroids, tricyclic antidepressants, neuroleptics, and methadone. Mrs. S. has two teenage children, and has been on disability from her job as a television personality for the past several months. She is Baptist and is an active member in her church.

Assessment of the Patient and Family

Through daily interactions with Mrs. S. and her family, the APN on the palliative care unit built a therapeutic relationship that focused on all dimensions of human suffering: physical, psychological, spiritual, and psychosocial. Despite the aggressive titration of pharmacotherapy being used to treat Mrs. S.'s pain, she continued to suffer from intense neuropathic discomfort. Her pain rating consistently was 8/10 or above on a visual analog scale, and over time her sense of despair about dying in such agony was increasing. In consultation with other IDT members, the APN was analyzing current research and consulting with other pain experts for novel approaches in treating neuropathic pain. The use of intravenous lidocaine has successfully worked in similar scenarios, and after critical analysis by the APN, the IDT decided to try this therapy. The APN presented all the literature regarding the use of intravenous lidocaine in refractory neuropathic pain to the hospital's quality committee. The committee granted permission for immediate use as long as the APN would commit to developing and implementing an institutional policy in the near future. The APN quickly developed an evidence-based guideline, as the neuropathic pain was escalating daily. The next step was to educate all team members, specifically the nursing and pharmacy staff, as well as the patient and family about the etiology, sequelae, and rationale for choosing this intervention. Mrs. S. received a test dose of the lidocaine and her pain decreased about 10% within 1 hour. Thus, the intravenous lidocaine was deemed appropriate to continue. Over the next days, her pain level decreased to 2/10. Respecting the value of non-pharmacological measures in relieving pain, the APN assisted in having Mrs. S. be offered massage and music therapy. She declined guided imagery.

While Mrs. S. was experiencing her pain crisis, the APN spent a lot of time with her, thus allowing an opportunity for Mrs. S. to express her feelings and fears. She revealed that she felt close to death and was struggling with guilt about one of her desires upon dying-that of spending her last minutes alone, if possible. She was fearful that this request would offend her very protective and involved family. But she had lived a very independent life and wanted to die that way. The APN listened, reflected, and assessed the situation and reported her findings to the IDT. Based on the APN's observations and recommendations, the IDT members set forth a plan to help Mrs. S. and her family deal with these very important issues. Social work and chaplaincy intensified their involvement.

Through interventions by the IDT, Mrs. S.'s family was learning to become more comfortable with respecting their mother's request and were working through their feelings of "abandoning" their wife and mother in time of need. This would continue to be a process.

With in-depth knowledge of family systems theory, the APN identified the need for the IDT to address the already actualized loss of Mrs. S.'s role within the family, including mother and wife. The APN consulted the bereavement counselor as an early intervention for high-risk grief status, as Mrs. S.'s family was still dealing with their loved one's request of dying alone.

Progressively, Mrs. S. showed signs and symptoms of nearing death. As her pain increased, the APN adjusted Mrs. S.'s pain regimen so that she would remain comfortable. The APN and the IDT increased support to Mrs. S.'s family to help them honor her wish at the time of death.

Discussion of the APN Role

Clinician. The APN utilized sophisticated and appropriate assessment strategies to evaluate pain and symptoms. The APN interfaced with other IDT members to develop and implement a comprehensive plan of care. The APN identified novel approaches to the treatment of neuropathic pain and developed hospital-based standards of care to reflect and support this treatment strategy, and executed interventions. Advanced clinical knowledge of complex pain syndromes and comfort measures to address symptoms was demonstrated through utilization of innovative, ethically sound, scientifically based practice.

Educator. The APN facilitated complex philosophical, ethical, and clinical management discussions, assisting the patient and family and all IDT members to achieve a positive outcome. The APN assessed the learning needs of Mrs. S. and her family and the entire staff. The APN presented scientifically based education on the following issues: 1) the management of neuropathic pain, 2) potential for role conflict, 3) actual loss/anticipatory grief, and 4) potential for high-risk bereavement. The APN educated other disciplines also, for example, the quality committee and pharmacy staff, through inservice and guidelines on the philosophy of palliative care and individualized treatment strategies, and most notably, the use of intravenous lidocaine for intractable neuropathic pain.

Researcher. The APN generated new knowledge through identifying research questions and by instituting novel approaches that address these questions. The APN investigated and integrated palliative care research strategies, for example, the use of intravenous lidocaine, to formulate an individualized plan of care for Mrs. S.

Collaborator. The APN mentored staff in bio-psychosocial and spiritual assessments and interventions. The APN built and preserved collaborative relationships, and identified resources and opportunities to work with palliative care colleagues. The APN facilitated the development and implementation of staff forums, inservices, physician/nurse collaboration, and quality committee consultation. The APN demonstrated the value of collaboration with the patient and family, the IDT, and other healthcare professionals in order to facilitate the best possible outcome.

Consultant. The APN consulted with the palliative care physician, palliative care colleagues, and quality committee representatives to determine the appropriate treatment strategies for meeting the needs of the patient and family. Also, the bereavement counselor was consulted after the APN identified the actualized loss experienced by Mrs. S.'s family. As a consultant, the APN was consistently available to the patient and family, IDT members, and other healthcare professionals to discuss and explain issues surrounding the palliative care philosophy. By maintaining a consistent presence with the patient and family and among IDT members, the APN helped to minimize decision-making conflicts. With advanced knowledge in the humanities, the APN through language and image gave expression to the experience of illness, death, grief, and human suffering.

CONTINUING PROFESSIONAL EDUCATION

Knowledge, public opinion, and changes in healthcare are generating rapid changes and developments in the area of how we understand and treat patients and families who face life-threatening illnesses. In order to fulfill the constantly expanding responsibilities of a palliative care nurse, the nurse is challenged to keep well informed of new developments in bioethics, symptom management, family care, and public policy. Various forums and educational resources are available to support the palliative care nurse in keeping abreast of evolving issues in palliative care. Participation in professional societies (e.g., Hospice and Palliative Care Nurses Association) and continuing education strategies (journals, national conferences, etc.) along with attainment of specialty certification (for instance, National Board for Certification of Hospice and Palliative Nurses) collectively enhances the palliative care nurse's ability to deliver quality bio-psychosocial and spiritual care for patients and families.

CONCLUSION AND FUTURE DIRECTION

Palliative care is an emerging specialty within healthcare, especially nursing. The philosophy and delivery of palliative care transcends all areas of nursing where suffering accompanies illness. The palliative care nurse is a true leader within the IDT and hence is in an ideal position to establish standards for consistent practice, foster education, and promote research. It is a professional privilege to be in the field of palliative care nursing, as it brings hopefulness to areas of end-of-life care that traditionally have been avoided: for example, ethics, pain, and human suffering. Equally applicable to the art of palliative care nursing practice is Thoreau (1943) prose in which he states: "It is something to be able to paint a picture, or to carve a statue, and to make a few objects beautiful. But it is far more glorious to carve and paint the atmosphere in which we work, to affect the quality of the day-this is the highest of the arts" (p. 90).

Case Study conclusion: Mrs. S's death occurred without pain and she was able to spend the last minutes of her life by herself, as requested. Through the coordinated efforts of the IDT, Mrs. S's family was able to begin to work through their feelings of having abandoned their loved one in the last moments of life and giving her a final gift: death by her terms with dignity, respect, comfort, and adoration. Mrs. S's family has agreed to participate actively in bereavement counseling to continue to work on the issues surrounding the death and how it impacts their grieving process.

EVIDENCE-BASED PRACTICE

There is paucity among research studies that demonstrate the importance of the nurse's role as a member of the interdisciplinary palliative care team. Further research is definitely warranted. Additionally, there is a modest amount of scientific data demonstrating the positive impact of an IDT on patient care. The data are summarized as follows:

- Gade et al. (2008) conducted a randomized controlled trial to measure the impact of an interdisciplinary palliative care service (IPCS) on patient satisfaction, clinical outcomes, and cost of care for 6 months post-hospital discharge. Five hundred and seventeen patients with life-limiting illnesses were included. The measures for the study included the Modified City of Hope Patient Questionnaire, total healthcare costs, hospice utilization, and survival. The study demonstrated that patients reported greater satisfaction with their healthcare experience and providers, had lower healthcare costs, and had fewer intensive care unit admission upon readmission.
- Jack, Hillier, Williams, and Oldham (2004) conducted an evaluation study which demonstrated that the input from a palliative care team resulted in improvements in patient's insight into their diagnosis. A nonequivalent control group design was utilized. One hundred cancer patients were investigated via a quota sample, where 50 patients received hospital palliative care team interventions and 50 patients received traditional care. Outcomes were assessed on three occasions via a self-report tool. A supplementary qualitative assessment was conducted.
- Jack, Hillier, Williams, and Oldham (2003) reported that hospital patients who utilized interventions from a palliative care team experienced a significantly greater improvement in their symptoms. A nonequivalent control group design was utilized using a quota sample to investigate 100 cancer patients. 50 patients received palliative care team intervention and 50 patients received traditional care. Data was collected using a self-report tool on three separate occasions."
- Schrader et al. (2002) conducted a hospital-based study which demonstrated that palliative care teams are beneficial and enhance end-of-life care experiences. A convenience sample of 50 hospitalized patients was used, various palliative care interventions were introduced, and data was obtained via self-reports. Statistically significant improvements were found in pain levels, non-pain symptoms, quality of life and perceptions of communication, and overall treatment.

REFERENCES

Beauchamp, T. L., & Childress, J. F. (1994). *The principles of biomedical ethics* (4th ed.). Oxford, UK: Oxford University Press.

Beauchamp, T. L. (2003). Methods and principles in biomedical ethics. *British Medical Journal, 29,* 269–274.

Block, S. D. (2007). Clinical and ethical issues in palliative care. *Focus, 5,* 393–397.

Bolmsjo, I. A. (2008). Review article: End-of-life care for old people: A review of the literature. *American Journal of Hospice and Palliative Medicine, 25,* 328–338.

Browning, D. M., & Solomon, M. Z. (2005). The initiative for pediatric palliative care: An interdisciplinary educational approach for healthcare professionals. *Journal of Pediatric Nursing, 20,* 326–334.

Bryant-Lukosius, D. (2004). Advanced practice nursing roles: Development, implementation and evaluation. *Journal of Advanced Nursing, 48,* 519–529.

Cairms, W., & Yates, P. M. (2003). Education and training in palliative care. *Medical Journal of Australia, 179* (1), 26–28.

Chulk, P. (2008).Clinical nurse specialists and quality patient care. *Journal of Advanced Nursing, 26,* 501–506.

Coyne, P. (2003). The evolution of the advanced practice nurse within palliative care. *Journal of Palliative Medicine, 6,* 769–770.

Crawford, G. B., & Price, S. D. (2003). Team working: Palliative care as a model of interdisciplinary practice. *Medical Journal of Australia, 179,* S32–S34.

Cummings, I. (1998). The interdisciplinary team. In D. Doyle, G. Hanks & N. Mac-Donald (Eds.), *Oxford textbook of palliative medicine* (2nd ed., pp. 3–8). Oxford, UK: Oxford University Press.

de Hennezel, M. (1997). *Intimate death.* New York: Vintage Books.

El Sayem, A., Swint, K., Fisch, M. J., Palmer, J. L., Reddy, S., Walker, P., et al. (2004). Palliative care inpatient service in a comprehensive cancer center: Clinical and financial outcomes. *Journal of Clinical Oncology, 22,* 2008–2014.

Ferrell, B., Connor, S. R., Cordes, A., Dahlin, C. M., Fine, P. G., Hurron, N., et al. (2007). The national agenda for quality palliative care: The national consensus project and the national quality forum. *Journal of Pain and Symptom Management, 33,* 737–744.

Gade, G., Venohr, I., Conner, D., McGrady, K., Beane, J., Richardson, R. H., et al. (2008). Impact of an inpatient palliative care team: A randomized control trial. *Journal of Palliative Medicine, 11,* 180–190.

Himelstein, M. D., Hilden, M. D., Morstad Boldt, M. S. & Weissman, M. D. (2004). Pediatric palliative care. *New England Journal of Medicine, 350,* 1752–1762.

Jack, B., Hillier, V., Williams, A., & Oldham, J. (2004). Hospital based palliative care teams improve the insight of cancer patients into their disease. *Palliative Medicine, 18,* 46-52.

Jack, B., Hillier, V., Williams, A., & Oldham, J. (2003). Hospital based palliative care teams improve the symptoms of cancer patients. *Palliative Medicine, 17,* 498–502.

Kapo, J., Morrison, L. J., & Liao, S. (2007). Palliative care for the older adult. *Journal of Palliative Medicine, 10,* 185–209.

Krammer, L. M., Muir, J. C., Gooding-Kellar, N., Williams, M. B., & von Gunten, C. F. (1999). Palliative care and oncology: Opportunities for oncology nursing. *Oncology Nursing Updates, 6*(3), 1–12.

Kuebler, K. (2003). The palliative care advanced practice nurse. *Journal of Palliative Medicine, 6,* 707–714.

Leslie, B., Adams, L., & Canter, J. S. (2002). Integrating an end of life curriculum into the internal medicine clerkship. *Journal of Palliative Medicine, 5,* 752–753.

Loscalzo, M. J., & Zabora, J. R. (1998). Care of the cancer patient: Response of family and staff. In R. K. Portenoy & E. Bruera, (Eds.), *Topics in palliative care* (Vol. 2, pp. 209–245). Oxford, UK: Oxford University Press.

Malloy, P., Sumner, E., Virani, R. & Ferrell, B. (2007). End-of-life nursing education consortium for pediatric palliative care (ELNEC-PPC). *American Journal of Maternal Child Nursing, 32,* 303–304.

Meier, D.E., Beresford, L. (2008). The palliative care team. *Journal of Palliative Medicine, 11,* 677–681.

Meier, D. E., Beresford, L. (2006). Advanced practice nurses in palliative care: A pivotal role and perspective. *Journal of Palliative Medicine, 9,* 624–627.

Merriam-Webster. (2008). *Merriam-Webster's collegiate dictionary* (10th ed.). Springfield, MA: Merriam-Webster.

Morrison, R., Maroney-Galin, C., Kralovec, P. D. & Meier, D. E. (2005). The growth of palliative care programs in United States Hospitals. *Journal of Palliative Medicine, 8,* 1127–1134.

Morrison, R., & Meier, D. E. (2004). Palliative care. *The New England Journal of Medicine, 350,* 2582–2590.

Mount, B., Hanks, G., & McGoldrick, L. (2006). The principles of palliative care. In M. Fallon & G. Hanks (Eds.), *ABC of palliative care* (2nd ed., pp. 1–4). Oxford: Blackwell publishing.

National Consensus Project. (2009). *Guidelines.* Retrieved 5/28/09 from http://www.nationalconsensusproject.org

Porchet, F. (2006). Interdisciplinary communication. In F. Steifel (Ed.), *Communication in cancer care* (pp. 81–90). Berlin, Heidelberg, New York: Springer.

Porter-O'Grady, T., Alexander, D. R., & Minkara, N. (2006). Constructing a team model: Creating a foundation for evidence-based teams. *Nursing Administration Quarterly, 30,* 211–220.

Rosen, E. J. (1998). *Families facing death: A guide for healthcare professionals and volunteers* (Rev. ed.). San Francisco, CA: Jossey-Bass.

Roy, D. J., & MacDonald, N. (1998). Ethical issues in palliative care. In D. Doyle, G. Hanks, & N. MacDonald (Eds.), *Oxford textbook of palliative medicine* (2nd ed., pp. 97–138). Oxford, UK: Oxford University Press.

Santa-Emma, P., Roach, R., Gill, M. A., Spayde, P., & Taylor, R. (2002). Development and implementation of an inpatient acute palliative care service. *Journal of Palliative Medicine, 5,* 93–100.

Schrader, S. L., Horner, A., Eidsness, L., Young, S., Wright, C., & Robinson, M. (2002). A team approach in palliative care: Enhancing outcomes. *South Dakota Journal of Medicine, 55,* 269–278.

Spross, J. A., & Baggerly, J. (1989). Models of advanced nursing practice. In A. B. Hamric & J. A. Spross (Eds.), *The clinical nurse specialist in theory and practice* (2nd ed., pp. 19–40). Philadelphia, PA: Saunders.

Strasser, F., Sweeney, C., Willey, J., Benisch-Tolley, S., Palmer, J. & Bruera, E. (2004). Impact of a half-day multidisciplinary symptom control and palliative care outpatient clinic in a comprehensive cancer center on recommendations, symptom intensity, and patient satisfaction: A retrospective descriptive study. *Journal of Pain and Symptom Management, 27,* 481–491.

Thoreau, H. D. (1971). Where I lived, and what I lived for. In J. Lyndon (Ed.), *Walden.* Princeton, NJ: Princeton University Press.

Twycross, R. (2003) *Introducing palliative care.* Oxford: Radcliff Medical Press.

Virik, K., & Glare, P. (2002). Profile and evaluation of a palliative medicine consultation service within a tertiary teaching hospital in Sydney, Australia. *Journal of Pain and Symptom Management, 23*(3), 17–25.

Von Gunten, C. F. & Lupu, D. (2004). Development of a medical subspecialty in palliative medicine: Progress report. *Journal of Palliative Medicine, 7*(2), 209–219.

Von Gunten, C. F., & Muir, J. C. (2000). Palliative medicine: An emerging field of specialization. *Cancer Investigation,*18, 761–767.

Development of the Specialty of Hospice and Palliative Care Nursing

Judy Lentz
Deborah Sherman

Key Points

- Nationally, there has been a growing interest in palliative and hospice care and an emphasis on the education of health professionals in this area.
- It is recognized that precepts underlying hospice care are essential principles for all end-of-life care.
- By developing and articulating the scope and standards of professional nursing practice, the specialty defines its boundaries, informs society about the parameters of nursing practice, and guides the development of rules and regulations for the specialty
- Standards of practice describe a competent level of generalist and advanced-practice registered nursing care as demonstrated by the nursing process, involving assessment, diagnosis, outcomes identification, planning, implementation, and evaluation
- Hospice and palliative nurses' professionalism is enhanced through membership in their professional organizations, certification in their specialty, and professional development through academic and continuing education.
- With the current nursing shortage and dire projections for the years ahead, the hospice and palliative specialty nursing organizations believe that all representatives of the nursing team must be competent.

Case Study: In May 2007 Marie graduated from an accredited masters level program as a nurse practitioner in geriatric care. Soon thereafter, Marie became a certified geriatric practitioner and was hired by a national for-profit agency. With a particular love of end-of-life care, Marie decided to enroll in a post master's palliative care program. Because of Marie's interest in the specialty and with the encouragement of her course instructor, Marie sought membership in the Hospice and Palliative Nurses Organization (HPNA). With 500 clinical hours in palliative care, Marie had achieved the required hours of practice in palliative care, so she sought the opportunity to become certified in hospice and palliative nursing by the National Board for Certification of Hospice and Palliative Nursing. Upon successful completion of this certification as an ACHPN, Marie was now positioned to seek new and expanded professional opportunities within the specialty of palliative care, an area of growing need. Through the HPNA special interest group listserv, Marie became aware of several job opportunities. Was she ready to submit her job application?

The scope of hospice and palliative care nursing continues to evolve as the science and art of palliative care develop. Hospice and palliative care nursing reflects a holistic philosophy of care implemented across the life span and across diverse health settings. In a matrix of affiliation, including the patient and family and other members of the interdisciplinary team, hospice and palliative care nurses provide evidence-based physical, emotional, psychosocial, and spiritual or existential care to individuals and families experiencing life-limiting, progressive illness. The goal of hospice and palliative care nursing is to promote and improve the patient's quality of life through the relief of suffering along the course of illness, through the death of the patient, and into the bereavement period of the family (Hospice and Palliative Nurses Association [HPNA], 2007). Relief of suffering and quality of life for individuals and families are enhanced by

- providing effective pain and symptom management;
- addressing psychosocial and spiritual needs of patient and family;
- incorporating cultural values and attitudes in developing a plan of care;
- creating a healing environment to promote a peaceful death;
- supporting those who are experiencing loss, grief, and bereavement;
- promoting ethical and legal decision making;
- advocating for personal wishes and preferences;
- utilizing therapeutic communication skills in all interactions;
- facilitating collaborative practice;
- ensuring access to care and community resources through influencing and developing health and social policy;
- contributing to improved quality and cost-effective services;
- creating opportunities and implementing initiatives for palliative care education for patients, families, colleagues, and community; and

- participating in the generation, testing, and evaluation of palliative care knowledge and practice.

The field of palliative care is one response to the changing profile of death in the 20th century, as it focuses on the prevention and relief of suffering through the management of pain and other symptoms and attention to the emotional, spiritual, and practical needs of patients and family from the early through the final stages of an illness (Field & Cassel, 1997). Palliative care builds upon the template of hospice care, with hospice care now recognized as a type of palliative care that is offered toward the end of life. Palliative care is the combination of active and compassionate therapies intended to comfort and support individuals who are living with and dying from life-threatening illness. During periods of illness and bereavement, palliative care strives to meet the physical, emotional, social, and spiritual needs of patients and their families. Palliative care may be combined with therapies aimed at reducing or curing illness, or it may be the total focus of care (Ferris & Cumming, 1995). Indeed, specialty organizations of hospice medicine and nursing have now incorporated palliative care in their titles (Sherman, 2001). The rise in hospice programs in the United States from 1 program in 1979 to more than 3,600 programs in 2008 and a rise in the number of patients and families served from 128,000 in 1985 to 885,000 in 2003 support the projection of future needs for hospice/palliative care services (National Hospice and Palliative Care Organization (NHPCO), 2003).

Hospice and palliative nursing is provided for patients and their families in a variety of care settings including, but not limited to, those such as acute care hospital units, long-term care facilities, assisted living facilities, inpatient, home, or residential hospices, palliative care clinics or ambulatory settings, private practices, and prisons. Practice settings for palliative and hospice care nursing are changing in response to the dynamic nature of today's healthcare environment.

Hospice and palliative nurses are licensed, registered nurses who are educationally prepared and licensed in nursing and are qualified for specialty practice at two levels-generalist and advanced. These levels are differentiated by educational preparation, complexity of practice, and performance of certain nursing functions.

Hospice and palliative licensed practical/vocational nurses are also educationally prepared and licensed but at a different level of complexity in their practice. Hospice and palliative nursing assistants are educationally prepared through local- and state-mandated processes to meet the requirements of the specific setting in which they function. These requirements differ significantly across the United States, although hours of educational requirements are specifically defined in the home care, hospice, and long-term care settings on a national basis. There are no licensure requirements for the nursing-assistant level of hospice and palliative caregiver.

According to an article entitled "History of the Hospice Nurses Association, 1986–1996" (Amenta, 2001), the founding of the Hospice Nurses Association occurred as follows:

> "... in spring 1986 a group of nurses attending the Third Western Hospice Nursing Conference sponsored by the Hospice Organization of Southern California in San Diego, frustrated by the failure of national groups to develop adequate standards and networking structures for hospice nurse, put out the call to start a national hospice nursing organization" (p. 13).

Membership in the organization grew rapidly. In 1998, the word "palliative" was added to the organization's name, now known as the Hospice and Palliative Nurses Association. By 2000, 2,800 nurses had joined this growing organization, with more than 1,000 new members added each year thereafter to date. With a pattern of continued growth, membership has reached nearly 10,000. The mission of HPNA relates to providing leadership in the specialty by

- promoting the highest professional standards of hospice and palliative nursing;
- studying, researching, and exchanging information, experiences, and ideas leading to improved nursing practice;
- encouraging nurses to specialize in the practices of hospice and palliative nursing;
- fostering the professional development of nurses, individually and collectively;
- responding to the changing needs of HPNA members and the population they represent; and
- promoting the recognition of hospice and palliative care as essential components within the healthcare system.

Within this mission are educational products and services designed for all levels of nursing practice.

Many of these educational services offer continuing education credits as well.

EVOLUTIONARY PERSPECTIVE OF HOSPICE AND PALLIATIVE CARE NURSING

Nationally, there has been a growing interest in palliative and hospice care and an emphasis on the education of health professionals in this area. Billings and Block (1997), at the early times of the specialty for palliative care, identified the following forces that have increased national attention regarding palliative care:

1) A growing interest in death and dying.
2) The development of hospice programs.
3) Increasing integration of pain and symptom management into conventional care.
4) Concern about the high cost of dying.
5) Increasing national focus on pain management.
6) Greater attention to the role of medicine in caring rather than curing.
7) National debates on physician-assisted suicide and euthanasia.

These factors combined to create a dramatically increased demand for healthcare providers, including nurses, who are educated at all levels to provide expert, comprehensive palliative and hospice care.

The landmark "Study to Understand Prognoses and Preferences for Outcomes and Risks of Treatment" (SUPPORT) (Support Study Investigators, 1995) highlighted an urgent need for healthcare professionals who were prepared and committed to improving the quality of life for seriously ill and dying patients and their families. The findings indicated a lack of communication between patients and their providers, particularly related to end-of-life preferences, aggressiveness of medical treatments, and a high level of reported pain by seriously ill and dying patients. The Support Study Investigators (1995) believed that improving the experience of seriously ill and dying patients requires an individual and collective commitment of healthcare providers, as well as proactive efforts at shaping the care giving process.

In 1997, the Institute of Medicine (IOM) released a significant report entitled "Approaching Death: Improving Care at the End of Life" (Field & Cassel, 1997). This report identified gaps of knowledge in many areas about caring for those at end of life. Based on this report, Field and Cassel reiterated that "the need for consensus and action to improve care for those approaching death is growing more urgent" (p. 17). On average, Americans live longer than they did in the 19th century, with more than 70% of the population dying after the age of 65. According to the Centers for Disease Control and Prevention, the average life expectancy in the United States is nearly 77 years (National Vital Statistics Report, Volume 56, Number 21, CDC accessed 10/29/08). Over the last 100 years, the leading causes of death have changed from primarily infectious processes to chronic illnesses experienced by an aging population. Although some people die suddenly and unexpectedly, the dying process for many has been extended, with some individuals-such as those with cancer-facing a steady and fairly predictable decline, while others have long periods of chronic illness punctuated by crises that are often fatal (Field & Cassel, 1997). The result is a national increase in the number of individuals who require palliative care. Although hospice and palliative care has been delivered mainly to patients with cancer, other patients with incurable diseases are also candidates for these services, including the growing number of elderly, those suffering from chronic diseases such as cardiovascular, pulmonary, neurological, and renal disease, as well as patients with AIDS (Doyle, Hanks, Cherney & Colman, 2001). More recently, the IOM collaborated with the National Cancer Policy Board and the National Research Council to release a follow-up report called "Improving Palliative Care for Cancer" (Foley & Gelband, 2001), which further supports the need for changes in care of the dying. The report details the under-treatment of distressing symptoms resulting from the continued deficiencies in the training of healthcare professionals. In the IOM report titled "Crossing the Quality Chasm: A New Health System for the 21st Century" (Foley & Gelband, 2001), the IOM argued that professional associations should commit to professional development and competency enhancement by developing curriculums, disseminating information, and promoting practice guidelines and standards related to hospice and palliative care.

In April 2004, the standards and guidelines of palliative care were defined by the National Consensus Project (NCP) Steering Committee in its Clinical Practice Guidelines for Quality Palliative Care. This document was the culmination of 2 years of collaboration by 20 representatives from five leading national hospice and palliative care organizations, specifically the American Academy of Hospice and Palliative Medicine, Center to Advance Palliative Care, Hospice and Palliative Nurses Association, National Hospice and Palliative Care Organization, and the former Last Acts organization. A need for consensus had been defined by practitioners to provide credible, broad-based guidelines for practice in an effort to standardize and improve the quality of palliative care in the United States. That need was affirmed when in the first 2 weeks following publication, 90,000 copies of the guidelines were downloaded from the National Consensus website (www.national-consensusproject.org).

Based on the National Consensus Project Guidelines, the National Quality Forum (NQF) (2006) released "A National Framework and Preferred Practices for Palliative and Hospice Care Quality" in recognition of the increasing services within the healthcare system. This report endorsed the framework of preferred practices to improve hospice and palliative care and has been utilized as the first step in developing quality measures (NQF, accessed 7/16/08). Both documents attempt to formalize the concept of palliative care by providing extended descriptions and definitions differentiating palliative care from other types of care, and each structures the theory and practice of palliative care into eight domains. The guidelines are for all settings in which the NQF framework has implications for reimbursement, development of quality measures, and accreditation. These documents are companion pieces serving to complement the process of improving palliative care quality (NCP, accessed 7/16/08).

One of the baseline assumptions of the NCP guidelines is that the qualifications of caregivers are determined by the organizations that grant professional credentials and programmatic accreditation. As a specialty organization, the Hospice and Palliative Care Nurses Association has identified the scope and standards of hospice and palliative care nursing and the competencies at all levels of nursing practice, specifically nursing assistants, licensed vocational nurses, professional registered nurses, and advance practice nurses.

EDUCATIONAL PREPARATION

It has been recognized that educational preparation for end-of-life care is inconsistent at best, and neglected for the most part, in both undergraduate and graduate curricula (American Association of Colleges of Nursing (AACN), 1997). In accordance with the International Council of Nurses' mandate that nurses have a unique and primary responsibility for ensuring the peaceful death of patients, the AACN, supported by the Robert Wood Johnson Foundation, convened a roundtable of expert nurses to discuss and initiate educational change related to palliative care. It was concluded that precepts underlying hospice care are essential principles for all end-of-life care. Such precepts include the assumptions that persons are living until the moment of death; that coordinated care should be offered by a variety of professionals with attention to the physical, psychological, social, and spiritual needs of patients and their families; and that care be sensitive to patient and family diversity. It was proposed that these precepts be foundational to the educational preparation of nurses. Based on these precepts, the document entitled "Peaceful Death" was developed, which outlined baccalaureate competencies for palliative and hospice care and content areas where competencies can be taught (AACN, 1997).

Emphasizing the role of nursing in end-of-life care, the American Nurses Association formulated a position statement regarding the promotion of comfort and relief of pain of dying patients, reinforcing nurses' obligation to promote comfort and ensure aggressive efforts to relieve pain and suffering. Specialized palliative care educational initiatives began in medicine and nursing, such as Education for Physicians on End of Life Care, known as EPEC; and the nursing initiative End of Life Nursing Education Consortium, known as ELNEC. The goal of ELNEC is to train nurse educators from associate and baccalaureate programs and continuing educational palliative care program supported by a grant from the Robert Wood Johnson Foundation to the AACN and the City of Hope Medical Center. The ELNEC curriculum has also been modified and specialized for geriatrics, pediatrics, and oncology.

A study conducted by Ferrell, Virani, and Grant (2000) revealed that only 2% of the text in nursing textbooks and teaching resources reflected content on end-of-life care. Initiatives are also underway in both medicine and nursing to revise medical and nursing textbooks to include palliative care content in licensing examinations. Most nursing curricula have been limited in terms of content or clinical experiences in end-of-life care, despite consensus reports, standards, and position statements from leading nursing specialty organizations indicating this need (Ferrell, Grant, & Virani, 2001).

Within the past 8 years, numerous palliative and hospice nursing-care resources have been published. Among the many are the following:

- *Textbook of Palliative Nursing* by Betty Ferrell and Nessa Coyle
- *Palliative Care Nursing: Quality Care to the End of Life* by Marianne LaPorte Matzo and Deborah Witt Sherman
- *Palliative Practices from A-Z for the Bedside Clinician,* 2nd edition, by Kim Kuebler and Peg Esper
- *Hospice Concepts: A Guide to Palliative Care in Terminal Illness* by Shirley Ann Smith
- *Hospice Care for Children* by Ann Armstrong-Dailey and Sarah Zarbock
- *Terminal Illness: A Guide to Nursing Care* by Charles Kemp
- *Nurse to Nurse Palliative Care* by Margaret L. Campbell
- *The Nature of Suffering and the Goals of Nursing* by Betty R Ferrell and Nessa Coyle
- *Pain Management, The Resource Guide for Home Health and Hospice Nurses* by Carol Long and Bonnie Morgan
- Numerous clinical resources from the Hospice and Palliative Nurses Association available through Kendall Hunt Publishers (www.hpna.org); and from the Oncology Nursing Society available through the Oncology Education Services (www.ons.org)

DEVELOPING THE SCOPE, STANDARDS, AND COMPETENCIES OF PALLIATIVE AND HOSPICE NURSING PRACTICE

By developing and articulating the scope and standards of professional nursing practice, the specialty defines its boundaries, informs society about the parameters of nursing practice, and guides the development of rules and regulations for the specialty. As in all nursing specialties, palliative care nurses must accept professional practice accountability and ensure that their practice remains within the scope of their state's Nurse-Practice Act, their professional code of ethics, and professional practice standards.

In order to provide quality hospice and palliative nursing care, standards have been defined by a credible body of peers who were charged with this responsibility. The standards of hospice care were defined by the National Hospice and Palliative Care Organization in 1986. The standards of hospice and palliative nursing practice were first defined by the Hospice Nurses Association in 1995, with subsequent revisions to the name of the organization to include palliative care. Scope and standards of hospice and palliative nursing care define the body of knowledge needed in terms of the standards of care and the standards of performance. Standards of care refer to the basic level of care that should be provided to all hospice and palliative care patients and families. Standards of performance for palliative and hospice care nurses describe the standards for activities related to quality of care, performance appraisal, education, collegiality, ethics, collaboration, participation in research, and resource utilization. Documents such as agency standards, guidelines, policies, procedures, and protocols may further direct the individual's performance. Standards are defined in broad terms to define the scope of the specialty of palliative and hospice care nursing.

The standards of palliative and hospice care nursing practice are authoritative statements described by the HPNA for the nursing profession, which identifies the responsibilities for which palliative and hospice care nurses are accountable. Standards reflect the values and priorities of palliative care nursing and provide a framework for the evaluation of practice. The standards are written in measurable terms and define the palliative and hospice care nurses' accountability to the public and the individual and family outcomes for which they are responsible.

The standards are divided into two sections: The Standards of Practice and the Standards of Professional Performance. Each section has identified criteria that allow the standards to be measured. Criteria include key indicators of competent practice. Standards remain stable over time as they reflect the philosophical values of the profession; however, the criteria should be revised to incorporate advancements in scientific knowledge, technology, and clinical practice. Criteria must be consistent with current nursing practice, and reflect evidence-based practice.

Standards of Practice (HPNA, 2007)

Standards of practice describe a competent level of generalist and advanced-practice registered nursing care as demonstrated by the nursing process, involving assessment, diagnosis, outcomes identification, planning, implementation, and evaluation. The development and maintenance of a therapeutic nurse-patient and family relationship is essential throughout the nursing process. The nursing process forms the foundation of clinical decision making and encompasses all significant actions taken by hospice and palliative care nurses in providing care to individuals and families. The precepts of nursing practice include the following:

1) Providing age-appropriate, culturally, ethnically, and spiritually sensitive care and support;
2) Maintaining a safe environment;
3) Educating patients and families to identify appropriate settings and treatment options;
4) Assuring continuity of care and transitioning to the next appropriate setting;
5) Coordinating care across settings and among caregivers;
6) Managing information and protecting confidentiality; and
7) Communicating promptly and effectively.

A fundamental practice focus for hospice and palliative care is the plan of care, which is developed with the patient and family as the unit of care and members of the interdisciplinary team. At the very minimum, the interdisciplinary team includes the physician, nurse, social worker, and clergy. Care responsibilities extend beyond the death of the patient and offers bereavement care to families for a minimum of 1 year.

Registered nurses at the generalist level have completed a nursing program and passed the state licensure examination for registered nurses. Registered nurses who practice in palliative care settings may provide direct patient and family care, and may function as educators, case managers, administrators, and in other nursing roles. Advance practice nurses develop and implement advanced plans of care based on the synthesis of complex health-assessment data. Advanced practice nurses are expert clinicians, leaders, educators, consultants, and researchers. The standards apply to both generalist and advanced practice nurses. There is specific notation of standards that apply only to the advanced practice nurse.

Standard 1: Assessment. The hospice and palliative registered nurse collects comprehensive data pertinent to the patient's health or the situation.

Standard 2: Diagnosis. The hospice and palliative registered nurse analyzes the assessment data to determine nursing diagnoses or issues.

Standard 3: Outcome Identification. The hospice and palliative registered nurse, in partnership with the interdisciplinary healthcare team, identifies expected outcome for a plan of care individualized to the patient or the situation.

Standard 4: Planning. The hospice and palliative registered nurse develops a plan of care that describes strategies and alternatives to attain expected outcomes.

Standard 5: Implementation. The hospice and palliative registered nurse implements the identified plan of care.

Standard 5A: Coordination of care. The hospice and palliative registered nurse coordinates care delivery.

Standard 5B: Health teaching and health promotion. The hospice and palliative registered nurse employs strategies to promote health and a safe environment.

Standard 5C: Consultation. The hospice and palliative registered nurse and the nursing role specialist provide consultation to influence the identified plan, enhance the abilities of others, and effect change.

Standard 5D: Prescriptive authority and treatment The advanced practice hospice and palliative registered nurse uses prescriptive authority, procedures, referrals, treatments, and therapies in accordance with state and federal laws and regulations.

Standard 6: Evaluation. The hospice and palliative registered nurse evaluates progress toward attainment of outcomes.

Standards of Professional Performance (HPNA, 2007)

Standards of professional performance and the associated measurement criteria describe competent professional role behaviors, including activities related to quality of practice, education, professional practice evaluation, collegiality, collaboration, ethics, research, resource utilization, and leadership. Hospice and palliative nurses must be self-directed and purposeful in seeking necessary knowledge and skills to develop and maintain their competency. Hospice and palliative nurses' professionalism is enhanced through membership in their professional organizations, certification in their specialty, and professional development through academic and continuing education.

Standard 7: Quality of practice. The hospice and palliative registered nurse systematically enhances the quality and effectiveness of nursing practice.

Standard 8: Education. The hospice and palliative registered nurse attains knowledge and competency that reflects current hospice and palliative nursing practice.

Standard 9: Professional practice evaluation. The hospice and palliative registered nurse evaluates one's own nursing practice in relation to professional practice standards and guidelines, relevant statutes, rules, and regulations.

Standard 10: Collegiality. The hospice and palliative registered nurse interacts with and contributes to the professional development of peers and colleagues.

Standard 11: Collaboration. The hospice and palliative registered nurse collaborates with the patient, the family, the interdisciplinary team, and others in the conduct of nursing practice.

Standard 12: Ethics. The hospice and palliative registered nurse integrates ethical provisions in all areas of practice.

Standard 13: Research. The hospice and palliative registered nurse integrates research findings into practice.

Standard 14: Resource Utilization. The hospice and palliative registered nurse considers factors related to safety, effectiveness, cost, and impact on practice in the planning and delivery of nursing services.

Standard 15: Leadership. Thehospice and palliative registered nurse provides leadership in the professional practice setting and the profession.

Standards of Care and Standards of Professional Performance are also written for the palliative- and hospice-licensed practical/vocational nurses and for the palliative and hospice nursing assistants. Variations to each standard are made to adapt to scopes of practice and statutory regulations.

Competencies

According to HPNA (2002b), competencies represent the "quantifiable knowledge, attitudes, and skills that practitioners demonstrate in the performance of safe, consistent, compassionate, state-of-the-art, evidence-based end-of-life care which conforms to the patients' and their families' wishes." This definition applies to all levels of nursing practice although the specific clinical judgments and core competencies vary with each level. The competencies for the palliative and hospice generalist and advanced practice nurse were initiated in 2001. Subsequently, competencies for the palliative- and hospice-licensed practical/vocational nurse and nursing assistant were also written.

Competencies must reflect the breadth of the standards, but are written in general domain statements with clinical judgments and core statements to demonstrate accomplishments of the particular domain of competence.

Why are competencies needed? The reason for competencies are discussed in the publication "Professional Competencies for Generalist Hospice and Palliative Nurses" (HPNA, 2001):

> "The use of standards and competencies and the process of accreditation are necessary and important strategies to meet stated goals. Identifying the intellectual, interpersonal, technical, and moral competencies needed to practice quality end-of-life care will help to ensure these standards are met. These competencies need to be outcome specific and therefore are more measurable than the objectives or goals of the past. Identified national competencies will be the benchmark to make explicit the areas of knowledge and skills a nurse needs in order to provide quality hospice and palliative care." (p. 2)

The basic competencies of palliative care nursing represent the knowledge, skills, and attitudes demonstrated when providing evidence-based physical, emotional, psychosocial, and spiritual care. The care is provided in a collaborative manner across the life span in diverse settings to individuals and families experiencing progressive illness. The generalist-level competencies and the related general statements are written as follows with special notation when applicable only for advanced practice nurses:

Clinical judgment. At the generalist level, the palliative and hospice nurse demonstrates critical thinking, analysis, and clinical judgment in all aspects of palliative and hospice care of patients and families experiencing life-limiting illness through the use of the nursing process to address the physical, psychosocial, and spiritual/existential needs of patients and families. At the advanced practice level, the palliative and hospice nurse must be able to respond to all disease processes with advanced clinical skills.

Advocacy and ethics. The palliative and hospice nurse incorporates ethical principles and professional standards in the care of patients and families who are experiencing life-limiting illnesses or progressive illness, as well as identifying and advocating for their wishes and preferences. Promoting ethical and legal decision making, advocating for personal wishes and preferences, and ensuring access to care and community resources through influencing or developing health and social policy are ways for the nurse to incorporate ethical principles and professional standards in the care of patients and their families.

Professionalism. The palliative and hospice nurse demonstrates knowledge, attitude, behavior, and skills that are consistent with the professional standards, code of ethics, and scope of practice for palliative and hospice nursing.

Collaboration. The palliative and hospice nurse actively promotes dialogue with patients and families, the healthcare team, and the community to address and plan for issues related to living with and dying from chronic, life-limiting progressive illness.

Systems thinking. The palliative and hospice nurse utilizes resources necessary to enhance quality of life for patients and families experiencing life-limiting progressive illness through knowledge and negotiation within the healthcare system.

Cultural competence. The palliative and hospice nurse demonstrates cultural competence by respecting and honoring the unique diversity and characteristics of patients, families, and colleagues in palliative and hospice care.

Facilitation of learning. The palliative and hospice nurse facilitates learning of patient, family, self, members of the healthcare team, and the community through the development, implementation, and evaluation of formal and informal education related to living with and dying from life-limiting progressive illnesses.

Communication. The palliative and hospice nurse demonstrates the use of effective verbal, nonverbal, and written communication with patients and families, members of the healthcare team, and the community in order to address therapeutically and convey accurately the palliative and hospice care needs of patients and families.

Advanced practice hospice and palliative nurses are held to the same competencies but at an advanced level because they exercise a high degree of critical thinking, analysis, and independent judgment, within the framework of autonomous and collaborative interdisciplinary practice. The advanced practice nurses are distinguished by their ability to synthesize complex data, implement advanced plans of care, and provide leadership in palliative and hospice care. The roles of the advanced practice hospice and palliative nurse include, but are not limited to, expert clinician, leader or facilitator of interdisciplinary teams, educator, researcher, consultant, collaborator, advocate, and administrator. Advanced practice palliative and hospice nurses who have fulfilled the requirements established by their state's Nurse-Practice Acts may be authorized to assume autonomous responsibility for clinical role functions, which may include prescription of controlled substances, medications, or therapies. To practice as an advanced practice palliative and hospice nurse, national certification in advanced practice palliative and hospice nursing is recommended, although it is recognized that the advanced practice palliative and hospice nurse may have concurrent advanced practice certification in another specialty.

Competencies for the licensed practical nurse focus on decision making instead of clinical judgment.

For the nursing assistant, clinical judgment is rooted in observation and reporting. Although the core competencies are very similar in all four levels of nursing, the criteria are specific to the various scopes of practice.

CERTIFICATION IN HOSPICE AND PALLIATIVE CARE NURSING

Incorporated in 1987, the Hospice Nurses Association (HNA) became the first professional nursing organization dedicated to promoting excellence in the practice of hospice nursing. Consistent with that goal, the HNA Board of Directors appointed the National Board for the Certification of Hospice Nurses (NBCHN) in 1992. A sister organization of HPNA is the National Board for Certification of Hospice and Palliative Nurses (NBCHPN). The mission of this organization is to promote a certification process that advances quality in the provision of hospice and palliative care.

In March of 1994, the NBCHN offered the first certification examination and the credential of Certified Registered Nurse Hospice (CRNH). A decade later, HNA recognized the similarity in the nursing practice of the hospice and palliative nurses, and expanded its name to embrace palliative nursing practice, becoming the Hospice and Palliative Nurses Association (HPNA). Hospice and palliative nurses were providing patient and family care in more diverse settings, and the fundamental nursing concepts developed in hospices were applied to other practice environments such as in acute-care hospitals, prisons, long-term care, and home care.

The results of the 1998 generalist hospice and palliative nurse Role Delineation Study, commissioned by NBCHN, scientifically demonstrated that only minor differences in practice activity existed between hospice and palliative nurses working in non-hospice settings. These differences correlated with requirements of the role or practice setting.

In 1999, the NBCHN became the National Board for Certification of Hospice and Palliative Nurses (NBCHPN), offering a new designation to recognize base competence in hospice and palliative nursing-Certified Hospice and Palliative Nurse (CHPN). For the licensed generalist, it is recommended to have a minimum of 2 years of clinical experience in palliative and hospice care. By 2008, nearly 10,000 registered nurses were certified as CHPNs.

Recognizing the need to offer an examination for advanced practice hospice and palliative nurses, in 2000 the NBCHPN began discussions with New York University and the American Nursing Credentialing Center (ANCC) to collaborate for this purpose. In an effort to expand the portfolio of examinations, NBCHPN successfully negotiated a buy-out of the partnership with ANCC effective December 2004 and has been successfully certifying these nurses as Advanced Certified Hospice and Palliative Nurses (ACHPN). Eligibility for this level includes having a current unrestricted registered nurse license; graduation from an accredited institution granting graduate-level academic credit for a master's or higher degree in nursing; and having a minimum of 500 hours of supervised advanced practice in palliative care as a Clinical Nurse Specialist or Nurse Practitioner. As of 2009, nearly 400 individuals are certified ACHPNs.

Through a commitment to a strategic plan to provide certification for all levels of caregivers, NBCHPN was funded by the Fan Fox and Leslie R. Samuels Foundation in October 2000 to certify nursing assistants in hospice and palliative care. Following development of the scope, standards, and competencies for the hospice and palliative nursing assistant, a role delineation study was completed, and the first hospice and palliative nursing assistant examination was offered in September 2001 and the credential of Certified Hospice and Palliative Nursing Assistant (CHPNA) was offered. To be eligible for the examination, the nursing assistant must have a minimum of 2,000 hours in palliative and hospice care as validated by the nursing supervisor. By 2008, more than 4,000 nursing assistants were certified as CHPNAs.

Continuing with the strategy of providing certification for all levels of caregivers, NBCHPN in 2002 began the process of developing the scope, standards, and competencies for the licensed practical/vocational hospice and palliative nurse. Using additional funds from the Fan Fox and Leslie R. Samuels Foundation, a Role Delineation Study for the hospice and palliative licensed practical/vocational nursing (LP/VN) was completed and the first examination offered in September 2004, conferring the credential of CHPLN. To be eligible for the examination, the palliative and hospice practical/vocational nurse must be licensed, and it is recommended to have 2,000 clinical hours in the prior 2 years. In 2008, over 1,100 CHPLNs had successfully completed the certification requirements.

Certification, as defined by the American Board of Nursing Specialties, is "the formal recognition of the specialized knowledge, skills, and experience demonstrated by the achievement of standards identified by a nursing specialty to promote optimal patient care," and the standards were approved by the American Board of Nursing Specialties (ABNS) Board of Directors in June 2003. The ABNS further defines standards for accrediting nursing examinations to ensure they are of the highest standard. NBCHPN's generalist and advanced practice nursing examinations have achieved accreditation by ABNS effective through 2011. The LPN and NA examinations are accredited through the National Commission for Certifying Agencies (NCCA) through 2012.

HPNA has written position statements supporting the certification of nurses and other qualified members of the nursing team in hospice and palliative care and encourages employers to actively support those individuals pursuing certification.

Certification is valued for the following reasons:

- Certificants achieve a *tested and proven competency* across the spectrum of hospice and palliative care;
- Certificants *increase their knowledge* of hospice and palliative care by seeking and maintaining certification;
- Certificants *demonstrate a commitment* to their specialty practice by pursuing certification;
- Certificants *demonstrate dedication to professional development* in their careers by attaining the credential;
- Certificants are *assets to themselves* because the commitment to certification improves patient outcomes, provides compensation incentives, and gains industrywide recognition;
- Certificants are *assets to their employers* because certification is a recognized quality marker by patients, physicians, providers, quality organizations, insurers, credentialers, and the federal government in an atmosphere of increasing awareness regarding quality in healthcare and appropriate utilization of services.

As of 2009, NBCHPN can proudly claim to be the only nursing specialty certification organization offering certifications for all levels of hospice and palliative care nursing staff. As hospice and palliative care needs increase, NBCHPN seeks to provide assurance of competency of all levels of the nursing staff who administer nursing care.

Case Study conclusion: Marie submits her application to a local academic university hospital system seeking a certified nurse practitioner within her state. Marie's friend from her graduate program who has not become certified ironically submitted an application to the same university hospital. As Marie proceeds through the interview process, she discovers the value of her achievement of certification. Marie is offered and accepts the position for which she interviewed. Later her friend shares her disappointment in not being hired. Marie recognizes the added value being certified offers.

FUTURE VISIONS FOR HOSPICE AND PALLIATIVE CARE NURSING

With the current nursing shortage and dire projections for the years ahead, the hospice and palliative specialty nursing organizations believe that all representatives of the nursing team must be competent. Therefore, four core curriculums, three scope/standards of practice, four competencies, and four examinations have been developed for all levels of nursing practice: advanced practice, generalist, licensed practical/vocational nursing, and nursing assistants. Hospice and palliative care is unique in this regard.

The National Consensus Project's Clinical Practice Guidelines for Quality Palliative Care (which can be viewed at www.nationalconsensusproject.org website) recommend that all palliative and hospice nursing care providers be educated and certified. Great progress has been made, with membership in the Hospice and Palliative Nurses Association more than tripling over the past 8 years to be nearly 10,000, and more than 16,000 nursing care providers certified across the four levels of nursing practice. However, this recommendation has not yet been actualized. When estimating the numbers of registered nurses, LP/VN, and nursing assistants employed in hospices, palliative care programs, long-term care facilities, assisted living facilities, and prisons, the hope is that many more hospice and palliative nurses will join HPNA and become certified by NBCHPN.

The vision for the future of advanced practice hospice and palliative care nursing was articulated in a monograph entitled "Promoting Excellence: A Position Statement From American Nursing Leaders in Palliative Care." This initiative was possible through the support of Dr. Ira Byock's Promoting Excellence in End of Life Care Program.

In the monograph, leaders in advanced practice palliative care nursing emphasize the role of advanced practice nurses in the national efforts to improve care and quality of life for Americans and their families living with advanced life-limiting illnesses. Leaders in the clinical professions, nursing educators, health service providers, healthcare payers, and public policy advocates are asked to take the following actions:

1) Professional organizations in nursing, medicine, hospice, and palliative are called to engage in dialogue about the APN and opportunities and strategies to advance the role.
2) Nursing educators must become knowledgeable about palliative care and develop continuing education programs that support hospice and palliative care nursing competencies.
3) Payers of healthcare services are called on to recognize the specialty of palliative care and provide APNs with adequate and consistent compensation that is commensurate with APNs' scope of practice, authority, and responsibility, regardless of practice setting.
4) The National Council of State Boards of Nursing and individual state boards of nursing are called on to work collaboratively and consistently to recognize the scope and standards of advanced practice palliative care nursing.
5) Healthcare systems or health service providers are asked to develop or expand practice opportunities for APNs in all settings that care for patients who may experience life-threatening illnesses.

6) Advanced practice nurses who practice in hospice and palliative care are called on to document and disseminate the outcomes of their practice experience and roles, engage in interdisciplinary research, and translate research findings into practice.

Although some progress has been made on each of these six action steps, continuing emphasis is needed. These recommendations will not be fully enacted and our vision for hospice and palliative care nursing will not be actualized only at the advanced practice level. Indeed, it will require the collective expression of passion and commitment to quality care across all levels of hospice and palliative care nursing and related constituencies to actualize our nursing potential and create the envisioned reality.

EVIDENCE-BASED PRACTICE

Buck, Joy. Negotiating Hospice and Palliative Nursing in the United States, 1978–2008.

Purpose. This study used the development of the American Hospice and Palliative Nurse Association (HPNA) as a case study to: 1) explore the motivations of its early and subsequent leaders; 2) investigate the processes by which they built core constituencies and negotiated intra- and interdisciplinary boundaries; and 3) analyze the impact of specialization on contemporary care for the dying.

Rationale/Significance. While scholarship on the politics of 20th century healthcare reforms is extensive, very few studies have analyzed the role of nurses and nursing within the policy arena. This study builds on previous research on care for the dying and nursing specialization and critically analyzes the processes by which early leaders defined, standardized, and specialized hospice and palliative nursing.

Methods. Primary data were collected and interpreted using blended social/policy history methods. Interviews with key hospice/palliative nursing leaders in the United States were conducted. Archival data were drawn from the HPNA organizational papers and correspondence and Congressional record, as well as from primary and secondary research data, and then analyzed within the historiographical framework of nursing specialization and 20th century healthcare reforms.

Results. Early HNA (now HPNA) leaders began organizing in the early 1980s in response to the lack of attention given to the standardization of hospice and palliative nursing practice by the National Hospice Organization. The founders and early leaders were radical thinkers, articulate and deeply committed to improving care for the terminally ill. The organization served as a vehicle for peer support, sharing "best practices," continuing education, and the development of standards and specialty certification. Some members were intricately involved with research and adeptly helped shape the policy agenda and reform debates. Yet, distinctions of class, gender, and disciplinary power often permeated their negotiations with other specialty and industry groups and limited the organization's ability to extend their influence beyond their ranks or determine national policy.

Conclusions. The standardization of hospice/palliative nursing served to improve the quality of care for many dying patients and their families. Yet, its specialization also served to sequester such care. As a state-sanctioned specialized model of care reserved for the dying, many individuals who might benefit from such care do not have access to it. Moreover, specialization served to reinforce a false dichotomy between care for the living and care for the dying. As a result, the integration of palliative care concepts into standard practice remains problematic.

CONCLUSION

Hospice and palliative nursing has a bright future. Although the specialty and nursing organization is still young, HPNA has established visibility, credibility, and recognition for hospice and palliative care nursing. An aggressive strategic plan for HPNA was developed in 2008 highlighting the newly approved research agenda, creative educational products and programs, and additional benefits for members. Additionally, HPNA plans to collaborate with other nursing specialties with the goal of being recognized as the leader and expert in palliative care nursing.

With the graying of America, demands for our specialty will grow. The work of the National Consensus Project under the leadership of the Hospice and Palliative Care Coalition (consisting of AAHPM, HPNA, CAPC, and NHPCO) will continue to challenge the delivery of palliative and hospice care in America. Quality indicators must be defined, earlier referrals to palliative and hospice care must be achieved, access to care must be addressed, and recognition of certification for advanced practice nurses leading to practice licensure and reimbursement must be ensured. Hospice and palliative nurses are being prepared and positioned to meet the challenges ahead.

REFERENCES

Amenta, M. O. (2001). History of the hospice nurses association. *Journal of Hospice and Palliative Nursing, 3,* 128–136.

American Association of Colleges of Nursing. (AACN) (1997). *Peaceful death document.* Washington, DC: Round Table Discussion on Palliative Care.

Billings, J. A., & Block, S. (1997) Palliative care in undergraduate medical education. *Journal of the American Medical Association, 278,* 733–736.

Doyle, D., Hanks, G., Cherney, N., & Calman, K. (2001). *Oxford textbook of palliative medicine.* New York: Oxford Medical Publications.

Ferrell, B. R., Virani, R., & Grant, M. (2000). *Analysis of end-of-life content in nursing textbooks. Oncology Nursing Forum, 26,* 869–876.

Ferrell, B. R., Grant, M., & Virani, R. (2001). Nurses urged to address improved end-of-life care in textbooks. *Oncology Nursing Forum, 28,* 1349.

Ferris, F., & Cummings, I. (1995). *Palliative care: Towards a consensus in standardized principles of practice.* Ottawa, Canada: Canadian Palliative Care Association.

Field M. J., & Cassel, C. K. (Eds.). (1997). *Approaching death: Improving care at the end of life.* Washington, DC: National Academies Press.

Foley, K. M., & Gelband, H. (Eds.). (2001). *Improving palliative care for cancer.* Washington, DC: National Academies Press.

Hospice and Palliative Nurses Association & American Nurses Association. (2007). *Hospice and palliative nursing scope & standards of practice.* Silver Spring, MD: HPNA.

Support Study Investigators. (1995). A controlled trial to improve care for seriously ill hospitalized patients: The Study to Understand Progress and Preference for Outcomes and Risks for Treatments (SUPPORT). *Journal of the American Medical Association, 274,* 1591–1598.

Sherman, D. W. (2001). Access to hospice care. *Journal of Palliative Medicine, 3,* 407–411.

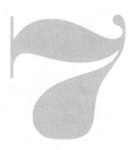

Ethical Aspects of Palliative Care

Judith Kennedy Schwarz
Anita J. Tarzian

Key Points

- Ethics involves decisions about right and wrong, which are influenced by our values.
- Nursing ethics involves clarifying moral uncertainty, resolving moral dilemmas, and coping with moral distress.
- Two major approaches to theoretical ethical analysis are deontological (duty-based) and teleological (consequence-based) systems of ethics.
- The major ethical principles of significance to nurses are respect for persons and autonomy, beneficence, nonmaleficence, and justice.
- Decisional capacity is task-specific, and differs from the concept of "mental competence."
- Surrogate decision-makers should strive to make a "substituted judgment" of what an incapacitated patient would have wanted. A "best interest" standard is used if it is unknown what the patient would have wanted.
- Advance directives may be helpful in identifying what a patient would have wanted when he or she no longer has decisional capacity.
- Minors still have rights to be included in end-of-life decision-making, depending on their decisional capacity and maturity.
- Parents or legal guardians of minors must make decisions within the medical standard of care.
- There is no moral distinction between withholding or withdrawing life-sustaining treatment.
- Decisions to withhold or withdraw life-prolonging interventions such as ventilators or artificial nutrition and hydration are not considered forms of "assisted suicide."
- Nurses should identify resources available to them to support ethical decision-making, including decision-making frameworks, ethics committees, the Nurses Code of Ethics, and expert colleagues.

Case Study: Mrs. Selano is a 78-year-old woman who has resided in a nursing home for the past five years. Due to end-stage dementia, she is totally dependent on the nursing home staff for all activities of daily living, is non-communicative, and receives nutrition through a feeding tube. She has no family, but has received consistent visits from Mrs. Jenkins, a close friend and former neighbor. Mrs. Selano has a living will stipulating that if she were terminally ill, she should be kept comfortable rather than be treated with aggressive life-prolonging medical technology. However, Mrs. Selano checked off on her living will that she would want artificial nutrition through tube feedings to keep her alive. Mrs. Jenkins served as a witness when Mrs. Selano signed the living will document. Mrs. Jenkins tells the nurse that Mrs. Selano would never have wanted to be kept alive in the state she is currently in—contracted into a fetal position, unable to meaningfully interact with others. She says that the lawyer did not fully explain what getting nutrition through a feeding tube might entail for someone with end-stage dementia. Instead, the lawyer presented this as something that might be implemented if Mrs. Selano was "hungry and couldn't eat." Mrs. Jenkins asks if the tube feedings could be stopped and Mrs. Selano allowed to die in peace.

Some decisions nurses make when providing end-of-life care seem particularly difficult; even experienced nurses may feel uncertain about whether they made the "right" decision. When the issue is what, all things considered, is the *right* thing to do, a moral or ethical question is asked. It is often exquisitely difficult to determine what the right response is when, for example, a terminally ill and suffering patient pleads with you to help speed her dying; you feel unable to help without causing her harm. An ethically hard case is one in which the good that you want to bring about can only be realized if the harm you seek to avoid is also brought about, that is, when benefiting the patient cannot be disentangled from harming (Cavanaugh, 1996).

Advances in scientific knowledge and developments in medical technology far exceed any social consensus about the circumstances for their appropriate use. The process of dying can now be prolonged almost indefinitely; this technological imperative (*can do* implies *ought to*) has given rise toan unprecedented array of professional, moral, and legal questions within healthcare. Many Americans fear the possibility of dying a painful, protracted, or undignified death, in an institutional setting, absent personal control or meaning (Schwarz, 2004a). Studies indicate that nurses also have concerns about how best to provide care for dying patients. Beckstrand, Smith, Heaston and Bond (2008) identified perceived obstacles to providing good end-of-life care in the emergency department (ED). These included ED nurses' work loads being too high to allow adequate time for patient care, poor ED design, and family members not fully understanding what "life-saving measures" means. Nelson et al. (2006) surveyed nursing and physician ICU directors about barriers to end-of-life care. The following barriers were identified most frequently: patient or family factors (such as unrealistic patient or family expectations); inability of patients to participate in discussions; lack of advance directives; clinician factors (such as insufficient physician training in communication); and institution or ICU factors (such as suboptimal space for family meetings and lack of a palliative care service).

Ethical aspects of end-of-life decision-making pose compelling challenges for nurses because they frequently involve conflicts among values, principles, and priorities of care; such conflicts require reasoned deliberation for their resolution. This chapter provides practicing nurses with the tools needed to identify and address the ethical issues in end-of-life care. In order to identify ethically relevant aspects of complex cases, nurses are encouraged to engage in values clarification and personal reflection. To address the ethical issues in end-of-life care effectively, nurses should use a decision-making framework that incorporates ethical theories, clearly defined moral concepts, and an understanding of the Code for Nurses (American Nurses Association [ANA], 2001).

Ethical and legal issues often seem intertwined in many end-of-life decisions. For example, the selection of who is permitted to speak for a person who is decisionally incapable is a legally determined question, but which treatment the decision maker chooses is often a moral issue.Often the most difficult clinicalconflicts occur at the junction of law and ethics, where an act that is illegal may seem morally required, or one that is legally required may seem morally inappropriate. Many of these cases resist satisfactory solutions. Although ethics and law function similarly in society in that they both sanction and guide behavior, they also differ in important ways. This chapter will focus on ethical issues in nursing care for those at the end of their lives.

Ethics and Ethical Theory

Ethics is a branch of philosophy that considers and examines the moral life. The word ethics comes from the

Greek *ethos,* and originally meant character or conduct; the word moral comes from the Latin *mores,* which means customs or habit (Davis, Aroskar, Liaschenko), Drought, 1997). *Ethics* and *morals* are frequently used interchangeably in nursing ethics to refer to conduct, character, and motivations involved in moral acts, although there are distinctions that are sometimes made between these terms.

The concept of morality is often used to refer to personally embraced concepts of duty, obligation, and principles of conduct. *Morals* is frequently used interchangeably with *values,* and refers in particular to values or principles of conduct to which one is personally and actually committed (Jameton, 1984). Use of the word ethics is distinguished by reflective thinking and practical reasoning, and often includes overarching, publicly stated sets of rules or principles, such as those found in professional ethics codes. Stanley and Zoloth-Dorfman (2001) note that ethics seeks to logically justify choices for right behavior and rules—particularly in situations that challenge established norms of behavior, or in those that require a new paradigm for judging behavior. These authors add that ethical inquiry—which seeks to interpret acts and to answer such questions as "What is the right thing to do?"—traditionally includes an evaluation of (1) the moral agent and his or her character, (2) the motive for the act itself, and (3) the effect of the action on others. *Normative* ethics seeks ways to answer questions about right and wrongor good or bad in situations that call for a moral decision. Nursing ethics is both normative and practical, in that it makes use of ethical theory and analysis to examine and resolve what *ought to be done* in situations involving moral conflict in nursing practice. *Bioethics* refers to the application of ethics and ethical analysis to moral and practical problems in biological sciences, medicine, and healthcare.

Values and Values Clarification

Values have been called the cornerstone of nursing's moral art (Uustal, 1987). Few aspects of our personal or professional lives are value free. Values are ubiquitous, although often unspoken and frequently unexamined; they determine the nature of our moral choices. Values are foundational to our notions of good and bad, and inform our understanding of what constitutes benefit and harm; thus they are instrumental to the ethical decisions we make. Because our values influence the choices we make, they may also bias our judgments about the worth of our own view and negatively influence our judgments about the merits of others choices; hence the need for values clarification. In the absence of reflection we may simply assume that others believe and would (should) do as we do. Uustal (1987) states that the price paid for unexamined values often includes "confusion, indecision, and inconsistency" (p. 149).

Values clarification is a process of self-reflection that helps individuals identify, consider, and articulate the belief, purposes, and attitudes they prize and that drive their actions. Beliefs about death and what makes life worth living, our conclusions about the nature and significance of truth, or the meaning of paths not chosen are all moral values. Fowler (1987) states that the purpose of values clarification is to assist individuals to identify those personal and professional values that influence behavior and their moral decision making. It is recognized that the essence of ethical conflict is the clash of values, principles, legal rules, and personal perspectives (Dubler & Liebman, 2004). The need for values clarification is an essential first step in moral decision-making.

Every nursing act that intervenes in the life of a patient has at least the possibility of enhancing or transgressing some value cherished by that patient. In situations of moral uncertainty or ethical dilemmas, questions of value will always be foundational. *Moral uncertainty* occurs when nurses are uncertain *if* a moral problem exists, are unsure about its nature, and are unclear which values conflict and which principles might facilitate clarification. These situations often occur in nursing practice. Moral uncertainty may occur when a patient seems to be suffering unnecessarily, is refusing pain medication, but is unwilling or unable to explain their reason for refusing your efforts to help.

Moral dilemmas occur less frequently and are understood as a situationin which two or more clear moral or ethical principles apply that support mutually inconsistent courses of action. Each alternative course of action can be justified by a moral rule or principle, but one can choose or satisfy only one course of action at the expense of *not* satisfying the other. The nurse who believes he or she is duty-bound both to preserve life and reduce suffering may experience a dilemma when preserving life causes intense suffering or when suffering can only be reduced by interventions that may shorten life. There is no satisfying right answer to an ethical dilemma, but one should utilize reasoned (principled) thinking in order to be able to provide a rationale for the decision reached.

The third type of moral problem is the experience of *moral distress,* an emotion that occurs when nurses have identified and know what right response is called for, but institutional or other constraints make it almost impossible to pursue the right course of action (Jameton, 1984). The repeated experience of moral distress can lead nurses to experience moral passivity, burnout, or to leave the profession (Cameron, 1997). Nurses who experience moral distress from institutional constraints on their ability to practice as morally autonomous clinicians must seek support from colleagues and from other institutional and professional resources such as institutional and nursing ethics committees and state nursing associations. The experience of organizational constraints on professional autonomy causes some nurse scholars to rhetorically ask whether nurses who face ethical dilemmas are able to be ethical (Davis, 1994).

Resources to assist the nurse to manage moral problems effectively will be included in subsequent sections of this chapter. However, whatever the conflict, knowing one's own values and being sensitive to the values of others is an essential first step in ethical nursing practice.

ETHICAL THEORIES

Moral theories are methods of determining what counts when a decision must be made, and offer a method for weighing or ranking considerations identified as morally relevant to that decision. More succinctly, an ethical theory provides a framework of principles within which an agent can determine morally appropriate actions (Beauchamp & Childress, 2008).

It should be noted that nurses regularly explore and resolve ethical questions in their practices without recourse to ethical theories and without a formal consideration of the nature of their foundational moral values. Yet, people hold different foundational views, which sometimes can heighten moral conflict and diminish the options for resolution. The following scenario by Benjamin and Curtis (1992) illustrates the role that ethical theories can play in facilitating or hampering decision making. The case involves the question of whether everything should be done to prolong the life of an elderly gentleman in a nursing home who is decisionally incapable. The staff must make the decision because there are no friends or family and no prior indication of his wishes. Person A argues that he should be treated because not to do so would violate the duty to protect and preserve life. Person B agrees that the man should be treated, but for a different reason. B argues that he should be treated because he is not in any pain, and although he is significantly cognitively impaired, he seems fairly content. In B's view, what one ought to do above all is to maximize happiness, and therefore the man's life should be prolonged. As presented, the question about whether to continue treatment can be answered without agreement about the nature of basic ethical values and with dissimilar ethical theories.

Suppose the facts are changed a little, so that the gentleman is experiencing intractable pain and distress. In this case, with her foundational commitment to maximizing happiness, B would revise her judgment and conclude that they should no longer strenuously attempt to extend the man's life. But this change in facts would be irrelevant to A, and her judgment that the patient's life should be prolonged would remain the same. This conflict is not likely to be resolved without further questions about the nature and justification of ethical principles that are the foundation to approaches of making ethical decisions.

Within bioethics, there are two major approaches to theoretical considerations—deontological and teleological systems of ethics. The deontological (from *deon*, Greek for duty), or Kantian, approach to ethics focuses on duties and obligations. Teleological theories (from *telos*, Greek for end) base the determination of whether an action is right or wrong on the action's consequences. These two ethical theories have been subject to criticism for their overreliance on unrelated and often conflicting principles in dealing with moral problems in healthcare (Clouser & Gert, 1990), and by feminist moral theorists for their oppressiveness and indifference to the particularity of relationships (Gadow, 1996). These theories continue to dominate the ethical arguments used to resolve moral problems in healthcare, and nurses must recognize them and be familiar with their use in decision making. These two theories will be described and contrasted to a decisional theory based on caring.

Deontological Moral Theory

A deontological, or Kantian, approach to decision making focuses on duty and obligations. Kantian deontology is attributed to the 18th-century moral philosopher Immanuel Kant. Deontologists maintain that whether an act is right or wrong depends upon the nature of the act itself when considered in terms of its inherent moral worth. Kant argued further that consequences can never make an action right or wrong. Duty-based theories hold particular duties to be fundamental and make use of principles or their derivative rules in order to guide decision making. An example of duty-based theories include natural law, which identifies a duty to obey God's will and requires that one shall not kill; and the rules of traditional medical morality derived from the Hippocratic tradition, which maintain that above all we should do no harm.

A deontological position requires commitment to the principle of universalizability, which means that once a moral decision is made, that same decision must be made in all similar situations. The essence of this position is that morality requires that we cannot make exceptions for ourselves. Thus, if the proposed action is one that would be wrong if done generally, then the particular action is also wrong—even when the specific action has no harmful consequences. Such rules as "it is always wrong to directly take innocent human life" are considered valid when they meet certain conditions, identified by Kant as categorical imperatives. Proposed by Kant as a means to resolve conflicts between rules and principles, this imperative means that for a rule to be valid it must be applicable to everyone universally. This principle can be illustrated as follows: If it is morally acceptable for me to act as I do for my patient (e.g., not charging for services, stealing medications for her use, skipping home visits, etc.), so must it also be acceptable for every other nurse to act similarly for his patients.

Another form of this categorical imperative requires that persons should always be treated (and valued) as ends in themselves, and never solely as means. Thus nurses are required to respect individuals and their beliefs regardless of consequences and they are similarly obliged to respect persons' autonomous choices. Kant identified these categorical imperatives as unconditional commands that are morally required and obligatory in any circumstance (Davis et al., 1997). Within this theoretical perspective, it is simply one's duty to obey categorical imperatives without any exceptions, without reference to the consequences of the act, and in the absence of external or guiding authority. The moral standard includes keeping promises, avoiding or preventing harm, and respecting persons; these are principles that are morally required and are consistent with the rules provided in our professional code of ethics. Fiester (2007) cautions that the trend to approach ethical decision-making using a "four principles" approach (i.e., weighing obligations toward beneficence, nonmaleficence, respect for persons and justice) predisposes clinicians to overlook other ethical obligations toward patients.

Teleological Moral Theories

Teleological theories determine an action to be right or wrong based on the consequences of the action. The most important teleological theory for contemporary healthcare is utilitarian ethics (Steinbock, Aaras & London 2002). Utilitarianism is best understood as a moral theory that asserts there is only one basic principle in ethics, the principle of utility, which declares that we ought always to produce the greatest possible balance of value over disvalue for the greatest number of persons (Beauchamp & Childress, 2008). This position assumes that one can weigh and measure harms and benefits and arrive at the greatest possible balance of good over evil for most people (Davis et al., 1997).

Utilitarians are disinterested in considerations of the agent's intentions, feelings, or convictions; all are viewed as irrelevant to the question of "What is the right thing to do?" In the same fashion, utilitarians regard the question of whether a proposed action conforms to established social norms or ethical codes as relevant only to the extent that conforming (or not) has a bearing on the achievement of happiness or value over unhappiness (Steinbock et al., 2002). At least in principle, utilitarians are able to provide definite answers to specific questions about how one ought to act. The question of whether it is ever morally permissible to be untruthful depends upon context and circumstances: in those situations where telling a lie would produce, overall, more happiness or value than unhappiness, then telling a lie would be morally justified.

As with deontological theories, there are two versions of this theory: an act-utilitarian is primarily concerned with the consequences of particular acts, while a rule-utilitarian is more concerned about the consequences of general policies. To illustrate the difference between these versions, imagine that a nurse is trying to decide if it would be morally right to help a terminally ill patient die. An act-utilitarian would try to determine which alternative in this particular situation would maximize happiness or minimize suffering, or both. The considerations included in making that determination would be the nature of the disease and the certainty of prognosis, the presence of a treatable depression, whether the patient really wanted to die or needed better palliative care, the impact in the patient's family, and professional repercussions for the nurse.

By contrast, a rule-utilitarian uses the principle of utility to formulate and justify moral rules, and the correct moral rules are those that promote the greatest happiness for the greatest number (Steinbock et al., 2002). In this particular case, the nurse would ask whether a general rule permitting assisted suicide would maximize happiness. Important considerations of this approach include questions about whether such a practice would put us on a slippery slope and threaten the lives of other terminally ill patients who do not really want to die but might feel obliged or are susceptible to being coerced. Thus a rule-utilitarian might agree that although helping this particular patient to die might maximize happiness (or minimize suffering) for the individual, it would still be wrong because of the larger negative consequences of a general policy permitting assisted suicide (Steinbock et al., 2002)

How would a Kantian resolve this nurse's problem? Steinbock et al. (2002) suggest that the categorical imperative gives less guidance—it functions only to tell us what *cannot* be done, and not what *should* be done. The principle of universalizability is just one value in Kantian ethics; the other mandate is respect for persons. The question would then be reframed: Does a policy of assisted suicide promote respect for persons or would such a policy lead to the devaluing of human life and to nonvoluntary killing of the weak, vulnerable, and poor?

Each of these theories has strengths and limitations, but neither ethical theories nor principles alone will provide a formula for resolving ethical questions. What they do provide is a framework for trying to reach workable solutions to complex and difficult questions (Steinbock et al., 2002).

Focus on Caring

An ethic of caring that focuses on relationships and responsibility is one aspect of the broader field of feminist ethics. This ethic stems in part from a criticism of traditional ethical theories as being biased in their representation of the experiences of men rather than women. Another dimension of feminist ethics is the analysis of oppression and dominance within relationships and social institutions. It is certain that power differentials between nurses (who are primarily women), physicians, patients, administrators, and payers illustrate just some of the relational inequalities that exist in most healthcare organizations (Davis et al., 1997). *Caring,* within the context of an *ethics of care,* refers to "care for, emotional commitment to, and willingness to act on behalf of persons with whom one has a significant relationship. Noticeably downplayed are Kantian universal rules, impartial utilitarian calculations, and individual rights" (Beauchamp & Childress, 2001).

The idea of an ethic of caring is particularly appealing to nurses because caring is considered to be the very foundation of their practice. Sara Fry, a nurse philosopher, proposed caring as a fundamental value for the development of a theory of nursing ethics (Fry, 1989). Care for others is a core notion in an ethic of care, and is evident in the ANA Code for Nurses (2001), which mandates respectful care of the individual as its core tenet.

In an ethic of care, the decision maker focuses on identifying actions that promote and maintain relationships, and views the patient as a unique individual within networks of relationships (Davis et al., 1997). Fry, Killen, and Robinson (1996) maintain that:

> ... the actions and judgments made using care-based reasoning must be measured against what it means to be 'caring' within the context of the responsibilities the decision maker has to others—care-based reasoning does not involve the application of abstract ethical principles to the situation or impartiality on the part of the decision maker.

Other scholars criticize the rejection of ethical principles as "an invitation to capriciousness" (Held, 1994). An ethic of care is not yet adequately developed to function as a conceptual theory for identifying "right" actions in morally troubling situations (Davis et al., 1997; Fry et al., 1996).

ETHICAL PRINCIPLES AND CONCEPTS

The major ethical principles of significance to nurses are respect for persons and autonomy, beneficence, nonmaleficence, and justice. The duties of veracity, fidelity, and confidentiality are moral rules derived from these principles that further guide and direct nursing actions. These moral rules are embedded in the provisions of the Code of Ethics for Nurses (ANA, 2001). One particular rule that resonates for nurses who care for patients at the end of life is the proscription that "nurses may not act with the sole intent of ending a patient's life even though such action may be motivated by compassion, respect for patient autonomy, and quality of life considerations."

There may be occasions when moral agents feel obliged to question these rules and their appropriateness in particular circumstances, and they may wish to "appeal" to a higher level of moral authority (Veatch & Fry, 1995). Perhaps a nurse may question whether it is *always* wrong to "act with the sole intent of ending a patient's life" and to ask whether other duties such as mercy and compassion might sometimes prevail. This higher level of authority within a moral framework consists of ethical principles.

Respect for Persons and the Principle of Autonomy

The most fundamental ethical principle within nursing practice is the principle of respect for persons. The first provision in the Code for Nurses (ANA, 2001) calls for nurses to "Practice with compassion and respect for the inherent dignity, worth, and uniqueness of every individual, unrestricted by considerations of social, or economic status, personal attributes, or the nature of health problems" (p. 7).

The principle of respect for persons is broader and more abstract than the principle that addresses individual autonomy and self-determination. Respect for persons requires that each individual be treated as unique and entitled to treatment that is respectful of his human dignity. It is this principle of respect for persons that requires particular justification before we are permitted to interfere with the plans, privacy, or behavior of autonomous adult persons, and specifically constrains *paternalistic* decisions made by health professionals for patients with decision-making capacity.

The concept of autonomy is multidimensional and in its broadest sense incorporates the following: Having a minimum of relevant information; Self-determined choice; Freedom to act on the basis of one's choices; and Self-governance (Yeo, Moorhouse, & Dalzeil, 1996a). Autonomous (or decisionally capable) persons determine their own course of action in accordance with a plan chosen by themselves. An autonomous action is understood as one done intentionally, made with understanding and without controlling influences that determine the action (Beauchamp & Childress, 2008).

How are nurses to understand and apply this principle? This principle guides nursing actions in that nurses are duty-bound to respect patients' autonomous choices in all situations unless this principle is overridden by another moral principle of greater weight or standing (Fry, 1987). Such would be the case when questions are raised about whether the choice is truly autonomous, whether the choice is perceived as harmful to the individual or others, and in other situations where autonomous choice is not possible. In these situations, the nurse's obligation to prevent harm to others or to benefit the patient may be determined to have greater moral weight. The example of intervening to prevent a suicide is not a good example of such a situation, because the rationale for preventing suicide is that the individual is not acting autonomously. Consider, instead, that a patient writes an advance directive stipulating that he not be fed—either artificially or by spoon feeding—in the event that he develops dementia and does not recognize family and friends. Imagine that he develops Alzheimer's that is in an advanced stage. The staff members at the nursing home where he is living would likely argue that to withhold freely accepted oral feedings from this patient would cause a greater harm to him than overriding his prior wishes that he not be fed, and may be construed as negligence on their part.

It is the principle of respect for persons and autonomy that is the foundation of informed consent. According to this rule, persons must be given sufficient, accurate, and complete information necessary to make informed decisions about treatment choices. This includes decisions to accept, refuse, or to terminate treatments, whether or not these treatments are necessary for sustaining or prolonging life.

Limiting Autonomy

Nurses who care for patients at the end of life may sometime wonder whether they ought to intervene to prevent harm that they fear may result from a patient's decision. Put another way, are clinicians ever justified in limiting or interfering with a person's autonomy? The two most frequently occurring ways that healthcare professionals infringe upon patient autonomy are through control of information (e.g., withholding, deceiving, or equivocating), or through preventing a patient from acting upon his or her choice (e.g., refusing to comply or assist, constraining, or forcing treatment) (Yeo, Moorhouse, & Dalzeil, 1996a). This type of interference, known as paternalism or parentalism, occurs often in healthcare and is done with the best of intentions; indeed, by definition it is understood as an intervention that is imposed for the patient's good or benefit.

In fact, paternalistic actions such as deception, breaking promises, or interfering with adult choices are violations of moral rules that are never morally permitted unless an adequate reason is provided. To justify such violations, philosophers Culver and Gert (1982) argue that we must determine whether we would publicly advocate this kind of violation in all similar situations. "If all rational persons would agree that the evil prevented by universally allowing this violation would be greater than the evil caused by universally allowing it, the violation is strongly justified" (p. 149). This would be a difficult standard to meet for those who presume justification exists for telling a lie based solely on the belief that doing so would benefit another. On the other hand, classic example given to justify lying is the case of a Dutchman who is hiding a Jewish family during World War II and lies to a Nazi officer to protect the Jewish family.

In considering circumstances when limitations on autonomy may be justified, "weak" paternalism is sometimes accepted to prevent persons from causing themselves seriousharm. In this view, one would be justified in interfering only to prevent a significantharm from occurring, but only when the person's conduct is substantially nonvoluntary or nonautonomous (Yeo, Moorhouse, & Dalzeil, 1996a). To justify this type of interference, one would have to demonstrate that the presumption of autonomy or self-determination is no longer held, and that the person's choices were in fact no longer autonomous or freely chosen. Under this rule, we would be clearly justified in intervening if we discovered a patient attempting to jump out of a hospital window.

"Strong" paternalism, by contrast, involves limiting or interfering with the self-determination of someone whose autonomy is not in question (i.e., an adult capable of rational decision-making) and is very rarely justified. For example, a decisionally capable person who at the end of her life makes a thoughtful and considered decision to stop eating and drinking would be seriously wronged or harmed if a clinician were to override her decision and insert a feeding tube or intravenous line to prolong her life. Paternalistic behavior, regardless of how good the motives or the size of the benefit gained or the harm avoided, violates the right of an adult to be treated as a person. To disregard a person's life plans and values in such a fashion is to show contempt for them as persons, or in Kant's terms, it is to treat them as mere means to an end, rather than as an end in themselves.

Before an act of paternalism can be considered justified, each of the following conditions must be present:

1) The patient's capacity for rational reflection must be significantly impaired. This (*autonomy* condition) must be clinically determined and substantiated.
2) The patient is likely to be significantly harmed unless interfered with (the *harm* condition).
3) It is reasonable to assume that the patient will, at a later time, with recovery of capacity for rational reflection, ratify or agree to the decision made to interfere (the *ratification* condition) (Benjamin & Curtis, 1992).

Questions About Capacity for Autonomous Choice

Patients should be assumed to have the capacity to make decisions for themselves unless there is clear evidence to the contrary (Beauchamp & Childress, 2008). Clinical judgments about a person's decisional capacity serve as a gatekeeping role in healthcare by distinguishing those whose decisions should be solicited and honored from persons whose decisions need not or should not be solicited or accepted (Beauchamp & Childress, 2008). Patient capacity is often neither completely present nor totally absent, as is particularly the case in some elderly persons who may evidence a level of capacity that waxes and wanes. When capacity waxes and wanes, caregivers should take advantage of opportunities to engage the patient in decision making and advance-care planning when their capacities are at their best (Lynn et al., 1999). Capacity is best understood as task-specific, in that a higher level of capacity is required for decisions associated with serious consequences (i.e., agreeing to a proposed surgical intervention) compared to decisions about choosing meals or where to eat them (Mezey, Mitty, & Ramsey, 1997). A capacity determination is a clinical judgment made by caregivers who know the patient best. When the consequences of the capacity determinations are particularly grave or the determination is contentious, clinicians may wish to seek a psychiatric consultation to assist in the capacity determination.

There are occasions when nurses may question whether a treatment choice reflects what the patient truly wants or whether their decision was informed and autonomous. Nurses may want to know whether the patient is capable of making an informed and autonomous choice and whether they should comply with a decision that seems inconsistent with previously stated wishes or values.

Assessing Decision-Making Capacity

A decisionally capable person is able to understand a proposed intervention (or its termination), deliberate regarding major risks and benefits, make a decision in light of that deliberation, and communicate the choice to others. The following is information that decisionally capable patients should understand:

- His or her condition for which the intervention is recommended.
- The nature of the recommended intervention.
- The risks and benefits of the recommended intervention, of alternative interventions, including no intervention or treatment.

Caregivers should determine the following:

- The patient acknowledges that treatment is recommended.
- The patient understands how the proposed treatment or lack of treatment can affect the quality of his life.
- The patient's decision is not substantially based on a delusional belief (Yeo, Moorhouse, & Dalzeil, 1996a, pp. 99–100).

These criteria are intended to establish whether the patient is capable of making a rational choice, and not whether the choice being made is rational.

Deciding for Others

If a patient lacks the capacity to make informed choices, other means must be identified for surrogate decision making. There are three standards for surrogate decision making: Written advance directives, substituted judgment, or best interest. These three standards are ordered so that advance directives have priority over the other two, and substituted judgment has priority over the best interest standard (Lynn et al., 1999). The best of all situations is a thoughtfully drafted advance directive applied by a surrogate decision-maker who knows the patient's values and wishes well.

The substituted judgment is a subjective standard that is ideally based on knowledge of the patient's wishes, values, views about particular interventions, and quality-of-life determinations. This standard allows the surrogate to decide as though the patient were speaking. Realistically, a surrogate's knowledge about the patient's goals and values is typically not entirely clear and decisive regarding a particular choice of treatment (Lynn et al., 1999). These authors state that "in practice, surrogate decision making for incompetent patients often has to draw on all three standards for decisions about an incompetent patient's care" (p. 273). The "best interests" standard is used when the patient's treatment wishes, or values, are unknown. Under these circumstances, the decision maker must objectively weigh the expected benefits and burdens associated with the treatment recommended by the healthcare team and determine what would be best for this patient.

Nurses have an important role to play in surrogate decision-making; the surrogate must be encouraged to focus on what the now incompetent patient would want if he or she were able to speak. It is often difficult for grieving family members to put aside their own distress about the implications of honoring patient preference, especially when the decision involves withholding or withdrawing life-sustaining treatments. While the patient retains capacity, he or she should be encouraged and guided by nurses to discuss end-of-life choices with family members or other potential surrogate decision makers. Nurses are well positioned to describe to patients and their loved ones the actual risks and benefits that are known to be associated with the use of interventions such as cardiopulmonary resuscitation, tube feedings, and mechanical ventilation. As Perrin (1997) notes, "advance directives are unlikely to have an effect on care if a healthcare provider, proxy or family member does not support and advocate for following the person's wishes" (p. 25). Yet, even when patients complete advance directives (ADs), clinicians observe that the ADs often are unavailable or not applicable in many of the clinical situations faced by seriously ill adults (Tonelli, 1996).

Use of advance directives

Researchers are beginning to investigate how advance directives actually function in various clinical settings, and are exploring whether the presence of an AD ensures compliance with patients' end-of-life wishes. For example, in a study by Tierney et al. (2001), investigators found that although discussions about ADs improved the "care satisfaction" of elderly patients with chronic illnesses, having completed a written living will did not increase the likelihood that family decision-makers would make treatment decisions that accurately reflected the patient's choice as stipulated in the AD.

A number of commentators agree that there are persistent difficulties associated with use of *written* directives that include incomplete information, the inability to anticipate future medical conditions, and uncertainty regarding the meaning and intent of written instructions (Fagerlin & Schneider, 2004). These problems of interpretation require clinicians to seek information from others in their attempt to determine what the patient "really meant" (Tonelli, 1996). Tonelli and others conclude that because of the limitations associated with use of written instructive directives, proxy or appointment directives are the preferred form of advance directive (Dexter, Wolinsky, Gramelspacher, Eckert, & Tierney, 2003; Perkins, 2000; Tonelli, 1996). Yet, surrogates also have difficulties accurately predicting the end of life treatment preferences of their spouses. Shalowitz, Garrett-Mayer, and Wendler (2006) reviewed 16 studies on surrogate accuracy published between 1966 and 2005 and found that, overall, surrogates are inaccurate 32% of the time . Perkins (2007) argues that advance directives promise more control over future care and end-of-life decisions than is possible to achieve. He concludes that "advance care planning must refocus from completing advance directives to preparing patients and families for the uncertainties and difficult decisions of future medical crises" (p. 51). Clearly, there is a need for further research to explore whether ADs facilitate good end-of-life care, and nurses are ideally situated to direct and participate in furthering understanding of the practical use o these documents.

In the absence of a thoughtful discussion that includes general end-of-life values and specific preferences about use of interventions such as artificial nutrition and hydration, the legally appointed surrogate may be poorly prepared to identify or implement treatment decisions that conform with the patient's actual end-of-life preferences. In addition, family stress associated with

decisions to withdraw life-sustaining treatments from decisionally incapacitated patients has been found to be high in the absence of a completed advance directive (Tilden, Tolle, Nelson, & Fields, 2001). Limerick (2007) identified the process that surrogate decision makers used when making decisions in an ICU environment to withhold or withdraw life-sustaining interventions from a loved one. This included evaluating the patient's past and future quality of life and rallying family support, developing relationships with the healthcare team and deciphering medical outcomes, and finding time alone to make a decision and then communicate it to those involved.

Beneficence and Nonmaleficence

Beneficence, known generically as doing good, is often hard to separate from nonmaleficence, or the duty not to inflict harm. Some philosophers argue that the principle of beneficence includes four rules:

1) One ought not to inflict evil or harm (what is bad).
2) One ought to prevent evil or harm.
3) One ought to remove evil.
4) One ought to do good or promote good (Frankena, 1973).

These rules are prioritized in that the first takes precedence over the second, which is in turn more compelling than the third, which takes moral precedence over the fourth, all things being equal (Frankena, 1973). Although, it can seem difficult in clinical practice to distinguish preventing harm from providing benefit, Benjamin and Curtis (1992) believe it is easier to get agreement on what constitutes harm than on what constitutes a benefit. When the duty not to inflict harm conflicts with the duty to provide benefit, there is agreement that, all things being equal, there is a greater obligation not to injure others than to benefit them (Beauchamp & Childress, 2008).

In healthcare, the principle of maleficence is understood as requiring clinicians to avoid intentionally causing patients unnecessary harm or pain, whether psychological or physical. The principle of nonmaleficence and none of its derived moral rules are absolute. We often do harm to patients in order to benefit them or to prevent a greater harm from occurring—administering chemotherapy to treat cancer is an obvious example. What is morally relevant is whether causing the harm is morally justified. Under most circumstances, death is considered a major harm; the question of whether causing death is ever justified is an issue of significance to nurses who provide care at the end of life.

Patients at the end of their lives may be particularly vulnerable to harm. They are harmed when they receive unwanted or unnecessary interventions, are overtreated with burdensome technological interventions that serve only to prolong dying, and also when treatments are withdrawn without their consent or agreement. Most certainly they are harmed when their pain is not managed adequately due to the nurse's fear that the patient's death might be hastened as a result of pain management with high-dose opiates. The Code of Ethics (ANA, 2001) stipulates that not only should nurses "not act with the sole intent of ending a patient's life," but also the requirement that "the nurse should provide interventions to relieve pain and other symptoms in the dying client even when those interventions entail risks of hastening death" (p. 8).

Balancing Good and Evil—The Principle of Double Effect

Any discussion that includes attempts to distinguish between harming and benefiting patients often includes the principle of double effect. Developed by Roman Catholic moral theologians in the Middle Ages, this principle is applied to situations in which it is impossible to avoid all harmful action and a decision must be made about whether one potentially harmful action is preferable to another (Quill, Dresser, & Brock, 1997). This principle is used to justify claims that the results of an act that would be morally wrong if caused intentionally are permissible if foreseen but unintended. The principle is often cited to explain why certain forms of care at the end of life that result in death are morally permissible and others are not (Coyle, 1992; Latimer, 1991; Quill, Lo, & Brock, 1997; Schwarz, 2004b, Truog, et al., 2008).

The traditional formulation of this principle stipulates that the following four conditions be met before an act with both good and bad consequences may be morally justified (Schwarz, 2004b):

1) The action itself must be good or at least morally indifferent.
2) The individual must sincerelyintend only the good effect and not the evil.
3) The evil effect cannot be the means to the good effect; and
4) There must be a proportionately grave reason for permitting the evil effect, that is, there must be a favorable balance between the good and the evil effects of action.

The first condition determines whether the potential action is ever permissible, while the second and third conditions are used to determine whether the potential harm is intentional or unintentional, either as a means or as an end in itself. The fourth condition requires the agent to compare the net good and bad effects of the potential act to determine which course produces an effect of proportionally greater good (Quill et al., 1997).

Nurses may appeal to this principle in morally difficult situations where it is not possible to benefit a patient by an action without at the same time causing harm. The classic example is that of the terminally ill pulmonary patient who is experiencing both great pain and a low respiratory rate. The treatment of choice, injecting morphine sulfate, will quell the pain but might also "quell" the respiratory rate. The nurse has a moral duty to prevent and remove evil (pain) that appears to conflict with the duty to benefit patients (protect and preserve life), a dilemma indeed. The answer to the question of whether the nurse may administer morphine is clearly yes. Applying the criteria of double effect illustrates why this is so:

1) The action of giving an injection of morphine is itself morally indifferent.
2) The intendedeffect is to relieve the pain, not to depress the respirations.
3) Respiratory depression is not the means by which the pain relief is obtained.
4) The relief of pain and the related reduction of suffering combine to provide a sufficiently important reason, or proportionately greater good than the harm that is incurred—respiratory depression and likely death (Schwarz, 2004b).

Although this moral analysis is consistent with the position found within the Code of Ethics (ANA, 2001), there are some who question the clinical usefulness of this principle as a guide to ethical decision making (Beauchamp & Childress, 2008). In particular, some clinical experts in palliative care challenge the purported "double effect" of opiate use in terminally ill patients, and describe the likelihood of a secondarily associated hastened death as an "over blown myth" (Manfredi, Morrison, & Meier, 1998, p. 139). Indeed, some studies have shown that opioids do not hasten death in terminally ill patients, particularly in patients who are not opioid naïve, due to acquisition of tolerance to an opioids respiratory depressant effect (Bakker, Jansen, Lima & Kompanje, 2008; Portenoy et al., 2006). Others caution that "using the [principle of double effect] to justify using opioids to treat pain in dying patients contributes to the belief in the double effect of pain medication, which in turn leads to fear of hastening death and the undertreatment of pain" (Fohr, 1998, p. 316).

Experienced palliative care nurses recognize that death sometimes occurs secondarily as an unintended though foreseen side effect of high-dose opiates used to manage refractory symptoms in dying patients. Despite the clear legal and moral consensus supporting the appropriateness of such interventions, when a patient dies immediately after a nurse provides additional analgesia, it can be a very disquieting experience. The fear of hastening death is well documented as one of the primary reasons nurses may be reluctant to provide adequate pain relief to suffering patients (Solomon et al., 1993).

Nurses are encouraged to also consult the ANA (1991) position statement on the promotion of comfort and relief of pain in dying patients. Nurses are supported in their obligation to provide "increasing titration of medication to achieve adequate symptom control, *even at the expense of life, thus hastening death secondarily*" (ANA, 1991, p. 1).

Justice. The last principle that may facilitate nurses' decisions about end-of-life care is justice, which is understood broadly as fairness. Justice involves the determination of what someone or some group is owed, merits, deserves, or otherwise is entitled to (Yeo, Moorhouse, & Donner, 1996b). At the societal (macro) level of resource allocation, the concept of justice includes questions of how scarce resources ought to be distributed and what should "count" as morally relevant differences between individuals in order to justify differences in treatment. Micro-allocation issues involve determining which particular person will receive a specific and limited resource. A number of criteria for making such selections include likelihood of medical benefit, random selection criteria, and present and future quality of life criteria (Yeo, Moorhouse, & Donner, 1996b). It is generally agreed that if a treatment will not medically benefit a patient, it is considered futile, and as such its use is morally and professionally unwarranted. Medically futile interventions should not be proposed or offered to patients or families. As an illustration of how questions of futility have been clinically addressed, Choi and Billings (2002) describe a Texas law cited by Fine and Mayo that attempts to remedy a situation that can occur when clinicians feel forced to provide medically inappropriate or futile care to terminally ill patients whose families insist that "everything be done" to avoid death. Under this Texas law, a detailed process of negotiation includes consultation with an ethics or medical committee; the option of family participation in the committee deliberations; and if the committee concludes that treatment is medically inappropriate, giving the family 10 days to transfer the patient, appeal to the courts, or accept that life support will be withdrawn. The concept of "medically inappropriate" treatment is broader than the concept of "medically futile" treatment. Both, however, involve analyzing probabilities of achieving a desired goal, and weighing proposed benefits against imposed burdens. For example, when considering whether cardio-pulmonary resuscitation (CPR) attempts would be medically futile, more recent research shows survival to hospital discharge in the 6%–7% range overall for patients with advanced cancer (Westphal, 2008). This is higher than the survival rate Schneiderman and Jecker (1995) proposed that a treatment should be considered medically futile if it has not achieved its intended goal in the last 100 cases. Nevertheless, Varon and Marik (2007) argue that obtaining Do-Not-Resuscitate (DNR) orders for patients with advanced cancer is medically inappropriate, whether or not it fits the definition for being medically futile.

At the individual level of end-of-life care, clinicians cite justice in support of claims for dying patients to receive access to a level of palliative care equal to that of curative care (Coyle, 1992). In the current era of cost containment and social injustice, some fear that those who are already marginalized and disadvantaged by poverty, chronic or terminal illness, old age, or by cultural and racial status or gender may feel a duty to die in order to spare families financial or emotional strain (Robinson, 1990; Bergner, 2007). Individual nurses or other healthcare professional will not resolve these complex issues at the bedside. However, many who advocate for U.S. health- care reform agree that cost must be considered in the allocation of healthcare resources (Emanuel, 2008). How to do this fairly requires interdisciplinary understanding and cooperative effort among all affected parties within society (American College of Physicians, 2008, Aroskar, 1987). Meanwhile, the Code for Nurses (ANA, 2001) stresses that the nurse's commitment is to particular patients, "unrestricted by considerations of social or economic status, personal attributes, or the nature of their health problem" (p. 7) and regardless of the cost of their care to society. The challenge for caregivers is to reach ethically supportable decisions that are fair to individual patients while using available resources responsibly.

ELEMENTS OF A DECISION-MAKING FRAMEWORK

When nurses must choose between alternative courses of action that seem equally unattractive, they experience an ethical dilemma. The decision will have significant implications for the well- being of the patient, involved family members, and for others affected by the choice. The nurse's ability to provide an ethically defensible rationale for decisions is recognized as a foundation to professional practice and the integrity of individual nurses (Davis et al., 1997). Rushton and Reigle (1993) argue in support of a shared decision-making model that promotes patient well-being and self-determination. According to this model, the health care team offers expert knowledge, treatment recommendations, and advice about medically available and appropriate options to the patient (patient family unit). The patient decides which option will best promote his or her life goals and values. The nurse is particularly well positioned to understand the values that inform patients'choices and to appreciate the context of the patient's whole life, including the patient/family unit; their cultural, religious, and spiritual affiliations; and other unique preferences. The nurse is a vitally important member of this decision-making team.

When a clinical problem is identified as ethical and conflicts in moral values or ethical principles are present, the following steps will assist the nurse to discuss, analyze, and successfully develop an ethically supportable decision:

1) Review the overall situation—identify what is going on in this case.
2) Gather all relevant facts about the patient and her or his contextual situation, including:
   i. significant medical and social history,
   ii. decision-making capacity, and
   iii. existence of any advance treatment directives— written, appointed, or verbal, and any pertinent institutional policies.
3) Identify the parties or stakeholders involved in the situation, including those who will be affected by the decision(s) made.
4) Identify relevant legal data, including both state and federal laws.
5) Identify specific conflicts of ethical principles or values. Identify and consider nursing guidelines and the profession's code and position statements.
6) Identify possible choices, their purpose, and their probable consequences to the welfare of the patient, who is the focus of primary concern. Identify and make use of interdisciplinary and institutional resources such as institutional and nursing ethics committees, ethicists, chaplains, social workers, and other experienced colleagues.
7) Identify practical constraints to decision making, for example, institutional, legal, organizational, political, and economic.
8) Take action if you are the decision maker and implementer of the decision(s).
9) Review and evaluate the situation after action is taken in order to determine what was learned that will help in the resolution of similar situations in patient care and policy development (Cassells & Gaul, 1998; Davis et al., 1997).

CONCEPTUAL CONFUSION AND DIFFICULT DECISIONS IN END-OF-LIFE CARE

The final segment of this chapter will explore issues of patient autonomy and decisions about end-of-life interventions that range from instances of allowing or permitting death, to hastening or intentionally causing death and how these decisions are understood by nurses.

Autonomy and the Refusal of Life-Sustaining Treatment

If the concept of autonomy means anything at all, it means the right to accept or refuse medical treatments. Decisions about the use or withdrawal of life-sustaining treatments (LST) are often complex and value-laden, in part because such decisions may forestall or hasten the time of death. Decisions regarding use of LST may also influence the patient's experience of the final stage of life by determining where death occurs, who is present, and whether the patient is able to communicate with loved ones (e.g., whether the patient is connected to a ventilator).

The concept of life-sustaining treatments includes any medical or nursing intervention, procedure, or medication, no matter how simple or complex, that is necessary for continued life. In the past, some treatments were considered ordinary and morally required, while others were called extraordinary and considered optional. This distinction between ordinary and extraordinary treatments has a prominent history within the Roman Catholic tradition and was used to determine whether a patient's refusal of treatment should be classified as suicide. Within that faith tradition, refusal of ordinary means was considered by some to be an unacceptable decision that was morally equivalent to an act of suicide (Beauchamp & Childress, 2008).

The terms *optional* or *non-burdensome treatments* include all medications, treatments, and operations that offer a reasonable hope of benefit and can be obtained and used without excessive expense, pain, or other inconvenience from the patient's perspective. *Extraordinary* (or *burdensome*) treatments are those that are very costly, unusual, difficult or dangerous, or do not offer a reasonable hope of benefit to the patient (Davis et al., 1997). What should be of moral concern for nurses is not what the intervention is, but whether the benefits of its continued use outweigh its associated burdens, as determined by the patient or surrogate decision-maker.

Withholding and Withdrawing Life-Prolonging Treatments

Many healthcare professionals and family members are more comfortable not initiating life-sustaining treatments than stopping them once begun. However, the question to be answered is whether this psychological fact has any moral significance (Beauchamp & Childress, 2008). Some clinicians regard withdrawing LST as "letting die," an act previously referred to as *passive euthanasia*, while others view withdrawing LST as an *act* that feelsmore like causing death, or killing. Withdrawing LST may be experienced as morally problematic for some nurses, particularly those who emphasize the "sanctity of life" and believe that continued life is an intrinsic good, regardless of burdens imposed by illness. However, nurses should be familiar with the legal and moral consensus that recognizes no moral distinction between withholding and withdrawing LST.

This consensus began to emerge in the early 1980s when a presidential commission was created to explore significant ethical issues in healthcare (President's Commission, 1983). One of their reports, entitled "Deciding to Forego Life-Sustaining Treatment,"maintains that "neither criminal nor civillaw—if properly interpreted and applied. . . forces patients to undergo procedures that will increase their suffering when they wish to avoid this by foregoing life-sustaining treatments" (p. 89). The commission further held that "the distinction between failing to initiate and stopping therapy—that is, withholding versus withdrawing treatment—is not in itself of moral (or legal) importance. A justification that is adequate for not commencing a treatment is also sufficient for ceasing it" (p. 61).

There is a clear ethical consensus that LST may be withheld or withdrawn under certain circumstances; in particular, when its use is against the patient's wishes (provided the patient is fully informed and freely consenting), when it will or has begun to harm the patient, or when it does not or will not benefit the patient in the future (Beauchamp & Childress, 2008). The ANA (1994b) position statement on assisted suicide similarly encourages nurses to honor the refusal of treatments that an informed patient does not want, either because they are deemed overly burdensome or because they will not benefit the patient. This position statement specifically notes that when nurses participate in decisions to forgo life-sustaining treatments or provide other interventions aimed at relieving suffering that have an associated risk of hastening death, these acts are ethically acceptable and do not constitute assisted suicide.

Withdrawing Artificial Nutrition and Hydration

Often the most difficult decisions about withholding treatments are those that involve simple noninvasive therapies, such as the use of antibiotics, and those that are symbolically linked to caring and nurturing interventions, such as providing food and fluids. "Artificial" or technologically provided nutrition and hydration must be distinguished from the oral provision of food and water. Although dying patients typically experience a decline in appetite as death nears, nurses should continue to offer fluids and food so long as patients indicate any interest or derive pleasure in eating or in drinking fluids. The administration of artificial nutrition and hydration is viewed differently. A moral and legal consensus concludes that artificial nutrition and hydration is a medical treatment that may be refused or withdrawn on the same grounds as any other medical intervention that is, on an estimation of its expected benefit or burden to the patient (Beauchamp & Childress, 2008). Ethical difficulties arise when it is unclear whether continued provision of nutrition is more beneficial or harmful to the patient.

A growing body of evidence suggests that routine use of artificial nutrition and hydration (ANH) in the care of terminally ill persons is unwarranted, and that providing ANH is unlikely to achieve the clinical outcomes for which it is most often employed, for example, to enhance comfort, prolong survival, and improve quality of life (Choi & Billings, 2002; Ersek, 2003; Suter, Rogers, & Strack, 2008).

In those cases where a patient is unable to make her or his wishes known, or is unable to evaluate the benefits or harms of refusing artificial nutrition and hydration, a surrogate decision-maker should be relied upon to determine what is in the patient's best interests. Nurses should know whether their state's legislative policy restricts or limits surrogates'rights to decide about the administrations of artificial nutrition and hydration. Many states have one or more explicit statutory provisions that require meeting a separate and more stringent standard before surrogates are permitted to refuse ANH (Seiger, Arnold, & Ahronheim, 2002).

From Letting Die to Assisted Dying

Nurses who regularly care for dying patients may experience requests for assistance in dying (AID) from patients or family members. Interest in clinician-provided assisted dying is thought, in part, to reflect an American public increasingly fearful of the process of dying, particularly the possibility of dying a painful, protracted, and undignified death that is absent from personal control or meaning (Schwarz, 2004a). Gallup's annual survey on Values and Beliefs, completed in May, 2007, found that, a majority (56%) of Americans believe doctors should be allowed to help a terminally ill patient commit "suicide" if the patient requests it. Most Americans also say doctors should be allowed by law to "end" a terminally ill patient's life by some painless means if the patient and family request it. Support for euthanasia has always been higher than support for doctor-assisted suicide. In the current poll, 71% favor euthanasia, while 27% oppose it (Carroll, 2007). Some commentators suggest that the option of voluntarily stopping eating and drinking (VSED) may be a preferable alternative to physician-assisted dying when suffering patients seek information about hastening death (Bernat, Gert, & Mogielnick, 1993; Terman, 2007). Other palliative care clinicians consider VSED to be an option of last resort for those whose suffering is intractable (Quill & Byock, 2000). Schwarz (2008) argues that nurses ought to respond to dying patients'questions about end of life options that may permit them to control their own dying; VSED is one such option that patients may legally choose.

The Oregon Death with Dignity Act (ODWDA)

Since 1997, physician-assisted dying has been a legally available end-of-life option in Oregon for terminally ill, decisionally capable citizens who make repeated, documented, voluntary requests for such assistance. In Oregon, a physician may write a prescription for a lethal amount of medication following a 15-day waiting period, between the first and second oral requests for assistance and after receiving a written request by the patient. The physician also must determine that the patient is terminally ill, decisionally capable, making an informed and voluntary request for assistance in dying, and that they have been informed about and referred to palliative and hospice care. A second consulting physician must confirm that the patient is in the terminal stage of disease and the absence of any impairment in judgment due to psychiatric or other psychological disorder like untreated depression.

Oregon physicians are required by law to explore and document the reasons for their patient's request for aid in dying, and to submit that and other demographic data to the Oregon Department of Human Services which publishes those data annually (http://egov.Oregon.gov/DHS/ph/pas/) Thus we know the following about those who used the law in 2007: almost 90% were diagnosed with cancer, most were between the ages of 55–64 (the median age, 65, was 5 years younger than the median age in previous years), there were, again, slightly more men than women (53.1%) and 90% of all patients died at home, were enrolled in hospice, and all had some form of health insurance.

During 2007, 85 prescriptions for lethal medication were written; 46 patients died after ingesting such medication, 26 died of their underlying disease, and 13 who had prescriptions were alive at the end of 2007. In addition, three patients with prescriptions from a previous year ingested the medications, thus a total of 49 deaths occurred during 2007 following self-administration of lethal medication. This corresponds to an estimated 15.6 deaths per 10,000 total deaths. Each year, approximately two thirds of those who receive prescriptions actually use them, which confirms the fact that only a small proportion of terminally ill Oregonians choose to hasten their deaths by using this law. Since the law was passed in 1997, a total of 341 pts have died using the ODWDA.

Oregon physicians report that, while their patients often have multiple reasons for their decision to hasten their death, the following three concerns are consistently reported: 1) Loss of autonomy, 2) Decreasing ability to participate in activities that make life meaningful, and 3) Loss of dignity. During 2007, more patients mentioned inadequate pain control (33%) than in previous years, despite the fact that almost 90% of these patients were receiving hospice care.

In summary, terminally ill Oregonians who choose to hasten their death under the provisions of the Death with Dignity Act, do so infrequently, and only after thoughtful consideration and careful planning. Such measured and considered steps in a process that requires at least two weeks to complete, seems to many to be distinct from acts of suicide that are frequently accompanied by impulsive, irrational, and often violent behavior. Perhaps in recognition of that distinction, in October 2006, the ORDHS, adopted a policy to stop using the terms "suicide" or "physician assisted suicide" when referring to the death of persons who use the ODWDA. That policy is consistent with the actual language in the law that specifically states that actions taken in accordance with the Act shall NOT constitute suicide, assisted suicide, mercy killing or homicide.

Increasingly, members of some professional organizations who work with dying patients have joined in the call for use of emotionally neutral language to describe the end-of-life choices made by decisionally capable, terminally ill persons who are considering hastening their dying deaths. In 2007, the American Academy of Hospice and Palliative Medicine (AAHPM) published a position statement on physician-assisted death that explained the reasons for their preferred use of the term physician-assisted death (PAD), stating that PAD more accurately captures the essence of the process than the more "emotionally charged designation of physician-assisted suicide." (www.aahpm.org/positions/suicide/html) This organization also took a position of "studied neutrality" on the question of whether PAD should be legally regulated or prohibited. Also in 2007, the American Medical Woman's Association published a position statement supporting the right of physicians to provide a competent, terminally ill pt with—but not administer—a lethal dose of medication and/or medical knowledge, so that the patient can, without further assistance, hasten his/her own death. They call this practice Aid in Dying.

No nursing organizations have taken a similar position. Indeed, in 2006, the Hospice and Palliative Nurses Association reconfirmed their opposition to the legalization of assisted suicide, and the American Nurses Association has yet to revise their 1994 position statement opposing nurse participation in assisted suicide that includes the frequently cited definition of such assistance as "making a means of suicide (e.g., providing pills or a weapon) available to a patient with knowledge of the patient's intention."

Nurses hold varied views about nurse participation in assisted dying and often justify their position by referring to their own clinical experience (Schwarz, 1999a). Crucial to most who argue in support of assisting in dying are duties of beneficence, compassion for irremediable suffering, and the obligation to respect the autonomy of competent persons (Daly, Berry, Fitzpatrick, Drew, & Montgomery, 1997). Some experienced hospice nurses argue for those "very occasional" patients who, despite receiving skilled palliative care, prefer death to the life they are left with (Stephany, 1994). Most participants in the study by Schwarz (2003, 2004a) maintained that if patients were decisionally capable, had received good end-of-life palliative care, and made a voluntary and informed decision to end their own lives, they had the right to do that, but patients did not have the right to a nurse's assistance in dying (Schwarz, 2004a).

The professional nursing organization opposes nurse involvement in both active euthanasia and assisted suicide; participation in either action is considered a breach of the Code for Nurses (ANA, 2001) and the ethical traditions of the profession. The justification for opposing nurse participation in active euthanasia is based on the principle of respect for persons, and nursing's historical commitment "to promote, preserve, and protect human life" (ANA, 1994a, p. 2). Opposition to assisted suicide is based on the nurse's "obligation to provide comprehensive and compassionate end-of-life care which includes the promotion of comfort and the relief of pain, and at times, foregoing life-sustaining treatments" (ANA, 1994b, p. 1). The rationale for opposing nurse participation in assisted dying refers to the profession's central moral axiom—respect for persons—as well as the duty to "do no harm." The ethic of care and the profession's covenant with society that historically has been to promote, preserve, and protect human life (ANA, 1994b) are also factors.

Ethical Issues in Gerontology

Medical research and technology have extended life spans which, together with the aging Baby Boomer generation, have shifted the population age demographics toward the older adult. Indeed, the fastest-growing age demographic in the U.S. is persons 85 years and older. While on the one hand this is a marker of success, on the other hand, it forces more complex decisions to be made about when, if ever, to place limits on the use of medical interventions for the older adult. Should the focus be on life-prolongation regardless of quality of life? How should decisions be made about allocating limited medical resources to older adults, who have less time to reap the benefits of expensive and potentially risky medical therapies? What obligations are owed to caregivers of the elderly, whose lives are often greatly impacted by the choices elders make about their health and living situation? While many embrace the *idea* of caring for their aging parents, the physical and emotional caregiving burden can be overwhelming, particularly when we consider the stressors experienced by the "Sandwich Generation"—those caring for both their own children and elder family members at the same time or in quick succession (Rogerson, 2005).

In discussing "ethics at the end of life," *end of life* usually serves as a euphemism for the process of dying and death. The term is generally reserved for those who are expected to die within a given time frame (e.g., less than six months) from an incurable, progressive disease. By this definition, the *end of life* is not restricted to the older adult. Yet, as one ages and surpasses his or her estimated life expectancy, mortality looms closer regardless of health status, causing most to include the older adult in discussions of "ethics at the end of life." This is likely what prompted one healthy 90 year old woman to tell her healthcare providers she was ten years younger than she was to ensure that they would not "give up too easily" in providing her medical care.

However, while some fear that doctors may "give up" too easily on their elderly patients, others suggest that the over-reliance on procedural, hi-tech medical diagnostics and interventions is creating more burden than benefit among the elderly. Such concerns, backed by research findings, have led to a movement known as "slow medicine," in which physicians stop to consider less aggressive alternatives before implementing high risk medical interventions that may reap limited rewards for the elderly. In the "slow medicine" approach, patients and families must be re-educated to resist the default option of emergency room visits and hospitalizations if they are not likely to achieve the desired goal of improving quality of life (Gross, 2008). Lynn and Goldstein (2003) also point out that the face of fatal illness has changed. Patients with chronic lung or heart disease, dementia, or even cancer, typically face many years of chronic illness and waxing and waning health before they die from the disease. Hence, Lyn and Goldstein use the term "chronic fatal illness" instead of "terminal illness." They advocate adjusting our approach to caregiving and end-of-life planning to accommodate this longer, less predictable dying trajectory.

The question of rationing is often raised when discussing hi-tech, expensive medical interventions that produce limited benefit. Could one conclude that individuals of a certain age should not be candidates for certain therapies, because they cannot reap enough benefit in their remaining years of life? It has been pointed out that age-based rationing already occurs in the U.S. through the Medicare program. That is, elders are *favored* in that they, unlike children in this country and the nonworking people who do not qualify for Medicaid, are assured of health care coverage. Some suggest that age-based rationing that would limit certain medical interventions (e.g., no renal dialysis or organ transplants, and certain other life-extending therapies, to those over a certain age) would be justified based on egalitarian and utilitarian arguments. The egalitarian argument is that individuals receive a greater investment of resources when they are young to allow them to be well-functioning citizens, with the understanding that as they get older, they will receive fewer resources to ensure that the next generation is able to enjoy the same investment of resources in their youth (Daniels, 1985). The problem with that argument is the same as the caveat mentioned above—not all citizens enjoy the same access to resources before they reach their senior years. Furthermore, Jecker (1991) argues that age-based rationing would unjustly disadvantage women, whose life opportunities may have been limited due to sex discrimination, who provide the bulk of child and family member caregiving, and who, comprising a greater percentage of older adults, would be subjected to age-based rationing more often than their male counterparts. And finally, there is evidence that age-based rationing already exists implicitly (Hurst, et al., 2006; Ward, 2000), and would only further disadvantage elder persons and erode their trust in the healthcare system (and further diminish the respect owed to them) if it were formalized through explicit rationing schemes.

A utilitarian argument for age-based rationing is based on poorer outcomes in older adults for certain medical interventions, based on available evidence such as "quality adjusted life years" (QALY) (Dolan, 2001). Yet, critics of this approach argue that age alone is an insufficient predictor of healthcare outcomes, and that if rationing of medical interventions were to be based on outcomes, such decisions should be made based on overall health indicators rather than age alone. (For a more in-depth discussion of the challenges inherent in using quality of life as an outcome measure, particularly for rationing purposes, see Dean, 1999.)

Many have observed that the U.S. culture is youth-oriented and does not afford the older adult the respect that other cultures bestow upon their elders we are a death-denying culture that seeks to defy individual mortality, and thus defy the aging process. Some argue that elders have a duty to accept the limits of their natural life span and avoid requests beyond that point for expensive life-extending medical technology (Callahan, 2000). However, most agree that the healthcare reforms needed in this country cannot be achieved through strict age-based rationing (what some refer to as "hard rationing"). Rather, instead of placing no limits on aggressive, life-extending medical technology while price-rationing the more effective, efficient, and humanistic primary care, we should re-envision our healthcare priorities to focus on quality, justice, and caring rather than life-extension alone. As Churchill wrote:

Most patients would not bankrupt their family and deny their children a fair start in life by striving for a last, expensive extension of their own lives. Neither should we extend our lives at the margins if by so doing we deprive nameless and faceless others a decent provision of care. And such a gesture should not appear to us as a sacrifice, but as the ordinary virtue entailed by a just, social conscience (Churchill, 1988, p. 647).

Clearly, decisions about withholding or withdrawing life-sustaining therapy at the end of life can weigh heavily on HCPs. However, the more seemingly mundane decisions about resource allocation for elder patients in the HCPs office or clinic may be the more difficult ones to reach consensus about what is just. A step in the right direction would be to put healthcare decisions in the hands of healthcare professionals and the inevitable rationing decisions in public forums where they can be debated and approached rationally, and compassionately.

Ethical Issues in Pediatrics

A cornerstone of ethics in pediatrics is recognizing the patient's and parent's input into medical decision-making throughout the developmental trajectory. From birth to the age of majority, the pediatric patient's involvement in their medical care evolves as they grow and mature. And parents, likewise, must respond to different obligations that accompany parenting an infant, toddler, child, and adolescent.

In pediatrics, as in other sub-specialties, many ethical issues and dilemmas are borne out of the increasingly complex medical technology that has evolved over recent decades. A growing number of neonates, for example, require the special services of a neonatal intensive care unit (NICU). This is partly due to higher risk pregnancies of women who delay pregnancy until later in life, and the increased reliance on artificial reproductive technologies that result in multiple gestation pregnancies (Goldenberg, Culhane, Iams, & Romero, 2008). Such pregnancies are more likely to result in premature births that require NICU support. The ensuing dilemmas were poignantly described in the seminal book, *Playing God in the Nursery* (Lyon, 1985). Many point to the NICU babies who beat the survival odds as "miracle babies" whose survival provides proof that pushing the boundaries of neonatal viability is worth the money and resources. Others suggest that providing life-saving NICU technologies to some severely compromised, extremely low-birth weight premature babies is tantamount to human experimentation (Chervenak, McCullough & Levene, 2007). Parents and healthcare providers must consider several important questions when considering whether to pursue life-saving technology for an impaired neonate. These include the following:

- Is there a reasonable chance that the infant will survive?
- If the infant survives, will (s)he have an acceptable quality of life?
- Will future required medical care entail a net benefit or harm to the child?
- When, if ever, is a life of severe physical and/or cognitive impairment worse than death?
- Are resources available to support the future medical needs of the child?

In addition, parents must consider their own beliefs and values, and how their decision will impact other family members. For example, some parents may feel that subjecting a severely impaired infant to aggressive medical therapy that may likely result in neurological devastation and dependence on intensive medical interventions throughout childhood not only imposes undue suffering on that child, but would also place an unacceptable burden on other children in the family, who would be deprived of parental attention. In contrast, other parents may believe that it is their obligation to prolong their child's life no matter what the outcome. You can see here that the former example leans more toward *consequentialism*—deciding what to do based on outcomes, whereas the latter example leans more toward *deontology*—deciding what to do based on moral duty, regardless of outcomes.

In the unique setting of the NICU and Labor and Delivery ward, parents do not have the final say about whether infants receive life-saving interventions. In the early 1980's, a case gained national attention involving an infant born with Down syndrome and esophageal atresia. The parents refused a routine surgical procedure to correct the deformity, resulting in the infant's otherwise preventable death. In response, the federal "Baby Doe" regulations were adopted by the Department of Health and Human Services to protect against discriminatory treatment toward babies and children with disabilities. The courts soon struck down the regulations, which hospitals protested as being overly restrictive. In 1984, Congress amended the Child Abuse Protection and Treatment Act (CAPTA) to help discourage disability bias from influencing life and death decisions, while also avoiding mandating hi-tech treatment for dying infants (Schwartz, 2008). According to CAPTA, a life-prolonging therapy may be withheld or withdrawn from an infant if it is considered to:

- merely prolong dying,
- not be effective in ameliorating or correcting all of the infant's life-threatening conditions,
- be futile in terms of the survival of the infant.

Because a baby's prognosis for survival may not be known immediately at birth, depending on state law, if an infant is born breathing, the healthcare providers may be legally obligated to administer life-saving interventions. However, despite the restrictions on foregoing life support at birth, palliative comfort care should always be an option for any neonate whose prognosis for survival is poor (Catlin & Carter, 2002, Kain, 2006).

For the most part, the same process for ethical decision-making applies to pediatric patients as to adults: consider the likely benefits and burdens of available choices, and act to minimize harm and maximize benefit. Children in general are considered to be "vulnerable persons" who must be protected. Generally, this involves a parent or legal guardian ("parent") making medical decisions for the child, with assent from the child obtained if he or she is capable. Ethical concerns in pediatrics often involve differences of opinion between providers, parents, and patients about the patient's course of treatment. Consider the case of Katie Wernecke. Katie was diagnosed with Hodgkin's lymphoma when she was 13 years old. Her oncologist gave her an 80% chance of survival with chemotherapy followed by radiation. However, Katie's parents wanted to forego the radiation to pursue an alternative treatment of Vitamin C infusions. How did the healthcare team respond? Children's Protective Services was involved, and Katie was placed with foster parents while she continued with her radiation. Ultimately, a judge ruled that Katie be allowed to return to her parents and pursue the alternative treatment, but only after she finished the recommended course of radiation. Some might advocate for a less adversarial way to resolve this conflict, to maintain Katie's family integrity and harmony at a time when she most needed it. However, such decisions are difficult when lives are at stake. As you can see, neither Katie nor her parents had boundless autonomy rights. The state intervened to ensure that Katie received the medical standard of care, which provided a good chance of putting Katie's cancer into remission. This is different from how the state handles a competent adult who refuses life-saving therapy. In that case, forced treatment would be considered a form of battery.

The state recognizes a competent adult's right to refuse life-saving therapy, but usually considers the state's interest in preserving life to trump autonomy rights when a child's life is at stake. Therefore, if a parent's request falls outside an acceptable medical standard of care, healthcare providers may be obligated to override the parent's request. Whenever possible, this should be approached using open channels of communication between the parents and healthcare team to avoid the need to involve the courts.

Conflicts may also ensue when the wishes of the parent and child differ. Consider a 14-year old who has advanced cancer with no hope of cure, but whose life may be prolonged with another course of chemotherapy. The patient tells the nurse she does not want the chemotherapy, that she is tired of fighting the cancer, and prefers to focus on being as comfortable as possible. The parents insist that the chemotherapy be started as soon as possible. In such a situation, the healthcare team has an ethical obligation to resolve this conflict and not proceed without the patient's assent to chemotherapy (Jacobs, 2005).

In rare cases, the rights of a "mature minor" to forego life-sustaining treatment are recognized. For example, if a 15-year old Jehovah's Witness demonstrates a clear and consistent commitment to forego blood products, an ethical argument could be made that this young person's autonomous choice should be respected, even if the risk of death is high. However, in most situations where death is likely and reasonably avoidable, and where parents refuse life-saving interventions for their minor child, healthcare providers opt to petition the court to mandate life-saving treatments.

Pediatric staff should familiarize themselves with their state's law regarding "emancipated minors." These are persons recognized by the courts as able to make their own medical decisions, even though they have not reached the legal age of majority (18 in most states). Criteria for emancipation vary from state to state, but typically include living independently from parents, having a child, and being on active duty in the armed forces. Minors are also allowed to obtain medical treatment for certain conditions without parental permission (e.g., birth control, and certain types of mental healthcare). The rationale for allowing these exceptions is that many teens may not seek needed medical intervention if they know a parent must be notified. Here, healthcare providers must continually weigh the dueling obligations that the principle of *respect for persons* demands—respecting a decisionally capable person's wishes, and protecting a vulnerable person from harm. Since a teenager's ability to make well-reasoned, mature decisions evolves over time, the degree to which his or her wishes and privacy should be respected is situation-specific. Regardless of who makes the final medical decision, children and adolescents should always be included in medical decision-making to the extent that their developmental level allows.

Barriers in the Practice Environment to Sound Ethical Practice

Nurses need to find ways to talk to each other and validate their experiences, tell their stories of despair or triumph, and share their experiences of moral uncertainty. Nurses may experience conflict between their own moral values and the values of the profession and they have the right to remain true to their conscientious moral and religious beliefs. Although prohibited from compromising legitimate patient choices or imposing their values on others, nurses who are ethically opposed to certain patient interventions will find support for their position in the Code for Nurses (ANA, 2001). They have the right to withdraw from providing care, assuming that arrangements can be made for the patient's safe transfer to the care of another.

It is undoubtedly true that some of the barriers that constrain nurses from participating in ethical decision-making are situations over which the nurse has no control. For example, most nurses practice as employees in healthcare organizations whose goals are business-oriented and whose focus is utilitarian (institutional values providing the greatest good for the greatest number). Nurses, by virtue of their education, experience, and moral commitment to caring, are focused on doing

good for individual patients. Conflict inevitably arises between the nurses' role as caregivers and patient advocates, institutional employees, and as clinicians expected to implement physicians' orders. The experience of being the nurse in the middle combined with the moral distress of being unable to do the right thing may result in nurse' perceiving that they are unable to act as morally autonomous agents.

Ethics Committees and Ethics Consultation Services

Ethical issues in clinical practice often involve life-or-death decisions, and such decisions give rise to a host of emotions and concerns. Just as physicians and patients turn to medical specialists and sub-specialists for advice and consultations on questions of medicine, healthcare professionals and patients may need to consult an ethics committee to discuss today's perplexing ethical issues. The overall role of an ethics committee is threefold. First, the committee may educate itself, the hospital administration, and the hospital staff about ethical issues occurring in our current healthcare environment. Second, the committee may participate in policy development. Third, the committee provides ethics case consultation. Ethics consultations are more timely, less adversarial, and more flexible than court proceedings as a way to resolve disputes. A recent survey found that 81% of U.S. hospitals have an ethics consultation service (Fox, Myers, & Pearlman, 2007). Ethics consultation is one mechanism by which a hospital may satisfy the Joint Commission's requirement to have a mechanism to address ethical issues that arise in patient care.

There are different goals that may be sought by ethics consultation. Bernard Lo (2004) identified the following: helping staff to identify and understand the specific ethical issues the case raises; improving communication between the patient, family, and healthcare team; providing emotional support to the health team members involved in a difficult case; offering "ethically justifiable" recommendations for how to resolve an ethical question or dilemma; and improving patient care by preventing patient care decisions that run counter to ethical guidelines and standards. In addition, Dubler and Liebman (2004) focus on the goal of conflict resolution through ethics consultation (Lo, 2000).

Another goal of ethics consultation may be, as Margaret Urban Walker (1993) suggests, to "protect moral spaces" within the healthcare setting. According to this view, burgeoning hi-tech, expensive medical technology—along with our fragmented healthcare system—has increased the complexity and burden of medical decision-making. Yet, healthcare providers have *less* time to grapple with this increasing complexity. Ethics consultations may provide one counter measure to this trend toward fast-paced decision-making by allowing patients, families, and healthcare providers to take a step back and reflect on the ethical issues involved before rushing to judgment about a particular case.

One issue of concern is that a majority of ethics committee members have been found to lack formal training in ethics (Fox et al., 2007). The American Society for Bioethics (1998) has identified core skills and knowledge competencies that ethics consultants (or consult services, collectively) should possess to effectively respond to consultation requests. Nurses should be knowledgeable about who serves on the ethics consultation service at their facility, how their competence is ensured, and how to access the service. Moreover, nurses should develop their own ethics knowledge and skills competencies to most effectively advocate for their patients.

Preventing Burnout

Nurses who care for dying patients often may find themselves in situations of ethical conflict; burnout is one potential consequence. To avoid the experience of burnout, nurses should seek support from peers, share experiences of uncertainty, and seek ethics advice and support for the development of skills in identifying and resolving ethical problems in clinical practice. It is most important for nurses to acknowledge their own suffering and sense of frustration in caring for patients at the end of life. For example, it can be very upsetting and discouraging to identify a treatment approach that appears to be in a patient's best interest but then be unable to implement it (perhaps due to disagreements among team members or family members about what's in the patient's best interests). Sometimes, with reflection, a morally acceptable compromise can be identified, one that preserves the underlying values of the concerned parties. Agreement to a trial of therapy and to reassess within a specified time can help resolve some of the uncertainty.

Hospitals and healthcare organizations that provide support systems for nurses that encourage and facilitate moral growth and understanding will employ nurses who are less likely to succumb to moral passivity. Nurses should be encouraged to create their own opportunities for support regarding end-of-life issues and may consider the following interventions:

1) Use of an ethics consultant can be a source of guidance and help nurses acquire the necessary skills for future application.
2) Multidisciplinary and nursing ethics committees should be available to nurses for case consultation regarding ethical conflicts. Nurses should be members and work in concert with professional colleagues. Multidisciplinary institutional ethics committees also develop institutional policies and guidelines and plan programs for the ethics education of staff members.

3) Interdisciplinary ethics rounds present an ideal opportunity for individuals working in different patient-care disciplines to discuss regularly troubling cases that may not require an immediate decision. Such meetings provide an opportunity for analysis, exploration, and sharing of different points of view. Thus, when ethical problems do occur, a foundation exists to provide guidance about the most effective way to respond.

CONCLUSION

Healthcare providers justifiably look for definitive answers when asking what the "right" thing to do is in a given situation. Sometimes, after sorting through the facts of a troubling case, the right way to handle the uncertainty or conflict becomes apparent. But often, there is no one "right" answer. Sometimes there is more than one response that can be ethically justified (as in the example of responding to a dying patient's request for assistance in hastening death). Other times, whatever course of action is taken requires compromising a core ethical principle, such as abiding by a patient's prior wish to be kept alive with aggressive medical technology, despite the pain and suffering it invokes with little apparent gain. Nurses should be encouraged to continue to provide compassionate care and a caring presence as they struggle together with patients, family members, and professional colleagues, in the attempt to identify what, all things considered, ought to be done in situations of moral conflict. In doing so, we are reminded that "to the extent that care of the dying draws us into their lives, we experience the gifts and deprivations of their own deaths and painfully anticipate the death of our loved ones and even ourselves" (Dixon, 1997, p. 297).

Nurses should continually seek to improve their ethics knowledge base by looking for learning opportunities. At a minimum, they should be familiar with ethical theories of deontology (duty-based ethics) and teleology (consequence-based ethics), ethical principles, and the concepts of decisional capacity, surrogate decision-making, advance directives, mature minors, consent versus assent, moral justifications for withholding and withdrawing life-sustaining treatment, and responding to requests for a hastened death. Nurses should access resources to assist them in ethical decision-making, such as institutional ethics committees, colleagues, and the Nurses Code of Ethics.

Case Study conclusion: How does one start in addressing the question of whether Mrs. Selano's tube feedings should be continued? Cassells and Gaul's "Ethical Assessment Framework" (1998) offers a guide. One of the first steps is to gather the relevant facts. What exactly does the living will document state? Was it properly witnessed and thereby legally valid? Why is it that Mrs. Jenkins thinks Mrs. Selano would benefit from having her tube feedings stopped at this time? Does she think that this has caused Mrs. Selano to suffer? One should involve other experts, as needed, to provide input in this fact-finding phase. In determining which options are ethically justifiable, one should consider how different ethical principles apply to the case. The two components of the principle of respect for persons are relevant—protecting vulnerable persons, and respecting the autonomy of competent adults. Regarding the latter, in considering whether Mrs. Selano's tube feedings should be continued, the nursing home staff is obligated to provide medical care that is consistent with Mrs. Selano's prior stated wishes. Mrs. Jenkins has cast doubt on the validity of Mrs. Selano's living will as it relates to tube feedings. However, given that stopping Mrs. Selano's tube feedings would hasten her death, and assuming that the living will is legally valid, Mrs. Jenkins' request alone would be insufficient to warrant stopping the feedings. This exemplifies the obligation to protect Mrs. Selano as a vulnerable person. One would need a good justification for withdrawing a medical treatment that would result in hastening a patient's death. This does not mean that Mrs. Selano's tube feedings should be continued beyond the point where they are no longer achieving their intended goal. If the tube feedings are considered medically ineffective (for example, they are no longer providing nutrition as evidenced by continued weight loss and increased residual gastric content and fluid back-up) it would be ethically justifiable for a physician to order them to be stopped based on this criterion. The nurse should discuss with Mrs. Jenkins what is being done to maximize Mrs. Selano's comfort and dignity. The hospice could be involved to help manage Mrs. Selano's end-of-life care. Just because Mrs. Selano has a tube feeding keeping her alive does not change the fact that she is dying from end-stage dementia, and deserves all the best that palliative care has to offer.

EVIDENCE-BASED PRACTICE

Review: Survival in cancer patients undergoing in-hospital cardiopulmonary resuscitation: a meta-analysis.

Reisfield, G.M., Wallace, S.K., Munsell, M.F., Webb, F.J., Alvarez, E.R., & Wilson, G.R. (2006). *Resuscitation, 71*(2), 152–60.

Question: Can cardiopulmonary resuscitation (CPR) attempts be considered medically futile for a patient with advanced cancer?

Data sources. National Library of Medicine's Medline database (1966–2005), using key words *CPR, resuscitation, cancer,* and *survival,* and by screening the cited references of the identified studies.

Study selection and assessment. Studies consisting of in-hospital cardiopulmonary arrests; adult patients; at least a subset of cancer patients; an outcome defined as survival to hospital discharge; identified numbers of cancer patients sustaining cardiopulmonary arrest and surviving until hospital discharge. Forty-two studies, in whole or in part, comprising 1707 patients mer the minimal inclusion criteria.

Outcomes. Proportion of survivors to hospital discharge

Main results. Overall survival to discharge was 6.2%. Survival in patients with localized disease was 9.5%, and in patients with metastatic disease was 5.6%. Analysis of data reported since 1990 reveals a narrowing of the survival gap, with survival rates in patients with localized disease of 9.1%, and in patients with metastatic disease of 7.8%. Survival in patients resuscitated on the general medical/surgical wards was 10.1%, while survival in patients resuscitated on intensive care units (ICUs) was 2.2%.

Conclusion. Overall survival of CPR to hospital discharge in cancer patients compares favorably to survival rates in unselected inpatients. Improved outcomes in recent years in patients with metastatic disease are likely to reflect more selective use of CPR in cancer patients, with the sickest patients deselected.

Commentary. The concept of medical futility has a wide scope of interpretations. One view suggests that a given intervention can be considered "futile" if there is less than a 1% chance that it will achieve its intended goal (Schneiderman, Jecker & Jonsen, 1990). The innovators of cardiopulmonary resuscitation (CPR) techniques cautioned physicians that the procedure was not meant to be used for all patients—rather, it should be applied selectively to patients who were likely to benefit from it. However, their caution was not heeded. The implementation of CPR on all patients who suffer cardiopulmonary arrest [in the absence of a Do-Not-Resuscitate (DNR) order] has given way to efforts to reduce the indiscriminate use of CPR (e.g., through the Patient Self-Determination Act of 1990 that encouraged the use of advance directives and discussions about end-of-life care planning between patients and physicians). The studies that Reisfield and colleagues identified before 1990 showed that resuscitation to hospital discharge was unsuccessful for all patients with metastatic cancer. This fueled effort in the 1990's to encourage patients with advanced cancer to agree to a DNR order. However, some physicians reasoned that if CPR is unsuccessful in achieving its intended goal for patients with advanced cancer, then offering them a choice for CPR attempts is disingenuous. Thus, some physicians have begun writing DNR orders for patients based on medical futility criteria (Cantor, et al., 2003). However, as Reisfield and colleagues has shown, post-1990 CPR survival rates have improved to 7.8% for patients with metastatic disease [although survival rates in the ICU (2.2%) are much lower than in the wards (10.1%)]. This is likely the result of both improved resuscitation techniques and selection bias (i.e., the subset of patients with metastatic cancer who had "full code" status and were thus excluded from the meta analysis could be different from the patients with metastatic cancer who had DNR orders precluding CPR attempts). Nevertheless, this evidence does not support the determination that a CPR attempt in a patient with metastatic cancer is medically futile, since a 7.8% chance of success is above the futility threshold that was established of less than 1%. This does not take into account other poor prognostic factors (which could lower the patient's success rate). It also does not address the question of whether the benefits of prolonging the patient's life outweighs the associated burdens.

Schneiderman, L. J., Jecker, N. S., Jonsen, A. R. (1990). Medical futility: Its meaning and ethical implications. *Annals of Internal Medicine, 112,* 949–54.

Cantor, M. D., Braddock, C. H., Derse, A. R., Edwards, D. M., Logue, G. L., Nelson, W., et al. (2003). Do-not-resuscitate orders and medical futility. *Archives of Internal Medicine, 163, 2689–2694.*

REFERENCES

American College of Physicians. (2008). Achieving a high-performance health care system with universal access: What the United States can learn from other countries. *Annals of Internal Medicine, 148,*55–75.

American Nurses Association. (ANA). (1991). *Position statement on the promotion of comfort and relief of pain in dying patients.* Washington, DC: American Nurses Association.

American Nurses Association. (ANA). (1994a). *Position statement on active euthanasia.* Washington, DC: American Nurses Association.

American Nurses Association. (ANA). (1994b). *Position statement on assisted suicide.* Washington, DC: American Nurses Association.

American Nurses Association. (ANA). (2001). *Code of ethics for nurses with interpretive statements.* Washington, DC: American Nurses Association.

American Society for Bioethics and Humanities. (1998). *Core Ccompetencies for Hhealth Ccare Eethics Cconsultation.* Glenview, IL: American Society for Bioethics & Humanities.

Aroskar, M. A. (1987). The interface of ethics and politics in nursing. *Nursing Outlook, 35,* 269.

Bakker, J., Jansen, T. C., Lima, A., & Kompanje, E. J. (2008). Why opioids and sedatives may prolong life rather than hasten death after ventilator withdrawal in critically ill patients. *American Journal of Hospice and Palliative Medicine, 25*(2), 152–154.

Beckstrand, R. L., Smith, M. D., Heaston, S., & Bond, A. E. (2008). Emergency nurses' perceptions of size, frequency, and magnitude of obstacles and supportive behaviors in end-of-life care. *Journal of Emergency Nursing, 34*(4), 290–300.

Beauchamp, T., & Childress, J. (2008). *Principles of biomedical ethics* (6th ed.). New York: Oxford University Press.

Benjamin, M., & Curtis, J. (1992). *Ethics in nursing* (3rd ed.). New York: Oxford University Press.

Bergner, D. (December 2, 2007). Death in the family. *New York Times Magazine,* http://www.nytimes.com/2007/12/02/magazine/02suicide-t.html. (Last accessed 10/07/08).

Bernat, J. L., Gert, B., & Mogielnick, R. P. (1993). Patient refusal of hydration and nutrition: An alternative to physician-assisted suicide or voluntary active euthanasia. *Archives of Internal Medicine, 153,* 2723–2728.

Callahan, D. (2000). *The Ttroubled Ddream of Llife.* Washington, DC: Georgetown University Press. Carroll, J. (May 31, 2007). Public divided over moral acceptability of doctor-assisted suicide. http://www.gallup.com/poll/27727/Public-Divided-Over-Moral-Acceptability-DoctorAssisted-Suicide.aspx

Cameron, M. E. (1997). Legal and ethical issues: Ethical distress in nursing. *Journal of Professional Nursing, 13,* 280.

Cassells, J., & Gaul, A. (1998, January). An ethical assessment framework for nursing practice. *Maryland Nurse, 6*(1), 9–12.

Catlin, A. & Carter, B. (2002). Creation of a neonatal end-of-life palliative care protocol. *Journal of Perinatology, 22*(3), 184–195.

Cavanaugh, T. A. (1996). The ethics of death-hastening or death-causing palliative analgesic administration to the terminally ill. *Journal of Pain and Symptom Management, 12,* 248–254.

Chervenak, F. A., McCullough, L. B., & Levene, M. I. (2007). An ethically justified, clinically comprehensive approach to periviability: Gynaecological, obstetric, perinatal and neonatal dimensions. *Journal of Obstetrics and Gynaecology, J Obstet Gynaecol. 27*(1), 3–7.

Choi, Y. S., & Billings, J. A. (2002). Changing perspective on palliative care. *Oncology, 16,* 515–527.

Churchill (1988). ADD

Clouser, K. D., & Gert, B. (1990). A critique of principlism. *Journal of Medical Philosophy, 15,* 219–236.

Coyle, N. (1992). The euthanasia and physician-assisted suicide debate: Issues for nursing. *Oncology Nursing Forum, 19,* 41–46.

Culver, C., & Gert, B. (1982). *Philosophy in medicine: Conceptual and ethical issues in medicine and psychiatry.* New York: Oxford University Press.

Daly, B. J., Berry, D., Fitzpatrick, J. L., Drew, B., & Montgomery, K. (1997). Assisted suicide: Implications for nurses and nursing. *Nursing Outlook, 45,* 209–214.

Daniels, N. (1985). *Just Hhealth Ccare.* Cambridge: The Press Syndicate of the University of Cambridge.

Davis, A. J. (1994). Selected issues in nursing ethics: Clinical, philosophical, political. *Bioethics Forum, 10,* 10–14.

Davis, A. J., Aroskar, M. A., Liaschenko, J., & Drought, T. S. (1997). *Ethical dilemmas and nursing practice* (4th ed.). Stamford, CT: Appleton & Lange.

Dean, A. M. (1999). The applicability of SERVQUAL in different health care environments. *Health Mark Q., 16*(3), 1–21.

Dexter, P. R., Wolinsky, F. D., Gramelspacher, G. J., Eckert, G. J., & Tierney, W. M. (2003). Opportunities for advance directives to influence acute medical care. *Journal of Clinical Ethics, 14,* 173–182.

Dixon, M. D. (1997). The quality of mercy: Reflections on provider-assisted suicide. *Journal of Clinical Ethics, 8,* 290–302.

Dolan, P. (2001). Utilitarianism and the measurement and aggregation of quality: Adjusted life years. *Health Care Analysis, 9*(1), 65–76.

Dubler, N. N. & Liebman, C. B. (2004). *Bioethics Mediation: A Guide to Shaping Shared Solutions.* New York: United Hospital Fund of New York.

Emanuel, E. J. (2008). The cost-coverage trade-off. "It's health care costs, stupid." *JAMA, 299*(8), 947–949.

Ersek, M. (2003). Artificial nutrition and hydration: Clinical issues. *Journal of Hospice and Palliative Nursing, 5,* 221–230.

Fagerlin, A., & Schneider. C. E. (2004). Enough: The failure of the living will. *Hastings Center Report 34*(2), 30–42.

Fiester, A. (2007). Viewpoint: Why the clinical ethics we teach fails patients. *Academy of MedicineAcad Med., 2007 82*(7), 684–689.

Hurst, S. A., Slowther, A., Forde, R., Pegoraro, R., Reiter-Theil, S., Perrier, A., et al. (2006). Prevalence and determinants of physician bedside rationing. *Journal of General Internal Medicine, 21,* 1138–1143.

Fohr, S. A. (1998). The double effect of pain medication: Separating myth from reality. *Journal of Palliative Medicine, 1*(4), 315–328.

Fowler, M. D. (1987). Introduction to ethics and ethical theory. In M. D. Fowler & J. Levine-Ariff (Eds.), *Ethics at the bedside: A source book for the critical care nurse* (pp. 24–38). Philadelphia: Lippincott.

Fox, E., Myers, S. & Pearlman, R. A. (2007). Ethics consultation in United States hospitals: A national survey. *The American Journal of Bioethics, 7*(2), 1–14.

Frankena, W. K. (1973). *Ethics* (2nd ed.). Englewood Cliffs, NJ: Prentice-Hall.

Fry, S. T. (1987). Autonomy, advocacy, and accountability: Ethics at the bedside. In M. D. Fowler & J. Levine-Ariff (Eds.), *Ethics at the bedside: A source book for the critical care nurse* (pp. 39–49). Philadelphia: Lippincott.

Fry, S. T. (1989). Towards a theory of nursing ethics. *Advances in Nursing Science, 11*(4), 9–22.

Fry, S. T., Killen, A. R., & Robinson, E. M. (1996). Care-based reasoning, caring and the ethic of care: A need for clarity. *Journal of Clinical Ethics, 7*(1), 41–47.

Gadow, S. (1996). Aging as death rehearsal: The oppressiveness of reason. *Journal of Clinical Ethics, 7*(1), 35–40.

Goldenberg, R. L., Culhane, J. F., Iams, J. D. & Romero, R. (2008). Epidemiology and causes of preterm birth. *Lancet. 371*(9606), 75–84.

Gross, J. (May 5, 2008). For the elderly, being heard about life's end. *New York Times,* http://www.nytimes.com/2008/05/05/health/05slow.html#. Last accessed August 31, 2008.

Held, V. (1994). Feminism and moral theory. In J. E. White (Ed.), *Contemporary moral problems* (4th ed., pp. 208–216). St. Paul, MN: West.

Jacobs, H. H. (2005). Ethics in pediatric end-of-life care: A nursing perspective. *Journal of Pediatric Nursing, 20*(5), 360–369.

Jameton, A. (1984). *Nursing practice: The ethical issues.* Englewood Cliffs, NJ: Prentice-Hall.

Jecker, N. S. (1991). Age-based rationing and women. *Journal of American Medical Association, 266*(21), 3012–3015.

Kain, V. J. (2006). Palliative care delivery in the NICU: What barriers do neonatal nurses face? *Neonatal Network, Neonatal Netw. 25*(6), 387–392.

Latimer, E. J. (1991). Ethical decision-making in the care of the dying and its application to clinical practice. *Journal of Pain and Symptom Management, 6,* 329–336.

Limerick, M. H. (2007). The process used by surrogate decision makers to withhold and withdraw life-sustaining measures in an intensive care environment. *Oncology Nursing Forum,Oncol Nurs Forum. 34*(2), 331–339.

Lo, B. (2000). *Resolving Eethical Ddilemmas: A Gguide for Cclinicians* (2nd ed.). Philadelphia, PA: Lippincott Williams & Wilkins.

Lynn, J., & Goldstein, N. E. (2003). Advance care planning for fatal chronic illness: Avoiding commonplace errors and unwarranted suffering. *Annals of Internal Medicine, Ann Intern Med. 138*(10), 812–818.

Lynn, J., Teno, J., Dresser, R., Brock, D., Lindemann Nelson, H., Kielstein, R., et al. (1999). Dementia and advance-care planning: Perspective from three countries on ethics and epidemiology. *Journal of Clinical Ethics, 10,* 271–285.

Lyon, J. (1985). *Playing Ggod in the Nnursery.* New York: W. W. Norton & Co.,

Manfredi, P. L., Morrison, R. S., & Meier, D. E. (1998). The rule of double effect. [Letter to the editor]. *Journal of the American Medical Association, 338,* 1390.

Mezey, M., Mitty, E., & Ramsey, G. (1997). Assessment of decision-making capacity: Nursing's role. *Journal of Gerontological Nursing, 23*(3), 28–35.

Nelson, J. E., Angus, D. C., Weissfeld, L. A., Puntillo, K. A., Danis, M., Deal, D., et al. (2006). End-of-life care for the critically ill: A national intensive care unit survey. *Critical Care Medicine,Crit Care Med. 34*(10), 2547–2553.

Perkins, H. S. (2007). Controlling death: The false promise of advance directives. *Annals of Internal Medicine, 147,* 51–57.

Perrin, K. O. (1997). Giving voice to the wishes of elders for end-of-life care. *Journal of Gerontological Nursing, 23*(3), 18–27.

Portenoy, R. K., Sibirceva, U., Smout, R., Horn, S., Connor, S., Blum, R.H., et al. (2006). Opioid use and survival at the end of life: A survey of a hospice population. *Journal of Pain & and Symptom Management, 32*(6), 532–540.

President's Commission for the Study of Ethical Problems in Medicine and Biomedical and Behavioral Research. (1983). *Deciding to forego life-sustaining treatment.* Washington, DC: U.S. Government Printing Office.

Quill, T. E. & Byock, I. R. (2000). Responding to intractable suffering: The role of terminal sedation and voluntary refusal of food and fluids. *Annals of Internal Medicine, 132,* 408–414.

Quill, T. E., Dresser, R., & Brock, D. W. (1997). The rule of double effect: A critique of its role in end-of-life decision making. *New England Journal of Medicine, 337,* 1763–1771.

Quill, T. E., Lo, B., & Brock, D. W. (1997). Palliative options of last resort: A comparison of voluntarily stopping eating and drinking, terminal sedation, physician-assisted suicide, and voluntary active euthanasia. *Journal of the American Medical Association, 278,* 2099–2104.

Robinson, B. (1990, Winter). Question of life and death: No easy answers. *Ageing International,* 27–35.

Rogerson, P. A. (2005). Population distribution and redistribution of the baby-boom cohort in the United States: Recent trends and implications. *Proceeding of the National Academy of Sciences, 25;–102*(43), 15319–15324.

Rushton, C., & Reigle, J. (1993). Ethical issues in critical nursing. In M. Kinney, D. Packa, & S. Dunbar (Eds.), *AACN's clinical reference for critical care* (pp. 8–27). St. Louis, MO: Mosby.

Schneiderman, L. J., & Jecker, N. S. (1995). *Wrong Mmedicine: Doctors, Patients, and futile treatment.* Baltimore: Johns Hopkins University Press.

Schwartz, J. (Spring, 2008). Considering baby doe rules. *Mid-Atlantic Ethics Committee Newsletter,* citing 42 U.S.C § 5106g(6).

Schwarz, J. K. (1999a). Assisted dying and nursing practice. *Image, 31,* 367–373.

Schwarz, J. K. (2003). Understanding and responding to patients' requests for assistance in dying. *Journal of Nursing Scholarship, 35,* 377–384.

Schwarz, J. K. (2004a). Responding to persistent requests for assistance in dying: A phenomenological inquiry. *International Journal of Palliative Nursing, 10,* 225–235.

Schwarz, J. K. (2004b). The rule of double effect and its role in facilitating good end-of-life care: A help or a hindrance? *Journal of Hospice and Palliative Nursing, 6,* 125–133.

Schwarz, J. (2008). I can't help you with that. *American Journal of Nursing, 108,* 11.

Seiger, C. E., Arnold, J. F., & Ahronheim, J. C. (2002). Refusing artificial nutrition and hydration: Does statutory law send the wrong message? *Journal of the American Geriatrics Society, 50,* 544–550.

Shalowitz, A. B., Garrett-Mayer, E., & Wendler, D. (2006). The accuracy of surrogate decision makers: A systematic review. *Archives of Internal Medicine,Arch Inter Med. 166,* 493–497.

Solomon, M., O'Donnell, L., Jennings, B., Guilfoy, J., Wolf, S., Nolan, K., et al. (1993). Decisions near the end of life: Professional views on life-sustaining treatments. *American Journal of Public Health, 83*(4), 14–22.

Stanley, J. K., & Zoloth-Dorfman, L. (2001). Ethical considerations. In B. R. Ferrell & N. Coyle (Eds.), *Textbook of palliative nursing* (pp. 663–681). New York: Oxford University Press.

Steinbock, B., Aaras, J. & London, A. (2002). *Ethical issues in modern medicine,* (6th Ed.). Columbus, OH: The McGraw-Hill Companies.

Stephany, T. M. (1994). Assisted suicide: How hospice fails. *American Journal of Hospice and Palliative Care, 10*(6), 1–5.

Suter, P. M., Rogers, J., & Strack, C. (2008). Artificial nutrition and hydration for the terminally ill: A reasoned approach. *Home Healthcare Nurse, 26*(1), 23–9.

Terman, S. A. (2007). *The best way to say goodbye: A legal peaceful choice at the end of Life.* Life Transitions Publications.

Tierney, W. M., Dexter, P. R., Gramelspacher, G. P., Perkins, A. J., Zhou, X. H., Wolinksy, F. D., et al. (2001). The effect of discussions about advance directives on patients' satisfaction with primary care. *Journal of General Internal Medicine,16*(1), 32–40.

Tilden, V. P., Tolle, S. W., Nelson, C. A., & Fields, J. (2001). Family decision-making to withdraw life-sustaining treatments from hospitalized patients. *Nursing Research, 50,* 105–115.

Tonelli, R. R. (1996). Pulling the plug on living wills: A critical analysis of advance directive. *Chest, 110,* 816–822.

Truog, R. D., Campbell, M. L., Curtis, J. R., Haas, C. E., Luce, J. M., Rubenfeld, G. D., et al. (2008). Recommendations for end-of-life care in the intensive care unit: A consensus statement by the American college of critical care medicine. *Critical Care Medicine, 36*(3), 953–963. Erratum in: *Critical Care Medicine, 2008 May, 36*(5),1699.

Uustal, D. B. (1987). Values: The cornerstone of nursing's moral act. In M. D. Fowler & J. Levine-Ariff (Eds.), *Ethics at the bedside: A source book for the critical care nurse* (pp. 136–170). Philadelphia: Lippincott.

Varon, J. & Marik, V. J. (2007). Cardiopulmonary resuscitation in patients with cancer. *American Journal of Hospice and Palliative Medicine, 24*(3), 224–229.

Veatch, R. M., & Fry, S. T. (1995). *Case studies in nursing ethics.* Boston: Jones and Bartlett.

Walker, M. U. (1993). Keeping moral space open. *Hastings Center Report, 23*(2), 33–40.

Ward, D. (2000). Ageism and the abuse of older people in health and social care. *British Journal of Nursing, 9*(9), 560–563.

Welch, S. B. (2008). Can the death of a child be good? *Journal of Pediatric Nursing, 23*(2),120–125.

Westphal, C. (2008). Is cardiopulmonary resuscitation medically appropriate in end stage disease? Review of the evidence. *Journal of Hospice & Palliative Nursing, 10*(3), 128–132.

Yeo, M., Moorhouse, A., Dalzeil, J. (1996a). Autonomy. In M. Yeo & A. Moorhouse (Eds.), *Concepts and cases in nursing ethics* (2nd ed., pp. 91–138). Peterbourough, Ontario, Canada: Broadview Press.

Yeo, M., Moorhouse, A., Donner, G. (1996b). Justice. In M. Yeo & A. Moorhouse (Eds.), *Concepts and cases in nursing ethics* (2nd ed., pp. 211–266). Peterbourough, Ontario, Canada: Broadview Press.

Legal Aspects of Decision Making in Palliative Care

Kathleen O. Perrin

Key Points

- An adult is presumed to have the ability to make his/her own healthcare decisions—including termination of life-sustaining technology—unless he/she is shown to be incapacitated by clinical examination or ruled incompetent by a court of law.
- Advance care directives are legal vehicles used by people to provide guidance to their healthcare providers concerning the care they would desire in the event they become incapacitated and cannot make their own decisions.
- Common forms of advance directives are living wills, Do-Not-Resuscitate directives, and durable powers of attorney for healthcare purpose documents.
- There are sometimes problems with advance directives, such as when they do not seem to apply to the patient's situation so that the healthcare team may be reluctant to follow them.
- In general, courts are hesitant to enforce advance directives.
- Conflicts among healthcare providers, patients and/or families about a patient's end-of-life care may be resolved by development of consensus about goals for care through listening, thoughtful discussion, multidisciplinary rounds, and ethics consultation.
- Many states now have intractable pain legislation either as part of their natural death act or as separate legislation that affirms dying patients' rights to adequate pain management.
- Nurses have essential roles in attaining ethically and legally appropriate end-of-life care. These roles include educating the patient and family about the patient's condition and legal end-of-life choices, identifying the patient's and family's wishes for end-of-life care, articulating the patient's and family's desires to other members of the healthcare team, and assisting the patient and family to obtain necessary and appropriate end-of-life care.

Case Study: Harriet Billings, a 76-year-old retired nurse, developed endocarditis and mitral valve dysfunction from an infected pacemaker lead. Harriet's past history included a 3-month hospital stay following mitral valve surgery 7 years earlier. She was overweight and had longstanding chronic lung disease but was precise in managing all her medications. Harriet had lived alone for the past 1 year following the death of her husband. She had recently updated her advance directive and Durable Power of Attorney for Health Care, reaffirming that she wanted to be intubated, have hemodialysis, and to have cardiopulmonary resuscitation, should they be necessary. In addition, she gave her brother power to make healthcare decisions for her should she become incapacitated.

Harriet was awake and able to understand what was occurring to her when the cardiac surgeon at her local hospital explained that her chances of surviving a second operation on the valve while she had endocarditis were slim. He stated that the infection was not responding to antibiotics, so surgery was necessary, but was also risky and could not be performed locally. He informed her that she had two choices: recognize that she was not likely to recover and forego surgery, or transfer to a teaching hospital and see if they were willing to operate. Harriet chose to transfer and have surgery.

Initially the surgery went well; Harriet was extubated 5 days after surgery and transferred to a stepdown unit. Then, Harriet respiratory arrested, was resuscitated, and required re-intubation. Following her cardiac arrest, Harriet developed renal failure and was started on hemodialysis with her consent. When it became apparent that Harriet was not going to tolerate extubation, she was asked if she wanted a tracheostomy, to which she immediately responded, "Yes." Harriet's brother and some of her friends asked the nurses, "Why are you still doing all this? She's been through it once already, isn't that enough?"

Introduction

Lay and professional communities throughout the world are struggling with bioethical and legal dilemmas brought about by the proliferation of medical technology. A heightened sense of self-determination and the decision making associated with the use of available life-sustaining technology, termination of life-prolonging treatment, patient-requested euthanasia, and assisted suicide have engendered bioethical and legal dilemmas in end-of-life care. Although these dilemmas have different ramifications for people, patient's well-being can best be served when healthcare professionals are able to collaborate with each other, the patient, and the family to set goals for patient care as the end of life approaches.

For nurses, in particular, end-of-life decision making is a moral as well as legal issue. The moral question of what is "right" or "best" for the patient, what ought to be done, and who is the best person suited to do the "right" or "best" thing evokes strong personal sentiments when discussing end-of-life care. These questions have the potential to provoke conflict among those involved in patient care—physicians, nurses, social workers, and others—and the questions for each are clouded by the individual's personal and professional ethics.

End-of-life questions pose a different dilemma for the family. Many times, families are faced with discussions regarding whether to stop treatment and allow the patient to die a natural death. Family members or patients may not understand that there are limits to how long and how well medical technology can sustain life. For example, most people do not realize how unlikely a person is to survive cardiopulmonary resuscitation (CPR). More importantly, family members may not be certain of what the patient would have wanted should she/he have been able to make the decision.

Knowledge of the patient's wishes is important since legal and ethical scholars agree that decisions about care at the end of life ought to be made in accordance with an individual's wishes, preferences, beliefs, and values. No one should be subject to medical care against his or her wishes. For the past 20 years in the United States, autonomy and self-determination have been the foundation for such decisions.

Nursing faculty, nursing students, and practicing nurses address ethical and legal issues including end-of-life care with patients and family members daily in clinical practice. With increased medical technology and competing interests of dying patients, their families, and significant others, the wish of many to die with dignity is a concern for healthcare professionals. Nurses are in a key position to address the escalation of bioethical dilemmas that result in wrenching situations for patients, families, providers, and the courts. Since the landmark cases of Karen Ann Quinlan (In re Quinlan, 1976) and Nancy Beth Cruzan (*Cruzan v. Director, Missouri Department of Health,* 1990), nurses, physicians, other healthcare professionals have shaped public policy regarding patient and surrogate participation in end-of-life decision making even when the patient is incapacitated and unable to make decisions.

LAW AND ETHICS: SAME OR DIFFERENT?

Law and *ethics* are similar in that they have developed in the same historical, social, cultural and philosophical soil (Davis, Aroskar, Liaschenko, & Drought, 1997). Black's Law Dictionary defines law as "that which is laid down, ordained, or established; a body of rules of action or conduct prescribed by controlling authority and having binding legal forces; and that which must be obeyed and followed by citizens subject to sanctions or legal consequences" (Garner, 2004, pp. 884-885). The law may be defined better as the sum total of rules and regulations by which a society is governed. Ethics, on the other hand, are informal or formal standards that guide how individuals or groups of people believe they ought to behave.

Law and ethics may differ in what they allow or require a person to do. For example, some actions may be legal yet not ethical. A historical example is the legality of slavery in the United States until the Civil War. More recently, a nurse in Oregon might legally have assisted a patient to commit suicide, although the American Nurses Association declared that such assistance was unethical. Other actions may be ethical but not legal. A historical example would be the development of the Underground Railroad to assist slaves fleeing to Canada. This dichotomy can occur because legal rights are grounded in the law and ethical rights are grounded in ethical principles and values. The law establishes rules that define a person's rights, obligations, and the appropriate penalty for those who violate it. Moreover, the law describes how government will enforce the rules and penalties. There are many laws that affect the practice of nursing, and nurses must be able to differentiate between ethical claims that suggest how a nurse should act and legal requirements for the nurse to act in specific ways or potentially incur sanctions.

Nursing and the Law

Legal and moral obligations are not new to nurses. The Nurse Practice Act, a legal statute regulating nursing, and the professional code of ethics are the foundations of nursing practice. Similarly, nurses are confronted with complex moral and legal questions on a regular basis when caring for dying patients: questions such as when does death occur? Does an individual have a right to choose death? Is there a difference between letting a person die and taking measures to hasten death? Do you disclose a terminal diagnosis to a patient? These are just a few of the ethical and legal issues in contemporary nursing.

Decision making at the end of life has been at the heart of many ethical-dilemma discussions and legal cases in bioethics in the past 25 years. Because nurses are legally responsible and accountable for the healthcare that patients and their families receive, nurses can no longer afford to view the questions of ethics and law as solely an academic exercise, nor should ethical and legal considerations of today's healthcare issues remain solely in the purview of the organization's ethics committee or risk-management departments. Nurses must understand the basic concepts of ethical decision making and know the relevant laws that address the current controversies to ensure that individual and societal rights and values are protected.

Informed Consent

Informed consent is not only a legal requirement but also a moral imperative. The legal requirement of informed consent is based on the value of patient autonomy and self-determination. Every human being of adult years and sound mind has a right to determine what shall be done with his or her own body (*Schloendorff v. Society of New York Hospital*, 1914). Accordingly, the fundamental goals of informed consent are patient autonomy and self-determination (*In re Farrell*, 1987). This goal is effectuated by allowing patients to make their own decisions about their healthcare based on their own values for as long as they are able.

A second goal of informed consent is to empower patients to exercise their right to autonomy rationally and intelligently (Meisel & Cerminara, 2001). There is no guarantee that providing patients relevant information about treatment will result in patients' making intelligent decisions, nor does it guarantee that they will use the information provided; however, without such a requirement, the likelihood of rational decision making diminishes (Meisel & Cerminara, 2001). The patient's right to consent presumes that the patient has sufficient information to make a reasonable decision.

Consent to treatment is only valid when the patient has the capacity to consent (Meisel & Cerminara, 2001). Competence is not the same as capacity, yet they are frequently considered to be synonymous. Competency to make healthcare decisions is a legal term that is determined only by a court. The law presumes that all adults are competent and have the ability to make their own decisions including those about healthcare, and the assumption is ordinarily correct (Meisel & Cerminara, 2001). To be considered competent, an individual must be able to comprehend the nature of the action in question and understand its significance. However, a patient need not be adjudicated incompetent to lack the capacity to consent to medical treatment (Meisel & Cerminara, 2001).

Capacity is determined not by the courts but rather by clinicians who assess functional capabilities to determine whether capacity is lacking. Incapacity is not determined solely by a medical or psychiatric diagnosis. Rather, decisional capacity within healthcare is determined via clinical assessment and the ability of the patient to give valid consent (Cooney, Kennedy, Hawkins, Hurme, & Balch, 2004).

The basic elements of a valid consent-the determination that a patient has sufficient decisional capacity to consent or refuse treatment-are based on the observation of a specific set of abilities. In order to have decision-making capacity, the patient must be able to understand the relevant information, appreciate the situation and its consequences, reason about treatment options, and communicate a choice (Appelbaum, 2007). Applebaum notes that the use of standardized questions can increase the reliability of raters determining a patient's capacity. He recommends the McArthur Competence Assessment Tool, which takes about 20 minutes to administer and score. However, he also suggests questions that are normally included when assessing each criterion to determine if a patient has the capacity to make a healthcare decision. Examples of the questions are as follows:

- Would you please tell me in your own words what your doctor told you about your current problem and its treatment?
- What is the treatment likely to do for you?
- What makes this treatment a good choice for you? Why is it better than any other one?
- Please tell me what you have decided to do.

Not all health decisions require the same level of decision-making capacity in order to make a valid decision. Decision-making capacity is not an "on-off switch" (Mezey, Mitty, & Ramsey, 1997); a patient does not either have it or not. Rather, capacity is usually viewed as task-specific; an individual may be able to perform some tasks adequately and may have the ability to make some decisions, but may still be unable to perform all tasks or make all decisions. The notion of "decision-specific capacity" assumes that an individual has or lacks the capacity for a particular decision at a particular time and under a particular set of circumstances (Mezey et al., 1997; Mitty & Mezey, 2004).

Special Concerns with Children: Assent Rather than Consent

In contrast to adults, children younger than 18 years of age are not considered to be legally competent and usually are not considered to be capable of giving fully reasoned consent. Therefore, in most cases parents and healthcare providers make healthcare decisions for children without the child's consent. Instead of giving consent, a child is asked to assent, that is to freely express an opinion in favor of a treatment. The child's assent about end-of-life care is deeply affected by the child's developmental and chronological age, since young children have limited understandings of illness and death.

Over the past 40 years, the thinking about children and medical decision making has evolved. Whereas at one time the decision was made for the child without explanation of the illness or consultation, now there is more likely to be a shared decision-making process in which children have more autonomy as they develop greater cognitive maturity. Preschool children are usually considered too young to make clearly rational decisions, so their parents are asked to make decisions for them based on the best interests' standard. When children reach school age, they are usually provided with information about their condition in a manner that they can understand. Although school-age children may express a preference and assent to treatment, parents and healthcare providers usually continue to be the primary decision makers since the child is not thought to have the capacity to make an informed decision yet. In contrast to this common belief and practice, a study by Hinds et al. (2005) found that children as young as 10 years dying from brain tumors could understand the potential treatment options and recognize that their death could be the consequence of their decision. Hinds et al. (2005) noted that these children usually based their decisions on their relationships with others and the risks that treatment imposed on themselves and others. Once a child enters adolescence, there is less controversy, and the adolescent often has the decision-making capacity of an adult. Harrison et al. (1997) recommend that the decision-making capacity of adolescents be examined in the light of their

- ability to understand and communicate relevant information;
- ability to think and choose with some independence;
- ability to assess the potential for benefit, risk, or harm, as well as to consider consequences and multiple options; and
- achievement of a fairly stable set of values.

Nurses can make a valuable contribution by ensuring that the informed-consent process is accurately met (Virani & Sofer, 2003). Nurses must become proficient in assessing decisional capacity and take an active role when the multidisciplinary team is determining decisional capacity. When nurses and other healthcare professionals assess capacity objectively, two types of mistakes can be avoided: first, mistakenly preventing persons who have the capacity to make healthcare decisions from directing the course of their treatment; and, second, failing to protect incapacitated persons from the harmful effects of their decisions (President's Commission, 1982). It is easy when a patient is very ill to let someone take over decision making for the person. However, as long as an adult patient has the capacity to make the decision, it is her/his right to do so. Nurses should make efforts to meet their legal and ethical obligations so that patients retain their rights to make decisions for as long as they are able.

Case Study follow-up: Harriet was aware of her surroundings, recognized that she would die if she were extubated, and had experienced two months of ventilation in the past. Although she was too weak to write and did not tolerate a speaking valve, she made her wishes clearly known. She wished to have a tracheostomy, and continue both ventilation and dialysis. She was not ready to die. Since all those involved in her care were convinced that Harriet was competent and had the capacity to make decisions for herself, neither her medical directive nor her durable power of attorney for healthcare came into effect. The care that she was receiving although extensive was believed to have the potential to benefit her and was not deemed to be futile. Thus, Harriet continued to make her own decisions about the amount and type of healthcare she desired.

The SUPPORT Study

Although in the case study, Harriet Billings wanted to continue to receive life-sustaining therapy, in many instances patients wish to discontinue interventions. Unfortunately, even with the increased attention to end-of-life issues in lay and medical publications, physicians are often unaware of their patients' preferences concerning end-of-life care. The Study to Understand Prognoses and Preferences for Outcomes and Risks of Treatment (SUPPORT) and its companion study the Hospitalized Elderly Longitudinal Project (HELP), which are both studies of seriously ill hospitalized patients, documented the lack of communication between physicians and their very ill patients about end-of-life issues (Knaus et al., 1995; SUPPORT Principle Investigators, 1995). The original SUPPORT study (SUPPORT Principle Investigators) and its offshoots documented the ineffectiveness of advance directives (Teno et al., 1994; Teno, Licks, et al., 1997; Teno, Lynn, et al., 1997), the effect of serious illness on patients and their families (Covinsky et. al., 1994, 1996), the lack of cost effectiveness of life-extending interventions at the end of life (Hamel et al., 1997), and the influence of patient age and race on decision making (Hamel et al., 1996, 1999; Phillips et al., 1996).

However, most importantly, the SUPPORT study (Support Principle Investigators, 1995) suggested that since physicians did not understand their patients' preferences about end-of-life care, they often continued aggressive, painful life-sustaining treatment beyond the time patients and their families believed was appropriate. Because of that, families indicated that patients spent a considerable amount of time during their last days and hours in pain. One of the reasons offered for such aggressive care at the end of life in the SUPPORT study was that it was not clear to the healthcare providers that patients were definitely dying until less than 48 hours before the patients' deaths. How then should a healthcare provider know when to counsel palliative care? How should a provider know when care was excessive for a patient?

Natural Death Acts

Natural Death Acts sprang from the belief that medical technology had made possible the artificial prolongation of patients' lives beyond their natural limits. Another underlying assumption of the Acts was that adults in the United States have the right to control decisions about how they live their lives as well as how they die. *The California Natural Death Act* was one of the first in the country. Originally enacted in 1975 and revised in 1992, it authorized people to sign a declaration directing that life-sustaining treatment be withheld or withdrawn should they become terminally ill or permanently unconscious if the administration of life-sustaining procedures would only prolong their dying process or unconscious condition.

Now, every state has a Natural Death Act explicitly allowing patients to refuse excessive medical care at the end of life. In addition, the Natural Death Acts in some states, such as Washington, specifically state that "physicians and nurses should not withhold or unreasonably diminish pain medication for patients in a terminal condition where the primary intent of providing such medication is to alleviate pain and maintain or increase the patient's comfort" [1992 c 98 § 1; 1979 c 112 § 2.]. Finally, most states also include in their Natural Death Act a provision that a person's right to control his or her healthcare may be exercised by an authorized representative who validly holds the person's durable power of attorney for healthcare.

However, as shown by the SUPPORT study (SUPPORT Principle Investigators, 1995), the presence of Natural Death Acts did not ensure that patients and their families were able to obtain the end-of-life care they desired. Guido (2006) states that the case of Nancy Cruzan, a young woman who remained in a persistent vegetative state following an automobile accident and whose family maintained that she would never have desired such technologically driven care, motivated Congress to enact federal legislation that would require states to make patients aware of their rights to have advance directives and to decide about their own care (*Cruzan v. Director, Missouri Department of Public Health*, 1990).

The Patient Self-Determination Act

The Patient Self-Determination Act (PSDA), which became effective on December 1, 1991, was the first federal law to focus on the rights of adults to refuse life-sustaining treatment. The act was motivated by concerns that in the absence of clear directives regarding their views on life-sustaining treatment, patients' views would not be respected when they became incapacitated. The PSDA requires that facilities participating in the Medicare and Medicaid program provide written information to individuals about their right to participate in medical decision making and formulate advance directives. The key provisions of the legislation are as follows:

With regard to the Patient Self-Determination Act, facilities must provide the following:

1) *Written information* to each adult individual concerning "an individual's rights under State law (whether statutory or as recognized by the courts of the State) to make decisions concerning such medical care, including the right to accept or refuse medical or surgical treatment and the right to formulate advance directives";
2) *Written policies* of the provider or organization respecting the implementation of such advance directives;
3) *Inquiry* as to whether a person has an advance directive;
4) *Documentation* in the patient's medical records whether the individual has executed an advance directive;
5) *Nondiscrimination,* that is, not to condition the provision of care or otherwise discriminate against an individual based on whether the individual has executed an advance directive;
6) *Compliance* with requirements of state laws respecting advance directives at facilities of the provider or organization;
7) *Education* for staff on issues concerning advance directives and provision for community education regarding advance directives.

PURPOSE AND TYPES OF ADVANCE DIRECTIVES

Since the PSDA was enacted, all states have Natural Death Acts and/or advance directive legislation. However, the specific types of advance directives, the formalities for executing a directive, and the requirement to alleviate pain and promote comfort at the end of life sometimes included within the directive vary from state to state.

Advance directives have several major purposes (Meisel & Cerminara, 2001). The first and perhaps most important is that they are a mechanism by which individuals who are currently competent indicate the type of healthcare they would desire should they lack decision-making capacity at some time in the future when a medical decision needs to be made. Directives provide guidelines to healthcare providers and family about the

kind of medical care the person would like to receive in advance of the need for that care. Advance directives generally are discussed in the context of the right to forgo life-sustaining treatments. However, they also may be used to direct the administration of specific treatments as they were in the case of Harriet Billings. Advance directives pertain to decision making about any kind of healthcare, and they may be executed by any adult as long as he or she possesses the requisite decision-making capacity.

The second purpose of advance directives is to provide guidance, especially to healthcare professionals, regarding how to proceed with decision making about life-sustaining treatment for a patient with diminished capacity. When patients lack decision-making capacity, a great deal of confusion can arise as to how healthcare decisions are to be made, who has the authority to make them, and what the treatment should be. Recently, Teno, Gruneir, Schwartz, Nanda, and Wetle (2007) found that bereaved family members of patients with advanced directives did report fewer concerns with communication with healthcare providers about treatment decisions and believed that the directives had facilitated the process.

The third purpose of advance directives is that they provide immunity from civil and criminal liability to healthcare providers when they act in good faith and in accordance with state statutes respecting advance directives (Meisel & Cerminara, 2001). Most litigated right-to-die cases end up in court because of the fear of liability. Statutory immunity provisions provide an impetus for clinical decision making by protecting healthcare professionals.

There are two broad types of advance directives. The first is the instructional directive, which has several subtypes including the living will, the medical directive, and the Do-Not-Resuscitate (DNR) order. Instructional directives usually give guidance about the type and amount of care that the person desires should she/he become incapacitated. The second type of advance directive is the durable power of attorney for health care (DPAHC), also known as the healthcare proxy. DPAHC documents usually identify an agent known as either a healthcare proxy or a durable power of attorney for health care (DPOA) to serve as a surrogate for decision making. This section will discuss each of these, as well as other relevant issues pertaining to advance directives.

Instructional Directives

Living wills. Instructional directives identify the amount and type of care that a patient would wish to receive if certain conditions are met. In the case of the living will, the patient affirms that if she/he is terminally ill, she/he does not wish to receive life-sustaining treatment(s). There are two major problems with the living will. First, it is not always clear when a person in dying. In the

SUPPORT (1995) study of seriously ill patients, many of the patients were still predicted to have a 50% chance of surviving for at least 2 months, 2 days before they died. Also, healthcare providers are reluctant to recognize that patients with some diagnoses, particularly heart failure, are dying (Forbes, 2001). Furthermore, the patient does not usually have the opportunity to refuse specific treatments. Despite these problems, patients who prefer to die at home do appear to benefit from having a living will. According to Degenholtz, Rhee, and Arnold (2004), patients with living wills were more likely to die in their place of residence than in a hospital and therefore probably less likely to receive aggressive care at the end of life.

Medical directives. Medical directives are more specific; they allow patients to specify their desires for or refusals of specific treatments under certain circumstances should the patient become incapacitated. For example, patients might indicate that they did not wish to be resuscitated (DNR) or would not want to be intubated, be ventilated, receive nasogastric feedings, or be dialyzed under specific circumstances such as becoming comatose. The major problem with medical directives that are not specific to a patient's illness is that the patient's situation may not be similar enough to the circumstance described in the advanced directive for anyone to determine how the patient would wish to be treated. Teno et al. (1997) found that directives were specific enough in only 3% of actual circumstances to guide decision making. Other problems with medical directives are that they do not allow advances in medical treatment, or the patient to change his/her mind about one of the interventions or situations without changing the directive. The medical directive may only represent the patients' desires for treatment at the time the directive was completed, not at the time treatment is being planned.

Do-not-resuscitate directives. In the United States, only about 20 to 30% of older adults have completed any type of advance directive, although in long-term care facilities three fourths or more of the residents may have a DNR order (Molloy et al., 2000). DNR orders represent the most common type of advanced planning done for adults in this country (Ghusen, Teasdale, & Jordan, 1997; Nolan & Bruder, 1997; Eun-Shim & Resnick, 2001). They are also often viewed as a "practical place to start" (Smith, Desch, Hackney, & Shaw, 1997) and are often the first step in considering treatment limitation at the end of life. When a DNR order is written, the patient or proxy designate and healthcare providers concur that if the patient is dying, the healthcare team will not make any attempt to stop the process or bring the patient back to life.

Originally, cardiopulmonary resuscitation (CPR) was established to be used with witnessed arrests, sudden death in the young, drowning, and predictable arrests, such as in anesthesia and cardioversion (Hall, 1996). In 1988, New York became the first state to enact DNR legislation requiring that consent to CPR be presumed; if physicians do not want to resuscitate patients, they must obtain patient's consent before writing such an order (Swidler, 1989). Many other states have enacted DNR legislation since New York did. The American Medical Association (1991) mandates that patients and families be consulted before a DNR order is written. Since then, all patients who have a cardiopulmonary arrest-for any reason, of any age, or with any condition-will have CPR performed in almost all hospitals or nursing homes in the United States unless there is a specific order written to the contrary (the DNR decision). With a policy of automatic resuscitation, obtaining a DNR order is critical if the patient wishes to avoid this type of treatment.

Most healthcare providers believe that it is quite reasonable for people, especially older adults, to forgo CPR because CPR is rarely successful when attempted on older adults. Buchanan (1998) estimated that 2 long-term care residents out of every 100 that receive CPR survive to hospital discharge, and they both would most likely have significant neurological impairments. Murphy, Murray, Robinson, and Campton (1989), in a study of older adults receiving CPR in hospital, rehabilitation, and long-term care settings, found 22% of patients survived the initial resuscitation attempt, but only 3.8% of the patients survived to hospital discharge. Banja and Bilsky (1993) had no patients survive to hospital discharge after resuscitation in a rehabilitation hospital. Survival rates post CPR for all age groups have stayed consistent for three decades at about 13% to as high as 18% (Schneider, Nelson, & Brown, 1993). Marik and Craft (1997) found that patients who survived to hospital discharge following CPR had one reversible condition, were otherwise healthy, and had suffered a sudden, unexpected dysrhythmia. Thus it seems very reasonable for adults with multiple chronic illnesses to forgo CPR.

The majority of clearly competent elders living in community or long-term care facilities would prefer not to be resuscitated if they were gravely ill and probably dying (Eun-Shim & Resnick, 2001; Wagner, 1984). However, elders who have moderate to severe impairment in daily decision making skills but are still alert and conversant may prefer CPR (O'Brien, Grisso, & Maislin, 1995). Molloy et al. (1996) state that there was no "gold standard" for determining when an older adult has the capacity to make decisions about end-of-life care and there is a lack of consensus about what tool ought to be used to measure capacity and who ought to administer the assessment. Eun-Shim and Resnick (2001) state that capacity must be clinically determined since the person must be shown to be able to understand and appreciate the consequences of their end-of-life treatment plan. Bradley, Walker, Blechner, and Wetle (1997) found that 48% of decisionally competent nursing home residents did not receive information about end-of-life treatment choices and advance directives, while 34% of partially or totally confused patients did.

What nurses need to know about DNR directives is that patients have a right to refuse CPR and may request DNR orders when they have the capacity to make the decision after they have been informed of the risks and benefits involved. Moreover, nurses need to know which patients have a DNR directive, the institutional policy and law governing the use of directives, the patient's wishes regarding interventions to be withheld, and their own values toward the decision to withhold treatment. The medical record should clearly indicate the terms of the directive and whether the terms accurately reflect the patients' current stated preferences.

Recently, Daly (2008) has called for nurses to be actively involved in advocating for the end of 'automatic' CPR. Daley reviewed the likelihood of success of CPR (most recently an 18% survival with only 14% having a favorable neurological outcome) and noted the difficulties of explaining to a patient and/or family that they are being required to refuse a treatment, which, although not likely to be of benefit, is still required. She proposes that the use of CPR should be restricted to "those patients who provide adequate informed consent and for whom CPR has a reasonable chance of success" (p. 378). All patients would have their CPR status assessed on admission, and in the absence of informed consent and a physician's order, CPR would not be attempted. Such a proposal would bring the use of CPR more clearly into the realm of other treatments and directives, and patients would be giving consent for treatment rather than non-treatment.

Durable Power of Attorney for Healthcare

The other broad category of advance directives is Durable Power of Attorney for Healthcare (DPAHC) documents. These documents permit individuals to designate another person to make healthcare decisions for them should they lose decision-making capacity. The person who is appointed by the patient to make decisions is called a healthcare proxy, healthcare agent, or surrogate or, in some states, a durable power of attorney (DPOA). The language used varies from state to state, and nurses should become familiar with their own state's language.

Usually, these directives allow greater flexibility and more relevance to the patient's specific situation than instructional directives since a DPAHC does not require that an individual know in advance all the decisions that may arise. In fact, a healthcare proxy can interpret the patient's wishes as medical circumstances change and can make treatment decisions as the need arises. While competent, the person should be encouraged to provide his/her proxy with guidance concerning the type of treatment she/he would like to receive. The advocacy group Aging with Dignity (2007) has promoted the Five Wishes public information campaign so that individuals have a format to discuss their wishes related to end-of-life care.

The five wishes are as follows:

The person I want to make care decisions for me when I can't

The kind of medical treatment I want or don't want

How comfortable I want to be

How I want people to treat me

What I want my loved ones to know.

Sometimes, patients do not have the capacity to answer these questions or envision end-of-life scenarios. Another advantage of a DPAHC noted by Molloy et al. (1996) is that the capacity required to designate a proxy is considerably less than that needed to envision scenarios and complete a medical directive. Thus, proxy designations may be more appropriate for people who, although competent, are having difficulty understanding options and making decisions about end-of-life care.

However, there are disadvantages to a DPAHC. The proxy designate may not realize all the responsibility that being a healthcare proxy entails and may have difficulty making a decision. The proxy may also confound his/her interests with those of the patient and fail to act in the patient's best interests (Perrin, 1997).

How should a proxy make an end-of-life decision for a patient? First and most important, the proxy should leave the decision to the patient until the appropriate time. Advance directives become effective only when it is determined that the individual is incompetent, lacks decision-making capacity, or requests that the proxy make the decisions for him/her. As long as the patient retains decision-making capacity and wishes to make the decision, his or her decisions govern. When the patient is deemed to lack decision-making capacity, the healthcare proxy is authorized to make treatment decisions on behalf of the patient. There are two ethically and legally acceptable ways by which a proxy might make a healthcare decision for an incapacitated patient, substituted judgment, and the best interests' standard.

In re Quinlan (1976), the courts recognized the use of substituted judgment for a family member declining the further use of mechanical ventilation for an incompetent patient. In such circumstances, the proxy makes the decision that she/he believes the patient would have made for himself or herself should she/he have had the ability to do so. Sometimes the decision is clear because the patient has discussed the matter with the proxy or commented about what she/he would want to do in the circumstance. Overall, studies show that even if flawed, patients' wishes and decisions expressed by healthcare proxies more closely approximate the patient's own treatment preferences than do decisions of physicians or others (Danis, Garrett, Harris, & Patrick, 1994; Emanuel, Emanuel, Stoeckle, Hummel, & Barry, 1994).

In situations where there is no clear and convincing evidence of what the person would have wanted or the patient has never been competent, the proxy will be called on to make decisions on the basis of what he or she believes to be in the best interests of the patient. Under this approach, it is impossible to analyze truly the proxy's decision based on the patient's right to self-determination. Rather, the effort is made to protect the interest of the patient and to carry out society's interest in providing appropriate healthcare for all.

Intractable Pain Legislation

Some states, such as Washington, contain a mandate for patient comfort and alleviation of pain at the end of life in their Natural Death Acts. Others have separate legislations regarding the management of pain at the end of life. Yet, all patients who suffer from pain, not just those who are dying, should be treated. The debate about patient-requested euthanasia and assisted suicide has drawn national and international attention to the fact that appropriate interventions can eliminate or drastically reduce the pain and suffering that many people experience. The need for appropriate types and amounts of pain medications was made clear in the U.S. Supreme Court ruling in *Vacco v. Quill* (1997). There is a relationship between pain and symptom management and the requests for assisted suicide (Foley, 1991).

Through the Federal Intractable Pain Regulation, the federal government in 1974 clarified the federal law that prohibits physicians from prescribing opioids to detoxify or maintain an opioid addiction. The regulation stated, in part, that the prohibitive regulations are "not intended to impose any limitation on a physician... to administer or dispense narcotic drugs to persons with intractable pain in which no relief or cure is possible or none has been found after reasonable effort" (Institute of Medicine [IOM], 1997). Similarly, some courts explicitly recognize that a patient's "right to be free from pain... is inseparable from their right to refuse medical treatment" (Meisel & Cerminara, 2001), and have granted immunity to healthcare providers who treat pain with strong doses of analgesic medications that inadvertently end the patient's life (McKay v. Bergstedt, 1990). Moreover, several states have enacted intractable pain statutes to encourage those who treat patients who are terminally ill and have intractable pain to manage the pain without threat of legal liability if the treatment results in the patient's death.

The IOM report "Approaching Death: Improving Care at End of Life, (1997), coupled with other palliative care literature, asserts that change must occur at many levels if we are to improve care for the dying. The development of intractable pain statutes is a good first step to the under-treatment of pain. However, they are imperfect and there are problems associated with intractable pain statutes that include the following:

1) They do not, in all cases, mark a clear area of medical practice in which physicians feel free to manage their patients' pain. The more specific laws, for example, those that set out detailed prescription practices, may actually afford physicians less leeway in the practice of medicine. Additionally, by carving out an area of pain treatment that is immune from discipline, there may be an implication that other forms of pain treatment should be subject to disciplinary review. However, physicians did obtain some measure of comfort that they would not be prosecuted for appropriate prescription of pain medications by the *Gonzales v. Oregon* decision that limited the Drug Enforcement Agency's (DEA) jurisdiction to actions involving drug trafficking (Kollas & Boyer-Kollas, 2007).

2) Even the strongest intractable-pain law is still limited by the term *intractable*. Many cases are ambiguous, and physicians may believe they must delay opioid treatment until pain is far enough along to be called intractable.

3) Finally, legal affirmations in these laws of the importance of pain control do not, in themselves, correct practice patterns or improve physician training. Laws could, however, encourage patients to expect diligence in pain relief, including use of generally effective medications. Medical boards could consider disciplining physicians who fail to apply proven methods of pain control (IOM, 1997). Additionally, Kollas and Boyer-Kollas (2007) observed that case law might be strengthening the requirement to relieve a patient's pain by establishing a new tort, failure to adequately manage pain. Not only have judges and juries repeatedly viewed pain in the dying patient as a compensatable injury, but recently plaintiffs have been able to "argue the tort of failure to appropriately manage pain by applying reasoning from *James v. Philhaven* and *Gaddis v. U.S.*" (Kollas & Boyer-Kollad, p. 1399).

Thus, healthcare system changes are needed to improve access to care and to eliminate barriers to effective treatment. Nurses need to educate patients and families about their right to adequate palliative care. In states where there are intractable-pain statutes, the PSDA requires all covered facilities to inform patients of their state law rights to adequate palliative care (Meisel & Cerminara, 2001). Healthcare providers need to "add the assessment of pain as the fifth vital sign" (Meisel & Cerminara, 2001), and national pain management standards ought to be followed (Joint Committee on Accreditation of Healthcare Organizations [JCAHO], 2000).

Combination Directives

A number of states have a single advance directive statute that combines elements of an instructional directive, a DPAHC, and possibly a pain management directive into a single document. A combination document arguably avoids many of the pitfalls of each document alone. If the instructions are too general, the healthcare proxy has the authority to determine whether instructions should be applied under the specific circumstances. If the instructions are too specific and do not address the particular situation at hand, the healthcare proxy has the discretion to apply them or not. Nevertheless, a discussion between the patient and the healthcare proxy should occur regardless of whether there is a DPAHC or a combination directive. Communication is the most effective way to ensure that the patient's wishes are known and that the healthcare proxy is prepared to follow the patient's directives.

Oral Advance Directives

Although a written advance directive is preferable, especially in the case of an emergency, courts view oral advance directives favorably, especially living wills. The courts either have enforced them per se or have heavily relied upon them in deciding whether to forgo life-sustaining treatment. Even when state statutes recognize written advance directives, oral directives have been found to be legally operative in a number of jurisdictions. The more specific the oral advance directive, the more likely it is to be enforced and have clinical and legal significance.

When made by individuals with full decision-making capacity, courts have considered patients' statements when making a decision to terminate life-prolonging treatments. Criteria for weighing these statements include the following (Furrow, Greaney, Johnson, Jost, & Schwartz, 2001):

- If the statements were made on serious occasions or were solemn pronouncements (were brought up when the parties were together);
- If they were consistently repeated;
- If they were made by a mature person who understood the underlying issues;
- If they were consistent with values demonstrated in other aspects of the patient's life (including the patient's religion);

- If they were made shortly before the need for the treatment decision;
- If they addressed with some specificity the actual condition of the patient.

Accordingly, such statements should be considered and documented by the healthcare providers when discussing advance directives with patients.

Family Consent Laws

Many people are under the impression that their family members will be allowed to make the proper decisions for them should the need arise and therefore see no need to execute a formal advance directive (Furrow et al., 2001). Traditionally, healthcare professionals and the courts have also relied on families to make healthcare decisions for family members throughout the years, without any legal authority. In 1982, the President's Commission concluded that given this practice, family decision making had gained and should be accorded legal acceptance. The commission pointed out five reasons why deference to family members is appropriate when done in consultation with the physician and other healthcare professionals:

1) The family is generally most concerned about the good of the patient.
2) The family usually is the most knowledgeable about the patient's goals, preferences, and values.
3) The family deserves recognition as an important social unit that, within limits, ought to be treated as a responsible decision maker in matters that intimately affect its members.
4) Especially in a society in which many other traditional forms of community have eroded, participation in a family often is an important dimension of personal fulfillment.
5) Because a protected sphere of privacy and autonomy is required for the flourishing of this interpersonal union, institutions and the state should be reluctant to intrude, particularly regarding matters that are personal and on which there is a wide range of opinion in society.

Motivated by concern over the formal legal status of family decision making in the 1980s, state legislatures recognized and began to regulate it by statute. In 1995, with the exception of New York and Missouri, the courts authorized family members and others close to the patient to make decisions (New York State Task Force on Life and the Law, 1995). In fact, the District of Columbia and 24 other states have statutes that explicitly grant family members and others close to the patient the right to make decisions for patients who lack capacity. Family consent statutes vary from state to state. Some have been added to state living-will statutes to provide an alternative mechanism for making life-sustaining treatment decisions for individuals who do not have an advance directive, while others are freestanding statutes that apply either to life-sustaining treatment or healthcare decisions generally.

Preference of Elders for Family Decision Makers

Elders are more likely to speak with a family member about end-of-life care than with a healthcare provider. This does not mean that they have completed a healthcare proxy or durable power of attorney for healthcare purposes. Rather, most elders have simply discussed their preferences for end-of-life care with at least one family member (High, 1993). When asked whom they believe knows them well enough and whom they would trust to make a healthcare decision for them, elders overwhelmingly (94%) choose family members, primarily spouses or adult children. Confidence and trust in family members to make any necessary decision for them may be a major reason older adults do not complete advance directives (High, 1994).

High (1994) believes that elders prefer family decision makers for a variety of significant and appropriate reasons. The family member has an inherent knowledge of the culture, values, and expectations of the patient and is usually concerned with the patient's welfare. In most instances, High believes, family members make a choice appropriately based on the patient's values and best interests. High suggests that there has been too much emphasis placed on disagreement and abuse within families and not enough on family empowerment and good-faith decision making. He suggests that elders' preferences for family decision makers ought to be recognized, and advance directives should only be encouraged for those who "have very specific or unusual preferences, do not want family to serve as substitute decision makers or have disagreements with family or have no family" (High, 1994, p. S17).

Elders say they have thought at least a "moderate amount" about who they would want to make healthcare decisions for them if they became incapacitated. Overwhelmingly, they would choose to have their families make such decisions without the benefit of a written directive (Nolan & Bruder, 1997; High, 1994). Although the elders in one study realized that having a written advance directive would help their families to know their wishes and possibly prevent guilt among family members over the decision, most elders still did not complete advance directives (Nolan & Bruder, 1997). These elders wanted their families to decide about end-of-life care based on their families' best judgments in the specific situation. Perhaps this is because these elders put their trust in their families and not in a piece of paper (High, 1993). Or, it might be because

elders believe that the family is the center of their lives (Blustein, 1999) and no individual can be completely autonomous; any decision made for one individual affects the entire family. In High's (1993) study, none of the elders stated they always expected to make their own decisions. Most elders realize that their families will be profoundly affected by providing or paying for their healthcare. Thus, elders may believe their families ought to have a significant role in determining what the most appropriate end-of-life care is.

Martin, Emanuel, and Singer (2000) emphasize that making a decision about end-of-life care ought to be done in a family context. They believe discussions with patients about end-of-life care "helps patients prepare for death, is influenced by personal relationships, is a social process and occurs within the context of family and loved ones" (p. 1672). They assert that the primary value of end-of-life care planning is to allow the patient and family to prepare for death and dying and to find ways to cope with the impending death. Thus, they believe that one reason patients may communicate about end-of-life issues with families more often than healthcare providers is that the discussion may help the family to resolve any outstanding issues and become ready for the patient's death.

Physician Involvement in Decision Making in Palliative Care

Although most adults have had discussions about end-of-life care preferences with at least one family member, few patients have had such discussions with their physicians (O'Brien, Grisso, & Maislin, 1995; Emanuel, Barry, & Stoeckle, 1991). Although, patients are willing and eager to engage in such a discussion, they believe it is not their role to initiate the discussion (Emanuel et al., 1991). Thus, they wait for their physicians to start the conversation; unfortunately, the physician usually does not.

Reasons physicians may be reluctant to initiate such conversations include the following:

- Personal discomfort with discussing death and dying (Ventres, Nichter, Reed, & Frankel, 1992). If the physician believes that the patient is dying because the physician has failed and there is no more that she/he can do, the physician is less likely to discuss CPR preference with the patient.
- Lack of physician education and experience in conducting such a conversation (Tulsky, Chesney, & Lo, 1995). Resident physicians learn early in the course of their education that various attending and older residents have differing views on how and when end-of-life discussions should occur. Unfortunately, according to Tulsky, resident physicians receive very little education in how to conduct a discussion about

end-of-life preferences and consequently they "often did not provide essential information" (p. 436).

- Fear that the patient will believe the physician has "given up on and is abandoning the patient" (Cotton, 1993). Some doctors say they have difficulty discussing end-of-life care without conveying a sense of hopelessness to the patient. Kohn and Menon (1988) state that physicians may be unwilling to bring up the issue until a crisis develops since they are afraid of unnecessarily alarming the patient.

- The physician may feel legally or morally bound to treat until death is proximate (Hanson, Tulsky, & Danis, 1997). About 10% of physicians believe they must treat all patients with maximal interventions and that to limit treatment is morally and ethically unacceptable. Another larger group of physicians believes that it is inappropriate to discuss treatment limitation until the patient is certainly going to die. Unfortunately, if discussion waits until the patient is definitely dying, the patient frequently no longer has the capacity to participate in decision making about her/his end-of-life care.

- Concern about the amount of time such a conversation will require (Emanuel, Barry, & Stoeckle, 1991). Some physicians fear that having discussions about end-of-life care planning, which are not reimbursable, may be very time consuming. Studies indicate that it takes approximately 10-16 minutes of physician time discussing with a patient and/or family for a DNR decision to be reached; this is often the first in a series of the end-of life decisions (Tulsky et al., 1995; Smith et al., 1997).

Although they do not tend to initiate end-of-life conversations with patients, most physicians (82%) believe it is their responsibility to begin the discussion (Markson et al., 1994) and to write the appropriate orders. Some physicians (Reckling, 1997) report they prefer nurses and other healthcare providers not discuss these issues with patients. The result is that healthcare providers and patients and families talk among themselves about appropriate end-of-life care, but do not talk with each other (Kohn & Menon, 1988). Less than a tenth of patients have spoken with their physicians when planning an advance directive, and the majority of patients with advance directives have never been asked by or told their physicians they have advance directives (Teno et al., 1997). Thus, unfortunately, conversations about end-of-life care among physicians, patients, and families usually do not occur until a crisis develops.

Researchers have documented concerns with how physicians engage in end-of-life care discussions in crisis situations. In Tulsky et al.'s 1995 study, conversations about resuscitation lasted about 10 minutes and

the resident physicians dominated the speaking time. Researchers did not believe that the information the residents provided to patients/families was adequate for them to make decisions about CPR. For example, only 13% of physicians mentioned the futility of CPR and the chance of the patient surviving. Additionally, residents did not allow patients or families many opportunities to ask questions and elicited information about the patient's values and goals in end-of-life care less than 10% of the time.

Hanson et al. (1997) had similar findings. They noted that since physicians tended to focus on treatment descriptions rather than listening to patient concerns, their understandings of patient preferences remained poor even after face-to-face discussions. They stated that physicians tended to be coercive in forcing their opinions. Markson et al. (1994) surveyed physicians who admitted that they would attempt to persuade patients to change decisions that they believed were not well informed (91%), medically reasonable (88%), or in the patient's best interest (88%). Ventres et al. (1992) concluded: "Physicians' presentation of opinions to patients are not neutral. Options are often presented in such a way as to influence DNR decision-making" (p.163) and communication strategies "may work to distance physicians from their patients at times when it is imperative for them to explore the values and wishes of the patient" (p. 165).

According to Ventres et al. (1992), there are three common prototypes physicians use to approach the discussion of DNR with patients and families. The first might be described as legalistic or technical. In this situation, the physician might ask, once the patient has become incapacitated, if the patient has an advance directive or has a healthcare proxy and if someone can produce the appropriate papers. In the second approach, the physician might admit there are no further medical treatments that might lead to a cure and ask patient or family what the patient would want for end-of-life care. In the third approach, the physician might mention there are legal requirements that CPR be attempted at the end of life unless a DNR order was written. The physician would next ask the patient's and/or family's opinion about the appropriateness of administering a painful and probably useless treatment.

Researchers have documented concerns with how physicians engage in end-of-life care discussions in crisis situations. In Tulsky et al.'s 1995 study, conversations about resuscitation lasted about 10 minutes and the resident physicians dominated the speaking time. Researchers did not believe that the information the residents provided to patients/families was adequate for them to make decisions about CPR. For example, only 13% of physicians mentioned the futility of CPR and the chance of the patient surviving. Additionally, residents did not allow patients or families many opportunities to ask questions and elicited information about the patient's values and goals in end-of-life care less than 10% of the time.

Hanson et al. (1997) had similar findings. They noted that since physicians tended to focus on treatment descriptions rather than listening to patient concerns, their understandings of patient preferences remained poor even after face-to-face discussions. They stated that physicians tended to be coercive in forcing their opinions. Markson et al. (1994) surveyed physicians who admitted that they would attempt to persuade patients to change decisions that they believed were not well informed (91%), medically reasonable (88%), or in the patient's best interest (88%). Ventres et al. (1992) concluded: "Physicians' presentation of opinions to patients are not neutral. Options are often presented in such a way as to influence DNR decision-making" (p.163) and communication strategies "may work to distance physicians from their patients at times when it is imperative for them to explore the values and wishes of the patient" (p. 165).

According to Ventres et al. (1992), there are three common prototypes physicians use to approach the discussion of DNR with patients and families. The first might be described as legalistic or technical. In this situation, the physician might ask, once the patient has become incapacitated, if the patient has an advance directive or has a healthcare proxy and if someone can produce the appropriate papers. In the second approach, the physician might admit there are no further medical treatments that might lead to a cure and ask patient or family what the patient would want for end-of-life care. In the third approach, the physician might mention there are legal requirements that CPR be attempted at the end of life unless a DNR order was written. The physician would next ask the patient's and/or family's opinion about the appropriateness of administering a painful and probably useless treatment.

Controversies in Decision Making in Palliative Care

When decision making involves withholding or withdrawing interventions that are prolonging a patient's life, it is not surprising that difficulties may arise. Some of the issues include the following:

- When is it certain that the patient is dying and further intervention is of limited benefit?
- Is the patient able to clearly identify what she would like done either by speaking herself or by the presence of instructions in an advance directive?
- If the patient has not spoken, is it possible to identify who the patient would want to speak for her?
- Does the patient or her proxy desire interventions that members of the health team believe are futile?

As noted earlier, the first issue is quite problematic for the members of the healthcare team, patient and family. It is usually not absolutely apparent that a patient is dying, even to experienced hospice nurses, until 24–48 hours before the patient's death. When the daughter of an elderly woman asked her mother's physician how much longer her mother might live, she was told, "Your mother is a determined woman. Any other person might only live 2 hours but she could live 2 hours, 2 days, 2 weeks or 2 months". Three months later the woman was still alive. It can be difficult to decide what care is most appropriate when time frames are so unclear.

It is also sometimes difficult to determine for certain what the patient really wants. Patients who are awake and aware, like Harriet in the case study, can be depressed, as she most likely was. The healthcare team was able to believe that she had the capacity to make an authentic decision by giving her a trial of an antidepressant. Sometimes there is no such easy resolution, and family, patient, and healthcare team members disagree about treatment.

Problems with Advance Directives

Advance directives were intended to clarify end-of-life decision making. However, there are a variety of problems with them. First, the public has not embraced the use of advance directives, and most Americans do not have one even though surveys demonstrate strong support for them(Larson & Tobin, 2000). The small number of patients who complete advance directives is alarming and is one of the factors that prevents them from being used effectively to guide end-of-life decisions. The literature suggests that more patients would complete advance directives if they had more information and assistance in completing them (Emanuel, Barry, & Stoeckle, 1991; Mezey, Ramsey, Mitty, & Rapport, 1997). To that end, a number of educational interventions have been implemented to address these issues. Notwithstanding, few interventions increased advance directive completion by more than 18% (Hare & Nelson, 1991; Rubin, Strull, Fialkow, Weiss, & Lo, 1994; Sachs, Stocking, & Miles, 1992), and many did not increase completion at all (Robinson, DeHaven, & Koch, 1993; Stiller et al., 2001). Even patients at higher risk of becoming decisionally incapable and who were more likely to understand the need for advance directives were not more likely to complete advance directives.

Fears that an advance directive permits providers to withhold care or will lead to substandard care may be at the root of the rejection of advance directives for some patients. People may be concerned that once an advance directive is completed and it contains a statement to withhold treatment, providers will devote less attention to their care and may withhold more treatment than was desired (Caralis, Davis, Wright, & Marcial, 1993; Patel, Sinuff, & Cook, 2004). In a study by Elder, Schneider, Zweig, Peters, and Ely (1992), some individuals feared that an advance directive might allow care to be withheld too soon and could result in a shirking of societal duties. One person commented that he would not want to hear, "Sorry, we don't have the time or money to treat you." This fear is not present among patients alone; nurses and other healthcare providers hold similar beliefs (Anderson, Walker, Pierce, & Mills, 1986; Davidson, Hackler, Caradine, & McCord, 1989; Louw, 2004).

Socioeconomic and cultural factors substantially influence decisions to complete an advance directive. Studies are confirming that people with less education, lower income, or who are African-American or Hispanic are less likely to formulate advance directives (High, 1993; Mezey, Mitty, Bottrell, Ramsey, & Fisher, 2000; Phipps et al., 2003; Robinson et al., 1993). Several explanations are plausible. Individuals with these sociodemographic characteristics are less likely to have regular access to care. For them, limiting any medical care would seem unnecessary because they already have too little, not too much. They are also less likely to have exposure to the concept of advance directives (Mezey et al., 1997).

The location and timing of when a patient receives information about advance directives is also important. It is well recognized that an acute episode or emergency admission is an inappropriate time to receive this information, yet this is the point at which most hospitals are fulfilling their responsibilities under the PSDA. Information may be better utilized during the preadmission period where patients can discuss advance directives in the comfort of their own homes. Alternatively, information can be presented as part of the discharge process when the impact of hospitalization is still new but without the distraction of acute symptoms.

Even when a patient has completed an advance directive, the directive may not be utilized because the healthcare team has not been made aware of its existence. A study of recently discharged hospital patients with advance directives documented that fewer than 15% were asked about an existing advance directive during their hospitalization, 60% of patients did not disclose to the hospital staff that they had a directive, and only 35% informed their physician about their advance directives (Mezey, Ramsey, et al., 1997). Though failure to communicate this information might be attributed to the patient's presumption that the directive would not be relevant for the hospital stay, selective disclosure may reflect a patient's misunderstanding or fear about use of the advance directive.

There is increasing concern in the medical community that the problem with advance directives may not be the flawed implementation of a sound concept but rather that advance directives are a fundamentally flawed concept (Perkins, 2007). Although Perkins believes there are some benefits of advance directives, primarily people might consider what they would want at the end of life and they remind physicians of the necessity of considering the patient's goals and desires at the end of life. He notes there are a series of problems. First among them is how few people have completed them. In addition, he notes that healthcare providers such as Jacobson et al. (1994) and Valente (2004) have expressed concerns about the patient's understanding of treatment options and thus the validity of the treatment choices the patient makes in the directive. A third problem Perkins believes is physician nonadherence. He notes that physicians may disregard directives because they conflict with hospital policy or family preferences, or because they do not appear to pertain to the current situation.

Most importantly though, Perkins (2007) believes that the use of advance directives is flawed because the "outcomes have consistently frustrated expectations" (p.54). He believes that most people do not have the experience to envision a wide variety of scenarios at the end of life and merely know that they would want a death with dignity. He also believes that advance directives promise a degree of control that is not possible when a patient is critically ill and it is not certain if the patient is dying. Decisions in such situations must be made quickly. Finally, he believes that advance directives may engender rather than limit disagreements between family members or family members and healthcare providers since the directives may be unclear and the proxy may be unprepared.

Conflict in Decision Making in Palliative Care

There are times when the healthcare team, patient, and family are not able to come to agreement about how to care for the dying patient. The patient, a member of the patient's family, or a member of the healthcare team may want to continue some or all of the lifesaving treatments even though the others involved in treatment decision making believe the patient is dying and treatments should be withheld or withdrawn (Perrin & Matzo, 2009).

By ensuring careful communication, instilling trust, and listening to the voices of the people involved in the decision, most of the time, when death is imminent, consensus can be reached about which life-sustaining interventions should be provided and which withheld so that the patient is able to die with dignity. However, sometimes consensus cannot be reached and conflict develops. One reason why conflict may develop is that trust was not established among the members of the multidisciplinary healthcare team, patient and family early in the hospitalization. If lack of trust is the primary reason the patient and family want to continue life-sustaining care, the healthcare team should act to reestablish trust before proceeding with a decision about end-of-life care. Disagreement about treatment may also result when decision makers do not share a common understanding of the patient's prognosis. Sometimes the conflict may result from a family member or a healthcare provider experiencing guilt about the care of the patient, there may be secondary gains for a family member from the patient remaining alive, or the patient may come from a religious tradition that does not permit the withdrawal of life-sustaining therapy. In such situations, it may not be possible to reach a consensus about limiting care (Perrin & Matzo, 2009).

Futile Care

The situation becomes especially complex when the patient or a family member demands an intervention that the healthcare team considers to be futile. Futility can be exceedingly difficult to define. In fact, one healthcare provider is said to have stated, "I can't define it but I know it when I see it." One possible definition is any treatment that is without any benefit to the patient. Since most treatments have the potential to provide at least minimal benefit, futility is not always apparent to all members of the healthcare team, the family and the patient (Pfeifer & Kennedy, 2006). This was the situation with Harriet Billings, the patient in the case study.

Case Study follow-up: Harriet had a tracheostomy inserted and continued on dialysis. She began to improve, was gradually weaned from the ventilator, and no longer required dialysis. After a 3½-month hospitalization, she was transferred to a rehabilitation center near her home. Three days after her transfer, when the aide went to awaken her in the morning, she was unresponsive. The rehabilitation facility had a copy of her durable power of attorney and immediately contacted a neurologist, the medical center from which she had been referred, and her brother. Since her advance directive clearly indicated that she wanted everything done, they anticipated her immediate transfer back to the medical center where she had been hospitalized.

Instead, Harriet was transferred to her local hospital where she was examined by the neurologist. On examination, Harriet was unresponsive, decorticate on her right side, and flaccid on her left. Her blood pressure had increased to 200/120 and she was hyperventilating. A CT scan revealed a large cerebral bleed. When the neurologist consulted with the medical center, they decided that there was little that the center could do that would benefit Harriet and she would not be transferred. Harriet's brother arrived and wondered why she was not being transferred and whether she needed to be intubated since she was breathing erratically.

Ethics Consultation

When the healthcare team, patient, and family cannot reach a consensus about the continuation of life-sustaining treatment, the issue should be referred to the hospital's ethics committee. The Joint Commission requires hospitals to have an ethics committee for discussion and consultation to aid in the resolution of such difficult issues. The consultation may be with a member or member(s) of the ethics committee; or the case may be presented before the entire committee. The goal of case consultations by ethics committees is to suggest ways to resolve disagreements in difficult situations.

Bernard Lo (1995) identifies five goals of ethics case consultations. First, the ethics committees can help the healthcare team identify and understand the specific ethical issues the case raises: for example, cases that involve questions about advance directives, surrogate decision making, or disputes over life-sustaining treatments. Healthcare providers need to think carefully and critically through the ethical issues themselves before they try to resolve disagreements with the patient or family. Second, the ethics committee can suggest how healthcare providers might improve communications with the patient and family. Poor communications and lack of communication among the healthcare providers and members of the team may be a problem that the ethics committee can identify and help resolve. Third, the committee may provide emotional support to the physician, nurses, and other health team members in a case. Fourth, the committee may offer specific recommendations to help resolve the dilemma. Most committees or consultants help the healthcare team analyze the ethical issues and facilitate discussions with patients and families, and then offer specific recommendations for resolving the dilemmas. Finally, the committees or consultants have a role in improving patient care. Patient care decisions do not necessarily need to change after consultations, nor is there a mandate that they must change. However, by participating in consultation, healthcare providers, patients, and families may feel that their concerns have been addressed and they may better understand the rationale for the treatment decision that is being proposed.

Unfortunately, not all cases can be resolved with an ethics consultation. In fact, a situation such as Harriet's, where an individual is requesting futile treatment, is one common reason why the healthcare team, family, and patient might not be able to come to consensus about goals for end-of-life care. Some states, such as Texas, have laws that delineate procedures that must be followed prior to, during, and after ethics committee deliberations about futile treatment. After reviewing the case, the ethics committee might recommend either supporting the continuation of life-sustaining therapy or limiting treatment. In Texas, if the ethics committee recommends discontinuation of life-sustaining treatment, the patient and proxy must receive written notification of a 10-day treatment limit with an option to request transfer to another facility. If they cannot find another facility to accept the patient, then the life-sustaining treatment is discontinued after the 10th day (Pfeifer & Kennedy, 2006).

Role of the Courts

There are times when disagreements concerning life-sustaining treatments give rise to litigation. Then, the institution's lawyer is well suited to advise and educate the healthcare team about litigation and should be available to answer questions about the legal process that the staff may encounter during litigation or to avoid litigation. Discussions with the lawyer may ease some of the fears and dispel some of the misconceptions that healthcare providers have about the law and litigation in this area. In addition, discussion with the lawyer may address the potential liability for members of the committee and available immunities.

In general, the courts are hesitant to become involved in litigation surrounding end-of-life care partially because they are reluctant to become involved in disputes about dying (Schneider, 2004). Schneider offers several reasons for this. First, the judicial process is not tailored to address issues with the speed required, and by the time that a decision to litigate has been reached the patient may have already died. In addition, such cases are usually very complex medically and the complexity may not be able to be untangled by the judicial process. Finally, "a suit to enforce a living will is usually a sign that horrible and irreconcilable differences polluted efforts to make decisions for a patient" (Schneider, p. 11). Or, as he summarizes, "In love and death alike, not all wrongs can be righted, and yet fewer can be righted by the law" (p 11). Thus, for the most part, the courts have allowed and occasionally encouraged the process in which healthcare providers, patients, and families work together to come to a consensus about what type of end-of-life care should be provided.

Role of the Nurse in Decision Making in Palliative Care

What then should be nurses' involvement in end-of-life decision making? According to the American Nurses Association (ANA), in a position statement revised in 1995, nurses have a responsibility to facilitate informed decision making about end-of life-care, including but not limited to the discussion of advance directives. The ANA also recognizes that nurses have roles as educators about end-of-life care and as patient advocates to ensure that appropriate end-of-life care is provided. Thus, nursing responsibilities in end-of-life decision making may predominate at two times: when a plan for end-of-life care is being developed, and when a plan for end-of-life care is being implemented.

The nurse may be involved in assisting a patient or resident to consider or plan for end-of-life care when the patient is admitted to a hospital or long-term care facility. Or, nurses, in their roles as educators, may encounter people in the community who wish to discuss end-of-life care planning. For example, some critical-care nurses are actively promoting end-of-life planning through television programs, group discussions, and community meetings. Most patients agree that it is when they are relatively well, which most believe they are even on hospital admission, that they ought to be considering end-of-life care planning (Nolan & Bruder, 1997).

The ANA concurs that nurses need not focus on completion of an advance directive during such discussions but instead ought to provide education about possibilities at the end of life and explore patients' values, wishes, and preferences. Davison and Degner (1998) suggest that a logical place to begin the discussion is determining how much control the person wishes to exert over his/her end-of-life care. They utilize a card-sort that establishes three categories of patient decision making. The three categories are as follows:

1) **Active.** The person might select "I prefer to make the final selection about which treatment I will receive." The patient might also choose to have the family make the final decision; a definitive choice for the family to decide is also seen as an active decision by the patient (p. 134).
2) **Collaborative.** The person would choose from the card sort: "I prefer that my doctor and I (or my family and my physician) share the responsibility for deciding which treatment is best for me."
3) **Passive.** The person would select a choice such as: "I prefer to leave all decisions concerning my treatment to my physicians." The person might suggest that the physician consult with the person or family for an opinion, but in this selection the final decision is the physician's alone.

Davison and Degner (1998) suggest that once it has been determined what role the patient wishes to assume in decision making and whom the patient wishes to include in the decision making, then it is the nurse's role to initiate appropriate discussion and education among decision makers.

Since most patients desire that they and their families have at least some input into end-of-life decisions, Davison and Degner recommend that the nurse next focus on identifying the patient's and families' goals and values, as well as their understanding of the possibilities and results of the use of life-sustaining technologies at the end of life. The nurse might begin such a discussion by saying:

> "I want you to imagine that you were diagnosed as having a terminal illness. By that I mean you were dying from the illness and would not be likely to get better no matter what treatment your doctor prescribed. What would matter to you; how would you like to be cared for at that time?"

This is the step that many physicians avoid. Although difficult, it is imperative that the healthcare provider listens actively to the patient's and family's concerns, questioning and clarifying what they desire, without the healthcare provider imposing his/her own values and goals. What the nurse is attempting to learn is what this person and his/her family believe they will value as the end of life approaches. Most elders have a strong tendency to favor limitation of treatment when they are unlikely to return to their baseline functioning or are probably dying (Gillick & Mendes, 1996), but this is not always true and some elders wish to continue to live until specific events occur or goals are reached. This is the nurse's opportunity to learn what the elder and family believe will probably be important as the end of life approaches.

After the patient's and families goals and values have been explored, the nurse should assess what they understand about the use of life sustaining treatment. According to Silveira, DiPiero, Gerrity, and Freudener (2000), a significant proportion of outpatients misunderstand options at the end of life. This is not particularly surprising since many Americans obtain their information about life-sustaining technology and end-of-life care from television. Diem, Lantos, and Tulsky (1996) documented that in reality-based television medical shows, nearly all patients survive CPR: while in fictional shows such as "ER", approximately 75% of patients survive CPR. This serious misinformation often needs to be dispelled before patients and families consider what types of life-sustaining interventions they would desire at the end of life.

According to the ANA, nurses have an important role in educating patients and their families about their options at the end of life. This includes a discussion of the experience and outcomes of such treatments as CPR and ventilation. The description of CPR should be accurate and include all of the elements of resuscitation (aeration with intubation, chest compressions, defibrillation, etc.). However, it is important that the nurse allow the patient and family to develop their own opinions and come to their own conclusions. Just as

physicians can color their discussions to patients and families with their perspectives on life-sustaining interventions, so can nurses. Many nurses have very negative remembrances of CPR (Page & Meerabeau, 1996), and it is quite possible for nurses to convey these impressions to their patients and the families. Nurses might begin discussion of specific preferences for life-sustaining treatments in a similar way to that which they began discussion of the patient's values and goals for end-of-life care, such as:

> "I want you to imagine that you are very close to dying and would not be likely to get better no matter what treatment your doctor prescribed. What type of medical interventions would you want us to try in an attempt to prolong your life and delay your death?"

The final step in the development of an end-of-life plan should involve interdisciplinary development of a plan. The meeting should involve at least the patient and physician but also family and other healthcare providers if the patient so desires and appropriate. At this meeting, the patient and family can clarify any questions they might have about end-of-life care options and develop a plan, possibly a written directive. Hopefully, the final plan would include the extent to which the patient desires to be involved in the decision making, the role she/he wishes her/his family or physician to play, the patient's goals or values for end-of-life care, any specific desires the patient has for specific interventions to be utilized or withheld at end of life, as well as a choice of healthcare proxy, if appropriate. The more physicians and other healthcare providers are involved in developing a plan for end-of-life care for a patient, the more likely the plan is to be followed when the patient becomes ill and a decision needs to be made.

Once the person becomes ill and enters the healthcare system, the ANA recommends that the nurse assume the role of advocate for the patient's end-of-life care preferences. On admission to a healthcare institution, the patient and family must be asked whether the patient has an advance directive and, if a directive exists, whether they can produce a copy of the directive. Before assuming the directive should come into effect, the nurse or another healthcare provider needs to inquire if the patient still wants the directive to take effect. As previously noted, many patients change their minds about portions of their advance directive as they age and their health status changes. However, only one member of the healthcare team needs to inquire of the patient about the patient's current thoughts and feelings. The spouse of one patient who had declined all life-sustaining technologies recalled his wife being asked by 13 healthcare providers in 24 hours if she had changed her mind. Communication among healthcare providers about advance directives is essential.

Communication between healthcare institutions is also essential. One major problem with existing advance directives is they are lost when the patient is transferred from one institution to another. If, as healthcare providers, we are asking people to complete advance directives prior to the development of an illness, we ought to be able to arrange for communication regarding the directive between facilities.

When directives exist, the nurse may use the directive to help families to understand and follow the choices laid out in the directive for a family member who has become gravely ill and is incapacitated. When a patient has stated in a directive that she/he wishes to have life-sustaining interventions such as CPR or intubation withheld, the family often feels relieved to know that they are not making the choice. Some families experience guilt over depriving a family member of even the smallest possibility of continued survival.

However, it is much more likely, when a patient becomes gravely ill suddenly, that if a directive exists, the patient's choices will not be clearly related to the specific circumstances the patient is experiencing or, most likely of all, that no advance directive exists. When the patient is gravely ill, it is often the nurse who notices first that death is approaching. Clear communication to the family and physician is essential at this time because the family frequently has not considered death as an alternative (Caswell & Omery, 1990). Families need adequate, consistent information in terms that they can understand. Woods, Beaver, and Luker (2000) describe this as having the family get the whole story. Norton and Talerico (2000) caution that families need healthcare providers to use words such as "death" and "dying"; vague language makes families become confused. It is especially important, as Norton and Talerico state, that healthcare providers not use terms like "better" when a patient's condition has temporarily stabilized but the overall prognosis is unchanged, because this leads to conflicting impressions among family members and family disagreement about treatment. Another term that confuses family members is "hope". Healthcare providers often use the term when there is hope for a good death or pain control: while for family members, hope primarily means survival. Norton and Talerico (2000) recommend that nurses be specific in identifying that they are hoping for a good death or pain control for the patient, not continued life.

When death appears imminent, nurses may introduce the discussion of withholding or withdrawing life-sustaining interventions, such as CPR, intubation, and ventilation. There are two common ways that nurses begin a discussion of these interventions (Norton & Talerico, 2000). One of them is as follows: The state requires that all people receive CPR (even when it is unlikely to be of any benefit to the person) unless a DNR order is written. This is often an easier way to begin the discussion if the family has not completely acknowledged that the patient is probably dying. However, it may prevent the family from acknowledging and discussing the nearness of the patient's death. Another common approach is to acknowledge that the patient is gravely ill, probably dying, and ask the family which vision of the patient's death would be in the patient's best interests: one in which they were surrounded by family with the lights lowered and were receiving medication for pain and symptom relief, or one in which they were surrounded by healthcare personnel who were providing CPR. A discussion of the likelihood of survival following CPR should also be included.

Most patients and families want to discuss end-of-life care with their nurse; but they need to hear the same message from the patient's physician. Thus, the nurse must be in communication with the physician about the elder patient's prognosis and the patient and family's preferences about end-of-life care. Hanson et al. (1997) note that one reason for delays in the withdrawal of patient treatments is that, although patient preferences are documented, they are not communicated to physicians so that the physicians actually appreciate the patient's wishes. When there are differences in expectations of patient outcome or confusion over the appropriateness of various therapies, interdisciplinary patient care conferences are very appropriate.

Discussion about CPR with families or patients in crisis cannot come as a barrage of questions all at once from multiple healthcare providers. It is best if the patient or family has some time to consider end-of-life care. Thus, often, withholding CPR is discussed first, and gradually questions concerning withholding or withdrawal of other life sustaining interventions are introduced.

As the ANA has stated in its position statement, it is the responsibility of nurses to facilitate informed decision making for patients at the end of life. This responsibility begins when the nurse has a patient consider what would be important to him or her at the end of life, continues with the nurse educating the person about end-of-life care options, and is completed when the nurse advocates for and delivers the type of care the patient desires at the end of her/his life. However, this process of communication about end-of-life care is not solely the responsibility of the patient and the nurse; it is an interdisciplinary process that includes at least the physician and family in addition to the patient and nurse.

Case Study conclusion: Harriet was admitted to the ICU of the local hospital. Her nurse remembered Harriet and her brother from Harriet's previous admissions. She recognized that the brother was unsure about what ought to be done for Harriet. She said to him, "Despite all that we have done for her, Harriet is dying now. There is nothing we can do to stop the dying process. However, we can keep her comfortable, I think that she would realize we have tried very hard to follow her directions. She asked you to be her healthcare proxy because she trusted you to know when the time had come to say 'it is time to stop doing things that will not help her and time to keep her comfortable instead'."

Harriet's brother agreed and she died peacefully an hour later.

CONCLUSION

Numerous factors make it likely that end-of-life decision making will continue to raise difficult issues for healthcare professionals, patients, and patients' families. The reasons that people do not complete advance directives and discuss end-of-life care, even after educational interventions, seem much more compelling than the reasons for completing them. Healthcare providers often do not have enough regular ongoing contact with patients, so patients do not feel comfortable discussing end-of-life issues or completing advance directives.

Instead of focusing on the actual number of advance directives completed, we should look at whether our activities are encouraging discussions of end-of-life care with patients and families. The evidence to date indicates that simply providing information encourages patients to talk about their preferences with family members and friends, that is, the people who will be making decisions in the event the patient loses decision-making capacity. Anything that encourages such conversations enhances patient autonomy and self-determination.

Advance directives, DNR orders, court and legislative actions, are all important mechanisms for nurses to consider when seeking ways to resolve the dilemmas that exist when caring for patients at the end of life. Nurses must have opportunities to think critically and articulate their views and positions on the dilemmas they face as individuals and as professionals. Ethics rounds, grand rounds, ethics colloquia, courses in basic nursing education, continuing education offerings, and conferences, all provide forums for nurses, students, faculty, and clinicians to enhance their ethical and legal awareness. The American Nurses Association Center for Ethics and Human Rights is one rich resource for nurses who seek consultation and ethics information.

Education can change nurses' comfort with and willingness to approach patients about advance directives. When they are well informed, they are more likely to initiate discussion about advance directives.

Physicians who are educated about directives are more comfortable with such discussions, have more discussions with their patients, and their patients complete more advance directives than do patients of noneducated physicians (Emanuel, von Gunten, & Ferris, 1999; Greenberg, Doblin, Shapiro, Linn, & Wenger, 1993; Robinson et al., 1993).

Education of healthcare providers about advance directives must be provided for all health professionals. This is not currently the case. For example, fewer than 50% of nursing homes in New York City provide ongoing education about advance directives for nurses, and less than one third provide education for physicians (Mezey, Ramsey, Mitty, & Rappaport, 1997). Much of the PSDA information available to institutions comes from legal departments, state departments of health, or from professional organizations (U.S. Department of Health and Human Services [DHHS], 1993). Although this study clearly indicates that nurses need basic information such as state and federal regulations concerning advance directives, education requires more than a description of the law and steps be taken in formulating directives. Nurses and other healthcare providers need to learn how to discuss advance care planning with patients and families; assess decisional capacity to execute a directive; identify methods to help patients analyze the benefits and burdens of decisions; and resolve conflicts among staff with different values and beliefs about end-of-life treatment. Education should also include the dissemination and discussion of treatment guidelines, attention to the psychology of decision making, and a dialogue between those who develop ethical recommendations and those who must carry them out at the bedside (Shapiro & Bowles, 2002; Solomon et al., 1993).

EVIDENCE-BASED PRACTICE

Review. Effects of knowledge and attitudes upon practices of nurses concerning advanced directives

Duke, G. & Thompson, S. (2007). Knowledge, attitudes, and practices of nursing personnel regarding advance directives. *International Journal of Palliative Nursing, 13*, 109-115.

Q: What are the knowledge, attitudes, and practices of nurses working in acute-care settings regarding advance directives (AD)?

Is there a relationship between nurses' education, length of experience, and their clinical practice setting and their knowledge, attitudes, and perceptions of ADs for their clients?

Is there a relationship between nurses' education, length of experience, and their clinical practice setting and their knowledge, attitudes, and perceptions of ADs for themselves and their own families?

Methods. Descriptive cross sectional study

Data sources. The Update on Advance Directives, a 40-item survey assessing attitudes practices, and knowledge regarding ADs developed by the authors with an internal consistency was utilized. Also included were six questions requesting demographic information and one open-ended question.

Study selection and assessment. A convenience sample of 108 of 283 eligible RNs and LPNs (39% response rate) working in two 350-450 bed acute care hospitals.

Main results. Nursing personnel reflected a lack of knowledge concerning federal and state laws as well as general information about advance directives. Nursing personnel had very low rates of completion of advance directives but most believed that such directives were valuable to the patient.

Conclusion. Nurses need more resources such as knowledge, administrative support, and physician support, as well as better communication tools, to facilitate advance planning for end-of-life care for patients.

Commentary. This study demonstrated that although nurses in Texas did understand the purpose of an advance directive, the majority could not identify what was included in the scope of comfort care in the Texas directive (pain medication), nor were they knowledgeable concerning the Texas requirements for the witnessing of an advance directive or where the directive for the patient ought to be located. Although the majority of nurses in the study believed that advance directives were of benefit to patients, the authors believed that the nurse's lack of knowledge affected their ability and to speak with a patient and family about an advance directive.

For correspondence. Gloria Duke (gduke@uttyler.edu)

Sources of funding. None provided.

REFERENCES

Aging with Dignity. (2007). *Five Wishes*. Tallahassee, Florida. http://www.agingwithdignity.org/5wishes.pdf

American Medical Association Council on Ethical and Judicial Affairs. (1991). Guidelines for the appropriate use of DNR orders. *Journal of the American Medical Association, 265,* 1868–1871.

American Nurses Association. (1996). *American nurses association position statement on nursing and the patient self-determination act* (pp.106–108). Compendium of ANA Position Statements. Washington, DC: American Nurses Association.

Appelbaum, P. (2007). Assessment of patients' competence to consent to treatment. *New England Journal of Medicine, 357,* 1834–1840.

Banja, J. D., & Bilsky, G. S. (1993). Discussing cardiopulmonary resuscitation with elderly rehabilitation patients. *American Journal of Physical Medicine and Rehabilitation,72* (3), 168–171.

Blustein, J. (1999). Choosing for others as a continuing life story: The problem of personal identity revisited. *Journal of Law and Medical Ethics, 27,* 20–31.

Buchanan, S. F. (1998). Guardians of care: Geriatrics and the law. *Clinical Geriatrics, 6* (12), 79–81.

Bradley, E., Walker, L., Blechner, J. D., & Wetle, T. (1997). Assessing capacity to participate in discussions of advance directives in nursing homes: Findings from a study of the patient self-determination act. *Journal of the American Geriatrics Society, 45* (1), 79–83.

Caralis, P. V., Davis, B., Wright, K., & Marcial, E. (1993). The influence of ethnicity and race on attitudes toward advance directives, life-prolonging treatments, and euthanasia. *Journal of Clinical Ethics, 4,* 155.

Casewell, D., & Omery, A. (1990). The dying patient in the critical care setting: Making the critical difference. *AACN Clinical Issues in Critical Care Nursing, 1* (1), 178–186.

Cooney, L. M., Kennedy, G. J., Hawkins, K. A., Hurme, S., & Balch, J. D. (2004). Who can stay at home? Assessing the capacity to choose to live in the community. *Archives of Internal Medicine, 164,* 357–360.

Cotton, P. (1993). Talk to people about dying-they can handle it, say geriatricians and patients. *Journal of the American Medical Association, 269* (3), 321–323.

Covinsky, K. F., Landefeld, S., Teno, J., Connors, A. F. Dawson, N. Youngres, S. et al. (1996). For the SUPPORT Investigators. Is economic hardship on the families of the seriously ill associated with patient and surrogate care preferences? *Archives of Internal Medicine, 156,* 1737–1741.

Covinsky, K. E., Goldman, L., Cook, E. F., Desbiens, N., Reding, D., Fulkerson, W. et al. (1994). The impact of serious illness on patients' families. *Journal of the American Medical Association, 272,*1839–1844.

Cruzan v. Director, Missouri Dept. of Health, 497 U.S. 261 (1990), 110 S. Ct. 2841 (1990).

Daly, B. (2008). An indecent proposal: Withholding cardiopulmonary resuscitation. *American Journal of Critical Care, 17* (4), 37–380.

Danis, M., Garrett, J., Harris, R., & Patrick, D. L. (1994). Stability of choices about life-sustaining treatments. *Annals of Internal Medicine, 120,* 567–573.

Davidson, R. W., Hackler, C., Caradine, D. R., & McCord, R. S. (1989). Physician attitudes on advance directives. *Journal of the American Medical Association, 262,* 2415–2419.

Davis, A., Aroskar, M., Liaschenko, J., & Drought, T. (1997). *Ethical dilemmas & nursing practice* (4th ed.). Stamford, CT: Appleton and Lange.

Davison, J., & Degner, L. F. (1998). Promoting patient decision making in life-and-death situations. *Seminars in Oncology Nursing, 14* (2), 129–136.

Degenholtz, H., Rhee, Y., & Arnold, R. (2004). Brief communication: The relationship between having a living will and dying in place. *Annals of Internal Medicine, 141,* 113–118.

Diamond, E. L., Jernigan, J. A., Moseley, R. A., Messina, V., & McKeown, R. A. (1989). Decision making ability and advance care directive preferences in nursing home patients and proxies. *The Gerontologist, 29* (5), 622–626.

Diem, S. J., Lantos, J. D., & Tulsky, J. A. (1996). Cardiopulmonary resuscitation on television: Miracles and misinformation. *The New England Journal of Medicine, 334* (25), 1578–1582.

Elder, N. C., Schneider, F. D., Zweig, S. C., Peters, P. G., & Ely, J. W. (1992). Community attitudes and knowledge about advance care directives. *Journal of the American Board Family Practice, 5*, 565–572.

Emanuel, E. J., & Weinberg, D. S. (1993). How well is the patient self-determination act working: An early assessment. *American Journal of Medicine, 95*, 619–627.

Emanuel, L. L., Barry, W., & Stoeckle, J. D. (1991). Advanced directives for medical care: A case for greater use. *New England Journal of Medicine, 324*, 889–895.

Emanuel, L. L., Emanuel, E. J., Toeckle, J. D., Hummel, L. R., & Barry, M. J. (1994). Advance directives: Stability of patient's treatment choices. *Archives of Internal Medicine, 154*, 209–217.

Eun-shim, N., & Resnick, B. (2001). End of life treatment preferences among older adults. *Nursing Ethics, 8* (6), 533–544.

Foley, K. (1991). The relationship of pain and symptom management to patient requests for physician-assisted suicide. *Journal of Pain and Symptom Management, 6*, 289.

Forbes, S. (2001). This is heaven's waiting room: End of life in one nursing home. *Journal of Gerontological Nursing*. 37–45.

Furrow, B., Greaney, T., Johnson, S., Jost, J. T., & Schwartz, R. (2001). *Hornbook on health law* (2nd ed.): Eagan, MN: West Group.

Ghusen, H., Teasdale, T. A., & Jordan, D. (1997). Continuity of do-not-resuscitation orders between hospital and nursing home settings. *Journal of the American Geriatric Society, 45*, 465–469.

Gillick, M., & Mendes, M. (1996). Medical care in old age: What do nurses in long term care consider appropriate. *Journal of the American Geriatrics Society, 44*, 1322–5.

Guido, G. (2006). *Legal and ethical issues in nursing* (3rd ed.). Upper Saddle River, NJ: Pearson/Prentice Hall.

Hall, J. (1996). *Nursing ethics and law*. Philadelphia, PA: Saunders.

Hamel, M. B., Phillips, R. S., Davis, R. B., et al. (1997). For the SUPPORT investigators. Outcomes and cost effectiveness of initiating dialysis and continuing aggressive care in seriously ill hospitalized adults. *Annals of Internal Medicine, 127*, 195–202.

Hamel, M. B., Phillips, R. S., Teno, J. M., et al. (1996). For the SUPPORT investigators. Seriously ill hospitalized adults: Do we spend less on older patients? *Journal of the American Geriatric Society, 44*, 1043–1048.

Hamel, M. B., Teno, J. M., Goldman, L., et al. (1999). Patient age and decisions to withhold life-sustaining treatments from seriously ill hospitalized adults. *Annals of Internal Medicine, 130* (4), 116–125.

Hanson, L. C., Tulsky, J. A., & Danis, M., (1997). Can clinical interventions change care at the end of life? *Annals of Internal Medicine, 126* (5), 381 (3rd ed.) 388.

Hare, J., & Nelson, C. (1991). Will outpatients complete living wills? *Journal of General Internal Medicine, 6*, 41–46.

High, D. M. (1993). Advance directives and the elderly: A study of intervention strategies to increase use. *Gerontologist, 33*, 342–349.

High, D. M. (1994, November/December). Families roles in advance directives. *Hastings Center Report, Special Supplement*, S16–S18.

Hinds, P. S., Drew, D., Oakes, L. L., Fouladi, M., Spunt, S. L., Church, C., et al. (2005) End-of-life care preferences of pediatric patients with cancer. *Journal of Clinical Oncology, 23*, 9146–9154.

Field, M., & Cassel, C. (Eds.) (1997). Approaching death: Improving care at the end of life. Washington, DC: National Academies Press. IOM (Institute of Medicine). (1997). Committee on End of Life Care. *In re Westchester County Medical Center (O'Connor)*, 72 N.Y.2nd 517, 531 N.E.2d 607, 534 N.Y.S.2d 886, rev'g 139 A.D.2d 344, 532 N.Y.S.2d 133 (1988). *In re Farrell*, 108 NJ 335, 529 A.2d 404 (N.J. 1987).

Knaus, W. A., Harrell, F. E., Lynn, J., et. al (1995). For the SUPPORT Investigators. The SUPPORT prognostic model: Objective estimates of survival for seriously ill hospitalized adults. *Annals of Internal Medicine, 122*, 191–203.

Kohn, M., & Menon, G. (1988). Life prolongation: Views of elderly outpatients and health care professionals. *Journal of the American Geriatrics Society, 36* (9), 840–844.

Kollas, C., & Boyer-Kollas, B. (2007). Evolving medicolegal issues in palliative care. *Journal of Palliative Medicine, 10*, 1395–1401.

Larson, D. G., & Tobin, D. R. (2000). End-of-life conversations: Evolving practice and theory. *Journal of the American Medical Association, 284*, 1573–1578.

Lo, B. (1995). *Resolving ethical dilemmas: A guide for clinicians*. Baltimore, MD: Lippincott, Williams, & Wilkins.

Lo, B., Rothenberg, K., & Vasko, M. (1996) Appropriate management of pain: Addressing the clinical, legal and regulatory barriers. *Journal of Law, Medicine and Ethics, 24*, 285–286.

Louw, S. (2004). Cultural issues in end-of-life decision making. *Age and Ageing, 33*, 212–213.

Marik, P. E., & Craft, M. (1997). An outcomes analysis of in-hospital cardiopulmonary resuscitation: The futility rationale for do not resuscitate orders. *Journal of Critical Care, 12* (3), 142–146.

Martin, D. K., Emanuel, L. L., & Singer, P. A. (2000). Planning for the end of life. *Lancet, 356* (9242), 1672–1677.

McKay v. Bergstedt, 106 Nev. 808, 801 P.2d 617 (Nev. 1990).

Meisel, A., & Cerminara, K. L. (2001). *The right to die: Vols.1 and 2: 2001 cumulative supplement*. New York: Aspen Law & Business.

Mezey, M., Mitty, E., Bottrell, M., Ramsey, G., & Fisher, T. (2000). Advance directives: Older adults with dementia. *Clinics in Geriatric Medicine, 16*, 255–268.

Mezey, M., Leitman, R., Mitty, E., Bottrell, M., & Ramsey, G. (2000). Why hospital patients do and do not execute an advance directive. *Nursing Outlook. 48* (4), 165–171.

Mezey, M., Ramsey, G., Mitty, E., & Rappaport, M. (1997). Implementation of the Patient Self-Determination Act (PSDA) in nursing homes in New York City. *Journal of the American Geriatrics Society, 45*, 43–49.

Mezey, M., Mitty, E., & Ramsey, G. (1997). Assessment of decision-making capacity: Nurse's role. *Journal of Gerontological Nursing, 23* (3), 28–35.

Mitty, E. L., & Mezey, M. D. (2004). Advance directives: Older adults with dementia. In M. Matzo and D. Sherman (Eds.), *Gerontological palliative care nursing* (pp. 118–131). St. Louis, MO: Mosby.

Mitty, E., Mezey, M., Ramsey, G., & Rappaport, M. (1996). Ethics committees and PSDA implementation in 100 nursing homes: Nursing home medicine. *Journal of the American Medical Directors' Association, 12*, 23–28.

Molloy, D. W., Guyatt, G. H., Russo, R., Goeree, R., O'Brien, B., Dedard, M. et al. (2000). Systematic implementation of an advance directive program in nursing homes. *Journal of the American Medical Association, 283* (11), 1437–1443.

Molloy, D. W., Silberfield, M., Darzins, P., Guyatt, G. H., Singer, P. A., Rush, B., et al. (1996). Measuring capacity to complete an advance directive. *Journal of the American Geriatrics Society, 44* (6), 660–664.

Murphy, P., Kreling, B., Kathryn, E., Stevens, M., Lynn, J. & Dulac, J. (2000). Description of the SUPPORT Intervention. *Journal of the American Geriatrics Society, 48*, S154–S161.

Murphy, D. J., Murray, A. M., Robinson, B. E., & Campton, E. W. (1989). Outcomes of cardiopulmonary resuscitation in the elderly. *Annals of Internal Medicine, 111* (3), 199–205.

New York State Task Force on Life and the Law. (1995). *A message about the family health care Decisions Act of 1995.* New York: Author.

Nolan, M. T., & Bruder, M. (1997). Patients' attitudes toward advance directives and end-of-life treatment decisions. *Nursing Outlook, 45* (5), 204–208.

Norton, S. A., & Talerico, K. A. (2000). Facilitating end-of-life decision-making: Strategies for communicating and assessing. *Journal of Gerontological Nursing, 26*(9), 6–13.

O'Brien, L. A., Grisso, J. A., & Maislin, G. (1995). Nursing home residents preferences for life sustaining treatments. *Journal of the American Medical Association, 274*(22), 1775–1779.

Pain Relief Promotion Act of 1999 (HR 2260).

Page, S., & Meerabeau, L. (1996). Nurses' accounts of cardiopulmonary resuscitation. *Journal of Advanced Nursing, 24,* 317–325.

Patel, R.V., Sinuff, T., & Cook, D. J. (2004). Influencing advance directive completion rates in non-terminally ill patients: A systematic review. *Journal of Critical Care, 19*(1), 1–9.

Pfeifer, G. M., & Kennedy, M. S. (2006). Understanding medical futility. *American Journal of Nursing, 106*(5), 25–26.

Perkins, H. (2007). Controlling death: The false promise of advance directives. *Annals of Internal Medicine, 147,* 51–57.

Perrin, K. O. (1997). Giving voice to the wishes of elders for end of life care. *Journal of Gerontological Nursing, 23* (3), 18–27.

Perrin, K., & Matzo, M. (2009). Caring for the ICU patient at the end of life. In K. Perrin (ed.) *Understanding the essentials of critical care nursing.* Upper Saddle River, NJ: Pearson/Prentice Hall

Phillips, R. S., Hamel, M. B., Covinsky, K. E., & Lynn, J. (2000). Findings from SUPPORT and HELP: An introduction. *Journal of the American Geriatrics Society, 48*(5), S1–S5.

Phillips R. S, Hamel, M. B., Teno, J. M., et al. (1996). For the SUPPORT Investigators. Race, resource use, and survival in seriously ill hospitalized adults. *Journal of General Internal Medicine, 11,* 387–396.

Prendergast, T. J., & Puntillo, K. A. (2004). Withdrawal of life support: Intensive caring at the end of life. *Journal of the American Medical Association. 288,* 2732–2740.

President's Commission for the Study of Ethical Problems in Medicine and Biomedical and Behavioral Research. (1982, March). *Deciding to forego life-sustaining treatment.* Washington, DC: U.S. Government Printing Office.

Pub. L. No. 101–508, '4206, 4751 [hereinafter OBRA], 104 Stat. 1388–115 to 117, 1388–204 to 206 (codified at 42 U.S.C.A. '1395cc(f) (1) & id. '1396a(a) (West Supp. 1994).

In re Quinlan, 70 N.J. 10, 355 A.2d 647 (N.J. 1976).

Reckling, J. (1997). Who plays what role in decisions about withholding and withdrawing life sustaining treatment. *Journal of Clinical Ethics, 8*(1), 39–45.

Robinson, M. K., DeHaven, M. J., & Koch, K. A. (1993). Effects of the patient self-determination act on patient knowledge and behavior. *Journal of Family Practice, 37,* 363–368.

Rubin, S. M., Strull, W. M., Fialkow, F., Weiss, S. J., & Lo, B. (1994). Increasing the completion of the durable power of attorney for health care. *Journal of the American Medical Association, 271,* 209–212.

Sachs, G. A., Stocking, C. E., & Miles, S. H. (1992). Failure of an intervention to promote discussion of advance directives. *Journal of the American Geriatrics Society, 40,* 269–273.

Schneider, C. (2004, July/August). Liability for life. *Hastings Center Report,* 10–11.

Schneider, A. P., Nelson, D. J., & Brown, D. D. (1993). In-hospital cardiopulmonary resuscitation: A 30-year review. *Journal of the American Board of Family Practice, 6*(2), 91–101.

Schloendorff v. Society of New York Hospitals, 211 N.Y. 125, 105 N.E. 92 (1914).

Shapiro, J., & Bowles, K. (2002). Nurses' and consumers' understanding of and comfort with the patient self-determination act. *Journal of Nursing Administration, 32,* 503–508.

Shapiro, R. (1996). Health care providers' liability exposure for inappropriate pain management. *Journal of Law, Medicine and Ethics, 24,* 360–364.

Silveira, M. J., DiPiero, A., Gerrity, M.S., & Freudener, C. (2000). Patients' knowledge of options in end-of-life care: Ignorance in the face of death. *Journal of the American Medical Association, 284* (19), 2483–2488.

Smith, T. J., Desch, C. E., Hackney, M. H., Shaw, J. E. (1997). How long does it take to get a "do not resuscitate" order? *Journal of Palliative Care, 13*(1), 5–8.

Solomon, M. Z., O'Donnell, L., Jennings, B., Guilfoy, V., Wolf, S. M., & Nolan, K. (1993). Decisions near the end of life: Professional views on life-sustaining treatments. *American Journal of Public Health, 83*(1), 14–23.

Stiller, A., Molloy, D. W., Russo, R., Dubois, S., Kavsak, H., & Bedard, M., et al. (2001). Development and evaluation of a new instrument that measures barriers to implementing advance directives. *Journal of Clinical Outcomes Management, 8*(4), 26–31.

SUPPORT Principal Investigators. (1995). A controlled trial to improve care for seriously ill hospitalized patients: The Study to Understand Prognoses and Preferences for Outcomes and Risks of Treatment (SUPPORT). *Journal of the American Medical Association, 274,* 1591–1598.

Swidler, R. (1989). The presumption of consent in New York State's do-not-resuscitate law. *New York State Journal of Medicine, 89,* 69–72.

Teno, J, Gruneir, A., Schwartz, Z., Nanda, A., & Wetle, T. (2007). Association between advance directives and quality of end of life care: A national survey. *Journal of the American Geriatrics Society, 55* 189–194,

Teno, J., Lynn, J., Phillips, R.S., Murphy, D., Youngner, S. J., Bellamy, P., et al. (1994). For the SUPPORT Investigators. Do formal advance directives affect resuscitation decisions and the use of resources for seriously ill patients? *Journal Clinical Ethics, 5,* 23–30.

Teno, J., Lynn, J., Wenger, N., Phillips, R. S., Murphy, D. P., Connors, A. F., et al. (1997). For the SUPPORT Investigators. Advance directives for the seriously ill hospitalized patients: Effectiveness with the patient self determination act and the SUPPORT Intervention. *Journal of the American Geriatrics Society, 45,* 500–507.

Teno, J. M., Licks, S., Lynn, J., et al. (1997). For the SUPPORT Investigators. Do advance directives provide instructions that direct care? *Journal of the American Geriatrics Society, 45,* 508–512.

Tulsky, J. A., Chesney, M. A., & Lo, B. (1995). How do medical residents discuss resuscitation with patients. *Journal of General Internal Medicine, 10* (8), 436–442.

Tulsky, J. A., Chesney, M. A., & Lo, B. (1996). See one, do one, teach one? House staff experience discussing do-not-resuscitate orders. *Archives of Internal Medicine, 156* (12), 1285–1289.

U.S. Department of Health and Human Services, Office of the Inspector General. (1993). *Patient advance directives: Early implementation experience* (OEI 06–91– 01130). Washington, DC: Author.

Vacco v. Quill, 521 U.S. 793, 117 S.Ct. 2293 (1997).

Valente, S. (2004). End-of-life challenges: Honoring autonomy. *Cancer Nursing, 27,* 314–319.

Ventres, W., Nichter, M., Reed, R., & Frankel, R. (1992). Do-not-resuscitate discussions: A qualitative analysis. *Family Practice Research Journal, 12*(2), 157–169.

Virani, R., & Sofer, D. (2003). Improving the quality of end-of-life care: Making changes at every level. *American Journal of Nursing, 103*(5), 52–60.

Wagner, A. (1984). Cardiopulmonary resuscitation in the aged: A prospective study. *New England Journal of Medicine, 310*(17), 1129–1130.

Washington v. Glucksberg, 117 S. Ct. 2258 (1997).

Wenger, N., Phillips, R., Teno, J., Oye, R., Dawson, N., Liu, H., et al. (2000). Physician understanding of patient resuscitation preferences: Insights and clinical implications. *Journal of the American Geriatrics Society, 48*(5), S44–S51.

Psychosocial Considerations

June 18

Candy had a friend from the neighborhood over when I arrived today. This woman was so eager to be of help to Candy and her family; apparently the whole neighborhood had rallied and were offering support by grocery shopping, preparing meals, house cleaning, and offering to watch the children. Candy's 5-year-old son was at his first sleepover and she was both pleased and sad that he felt comfortable leaving her to stay with a friend. She talked about how involved her husband was with her and the situation that they were in. She said they laughed about the sounds that came from her colostomy and how she could talk to him about the decisions she had to make regarding her care. Her therapist had talked with the children to determine their feelings and ideas about what was happening and helping them to deal with their

mother's illness. Candy did say that she has not talked to them about dying because she was not ready to talk about it herself. She was still struggling with her loss of function and role changes, now that she did not have the energy to care physically for her children.

Yet, Candy was still hoping for a cure. As a nurse, I knew that at some point the hope would change from a hope of cure to the hope for a comfortable death, free of pain and surrounded by those who loved her. I could only imagine her feelings of loss and grief. I, too, pushed the thoughts of death from my mind. Because I was close to her age, I became increasingly aware of my own mortality. As Candy told me how her children snuggled close to her in bed, I felt incredibly saddened by the thought of her death, and the idea that her children would lose their mother. I imagined the pain of my children, if I were to die.

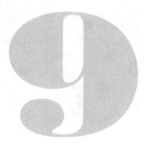

Communicating with Seriously Ill and Dying Patients, Their Families, and Their Health Care Providers

Kathleen O. Perrin

Key Points

■ Conveying or discussing "bad news" requires preparation—locating a private place for the conversation, asking the patient or family to have a significant other present, having as much information available as possible, and practicing what will be said.

■ Patients and their families may respond to "bad news" with disbelief, anger, or denial. Nurses and nursing students should practice their reactions to these defense mechanisms.

■ Nurses may inappropriately block patient or family communication by ignoring what the patient or family member has to say, offering elaborate explanations or inappropriate advice, and providing their opinions without being asked.

■ Nurses may assist patients and their families to decide what is important to them while the patient is dying by asking the patient, "What would be left undone if you died sooner rather than later".

■ Byock believes that it is essential that patients, their families, and significant others find time before the patient dies to say to each other "Please forgive me; I forgive you; Thank you; and I love you".

■ It is imperative that nurses demonstrate to patients and their families by their words and deeds that healthcare providers will not abandon the patient after a decision has been made about end-of-life care.

169

Case Study: Gloria Richards, an 82-year-old woman with severe chronic obstructive lung disease, consented to surgery for an intestinal obstruction. Following the surgery, she required re-intubation in the PACU and was transported to the ICU for posoperative care. Although she was being ventilated with low tidal volumes, shortly after her arrival in ICU, several blebs burst in her lungs, she developed creptius from her chin to her waist, and required multiple chest tubes. This marked the beginning of a difficult postoperative course. Three weeks after surgery, her chest tubes could finally be removed. However, she remained intubated and every effort to wean her from the ventilator resulted in her becoming hypoxic and unresponsive.

After her first week in the ICU, Gloria was awake and responsive during the day. She was able to mouth words to the staff and was involved in developing her plan of care. Although Gloria was able to communicate her wishes clearly, communicating with her was very time consuming. During the second week, Gloria announced that she "was fed up." She believed she was not improving and said she either wanted to get better or have the ventilator removed. Gloria had been living with her brother who had died 6 months before her hospitalization, so there was concern among members of the healthcare team that she was depressed. During interdisciplinary rounds, a trial of an antidepressant was proposed and Gloria and her niece, her next of kin, agreed to the plan. However as time progressed, Gloria indicated that she was "tired of all this and did not want it anymore." She wanted to know what was happening to her and if she was likely to get better.

Introduction

Like Gloria in the case study, seriously ill or dying patients and their families want their healthcare providers to communicate prognoses and treatment options with honesty (Furukawa, 1996; Parker et. al., 2007) and caring (Czerwiec, 1996; London & Lundstedt, 2007). In 1995, The Study to Understand Prognoses and Preferences for Outcomes and Risks of Treatment (SUPPORT) demonstrated that this discussion does not occur as often as families and hospitalized patients would prefer. Despite years of effort to improve end-of-life communication, the SUPPORT finding was reaffirmed in 2007 when in a study by Sullivan et al. only 33% of physicians reported that anyone on the healthcare team had spoken with hospitalized patients identified as likely to die about the possibility of dying. However, in the same study, majority of physicians did report that a few days before the patient's death, someone had spoken about the likelihood of death with the patient's family. Because most Americans die in hospitals, the absence of such discussion is a major shortfall in the care of dying Americans. Moreover, even for patients who are cared for at home and referred to hospice, discussion, and preparation for death are often avoided until hospice referral. Because most patients are not referred to hospice until the last weeks of their lives, this means that discussion of end-of-life care is often postponed as in Gloria's situation until it is unavoidable.

According to Servaty, Krejci, and Hayslip (1996), healthcare providers with less anxiety about death are more likely to talk meaningfully with dying patients. In their study, nursing students were less anxious and more willing than other college students and beginning medical students to communicate with dying people. Thus, they reasoned, nursing students may be responsive to educational endeavors to promote honest, caring communication with patients and families at the end of life. This chapter will explore ways to encourage both nursing students and graduate nurses to facilitate communication with dying patients, their families, and their healthcare providers.

In addition to patients and their families benefiting from communication with nurses at the end of life, the nurses may also benefit. Stiles (1990) described seven types of personal growth that nurses dealing with dying patients felt they experienced as "gifts" from their patients. These included learning to confront their own mortality, learning about self, developing a faith in self and in a higher being, transcending their limitations, learning realistic expectations, and clarifying personal responsibility. Although experienced nurses perceived these opportunities for personal growth as gifts from their patients, undergraduate nursing students may be more distressed by them. Ways in which nursing faculty members might assist undergraduate nursing students to enrich themselves by working with dying patients will also be explored in this chapter.

This chapter will be organized according to the phases of the therapeutic relationship because in many ways the phases of therapeutic relationship—introductory, working, and termination—parallel to the dying trajectory. When appropriate in the phases, distinctions will be made between the roles and educational needs of the undergraduate nursing student, the nurse with an undergraduate degree, the advanced practice nursing student, and the nurse with an advanced practice degree.

INTRODUCTORY PHASE

During the introductory phase of the therapeutic relationship, the nurse and patient open the relationship, begin to clarify and define the problem that has brought the patient in contact with the nurse, and begin to define their relationship.

Opening the Relationship

For the nursing student, the components of this phase include conveying respect for the dying patient and his or her family as well as establishing a trusting relationship. These constituents are no different from their establishment in any therapeutic relationship. The student should introduce herself or himself to the patient and identify how the student will be involved in the patient's care. The nursing faculty member ought to note if the student caring for a dying patient seems unusually reluctant to engage in care of that patient. If the student appears hesitant, the faculty member might demonstrate by introducing himself or herself to the patient that this portion of the relationship is no different merely because the patient is dying. At this very early stage in the relationship, the student, or any healthcare provider, probably ought to avoid discussing the subject of death and dying unless the patient brings up the topic (Byock, 1997).

In contrast, it may be the responsibility of the advanced practice nurse to explain to a patient that the patient is severely ill and may be dying during one of their initial meetings. It would always be preferable that the advanced practice nurse and patient have had an opportunity to establish a trusting relationship before the advanced practice nurse is required to deliver such bad news to the patient. However, in today's fast-paced healthcare environment, especially in emergency departments and critical care units, that is not always possible.

Conveying bad news requires thought and preparation. When preparing for the discussion, Buckman, Lipkin, Sourkes, and Tolle (1997) recommend that the healthcare provider locate a private place for the discussion, ask the patient to have a family member or friend present, have all information available to explain to the patient, and practice what she or he is planning to say. Buckman et al. (1997) suggest that after any introductions are made to the patient and family the patient be asked if it would be permissible to tape the interview. They state that taping the interview and providing the tape to the patient when the interview is finished enhances the patient's long-term adjustment. The steps recommended by Buckman (1992) for breaking bad news are listed in Table 9.1. Although these steps have been advocated and circulated for years, there is little consistent, good quality evidence to support any interventions to convey "bad news" and they are recommended either on the basis of limited

9.1 | Breaking "Bad News"

- Get the context right.
- Find out what is already known.
- Find out how much information the patient and/or family wants to know.
- Share the information, starting from their viewpoint and step by step bring their understanding closer to the medical facts.
- Respond to their reactions using an empathetic approach.
- Explain the treatment plan and prognosis, summarize, and make a contract.

Source: How to Break Bad News: A Guide for Health Professionals by Buckman (1992).

quality patient-oriented evidence (B level) or consensus and expert opinion (C level) (Barclay, Blackwell, & Tulsky, 2007; Ngo-Metzger, August, Srinivasan, Liao, & Meyskens, 2008).

Buckman et al. (1997) and Barclay et al. (2007) recommend starting the interview by finding out what the patient knows or suspects. Often the patient has a preconception of the problem and it may be necessary not only to convey bad news but to counter the patient's and family's misconceptions of the situation. In numerous studies, families have indicated that prognosis should be conveyed in an honest, caring manner but that they need to be prepared for a poor prognosis and it should be tempered with hope rather than delivered bluntly (Barclay, Blackhall, & Tulsky) .

Not all patients want to know the extent of their illness. Therefore, Ngo-Metzger et al. (2008) recommend that patients be asked directly and at the start of the interview how much information they want to know about their prognosis. Kagawa-Singer and Blackhall (2001) note that people from other cultures may not emphasize autonomy as much as Americans do. In some cultures, it is the members of the family and not the individual who learn the prognosis and agree to a plan of care. To uncover the desires of such patients and families, Kagawa-Singer and Blackhall suggest utilizing the following question: "Some patients want to know everything about their condition, others prefer that we talk with their families. How would you like to get information?" (p. 2995).

Before actually stating the problem, Buckman et al. (1997) suggests foreshadowing the news in simple language such as "I'm sorry, I have some bad news for you." They suggest that the situation then be explained in simple terms that are understandable to the patient. Patients and families consistently identify the use of medical jargon as a major deterrent to their understanding of the prognosis. After conveying the information in understandable terms, Buckman et al. (1997) recommends something that can be very difficult for the beginning practitioner—silence. During the period of silence, the patient will have an opportunity to absorb the information, react, and ask questions.

After the information is conveyed to the patient and the patient has had a chance to react, Buckman et al. (1997) suggest an empathetic approach. This implies that the person conveying the bad news should first identify the emotion that the patient is experiencing and identify the origins of the emotion. Then, the nurse should respond in a way that tells the patient that the nurse understands what the patient is experiencing. This means the nurse should "reflect, name, and legitimize the patient's feelings" (Buckman et al., 1997 p. 63). For example, the nurse might say, "I can see that this has really upset you. Was that something that you weren't expecting" (Radziewicz & Baile, 2001, p. 952).

The final step in breaking bad news is providing an initial explanation of potential treatments and prognoses. Later in the therapeutic relationship, the advance practice nurse may become involved in empowering the patient to be an active participant in the decision-making process about treatment and developing an agreement about care. At this stage, the possibilities are usually just described to provide the patient and family with an opportunity to begin thinking about goals of treatment. Before the interview is complete, the advanced practice nurse should summarize the discussion for the patient.

Gordon, Buckman, and Buckman suggest using the SPIKES mnemonic as a tool to remember the steps for delivering bad news to patients and families. This mnemonic summarizes the steps previously described and is displayed in Table 9.2.

9.2 SPIKES Mnemonic

S Set up	Set up an interview with the patient and family
P Perception	Find out what the patient and/or family understand about the prognosis
I Invitation	Ask who should be provided with the prognosis
K Knowledge	Convey the bad news to the appropriate person in a manner that s/he can understand
E Emotions	Empathize with the person's emotions
S Summary and strategy	Summarize the discussion and have the person begin to think about a plan of care

Source: Gordon, Buckman, and Buckman (2007). "Bad news" communication in palliative care: A challenge and a key to success. *Annals of Long-Term Care, 15*(4), 32–38. American Geriatrics Society, reprinted with permission.

Tulsky, Chesney, and Lo (1996) recommend that a new practitioner be observed several times and offered feedback before being allowed to discuss bad news without supervision. Emanuel (1998) suggests the new practitioner be provided with talking points so that all of the appropriate information is covered. Latimer (1998) describes criteria for ethical communication of information that might be used to evaluate the communication skills of a beginning practitioner. To be ethical, according to Latimer, communication should be timely and desired by the patient. Information must be accurate. Words should be understandable to the patient and family and information must be conveyed in a gentle, respectful, and compassionate manner.

There is developing awareness that an individual healthcare provider should not confront a patient and family with bad news without informing other members of the healthcare team of the details of the discussion (Davis, Kristjanson, & Blight, 2003; Fallowfield & Jenkins, 2004; Larson & Tobin, 2000; Pattison, 2004). Unfortunately, more than 80% of physicians in a study by Ptacek, Ptacek, and Ellison (2001) did not have another healthcare provider accompany them when they delivered bad news. When individual providers provide bad news to patients and families without informing the other members of the healthcare team, lack of communication can be a significant barrier to quality end-of-life care (Yabroff & Mandelblatt, 2004). Patients and families who are anxious often do not hear or understand bad news the first time they hear it. Nurses describe feeling caught "in the middle" or "going in blind" when they do not know what a patient has been told and the patient or family is requesting further information or explanations (Davis et al., 2003). In order to improve communication and develop an alliance among healthcare providers, patient, and families, Pattison (2004) suggests a policy change requiring that a senior or primary nurse be present when such discussions are initiated in the hospital.

Clarifying the Problem

There are several components to the phase of clarifying the problem. They include facilitating the patient's expression of emotions, identification of what the patient and family believe are problems, and identifying and responding to the patient's and family's concerns about care. Nurses at all levels should be expert in assisting patients to clarify what they believe are their significant healthcare-related concerns.

When the healthcare provider delivering the bad news has not informed the other members of the healthcare team about the discussion, it is often difficult for a nurse to identify if a patient has received bad news or when the patient is prepared to discuss such news. May (1995) suggests that if the nurse was present at the interview when the bad news was delivered, the patient will feel free to initiate a conversation when the patient is ready. If the nurse was not present during the interview, but suspects such an interview has occurred, the nurse might say to the patient, "I noticed the physician [or advanced practice nurse] was speaking with you. What did she have to say?" Larson and Tobin (2000) suggest asking a more general question such as, "How is this hospitalization going for you and your family?" or "What has been the most difficult thing about this illness for you?" (p. 1574). May (1995) emphasizes that the nurse should not initiate such a discussion unless the nurse is able to sit down and actively listen to the patient. Initiating a discussion of patient concerns or problems requires that the nurse has strong facilitative communication skills and be able to put aside other competing demands for her or his time.

May (1995) warns that when a nurse asks a patient how the patient feels, the patient usually responds by describing her or his physical condition. Thus, if a nurse wants information about the person's psychological concerns, the question will need to be phrased somewhat differently. Byock (1997) began using the phrase, "How are you feeling within yourself?" after he had noticed that hospice workers in England successfully cut though defenses and learned how the patient was feeling when they were asked that question. He suggests it as a way of getting immediately to the heart of the patient's concerns. Emanuel (1998) recommends several questions including the following: "During the last few weeks how often have you felt downhearted or blue?" "What do you believe is bothering you?" "Who are you able to confide in?"

Wilkinson (1991) examined factors that influenced how nurses communicated with cancer patients. She concluded that, in general, nurses had difficulty employing facilitative communication with patients with cancer. She noted that nurses frequently used blocking techniques when dealing with patients who had had a recurrence of their cancer. Because these blocking techniques prevented the nurses from identifying patient concerns, the nurses obtained only a superficial nursing assessment and planned nursing care based on assumptions rather then on actual patient concerns.

Wilkinson (1991) identified three groups of nurses who used different methods to block patient communication. These were ignorers, informers, and mixed responders. *Ignorers* ignored patient cues to talk about specific problems or issues throughout the interview. These nurses changed the subject, engaged in conversation with the patient's relative, or began social chitchat to avoid emotionally laden conversations. *Informers* were nurses who gave elaborate explanations of procedures, offered inappropriate advice, or stated their opinions without being asked. These nurses indicated that providing such detailed, unasked for information allowed them to maintain control of the situation

and avoid difficult or emotionally laden conversations (Wilkinson, 1991). *Mixed responders* were the largest group of nurses in Wilkinson's study. They utilized both facilitative and blocking responses, attempted to understand patient problems, and were more aware of their blocking behaviors when questioned about them.

Although they had been taught facilitative communication, most of the practicing nurses in Wilkinson's 1991 study were unaware that they were blocking their patients' attempts to communicate important needs and concerns until they listened to an audio tape and discussed their responses. Nursing students need experiences in communicating with dying patients, with opportunities to have their interactions evaluated by a nursing faculty member in order to develop proficiency in communication with seriously ill patients. An audiotape allows the faculty member a complete, accurate record of the verbal component of the communication between the student and patient. The patient's consent for taping must be obtained and in some circumstances the Institution Review Board (IRB) of the facility may also need to provide approval. The faculty member then may use the tape as a tool to discuss student responses as well as possible facilitative alternatives. Heaven and Maquire (1996) noted that demonstration with audiotaping and feedback improved the facilitative communication skills of registered nurses. However, since the improvement was not to a statistically significant extent, further study of this approach is warranted.

Moreover, taping is often not possible. On occasion, the faculty member may be present during the student's interview with the patient. This has the advantage of allowing the faculty member to observe the nonverbal behavior of the student and patient as well as the verbal. In many circumstances it permits the faculty member to provide immediate feedback to the student. If direct observation is not possible, then student journals or verbatim process recordings can be used to allow faculty to help students develop an ability to facilitate rather then block communication with seriously ill patients.

Slightly less than a quarter of the nurses in Wilkinson's 1991 study used primarily facilitative communication techniques when interviewing cancer patients. Nurses who used these techniques were able to do so no matter how ill the patient was or how emotionally laden the material to be divulged. By employing such standard facilitative communication techniques as active listening, use of open-ended questions, reflection or clarification of patient concerns, and empathy, they were able to obtain a more in-depth understanding of their patients' problems and concerns. In "An Interview with Dr. Stuart Farber," (1999) Farber states that patients and families most welcomed and remembered interactions with nursing staff that were personalized to the needs of the individual patient and family.

Yabroff and Mandelblatt (2004) emphasize that it is not only healthcare providers who may establish barriers to good communication and optimal patient care. Patients and families may also establish such barriers by their inability to confront death and their utilization of defense mechanisms like disbelief, anger, and denial. Radziewicz and Baile (2001) describe ways that the nurses might recognize and respond therapeutically to each of these behaviors. They define disbelief as "the patient or family's attempt to make sense of what they have heard" (p. 952). They recommend the nurse respond to the patient's disbelief by saying something like, "Accepting such a serious illness must be hard because you have taken such good care of yourself" (p. 952). They believe that anger can be one of the most difficult emotions for an inexperienced nurse with an undergraduate degree to deal with especially since it may be targeted at healthcare providers. Radziewicz and Baile recommend that the nurse realize the anger is often masking another strong emotion such as fear or disappointment. So, the nurse might respond to the angry patient or family member by saying, "I can see how frightening this is for you. Do you want to tell me more about it?" (p. 952).

Radziewicz and Baile (2001) define denial as the patient's refusal to believe bad news, saying that the news is a mistake and not real. Block (2001) notes that denial is a natural response that may be helping the patient to deal with the illness and should be respected. Radziewicz and Baile believe the nurse should not argue with the patient or family who is expressing the denial, should acknowledge the difficulty in accepting the truth, suggest a possible reason for the difficulty, but avoid continuing any blaming or feeling of mistake (Radziewice and Baile, p. 953). For example, a family member might say, "The doctors don't know what they're talking about. My father is going to be fine! He's going to walk again. I don't want anyone to tell me otherwise." The nurse might respond, "It must be difficult believing something so unimaginable could be happening when everything was fine a few days ago." Block agrees with this approach unless the patient is one of the 10% of patients who is in severe denial and the denial is likely to cause problems. In such a circumstance, Block recommends challenging the patient's denial to achieve a greater good. The nurse might say, "I know that making a decision about this is extremely painful, yet if we don't make plans now, we may lose that chance" (Block, 2001, p. 953).

Ambuel, (2003), Farrell, Ryan, and Langrick (2001), and Rosenbaum and Kreiter (2002) have demonstrated that healthcare providers can learn to respond to such patient and family behaviors by role-playing case studies. Some authors suggest scripted case studies, others establish a general style of patient/family behavior and allow the healthcare participants to practice a variety of responses. In either instance, after role-playing,

healthcare providers indicate more confidence in their abilities and greater willingness to communicate with patients who have received bad news. Nursing faculty members can incorporate case studies in undergraduate or graduate nursing education programs that require nursing students to role-play responses to patient and family defense mechanisms of disbelief, anger, or denial.

It is also important to realize that just because the topic is dying and the problems are serious, the talk does not always need to be solemn. Langley-Evans and Payne (1997) noted that lighthearted talk about illness, symptoms, bereavement, and personal mortality was quite valuable to outpatients in a palliative day-care center. What was important was the nursing staff created an atmosphere that facilitated rather then blocked patients' disclosure of their concerns. Table 9.3 lists essential nursing communication behaviors for both the undergraduate and graduate nurse.

Nursing administrators can do a great deal to encourage nurses to communicate with dying patients. Studies by Booth, Maguire, Butterworth, and Hillier (1996) and Wilkinson (1991) found the major predictor of nursing staff's use of facilitative communication with patients with cancer or in hospice was the supportiveness of the nurses' supervisor. In the study by Wilkinson, the ward sisters (unit managers) who took assignments, cared for patients, and demonstrated facilitative communication with patients to their staff had staff who were more likely to communicate therapeutically with their patients. These same ward sisters also encouraged their nurses to work autonomously and make decisions about nursing care. They had negotiated with the physicians who admitted patients to their units to obtain permission for the nurses to talk truthfully with any patient who requested information about her or his prognosis or treatment.

Advanced practice nurses need to have excellent facilitative communication skills. They must be able to communicate with patients individually but they must also be able to demonstrate to staff members ways to communicate with difficult patients and families. The advance practice nurse's efforts to create an environment where communication between patient and nurse is valued is essential to developing the communication skills of the nurse with an undergraduate degree. Although theory is important, practice with evaluation or supervision by a skilled practitioner is what allows an advanced practice nurse to develop such a level of mastery of facilitative communication skills.

Structuring and Formulating the Care Agreement

There are several components to this phase of the therapeutic relationship. In any therapeutic relationship, the nurse and patient should be continuing to develop trust

9.3 | Essential Behaviors

BASIC	ADVANCED
Interpreting "bad" news	Conveying "bad" news
Listening to clients' and families' concerns about EOL care	Initiating the discussion of EOL treatment options
Reviewing EOL treatment options	Promoting a supportive unit environment
Assisting patients, families, and HCPs to make EOL decisions	Determining with other HCPs that patient is dying
Advocating for patient's choices at EOL	Initiating discussion of EOL treatment withdrawal
Implementing EOL treatment withdrawal	Establishing palliative care contract
Preparing patient and family for physical signs of impending death	Dealing with families in crisis after a sudden unexpected death
Smoothing the passage	Presenting organ donation options
Being with patient and family during the dying process	
Consoling the bereaved family	

during this phase, coming to an agreement about the frequency of meetings, and developing goals for care and relationship. At this point in a dying patient's care, advanced practice nurse might initiate a discussion of the patient's treatment goals. Murphy and Price (1995) emphasize that the nurse should avoid using any phrase that resembles "There is nothing more that we can do." Ngo-Metzer et al. (2007) place "There is nothing more we can do" foremost in the commonly misconstrued phrases used in end-of-life discussions with patients. Although the phrase may be intended by the healthcare provider to convey that the patient's disease will progress and the patient will eventually die, it often implies to the patient and family that the healthcare team will abandon the patient.

Instead of focusing on what will not be done, the patient, family, and members of the healthcare team should begin to identify goals for patient care. Patients and families recall feeling supported by healthcare providers when they were told something like, "We promise we will work with you to manage your symptoms and we will stay with you as your disease progresses. We can set goals for this portion of your life together."

Farber ("Interview," 1999) identified a number of possible goals that a dying patient might choose. These included living to the last possible second, living until the burden becomes too great, living at home with family, avoiding medical interventions, living as comfortably as possibly until death, and

avoiding medical treatments unless they have meaningful outcomes. Once a goal has been identified, the healthcare team, patient, and family can begin to identify interventions that achieve that goal.

Unfortunately, there has been limited improvement since Cotton (1993) noted that many physicians avoid initiating discussions about end-of-life treatment with their patients for fear the patients will become depressed or distrustful of the physicians'' willingness to care for them. Often physicians of dying patients will delay the conversation until the patient is unresponsive and the family must be consulted (Shmerling, Bedell, Lilienfeld, & Delbanco, 1988; Sullivan et al., 2007). In fact, patients, especially elders, want to identify goals and interventions for end-of-life care and are relieved when the subject is broached. Most Americans do not have an advance directive, yet as long as they are competent, it is their right to have the deciding voice in the type of healthcare they receive. When the members of the healthcare team avoid discussing the goals of end-of-life care until the patient is unresponsive, the patient is deprived of the right to determine appropriate end-of-life care.

The role of the nurse is usually to interpret medical information into terms the patient can understand and repeatedly explain the end-of-life treatment options to the patient. Patients and families often indicate that listening to the healthcare provider's explanation of a patient's prognosis and possibilities for treatment is like trying to understand a foreign language. In addition, most patients and their families experience stress when they receive bad news. Thus they are unable to hear or retain much of what has been said to them. Being able to repeatedly replay the taped information is one of the reasons a tape recording of the initial interview may be beneficial for some patients and families (Buckman et al., 1997). However, most of the time, it is the responsibility of the nurse to translate medical jargon into "lay terms" the patient can comprehend and to reinforce the information regularly. The nurse might try a variety of teaching strategies, such as diagrams or written explanations, to help the patient and family understand the information. Treece (2007) recommends acknowledging that the information is complex to prevent the patient and family from feeling inadequate and asking them to explain what they understand. It is essential that nurses determine not only what treatment the patient believes she wants but also what she believes will happen if she has the treatment that she wants as shown in the following portion of the case study.

Case Study follow-up: By the end of the third week, Gloria Richards was more adamant that she wanted the ventilator and endotracheal tube removed. Gloria's niece was scheduled to arrive for a discussion with the interdisciplinary team after she finished work one Tuesday. That morning a student nurse and new graduate were caring for her. While giving Gloria her morning bath, the nurse said to her: "Gloria, we'll be meeting this afternoon to talk about your plan of care; would you tell me again what you would like to have done."

"I want this tube out now," she mouthed.

"Would you please tell me what you believe will happen if we take out the tube?" the nurse asked. "It will be harder for me to breathe and I probably will die but I have had it," replied Gloria.

Shortly after, Gloria's primary care physician arrived. He asked what she wished to have done and informed her that she would most likely die if the healthcare team followed her wishes. Gloria reaffirmed that she wanted to be extubated.

WORKING PHASE

During the working phase of the therapeutic relationship, the nurse explores and understands the patient's feelings and expectations, elaborates on the goals of treatment developed in the previous phase, and facilitates or takes actions that the patient desires. In this case, feelings and expectations explored relate to the dying process and goals include defining what the patient believes constitutes dying well.

Exploring and Understanding Patient Feelings and Expectations About Death and Dying

Nurses should be able to assist a patient to define what she or he believes constitutes dying well or represents a good and timely death. Quill (2000) recognizes that healthcare providers often do not agree about appropriate indications to begin a discussion with patients and families about end-of-life care. Although he believes the discussion should begin sooner, he states it is urgent to have such a discussion with patients who are facing imminent death, are talking about wanting to die, are inquiring about hospice, have been hospitalized for severe progressive illness, or are suffering out of proportion to the prognosis. Quill suggests beginning the conversation with a question such as "What would be undone if you were to die sooner rather than later?" (p. 2504). Quill believes this question subtlety conveys the message that time may be short and plans ought to be made now. Griffie, Nelson-Martin, and Muchka (2004) suggest a different question that conveys a similar message "Now that we've discussed the uncertainty of your situation, what's most important to you?" (p. 51).

Nurses should be involved in helping to identify with the patient which issues would be most important to address so the patient might die well. Some of the issues that may be important to patients at the end of life include participating in those end-of-life rituals that provide meaning to the patient and family, completing unfinished business, resolving relationship concerns with family and friends, and carrying out a life review. Once the issues are identified, members of the healthcare team may assist in addressing them.

The nurse will need to inquire of the patient and family about any end-of-life customs or rituals that provide meaning to them. Because a range of responses occurs within cultural and religious groups (Kagawa-Singer & Blackhall, 2001; Mazanec & Tyler, 2004), it is imperative that the nurse not assume specific rituals will be of significance to a patient and family simply because they are members of a particular ethnic or religious group. The nurse might want to inquire: "What is your faith or belief? "Is there a religious or ethnic community that is a source of support for you? Would you like me to notify the community or arrange for something for you?" Once these customs or rituals have been identified, Mazanec and Tyler (2004) state they should be integrated into the plan of care for the dying patient.

If it is necessary to use an interpreter to have a discussion with a patient about end-of-life care, the use of a professional interpreter is supported by grade A evidence. A meeting with the interpreter prior to the discussion is recommended to plan the approach for the discussion, to identify cues for stopping points, and to decide how much should be disclosed before stopping. During the discussion, the healthcare provider needs to continue to respond to the nonverbal cues that the patient and family display and convey empathy. Following the discussion, it is recommended that the healthcare team meet the interpreter to clarify any misunderstandings (Barclay et al., 2007).

Patients may have a wide variety of unfinished business. Often these issues are related to the patient's age and developmental level. For example, a teenager might want to graduate from high school or an older adult might want to witness the arrival of a first grandchild. To identify what business, if any, the patient would like to complete, the nurse might ask, "If you were to die soon, what would be left undone?" or "Is there some event that would add a great deal of meaning to your life? What do we have to do so that event can take place?" Once the issue has been identified, rules might need to be bent (e.g., a child be allowed to participate in graduation ceremonies without completing required coursework, a grandchild or pet allowed into an intensive care unit), resources expended, or help mobilized to permit the event to happen.

Patients may need both time and assistance to resolve relationship problems with their family and friends. Byock (2004) advocates that patients and their families make every effort to say four things to each other as they prepare to say farewell: "Please forgive me; I forgive you; Thank you; and I love you"(p. 5). He believes that saying these four things "offers essential wisdom for completing a lifelong relationship before a final parting." When dying people "can reach out to express love, gratitude, and forgiveness . . . they consistently find that they, and everyone involved, are transformed for the rest of their lives, whether those lives last for decades or just days" (p. 7).

Emanuel (1998) notes that some patients seem to be able to postpone dying so that they can complete their family business. Often deaths occur after important events such as birthdays or holidays. One woman who was dying from respiratory failure asked to have her life prolonged by whatever means necessary until her estranged daughter, whom she had not seen in 10 years, arrived from across the country. After the daughter's arrival, arrangements were made for counseling sessions for the mother and daughter. Two days later, the mother died with the daughter present, holding her mother's hand.

Life review is another important part of both the aging and the dying process. According to Butler ("Roundtable Discussion," 1996), life review is a normal developmental task of the later years characterized by the return of memories and past conflicts. In some cases, this can contribute to psychological growth, including the resolution of past conflicts, reconciliation with significant others, atonement for past wrongdoing, personality integration, and serenity (p. 42).

Mazanac and Tyler (2004) encourage nurses to participate in patients' life reviews. They believe that when patients are encouraged to tell their life stories, the patients are often able to recognize meaning and purpose in their lives. Being present with the patient while the patient begins a life review means a commitment on the part of the nurse to listen actively and devote time to the patient. This is a skill that all nurses ought to have, although it does not require the presence of a nurse or even a professional for the patient to conduct a life review. Life review can provide the patient with a powerful way to work out family relationships and gain a sense of inner peace.

Talking with Patients Across the Life Span and Their Families About Death

A nurse caring for a dying child must establish a trusting relationship with the child and its parents. Novice nurses should be especially aware of their emotions and though empathizing with the family should avoid burdening them with their own emotions (Buckman et al., 1997). Children want to know varying amounts of information about their illness. However, most children want to have an appreciation of how the illness will affect the way they will be able to live their lives. Like adults, however, children vary in how much information they are able to understand and absorb even when it is presented at an appropriate level. Young children's verbalization about their potential death can vary across a continuum and may be fluid over time (Buckman et al., 1997). At one end of the continuum, children will state that they are very sick or have a bad disease but will not mention death. Often, children younger than 7 or 8 years of age view death as temporary and reversible, happening only to others and perhaps caused by previous thoughts and actions (Freyer, 2004). Other children may mention an uncertainty about living but will not allude to dying. At the far end of the continuum, usually when the child is older than 7 or 8, the child may understand the central aspects of death and may state that she or he could die from this illness. Freyer believes that children today are more insulated from death than in the past and are more likely to learn about death from television and video games than from real-life occurrences. In order to understand children's concerns, the advance practice nurse might utilize play therapy or drawing with various colors to help children express their emotions, fears, and realizations about death.

Adolescents, especially ones who have been chronically ill, usually have an accurate understanding of death and are able to verbalize its personal significance as well as it its effect on others. Freyer (2004) notes that adolescents "who are medically experienced often demonstrate remarkable insight into their illnesses, prospects for survival, and preferences for how they wish to spend their remaining time" (p. 383). Due to this insight, "adolescents older than 14 are usually assumed to have functional competency to make binding medical decisions for themselves, including decisions relating to the discontinuance of life-sustaining therapy and end of life issues" (Freyer, 2004, p. 383). Freyer emphasizes it is essential that a truthful, honest relationship be established with the adolescent from the very beginning. He believes this can be accomplished if healthcare providers establish an agreement with the adolescent to share all relevant information with the adolescent as soon as it is available and the adolescent agrees to ask all questions, no matter how trivial. In order to assure that the adolescent feels free to ask all his or her questions, the nurse will want to assure that the nurse has time to spend speaking with the adolescent alone, without either parent present.

Freyer (2004) notes that because most adolescents really do not believe they can ever die, they may talk about death and plan for their eventual death in ways that seem contradictory. At one moment they may be making plans for termination of chemotherapy and a few moments later they may be talking about attending an event that is years in the future. The nurse may want to help the adolescent arrange to attend important life events (e.g., school prom or graduation) in the near future while helping the adolescent recognize and accept his or her deteriorating condition.

Because there was not sufficient evidence to guide communication with parents of dying children, in 2003, the Institute of Medicine put out an urgent call for descriptive research on the process (Hendricks-Ferguson, 2007). This was designed as a first step prior to developing intervention studies. As more studies are circulated and published, more evidence-based interventions should be available to guide the communication between healthcare providers and the parents of dying children.

It has been shown that parents of seriously ill, possibly dying children may have difficulty making sense of what is being said or experienced (Anderson & Hall, 1995). They may feel unable to make decisions, especially if they believe that both minor and major decisions are needed simultaneously. At times, according to Anderson and Hall (1995), the parents may feel they cannot differentiate between decisions that merely involve personal preference and ones that have grave implications. They may need help from nurses untangling these concrete issues but also in dealing with more philosophical ones such as how to determine the line between what is best or right for their child and what is best or right for them.

Nurses can help these families by reminding them that "forced or hasty decision making may cause them to abrogate responsibility because they have not had an opportunity to understand the issues, their feelings

or their roles" (Anderson & Hall, 1995, p. 16). Experienced nurses can assist the parents to understand the issues, express their feelings, and delineate their roles so that the parents can be actively involved in the decision-making process for their children.

Most importantly, nurses should assure that end-of-life care discussions with parents are sensitive and caring. In a descriptive study by Hendricks-Ferguson (2007), 50% of parents believed that healthcare providers conveyed a recommendation that their child be referred to hospice in an uncaring or insensitive manner. This happened when a healthcare provider said something like: "We can treat your child but it will convey no benefit". In contrast, 17% of parents who felt the recommendation to hospice was conveyed in a caring manner were told, "We have a wonderful hospice team and we will be sure that your child is at peace." Multiple studies of family members of both dying adults and children have indicated that at least as important as the content that is provided is the sensitivity with which the content is conveyed.

Young or middle-aged adults who are dying may feel they have a great deal of unfinished business or many unresolved relationships. The dying patient may need professional assistance in dealing with anger at leaving so much undone. A parent who is dying and leaving young children behind may need assistance from a nurse to find ways to leave mementos or lasting words of wisdom for the children. Some dying parents pick out special Christmas mementos in July for their children. One mother made 12 audio-tapes with words of love and encouragement for her only child, one for each year until he would reach age 21.

Older adults are often perceived by healthcare providers as having lived a full life and being prepared to die. Yet, according to Cavendish (1999), nurses should assess all elders' quality of life prior to the illness and realize that many have the potential for additional healthy, happy years. Farber ("Interview," 1999) states that adults over the age of 70 usually do not believe they have a choice in healthcare treatment. When asked how they had made decisions, they answered, "What do you mean? The doctor told us what to do and we did it." Elders in a study by Schroepfer (2007) on sources of suffering at the end of life indicated that being excluded from discussions and decisions about pain management or withdrawal of treatment resulted in their experiencing unnecessary pain and suffering. Nurses, especially advance practice nurses, need to assist elders in participating in their treatment decisions whenever they appear to desire a decision-making role. Finally, life review is particularly important for the dying elder ("Roundtable Discussion," 1996), so time and a compassionate listener should be allotted to this important activity. A nurse might be this compassionate listener or the nurse might delegate another individual for this task.

Facilitating and Taking Action

There are several components of this phase. The first part is determining that the patient will die soon. The nurse may be involved with other healthcare providers in deciding when the patient is entering the active dying phase, while the advanced practice nurse, in some circumstances, may participate in the decision that further treatment is futile when the patient is clearly dying. According to Cassem (Stein, 1999), nurses are the people who guide patients along the path to a peaceful death by recognizing when the patient is suffering needlessly because of inappropriate aggressive treatment. The physician, in some settings, may be the last to realize the patient is dying. Therefore, it becomes incumbent on nurses to relay their impressions to the physician and possibly to the family. The SUPPORT (1995) study indicates that there have been e problems in the way such information is communicated in hospital settings.

Griffie et al. (2004) note that it may be necessary for nurses to act as go-betweens between patients and physicians when there is disagreement about whether a patient is dying and what type of end-of-life care should be provided. They argue that initiating a discussion of end-of-life care should be part of standard nursing practice. Crucial elements for nurses to establish effective communication with physicians during disagreement about end-of-life care include:

- assessing the patient by learning the details of the situation and identifying any questions that the nurse or patient has prior to contacting the physician,
- focusing on the patient's and family's desires and concerns while indentifying their readiness for additional information
- identifying medications or interventions that the nurse and/or patient believes might be effective, recommending them to the physician, and providing a rationale for their use,
- respectfully questioning interventions chosen by the physician with which the nurse, patient, or family does not agree.

An example of a student nurse communicating with a physician about her patient's wishes is shown in the continuation of the case study.

Case Study follow-up: By midmorning, when multidisciplinary rounds were in progress, Gloria Richards' nurse's other patient needed to be prepared for emergency surgery and there were several other events occurring in the ICU. The student nurse represented the nursing team at multidisciplinary rounds. The intensivist was hurrying due to the multiple events in the unit and did not have time to have a discussion with the patient. He announced he was concerned that no one was present who had assessed and could voice Gloria's wishes about end-of-life care so he wanted to postpone the family meeting planned for the afternoon. He was deeply concerned that Gloria might not understand the repercussions of her decision. The student responded, "Both Gloria's primary nurse and primary physician spoke with her this morning about her desires. She told each of them separately that she wanted the endotracheal tube and ventilator removed and that she understood that she would probably die when they were discontinued. Repeatedly this morning she has said she has had enough and asked when the meeting and removal would occur." The intensivist agreed to hold the meeting later in the afternoon.

Determining and agreeing that the patient is dying is extremely important, because most deaths in the United States occur in hospitals and all patients in hospitals must receive cardiopulmonary resuscitation (CPR) unless the physician or advance practice nurse has written a Do Not Resuscitate (DNR) order. Once there is a determination that the patient is dying, the physician or advanced practice nurse should discuss a DNR order with the patient, family, and other healthcare providers.

There are two common mistakes that inexperienced practitioners make when discussing a DNR order. The first is to ask "Do you want everything done?" Most laypersons do not assume "everything" means compressing the chest of a person who has already died. They assume it means comfort, care, and support. So, they often answer yes when they really would not want CPR. The second mistake is to use the words "There is nothing more we can do." Although the patient is dying and medical interventions will not prevent the death, there is much that healthcare providers can do to help the patient die well. The role of the advanced practice nurse is to initiate this discussion using Latimer's (1998) criteria for ethical communication described earlier and

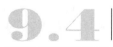 | Criteria for Ethical Communication of Information

- The communication should be timely and desired by the patient.
- The information must be accurate.
- The words should be understandable to the patient and family.
- The information must be conveyed in a "gentle, respectful, and compassionate manner."

Source: Ethical Care at the End of Life, by Latimer (1998).

listed in Table 9.4. However, Tulsky et al. (1996) stress that new practitioners, such as residents and advanced practice nursing students, should be evaluated by skilled professionals before being allowed to attempt such a discussion on their own.

The nurse is usually the staff member to whom the patient and family turn to discuss exactly what a DNR order is and what the ramifications are likely to be for the patient (Peel, 2003). If that nurse was not present for the discussion, he or she might use the question, "I noticed the physician [advanced practice nurse] was speaking with you. What did she say?" The nurse might follow that with, "Many people have questions about what this means for them. What questions do you have?" Most people want reassurance that they are not forgoing an intervention that is likely to offer them benefit. Because only about 12% of all patients survive from CPR to hospital discharge, this reassurance is easy to provide.

As noted previously, the nurse is often the guide on the path to a peaceful death (Stein, 1999). This role is important because the decision to forgo CPR is merely the first of many decisions the patient and family may need to make about end-of-life care. After deciding to forgo CPR, the patient and family might choose to forgo any further curative therapy or might opt to have only comfort measures provided for the patient. Palliative care decisions may need to be made that involve the amount of pain medication the patient desires and whether the patient wishes to receive medical interventions for hydration and nutrition or even to continue eating and drinking. Nurses who are caring for a dying patient should be able to describe the benefits and burdens of each of these therapies to the patient. They should also be able to facilitate patient and family decision-making about these choices through effective communication.

The nurse may be responsible for advocating for the patient's wishes for end-of-life care and communicating them to the family and other healthcare providers. This is easier if the patient has verbally expressed a preference to the nurse and is willing to state that preference to the physician and family. It may be more difficult when the nurse, physician, and family are trying to interpret an advance directive that does not fit the patient's situation precisely, when the person who has the durable power of attorney for healthcare purposes is not clear about the patient's wishes, or when there is no advance directive. Harlow, in "Family letter writing" (1999), recommends that the family or proxy consider the following:

1) What type of person was the patient?
2) Did the patient ever comment on another person's situation when they were incapacitated or on life support?
3) Did the patient relate those experiences to his or her own personal views for herself or himself?
4) What vignettes can you recall from the patient's life that illustrates her or his values and beliefs?

In "Family letter writing" (1999), Harlow then asks the family to write a letter incorporating the answers to these questions. He believes that the process is almost a spiritual one for the families that often brings them closer together. It helps them to review and clarify the person's life and understand what was meaningful to the person. Harlow notes that family letter writing may be "experienced by the family as a last act of commitment and caring toward their loved one." The nurse may be the person who encourages the family to begin such an activity.

Either in conjunction with family letter writing or alone, family conferences are often convened to help the patient, family, and healthcare team reach a decision about end-of-life care. According to Griffie et al. (2004), it is essential to identify the purpose of the conference beforehand. It is also necessary to determine where the meeting should be held. If the patient is able to participate, it may need to be in the patient's room. Some healthcare providers argue that the meeting should always be in the patient's room since it makes everyone consider the patient in the decision. Others believe that if the patient cannot participate then the meeting should be held in a comfortable, private setting away from the patient. If the patient is incapacitated, whoever is the patient's legal decision maker should be present as well as the people that the patient considers to be family.

After the purpose of the meeting has been identified and participants have been introduced, Randall (2008) suggests healthcare providers focus on specific behaviors that can enhance family satisfaction during a conference. These behaviors include the following:

- Assuring the family the patient will not be abandoned by the healthcare team
- Assuring the family the patient will not suffer and
- Providing support for the family's decision whatever the family decides.

Furthermore, Randall recommends that healthcare providers use the mnemonic VALUE to guide their communications with families during the conference. The behaviors described in the VALUE mnemonic have been shown to improve communication between healthcare providers and the families of intensive care patients. The mnemonic stands for the following:

V... Value family statements.
A....Acknowledge family emotions.
L... Listen to the family.
U....Understand the patient as a person.
E....Elicit family questions.

Once a decision is made to limit further aggressive, curative treatment, the nurse may be involved in establishing a palliative care understanding with the patient and family. This is an understanding of what the healthcare team will do for and with the patient and family. Byock (1997) offers the following version of a commitment between the healthcare team and a dying patient:

We will keep you warm and we will keep you dry. We will keep you clean. We will help you with elimination, and your bowels and your bladder function. We will always offer you food and fluid. We will be with you. We will bear witness to your pain and your sorrows, your disappointments and your triumphs; we will listen to the stories of your life and remember the story of your passing (p. 247).

Although the advance care nurse or physician may be the person who establishes this palliative care understanding, it is the nurse with an undergraduate degree who is responsible for assuring that it is carried out. It is imperative that the nurse demonstrates by words and deeds that the healthcare providers will not abandon the patient after end-of-life choices are made; that instead, nurses and other healthcare workers will provide the care the patient needs or will teach and assist family members or friends to provide the care and support the patient requires while dying.

TERMINATION PHASE

During this phase in the therapeutic relationship, the nurse, family, and patient prepare for the end of the relationship, accept the feelings of loss, and review or evaluate what has occurred. As a patient is dying, this phase may entail withdrawing medical interventions, preparing the patient and family for the physical signs of impending death, smoothing the passage, consoling the bereaved family, exploring personal reactions, and evaluating nursing responses.

Withdrawing Medical Interventions

During the termination phase, medical interventions, such as ventilators, IV fluids and nutrition, or dialysis may be withdrawn. The nurse reassures the family that withdrawing such aggressive medical interventions from the dying patient is acceptable to most of the major religious and ethical traditions. The nurse demonstrates that despite the withdrawal of curative measures, the healthcare team will remain present and will provide aggressive comfort measures and respect the patient's individuality.

Preparing the Patient and Family for Physical Signs of Impending Death

The nurse will need to be able to explain the final stages of the dying process to the patient and family. A family that does not understand the dying process may become anxious and feel unable to cope with the patient's care. The nurse may initiate the discussion by stating, "There are some common signs and symptoms that identify when a person's life is coming to an end. Not all of the signs occur in every person nor do they happen in the same sequence in each person. But it might be helpful if we talk about what may be occurring soon and what you may need or want to do."

Smoothing the Passage

As death approaches, patients may display a variety of typical behaviors. Nurses educated at the undergraduate and graduate levels should be able to explain these behaviors to family members and assist families and dying patients to communicate with each other during the patient's last days and hours. According to Callanan (1994), when a patient is approaching death, she or he may begin to speak in symbolic language. The patient might say, "Oh, here are my mother and brother-in-law, they've come to get me. We have to catch the train." Or, "It's a beautiful place that I'm going to now." Callanan cautions that the family may fear the patient is "losing his mind" or believe she or he is reliving the past. In actuality, it is believed that the patient is preparing to detach from this life. Callanan suggests that nurses should help the family listen to the patient's statements and respond with gentle open-ended questions such as, "When does the train leave?" The family should be discouraged from trying to reorient the patient ("Your mother died years ago") or contradicting the patient ("You're not going anywhere!").

Close to the moment of death, the patient may appear more withdrawn, almost detached from the surroundings. The nurse should inform the family that although the patient may appear unresponsive, they should still communicate verbally with the patient because the patient can probably still hear what people in the room are saying. The family may want to say Good-bye or one of the four things that Byock (2004) believes matters most-"Please forgive me; I forgive you; Thank you; and I love you"-if they have not done so already. This might be a time for the family to recount some favorite memories that illustrate what the dying person meant to them. A member of the family might say, "We will miss you, but we will always love you and we understand that it is time for you to go." Or, a family member or close friend might simply be present with the dying person, sitting nearby, holding the person's hand or lying next to the person and embracing him or her.

It is the role of the nurse to help the patient and families find an appropriate way to express their feelings and to smooth the patient's passage from this life. Individuals take their own time dying, and each death occurs at its own pace. The nurse may need to help the patient's family understand how idiosyncratically and sometimes how slowly the final moments may pass.

Consoling the Bereaved Family

Nurses need to be able to console families through the bereavement process. If the family has not been present during the death, the nurse will want to prepare the body and attempt to create a peaceful environment for the family to view the deceased. Because the nurse is often the professional present at the death or the one who views the body with the family, the nurse will need to demonstrate an acceptance of death and display respect for the deceased. If the family was not present for the death, the members may want a description of the patient's last moments. The nurse should respond both tactfully and truthfully. If it is true, saying to the family, "She was not alone" or "He seemed to be at peace" may be a great source of comfort to the family.

Although students in and recent graduates often are worried about what they ought to say to the family at this time, bereaved families usually are more in need of someone to listen to them. Thus, one of the major roles of the nurse at this time is active, compassionate listening. Short statements like "I'm sorry" and "I'll keep you in my thoughts or prayers" may be helpful but the nurse usually does not need to say much. Trivializing statements such as "She is better off now" or "I know just how you feel" are inappropriate. Depending on the nurse's relationship with the family, a hug might be helpful to both the family and the nurse. The nurse's expression of emotion through tears is not unprofessional when it is an expression of the attachment between the nurse and the patient.

When the death is sudden and unexpected, it is often more difficult for both the healthcare providers and the family to understand. It is usually the physician or the advance practice nurse who conveys the fact of the death to the family. Buckman et al. (1997) recommend a simple unequivocal statement that the patient (her or his name should be used) has died and the cause stated. Then the healthcare provider should remain silent and allow an opportunity for the family to respond and ask further questions. A truthful statement that the advance practice nurse is sorry helps some families. Though some people prefer a human touch at this point, others may withdraw in grief. When the initial response has subsided, Buckman recommends focusing on the needs of the family, determining if they need to phone anyone or if they would like an opportunity to view the body. If there is a possibility of organ donation, the advance practice nurse would broach the subject at this time.

Review of the Relationship, Exploration of Personal Feelings, and Evaluation of Nursing Responses

Although not a specific step in the therapeutic relationship, it is always wise following the termination of a relationship for the nurse to review the process to explore her or his feelings and evaluate her or his behavior. A nursing student encountering his or her first experience with death may need to explore it with the faculty member or preceptor after the patient and family has been cared for. Ambuel (2003) suggests that a faculty member or preceptor who is debriefing a student should include questions such as: What went well?; What was difficult?; What did you learn from this experience that will influence your work with patients and families in the future? In most circumstances, it is helpful for the student to be involved in preparing the body and talking with the family. For the first experience with death, it is helpful if a nursing faculty member or an experienced nurse prepares the body with the student. While preparing the body, most undergraduate nursing students find it helpful if the faculty member provides simple factual statements of how the body changes after death. Many students will remark how different the deceased seems once the suffering is over and life has departed.

Nursing students often state that listening to the family helps them to find some meaning in the dying experience. If the death has been anticipated, the family will frequently discuss how the patient felt in the last few days and weeks and will often convey a sense of relief that the patient is no longer struggling. The family may review the person's life and help the student to realize that it had reached its natural end.

When the death is sudden and unexpected, nursing students often are distraught. This is especially true if the patient was close to their own or their parents' ages. A review of what happened to the patient with an emphasis on how the healthcare team responded may at least help the student realize there was no way in which the healthcare team could have prevented the death. Later, many nursing students and nurses question why the person had to die at this time in his or her life. Active listening by the nursing faculty member or perhaps the hospital chaplain is most likely to assist the student to come to some understanding of the death.

Novice nurses may idealize death; they may want each experience to be mystical and transcendent. However, death, like birth, is both messy and difficult as well as beautiful and transcendent. Learning to live and care within the realm of what is possible for people at the end of their lives is often difficult for the nursing student and the new graduate. Nursing faculty should help the student recognize the realities that shaped the way in which this particular patient died and identify factors that the student would want to modify when caring for future patients.

CONCLUSION

When nurses communicate with their dying patients and the families, they have a clearer understanding of their patients' needs and goals at the end of life. Once these goals are established, the nurse may assist the patient in dying well. That death might include limited technology, symptom relief, life review with resolution of past uncompleted business, and the presence of loving family and friends. Or it might involve fighting for the last breath, remaining alive until the last possible second, using the latest medical technology. However, without thoughtful communication with the patient and family, the nurse cannot be sure which course to take to help the patient die well.

Case Study conclusion: By early afternoon, Gloria announced she was tired of waiting and disconnected the ventilator from her endotracheal tube. Her nurse explained that her niece would be arriving soon for a short discussion so that the niece would understand Gloria's wishes and so she could say goodbye. Gloria wanted to know the precise time. An hour later, Gloria attempted to disconnect the ventilator again and said, "It's time." The nurse explained it was only 3 o'clock and her niece wasn't coming until after 4 and turned Gloria so she could see the clock in the room. The niece arrived promptly at 4 and a conference of persons that included the patient, her niece, the nurse, the intensivist, and a social worker took place at the patient's bed side. The nurse asked the patient against if she wanted the tube and ventilator removed. Her niece asked if she was certain, and the patient nodded emphatically yes. An hour later a morphine drip had been started, Gloria was extubated, and her niece was sitting at her bedside with the lights in the room dimmed holding her hand. Within an hour Gloria was unresponsive and she died peacefully later that evening.

EVIDENCE-BASED PRACTICE

Review: Preferences of older American veterans for communication about end-of-life

Rodriquez, K., & Young, A. (2005). Perspectives of elderly veterans regarding communication with medical providers about end-of-life care. *Journal of Palliative Medicine, 8,* 534–544.

Q: What are the perspectives of older veterans concerning communication with healthcare providers about end-of-life care?

Data sources. Audiotapes of responses to open-ended questions from a semistructured interview. The audiotapes were transcribed, coded, and analyzed using qualitative content analysis.

Study selection and assessment. Male and female veterans 60 years of age or older who were ambulatory and living in the community while receiving outpatient care from an urban Veterans Administration (VA) Medical Center were included. Participants were excluded if they could not read or speak English, were acutely ill, or were cognitively impaired.

Outcomes: Patient preferences concerning end-of-life communication

Main results. Seven essential elements of advice for healthcare providers emerged: engage in strategies to ensure patient understanding, communicate honestly and truthfully, develop a compassionate bedside manner, treat others as you would want to be treated, provide empathic care, take the time needed to communicate, and determine patient information and decision- making preferences.

Conclusion. Effective end-of-life discussion with patients requires attention to content, process, and perception of the patient-provider communication.

Commentary. Since Buckman began discussing how healthcare providers ought to convey bad news in 1992, there have been numerous articles suggesting what healthcare providers ought to do. However, according to Barclay et al. (2007) and Ngo-Metzger et al. (2008) there has little consistent, good quality evidence to support these interventions and they are recommended either on the basis of limited quality patient-oriented evidence (B level) or consensus and expert opinion (C level). This was a pilot study to identify how healthcare providers can communicate with patients about end-of-life care to the patients satisfaction. It provided early validation of some of the strategies suggested by Buckman and others. However, the authors did caution that end-of-life communication is not a "one size fits all" phenomenon and the healthcare provider will require skill, patience, and sufficient time to understand the specific patient and communicate with him/her to the patient's satisfaction.

For correspondence. Keri L. Rodriquez PhD, Center for Health Equity Research and Promotion, VA Pittsburgh Healthcare System (151-C), University Drive C, Building 28 Room 1A129, Pittsburg, PA 15240-1000, Keri.Rodrigues@med.va.gov

Sources of funding. None identified

Barclay, J., Blackwell, L., & Tulsky, J. (2007). Communication strategies and cultural issues in the delivery of bad news. Journal of Palliative Care Medicine, 10, 958–77.

Buckman, R. (1992). *How to break bad news: A guide for health professionals.* Baltimore: Johns Hopkins Press.

Ngo-Metzger, Q., August, K., Srinivasan, M., Liao, S., & Meyskens, F. (2008). End-of-life care: Guidelines for patient-centered communication. *American Family Physician, 77,* 167–174.

REFERENCES

Ambuel, B. (2003). Delivering bad news and precepting student/resident learners. *Journal of Palliative Medicine, 6,* 263–264.

Albom, M. (1997). *Tuesdays with morrie.* New York: Doubleday.

Anderson, B., & Hall, B. (1995). Parents perceptions of decision making for children. *Journal of Law, Medicine and Ethics, 23*(6), 15–19.

Barclay, J., Blackwell, L., & Tulsky, J. (2007). Communication strategies and cultural issues in the delivery of bad news. *Journal of Palliative Care Medicine, 10,* 958–77.

Block, S. (2001). Psychological considerations, growth, and transcendence at the end of life: The art of the possible. *Journal of the American Medical Association, 285,* 2898–2904.

Booth, K., Maguire, P. M., Butterworth, R., & Hillier, V. F. (1996). Perceived professional support and the use of blocking behaviors by hospice nurses. *Journal of Advanced Nursing, 24,* 522–527.

Buckman, R. (1992). *How to break bad news: A guide for health professionals.* Baltimore: Johns Hopkins Press.

Buckman, R., Lipkin, M., Sourkes, B., & Tolle, S. (1997, June 15). Strategies and skills for breaking bad news. *Patient Care, 6,* 61–66.

Byock, I. (1997). *Dying well: Peace and possibilities at the end of life.* New York: River-head Books.

Byock, I. (2004). *The four things that matter most: A book about living.* New York: Free Press.

Callanan, M. (1994). Farewell messages. *American Journal of Nursing, 94* (5), 19–20.

Cavendish, R. (1999). Improving care for the elderly. *American Journal of Nursing, 99*(3), 88.

Cotton, P. (1993). Talk to people about dying: They can handle it, say geriatricians and patients. *Journal of the American Medical Association, 269,* 321–323.

Czerwiec, M. (1996). When a loved one is dying: Families talk about nursing care. *American Journal of Nursing, 96*(5), 32–36.

Davis, S., Kristjanson, L. J., & Blight, J. (2003). Communicating with families of patients in an acute hospital with advanced cancer. *Cancer Nursing, 26,* 337–345.

Emanuel, E. J. (1998). The promise of a good death. *Lancet, 351* (9114, Suppl.), S1121–1126.

Fallowfield, L., & Jenkins, V. (2004). Communicating sad, bad, and difficult news in medicine. *Lancet, 363,* 312–319.

Family Letter Writing: An Interview with Nathan Harlow. (1999). *Innovations in end of life care: An international on-line forum for leaders in end of life care.* Retrieved 6/12/2000 from http://www2.edc.org/last-acts/featureinn.asp

Farrell, M., Ryan, S., & Langrick, B. (2001). Breaking bad news within a pediatric setting: An evaluation report of a collaborative education workshop to support health professionals. *Journal of Advanced Nursing, 36,* 763–775.

Freyer, D. (2004). Care of the dying adolescent: Special considerations. *Pediatrics, 113,* 381–388.

Furukawa, M. M. (1996). Meeting the needs of the dying patient's family. *Critical Care Nurse, 16*(1), 51–62.

Griffie, J., Nelson-Marten, P., Muchka, S. (2004). Acknowledging the 'elephant': Communication in palliative care. *American Journal of Nursing, 104,* 48–57.

Gordon, M., Buckman, D., & Buckman, S. (2007). "Bad news" communication in palliative care: A challenge and a key to success. *Annals of Long-Term Care, 15*(4), 32–38.

Heaven, C. M., & Maguire, P. (1996). Training hospice nurses to elicit patient concerns. *Journal of Advanced Nursing, 23,* 280–286.

Hendricks-Ferguson, B., (2007). Parental perspectives of initial end of life care communication. International *Journal of Palliative Nursing, 13,* 522–531.

Interview with Dr. Stuart Farber, Living with a serious illness: A workbook for patients and families. (1 999). *Innovations in end of life care: An international on-line forum for leaders in end of life care.* [on-line] Available: http://www2.edc.org/lastacts/feature inn. asp

Kagawa-Singer, M, & Blackhall, L. J. (2001). Negotiating cross-cultural issues at the end of life: "You got to go where he lives." *Journal of the American Medical Association, 286,* 2993–3000.

Langley-Evans, A., & Payne, S. (1997). Lighthearted death talks in a palliative day care context. *Journal of Advanced Nursing, 26,* 1091–1097.

Larson, D. G., & Tobin, D. R. (2000). End of life conversations: Evolving practice and theory. *Journal of the American Medical Association, 284,* 1573–1577.

Latimer, E. (1998). Ethical care at the end of life. *Canadian Medical Association Journal, 158,* 1741–1745.

London, M., & Lundstedt, J. (2007). Families speak about inpatient end of life care. *Journal of Nursing Care Quality, 22,* 152–158.

May, C. (1995). To call it work somehow demeans it: The social construction of talk in the care of the terminally ill patients. *Journal of Advanced Nursing, 22,* 556–661.

Mazanec, P., & Tyler, M. K. (2004). Cultural considerations in end-of-life care: How ethnicity, age, and spirituality affect decisions when death is imminent. *Home Healthcare Nurse, 22,* 317–324.

Murphy, P. A., & Price, D. M. (1995). ACT: Taking a positive approach to end of life care. *American Journal of Nursing, 95*(3), 42–43.

Ngo-Metzger, Q., August, K., Srinivasan, M., Liao, S., & Meyskens, F. (2008). End of life care: Guidelines for patient-centered communication. *American Family Physician, 77,* 167–174.

Parker, S., Clayton, J., Hancock, K., Walder, S., Butow, P., Carrick, S., et. al. (2007). A systematic review of prognostic/end of life communication in adults in the advanced stages of life-limiting illness: patient/caregiver preferences for content, style, and timing of information. *Journal of Pain and Symptom Management, 34,* 81–93.

Pattison, N. (2004). Integration of critical care and palliative care at the end of life. British Journal of Nursing, 13(3), 132–139.

Peel, N. (2003). The role of the critical care nurse in the delivery of bad news. *British Journal of Nursing, 12,* 966–971.

Ptacek, J. T., Ptacek, J. J., & Ellison, N. M. (2001). "I'm sorry to tell you. . . ." Physicians's reports of breaking bad news. *Journal of Behavioral Medicine, 24,* 205–217.

Quill, T. E. (2000). Initiating end-of-life discussions with seriously ill patients: addressing the elephant in the room. *Journal of the American Medical Association, 284,* 2502–2507.

Randall,J. (2008). Caring for patients with critical illness and their families: The value of the integrated clinical team. *Respiratory Care, 53,* 480–487.

Radziewicz, R., & Baile, W. F. (2001). Communication skills: Breaking bad news in the clinical setting. *Oncology Nursing Forum, 28,* 951–953.

Rosenbaum, M. E., & Kreiter, C. (2002). Teaching delivery of bad news using experiential sessions with standardized patients. *Teaching and Learning in Medicine, 143*(3), 144–149.

Roundtable Discussion: Part 2. (1996). A peaceful death: How to manage pain and provide quality care. *Geriatrics, 51(6)*, 32–42.

Schroepfer, T. (2007). Critical events in the dying process: The potential for physical and psychosocial suffering. *Journal of Palliative Medicine, 10*, 136–147.

Servaty, H. L., Krejci, M. J., & Hayslip, B. (1996). Relationships among death anxiety, communication apprehension with dying and empathy in those seeking occupations as nurses and physicians. *Death Studies, 20*, 149–161.

Shmerling, R. H., Bedell, S. E., Lilienfeld, A., & Delbanco, T. L. (1988). Discussing cardiopulmonary resuscitation. *Journal of General Internal Medicine, 3*, 317–321.

Stein, C. (1999). Ending a life. *Boston Globe Magazine, 13*, 24, 30–34, 39–42.

Stiles, M. K. (1990). The shining stranger: Nurse-family spiritual relationship. *Cancer Nursing, 13*, 2235–2245.

Sullivan, A., Lakoma, M., Matsuyama, R., Rosenblatt, L., Arnold, R., & Block, S., et al. (2007). Diagnosing and discussing imminent death in the hospital: A secondary analysis of physician interviews. *Journal of Palliative Medicine, 10*, 882–893.

SUPPORT Principal Investigators (1995). A controlled trial to improve care for seriously ill, hospitalized patients: The study to understand prognoses and preferences for outcomes and risks of treatments (SUPPORT). *Journal of the American Medical Association, 274*, 1591–1598.

Treece, P. (2007). Communication in the intensive care unit about the end of life. *AACN Advanced Critical Care, 18*, 406–414.

Tulsky, J. A., Chesney, M. A., & Lo, B. (1996). See one, do one, teach one? House staff experience discussing do-not-resuscitate orders. *Archives of Internal Medicine, 156*, 1285–1289.

Wilkinson, S. (1991). Factors that influence how nurses communicate with cancer patients. *Journal of Advanced Nursing, 16*, 677–688.

Yabroff, K. R., & Mandelblatt, J. S. (2004). The quality of medical care at the end of life in the USA: Existing barriers and examples of process and outcome measures. *Palliative Medicine, 18*, 202–216.

10

Family Caregivers

Kay Blum

- Structure, purpose, function, and symbolism are categories of family definitions; but each family is individually defined by the members.
- Family caregivers and carerecipients are a unit when considering care requirements and care planning.
- Careful, systematic family assessment should be the basis and foundation of all care planning for palliative care.
- Caregivers can easily become overwhelmed by the magnitude of the work that their commitment entails leading to depression and self-neglect.

Case Study: DL is a 54-year-old man with chronic heart failure (CHF), emphysema, and prostate cancer. He lives alone in a house his family has owned for generations. His wife died 4 years ago in a motor vehicle crash while riding with DL when he was drinking. He has 4 daughters and a son who do not speak to him regularly or see him except at holiday family gatherings, although they live in the same city. His great niece and her family live 3 houses from his and she checks on him daily, cleans his house, and takes him to medical appointments. He was just discharged from the hospital after an exacerbation of his CHF caused by not taking his medication. He has been showing signs of cognitive dysfunction with mild memory loss. He becomes short of breath with minimal activity but refuses to give up his home or live with his niece.

DL's niece is 32 and is a single parent with children who are 3 months, 6 years, and 16 years old. She works as a school crossing guard mornings and afternoons. The 16-year-old has a learning disability and is frequently in trouble in school for acting out and has anger management problems. He spends a lot of time hanging out with friends who are gang members (although he is not a member of any gang) and uses drugs from time to time. He has started stealing from his mother's purse to buy marijuana.

INTRODUCTION

Family is a cultural, legal, sociological, and individually defined concept. Traditional definitions of family include what we refer to as a nuclear family—father, mother, and one or more children—or the extended family which adds grandparents, aunts, uncles, and cousins. In the past people grew up and lived in the same community for a lifetime in close contact with that extended family. Family members counted on each other for help and there was usually someone or more than one member who was available to help with the care of children or older family members. This was usually a wife, mother, grandparent, or other family member usually female. After World War II more and more women moved into the workforce and a new childcare industry emerged. Social forces such as job mobility, air travel, increased divorce rate and an increase in cohabitation instead of marriage that accelerated during the 1960s and 1970s impacted the definition of family as well as the availability of family members to help each other. At the same time advances in healthcare extended the longevity of humans, and also increased the number of people living with chronic diseases that were untreated or unheard of when early definitions of family were valid. Today blended families, those with parents who are on their second or more marriages with children from previous marriages blended into new families as well as single parent families, same-sex families and childless by choice families are more common. Extended families are either smaller or in other locations and often have limited contact with each other. Legal and illegal immigration has led to communities of immigrants who often live in fear, do not speak English and delay healthcare because of limited resources or fear of deportation.

Homelessness and the increase of people with mental illness living on the street without support or family connections have created another community with family-like qualities and characteristics. These forces along with the aging of the population and the incidence of chronic illness have increased the need for family caregivers and have changed the way we look at family and their involvement in the care of individuals (http://family.jrank.org/ accessed May 20, 2009).

What then is a family? There are legal, social, political, cultural, and theoretical definitions of family. These definitions are more or less helpful depending on the purpose of the definition. The Marriage and Family Encyclopedia is an online reference that brings together a variety of references and writings related to structure, function, and meaning in research and clinical practice related to families (Family Theory—Meaning of Family accessed May 20, 2009). Within the discussions in this reference are classification systems and conceptual frameworks to assist in the understanding of family. Four categories of definitions are presented. First, structural definitions describe families based on membership and relationship between the members. An example of a structural definition is "a single mother and her children" or "first degree relatives including step- and half-siblings which would include a father a mother and all their collective children".

A second category for defining families is functional. If the function of families is to procreate and then nurture children, then the evaluation of family function is based on the number and/or quality of children produced. A childless by choice family would be dysfunctional in this definition. A third meaning of family is based on interactions within the family group. It looks at what members do, what is the power dynamic and how do the members relate to each other? This broad category would allow for work-groups or societies to be defined as family as well as a group of friends who view themselves as a family.

The fourth pattern of family definitions is a symbolic representation and is defined by the individual family usually using stories or symbols to define membership. This might include a house that has housed generations often with many of the members being born there or a piece of land or some other symbol or experience that holds the family unit together.

Most definitions are a combination of these categories. Merely naming the members of a family related by blood or legal arrangements such as adoption or guardianship is the most common but it defines only a portion of groups who define themselves as families based on their purpose and relationship. Friends and domestic partners, with or without legal sanctions, often depend on each other and have the expectations of loyalty, love and help that one usually associates with blood relatives and of nuclear families. Even though they are in decline, the nuclear and to some extent the extended family of history are considered the norm legally, politically and in medicine where patient's families are included in the plan of care.

Myths about the family have persisted in the approach we take to patients and families. The first is that family members have the best interests of the patient in mind. This assumption persists in the face of reports of domestic violence, elder and child abuse, neglect and abandonment. The second is the belief that children, especially female children, have an obligation to care for chronically ill or impaired family members, especially elders. This expectation is shared by family, medical providers and cultural norms irrespective of the burden this places on that person in addition to their other family and work responsibilities.

For the purposes of this discussion, a family is two or more people who have come together for a self-defined common purpose. That purpose may be procreation or it may be simple companionship but the persons involved view themselves as family with the bonds and responsibilities one expects from a family of origin or blood relationship. A family caregiver is a member of this family who has chosen or who has been designated as the caregiver for one or more family members who cannot manage normal activities of daily living without help. The requirement for help may reflect physical or mental limitation.

FAMILY CAREGIVERS

The statistics related to family or informal caregivers as they are often referred to are staggering. The Family Caregiver Alliance reports that there are 52 million caregivers for recipients 20-years old or older who have chronic illness or disability (http://www.caregiver.org/caregiver/jsp/content_node.jsp?nodeid = 439 accessed May 20, 2009). Thirty-four million caregivers care for adults 50-years old or older, 8.9 million of them care for these adults who also have dementia. Fifty-one to seventy-five percent of caregivers are female although an increase of 50% was noted among men caregivers for the 10 years from 1984 to 1994. Women caregivers are more likely to suffer from anxiety and depression or other emotional disturbances related to care giving. The average age of caregivers for persons 65 and older is 63 years. Caregiver age increases with the age of the recipient. Almost half of caregivers are children of the recipients followed by spouses or other relatives when the person is 65 or older. Nonrelative caregiver estimates range from 8% to 24%. Most caregivers are employed full or part time (60%) and 48% are employed full time in addition to their informal caregiving. Twenty percent, or 1 in 5, provide 40 hours or more of care to someone 65 or older. Severe dementia increases the average caregiving time to >46 hours per week. The duration of care can range from less than a year to over 40 years. Forty-two percent of caregivers live within 20 minutes of the recipient but 15% live more than an hour away.

Abaya (1999) has coined the term "The Sandwich Generation®" to describe the caregivers sandwiched between caring for elder parents or grandparents and spouses and/or children of their own. These caregivers are pulled in both directions and often have jobs as well as these dual responsibilities. They are typically middle-aged women who are overwhelmed with responsibility and acting out of duty who, in the process of caring for others, neglect themselves because there are competing demands for their time leading them to put themselves last.

THEORETICAL FRAMEWORKS

How then does one begin to study and intervene to promote creative and supportive relationships where both the patient and the caregiver benefit? A number of frameworks have been proposed. (Ingoldsby, Smith, & Miller 2004; Bahr & Bahr, 2001; Grey, Knafl, & McCorkle 2006; Tsai 2003) Traditional family theories are useful for examining family structure and dynamics. The evolution of philosophical perspectives are reflected in the emergence of new family theories such as feminist family theory, symbolic interactionism, conflict theory, family stress theory and crisis framework to name a few.(Ingoldsby et al., 2004) Bahr and Bahr (2001) have taken family theory a step further in exploring the concept of self-sacrifice and its meaning in the family. They take this stance in opposition to the theories that stress individual choice and the primacy of the individual over the good of the whole. They assert that self-sacrifice in the interest of the family is viewed as a virtue for men/fathers and a defect in women/mothers. They go on to say that love is the motivation for this sacrifice manifested as selfless generosity and contrasts with the ethic of personal gain that characterizes social relationships outside the family.

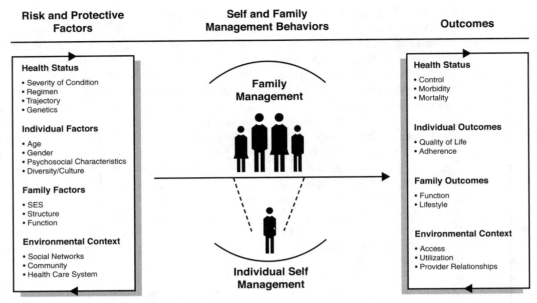

Figure 10.1 Self and Family Management Framework
Adapted from *Nursing Science Quarterly* 2006 by Grey, M., Knafl, K., & McCorkle, R., with permission from Elsevier.

Grey et al. (2006) developed a theoretical model of self and family management of chronic conditions. The model (Figure 10.1) is a Structure/Process/Outcome type model that defines structural elements of health status, individual factors, family factors, and environmental context that characterize the burdens and resources that impact both family processes and individual activities that are directed at management of chronic conditions. These management processes result in outcomes that correspond to the structures in that they include the same categories, namely health status, individual outcomes, family outcomes and environmental context. Their framework is proposed as a means of identifying gaps in the research literature in relation to individual and family factors in successful management of chronic conditions.

Tsai (2003) has developed a middle-range theory of caregiver stress. This theory reflects the philosophy and framework of the Roy Adaptation Model. The model and subsequent theory is an input/process/output type model (Figure 10.2) that makes four assumptions.

1) Caregivers can respond to change.
2) Caregivers' perceptions determine how they respond to environmental stimuli.
3) Caregivers' adaptation is a function of their environmental stimuli and adaptation level.
4) Caregivers' effectors—for example physical function, self-esteem/master, role enjoyment and marital satisfaction— are results of chronic caregiving. (Tsai, p 139).

These models have yet to be tested sufficiently to determine their usefulness in studying caregivers and caregiving behaviors and stresses. Family caregiving, and informal caregivers in general, are complex; and the dynamics of the relationships involved, as well as family history, social evolution, legal challenges, and medical advancement, make decision-making a challenge. How then should we view the commitment of family caregivers? Are these activities and responsibilities a reflection of duty and obligation derived from social and cultural definitions of family? Are the activities and responsibilities acts of love and self-sacrifice manifesting generosity? Are these activities and responsibilities merely the reflection of social, political, economical, and medical realities of the time and environment in which we live? Given the economic conditions we currently live under, is there an ethical or legal obligation of society to care for people in our communities who have chronic illnesses or disabilities? If so, how will we distribute our limited resources to support those family caregivers who are already committed to the care of one or more family members and find ways to help those who do not have family or friends to depend on?

REWARDS AND BURDENS OF CAREGIVING

"Life is Hard." So opens Scott Peck's "The Road Less Traveled" (1978). His acknowledgement of this fact is balanced by his assertion that it is this difficulty that makes life meaningful and contributes to the growth and enlightenment of the individual. Life is indeed hard for many if not all of the persons caring for a loved one with a chronic disease or disability. Whether the caregiver gives out of duty or out of generosity, the work and the time commitment can be grueling. The life one

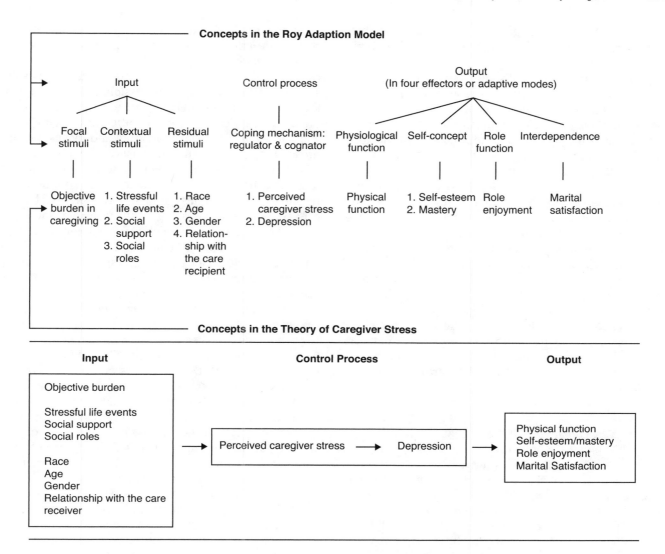

Figure 10.2   A middle-range theory of caregiver stress
Adapted from *Nursing Science Quarterly* 2003, with permission from Elsevier.

leads while incorporating the caregiver role is one of great paradox and irony.

A review of the literature in the area of family or informal caregiving produces volumes of studies, reviews, and opinions on the stresses and burden of the caregiving role. While these documents are valuable and timely in describing the work and proposing intervention, they miss the opportunity to address or describe the rewards and satisfactions that come from the role and from the giving. Certainly the rewards exist because they have been described by caregivers. (Grant, Ramcharan, McGrath, Nolan, & Keady, 1998; Narayan, Lewis, Tornaotre, Hepburn, & Corcoran-Perry, 2001; Schumaker, Beck, & Marren 2006; Neff, Dy, Frick, & Kasper 2006). Caregivers describe feelings of satisfaction of a job well done, a sense of giving back for care and nurturing they received themselves. There is a sense of satisfaction as well because of the gratitude

and acknowledgement of the person who receives the care and/or other family members. For some caregivers there may even be financial gain. The child or sibling who cares for a dying family member may inherit all or more of the family member's estate than those less involved in the care. This may or may not be a motivation for the care, but may also be part of a negotiation prior to or at the beginning of care.

By contrast, a Pubmed search on just the term "Caregiver Burden" returns 878 articles (as of May 21, 2009). Study after study looking at the burdens of caregiving document anxiety and depression. These components of burden are compounded by physical, mental, and compassion fatigue. Particularly in situations where dementia complicates physical disability or chronic illness, isolation, physical dependency, and even violence may characterize the world of the caregivers. (Jackson, Turner-Stokes, Murray, Morven, & Mcpherson, 2009).

Jackson and colleagues go on to point out that caregivers for younger persons who have traumatic brain injury describe greater burden, and worse quality of life, than those caring for family members with dementia. Perhaps some of this distress is related to the younger age of brain-injured persons compared to those with dementia. This has great significance due to the significant number of young people returning from the wars in Afghanistan and Iraq and returning to civilian life and the care of family members.

Given that half of all caregivers work full time at jobs outside the home and that, especially older and demented persons average > 40 hours of care each week, it is no surprise that caregivers are overwhelmed by just the quantity of work required. If there is little or no help with their own household, or a lack of support from their spouse or children, the caregiver can be overcome by despair and hopelessness. Competing responsibilities and obligations can leave the caregiver feeling like they are on a treadmill that never ends. Family dynamics can improve or exacerbate the primary caregiver feelings of despair. If the despair is compounded by financial hardship stresses may tear the family apart.

> **Case Study follow-up:** DL's condition is worsening. His cognitive dysfunction has led to his missing medication. Whether it is a problem of memory or understanding is irrelevant. His medication regimen is complex and he needs supervision to ensure the medication is apportioned correctly and that he remembers to take it. His niece lives close by and does not work full time. This advantage is countered by the attention her children need, especially her teenage son who is getting into trouble with stealing, drugs, and acting out in school. These competing responsibilities will increasingly demand more of her time and attention. She is not getting any help from DL's children who have essentially abandoned him. She is also at risk for financial hardship if she takes on more responsibility for her uncle.

FAMILY ASSESSMENT

The Family Caregiver Alliance (FCA) sponsors the National Center on Caregiving (http://www.caregiver.org accessed May 20, 2009). They sponsor programs for family and informal caregivers as well as providers working toward family-oriented care that makes provider, family, or patient partnerships a reality. Speaking at the National Consensus Development Conference for Caregiver Assessment Carol Levine (Family Caregiver Alliance, 2006a) and Dan Ahern (Family Caregiver Alliance, 2006b) spoke poignantly about their experiences

as caregivers. Their experiences were very different but equally descriptive of the world in which caregivers must navigate. Ahern points out how quickly one's life can change forever and how critical it is to have the support of family and of professionals in the care of loved ones; but ultimately it is an act of love to care for them. Levine's experience was different in many ways and she vividly describes the cruel and insensitive approach of the nurses and therapists at the rehab facility where her brain-injured husband was living. She felt there was no helpful assessment of her commitment, resources, or willingness to be a part of her husband's care although she was doing all she was able. She experienced only judgment, which was rigid and subjective as providers sought a "one-size-fits-all" approach to family caregiving. Her experience is validated in many ways by Thomas (2006) whose young husband was also brain injured changing both their lives forever.

One thing is clear, a "one-size-fits-all" approach to caregivers is at best not helpful and at worst destructive. How then does one begin to take a more helpful path in working out the partnership that will lead to successful caregiving for both the caregivers and the care recipients? That path begins with a caregiver assessment.

Caregiver assessment is a structured, systematic evaluation of the caregiver and the relationship with the carerecipient for the purpose of matching resources with needs and promoting the well-being of both the caregiver and the carerecipient. The FCA website is a treasure of resources for caregivers and providers alike. A section on caregiver assessment provides a comprehensive plan for how and when to perform the assessment and the content (Table 10.1). Exhibit 10.1 lists some resources for identifying appropriate assessment tools.

The advantages of assessment as a basis for accessing services and support are many, but Zarit (Family Caregiver Alliance, 2006c) outlines some specific benefits. The first is the identification of problems in the caregiving context including but not limited to interpersonal, relational, situational, or financial problems. These problems may be potential or actual. The second advantage is the clarification of roles and responsibilities for family members as well as a clear estimate of the

EXHIBIT 10.1: ASSESSMENT TOOL

(http://www.caregiver.org/caregiver/jsp/content_node.jsp?nodeid=1709)
http://www.familyassessmentform.com/
http://humanservices.ucdavis.edu/resource/practice/assessment.asp
Assessment Tools by State
http://www.caregiver.org/caregiver/jsp/content_node.jsp?nodeid=1717
Annotated Bibliography of Assessment References
http://www.caregiver.org/caregiver/jsp/content_node.jsp?nodeid=1719

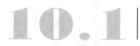

10.1 | Recommended Domains and Constructs for Family Assessment

DOMAIN	CONSTRUCTS
CONTEXT	■ Caregiver relationship to care recipient ■ Physical environment (home, facility) ■ Household status (number in home, etc.) ■ Financial status ■ Quality of family relationships ■ Duration of caregiving ■ Employment status (work/home/volunteer)
CAREGIVER'S PERCEPTION OF HEALTH AND FUNCTIONAL STATUS OF CARE RECIPIENT	■ Activities of daily living (ADLs; bathing, dressing) and need for supervision ■ Instrumental Activities of Daily Living (IADLs; managing finances, using the telephone) ■ Psychosocial needs ■ Cognitive impairment ■ Behavioral problems ■ Medical tests and procedures
CAREGIVER VALUES AND PREFERENCES	■ Caregiver/care recipient willingness to assume/accept care ■ Perceived filial obligation to provide care ■ Culturally based norms ■ Preferences for scheduling and delivery of care and services
WELL-BEING OF THE CAREGIVER	■ Self-rated health ■ Health conditions and symptoms ■ Depression or other emotional distress (e.g., anxiety) ■ Life satisfaction/quality of life

CONSEQUENCES OF CAREGIVING	■ Perceived challenges
	  ☐ Social isolation
	  ☐ Work strain
	  ☐ Emotional and physical health strain
	  ☐ Financial strain
	  ☐ Family relationship strain
	■ Perceived benefits
	  ☐ Satisfaction of helping family member
	  ☐ Developing new skills and competencies
	  ☐ Improved family relationships

SKILLS/ABILITIES/ KNOWLEDGE TO PROVIDE CARE RECIPIENT WITH NEEDED CARE	■ Caregiving confidence and competencies ■ Appropriate knowledge of medical care tasks (wound care, etc.)
POTENTIAL RESOURCES THAT CAREGIVER COULD CHOOSE TO USE	■ Existing or potential strengths (e.g., what is presently going well) ■ Coping strategies ■ Financial resources (health care and service benefits, Entitlements such as Veteran's Affairs, Medicare) ■ Community resources and services (caregiver support programs, religious organizations, volunteer agencies) ■ Formal and informal helping network and perceived quality of social support

Source: Family Caregiver Alliance (2006). *Caregiver Assessment: Principles, Guidelines and Strategies for Change.* Report from a National Consensus Development Conference (Vol. I). San Francisco: Author.

resources available versus those that will be needed to provide the required care. The assessment can also reveal actual and potential stresses that can be intervened with before they reach overwhelming and incapacitating anxiety and depression leading to despair. The structured and systematic nature of a good caregiver assessment assures that important aspects will not be missed and that a comprehensive approach is implemented.

Zarit (Family Caregiver Alliance, 2006c) goes on to address models and instruments that can be used as a basis for the caregiver assessments who research caregivers and caregiving. He approaches this study from a stress/coping model and the details of his recommendations are beyond the scope of this discussion. The Pearlin Stress Process Model (Pearlin, Mullan, & Skaff, 1990) and a number of stress and coping measures are compared and are helpful for researchers studying stress in caregivers. This model is an alternative to the Nursing models described earlier.

The Pearlin Stress Process Model addresses the experience of caregiving including caregiving transitions and transitional events that occur from one phase of the illness trajectory to another and one stage of caregiving to another. According to Pearlin et al. (1990), the five major components in caregivers' experience, include:

Caregiving context. Which includes sociodemographic characteristics of the caregiver and patient, history of illness, history of caregiving, and caregiving living arrangements.

Primary stressors. Which arise directly from the patient's illness and may include the patient's symptoms or impairment, ability to perform activities of daily living, cognitive deficits, and behavioral problems, as well as stressors such as caregiver burden, including the subjective assessment of the degree to which the caregiver perceives each event, including possible role overload (time and energy), role captivity (trapped in the caregiving role) and the loss of relationship (lost intimacy and social exchanges).

Secondary stressors. Which include tension and conflict in maintaining other roles in one's life such as employment and family relationships; interruptions in other areas of the caregivers' life, intrapsychic strains which erode a person's self-concept such as sense of caregiver mastery and competence

Resources. Which include social, financial, and the internal resources which increase the ability to manage stressful experiences, including social support which involves information, material, or financial support, as well as instrumental and emotional support, and *perceived gains* of the caregiving experience.

Outcomes. Which include positive and negative health outcomes related to caregivers.

There is a limited focus on family caregivers as "recipients of care," despite the palliative care precept that patients and families are the unit of care (National Consensus Guidelines for Quality Palliative Care, 2009). The collaborating oncologists involved in this study have emphasized their concern for family caregivers of patients with pancreatic cancer and the importance of identifying the experience of caregivers, and associated needs. They believe that the findings of this mixed methods study will result in cancer phase and transition- specific interventions to promote caregivers' physical and emotional health and quality of life which has personal, social, and institutional implications.

Guberman (Family Caregiver Alliance, 2006d) discusses the nature of caregiver assessment from a clinical not research perspective. She acknowledges a number of purpose driven definitions of caregiver assessment. Caregiver assessment can be used for determining eligibility for services, identifying unrecognized or subtle problems that might not be obvious although they have great impact on successful caregiving. The assessment process also allows for the development of a strong, trusting, therapeutic relationship between the clinician and the caregivers. Guberman goes on to describe a number of tools that can be used to perform the assessment although little consensus exists as to the best strategy. She asserts that the best assessments would include all caregivers and would include the carerecipients, both assessed by the same provider in the caregivers' home or another place where the caregiver feels safe to discuss all aspects of the situation.

FAMILY STRENGTHS PERSPECTIVE

The family strengths perspective asserts that if one examines families for the identification of problems, one will find only problems, but if the search is for strengths then strengths will be found that will provide the means of dealing with any problems that co-exist (http://family.jrank.org/pages/593/Family-Strengths-Family-Strengths-Perspective.html accessed May 22. 2009). The goal should be to identify strong families and provide means of developing the strengths of families who are struggling. Table 10.2 describes the qualities that reflect strength in families. The focus on family strengths does not deny the presence of stressors or perceived burden; rather it offers a focus on the resources any family can develop and use in reducing the negative effects of stressors and burden.

CARING FOR THE CAREGIVERS

When one thinks of Palliative Care, one naturally thinks of ease of symptom burden, end-of-life discussion and preparation and ultimately preparation for death. These are valuable associations and are at the heart of palliative care. They focus primarily though on the care recipient rather than the caregiver and the dyad that is formed out of this caring commitment. (Lingler, Sherwood, Crighton, Song, & Happ, 2008). The National Consensus Project Guidelines for Palliative Care (2009) states:

10.2 | Qualities of Strong Families

CATEGORIES	QUALITIES
APPRECIATION AND AFFECTION	■ Caring for each other ■ Friendship ■ Respect for individuality ■ Playfulness ■ Humor
POSITIVE COMMUNICATION	■ Sharing feelings ■ Giving compliments ■ Avoiding blame ■ Being able to compromise ■ Agreeing to disagree
SPIRITUAL WELL-BEING	■ Hope ■ Faith ■ Compassion ■ Shared ethical values ■ Oneness with humankind
COMMITMENT	■ Trust ■ Honesty ■ Dependability ■ Faithfulness ■ Sharing
TIME TOGETHER	■ Quality time in great quantity ■ Good things take time ■ Enjoying each other's company ■ Simple good times ■ Sharing fun times
ABILITY TO COPE WITH STRESS AND CRISIS	■ Adaptability ■ Seeing crises as challenges and opportunities ■ Growing through crises together ■ Openness to change ■ Resilience

Adapted from: http://family.jrank.org/pages/593/Family-Strengths-Family-Strengths-Perspective.html

The uniqueness of each patient and family is respected, and the patient and family constitute the unit of care. The family is defined by the patient or, in the case of minors or those without decision-making capacity, by their surrogates. In this context, family members may be related or unrelated to the patient; they are individuals who provide support and with whom the patient has a significant relationship. The care plan is determined by the goals and preferences of the patient and family, with support and guidance in decision-making from the healthcare team (p. 9).

There is agreement that many times caregivers simply burn out over the course of caregiving. Physical, emotional, compassion fatigue sets in, the caregivers have no reserve to care for the recipients, much less themselves. This leads to neglect of their own needs and health and the development of depression and other emotional complications as well as physical illness. Often caregivers are unaware of resources available to them or simply lack the energy to seek them out and then wade through all the red tape involved in documenting eligibility for the help. The financial hardships that develop over time are an added burden. There is also agreement that palliative care nurses, case managers,, and therapists can break this cycle by advocating for the caregivers as well as the carerecipients. What is less clear is why so many family caregivers fail to have access to these supports and services. It is too easy to fault the assessments of family resources. Assessment is critical as has been presented earlier, however assessment without intervention is impotent and of questionable value.

After one has completed careful family assessment, identification of the family strengths and weaknesses that will have an impact on the caregiver and/or the carerecipient and their relationship should be identified, clustered, and organized in a way that they reflect the priorities and function of the dyad. Generally, strategies can be successful by addressing four general areas.

1) Setting realistic goals.
2) Having difficult discussions.
3) Finding help.
4) Negotiating expectations.

Setting realistic goals. Setting realistic goals involves the identification of key tasks and responsibilities and then priorities for what must and can be accomplished in an hour, a day, or a week. It means looking honestly at the chronic disease or disability that is the focus of palliative care and estimating the level of functioning and participation the caregiver can expect from the care recipient. Will that husband with the stroke regain any ability to swallow? Will the mother with progressive, accelerated memory loss maintain the ability to dress herself? While the answers to these questions may seem obvious to the provider who lacks the history, hope, and desire of the caregiver; the caregiver sees improvement everywhere. The objective observer sees only the reality of permanent dysfunction. If the caregiver can come to see the situation realistically, then goal setting is easier, but more commonly, the caregiver exhausts themselves trying to reach the unrealistic goals and the expectation that they will be able to handle all the care required. It is just as important to be there for the caregiver when they reach the place where they can no longer cope with the enormity of the commitment they have taken on. It is critical to have a safe, non-judgmental place to come to and admit the need for help.

Having difficult discussions. Difficult discussion often brings to mind end-of-life discussions, but there are many areas of life that are difficult to discuss for reasons of history, family dynamics, cognitive dysfunction or embarrassment. Chances are that the more difficult the discussion, the more important it is to have that discussion. The imminence of dying often breaks down years of barriers to open, honest communication leading to a restoration of family relationships (Branum, 2002). There is always the possibility that fissures in family structures will become vast crevices, but the potential for healing makes some discussions worth having. Financial discussions may be just as difficult as healing and end-of-life discussions. When a parent or sibling lacks the cognitive ability or judgment to handle their own finances, the rational thing to do is manage those components for him/her. However, the care recipients may not see the rationality of that action, particularly if they are paranoid or psychotic.

Difficult discussions require extensive planning and careful selection of place and time. It is best to be very direct with short, simple sentences (Ngo-Metzger, Srinivasan, Solomon, & Meyskens 2008). It is good not to try to accomplish too much in any one meeting, taking time to work through issues with as little defensiveness and blame as can be accomplished. It is hard to lay aside years of pain and resentment and some of the apologies and forgiveness will need repeating. Forgiveness is a process.

Finding help. There are two categories of finding help. First, and possibly most straight forward is help that is available through social programs, support groups, and organizations. There are specific criteria for medicare, medicaid, food stamps, even meals-on-wheels. It may be difficult for caregivers to navigate the endless maze of programs and program rules, but help from a case manager or social worker can facilitate this process. Support groups exist for both caregivers and for caregivers and recipients related to diagnosis, disabilities, and specific causes and charities associated with chronic disease and disabilities. For caregivers, simply entering the term "Family Caregivers" into Google returned 4,140,000 potential results. Most notable of those results and in the first 10 returned were the Family Caregiver Alliance, the National Family Caregivers Association, and the Family Caregiver Support Network. Exhibit 10.2 is a sampling of organizations that exist to support family and informal caregivers.

The second and more difficult task of finding help may be exacting the cooperation and contribution of other family members in the care of the recipient. Family history and dynamics may make this impossible even with difficult discussions directed at resolving conflicts that fester with anger and resentment and/or blame for past experiences. It may be impossible and inappropriate to request some family members to overcome past abuse that they have finally resolved in order to provide care for the source of their abuse.

EXHIBIT 10.2: CAREGIVER SUPPORT WEBSITES

- National Family Caregivers Association
  www.nfacares.org
- Family Caregiver Alliance
  www.caregiver.org
- Family Caregiving 101
  www.familycaregiving101.org
- Family Caregivers Support Network
  www.caregiversupportnetwork.org
- The Family Caregiver Web
  www.familycaregiverweb.com
- Caregiving.com
  www.caregiving.com
- American Red Cross
  https://www.crossnet.org/services/hss/care/family.html
- Family Caregiver Handbook
  web.mit.edu/workplacecenter/hndbk/
- Caregiver
  www.ala.gov/AoARoot/AoA/programs/HCLTC/caregiver/index.aspx

This is not an exhaustive list and there are state specific programs available. These sites were active on May 22, 2009.

Negotiating expectations. The most difficult of the four categories of intervention may be negotiating expectations. It depends so much on the other three and time to deal with the realities of caregiving and the development of a trusting relationship with the case manager or palliative care nurse. Caregivers often take on more than one person can honestly accomplish (Stajduhar & Davies 2005). Whether out of love, duty or self-interest, the tasks of caring for someone who is physically and/or psychologically dependent may not appear overwhelming until the caregiver tries to get them all accomplished alone in the course of one day (Penson et al., 2007). Even if their caregiving activities are not accomplished in addition to a 40+ hour a week job and nuclear family responsibilities, it can be exhausting and mind-numbing. Some caregivers will persist in spite of pleading from family and friends to get help or give up some of the tasks. Release from the responsibilities comes only after the death of the carerecipient. Even placement in a long-term care facility may not release the caregiver from self-imposed responsibilities.

For others the reality of the responsibilities sinks in quickly and they seek help from family, professional agencies, or through placement in a long term care facility. There is always some degree of guilt associated with this decision but some will deal with their guilt in healthy ways; some will not.

For some, the despair and hopelessness that come from this sense of being overwhelmed with work and responsibilities, lack of support and acknowledgement if not appreciation can be manifested in abuse. It would be naive to say there are no mean and naturally abusive people who become caregivers for whatever reason. I have to believe though that they are a definite minority. What then could cause a kind, well-meaning caregiver, who has made a commitment to the care of a family member go on to starve, slap, pinch, demean, or threaten an elder or disabled family member? Some instances can be explained by despair and hopelessness that leads to acting out on the perceived source of the despair; anger that becomes resentment and develops into rage; too few resources to meet the demands of the caregiving. A few will have mental illness themselves that manifests in stressful situations such as extreme caregiving. These are potential explanations, not excuses. Consequently, the palliative care nurse or case manager must be vigilant for signs of abuse even in situations where everything seems to be going well. Abuse may be a call for help; it may be a manifestation of evil but regardless, it must be identified and stopped. It may take all the negotiating skill of the nurse to protect the care recipient while also getting help for the abuser.

Case Study conclusion: The palliative care nurse and case manager jointly interviewed DL and his niece at DL's home. Careful questioning revealed that DL had broken off relations with his children after their mother's death because he felt guilty for driving intoxicated. He was not injured in the accident that took his wife's life. He felt his children blamed him and although he blamed himself, he could not bear his children's feelings. The niece, who keeps close contact with DL's children, says that the daughters are concerned about their father and would like to restore relations. His son does indeed blame his father for his mother's death and does not want to be involved.

DL recognizes that he is forgetful about taking his medication even though he knows that the medication keeps his CHF controlled and him out of the hospital. His scores on the MMSE and the Beck depression inventory suggest that he is quite depressed, but his MMSE score of 28 suggests that he does not have early dementia. He has agreed to meet with his daughters and niece together and discuss their differences and to speak to his doctor about treatment for his depression. The niece recognizes that her own children are in need of more of her attention and is willing to relinquish her responsibilities for her uncle to his daughters and be available to him for emergencies and social visits. Since he is a veteran as well as disabled, he is eligible for a number of services that he was not aware of to help him with activities of daily living and housekeeping, enabling him to continue living independently in his home.

CONCLUSION

Palliative care is care that alleviates suffering when cure is not possible. Physical, emotional, and psychological suffering have meaning when they add meaning to our lives but so much of the suffering we are exposed to serves no meaningful purpose. As formal, educated caregivers we seek to provide support and nurturing to those informal caregivers who bear the brunt of the work and sacrifice that is necessary to care for those with chronic illness and disability. Extensive research has shown what a burden this can be, but also how rewarding it can be as well. Our job is to help caregivers and recipients balance resources so that the burden does not consistently outweigh the reward. This is a difficult task in itself and requires a careful assessment of the resources and skills of the caregivers so they can be matched with the tasks they will have to perform as well as the advocacy, perseverance, and stamina they will need to meet their goals. We can influence their expectations to help keep them from becoming overwhelmed by the enormity of what they may have taken on. No simple task in itself.

No human care can give endlessly without some reciprocity within the caring relationship. Family caregivers must perceive some acknowledgement and/or appreciation for the commitment and hard work they do for the care recipient. As professional caregivers we are no less in need of the same things in the therapeutic relationships we form.

EVIDENCE-BASED PRACTICE

Schulz, R., Czaja, S.J., Lustig, A., Zdaniuk, B., Martire, L.M., and Perdomo, D. (2009). Improving quality of life of caregivers of persons with spinal cord injury: A randomized controlled trial. *Rehabilitation Psychology, 54*(1), 1–15.

Problem. Caregivers of individuals with spinal cord injury (SCI) report high levels of depression and burden. As those individuals and their caregivers age, the effects of aging, multiple co-morbidities and chronic disease complicate the care required and increase caregiver burden potentially decreasing quality of life for both.

Design. Randomized, Controlled Trial

Sample/Setting. 173 Caregiver/Care Recipient dyads randomized to three conditions of "Dual Treatment," "Caregiver Only," and "Control." 86% completed the 12-month follow-up. The interventions were delivered at the caregiver's/care recipient's home and vial computer telephone technology system over a 6-month period. All participants were assessed at home and at 6 and 12 months after baseline. Assessors were blinded to treatment condition at the follow-up assessments.

Methods. Caregiver-only intervention: "Provided caregivers with knowledge and cognitive/behavioral skills to reduce environmental and personal stress, improve health and self-care, enhance access to formal and informal support and improve emotional well being" (pp. 3–4). **Dual-target intervention:** The dual-target intervention condition was designed to complement the caregiver-only intervention and targeted both the caregiver and the individual with SCI. The caregiver component intervention was identical to that of the caregiver-only condition" (p. 4). **Information-only control group:** "Caregivers who were randomly assigned to the control condition received the same standardized packet of written information on caregiving as the participants randomly assigned to the active intervention conditions" (p. 4). Measures of depressive symptoms, social support/integration, self-care problems, physical health symptoms were measured in both caregiver and recipient and in addition caregiver burden was measured in caregivers only at baseline, 6 months, and 1 year. These were combined with baseline demographic variables for analysis. Analysis was of change scores from baseline for the psychosocial measures. Among 6-month changes were very small so only 1-year changes were reported.

Results. Multivariate ANOVA results indicated that there were no differences in the measures between the three groups at baseline. ANOVA's demonstrated significant superiority of the Dual-Target Intervention over the control group ($p = .049$) and over the Caregiver-Only group ($p = .033$). Univariate analysis showed the dual target superior to the control for physical health symptoms and superior to the caregiver-only group for depression and physical symptoms. Effect sizes were small to moderate.

Implications. Education and intervention directed at both the caregiver and recipient together is more effective in controlling physical and depressive symptoms. Limitations to this study include the use of difference scores rather than a repeated measures design that offers better control of Type II errors. The numbers of couples in minority racial groups and in different socio-economic and educational categories limited the ability to examine these differences that have been shown in other studies to affect the measured outcomes.

REFERENCES

Abaya, C. (1999, January 17). A survival course for the sandwich generation. *The New York Times*. Section 14NJ, 4.

Bahr, H. M., & Bahr, K. S. (2001). Families and self-sacrifice: Alternative models and meaningsfor family theory. *Social Forces, 79*(4), 1231–1258.

Branum, K. (2002). Healing in the context of terminal illness. In P. B. Kritek (Ed.), *Reflections on healing: A central nursing construct*. Sudbury, MA: Jones and Bartlett.

National Consensus Project for Quality Palliative Care (2009). *Clinical practice guidelines for quality palliative care [www.nationalconsensusproject.org]*

Family Caregiver Alliance. (2006). *Caregiver assessment: Principles, guidelines and strategies for change*. Report from a National Consensus Development Conference (Vol. I). San Francisco: Author.

Family Caregiver Alliance. (2006a). *Caregiver assessment: Voices and views from the field*. Report from a National Consensus Development Conference (Vol. II). San Francisco: Carol Levine.

Family Caregiver Alliance. (2006b). *Caregiver assessment: Voices and views from the field*. Report from a National Consensus Development Conference (Vol. II). San Francisco: Dan Ahern.

Family Caregiver Alliance. (2006c). *Caregiver assessment: Voices and views from the field*. Report from a National Consensus Development Conference (Vol. II). San Francisco: Steven H. Zarit.

Family Caregiver Alliance. (2006d). *Caregiver assessment: Voices and views from the field*. Report from a National Consensus Development Conference (Vol. II). San Francisco: Nancy Guberman.

Grant, G., Ramcharan, P., McGrath, M., Nolan, M., & Keady, J. (1998). Rewards and gratifications among family caregivers; towards a refined model of caring and coping. *Journal of Intellectual Disability Research, 42*, 58–71.

Grey, M., Knafl, K., & McCorkle, R. (2006). A framework for the study of self and family management of chronic conditions. *Nursing Outlook, 54*(5), 278–286.

Ingoldsby, B. B., Smith, S. R, & Miller, J. E. (2004). *Exploring family theories*. Los Angeles: Roxbury Publishing Company.

Jackson, D., Turner-Stokes, L., Murray, J., Morven, L., & Mcpherson, K. M. (2009).

Acquired brain injury and dementia: A comparison of carer experiences. *Brain Injury. 23*(5), 433–444.

Lingler, J. H., Sherwood, P. R., Crighton, M. H., Song, M. K., & Happ, M. B. (2008). Conceptual challenges in the study of caregiver-care recipient relationships. *Nursing Research, 57*(5), 367–372.

Narayan, S., Lewis, M., Tornaotre, J., Hepburn, K., & Corcoran-Perry, S. (2001). Subjective responses to caregiving for a spouse with dementia. *Journal of Gerontological Nursing, 27*(3),19–28.

Neff, J. L., Dy, S. M., Frick, K. D., & Kasper, J. D. (2007). End-of-life care: Findings from a national survey of informal caregivers. *Archives of Internal Medicine, 167*, 40–46.

Ngo-Metzger, Q., Srinivasan, M., Solomon, L., & Meyskens, F. L. (2008). End-of-life care: Guidelines for patient-centered communication. *American Family Physician, 77*(2), 167–174.

Pearlin, L. I., Mullan, J. T., & Skaff, M. M. (1990). Caregiving and the stress process: An overview of concepts and their measures. *Gerontologist, 30*(5), 583–594.

Peck, M. S. (1978). *The road less traveled*. New York: Simon and Shuster, Inc.

Penson, R. T., Gu, F., Haris, S., Thiel, M. M., Lawton, N., Fuler, A. F., et al. (2007). Hope. *The Oncologist, 12*(9), 1105–1113.

Schumaker, K., Beck, C. A., & Marren, J. M. (2006). Family caregivers: Caring for older adults, working with their families. *AJN, 106*(8), 40–50.

Stajduhar, K. I., & Davies, B. (2005). Variations in and factors influencing family members' decisions for palliative home care. *Palliative Medicine, 19*, 21–32.

Thomas, A. (2006). *A three dog life*. New York: Houghton-Mifflin Co.

Tsai, P. F. (2003). A middle-range theory of caregiver stress. *Nursing Science Quarterly, 16*(2), 137–145.

11

Loss, Suffering, Grief, and Bereavement

Mertie L. Potter

Key Points

- Loss and suffering are universal experiences that occur across the life span.
- Traditional grieving theories view the process in stages with closure or resolution; some contemporary theories view the process as nonstaged and ongoing.
- Although culture and ethnicity may influence an individual's views on living with and dying from life-threatening illness, individuals must be recognized as unique and encouraged to grieve as best suits them.
- The nurse is on his/her own journey along with patients and their families and significant others who are facing living with and dying from life-threatening illness.
- Nursing presence is an important aspect that can enhance healing in others who are grieving.

Case Study: Roberto Carballo, a 69-year-old widower, is hospitalized in a medical surgical unit of a large west coast teaching hospital. Mr. Carballo is suffering from septicemia and a gangrenous lower right extremity (LRE) resulting from a five-decade history of having diabetes mellitus (DM). Mr. Carballo's physician feels that Mr. Carballo will not survive amputation of his gangrenous LRE, nor is he responding well to a number of different antibiotics. Mr. Carballo has stated that he thinks he is nearing his time and he is ready to join his beloved wife Carmelita, who died 6 months earlier.

Mr. Carballo has three adult children: Isabella, a single 47-year-old bookkeeper; Kasandra, a 44-year-old mother of 7-year-old Teresa and 5 year-old Alberto; and Roberto Carballo, Jr. (Bob), a divorced 39-year-old navy captain. Mr. Carballo's two daughters live in the area and take turns staying at their father's bedside. The grandchildren visit Mr. Carballo briefly each day, are curious about "all the tubes in Lito" (Spanish nickname for grandfather), and ask many questions about what is happening to their grandfather. Bob is stationed in Guam, has no children, and is kept updated by Kassandra on their father's condition.

Loss and Suffering

Like 7-year-old Teresa and 5-year-old Alberto, I was very moved by two deaths in my early childhood: my grandmother's and a little bird's. I was 6 years old. My sister and I were doing our nightly routine. My mother came into our room and sat down on my bed. Mom was crying. She had just received a phone call from "way far away" (my 6-year-old mind's concept of distance) that my grandmother had died. Although I had seen my grandmother only a few times in my young life, I felt very connected to her. I loved her very much, because I felt cherished by her. I also knew my mom and dad loved her greatly, and that Grammie had been sick for a long time. Mom answered our questions and prayed with my sister and me. After my mom and big sister left the room, I remember that I "talked to" Grammie out my bedroom window. I said, "I don't know if you can hear me, but I love you a lot and will miss you." I felt sad and cried. I waited, half expecting to hear an answer from her; it was okay when I did not. It was our little good-bye with one another. I felt secure that she was in Heaven and that Heaven seemed like a good place for her to be if she were dead and no longer on earth. I felt at peace.

The other striking memory related to death occurred at the same period. My sister and I were playing in one of our favorite pine-needle-laden spots on our farm. We came upon a dead robin. We were horror-struck to see this beautiful creature lifeless on the ground. We ran and got a dustpan and gently scooted the bird onto it with a little pine branch. We dug a hole, wrapped the bird in a paper towel, respectfully placed it in a shoebox, and laid the bird to rest in its grave. We read Scripture, sang a hymn, and prayed for the bird. I was very grateful I had an older sister who knew how to conduct a proper funeral service for this dear little creature. We were both sad and cried. That also was the first time I remember questioning if animals have souls and where they go when they die.

Loss and suffering are major experiences along life's journey. How one learns to accept, adapt to, and advance through these experiences determines how the individual will move through life itself. Are losses and suffering perceived as natural, functional, growth-promoting, and normal dimensions in and transitions through life, or are they perceived as unnatural, dysfunctional, harmful, and abnormal circumstances to be avoided?

Living With and Dying From Life-Threatening Illness

Case Study follow-up: On day 5, Mr. Carballo becomes unconscious. His physician approaches the daughters about a Do-Not-Resuscitate (DNR) order. Isabella does not want their father "to suffer any longer" and wants to go forward with the DNR order. Kasandra informs Mr. Carballo's primary nurse, Jake, that she wants Mr. Carballo kept alive for as long as possible and thinks her sister just wants him to die. Kasandra indicates she has been in touch with their brother, Bob, and is trying to convince him to come "make things right with Dad so Dad can die in peace when it is his time." On day 6 a feeding tube is inserted to provide nourishment for Mr. Carballo.

"Losing, leaving, and letting go" are normal processes that help individuals grow (Viorst, 1987, p. 3). However, contemporary grief theorists suggest that grief may be an ongoing experience in which one connects with the lost relationship via memories, heritage, or spirit, rather than severs the relationship (Moules, Simonson, Fleiszer, Prins, & Glasgow, 2007; Moules,

Simonson, Prins, Angus, & Bell, 2004). Loss and suffering are inescapable dimensions of life. How an individual transitions through loss and suffering is what remains variable. When planning the patient's care, it is important for the nurse to note how the patient with a life-threatening illness and significant others view loss, suffering, and living with and dying from such an illness. It also is important for nurses to examine their own beliefs related to these life experiences. Developing awareness of and attending to each person's perspective is key in formulating successful interventions.

Provision of nursing care takes place within a person's cultural context. Having an awareness of a patient's cultural background, as well as their usual cultural interventions, is both helpful and important. Variations within specific cultures exist, so it is important to discern with a patient and significant others what specific customs and rituals around death and grief are important and preferred (Choi & Lee, 2007; Clements et al., 2003; Mystakidou, Tsilika, Parpa, Katsouda, & Vlahos, 2003). Holloway (2006) considers death to be a leveler in the context of culture; death causes individuals to face the common humanity of mankind. However, nurses must explore the individual's specific view of dying and death while considering the individual's view of self within a given culture or ethnicity.

Narayanasamy (2006, p. 841) details an "ACCESS" model of transcultural nursing. (See Table 11.1.)

The living–dying interval often is a time of great uncertainty and questioning. Patients may question, "Why? Why me? Why now?" Patients often seek answers to questions related to the meaning of life, the meaning of suffering, the meaning of death, and the meaning of loss. This may be a time of opportunity for the patient to grow and sense a greater wholeness than

ever before in spite of an acute awareness of loss, suffering, and grief. Patients living with and dying from a life-threatening illness need to focus on what they are able to do rather than on what they cannot do.

Grief is considered by clinicians in both traditional and contemporary views as work. Grief work involves cognitive and emotional realms. At the heart of grief is "excruciating sorrow," and at the core of grief work is "spiritual comfort" and "spiritual healing" (Moules et al., 2007, p. 127).

The Nurse's Role

Case Study follow-up: Jake has been Mr. Carballo's primary nurse for 5 of the 6 days he has been hospitalized so far. During that time, he has witnessed the tension that exists between the two daughters and that surrounds Mr. Carballo's relationship with his son. Jake hopes silently that a DNR not be initiated, because he wants Mr. Carballo's son to come while his father is alive. Jake has not expressed his feelings to the sisters but soon realizes he is over-identifying with Roberto Carballo, Jr. Jake sets up an appointment to meet with his supervisor to process his feelings. Jake shares with his supervisor that he did not get an opportunity to reconcile with his own father before he died 2 years ago.

Nurses meet individuals across the life span and often at the crossroads of their suffering and loss. Regardless of the setting, nurses are in a unique position to help individuals and their significant others who may be in physical, emotional, social, and spiritual pain related to suffering and loss. The nurse has a broad-based background in providing competent nursing care to individuals across the health/illness continuum. The breadth and depth of each nurse's skills in the specific area of giving care to those living with and dying from terminal illness will be dependent upon numerous factors. Some of these include the nurse's personal beliefs and values, life experiences (professional/nonprofessional), level of comfort with death and dying, educational level, licensure, and interest in this area.

Every nurse must be committed to providing patients, either directly or indirectly, quality care at the end of life. Critical to helping the nurse fulfill this obligation is a degree of comfort in dealing with death and dying. Student nurses need experience and support coping with dying and deceased patients. One student nurse shared how traumatic it was for her during her senior preceptorship to be left alone while providing her first postmortem care; the staff member assisting her had to step out of the room temporarily. The student nurse expressed frustration with herself that

11.1 | Transcultural Nursing

Assessment	Focus on cultural aspects of clients' lifestyle, health beliefs and health practices
Communication	Be aware of variations in verbal and non-verbal responses
Cultural negotiation and compromise	Become more aware of aspects of other people's culture as well as understanding
Establishing respect and rapport	A therapeutic relation which portrays genuine respect for clients' cultural beliefs and values is required
Sensitivity	Deliver diverse culturally sensitive care to culturally diverse groups
Safety	Enable clients to derive a sense of cultural safety

she felt "frozen" and "scared" until the staff member returned. Processing this experience with her faculty member helped her.

Knowledge of the process of dying and the degree of comfort in dealing with others who are experiencing death and dying are two important areas in which the advanced practitioner's education, experience, and expertise will provide more depth in discerning the special needs of the patient. Furthermore, the advanced practice nurse's skill level is more appropriate for dealing with high-risk and complicated situations.

A number of endeavors have been supported to enhance end-of-life care and further education around death, grief, and bereavement. One project is the End of Life Nursing Education Consortium (ELNEC) funded by the Robert Wood Johnson Foundation. Nurses involved with the ELNEC project developed a curriculum to improve end-of-life nursing care. Nurses are taught interventions that assist patients and families experiencing loss, grief, death, and bereavement, particularly in relation to effective and supportive communication strategies (Matzo & Sherman, 2006; Matzo et al., 2003).

Communication may be impaired or even unintelligible in the dying patient. In such circumstances, the nurse needs to inform the patient that the nurse is attempting to understand. It also is important that the nurse convey an understanding of how difficult it must be for the patient not to be able to communicate and that the nurse will make every effort to meet the patient's needs.

Living with and dying from a life-threatening illness can thrust a patient into a sense of uncertainty. Each patient must be allowed to live and die in his or her own way. The nurse may assist patients to express what this way is and help them regain some semblance of control (Ferrell & Coyle, 2008). Nurses must be educated to promote holistic care, recognizing that quality-of-life issues that are important to dying patients include finding peace of mind, having a voice and being heard, finding meaning, experiencing comfort, and seeking spiritual understanding (Ferrell & Coyle, 2008).

Fostering patterns that are health-promoting and positive for individuals is the ideal in nursing care. Unhealthy patterns need to be identified and interventions provided to promote health and healing even as death approaches.

Experience of Loss and Suffering Across the Life Span

At birth, an infant is thrust or pulled into a new environment through expulsion and separation from the mother's womb. The infant has no control over this experience. A fairly traumatic transition takes place; one no longer is in the safe and warm environment that provided nourishment and protection during this critical developmental stage. The infant now has to adjust to a new home. This new environment includes the experiences of suffering and loss.

Nearing the sixth month, the infant usually develops an acute awareness of separation from the mother or mother figure. This state is referred to as "separation anxiety." This keen awareness of loss may initiate a rudimentary development of death awareness (Backer, Hannon, & Gregg, 1994). This hypothesis is based on Bowlby's (1980) model of attachment between mother and infant and the infant's experience of separation from the mother. As the individual continues to develop, suffering and loss continue to occur. Generally, this occurrence causes the individual to move from a dependent state to an interdependent state and then to an independent state. In some cases, usually due to more loss and suffering, the individual may return to a dependent or interdependent state prior to death. Thus, life often involves a rhythm of change, interfacing with suffering and loss, from the time an individual is born.

Children under the age of 2 usually have a sense of separation but little understanding of the concept of death. For children between 2 and 5 years of age, death is seen as a transient state but not a permanent event.

Between 6 and 10 years of age, children begin to grasp the reality of death (McIntier, 1995). Adolescents conceptualize death in a way similar to adults; namely, they are mortal and will eventually die. As the adolescent comes to terms with his or her individuality and increasing independence, there is an increasing awareness of one's own mortality. Although death is considered a future event to adolescents and young adults, death anxiety is more evident than at earlier ages. Middle-aged adults and older adults are more aware and accepting of death. However, no assumptions can be made concerning any age group, and the previous remarks are generalizations. Each individual's response to death is unique (Rando, 1984) (see Table 11.2 for developmental views of death).

Theoretical Underpinnings and Theories on Death and Dying

Stage theory of grief, although widely accepted, has been empirically tested only recently (Maciejewski, Zhang, Block, & Prigerson, 2007). This longitudinal study consisted of 233 individuals experiencing grief after the loss of a family member to natural causes. The stages encompassing disbelief, yearning, anger, depression, and acceptance attained peak values in the given sequence when rescaled but not in expected sequencing when examined for most frequently endorsed at initial checkpoints. An interesting finding was that the first four negative indicators all reached maximum values within a 6-month period (disbelief – 1 month;

11.2 | Developmental Views of Death

DOMAIN	STAGE OF DEVELOPMENT	TASK/AREA OF RESOLUTION
Birth – 2 years	Infancy	Sense of separation; no concept of death
2 – 5 years	Early childhood	Death is transient, not permanent state
6 – 10 years	Late childhood	Beginning awareness of the reality of death
13 – 25 years	Adolescence— young adulthood	Similar to adult view— realization of mortality and eventual death; death anxiety more evident; death perceived as a future event
26 – 65 years	Middle-aged and older adults	More aware and accepting of death

Adapted from McIntier, T. M. (1995). Nursing the family when a child dies. *RN, 2,* 50–55.

yearning – 4 months; anger – 5 months; and depression – 6 months). Acceptance increased throughout the entire 24-month observation period.

As will be reviewed, Freud (1957), Lindemann (1944), Engel (1964), Glasser and Strauss (1965), and Kubler-Ross (1969) developed classical work related to dying and death. Pattison (1977), Bowlby (1980), Worden (1991), and Rando (1984) broadened knowledge in the field with their work. More recent writings by Corr (1992), Buckman (1993), Evans (1994), Copp (1997), and Mallinson (1999) have challenged, as well as added to, previous theoretical information. New information relevant to theories on death and dying is expanding rapidly. Contemporary research on death and dying views the time frame for grief resolution in a less restrictive way than earlier writings. Although different in some ways, most of the authors demonstrate a similar thread and core knowledge related to grief work that is helpful to both the beginning clinician and the advanced practitioner.

Freud (1957) brought the concept of grief work to the forefront after examining his personal feelings and societal observations following the mass losses brought about by World War I. Freud saw grief as a necessary process to assist an individual in adapting to loss. He also felt that an individual needed to free himself or herself from attachment to the "lost object."

Lindemann (1944) studied bereavement in individuals who were survivors of the Coconut Grove Hotel fire in Boston (as well as their close relatives); patients who lost a relative while in treatment; relatives of members of the service; and relatives of patients who died while in the hospital. He determined that common physical symptoms, affective symptoms, behavioral manifestations, and physiological changes accompanied each grief experience. Lindemann also first alluded to anticipatory grief in relation to women anticipating the potential death of significant males in their lives during World War II.

Engel (1964) cited three stages through which one progresses in uncomplicated bereavement: shock and disbelief; developing awareness; and restitution and recovery. Engel pointed out that denial predominates initially and helps prevent the individual from being totally overwhelmed. During the second stage, the individual may express guilt and cry. Finally, thoughts and memories of the deceased are discussed, and behaviors of the deceased may be displayed by the bereaved.

Glasser and Strauss (1965) examined different contexts related to caregivers and patients regarding knowledge about a patient's dying. They suggested that there are four states of awareness related to dying: closed awareness, suspicion awareness, mutual pretense awareness, and open awareness. In the first context, i.e., closed awareness, caregivers are aware that the patient is dying but keep that information from the patient. In suspicion awareness, the caregivers know that the patient is dying, but the patient only suspects he is dying. The patient is ambivalent about wanting to know and not wanting to know that he is dying. In the mutual pretense context, both the caregiver and the patient act as though they do not know the patient is dying, but both know that the patient is. Within the context of open awareness, there is a sharing of knowledge, information, and communication about the patient's dying between the caregiver and the patient (Glasser & Strauss, 1965; Rando, 1984).

Kubler-Ross (1969) studied more than 200 patients diagnosed with terminal cancer. Her work was pivotal in theorizing that individuals move through (not necessarily sequentially) five phases when trying to cope with pending death. These five stages are denial and isolation, anger, bargaining, depression, and acceptance. In the denial and isolation phase, an individual experiences shock and disbelief. A comment such as "I don't believe this is happening" may be made. During the anger phase, the individual questions "Why me?" Anger often is displaced. The individual may try to rationalize during the bargaining phase by pleading or regretting, "Yes, me, but . . . ." Bargaining is an attempt to postpone death and extend life. It involves self-imposed deadlines. During the depression phase, the individual may express feelings of guilt or sadness, such as "Yes, this is happening to me." There often is an awareness of great loss for the patient. In the acceptance stage, the struggle is over. The individual has come to accept his imminent death and is ready to let go and move on. A comment such as "My time is close; it's all right now" may be made.

Pattison (1977) was the first to focus on a model that examined the "living-dying interval." Pattison defined that interval as existing between knowing that death was imminent and the actual point of death. He incorporates three clinical phases within the living-dying interval: acute crisis phase, chronic living-dying phase, and the terminal phase. During the acute crisis phase, the patient is confronted with the knowledge that a process beyond his control influences his death. The chronic living-dying phase involves an acute awareness of living and dying simultaneously. Last, the terminal phase commences when the patient starts withdrawing from the outside world. There is an internal awareness that he must conserve his energies for himself.

Bowlby (1980) described four phases of bereavement: numbness; yearning and searching; disorganization and despair; and reorganization. His theory is based on an attachment model in which the child must separate from the mother. The process includes 1) shock and disbelief related to the loss (numbness); 2) protest involving an attempt to regain the lost object (yearning and searching); 3) an intense sense of despair in which the individual tries to regain the lost object (disorganization and despair); and 4) completion of the mourning when the individual stops searching and develops new relationships (reorganization) (Evans, 1994).

Worden (1991) refers to four tasks of mourning: accepting the reality of the loss; experiencing the pain of grief; adjusting to an environment in which the deceased is not there; and emotionally relocating the deceased and moving on with life. Mourning may become maladaptive if an individual's response is to avoid, distort, amplify, or prolong grief (Kissane & Bloch, 2002).

Rando (1984) cites six processes of mourning or grief work: recognizing the loss; reacting to the separation; recollecting and re-experiencing the deceased and the relationship in a realistic way; relinquishing old attachments to the deceased and the assumptive world; readjusting to move adaptively in the new world without forgetting the old; and reinvesting. Rando (1984) considers that complicated grief may exist if there is compromise, distortion, or failure of one or more of the six "R" processes occurring after consideration of the amount of time since death.

As mentioned, Corr (1992), Buckman (1993), and Copp (1997) developed more contemporary theories. Corr expanded the theoretical premise of task work postulated by Pattison (1977) and Kalish (1979) to include four major areas of task work in coping with dying, specifically physical, psychological, social, and spiritual loss. Addressing physical tasks involves meeting bodily needs satisfactorily and minimizing the individual's physical distress. Working through psychological tasks maximizes the individual's psychological security, autonomy, and richness of living. In order to meet social tasks, interpersonal attachments of significance must be sustained and enhanced, as well as assisting the individual to explore social implications of dying. In addition, spiritual task work involves determining and affirming sources of spiritual energy, which, in turn, stimulate hope.

Buckman (1993) promoted the concept that grief is more characteristic of the individual than of the individual's progression through particular grief stages. The second major point made by Buckman is that an individual's movement during the grieving process is dependent upon resolution of various issues related to emotions rather than changing from one emotion to another, as in Kubler-Ross's model. Additionally, Buckman addressed other responses to dying, such as fear of dying, guilt, hope, despair, and humor (Buckman, 1993).

Copp's (1997) work with dying individuals and the nurses caring for them examined two additional dimensions that seem to occur within the dying individual: readiness to die and a body-person split. Copp observed many direct and indirect actions between patients and nurses: protecting and letting go; watching and waiting; and holding on and letting go. Copp further noted a distinct reference by nurses and patients to the body as separate from the self in relation to patients who were nearing death. A dying individual's personal acceptance of imminent death and physical condition determined the individual's readiness to die. The states of readiness included 1) person ready, body not ready; 2) person ready, body ready; 3) person not ready, body ready; and 4) person not ready, body not ready. One major thrust of Copp's (1998) work is that the dying experience impacts everyone who is involved with the dying patient.

Theories are emerging that demonstrate the ongoing process and complexity of reconstructing meaning for individuals who have experienced a loss versus traditional linear stage theories (Pilkington, 2008). These theories are supported through qualitative studies, such as those related to parents dealing with loss of an infant through the Sudden Infant Death Syndrome (SIDS) (Krueger, 2006).

Florczak (2008) incorporates Parse's (2007) humanbecoming theory in her contemporary conceptualization of grief. Florczak's views vary from traditional ones in that she asserts: 1) the loss is maintained, not severed; 2) a changed meaning about the loss occurs; and 3) sorrow persists related to unfamiliar-familiar patterns being woven into one's life related to the loss (2008).

In contemporary grief theory, grief is seen as dynamic, individualized, pervasive, ongoing, and normative (Cowles & Rodgers, 2000). Contemporary theorists address masculine and feminine differences in grieving (McCreight, 2004; Thomas, 2004; Baum, 2003).

As Pilkington (2006) points out, many of the studies done in relation to humanbecoming theory are qualitative. Thus, they are not generealizable. However, they provide knowledge for nurses to better understand the importance of presence and to better relate to those who are grieving. Although sorrow related to the loss may continue, the meaning attributed to the loss may change as the individual continues to journey through the process of separating-connecting (Florczak, 2008).

DIMENSIONS OF LOSS, SUFFERING, GRIEF, AND BEREAVEMENT

Definitions

Loss. Loss is defined as "the condition of being deprived or bereaved of something or someone" (*American Heritage Dictionary*, 2006, p. 1034). Losses can be actual, potential, physical, or symbolic. Loss related to health, function, roles, relationships, and life itself is the central focus of this book. Losses other than the death of the loved one are referred to as secondary losses (Rando, 1984).

Mitchell and Anderson (1983) describe six types of loss: materialistic, relational, intra-psychic, functional, role, and systemic. Material loss involves separation from a physical object or surroundings. In relationship loss, an individual no longer has the ability to relate to another individual. Intrapsychic loss impacts an individual's self-image through loss of what might have been changed perceptions, lost emotions (i.e., faith, hope, or courage), or emotions that result when a major task has been completed successfully. Functional loss occurs through bodily decline or deterioration in illness or aging. Role loss results when an individual changes or loses (e.g., healthy person to terminally ill person) a customary role or acquires a new role (e.g., patient). Systemic loss involves the loss of contact with customary behaviors or functions within a system, such as absence from a usual work environment or home environment.

Loss can be primary or secondary. Primary loss refers to the initial loss (whether of health for the patient or possibly loss of the patient through death for the significant others). Secondary losses stem from the initial loss. As a result of being diagnosed with a terminal illness, the patient also may experience secondary losses of roles, job, income, etc. Significant others may experience secondary losses of roles, income, their own health, and so forth.

> **Case Study follow-up:** Mr. Carballo's family members and caregivers are experiencing "anticipatory grief," as they watch Mr. Carballo's condition decline. His gangrenous LRE is becoming much worse. He is not responding to any treatment attempts.

Suffering. Suffering is defined as "the condition of one who suffers: the bearing of pain or distress" (*American Heritage Dictionary*, 2006, p. 1730). Suffering impacts a patient's body, mind, and spirit. Cassell (1991) defines suffering as "the state of severe distress associated with events that threaten the intactness of person" (p. 33). Cassell recognizes the importance of human suffering within any of the human dimensions, such as body, mind, and spirit. He also advocates asking individuals about the presence or absence of suffering because suffering is a very individualized experience and may result from treatment, as well as from the disease process or a number of other events. Ferrell and Coyle (2008) assert that relieving suffering is the crux of nurses' professional work.

According to Georgesen and Dungan (1996), the presence of pain compounds suffering and results in spiritual distress. Pain is a frequent companion of terminal illness. Suffering can be present with or without the presence of pain. Suffering, however, cannot be treated or managed like pain. Suffering is a personal experience. Framing suffering in a religious, philosophical, or personally meaningful perspective can help patients endure it better (Rando, 1984). Physical pain is associated with psychological, social, and spiritual distress; pain that continues without meaning results in suffering (Ferrell and Coyle, 2008).

Suffering can be acute or chronic. Acute suffering occurs when the patient is in crisis and confronted with an immediate loss. Chronic suffering results from the longer term realization and impact of a loss that carries a great deal of significance for, and meaning to, the patient. The patient with a terminal illness may experience only one type of suffering, both types at different times, or both simultaneously. Intervention involves trying to understand the patient's suffering and trying to help the patient cope effectively with suffering. Key to helping the suffering patient is attempting to understand the meaning of the suffering and attempting to comfort and sustain the individual through it.

Similar to chronic suffering is the middle-range nursing theory of chronic sorrow introduced by Eakes, Burke, and Hainsworth (1998). Chronic sorrow is viewed as normal in response to the recurrent experience of ongoing, significant loss that may be actual or symbolic or both. Major concepts within this theory relate to the following: losses, disparity between reality and idealism, trigger events or milestones, and an individual's internal and external means of managing reoccurring grief that accompanies chronic sorrow. One of the key antecedents to chronic sorrow, namely disparity between the individual's current reality and idealized reality, is what differentiates chronic sorrow from chronic suffering. An individual experiencing chronic suffering does not necessarily face disparity with chronic suffering.

> **Case Study follow-up:** Mr. Carballo groans occasionally. His daughters Isabella and Kasandra ask Jake, the nurse, if Mr. Carballo is in a lot of pain. Jake assures them he will do a thorough pain

assessment and ask for more pain medication if needed. Isabella tells Jake she cannot bear to see Mr. Carballo in physical pain and that she saw her mother suffer "a painful death at home when she had a heart attack."

Grief. Grief is defined as "deep mental anguish, as that arising from bereavement" (*American Heritage Dictionary*, 2006, p. 772). Rando (1984) describes grief as a normal reaction to the perception of loss. Grief is generally a transitory, acute state in response to loss with the possibility that the individual's ability to function may be disrupted temporarily. In addition, the individual may be distracted, disoriented, distressed, or all of these (Mallinson, 1999). Feelings that may accompany grief include anger, shame, helplessness, sadness, guilt, despair, relief, peacefulness, calm, and release (McCall, 1999). Charleton (2003) asserts that stages of grieving might include any or all of the following: "distress, shock, denial, anger, feeling 'low in spirits,' depression, resignation, acceptance, resolution" (p. 671).

Common grief responses are listed in Table 11.3. These responses may involve physical, psychological, and spiritual/sociocultural responses. They may have aspects that seem contradictory in nature. The impact of grief can be extensive and pervasive. Anticipatory grief, those feelings of grief experienced prior to an expected loss, generally assists individuals in working through depression related to the upcoming death, rehearsing of the death, adjusting to the consequences of the death, and having an increased concern for the terminally ill (Fulton & Fulton, 1971). Rando (1984) views anticipatory grief as also allowing for gradual absorption of the reality of the loss, helping resolve unfinished business, changing assumptions about life and identity, and making future plans.

Evans (1994) challenges the belief that anticipatory grief experienced prior to death is the same process as the conventional grief experienced in the postdeath period. Evans proposes the use of the label "terminal response" to describe the process that occurs between diagnosis of terminal illness and death. Differences noted between pre and postdeath grieving include the following: 1) anticipatory grieving ends at the time of death, whereas conventional grieving can go on indefinitely;

11.3 | Grief Responses

PHYSICAL	PSYCHOLOGICAL	SPIRITUAL/ SOCIOCULTURAL	DICHOTOMOUS NATURE
■ Shortness of breath ■ Insomnia ■ Loss of appetite ■ Loss of sleep ■ Energy loss ■ Greater susceptibility to illness ■ Sighing ■ Nervousness and restlessness ■ Sensation of something in the throat ■ Feelings of emptiness or heaviness ■ Heart palpitations ■ Crying ■ Psychomotor retardation ■ Decreased libido or hypersexuality ■ Weight loss	■ Depression ■ Anxiety ■ Guilt ■ Anger and hostility ■ Anhedonia ■ Self-reproach ■ Low self-esteem ■ Helplessness and hopelessness ■ Sense of unreality ■ Suspiciousness ■ Interpersonal problems ■ Imitation of the deceased's behaviors ■ Idealization of the deceased ■ Ambivalent feelings about the deceased	■ Spiritual pain and suffering ■ Spiritual loneliness ■ Fear of God, the unknown, and/or the future ■ Feelings of failure and guilt ■ Feelings of unfairness and anger ■ Loss of transcendence ■ Hopelessness ■ Search for meaning ■ A need for love and hope ■ A sense of forgiveness ■ Participation or lack of participation in formal religious group ■ Views related to use of "extraordinary" life-prolonging measures ■ Beliefs related to afterlife ■ Handling of the body after death ■ Rituals performed after death	■ Universal/individual ■ Benign/malignant ■ Life-giving/life-requiring ■ Active/passive ■ Internal/external ■ State/process ■ Heart/head ■ Inarticulate/poetic ■ Celebration/bereavement

Adapted from Lindemann (1944); Rando (1984); Stuart & Sundeen (1991); Pritchett & Lucas (1997) p. 203; Kazanowski (2006) p. 114; Moules et al. (2007) p. 122.

and 2) anticipatory grieving increases as death draws nearer, but conventional grieving usually diminishes in intensity with time.

> **Case Study follow-up:** Talking with his supervisor helped Jake deal with some of his unresolved grieving issues related to his own father's death. When Jake goes home after his 3–11 p.m. shift, his sixth shift of providing care for Mr. Carballo, Jake takes out pictures of his father and him. He cries about the loss of his father for the first time since his father's death.
>
> Jake purposes to make sure Mr. Carballo's family members are offered resources that might help them deal with their father and grandfather's pending death. He recalls how pained Isabella appeared the night before and purposes to suggest she talk with the spiritual care advisor connected with his unit. He also decides to talk with Kasandra about any needs she or her children might have in relation to Mr. Carballo's care and pending death.

Bereavement. Bereavement is defined as the state of being bereaved, which is to be left "desolate or alone, especially by death" (*American Heritage Dictionary*, 2006, p. 170). Rando (1984) describes bereavement as the state of having suffered a loss. McCall (1999) describes bereavement as the "overall reaction to the loss of a close relationship" and sees it as a description of various "patterns, phrases, and/or stages that an individual goes through when grieving" (p. 42). Mallinson (1999) depicts bereavement as the long-term process of the survivor's accommodating his or her life without the loved one. Bereavement is a major life event that can result in an individual's having impaired health (Charleton, 2003).

Mourning, grief, and bereavement. Mourning, grief, and bereavement often are used interchangeably. Mourning often encompasses a sociocultural dimension and involves customs and rituals that are influenced by sociocultural and religious beliefs and values. Rando (1984) differentiates among the three in the following ways: 1) grief is the response to the perception of loss and is a transitional phase in the overall process of mourning; 2) mourning is the intrapsychic processes initiated by loss; and 3) bereavement is the state of having suffered a loss (pp. 15–16).

> **Case Study follow-up:** Jake decides that he is going to write a letter of reconciliation to his father, go to his father's grave on his next day off, and read it to his father. He tells his supervisor the next day how helpful her suggestions to him were.

Meaning of the Relationship and Significance to Loss and Suffering

The intensity of loss for the dying patient and his/her significant others relates directly to each individual's perceptions of how close the relationship is and how great the loss of this relationship will be. The significance of the relationship impacts how the individual will interpret the loss and the accompanying suffering. The meaning that the patient, significant others, and nurse assign to loss and suffering also will determine how each individual faces the patient's dying and death. Interpretation of loss and suffering is unique to each individual and to each individual's particular circumstances.

Relationships fall into three categories: social, intimate, and therapeutic (Brady, 1997). Social relationships incorporate the everyday contacts individuals have, such as work colleagues and casual friends. Both individuals in this type of relationship are attempting to have their needs met. There is no particular goal within this relationship. Intimate relationships imply commitment by both individuals to one another. Therapeutic relationships involve goal-directed interaction with the purpose of helping one individual obtain an anticipated outcome to meet an identified need and facilitate growth.

The degree of intimacy and involvement within a relationship is not necessarily dependent upon the relationship's being a long-term one versus a short-term one or a blood relationship versus a non-blood relationship. Many factors determine how an individual will view his or her relationship with another individual. Some of these factors include respect, responsibility, commitment, compatibility, values, biases, beliefs, and time.

The stage of growth and development of the individual with terminal illness influences his or her ability to cope with the loss, suffering, and grief related to terminal illness. The stage of growth and development of significant others and the nurse also determine their ability to cope with the loss, suffering, grief, and bereavement related to the patient with a terminal illness. In addition, the stages of growth and development for all three groups (patient, significant others, and nurse) significantly impact how each will deal with the other.

Two of the most difficult aspects of a terminal illness are the accompanying uncertainty and unpredictability. These two factors may stress the relationships between the patient, the significant others, and the nurse. For some individuals, not knowing what is going to happen to the patient and when it might happen are difficult and unbearable aspects of coping with the patient's terminal illness.

Balancing aspects of "getting through it" and "accepting that it will take time and a lot of hard work" were critical in a study involving 39 families who each had a child diagnosed with cancer (Woodgate & Degner, 2003, p. 117). In addition, support from the family unit was considered most important for helping maintain one's spirit and keeping the family together. Families wanted to share the entire experience of their children's having cancer and not focus on symptomatology.

Some terminal conditions, such as HIV/AIDS, may not be discussed by the patient or significant others who fear stigma or repercussions. In such situations, it is imperative that the nurse understands and be ready to assist the patient and significant others in sharing the pain associated with these conditions.

Nurses, patients, and caregivers assigned similar meaning to pain in a study of patients with cancer (Ferrell, Taylor, Sattler, Fowler, & Cheyney, 1993). Although both nurses and patients viewed pain as a challenge, nurses saw the challenge to eliminate pain, whereas patients saw the challenge to live with the pain in order to obtain vitality. Caregivers greatly empathized with the patient's pain and experienced personal suffering and grief. Grief was triggered by pain, as it represented death to the caregivers.

Furthermore, an individual's view of change itself will help determine how that individual will accept loss and suffering related to his/her terminal illness. Has the individual's pattern been to welcome and embrace change or resist and fear change? The answer to that question can assist the nurse in implementing care that will help the patient and significant others to grow through the loss and suffering associated with the patient's terminal illness. Knowledge of change theory can help the advanced nurse facilitate acceptance of, and growth through, loss and suffering for the patient, significant others, and the nurse. Knowing the benefits and risks of change, change strategies, and resistance to change can help the nurse maximize the many changes within the patient's life.

ASSESSMENT—WHERE AM I (THE NURSE) ON THE JOURNEY?

In order to be an effective caregiver to the dying patient and the significant others, nurses must come to terms with their own mortality and views on dying and death. Death is an inevitable outcome of life for each individual. The death of a patient with a terminal illness forces the nurse to acknowledge that a cure cannot always be achieved. Fear related to death and dying is normal. Likewise, issues related to grief and bereavement during the death and dying process also are normal and even necessary for healthy adaptation to the preceding loss and suffering.

In American culture, individuals generally believe that explanations for dying always should be given. Furthermore, Americans feel that options to deal with the dying process always should be available (Kazanowski, 2006). This widely held belief impacts the nurse, as well as the patient and significant others, in relation to high expectations of cure, treatment, care, and avoid-

ance of a painful death. This approach is considered by some to be the "medicalization of human mortality"; this approach has limitations, however, because it cannot address psychological and spiritual factors associated with the suffering related to dying (Kissane & Bloch, 2002[S1], pp. 78–79).

Nurses are encouraged to maintain composure when caring for patients. However, professionalism for the nurse within this context does not require that the nurse deny emotional engagement with the patient and significant others during the dying process and bereavement period. It does require, however, that the nurse's needs be subordinate to the needs of the patient and significant others. Constructive self-disclosure of feelings by the nurse may role-model to others a healthy process of acknowledging and resolving the suffering of loss. The nurse may or may not actually cry with the patient and significant others. If crying occurs, the nurse needs to be able to direct this situation into a meaningful and positive one for the patient and significant others. Empathy appropriately shared in this manner may well be described as a "therapeutic tear."

Lewis (1998) describes a strategy used to assist nursing students in working with patients and significant others who are experiencing loss and grieving. The learning activity is called "Culture and Loss: A Project of Self-Reflection." Student nurses are requested to examine how their culture handles loss, to prepare a creative presentation for a small group of peers on how their culture responds to loss, and to describe to their class the meaning of their project and how it connects to their culture. Goals for implementing this strategy are identifying personal responses to loss, recognizing differing responses to loss and the influence of individual and cultural factors, and learning skills related to supporting individuals who are grieving.

Spencer (1994) examined which strategies were helpful to nurses in dealing with their own grieving. The most significant strategy noted was the nurse's informal network of peer group support. In addition, the nurses recommended formal group support and increased grief resolution training. When a team is involved, it is helpful to provide an opportunity for staff members to have open communication and to sustain and care for one another (Leichtling, 2004). There are numerous other health-promoting strategies to help the nurse cope with caring for dying patients. These include regular exercise, good nutrition, diversional activities, focus on caring rather than curing, emphasizing the positive dimensions of the nurse's role, and recalling positive experiences with families (Pritchett & Lucas, 1997).

Advances in technology have prolonged dying and death in our culture. As a result, advance directives have taken on greater significance in relation to end-of-life care. Studies have indicated that patients who have prepared advance directives select palliative care more frequently, are more accepting of death, and have less expensive care and less aggressive treatment (Danis, 1998).

There are incongruences between the ideal and reality in end-of-life care. First, clinicians are expected to be able to predict the expected time of death for a terminally ill patient; however, this involves a great deal of uncertainty. Goals of care may need to change quickly as the patient's condition changes or therapeutic trials fail. Second, it is expected that the patient's clinicians know the patient's wishes concerning dying and death. In reality, organizational factors may impact the patient's care more than the patient's wishes during the end-of-life process. Third, it is thought that the patient's care is well coordinated. Often this is not the case because some intensive-care facilities are staffed with their own primary care providers who may not know the patient admitted with a terminal illness. Therefore, it is important for the nurse to work closely with the patient and the significant others concerning the patient's priorities and wishes. Finally, the measurement of goals and outcomes may not be congruent. Measures of care for dying patients usually focus upon the frequency of DNR orders and lengths of time a patient spends on life support or in a coma. It may be more important to patients and significant others to examine issues related to pain management and satisfaction with care (Danis, 1998).

Confronting death with a terminal illness is difficult, painful, and complex. Nurses need to be strong advocates for satisfactory pain management. Keeping abreast of the patient's treatment wishes (which may change during the dying process) and coordinating care between facilities and providers also are important.

Personal Experiences with Death

Personal experiences with dying and death influence how nurses give care to those who are dying and their significant others. For example, examining personal experiences can help nurses understand their own fears and anxieties related to dying and death. Understanding the meaning and significance of relationships helps put the loss in perspective. The nurse's ability to articulate feelings regarding a good or bad death is important when working with individuals who are dying. Exploring individual values and biases can enhance the nurse's competence; this helps the nurse better understand individual's healthcare attitudes and behaviors (Warren, 1999).

Kazanowski, Perrin, Potter, and Sheehan, (2007) developed a course in which student nurses examine their personal losses in a progressive manner, both in terms of the level of difficulty and level of disclosure. The intent of the course is to assist students in coping with the suffering of patients with whom they are working, as well as the suffering they are experiencing themselves in witnessing such suffering.

Offering one's presence to patients, families, and significant others affects nurses. The impact on a nurse researcher, supervisor, and two transcribers was examined in addition to data obtained from the original sample group of 38 pregnant women in a grounded theory study exploring their experiences after hearing they had a diagnosis of fetal abnormality (Lalor, Begley, & Devane, 2006). The three themes that emerged were: bearing to watch, bearing to listen, and bearing to support. Painful stories cause strong emotional reactions to those interacting with such information (Lalor, Begley & Devane, 2006). Nurses identify sources of suffering for patients and offer their presence to help patients move through the suffering (Ferrell & Coyle, 2008).

Use the following exercises to help you expand your self-understanding in relation to loss and suffering, dying and death, and grief and bereavement.

Self-Reflective Questions

- What experiences have you had with death? Describe your earliest memory of death. Was anything positive about it? Was anything negative about it? Have you experienced what you would call a "good death?" Have you experienced what you would describe as a "bad death?"
- Can you picture yourself helping someone who is dying? How? What do you have to offer that is special and unique?
- Relate what you believe happens when someone dies. What do you fear about death? What do you fear about your own death?
- Assume you have just received news that you have been diagnosed with a terminal illness. What would be the most difficult things for you to have to give up during this time?
- How do you feel about cultural attitudes or behaviors that may be different from your own?

ASSESSMENT—WHERE IS THE PATIENT AND FAMILY ON THIS JOURNEY?

Living with and dying from a terminal illness can be best understood within the context of a continuum. One generally does not remain on a fixed point along the continuum. Like one's view of health and illness, living with and dying from terminal illness is a dynamic and fluid experience in which the individual moves back and forth across the continuum.

Reactions to dying and death vary across the life span. They also are dependent upon physical, psychological, spiritual, and sociocultural factors that impact the individual's sense of wellness. Physiological change can lead to sequelae of loss: function, body image, self-esteem, sexuality, and role competence. Furthermore, interfacing of the various factors has the potential to result in grief over lost health (Talerico, 2003). The living-dying interval occurs from the time death is acknowledged as imminent to the point of the actual death. A difficult task during this period is continuing to treat the individual as still living and as a person and not just a patient. Tasks that the individual needs to attend to are arranging his or her affairs; coping with loss (loved ones and self); attending to future care needs; planning remaining time; confronting loss of self and identity; facing one's own death encounter; deciding whether to succumb to or resist the dying process; and struggling with the psychosocial problems of dying. Some of the issues for the individual during this period include treatment choices, remissions and exacerbations, expression of sexuality, financial pressures, employment concerns, struggle for control, and suffering (Rando, 1984).

Depending on level of maturity, the patient may be confronted with the meaning of life, relationship with God and others, and the reality of death (Georgesen & Dungan, 1996). In addition, the patient may face losses related to independence, control, work, physical comfort, a sense of normalcy, sexual activity, and usefulness when living with a life-threatening condition (Ferrell et al., 1993). For example, it may be difficult for older adults who have served as caregivers to receive care from another because of loss of independence. An aid to this transition of caregiving may be to enable older adults to focus on ways they can affirm the individuals now serving as caregivers to them (Talerico, 2003).

Once rapport has been developed, the nurse may suggest that the patient and the patient's significant others consider attending a support group. Support groups have been found to be particularly helpful for significant others facing traumatic (e.g., loss of a child) or stigmatized (e.g., acquired immunodeficiency syndrome) deaths, as well as for individuals who themselves are dying (Callanan & Kelley, 1992; Goodkin et al., 1999; McCreight, 2004; Rando, 1984, Vigil & Clements, 2003).

Individual Needs

During the illness/dying trajectory, the nurse needs to assess the patient's immediate and specific needs. Certain simple pleasures may be more important to the patient than a nurse-perceived need for oxygen. For a peaceful death, a patient may need the comfort and joy that a treat, such as food or music, may represent. Asking the patient (or significant others if the patient is unable to respond) what the immediate and specific needs are may bring insight as to what intervention is needed to help the patient be more comfortable.

Maintaining some control is especially important during this time, as the patient may have had to relinquish control in many areas. Moreover, having

control over pain is critical. Patients with a terminal illness and their significant others fear lack of pain control during end-of-life care (Ferrell & Coyle, 2008; Danis, 1998).

Having a sense of order and a sense of closure in personal affairs are important aspects to address with the patient also. Sharing what one needs to say to others, through direct contact (e.g., in person or phone) or indirect contact (e.g., written communication), may help the patient have a more peaceful death.

Sensitivity to the patient's leading in this area is critical.

Areas of Assessment

Use the following questions to assess the patient on the journey living with and dying from a terminal illness in relation to loss and suffering, dying and death, and grief and bereavement.

- How do you view your illness?
- What is the meaning of your illness to you?
- What fears or concerns do you have regarding your illness?
- In what ways are you experiencing loss and suffering?
- Are there any unresolved issues or business that need to be resolved?
- Do you have any specific fears about dying and death in general? About your own dying and death?
- What concerns do you have for others now and after your death?
- What helps you maintain a sense of hope during difficult times?
- What specific needs do you have at this time?
- In what ways might I be most helpful to you in meeting those needs?

ASSESSMENT—WHERE ARE THE SIGNIFICANT OTHERS ON THE JOURNEY?

Healthy spouses of terminally ill cancer patients were studied (Siegel, Karus, Raveis, Christ, & Mesagno, 1996). Men were found to be more at risk for depressive symptoms than women if they were parents of school-aged children. Part of this could be due to their having less of a social network than women in general, and part may be due to their having to assume additional parenting responsibilities as the result of their spouse's illness and subsequent death. Overall adjustment was better for well spouses and inversely proportional to the number of children in the household. Work was perceived as both a stressor due to the demands of the job and as a stress buffer due to the potential emotional support, sense of control, and predictability it may provide for the significant other. Masculine and feminine differences have been explored more recently, as well, indicating that feminine grieving involves more talking, helpseeking, and social involvement than masculine styles of grieving, which involves solitude, self-medicating, and expression of grief through activities (McCreight, 2004; Thomas, 2004; Baum, 2003).

Elderly males have been found to be at increased risk for suicide after the death of a spouse (McCall, 1999). In general, older adults face multiple losses for numerous reasons including declining health with increasing age (Talerico, 2003).

Sherman (1998) refers to the reciprocal suffering inherent in being a family member or significant other of a patient diagnosed with a terminal illness. This suffering results from the expectations and responsibilities placed upon the significant other to care for the patient, the mutual experience of intensified needs brought about by the patient's illness, and the often rapidly changing needs of both the patient and the significant other. Quality-of-life issues arise for the family members and significant others, as well as for the patient.

Koop and Strang (1997) reviewed a number of studies to determine correlates of greater satisfaction in families of patients with a terminal illness. They found higher satisfaction in families in which there had been psychosocial support from the nurse, fulfillment of basic needs, high frequency of home visits, support at night, connection to other services, visits to the bereaved caregiver, choices in treatments, privacy during hospitalizations, treatment of respiratory symptoms, the presence of professional caregivers (especially if the patient is at home), and participation in a hospice program.

There is interdependence between the patient, the significant others, and the nurse in relation to providing optimal care for the patient with a terminal illness. The nurse can maximize the positive aspects of this interdependence by recognizing and affirming the patient's significant others, incorporating them into the patient's care as desired by the patient, and assisting the significant others in their loss, suffering, and grief related to the patient's dying and death. Kissane and Bloch (2002[S2]) recognized the influence of family in Reiss' (1990) study on renal disease, claiming, "This research highlights the potential influence of the family on both the course of illness and survival" (p. 26). Woodgate and Degner (2003) note in their research of children with cancer that, "It is important for those involved in the care to recognize that maintaining the family unit was equally important to families as was beating the child's cancer" (p. 117). In addition, the patient's significant others will experience bereavement issues once the patient dies. Research by Jordan and Neimeyer (2003) demonstrates that "With the help of family and friends, apparently most mourners are able to work through and integrate their losses relatively well" (p. 772).

How does one know when the patient is ready to die? Four types or stages of death occur, usually in the following order: social death, psychological death, biological death, and physiological death (Sudnow, 1967). Social death marks the narrowing of the patient's world, as he has known it. This is a highly individualized stage that is dependent upon the patient's level of involvement versus detachment in his social world. Psychological death is a death of the patient's personality. Relationships change. The patient withdraws and distances himself or herself from others. Terminal illness places demands that result in the patient's becoming regressed and dependent. Biological death involves the loss of consciousness and awareness on a self-sustaining basis; the patient may be on life supports at this point. Finally, physiological death occurs. All vital organs cease to function (Rando, 1984). At this point, a nurse or physician (depending upon state law) pronounces death. The moment of finality has arrived. Life as the patient and the significant others knew it for the patient has ceased.

Relationships

Support from significant others can aid in decision making and acceptance of death for a patient with a terminal illness. Patients and their significant others may determine together whether they want to pursue life-sustaining procedures or to forgo them in light of the uncertainty and potential trauma that surround the situation. Close communication with the nurse during end-of-life care is essential because the needs of the patient and care planned for him are apt to change rapidly. Patients and their significant others may change their minds concerning treatments depending upon the patient's level of consciousness, the patient's pain level, both the patient's and significant others' fear levels, additional troublesome symptomatology for the patient, failure of therapeutic trials, and the level of support and contact between the patient and his significant others (Danis,1998).

Significant others who care for a terminally ill patient are faced with increased feelings of powerlessness, anger, and grief when the patient's pain is unrelieved (Ferrell & Coyle, 2008; Ferrell et al., 1993). Danis (1998) found that families of deceased patients indicate that more attention should be given to analgesia and communication in end-of-life care. Significant others may or may not provide direct care to the patient. They may have other resources, hired or voluntary, to provide caregiving to the patient. If significant others are providing care, they will be at risk for burnout or fatigue. A proactive approach in order to prevent this should be in place in the patient's care plan.

Areas of Assessment

- Determine with significant others what they perceive as the patient's needs.
- Provide education in pain assessment and pain management strategies.

- Assess how the significant others feel they are doing and what degree of loss and suffering they are currently experiencing.
- What types of secondary losses are being experienced or anticipated as a result of the primary loss (i.e., anticipatory death or actual death of the patient)?
- Determine the level of emotional support needed.
- Ascertain if spiritual support is desired.
- Assure significant others that they are not an imposition to professionals who also are providing care for the patient.
- Identify available resources to help significant others care for the patient.
- Encourage significant others to grieve in whatever ways are best for them.

NORMAL GRIEF

Grief is a normal response to loss. Grief may become manifest in feelings, physical sensations, cognition, and behaviors (see Table 11.3). Psychological, sociocultural, and physical factors influence the grief reaction. The nurse needs to assess which factors are influencing the significant others. Rando (1984, pp. 43–57) addresses these influences as follows:

Psychological factors:

- Significance of the loss
- Attachment level
- Family role of the deceased
- Individual coping behaviors, such as avoidance, distraction, preoccupation, impulsivity, rationalization, intellectualization, prayer, and connection with others
- Intelligence and maturity levels
- Previous experience with death and loss
- Conditioned sex roles
- Age of the individual grieving
- Age and characteristics of the deceased
- The death of a parent representing loss of the past
- The death of a spouse representing loss of the present
- The death of a child representing loss of the future (The death of a child may be the most difficult death to handle.)
- Unattended business between the griever and the deceased
- Perception of fulfilled life for deceased
- Circumstances related to death including location, type, reason, and preparedness
- Timing of the death (Is the death psychologically acceptable?)
- Perception of death's prevention
- Sudden or anticipated death
- Chronic versus acute illness
- Impact of anticipatory grief on the relationship with the dying patient
- Impact of secondary losses
- Additional stresses or crises

Social factors:

- Level, acceptance, timing, and duration of support
- Religious, sociocultural, ethnic, and philosophical backgrounds
- Bereaved's educational, economic, and occupational status
- Positive or negative funeral rituals.

Physiological factors:

- Positive and negative impact of medications
- Need for nutrition, sleep and rest, exercise, and physical health

In addition, grief may be mistaken for un-diagnosed depression. A way to distinguish between the two is to note whether the individual in question is able to experience pleasure. Grieving individuals can experience pleasure; depressed individuals often have difficulty experiencing pleasure and may lose morale and hope (Kissane & Bloch, 2002).

CHILD'S EXPERIENCE OF LOSS

The death of a parent impacts a child greatly. Family life and daily routine are disrupted permanently. A child may have a depressed mood, cry, be sad or irritable, withdraw, or have sleep disturbances during the first 4 months after the loss of a parent. Physical, behavioral, and emotional responses occur immediately for young children. Although infants and toddlers are not at a developmental stage to be able to comprehend loss or death, they are distraught that someone important to them is absent (Hames, 2003). A child's reaction may be impacted by individual personality factors, sociocultural factors, the child's age, child's history, child's religious beliefs, family dynamics, family's socioeconomic status, sex of the child and the remaining parent, additional stress in the child's life, parental substitutes, nature of the death, and how the child was notified (Geis, Whittlesey, McDonald, Smith, & Pfefferbaum, 1998).

Children who have lost a parent, especially by suicide, are at risk for anxiety, depression, and social problems. Regression may occur temporarily. Having a baseline of a child's behaviors is important when discerning whether there is a serious problem. Suicide bereavement is compounded by the stigma and lack of social support oftentimes in such circumstances (Mitchell et al., 2007)

Caregivers must recognize the importance of age in relation to a child's ability to experience loss and grief. Saldinger, Cain, and Porterfield (2003) note that children may have a very difficult experience with anticipatory grief if they are expected to demonstrate levels of "self-sacrifice" that exceed their "levels of maturity" (p. 175). The ELNEC curriculum provides a table of children's ages and expected grief reactions that can be valuable to caregivers (see Table 11.4).

11.4 | Grief and Bereavement in Children

BIRTH TO 6 MONTHS		
CHARACTERISTICS OF AGE	**VIEW OF DEATH AND RESPONSE**	**WHAT HELPS**
Basic needs must be met, cries if needs are not met. Needs emotional and physical closeness of a consistent caregiver. Derives identify from caregiver. View of caregiver as source of comfort and all needs fulfillment.	Has no concept of death. Experiences death like any other separation—no sense of "finality." Nonspecific expressions of distress (crying). Reacts to loss of caregiver. Reacts to caregiver's distress.	Progressively disengage child from primary caregiver if possible. Introduce a new primary caregiver. Nurturing, comforting. Anticipate physical and emotional needs and provide them. Maintain routines.
6 MONTHS TO 2 YEARS		
CHARACTERISTICS OF AGE	**VIEW OF DEATH AND RESPONSE**	**WHAT HELPS**
Begins to individuate. Remembers face of caregiver when absent. Demonstrates full range of emotions. Identifies caregiver as source of good feelings and interactions.	May see death as reversible. Experiences bona fide grief. Grief response only to death of significant person in child's life. Screams, panics, withdraws, becomes disinterested in food, toys, activities. Reacts in concert with distress experienced by caregiver. No control over feelings and responses; anticipate regressive behavior.	Needs continual support, comfort. Avoid separation from significant others. Close physical and emotional connections by significant others. Maintain daily structure and schedule of routine activities. Support caregiver to reduce distress and maintain a stable environment. Acknowledge sadness that loved one will not return—offer comfort.
2 YEARS TO 5 YEARS		
CHARACTERISTICS OF AGE	**VIEW OF DEATH AND RESPONSE**	**WHAT HELPS**
Egocentric. Cause-effect not understood. Developing conscience. Developing trust. Attributes life to objects. Feelings expressed mostly by behaviors. Can recall events from past.	Sees death like sleep: reversible. Believes in magical causes. Has sense of loss. Curiosity, questioning. Anticipate regression, clinging. Aggressive behavior common. Worries about who will care for him/her.	Remind that loved one will not return. Give realistic information, answer questions. Involve in "farewell" ceremonies. Encourage questions and expression of feelings. Keep home environment stable, structured. Help put words to feelings; reassure/comfort. Reassure child about who will take care of him/her; provide ways to remember the loved one.

The degree of attachment also impacts how a child will respond to the loss of a parent. Stroebe (2002) found that individuals who had a more secure attachment to the lost figure had a more fluid movement between loss and restoration orientations and experienced less complications with grieving.

Case Study follow-up: Teresa, age 7, and Alberto, age 5, had been at their Lita's (Spanish nickname for grandmother) wake about 6 months earlier. They remembered that her body was "cold" and "hard" when they touched her. Both Teresa and Alberto put one of their favorite toys in the coffin to take with her in "her new home in Heaven." Teresa remembered how Lita used to take their faces in her hands and tell them how much she loved them. She was sad and cried at Lita's wake. Alberto did not seem to grasp totally what was happening but started to cry when he saw Teresa crying and had asked when Lita would wake up.

Children often experience separation anxiety after the death of a parent. Coming to terms with surviving in a world without the presence of the deceased parent can be traumatic for the child. Secondary to that trauma may be the additional stress of observing a surviving parent cope with the loss or the anticipated loss if such were the case (Saldinger et al., 2003). Nurses can help a dying parent communicate with children who will be left behind; this can enhance meaning and comfort to the dying by making a contribution to their child's journey with grief. Likewise, a surviving parent inadvertently becomes a role model for grieving to children left behind by a deceased parent (Hames, 2003).

If a child loses a sibling, other issues, such as guilt, ambivalence, denial, increased vulnerability, and fear for his/her own well-being, may arise. Parental response to surviving siblings helps determine the child's adjustment. Similar responses may occur for adolescents with possible reframing of the adolescent's self-concept, self-identity, and family role (Geis et al., 1998). Tasks that occur for all siblings of a deceased child, regardless of age, include grieving the deceased sibling, coping with family changes, realigning relationships, and attempting to understand the meaning of the tragedy within the family (Kiser, Ostoja, & Pruitt, 1998). Research related to the loss of a sibling through suicide indicated that younger siblings living at home experience a more difficult time than either older siblings or parents; intervention resources frequently are focused upon parents (Dyregrov & Dyregrov, 2005).

Areas of Assessment

- How is the child functioning socially according to his or her developmental level? What is the child's involvement in relationships, recreation, and routines?
- Is the child exhibiting any changed behaviors?
- What is the child's predominant mood (sad, withdrawn, hyperactive, angry)?
- How does the child express his or her suffering or "pain" related to the loss?
- What does the child feel might help make the "pain" better (besides the return of the lost loved one)?

FAMILY CAREGIVING—PARENTAL EXPERIENCE OF LOSS

Living with dying can tax a patient and his significant others economically, as well as physically, spiritually, and psychologically. Often, the patient or his significant others lose work time because of the patient's care requirements. Additional expenses may arise with treatments, hospitalizations, or other hidden expenses, such as transportation, child care, out-of-home food purchases, lodging, and so forth. Dying patients often experience much stress because of the financial burdens that fall upon the significant others (Rando, 1984). If the nurse feels unprepared to counsel the patient and significant others in this area, it is imperative to refer them to someone who can.

The loss of a child often is devastating to the parents and to the family. Parents feel responsible for their child's health, well-being, and safety. In the case of a newborn with a serious condition, there is accompanying parental blame and guilt for the infant's condition. Parents must grieve the healthy, "normal" child they lost in addition to the anticipated death of the infant.

Parents usually do not expect their child to die. This is true even in the case of adult children who die before parents. Older adults may experience "survivor guilt, powerlessness, and loss of religious faith"; the deceased child may be idealized, which can complicate grief resolution (Talerico, 2003, p. 14).

Grief related to the loss of a child is apt to be severe and complicated. Anniversary events and developmental milestones for the deceased child reopen the grief experience throughout the parents' lifetime (Kiser et al., 1998). Acknowledging that their lives have changed forever is part of the grief resolution that takes place for

parents; however, recovery from the death of a child is a lifelong process (Geis et al., 1998). For the single parent, aloneness may be magnified (Backer et al., 1994). Controversy exists about parents' viewing prenatally deceased infants and stillborn infants; in general, viewing the body is thought to help with grieving (Haas, 2003). Nurses must be sensitive to family members' readiness and wishes related to viewing the body of their deceased loved one.

Areas of Assessment

- How has your loved one's illness impacted your life?
- In what ways will you remember your child who died?
- What is the most significant type of suffering you are experiencing right now?
- What are your specific needs at this time and how can I help you meet them?

GERONTOLOGIC GRIEF

Parker et al., (2002) have asserted that successful aging involves achieving competency in four distinct areas. They include the following:

- Engaging in life actively
- Maximizing cognitive and physical function
- Preventing disease and disability
- Experiencing spirituality in relation to developmental processes.

However, what happens when one does become ill, either physically or mentally, or acquires chronic illness and/or disability? Hardiness can assist older adults as they age with diagnoses, such as HIV; hardiness includes factors, such as control, commitment, and challenge (Vance, Burrage, Couch, & Raper, 2008). Obstacles may become perceived as opportunities. Although there are conflicting reports, more research is needed to determine if an association exists between hardiness and immunological responsiveness in adults with HIV (Vance et al., 2008).

Recognizing whether an older adult is grieving or depressed is important. Although an older adult may deny feeling sad or depressed, it is important to look for additional signs of depression, such as the following:

- Complaints of unexplained aches and pains
- Expressions of hopelessness or helplessness
- Symptoms of anxiety
- Memory impairment
- Loss of pleasure
- Decreased movement
- Irritability
- Forgetful of meals, personal hygiene, or taking medications (Segal, Jaffe, Davies, & Smith, 2007).

RISK FACTORS FOR COMPLICATED GRIEF

Predicting bereavement outcomes is difficult because the subjects are considered to be a vulnerable study population. A balance between the need for protection and the benefits of participation must be attained. Studies increasingly suggest that the greatest predictor of well-being during bereavement is prior well-being (Koop & Strang, 1997). The persistence of what some perceive as negative emotions of grieving, namely, disbelief, yearning, anger, and depression, may be an additional predictor of the need for intervention (Maciejewski et al., 2007).

Although each individual's grieving is unique, the bereavement process may be functional or dysfunctional, adaptive or maladaptive. The time for grief resolution has varied from peaks at 4 months to as long as 3 years (Lev & McCorkle, 1998). Prolonged reactions occur in approximately 15% of the bereaved. These prolonged reactions range from exaggerated normal reactions to abnormal grief reactions. Furthermore, grief may be unresolved or compounded if a loss or losses occur within a community of individuals where the losses are minimized or ignored; this may result in further complications with subsequent losses (Talerico, 2003).

Backer et al. (1994) describe three basic types of complicated grief reactions: delayed, inhibited, and chronic grief. In delayed grief, the grief is triggered by the loss of someone or something else. There is minimal impact in this situation. For example, someone whose father has recently died may experience delayed grief related to the death of the individual's mother 10 years prior to the father's death. The individual has never experienced full grief for the death of the mother until the death of the father. His death triggers the deeply felt but unexpressed loss of the mother. Inhibited grief occurs when an individual never grieves. It also may occur if the individual feels great distress related to a lost relationship. This type of grief becomes complicated if another condition develops related to the unfelt grief. Last, chronic grief exists when the grieving is unending, and the intense yearning for the lost relationship continues. A cause for this type of grief could be unspeakable deaths, such as those due to AIDS or suicide.

Rando (1984) addresses delayed, inhibited, and chronic grief reactions but also includes absent grief, conflicted grief, unanticipated grief, and abbreviated grief in her list of complicated grief types. Absent grief is characterized by a total lack of grief emotions and processes of mourning. Conflicted grief involves an amplification of the characteristics of normal grief partnered with a suppression of other manifestations of normal grief. Unanticipated grief takes place after an unexpected loss that the individual cannot grasp. Abbreviated grief is normal grief that lasts a short period of time because of swift replacement of the lost individual or lack of attachment to the lost individual. One study (Prigerson et al., 1997) identifies grief involving

trauma and separation as traumatic grief and indicates that psychiatric sequelae, such as traumatic grief, puts bereaved individuals at risk for complicated grief.

Families grieve in a unique way. Family members all fill unique roles. A lost family member means the family must reassign the lost role. Likewise, families may distort circumstances through idealization, blame, anger, or despair. Families who do not share their grief may experience poor coping or breakdown (Kissane & Bloch, 2002).

There are a number of individuals at risk for complicated grief after the death of an individual with a terminal illness. These include spouses, parents, those experiencing the loss of loved ones through unspeakable deaths, and those with a psychiatric history. Male spouses are more at risk than female spouses because of more limited social networks. Men often feel responsible to be the stronger partner (McCreight, 2004). In her study related to pregnancy loss, McCreight (2004) also found that men did not experience bereavement through "an intellectualization of the process of grief" (p. 346), but rather experienced loss on an emotional level. Furthermore, single parents are at higher risk because of less support. In addition, those diagnosed with depression are at the highest risk for complicated grief (Kurtz, Kurtz, Given, & Given, 1997).

Work done by Pennebaker, Mayne, and Francis (1997) indicates that language usage can help to impact bereavement outcomes in a positive way. Encouraging individuals to talk about traumatic events forces a disorganized event and emotions to become more organized, coherent, and insightful. Over time, the use of insight and causation words in relation to the event and its accompanying emotions helps cognitively reframe the experience, which results in more adaptive outcomes.

Frank, Prigerson, Shear, and Reynolds (1997) postulate that individuals experiencing prolonged periods of distress (for several months) and exhibiting criteria for major depressive episodes are undergoing traumatic grief reactions. They advocate treatment interventions that involve re-experiencing the moment of death, saying good-bye to the deceased while still retaining special memories of the person, and gradually being exposed to situations that the bereaved has avoided since the deceased's death. The outcome of this traumatic grief treatment has been reduced subjective distress. They do not advocate for pathologizing or treating brief periods of bereavement-related distress.

A number of factors were examined in a study attempting to predict depressive symptomatology in the post-bereavement period (Kurtz et al., 1997). Pre-bereavement depressive symptomatology scores, levels of support from friends, and caregiver optimism were most predictive of post-bereavement depressive symptomatology. The link between pre-bereavement and post-bereavement depressive symptomatology scores was anticipated. The role of optimism is important for nurses to capitalize on and strengthen when working with significant others. The connection between high social support in the pre-bereavement period from friends and post-bereavement depressive symptomatology was strong. This phenomenon could be caused by altered or lost relationships due to the dying and death of the spouse. Possibly, friends experience a social death before the physical death of the bereaved's spouse.

Poor bereavement outcomes are likely to occur if the death is unexpected, untimely, or traumatic for the bereaved, such as with homicide or suicide (Vigil & Clements, 2003). Moreover, maladaptive grieving may occur if the significant other had an ambivalent or dependent relationship with the deceased, perceives their social networks as unsupportive, and is experiencing concurrent loss. Family coping styles that negatively impact outcomes are 1) hostile (high conflict, low cohesiveness, and poor expressiveness); 2) sullen (limited but less in comparison with the hostile group); and 3) intermediate (intermediate cohesiveness and low control and achievement orientation). Additional correlates for poor outcome include use of medications or alcohol, concern for self, level of contentment, and not viewing the deceased's body. Positive bereavement outcomes are more likely to occur in families who are supportive (high cohesion) and resolve conflict well (Kissane, Bloch, & MacKenzie 1997[S3]).

In more dysfunctional grieving situations, the advanced nurse practitioner must treat symptoms of pathological grief. Three major symptom categories of pathological grief would be intrusion, denial, and dysfunctional adaptation (Horowitz, Bonanno, & Holen, 1993). Spending long periods idealizing the memory of the deceased is a sign of an intrusive thought process. Living as if the deceased were still alive for more than 6 months is evidence of denial. Minimal dysfunction is evidenced in having difficulty making decisions, whereas major dysfunction is evidenced in more severe impairments. Such severe dysfunctional parameters would involve extreme fatigue or somatic symptoms that last more than 1 month; inability to resume work, other interests, routines, and other responsibilities after more than 1 month; and reluctance to develop new relationships after 13 months of grieving (Lev & McCorkle, 1998, p. 147).

Use the following exercises to expand your understanding of helping the patient's significant others on their journey with the patient who is living and dying with a terminal illness in relation to suffering and loss, death and dying, and grief and bereavement:

Exercise I—Discuss how you might feel and what you might do if you were the nurse who walked into a patient's room just as he has died and his family or significant others are there.

Exercise II—A family member who has been estranged from the dying patient on your floor is in the room as you come in to check on the patient who is unconscious. The family member says, "He wasn't a very good father. He abused my sister and me. I'll be glad when he's dead." How would you respond to this family member?

Exercise III—You are the clinical nurse specialist heading up the first meeting of nursing staff since a patient on your floor died from cancer. What would be your objectives for the meeting?

CONTEXT OF CAREGIVING AND RELATED INTERVENTIONS

Working with the patient who is living with and dying from a terminal illness and that person's significant others requires compassion, skill, energy, sensitivity, and patience. Compassion promotes a positive connection between the nurse and the patient and the significant others. Skill gives the nurse credibility in working with them. Energy, often in the form of providing hope for the moment, moves the patient and significant others forward when they feel like giving up. Sensitivity enhances understanding and rapport in the relationships. Patience allows individuals the time needed to face and plan for an uncertain and unpredictable future.

The nurse attempts to help meet the needs of the patient and the significant others. Addressing immediate needs may take on greater significance with the patient experiencing a terminal illness than addressing either short-term or long-term needs. Values, control issues, and goals of both the patient and significant others need to be taken into consideration, addressed directly, and handled tactfully and sensitively.

The nurse has a unique window into the patient's circumstances. Depending on the setting, nurses may provide 24-hour care. Even if nursing coverage is not for 24 direct-care hours, nursing care may be accessible for that period. Generally, it is the nurse who gets the most consistent, current, and constant view of what is actually happening with the patient and significant others. With few exceptions, the nurse usually is the most readily available and informed team player to help coordinate the patient's care.

Developing goals with the patient and family provides some stability and security during this time. It can empower the patient and the significant others to take an active role in planning the patient's remaining earthbound journey, uncertain and unpredictable as it may be. Furthermore, it helps set the stage for the continuing connection between the nurse and the patient's family in the bereavement period following the patient's death.

Nurse

Nurses care for themselves by seeking support from colleagues, ensuring time for themselves by maintaining healthy boundaries with the patient and significant others, and tending to their own physical, emotional, sociocultural, and spiritual needs. After a patient's death, nurses may work through their grief by attending the memorial service or funeral for the deceased patient if this is deemed acceptable by the nurse's employing agency policy and the deceased patient's family. Sending a sympathy card to significant others, doing follow-up bereavement work with significant others, and reminiscing about the deceased patient with empathic colleagues usually help nurses in dealing with their own grief.

> **Case Study follow-up:** Jake met once more with his supervisor and felt better able to be objective again. Jake affirmed Isabella and Kasandra in their care and concern for their father and Kasandra in her concern for their brother. He suggested to Mr. Carballo's daughters that it might be helpful to meet with the unit's spiritual care advisor to help them as they traveled on this difficult journey of watching their father dying. Jake also suggested they meet with the medical ethics committee to explore the best ways to make decisions concerning their father's care. He also shared with them that he thought their bringing in pictures of Mr. and Mrs. Carballo had been meaningful to him in providing care for Mr. Carballo. He asked if there were anything he could do for them and said he would be available to talk with them if they wished.

Nursing Interventions

Nurses are accustomed to action-oriented, "doing for" interventions. However, when intervening with the patient with a terminal illness, the nurse's role may be less action-oriented. At the end of life, nursing interventions involve more "being with" the patient and "caring" instead of "doing for" the patient and "curing" (Rando, 1984).

Given that so many American deaths occur in hospitals, the nurse is most likely to be with the patient and significant others at the exact time of death. Becoming comfortable with viewing the dying and death process, touching the deceased's body, talking with significant others about the death and their feelings, and dealing with the patient's death among staff are important aspects with which the nurse will be confronted.

The nurse's relationship with the patient will be critical in determining how she or he handles grief and bereavement in relation to the patient's dying and death. Was it a short-term nurse-patient relationship or did the nurse have a professional relationship with the patient for an extended period of time? In addition, how comfortable does the nurse feel sharing feelings, and how appropriate is it to share feelings with the patient? Nurses need to answer for themselves what the goal is of sharing their feelings and what the expected outcome is of doing so before proceeding.

Johns (2007) contends that reflection is a helpful practice to respond to a patient's suffering. He suggests that reflection should be structured and guided to maximize benefits and deepen attainment of the kind of healthcare provider one wants to be during a patient's suffering. He also encourages construction of the story that is taking place to discover meaning and insight related to the total experience.

Level of intervention by the nurse will be based on professional skills, theoretical background, and clinical setting. The nurse will develop therapeutic relationships; ensure the patient's physical comfort to maintain function; explore the meaning of physical suffering and loss with the patient and significant others; reframe the patient's limitations to identify areas of value that will enhance the patient's quality of life; encourage patient and significant others' attendance at support groups; and identify and maximize prior coping skills of the patient and the significant others. Advanced practice nurses will offer more intensive and extensive interventions for grieving and bereavement needs and be involved in conducting or participating in research studies. For example, the advanced practice nurse may prescribe various medications, offer individual or family counseling, lead a bereavement group, or conduct research on quality of life and quality of dying outcomes.

Patient

Each patient who is living with and dying from a terminal illness is unique. His or her experiences living with and dying from terminal illness also are unique. A critical factor in promoting good nursing care of this patient and significant others is affirming this uniqueness. Affirming the individual's growth and wholeness during this difficult living-dying interval is critical (Georgesen & Dungan, 1996; Talerico, 2003). Empowering patients to integrate the living-dying experience and optimize their quality of life will affirm the patient further.

For example, the patient is affirmed when the nurse acknowledges the patient's level of acceptance of dying and death. The patient's acceptance or denial may seem selective at times. In reality, varying levels of acceptance or denial may serve an adaptive function in which only specific aspects of dying are tolerable at a given point in time. The patient is aided when the nurse accepts and supports the patient's coping in this way to deal with the extensive and intensive challenges during the living-dying interval (Kastenbaum, 1997). False reassurances prevent patients from accepting reality; the nurse must be honest and not foster false pretenses (Matzo et al., 2003).

Medical science has limitations, and often patients feel dehumanized during some medical procedures. In addition to addressing comfort needs, patients need assurance that their humanity will be respected and valued. The nursing profession has reawakened to the importance of integrating spiritual care within total patient care. Patients have indicated that their spiritual needs are best met through nurses' listening to, talking with, supporting religious practices of, and being with them (O'Neill & Kenny, 1998). Even in the midst of suffering through the loss of physical well-being, patients may sense spiritual well-being. Buckwalter (2003) refers to "moments of ministry" or "ministry of the moment" as those times when nurses or others assist patients in a "holy moment of connection," especially for someone who may be experiencing profound memory loss (p. 22). If a nurse feels inadequate or uncomfortable assisting dying patients in this area in any way, a pastoral care referral may be indicated. In addition, the patient may desire to have clergy closely involved even if the nurse is comfortable meeting the patient's spiritual needs.

Saying good-bye is painful for the patient with a terminal illness, for his significant others, and for the nurse. Discerning when (timing) and how (tone) to say and facilitate others' saying good-bye takes sensitivity (touch, emotional, and, physical) and skill (training/technique) on the nurse's part. This intervention can be illustrated as follows:

Discernment of readiness to facilitate good-byes = nurse sensitivity (touch) + skill (training/technique) + when (timing) + how (tone)

An important question to ask when caring for the patient who is dying from and living with a terminal illness is "What type of patient has the disease, rather than what type of disease does the patient have?" (Harris, 1991, p. 111). Respecting and affirming the patient as a unique and valuable human being will help promote wholeness during a time of brokenness. As the individual is faced with imminent death, she or he must reorient her or his life to adapt to this realization and the accompanying losses. Minimizing losses due to isolation, rejection, and loss of control can decrease the individual's suffering (Rando, 1984). Optimizing patients' strengths is essential in helping them achieve the quality of life they would like to pursue in this living-dying interval.

Chronic sorrow is the "periodic recurrence of permanent, pervasive sadness or other grief related feelings associated with a significant loss" (Eakes et al., 1998, p. 179). Chronic sorrow may be triggered if the individual senses a disparity with norms. For example, the individual may feel different from others. Situations such as hospitalization accentuate this discrepancy to the individual. Both patients and significant others may experience chronic sorrow.

Counseling can assist individuals with chronic sorrow by helping the individual anticipate trigger events and reinforce effective internal and external management strategies. Internal strategies would be continuing involvement in interests and activities, having a positive attitude, focusing on one day at a time, and emphasizing the positive aspects in the individual's life. External

strategies are those provided by healthcare professionals that view chronic sorrow as a normal experience for individuals dealing with chronic, life-threatening illness. Interventions found to be helpful by patients and their significant others include listening, being supportive and reassuring, addressing feelings, and affirming the uniqueness of each patient and significant other (Eakes et al., 1998). The nurse may advocate for a patient with a terminal illness by employing the following interventions: advancement of grief work, encouraging health-promoting strategies despite a compromised health state, making referrals, meeting with significant others, utilizing cognitive reframing of negative patterns, and engaging the patient in individual or group therapy to work through unresolved situations. The nurse may be asked to work with support staff and significant others to help them accept, support, and devise strategies to work with a patient or significant other who has a dysfunctional approach to suffering and loss.

However, the most meaningful "intervention" that may be provided to a patient with a terminal illness is the gift of presence. Presence validates one's existence amidst the experience of suffering (Lavoie, Blondeau, & De Koninck, 2008).

Family and/or Significant Others

The term "family" will be used to represent both family and significant others. The family of a patient dying from and living with a terminal illness experiences great turmoil and disequilibrium. Often, the illness becomes the focal point of family activity and organization. If the patient is a child and has siblings, the family struggles at maintaining life within the household, as well as preparing for the death of one of its members. The child simultaneously may be growing in many ways while dying in others. Treatment programs and appointments may consume much of the family's energy, possibly for extended periods. Helping the family maintain a sense of normalcy and balance throughout this period will be an important task for the nurse. Keeping the family as involved as possible in the patient's care applies to the patient with a terminal illness of any age (Matzo et al., 2003; Rando, 1984).

The question of where the patient and family would like the anticipated death to occur must be answered. With shortened hospital stays, families have been forced to assume extended and at times intensive care responsibilities for the dying patient in addition to their usual role expectations and demands. Helping the patient and family decide where and when care will take place becomes an important goal (Lev & McCorkle, 1998). The patient may wish to die at home, in a hospice setting, in a hospital, or another setting. Assisting the patient and family to communicate what they each can handle at different stages of the patient's dying will be critical.

A family's response to the patient's death is as unique as the individuals making up the family constellation. A family may seek or need to be referred for counseling if maladaptive symptoms develop. Family bereavement therapy involves assessing the circumstances related to the family member's death; the role of the deceased in the family before and after death; timing of the death in relation to family member's stage of growth and development; previous and current levels of family functioning; the context of the death; and the meaning assigned by the family to the death (Kiser et al., 1998, p. 97). There is little scientific evidence related to the impact of formal interventions with those bereaved; one reason for this may be that uncomplicated grieving resolves on its own (Jordan & Neimeyer, 2003). Jordan and Neimeyer further assert there is more evidence to support relational contexts of therapy (i.e., friends and family) over medical interventions (i.e., psychology or psychiatry) for those bereaved because those aspects promote hope and learning new coping skills.

However, the nurse must now focus attention on helping significant others begin the tasks of bereavement: accepting the reality of the loss, experiencing the pain of grief, adjusting to an environment without the deceased and reinvesting energy into other relationships (Worden, 1991). Backer et al. (1994, p. 165) have identified guidelines for counseling the bereaved as follows:

1) Help actualize the loss by talking about the loss.
2) Identify and express feelings related to the loss.
3) Help the bereaved in decision making.
4) Facilitate emotional withdrawal and development of new relationships.
5) Provide time to grieve and be cognizant of holidays and anniversary dates.
6) Reassure the bereaved that their behavior is normal and that they are not abnormal because of their feelings.
7) Allow for individual differences in the bereavement process.
8) Provide support.
9) Examine individual defenses and coping styles (be aware of problems with alcohol or other substance abuse).
10) Identify pathological behaviors and refer to treatment.

The length of time for intense grief to be resolved varies from individual to individual. As long as the bereaved's grieving behavior does not interfere significantly with their physiological or psychosocial functioning, it is not considered abnormal. In general, intense responses to grief generally subside in about 6 to 12 months (Rando, 1984). Grieving, however, continues throughout the bereaved's life. The loss, in some cases, may be replaced, but in all cases, it is never recovered.

Grief can inflict a woundedness of spirit, much different than a physical wound, that calls for the nurse to wait patiently versus debride quickly and that allows the body and soul to heal (Moules et al., 2007).

The living-dying interval comes to an end with the death of the patient, yet how does one know when grieving ends, or in a contemporary view, if grieving is moving forward, for the bereaved? Parkes and Weiss (1983) identified 10 major areas for assessment of recovery:

1) Functioning has returned to a level equal to or better than before bereavement.
2) Outstanding problems are being solved.
3) Acceptance of the loss has occurred.
4) Socialization is as effective as before the death.
5) The future is viewed positively and realistically.
6) General health is at pre-bereavement level.
7) Anxiety or depression levels are appropriate.
8) Guilt or anger levels are appropriate.
9) Self-esteem levels are appropriate.
10) Coping with future loss is feasible.

The process of bereavement varies from individual to individual. For some, total resolution may never occur (Krueger, 2006; Rando, 1984) or may occur in ways unfamiliar to the nurse. Through appropriate interventions, the nurse can help the bereaved adapt to their loss in a way that will foster their growth and wholeness as well. The nurse might determine with the bereaved if she/he is in a loss-oriented process or a restoration-oriented process and adapt nursing interventions accordingly (Stroebe & Schut, 2001).

CONCLUSION

Living with and dying from a terminal illness results in many losses—for the patient, for the family, and for the nurse. Terminal illness can occur over an extended period or a brief period. The nurse functions as both facilitator and participant in this process. The nurse also can add objectivity while the patient and family resolve many feelings, issues, and decisions related to the living-dying experience.

This period frequently involves suffering in multiple dimensions. The nurse can utilize technical skills to alleviate certain attributes of the suffering, such as the patient's physical pain. When these technical skills are accompanied by the nurse's sensitivity, compassion, empathy, and presence, the patient and family are better equipped to face the other attributes of suffering as well. Thus, the nurse, as a caring professional, may contribute meaningfully to the health and wholeness of the patient and his/her family through one of life's most challenging and difficult transitions.

Case Study conclusion: On day 10, Mr. Carballo went into cardiac arrest. Isabella and Kasandra were in the room at the time and called for help. There was no DNR recorded for Mr. Carballo at that time. He underwent cardiopulmonary resuscitation (CPR) and cardioversion. He sustained two fractured ribs and a punctured liver during that procedure. Mr. Carballo was placed on a respirator.

Isabella and Kasandra expressed guilt to Jake. Jake encouraged the daughters once again to see the medical ethics committee. Jake reported to his supervisor that he also felt guilty that he had not insisted that the daughters go to the medical ethics committee sooner. Jake's supervisor reminded Jake of patient/family choice in such matters and reminded him of the good care he was providing for Mr. Carballo and his family, including giving them constructive options for Mr. Carballo's care.

Isabella and Kasandra met with the medical ethics committee on day 11. They concurred with the committee's recommendation to have a DNR order placed in Mr. Carballo's chart. They discussed the possibility of withdrawing Mr. Carballo's respirator, but could not make a decision about that during the meeting.

Isabella and Kasandra also requested an appointment with the unit's spiritual advisor and met with her on day 12. They worked on feelings of anger related to their brother Bob's decision not to come until after Mr. Carballo's death. They discussed their discomfort about withdrawing the respirator but were thinking they might do so the next day.

On day 12, Isabella and Kasandra met at 8:00 a.m. in Mr. Carballo's room. They told him they loved him and that they did not want to see him suffer any more. They told him they hoped he would understand why they were going to withdraw his respirator. They each kissed him on the forehead and said a personal good-bye. They turned to go to the nurses' station, heard an alarm, looked up, and saw a straight line on the cardiac monitor. They immediately called for a nurse. Mr. Carballo was pronounced dead on day 12 at 8:17 a.m. The daughters looked at each other, hugged one another, and cried.

Jake was off duty that day. One of his colleagues called him, but he did not receive the message on his home phone machine until later that night. He sat in his favorite chair and reflected on the care he had given Mr. Carballo and his family. In a few days, Jake was part of a medical ethics review of Mr. Carballo's care in terms

of how the facility could handle such situations better in the future.

Roberto Carballo, Jr. wrote Jake a letter thanking him for the care he heard Jake had provided for his father and family members. He said he did not want to go into details but felt it was best that he not see his father or his sisters before Mr. Carballo's death. He said he hoped Jake would understand.

Teresa and Alberto each selected another favorite toy that they placed in "Lito's" casket. They told each other that "Lito doesn't look like Lito, but he's with Lita in Heaven now."

EVIDENCE-BASED PRACTICE

Review: The soul of sorrow work: Grief and therapeutic interventions with families.
Moules, N. J., Simonson, K., Fleiszer, A. R., Prins, M., & Glasgow, B. *Journal Family of Nursing, 13,* 117–141.

Q: What is the work clinicians do in helping families experiencing grief?

Data sources. Hermeneutic interpretive inquiry by means of interviewing six participants. Interviews were transcribed verbatim and analyzed interpretively in order to achieve a collective hermeneutic understanding of the data.

Study selection and assessment. Three clinical practice exemplars and three willing family members with whom the clinicians had worked. The setting was the Calgary Health Region Grief Support Program, Calgary, Alberta, Canada. Two clinicians were women; one was a man. All were Caucasian, whose experience ranged between 5 and 26 years. Educational background of the clinicians included a social worker with a bachelor's degree, a psychologist with a master's degree, and a clergyman. Family members were all women, ranging in age from 30 to 55 years of age with experience of losses from 2 to 8 years.

Outcomes. Grief has an inarticulate and changing nature to it. Clinicians working with those bereaved do not follow models as much as they follow maps based upon experience and a willingness to journey "off the map" if necessary.

Main results. All grief is complicated and falls in between a number of areas (e.g., it is both universal/individual, active/passive, internal/external, etc.). Grief may involve struggle that may be identified by anger, guilt, and/or identity. Grief often is pathologized by society and forced into stages inaccurately. The core of grief and grief work is spiritual in nature, involves soul work, and is ongoing in nature.

Conclusion. Grief work involves a "recollection of connections." Clinicians enhance healing in those grieving by journeying with them in their suffering and sorrow work.

Commentary. Traditional and well-accepted grief work addresses specific stages of grieving, namely denial, anger, bargaining, acceptance, and resolution. Different types of grieving in traditional framework include anticipatory, delayed, distorted, and complicated grieving.

In contrast, current nursing literature challenges stage theory of grief by asserting that grief is ongoing and that the meaning one attributes to loss changes constantly. Many of these assertions are based upon humanbecoming theory, science of unitary human beings, and the Neuman Systems Model (Pilikington, 2008).

Floczak (2008) postulates that the sorrow of loss continues while the meaning of loss constantly changes. Likewise, the concept of instilling hope in clients with enduring circumstances is supported through open-ended grieving rather than time-limited grieving.

For correspondence. Nancy J. Moules, RN, Ph.D., Faculty of Nursing, University of Calgary, 2400 University Drive NW, Calgary, Alberta, Canada T2N 1N4; email: njmoules!ucalgary.ca

Sources of funding. University of Calgary and Faculty of Nursing, Calgary, Alberta, Canada

Floczak, K. L. (2008) The persistent yet everchanging nature of grieving a loss. *Nursing Science Quarterly, 21,* 7–11.

Pilkington, F. B. (2008). Expanding nursing perspectives on loss and grieving. (2008). *Nursing Science Quarterly, 21,* 6–7.

REFERENCES

American Heritage Dictionary of the English Language (4th ed., new updated edition) (2006). Boston: Houghton Mifflin Company.

Backer, B. A., Hannon, N. R., & Gregg, J. Y. (1994). *To listen, to comfort, to care: Reflections on death and dying.* Albany, NY: Delmar.

Baum, N. (2003). The male way of mourning divorce: When, what, and how. *Clinical Social Work Journal, 31*(1), 37–67.

Bowlby, J. (1980). *Attachment and loss: Loss, sadness and depression* (Vol. III). New York: Basic Books.

Brady, P. F. (1997). The therapeutic relationship. In B. S. Johnson (Ed.), *Psychiatric-mental health nursing: Adaptation and growth* (4th ed., pp. 49–57). New York: Lippincott.

Buckman, R. (1993). Communication in palliative care: A practical guide. In D. Doyle, G. W. C. Hanks, & N. Macdonald (Eds.), *Oxford textbook of palliative medicine* (pp. 47–61). Oxford, England: Oxford Medical.

Buckwalter, G. (2003). Addressing the spiritual and religious needs of persons with profound memory loss. *Home Healthcare Nurse, 21*(1), 20–24.

Callanan, M., & Kelley, P. (1992). *Final gifts.* New York: Poseidon Press.

Cassell, E. (1991). *The nature of suffering and the goals of medicine.* New York: Oxford University.

Charleton, R. (2003). Managing bereavement. *Practitioner, 247,* 6[S5]), 671–674.

Choi, Y.-J., & Lee, K.-J. (2007). Evidence-based nursing: Effects of a structured nursing program for the health promotion of women with Hwa-Byung. *Archives of Psychiatric Nursing, 21*(1), 12–16.

Clements, P. T., Vigil, G. J., Manno, M. S., Henry, G. C., Wilks, J., Das, S., et al. (2003). Cultural perspectives of death, grief, and bereavement. *Journal of Psychosocial Nursing, 41*(7), 18–26.

Copp, G. (1997). Patients' and nurses' constructions of death and dying in a hospice setting. *Journal of Cancer Nursing, 1*(1), 2–13.

Copp, G. (1998). A review of current theories of death and dying. *Journal of Advanced Nursing, 28,* 382–390.

Corr, C. A. (1992). A task-based approach to coping with dying. *Omega, 24*(2), 81–94.

Cowles, K., & Rodgers, B. (2000). The concept of grief: An evolutionary perspective. In B. Rodgers and K. Knafl (Eds.), *Concept development in nursing* (pp. 103–117). Philadelphia: W. B. Saunders.

Danis, M. (1998). Improving end-of-life care in the intensive care unit: What's to be learned from outcome research? *New Horizons, 6*(1), 110–118.

Dyregrov, K., & Dyregrov, D. (2005). Siblings after suicide: "The forgotten bereaved." *Suicide and Life-Threatening Behavior, 35*(6), 714–724.

Eakes, G. G., Burke, M. L., & Hainsworth, M. A. (1998). Middle-range theory of chronic sorrow. *Image: Journal of Nursing Scholarship, 30,* 179–184.

Engel, G. L. (1964). Grief and grieving. *American Journal of Nursing, 64,* 93–98.

Evans, A. J. (1994). Anticipatory grief: A theoretical challenge. *Palliative Medicine, 8,* 159–165.

Ferrell, B. R., & Coyle, N. (2008). The nature of suffering and the goals of nursing. *Oncology Nursing Forum, 35*(2), 241–247.

Ferrell, B. R., Taylor, E. J., Sattler, G. R., Fowler, M., & Cheyney, B. L. (1993). Searching for the meaning of pain. *Cancer Practice, 1,* 185–194.

Florczak, K. (2008). The persistent yet everchanging nature of grieving. *Nursing Science Quarterly, 21*(1), 7–11.

Frank, E., Prigerson, H. G., Shear, M. K., & Reynolds, C. F. (1997). Phenomenology and treatment of bereavement-related distress in the elderly. *International Clinical Psycho-Pharmacology, 12*(Suppl. 7), S25-S29.

Freud, S. (1957). The disillusionment of the war. In J. Strachey (Ed.), *The complete psychological works of Sigmund Freud,* Vol. 14, (pp. 1914–1916). London: Hogarth Press and the Institute of Psychoanalysis.

Fulton, R., & Fulton, J. A. (1971). A psychosocial aspect of terminal care: Anticipatory grief. *Omega, 2,* 91–99.

Geis, H. K., Whittlesey, S. W., McDonald, N. B., Smith, K. L., & Pfefferbaum, B. (1998). Bereavement and loss in childhood. *Child and Adolescent Psychiatric Clinics of North America, 7*(1), 73–85.

Georgesen, J., & Dungan, J. M. (1996). Managing spiritual distress in patients with advanced cancer. *Cancer Nursing, 19,* 376- 383.

Glasser, B. G., & Strauss, A. L. (1965). *Awareness of dying.* Chicago: Aldine.

Goodkin, K., Blaney, N. T., Feaster, D. J., Baldewicz, T., Burkhalter, J. E., & Leeds, B., et al. (1999). A randomized controlled clinical trial of a bereavement support group intervention in human immunodeficiency virus type I-seropositive and seronegative homosexual men. *Archives of General Psychiatry, 56*(1), 52–59.

Haas, F. (2003). Bereavement care: Seeing the body. *Nursing Standard, 17*(28), 33–37.

Hames, C. C. (2003). Helping infants and toddlers when a family member dies. *Journal of Hospice and Palliative Nursing, 5,* 103–112.

Harris, J. M. (1991). Death and bereavement. *Problems in Veterinary Medicine, 3,* 111–117.

Holloway, M. (2006). [AN6]Death the great leveler? Towards a transcultural spirituality of dying and bereavement. *Journal of Clinical Nursing, 15*

Horowitz, M. J., Bonanno, G. A., & Holen, A. (1993). Pathological grief: Diagnosis and explanation. *Psychosomatic Medicine, 55,* 260–273.

Johns, C. (2007). Toward easing suffering through reflection. *Journal of Holistic Nursing, 25*(3), 204–210.

Jordan, J., & Neimeyer, R. (2003). Does grief counseling work? *Death Studies, 27,* 765–786.

Kalish, R. A. (1979). The onset of the dying process. In R. A. Kalish (Ed.), *Death, dying, transcending* (pp. 5–17). New York: Bay-wood.

Kastenbaum, R. A. (1997). *Death, society, and human experience.* Boston: Allyn and Bacon.

Kazanowski, M. (2006). End of life care. In D. D. Ignatavicius, M. L. Workman, & M. A. Mishler (Eds.), *Medical-surgical nursing: Critical thinking for collaborative care* (5th ed.). St. Louis, MO: Elsevier Saunders.

Kazanowski, M., Perrin, K, Potter, M., & Sheehan, C. (2007). The silence of suffering. *Journal of Holistic Nursing, 25*(3), 195–203.

Kiser, L. J., Ostoja, E., & Pruitt, D. B. (1998). Dealing with stress and trauma in families. *Child and Adolescent Psychiatric Clinics of North America, 7*(1), 87–103.

Kissane, D. W., Bloch, S., & McKenzie, D. P. (1997). Family coping and bereavement outcome. *Palliative Medicine, 11,* 191–201.

Kissane, D. W., & Bloch, S. (2002). *Family focused grief therapy.* Philadelphia: Open University Press.

Koop, P. M., & Strang, V. (1997). Predictors of bereavement outcomes in families of patients with cancer: A literature review. *Canadian Journal of Nursing Research, 29*(4), 33–35.

Krueger, G. (2006). Meaning-making in the aftermath of sudden infant death syndrome. *Nursing Inquiry, 13*(3), 163–171.

Kubler-Ross, E. (1969). *On death and dying.* New York: Macmillan.

Kurtz, M. E., Kurtz, J. C., Given, C. W., & Given, B. (1997). Predictors of post-bereavement depressive symptomatology among family caregivers of cancer patients. *Support Care Cancer, 5*(1), 53–60.

Lalor, J. G., Begley, C. M., & Devane, D. (2006). Exploring painful experiences: Impact of emotional narratives on members of a qualitative research team. *Journal of Advanced Nursing 56*(6), 607–616.

Lavoie, M., Blondeau, D., & De Koninck, T. (2008). The dying person: An existential being until the end of life. *Nursing Philosophy, 9,* 89–97.

Leichtling, B. (2004). Dealing with dying, death and grief. *Caring: National Association for Home Care Magazine, 23*(1), 38–39.

Lev, E. L., & McCorkle, R. (1998). Loss, grief, and bereavement in family members of cancer patients. *Seminars in Oncology Nursing, 14,* 145–151.

Lewis, M. L. (1998). Culture and loss: A project of self-reflection. *Journal of Nursing Education, 37,* 191–201.

Lindemann, E. (1944). Symptomatology and management of acute grief. *American Journal of Psychiatry, 101,* 141–148.

Maciejewski, P. K., Zhang, B., Block, S. D., & Prigerson, (2007). H. G., An empirical examination of the stage theory of grief, *Journal of American Medical Association, 297,* 716–723.

Mallinson, R. K. (1999). Grief work of HIV-positive persons and their survivors. *Nursing Clinics of North America, 34,* 163–177.

Matzo, M. L., & Sherman, D. W. (2006). *Palliative Care Nursing: Quality Care to the End of Life* (2nd ed.). NY: Springer Publishing Company.

Matzo, M. L., Sherman, D. W., Lo, K., Egan, K. A., Grant, M., & Rhome, A., et al. (2003). Strategies for teaching loss, grief, and bereavement. *Nurse Educator, 28*(2), 71–76.

McCall, J. B. (1999). *Grief education for care-givers of the elderly.* New York: Haworth Pastoral Press.

McCreight, B. S. (2004). A grief ignored: Narratives of pregnancy loss from a male perspective. *Sociology of Health & Illness, 26*(3), 326–350[S7].

McIntier, T. M. (1995). Nursing the family when a child dies. *RN*[AN8], *2,* 50–55.

Mitchell, A. M., Wesner, S., Garand, L., Gale, D. D., Havill, A., & Brownson, L., et al. (2007). A support group intervention for children bereaved by parental suicide. *Journal of Child and Adolescent Psychiatric Nursing, 20*(1), 3–13.

Mitchell, K. R., & Anderson, H. (1983). *All our losses, all our griefs.* Philadelphia: Westminster Press.

Moules, N. J., Simonson, K., Fleiszer, A. R., Prins, M., & Glasgow. (2007). The soul of sorrow work: Grief and therapeutic Interventions with Families. *Journal of Family Nursing, 13*(1), 117–141.

Moules, N. J., Simonson, K., Prins, M., Angus, P., & Bell, J. M. (2004) Making room for grief: Walking backwards and living forward. *Nursing Inquiry, 11*(2), 99–107.

Mystakidou, K., Tsilika, E., Parpa, E., Katsouda, E., & Vlahos, L. (2003). A Greek perspective on concepts of death and expression of grief, with implications for practice. *International Journal of Palliative Nursing, 9,* 534–537.

Narayanasamy, A. (2006). The impact of empirical studies of spirituality and culture on nurse education. *Journal of Clinical Nursing, 15*(7), 840–851.

O'Neill, D. P., & Kenny, E. K. (1998). Spirituality and chronic illness. *Image: Journal of Nursing Scholarship, 30,* 275–280.

Parker, B., Alex, L., Jonsen, E., Gustafson, Y., Norgber, A., & Lundman, B., et al. (2002.) Resilience, sense of coherence, purpose in life and self-transcendence in relation to perceived physical and mental health among the oldest old. *Aging and Mental Health, 9,* 342–362.

Parkes, C. M., & Weiss, R. S. (1983). *Recovery from bereavement.* New York: Basic Books.

Parse, R. R. (2007). The humanbecoming school of thought in 2050. *Nursing Science Quarterly, 20,* 308–311.

Pattison, E. M. (1977). *The experience of dying.* New York: Simon and Schuster.

Pennebaker, J. W., Mayne, T. J., & Francis, M. E. (1997). Linguistic predictors of adaptive bereavement. *Journal of Personality and Social Psychology, 72,* 863–871.

Pilkington, F. B., (2006). Developing nursing knowledge on grieving: A human becoming perspective. *Nursing Science Quarterly, 19*(4), 29–303.

Pilkington, F. B. (2008). Expanding nursing perspectives on loss and grieving. *Nursing Science Quarterly, 21*(1), 6.

Prigerson, H. G., Bierhals, A. J., Kasl, S. V., Reynolds, C. F., Shear, M. K., Day, N., et al. (1997). Traumatic grief as a risk factor for mental and physical morbidity. *American Journal of Psychiatry, 154,* 616–623.

Pritchett, K. T., & Lucas, P. M. (1997). Grief and loss. In B. S. Johnson (Ed.), *Psychiatric mental health nursing: Adaptation and growth* (4th ed., pp. 199–218). New York: Lippincott.

Rando, T. A. (1984). *Grief, dying, and death*. Champaign, IL: Research Press.

Reiss, D. (1990). Patient, family, and staff responses to end-stage renal disease. *American Journal of Kidney Disease, 15,* 194–200.

Saldinger, A., Cain, A., & Porterfield, K. (2003). Managing traumatic stress in children anticipating parental death. *Psychiatry, 66,* 168–181.

Segal, J., Jaffe, J., Davies, P., & Smith, M. (2007). Depression in older adults and the elderly: Recognizing signs and getting help. Retrieved October 14, 2008, from http://www.help-guide.org/mental/depression_elderly.htm.

Sherman, D. W. (1998). Reciprocal suffering: The need to improve family caregivers' quality of life through palliative care. *Journal of Palliative Medicine, 1,* 357–366.

Siegel, K., Karus, D. G., Raveis, V. H., Christ, G. H., & Mesagno, F. P. (1996). Depressive distress among the spouses of terminally ill patients. *Cancer Practice, 4*(1), 25–30.

Spencer, L. (1994). How do nurses deal with their own grief when a patient dies on an intensive care unit and what help can be given to enable them to overcome their grief effectively? *Journal of Advanced Nursing, 19,* 1141–1150.

Stroebe, M. S. (2002). Paving the way: From early attachment theory to contemporary bereavement research. *Mortality, 7,* 127–138.

Stroebe, , M. S., & Schut, H. (2001). [AN9]Meaning making in the dual process model of coping with bereavement. In *Meaning reconstruction and its experience of loss,* R. A. Neimeyer (Ed.).

Stuart, G. W., & Sundeen, S. J. (1991). *Principles and practices of psychiatric nursing*. Boston: Mosby Year Book.

Sudnow, D. (1967). *Passing on: The social organization of dying*. Englewood Cliffs, NJ: Prentice-Hall.

Talerico, K. A. (2003). Grief and older adults. *Journal of Psychosocial Nursing, 41*(7), 12–16.

Thomas, S. P. (2004). Men's health and psychosocial issues affecting men. *The Nursing Clinics of North America, 39*(2), 259–70.

Vance, D. E., Burrage, J., Couch, A., & Raper J. (2008). Promoting successful aging with HIV through hardiness. *Journal of Gerontological Nursing, 34*(6), 22–29.

Vigil, G. J., & Clements, P. T. (2003). Child and adolescent homicide survivors: Complicated grief and altered world-views. *Journal of Psychosocial Nursing, 41*(1), 30–39.

Viorst, J. (1987). *Necessary losses*. New York: Ballantine Books.

Warren, B. J. (1999). Cultural competence in psychiatric nursing: An interlocking paradigm approach. In N. L. Keltner, L. H. Schwecke, & C. E. Bostrom (Eds.), *Psychiatric nursing* (3rd ed., pp. 98–148). Boston: Mosby.

Woodgate, R., & Degner, L. (2003). A substantive theory of keeping the spirit alive: The spirit within children with cancer and their families. *Journal of Pediatric Oncology Nursing, 20,* 103–119.

Worden, J. W. (1991). *Grief counseling and grief therapy: Handbook for the mental health practitioner*. New York: Springer.

Physical Aspects of Dying

July 3, 2004

Up until this last week Candy has been relatively independent with her activities of daily living. She was having occasional right sided chest pain, which she rated as a "3" in intensity, but was relieved by 2 Percocet. In the past week, the pain increased in frequency and intensity, and she had dyspnea at rest. In the past three days, Candy became very weak, with no appetite, and she spent most of her time sitting in her "Lazy Boy" chair. Because of her increase in symptoms, I called her daily and visited her every other day. She was extremely lethargic and her husband told me that she became very short of breath on ambulation to the bathroom.

Lethargy and loss of appetite in a person with advanced cancer are common physical symptoms associated with the process of dying. The fact that she was having an increase in symptoms of pain and dyspnea was further evidence that she was nearing death. I called her doctor and asked for a standing order for liquid Morphine and Ativan. I showed Candy and Ron how to administer 5 mg. of the morphine in her cheek and recommended repeating the medication dose in 15 minutes if it wasn't effective, and to take the prescribed rescue dose if she experienced heightened pain or shortness of breath.

Today was the first time in the year that I have known Candy that she mentioned dying. I held her hand while she cried and told me how surprised she was that the end was coming so quickly. I suppose these things are surprising when it is clear that the disease will not be cured. Candy asked me to promise her that she would not suffer at the end; it was such a poignant moment. As I hugged her, I told her I would be with her till the end. With the support of members of the Hospice/Palliative Care team, Candy's pain and symptoms were alleviated, and the emotional and spiritual needs of Candy and her family were being addressed.

July 4, 2004

When I arrived at Candy's house today, I saw that her level of consciousness had significantly declined. She had not had any oral intake for two days, and was only responding occasionally to her name. Her skin was cool and starting to become mottled. Ron said he had given Candy 4 rescue doses of 10mg. of morphine since yesterday. She appeared comfortable and peaceful, with no evidence of grimacing or restlessness, which may indicate pain. Candy did not appear to have difficulty breathing, but her breaths were slow and shallow, and there was a rattle in the back of her throat. I explained that this noise was from secretions in the back of her throat, but that it is usually not distressing to the patient.

I told Ron that Candy was actively dying and held him as he cried. I suggested to him that he get the children if he wanted them to be with her as she died. They came in and crawled into the bed with their mom and lay in her arms for the last time. Ron put his arms around them all, as they prayed together. I was thinking what a good job Candy had done with her kids that they were so comfortable to be with her during this time; I don't know where Ron got his strength to support his family in this way. The love and faith were almost palpable. I stayed at the foot of her bed and did Reiki on Candy's feet, something she had always liked me to do during my visits. She opened her eyes, looked at each of us, stopped breathing, and died.

Ron held the children and told them what had happened. Fortunately, there were family and friends in the house to be with the children, as Ron stayed with me to bathe Candy's body. He wanted to do this final act for her because she never liked to leave the house looking "messy." He talked to her as we prepared her to leave her home for the last time.

As I reflect on this nursing experience, I realize the importance of the relationship that we developed over time. The family members allowed me to care for them at one of the most vulnerable times of their lives. I learned so much from Candy about life, living, and ultimately about dying. These are gifts given to us by our patients at the end of life. Palliative care nursing transcends traditional care-giving experiences. In a very intimate way, nurses co-journey with their patients and families experiencing life-threatening illness and help them to live as fully as possible until death. With the knowledge and skills to alleviate the physical, emotional, social, and spiritual pain and suffering, and by bearing witness to the precious moments of life as patients and their families say their last goodbyes and express eternal love, nurses experience the joy and rewards of hospice/palliative care nursing. Through competent and compassionate care at the end of life, nurses can make a difference in the quality of life and quality of dying for their patients and their families.

12

Cancer

Amy E. Guthrie
Polly Mazanec

Key Points

- Cancer affects all ages.
- The overall incidence and prevalence of cancer has increased with individuals living with cancer as a chronic illness.
- Treatment options have improved in survival benefits, toxicity, and palliation.
- Symptoms associated with the disease and the toxicities of treatment require a commitment to an interdisciplinary model of care throughout service delivery locations.
- Palliative care regards the cancer patient and family as the focus of care and treats physical, psychosocial, spiritual, and bereavement needs.

Case Study: Mr. J. is a 42-year-old Caucasian male who was diagnosed with Stage IV T3 N2 M1 colon cancer in May 2006. He underwent a right hemicolectomy and multiagent chemotherapy of erlotinib and FOLFOX. His past medical/surgical history was unremarkable. Current medications included oxycodone 5 mg p.o. every 2 hr as needed for pain and ondansetron 8 mg p.o. every 6 hr as needed for nausea and vomiting. He was being cared for at a comprehensive cancer center.

Physical examination at the time of chemotherapy initiation revealed a slightly overweight Caucasian male in no acute distress. Vital signs: afebrile, pulse 76 beats/min, regular rate and rhythm, respirations 16 breaths/min, blood pressure 126/82. Cardiac exam, S1, S2, no S3 or S4, no murmurs, no edema, pulses 2 + throughout, no bruits. Lungs clear to auscultation. Abdominal exam revealed soft, nontender abdomen, well-healed surgical scar, bowel sounds present in all four quadrants, liver nontender, palpated to be 14 cm. No palpable masses, no lymphadenopathy. Musculoskeletal exam unremarkable. Neurological exam grossly intact.

Mr. J. worked as a tool and die maker and lives in the area with his wife of 5 years. He has a child aged three and four step children. His first wife's husband died 4 years ago from cancer, after their divorce. The children have become very attached to Mr. J. Mrs. J. has a strong religious devotion to the Roman Catholic faith; however, Mr. J. is struggling with his spirituality and has no religious affiliation.

Questions that the nurse should consider are:

1) What is the best palliative care practice model for Mr. J.'s plan of care?
2) What are the benefits and burdens of continued chemotherapy treatment for Mr. J.?
3) What support is needed to help Mr. J. and his family cope with his diagnosis, treatment, disease progression, and loss, grief, and bereavement?
4) How can the nurse support Mr. J. during his spiritual crisis?

Introduction

Cancer is a devastating diagnosis that many individuals associate with death. Upon initial diagnosis, individuals embark on a treatment journey that is overwhelming with medical jargon, new healthcare providers, unknown outcomes, and fluctuations of hope amidst the distressing effects of the disease and its treatment. Although people are living longer with cancer, and some cancers can be considered chronic in nature, living with cancer can provoke anxiety and a loss of control for the patient and family. Individuals living with cancer rely on family or chosen support people to assist them for physician office visits and treatment, contribute additional ears to absorb disease and treatment information, and provide physical and emotional support for treatment and possibly end-of-life (EOL) care. Oncology healthcare providers work with a heterogeneous patient population attempting to provide the patient and family with clear communication, the most effective treatment methods, and a healthy balance of hope for the future.

Despite continuous improvement in treatment efficacy and survival outcomes, cancer remains the second leading cause of death for both genders and throughout the lifespan. Adult cancer is second to heart disease while pediatric cancer is second to accidental death in most age groups through adolescence (Djulbegovic et al., 2008; Aldridge & Roesch, 2007; Wolfe, Friebert, & Hilden 2002). The American Cancer Society (ACS) estimated 1.4 million new cases of all cancer sites in 2007. However, a new cancer diagnosis is no longer synonymous with a limited life expectancy, and could possibly mean a future navigating a cancer treatment system and living with the chronicity of survival. Historically, palliative care for cancer patients was mainly contained within hospice care. Now, cancer specialists are incorporating the precepts of palliative medicine and an interdisciplinary approach to patient care. Due to medical and nursing certifying boards regulating the specialty of palliative medicine and palliative care, the increasing number of healthcare professionals certified in palliative care offers more options for the supportive care of cancer patients actively involved in curative treatment, receiving expensive physiological supportive treatment, and eventually facing imminent death (Gelfman, Meier, & Morrison, 2008; Griffin, Koch, Nelson, & Cooley, 2007; Kuebler, Lynn, & Rhohen, 2005).

For the majority of 20th century patients, cancer was more likely to be diagnosed in a later stage, treatment was largely ineffective, and death usually resulted within a few months. Today, roughly half of all cancer patients will die of their disease (Kuebler et al., 2005). The care of cancer patients has evolved in the last 20 years not only as a result of changes in treatment efficacy, but also due to the interdisciplinary model of support currently incorporated in care. Healthcare consumers prefer honest and more complete information pertaining to diagnosis, prognosis, symptom burden, and survival benefits related to treatment. As a result, healthcare professionals are learning more compassionate communication skills and recognizing the importance of shared decision-making with the patient, family, or family of choice (Surbone, 2008; Kuebler et al., 2005). Throughout the various stages of cancer, the needs of the patient and family are complex requiring special attention to physical, psychological, social, and spiritual distress. Arrangements for an appropriate care setting and adequate care giving support throughout treatment and at EOL requires knowledge of specialized treatment providers, available alternatives, and an experience-based understanding of how best to match the needs of the patient and family living with cancer (Griffin et al., 2007). Even though many cancer specialists are experienced in EOL care and consider it germane to their practice, the specialty of palliative care is emerging as an interdisciplinary specialty with strong support for patient, family, and the clinicians involved in cancer management. Evidence suggests that palliative care teams assisting in cancer care improve patient care and reduce costs to the family and healthcare system by cultivating an equal exchange of information matching the goals of the patient with treatments offered (Gelfman et al., 2008). In addition, palliative care teams support the clinicians working so closely with a patient population living with a life-threatening disease by providing emotional and educational support. Where multiple clinicians representing different specialties are involved, palliative care teams provide the hub of communication and specialized spiritual and bereavement support of patients, families and clinicians that cancer care requires. Palliative care should be integrated into every cancer patient's treatment, including those pursuing curative or life-prolonging therapies, and whether or not palliative care specialist teams are available, cancer treatment teams should receive education in the essentials of palliative care (Griffin et al., 2007).

Future implications for cancer care will include supporting patients through complex treatments offered in a variety of treatment locations and supporting late effects of treatment as seen with survivorship. Young and old, it is important to note that the stage of growth and development, familial support, physiological stamina, psychological reserve, and community resources all present significant consideration for the treatment of adults and children living with cancer.(Aldridge & Roesch, 2007; Matsuyama, Reddy, & Smith, 2006). The National Institute for Health and Clinical Excellence (NICE, 2005) and the National Collaborating Centre for Cancer (NCC-C, 2005) have issued guidelines standardizing care services for children and young people with cancer in England and Wales. Key recommendations include the following: 1) Care for children and young adults up to 19 years of age should be provided in age-appropriate facilities; 2) Children and young adults must have access to treatment specific clinical expertise; 3) All aspects of cancer care for children and young adults should be provided by appropriately trained staff, and 4) Children, young adults, and their families should be supported by expert healthcare providers to coordinate care across the continuum of disease providing age and culture appropriate information (NICE, 2005).

INCIDENCE AND PREVALENCE

Pediatric and Younger Adult

It is estimated that roughly 11,000 children under the age of 15 in the United States will be diagnosed with some form of cancer in 2008. This is an increase in prevalence in the past 20 years, yet due to considerable advances in treatment, 80% of those children could experience a long-term remission representing a 30% increase in the 5-year survival rate between the 1970s and late 1990s (ASC, 2008; Aldridge & Roesch, 2007). The sites of cancers that occur in children contrast greatly from those affecting adults. Leukemias (acute myelogenous and acute lymphocytic) account for approximately 33% of all childhood cancers, brain, and nervous system cancers make up about 21% of childhood cancers, while neuroblastoma is the most common (7.3% of all childhood cancer types) solid tumor outside of the central nervous system. Despite advances in early detection and treatment, about 1,500 children will die from cancer in 2010 (ASC, 2008; Aldridge & Roesch, 2007).

Adult

According to the ACS, the most frequent diagnozed adult cancer cases considering all sites are female breast, prostate, lung, and colorectal (Figure 12.1). These four most commonly occurring cancers will be the physiological focus of this chapter. It is estimated that over 200,000 adult Americans will be diagnosed with lung cancer in 2007, and over 150,000 adult Americans will die of the disease within that same year. Estimated incident rates for new prostate and female breast cancer cases are similar while colorectal cases affecting both genders reaching over 140,000 individuals in the

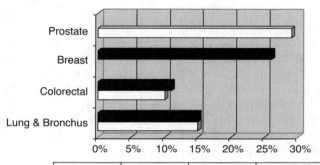

	Lung & Bronchus	Colorectal	Breast	Prostate
■ Women	15%	11%	26%	
□ Men	15%	10%		29%

Figure 12.1   Leading sites of new cancer cases–2007 (estimated).
Source: American Cancer Society, Inc. Surveillance Research © 2007.

year 2007 (ACS), 2008). The total 2007 estimated cancer death rate representing all sites could equal over 650,000 individuals in the Untied States.

Older Adult

The greatest impact of cancer is seen in the older adult population, since 60% of new cancer incidences, and 69% of all cancer deaths occur in individuals 65 years and older (Terret, Sulian, Naiem, & Albrand, 2007). The relationship between increasing age and the development of cancer is attributed to cancer growth characteristics (age-related cellular mutations) and the biophysical environment (pro-oncogenic changes in the tissue milieu) allowing mutant cells to survive, proliferate, and express their neoplastic phenotype. First, cancer cells take time to proliferate; this growth may not be apparent until the later stages of life. Second, a changing physical environment contributes to the programed cell death of healthy cells and the propagation of cancer cells. As a result, older adults are at increased risk for cancer (Extermann & Hurria, 2007; Terret et al., 2007; Repetto et al., 2003).

PATHOGENESIS

The etiology of cancer is multifactorial, with genetic (nonmodifiable), environmental (modifiable), medical (modifiable), and lifestyle (modifiable) factors interacting to produce a given malignancy. Knowledge of cancer genetics is rapidly improving our understanding of the biologic aspects of cancer, helping to identify at-risk individuals, furthering the ability to characterize malignancies, establishing treatment tailored to the molecular fingerprint of the disease, and leading to the development of new therapeutic modalities including early detection. As a consequence, this expanding knowledge base has implications for all aspects of cancer management, including prevention, screening, and treatment.

Malignant tumors are produced by a synergy between the accumulation of mutations and tissue changes that support the survival of mutant cells (Terret et al., 2007). Factors that cause or facilitate cancer development include chemical mutagens, radiation, free radicals, genomic instability, inherited cancer susceptibility, telomere shortening, and altered cellular environment. Factors such as smoking, diet, physical activity, and weight control are known modifiable risk factors that alter cellular environment and influence the proliferation of cancer cells. Carcinogenesis works in a stepwise progression in which a normal cell undergoes transformation to a malignancy. Steps include initiation, promotion, premalignant progression, and finally, malignant conversion. The complete explanation of these steps is outside the scope of this chapter; however, this information provides a framework for further discovery and detailed understanding. Occasionally, family members will question the cause of cancer when a loved one is diagnosed; however, further investigation usually reveals an existential concern that a genetic explanation may not satisfy.

DISEASE TRAJECTORY

Breast Cancer

Breast cancer is the most frequently occurring female malignancy in the United States with approximately 182,460 new cases of invasive breast cancer each year. An additional 67,770 women will be diagnosed in 2008 with the noninvasive form of breast cancer, carcinoma in situ. Estimated death occurrence is expected to reach over 40,000 women in the year 2008 (ACS 2008). More than 50% of all new cases occur in women 65 years and older. The frequency of breast cancer in women over the age of 70 is 300 out of 100,000, and 430 out of 100,000 over 80 years of age (Hampton, 2008b; Litsas, 2008).

Breast cancer is a complicated disease representing a highly heterogeneous patient population. Breast cancer originates in two separate cell types: Ductal and lobular. Ductal cancers are the most common with invasive ductal cancer representing 70%–80% of all ductal cancer cases. Lobular breast cancer rarely occurs alone, is more hormonally influenced, and occurs predominately in premenopausal women. Breast cancer affecting the breast nipple is Paget's disease and is associated with intraductal or invasive ductal carcinoma. Breast cancer can be estrogen receptor (ER+) positive or negative (ER–) and progesterone receptor (PR+ or –) positive or negative. Most breast cancers are hormone sensitive while nonhormone sensitive breast cancers are found to be the faster growing of the two. Generally speaking, the goal of treatment for women with early stage breast cancer is to prevent death and re-occurrence while minimizing side-effects from treatment. The goal for women diagnosed with late-stage or metastatic breast cancer is to maintain quality of life (QOL), control the disease, and extend survival time (Hampton, 2008b; Holcomb, 2006).

Pathogenesis involves DNA mutation by genetic alterations or environmental agents, probably occurring early in life. Only 5%–10% of all breast cancers are inherited and carry the breast cancer specific gene. Growth factors then increase the growth rate of those mutated cells, and finally, progressive alteration of specific oncogenes, or the loss of suppressor genes lead to advanced metastatic disease (Robinson & Huether, 1998). The environment for breast cancer growth in older women is not as favorable as that of younger women because of the decrease of stimulating growth factor specifically for breast cancer and diminishing mononuclear cell reactions. Breast cancer in the older woman tends to be more differentiated and rich in hormone receptors than in young women. This renders nonmetastatic tumors more receptive to treatment. Thus, rather than treating cancer based on the patient's age, it is essential to treat each tumor individually, addressing the characteristics of the tumor and the desires of the patient (Balducci & Extermann, 2001).

Signs/symptoms/staging. Most generally, breast cancer presents as a painless lump, other signs include palpable axillary nodes, dimpling, or bone pain due to metastasis. Breast cancer is evaluated with mammography, percutaneous needle aspiration, biopsy, and hormone receptor assays. Treatment is determined by cell type, stage, growth rate, and hormone responsiveness. The TNM classification system evaluates primary tumor size (TX to T4), regional lymph nodes (NX to N3), and distant metastasis (MX to M1), while staging from 0 to IV is used in addition to the TNM determination. Staging levels increase with tumor size and node involvement; stage IV is the only stage that represents metastasis. Rate of growth can be determined by S-phase or Ki-67 tests (Holcomb, 2006; Robinson & Huether, 1998).

Disease management. Treatment options include lumpectomy, simple mastectomy with sentinel node biopsy, radical mastectomy, radiation (external and brachytherapy), systemic therapy (chemotherapy and hormonal therapy), adjuvant therapy (prior to surgery to reduce tumor size and burden). A bone scan and computed tomography of abdomen and chest are performed to rule out metastasis.

Surgery. Surgical procedures for breast cancer include: lumpectomy, quadrant excision, partial mastectomy, total or simple mastectomy, modified radical mastectomy, and radical mastectomy (Robinson & Huether, 1998). Options available for the surgical management of stage I or II breast cancer are lumpectomy with removal of axillary lymph nodes, mastectomy with the removal of the axillary lymph nodes, radiation therapy, chemotherapy, or hormone therapy. The treatment is typically multimodal (Holcomb, 2006).

Axillary node involvement is the most important prognostic indicator for the breast cancer patient. Historically, many medical authorities suggest testing at least 4 nodes at the time of surgery; however, others recommend testing the sentinel node to accurately indicate lymph node involvement. Adequate nodal removal is not commonly offered to older adults, which may lead to inadequate adjuvant therapy (Holcomb, 2006; Robinson & Huether, 1998). Treatment for DCIS includes excision of the tumor, radiation, and/or tamoxifen. High dose chemotherapy has been shown to increase survival rates up to 6 months, however, is not considered a curative treatment option at this time for the older adult with multiple co-morbidities (Coyne, Lyckholm, & Smith, 2006). Estrogen receptor (ER)-positive breast cancer is responsive to Tamoxifen

(a nonsteroidal selective estrogen receptor modulator) treatment, significantly reducing the long-term risk of reoccurrence (Litsas, 2008). Treatment for stage III (locally advanced tumors) does not usually involve curative surgery due to the poor prognosis associated with this stage. Conversely, a combination of surgery, chemotherapy, and radiation would be an option for local control of the tumor, since many locally advanced tumors carry the likelihood of metastasis (Hunter-Dorcas, 1991). Inhibition of the aromatase system using third-generation aromatase inhibitors and inactivators has shown statistically significant improvement in survival benefit for patients with advanced breast cancer as compared with standard hormonal treatment (tamoxifen or progestagens) (Litsas 2008; Mauri, Pavlidis, Polyszos, & Ioannidis 2006).

Radiation therapy. External beam radiation and brachytherapy are current radiotherapies recommended for the treatment of breast cancer. External radiation is the typical radiation therapy given after lumpectomy and is given to the entire breast with an extra dose ("boost") to the site of the tumor from an external source. Treatment course could last up to 6–7 weeks with daily treatments. Brachytherapy is internal radiation or interstitial radiation. Radioactive materials, or "seeds," are placed in or near where the tumor was removed. They may be placed in the lumpectomy site to augment the radiation dose in addition to external beam radiation therapy (Holcomb, 2006).

Older women assessed with adequate functional reserves tolerate radiation as well as their younger counterparts. However, radiotherapy can be problematic for the older patient with cognitive impairment since the procedure requires immobilization, which could concern the patient to the point of anxiety (Balducci & Extermann, 2001).

Hormonal therapy. The addition of tamoxifen provides optimistic results towards longevity, and is considered first-line treatment for endocrine therapy, regardless of node involvement (Aebi & Pagani, 2007; Mackay, 2000). When used in premenopausal women for 5 years or longer, the recurrence rate dropped 40%, and the mortality rated dropped 32% (Aebi & Pagani 2007). Systemic adjuvant treatment of breast cancer is most useful for women with a life expectancy of two or more years. Tamoxifen therapy extends over a 5-year period and therefore may not be considered an option for the frail older adult (Litsas, 2008; Balducci, & Extermann, 2001).

Chemotherapy. Factors to be evaluated when considering chemotherapy include: physical well- being, staging, tumor type, comorbidity, patient preference, and drug efficacy in the older adult (Balducci & Extermann, 2001). Tumors rich in hormone receptors are less sensitive to chemotherapy than tumors poor in hormone receptors. The international breast cancer study group concluded that overall survival benefits from chemotherapy decreased as age increased, and was nonexistent in ages over 65 (Aebi & Pagani, 2007; Balducci & Extermann, 2001). However, reports show that chemotherapy increases survival rates of older women significantly when compared to those who are not treated as long as frequent dose adjustments are made for toxicity. Low-dose taxines, Capecitabine, Navelbin, Gemcitabine have low toxicity indices, when dosed appropriately (Balducci & Extermann, 2001). The controversy over chemotoxicity in older adults is a result of the heterogeneous population and the underrepresentation of older adults in clinical trials.

Palliative care for breast cancer. Treatment of women with advanced breast cancer is palliative in its intent. There are no data at this time from controlled trials comparing chemotherapy to best supportive or palliative care. No single regimen has been identified as the gold standard for disease control or symptom management. Literature shows that tumor shrinkage from chemotherapy can benefit some women suffering from tumor burden, yet side-effect profiles include nausea, vomiting, and myelosuppression have been reported with high symptom burden. A complete discussion regarding benefits versus burden should precede undergoing treatment (Archer, Billingham, & Cullen, 1999).

Prostate Cancer

Prostate cancer is the second leading cause of cancer death in men in the United States with an estimated frequency of 28,660 in 2008 (ACS, 2008). The ACS (2008) estimates 186,320 newly diagnosed cases in the year 2007. Prostate cancer is common in America, North America, and Northwestern Europe; conversely, it is rare in Asia, Africa, and South American populations. Incidence rates remain highest in African American men. Risk factors for prostate cancer include age, race, family history, and dietary factors (ACS, 2008; National Cancer Institute, 2007).

Over 95% of prostate malignancies are adenocarcinomas, primarily occurring in the periphery of the prostate. Grading systems represent the glandular pattern, degree of differentiation, or a combination of the two (Robinson & Huether, 1998). The cancer cells metastasize via posterior local extension, lymphatic system, and blood vessels to distant lymph nodes, bone, liver, lungs, and adrenal glands. The most common sites of bone infiltration are pelvis, lumbar and thoracic spine, femur, and ribs. The 5-year survival rate for localized prostate cancer is 98%, and 78% for all prostate cancers. These figures do not factor co-existing conditions that may affect prognosis (Robinson & Huether, 1998).

Signs/symptoms/staging. Early and localized stages of prostate cancer generally do not present with symptoms. Hallmark symptoms that occur more frequently in advanced stage cancer are usually associated with urinary outlet obstruction: frequent urination; urinary hesitancy, inability to urinate; nocturia; and dysuria. Impotence, painful ejaculation, bloody urine or semen, frequent pain, stiffness in lower back, hips, or upper thighs are additional symptoms signifying malignancy. Due to the fact that many of these symptoms can be caused by other factors, it is common for men to postpone medical consultation. Symptoms of malignant prostate disease usually do not subside, which distinguishes prostate cancer from benign disease. In advanced disease, upper urinary tract ureter and rectal obstructions are possible. If rectal obstruction occurs, bowel obstruction or difficult defecation will follow (Darmber & Aus, 2008; Ryan & Small, 2006).

Digital rectal exam, prostate-specific antigen blood test, and tissue biopsy are the three most effective diagnostic procedures; however, physicians and medical groups may not agree on when men should be routinely screened. Diagnosis of prostate cancer is confirmed by transrectal ultrasonography, intravenous pyelogram, and possibly cystoscopy. Biopsy is completed after the tumor has been visualized and when cancer is suspected.

Disease management. Treatment depends on age, life expectancy, overall health status, PSA level, Gleason score, and tumor size and spread (as indicated by the TNM classification system). If factors appear favorable, the stage of neoplasm determines the treatment. After initial diagnosis, grading is done to evaluate tumor growth rate. The Gleason grading is the most used grading scale, using numbers 1–5, with 1 signifying the lease aggressive form with tissue cells looking normal. The numbers refer to the appearance and activity of the cancer cells and are useful in determining the most effective treatment options. The Gleason score adds the grades of the two most prevalent patterns of the cells. Scores may range from 2, representing nonaggressive cancer, to 10, signifying the most aggressive with the greatest potential of spread. Historically, treatments have increased curative rates in many men with early and localized tumors, while treatments for more advanced disease are more beneficial to shrink tumors larger in size, palliate symptoms, and possibly increase survival time (Darmber & Aus, 2008).

Expectant management is referred to as "watchful waiting" and involves watching for new signs and symptoms of disease progression between regular checkups and testing. At the onset of symptoms, hormonal treatment is initiated. Deferring treatment is only beneficial for Stage I and II cancers, since it postpones the undesirable side effects of hormonal therapy. In order to lengthen survival rates, hormonal treatment following a radical prostatectomy should be done immediately (Pignon et al., 1997).

Surgery. Surgery, prostatectomy, is most effective for individuals with poorly differentiated tumors. As a result of a stratified analysis Merglen et al., (2007) recommend surgery for young patients with high Gleason scores. For the most part, the prostate cancer patient population represents a statistically diverse group and is considered highly heterogeneous due to the various grades, cellular responses, and sizes of tumors presenting in trials. Since surgical intervention can result in impotency and incontinence, it is important that treatment discussions involve the spouse or significant other in order to enhance emotional coping and physical healing (Merglen et al., 2007; Willert & Semans, 2000).

Radiation. Radiation therapy is offered as two different therapeutic approaches: 1. External beam—external application, and 2. Brachytherapy—internal application of radioactive materials placed directly in the prostate. It is important to note that the effects of radiotherapy to the pelvis can be menacing and unyielding. Complications related to radiotherapy include gastrointestinal toxic effects, genitourinary toxic effects, urinary incontinence, erectile dysfunction, and mortality. Many men diagnozed with prostate cancer are older adults and treatment burden may be overwhelming if the patient's condition is compromized by comorbidity or the presence of a geriatric syndrome (Damber & Aus, 2008). Patients with hypertension, diabetes mellitus, and pelvic inflammatory disease are not considered candidates for radiation therapy (Pignon et al., 1997).

Hormone therapy and palliative care for prostate cancer. For most men who are at high risk for systemic failure, hormonal therapy is recommended before metastatic disease is confirmed. Androgen-ablative therapy has been the mainstay for advanced prostate cancer since the 1940s. Approximately 70–80% of treated individuals will receive cancer specific system relief including bone pain from metastatic disease. The side effect profile associated with endocrine manipulation is mild compared to other anticancer therapies. Studies show that immediate hormonal therapy delays disease progression, yet not without cardiovascular toxic effects. Therefore, hormonal therapy is delayed until symptomatic progression is evident (Damber & Aus 2008). Until recently, cytotoxic chemotherapy was regarded as ineffective; however, recently is considered second and third-line treatment for hormone refractory prostate cancer. Two large clinical trials have shown improved survival in men with hormone-refractory disease comparing docetaxel used alone or in combination with extramustine to mitoxantrone and corticosteroids. This treatment is still considered palliative in nature and the gastric/cardiotoxic side effect profiles may not make the treatment option desirable to many men (Armstrong & Carducci, 2005; Damber & Aus, 2008). Zoledrunic acid, a bisphosphonate, was approved for use in men with hormone refractory

metastatic disease to reduce bone pain. Long-term use of the bisphosponate has recently been shown to cause osteonecrosis of the jaw (ONJ) causing alarm and caution in its use (Ryan & Small, 2006).

Lung Cancer

Lung cancer remains the leading cause of cancer death in men and women in the United States and around the world. In 2008 in the United States, 213,020 new cases and 161,840 deaths are projected (Jemal et al., 2008). The incidence has reached a plateau in women and declined in men, reflecting the trends in smoking patterns over the past few decades (Dubey & Powell, 2008). Most individuals who are diagnozed with lung cancer are former, rather than current tobacco smokers. Only 10% of lung cancers occur in individuals with no prior smoking history (Dubey & Powell, 2008). The overall 5-year survival rate is 15%, reflecting the poor prognosis associated with this disease (National Cancer Institute, 2007).

Lung cancer is divided into two main groups, non-small cell lung cancer (NSCLC) and small cell lung cancer (SCLC). NSCLC accounts for more than 80% of all lung cancers and is further characterized by histology as squamous cell carcinoma, large cell carcinoma, and the most prevalent type, adenocarcinoma (NCI, 2007). SCLC (17% of lung cancers) has a very aggressive clinical course and poorer prognosis than NSCLC. It is classified as limited stage or extensive stage and is usually detected at a more advanced stage, growing rapidly, and metastasizing early in the disease trajectory.

The disease trajectory for lung cancer is different depending on the staging and in NSCLC, depending on the sensitivity to newer treatments of targeted agents. If treated, locally advanced NSCLC (Stage IIIA or B) has a median survival of 16–17 months and Stage IV NSCLC has a median survival of 12.5 months (Sandler et al., 2005). Individuals with limited and extensive stage disease SCLC who are treated have a median survival of 18–24 months and 7–11 months respectively.

About one third of surgically resected NSCLC recur in the ipsilateral and contralateral lung, and can metastasize to various sites including bone, liver, adrenal glands, and brain. More than 80% of recurrences occur within 2 years and are complicated by distressing symptoms. Individuals with SCLC are at risk for brain metastases; however, prophylactic cranial irradiation significantly decreases the occurrence and improves 1-year survival in extensive stage disease (Slotman et al., 2007).

Signs/symptoms/staging. A tissue diagnosis and staging work up determines the type and extent of disease. Accurate staging is critical to determine if surgery would be appropriate. Positron emission tomography/computer tomography (PET/CT) combined with cranial imaging is more accurate in identifying metastatic disease than conventional imaging (CT scan of chest, abdomen, and pelvis, bone scan, and cranial imaging) in NSCLC (Hampton, 2008a). In NSCLC staging, the TNM classification groups patients according to size and extent of the tumor (T), the lymph node involvement (N), and the presence or absence of metastatic disease (M). Seventy-five percent of patients with NSCLC have locally advanced or unresectable stage IV disease at the time of diagnosis (Walker, 2003). SCLC is considered a systemic disease at diagnosis and has its own staging system. Two thirds of SCLC patients have metastatic disease at diagnosis (NCCN, 2008a). Once staging is completed, the treatment plan is individualized and based on staging classification, lung cancer genomics, biomarkers, which predict outcomes and treatment responses, the patient's ability to tolerate treatment, and the patient's performance status (Dubey & Powell, 2008).

Disease management. Because SCLC is considered a systemic disease, surgery is not an option. However, surgical resection remains the only potential curative treatment for patients with NSCLC presenting with surgically resectable disease. Surgery is recommended for all adults with a good performance status. There is no difference in overall survival between younger and older individuals (Yamamoto et al., 2003). Newer surgical techniques, such as the video-assisted thoracic surgery (VATS), have provided a minimally invasive approach with similar long-term survival rates as the thoracotomy (Molina, Yang, Cassivi, Schild, & Adjei, 2008). Current standard of care includes adjuvant chemotherapy for resected early stage disease and studies of adjuvant, targeted therapies in this population are underway (NCCN, 2008a). For Stage IIIA NSCLC, a trimodality approach (chemotherapy with concurrent radiation followed by surgery) improves progression-free survival (Albain et al., 2005).

Radiation therapy. Radiation therapy is an important treatment modality in inoperable regional NSCLC and in SCLC. It is also used as an alternative for older patients with NSCLC who are not considered surgical candidates due to comorbid disease states, or for those who decline surgery. Combined modality treatment with radiation therapy and chemotherapy in patients with nonresectable stage IIIA and IIIB NSCLC and limited stage SCLC is the standard of care for physiologically fit individuals. In patients receiving radiotherapy alone, authors of a Cochrane review of 14 randomized trials of palliative radiotherapy to the chest concluded that the majority of patients with advanced NSCLC could be treated with short courses of palliative radiotherapy (one to two fractions) (Lester, Macbeth, Toy, & Coles, 2006). This practice would greatly decrease treatment burden for patients and families. Radiation has a major role in palliation of symptoms, in particular the pain associated with bone metastases, in managing dyspnea and hemoptysis from tumor invasion, and in

controlling signs and symptoms associated with brain metastases (seizures, confusion, nausea and vomiting, and headache) (Kvale, Selecky, & Prakash, 2007).

Chemotherapy. Chemotherapy has had some promising survival benefit as adjuvant therapy for high risk stage I, Stage II, and select stage III NSCLC (NCCN, 2008a). Chemotherapy and targeted therapies are the mainstay in advanced NSCLC. Standard chemotherapy includes one of a number of chemotherapy doublet combinations given for four cycles. Doublet therapy, combining a platinum-based drug with vinorelbine, gemcitabine, or a taxane, has been shown to be more effective than single agents or best supportive care for first line therapy (Obasuju et al., 2007). Concurrent chemoradiotherapy is superior to sequential treatment, but has an increased toxicity (Curran et al., 2003). Single agent chemotherapy is preferred for patients who have a poor performance status and multiple comorbidities. In individuals who have progressed on platinum-based therapy, second-line therapy includes docetaxel and pemetrexed. Predictive modeling, tailoring chemotherapy to individuals with overexpression of specific genes, is an exciting new area that holds promise for improving response and overall survival (Walker, 2003).

SCLC is a systemic disease; therefore, treatment options are usually limited to chemotherapy and/or radiation. Chemotherapeutic regimens for limited stage disease consist of concurrent combination chemotherapy and radiation, followed by prophylactic cranial irradiation which can increase survival by about 5% (Jassem, 2007). This regimen is difficult to tolerate due to side effects associated with the toxic chemotherapeutic agents such as cisplatin and etoposide and the burden of concurrent chemoradiation. Targeted agents have not been shown to be effective.

Extensive stage SLCL is treated with etoposide/cisplatin, etoposide/carboplatin, and irinotecan/cisplatin (NCCN, 2008a). Slotman et al. (2007) demonstrated that prophylactic brain irradiation in patients with extensive SCLC who responded to chemotherapy reduces the incidence of symptomatic brain metastases and prolongs disease-free and overall survival. The debate continues as to whether highly toxic combination chemotherapy is appropriate for elders. Studies of elder patients to date suggest that they can derive benefit from treatment for SCLC; however, the limited data available supports the need to include this age group in future large SCLC clinical trials.

Targeted therapies are aimed at specific tumor pathways. The antiepidermal growth factor receptor (EGFR) inhibitor erlotinib reduces proliferation and survival of tumor cells by inhibiting tyrosine kinase. Bevacizumab, a recombinant monoclonal vascular endothelial growth factor (VEGF) monoclonal antibody prohibits angiogenesis, the development of the tumor's vascular supply which provides needed oxygen and nutrients once the tumor reaches 2–3 mm in diameter.

Blocking angiogenesis limits local and systemic metastases. Targeted therapies are being used in combination with chemotherapies or as second line treatment. As second-line therapy, erlotinib is especially effective in a subpopulation of females, nonsmokers, individuals who are of East-Asian descent, and those who have a histology of adenocarcinoma (Besse, Ropert, & Soria, 2007). Recently, bevacizumab has been shown to be effective in combination with platinum-based chemotherapy for nonsquamous cell advanced NSCLC (NCI, 2008b). Additional targeted agents such as cetuximab, an EGFR inhibitor and sunitinib and sorafenib, anti-VEGF receptor agents, are currently in trial (Besse et al., 2007; Walker, 2003).

Colorectal Cancer

The estimated new cases of colorectal cancer in the United States in 2008 are 108,070 colon cancer cases and 40,740 rectal cancer cases (Jemal et al., 2008). The projected combined death rate (49,960) has declined over the past 10 years with improved screening procedures and significant advances in surgery, radiation, and chemotherapy (Wolpin, Meyeerhardt, Mamon, & Mayer, 2007). Colorectal cancer (CRC) ranks fourth as the most common noncutaneous malignancy in the United States and is the second leading cause of cancer death. It is a disease of aging, as the median age of individuals with newly diagnosed CRC is 70 years (Rosati & Bilancia, 2008). In minorities, particularly African Americans, cancer-related mortality remains higher than in Caucasians (65% vs. 55%) (Wolpin et al., 2007).

Colorectal cancer is difficult to diagnoze at an early stage because patients are usually asymptomatic early in the disease process (ACS, 2008). Screening to detect polyps and cancer is important for all those deemed to be at risk and for those over the age of 50. Diagnosis of colorectal cancer in the older adult is especially challenging because many of the common changes of aging in the gastrointestinal tract can prevent early detection. For example, constipation, change in bowel patterns and fatigue may be inaccurately attributed to the aging process.

Approximately 50% of patients present with hepatic metastases or develop them during the course of the disease (Pawlik, Schulick, & Choti, 2008). Because the portal vein drains blood supply from the colon, the liver is the most common site of metastasis for advanced disease. Isolated lung or liver metastases may be resected in later stage disease (Engstrom et al., 2007). As the disease progresses, patients may experience bowel obstruction. Widespread metastases to abdomen (carcinomatosis), lung and/or liver is often the cause of death.

Signs/symptoms/staging. Most cancers of the bowel are moderately or well-differentiated adenocarcinomas. These cancers usually develop as a result of progressive colonic polyp mutations (Engstrom et al., 2007). Screening for and removal of potentially malignant polyps can prevent development of metastatic disease. TNM staging has been modified to correspond with the Astler-Coller Dukes system. This staging process evaluates the depth of bowel wall penetration by the tumor, lymph node involvement, and presence of distant metastasis. The accuracy of the staging in high risk Stage II and III is associated with the number of nodes surgically removed (Engstrom et al., 2007). Staging ranges from Stage I to Stage IV, with overall survival declining from greater than 90% to less than 10% for Stage IV disease (Meyerhardt & Mayer, 2005).

Disease management. A complete staging workup includes a physical exam, pathologic tissue review, colonoscopy, baseline computed tomography of the chest, abdomen and pelvis, complete blood count, chemistry profile, and carcinoembryonic antigen (CEA) determination.

Surgery. For resectable colon cancer, surgery remains the standard treatment. Tumor location, blood supply, and lymph node patterns in the area of cancer determine the extent of resection. Examination of a minimum of 12 lymph nodes is necessary for accurate staging (Engstrom et al., 2007). Laparoscopic advances have allowed the use of minimally invasive surgical procedures to resect colon cancers without increasing recurrence rates (Clinical Outcomes of Surgical Therapy Study Group, 2004). Early mobility, return of pulmonary function, and decreased ileus and adhesion formation have made this procedure desirable for many patients, especially those with advancing age and comorbid illnesses (Baker, 2001).

Surgical management of rectal cancer involves resection with preservation of anorectal sphincter function, and sexual and urinary function whenever possible (Engstrom et al., 2007). Preoperative combined modality therapy (chemotherapy and radiation) has resulted in significant reductions in tumor size and decreased rates of local recurrence in rectal cancer. However, it is associated with increased toxicity when compared to surgery alone (Bosset et al., 2006).

Radiation therapy. The role of radiation therapy is not well defined for colon cancer, but more studies are needed, as completed studies are underpowered (ACS, 2008). Debate over the value of pre- or post-surgical radiation therapy for rectal cancer continues. Although preoperative and postoperative radiotherapy has been shown to reduce local recurrence when compared to surgery alone, neither intervention resulted in a statistically significant improvement in overall survival (Kapiteijn et al., 2001). Preoperative chemoradiotherapy doubled the rate of rectal sphincter sparing operations and lowered the rates of local recurrence, acute toxicity, and long term toxicity (Sauer et al., 2004).

Chemotherapy. Current guidelines for adjuvant therapy do not recommend chemotherapy for individuals with Stage II disease. However, patients with advanced colorectal cancer do have a survival benefit from newer chemotherapeutic regimens and targeted agents. Current therapy includes bevacizumab, the VEGF blocker, plus FOLFOX infusional 5-FU, leucovorin, oxaliplatin, FOLFIRI (infusional 5-FU, leucovorin, and irinotecan), capecitabine, or 5-FU/LV. The two EGFR monoclonal antibodies, cetuximab and panitumumab, have also been shown to be effective. Genotyping of tumors may help to predict which therapy would be most beneficial to an individual. For example, patients with advanced colorectal cancer who do not have a mutated form of the gene KRAS may benefit from cetuximab and chemotherapy (McBride, 2008). Overall survival is improved with single agent cetuximab when other treatments have failed (Jonker et al., 2007).

CANCER COMORBIDITIES

For many years, lung cancer risk has been associated with chronic obstructive pulmonary disease (COPD) (Dubey & Powell, 2008), and tobacco smoke. Smokers are also known to be at risk for coronary artery disease, peripheral vascular disease, and stroke. These comorbidities may affect the performance status of individuals with lung cancer, limiting treatment options and increasing symptom burden.

Individuals at high risk for colorectal cancer are those with a first degree family history of CRC and women with a personal history of ovarian, endometrial, or breast cancer. Two major conditions that are known to have a genetic pre-disposition to CRC are familial adenomatous polyposis (FAP) and hereditary nonpolyposis colorectal cancer (HNPCC) Comorbidities often linked to CRC are the inflammatory bowel diseases including ulcerative colitis and Crohn's disease. FAP, HNPCC and inflammatory bowel diseases constitute about 10%–15% of CRC cases. Comorbid conditions that have been identified as increasing the risk of CRC are obesity, sedentary lifestyle, diet high in fat, smoking, and alcohol consumption (> 4 drinks per week) (ACS, 2008).

Frailty at any age adds a risk factor to cancer morbidity and anticancer therapies often decreases the patient's functional level allowing for catabolic syndrome, muscle wasting, and infection secondary to immobility. Paraneoplastic Syndromes are syndromes associated with tumor growth and anticancer therapies. To name a few, superior vena cava syndrome (SVCS) occurs within lymphoma, lung, and breast cancer. Deep vein thrombosis (DVT) and Pulmonary embolism (PE) are blood clots commonly occurring in solid tumor cancers and increase in frequency with anticancer therapies. Spinal cord compression occurs in cancers with systemic tendencies. All require expert assessment and rapid management.

COMMON ASSOCIATED SYMPTOMS OF CANCER

Palliative care is best initiated at the time of a cancer diagnosis, especially for patients with a life-limiting cancer. Many individuals experience symptoms that interfere with QOL at the time of diagnosis as well as other points in time along the disease trajectory. Hoffman, Given, von Eye, Gift, and Given (2007) have identified a symptom cluster of pain, fatigue, and insomnia in patients who are newly diagnozed and undergoing chemotherapy. Pain, dyspnea, fatigue, weight loss, and cough are commonly associated with lung cancer. Pain may occur as a result of tumor infiltration into lung parenchyma, the brachial plexus, spinal cord, bone metastasis, or brain metastasis-producing headache. Dyspnea occurs in as many as 55 % of lung cancer patients, and in up to 80% of patients at the EOL (Becze, 2008). Interventions for dyspnea have been reviewed, critiqued, and summarized by the Oncology Nursing Society's Putting Evidence Into Practice (PEP) Dyspnea Intervention Project Team (DiSalvo, Joyce, Tyson, Culkin, & Mackay, 2008). Fatigue has been described a very distressing symptom of the disease and treatment. Potentially treatable causes such as anemia should be identified and addressed.

More than 95% of individuals with lung cancer are symptomatic at the time of diagnosis (Kvale et al., 2007). Common symptoms such as cough, dyspnea, dysphagia, hoarseness, fatigue, and weight loss are frequently attributed to comorbid illnesses and are often ignored. Unfortunately with lung cancer, these common symptoms usually are the result of locally advanced or metastatic disease. Symptoms may be present as a result of primary cancer itself (dyspnea, wheezing, cough, hemoptysis, chest pain), from locoregional metastases within the chest (superior vena cava syndrome, pleural effusions, ribs, and pleura), or from distant metastases (back pain, metastases to brain, spinal cord or bone) (Kvale et al., 2007).

Depending on the type of treatment received, there may be additional symptoms experienced. For example, persons receiving radiation therapy may have new or increased dysphagia because of the location of the treatment field. Individuals receiving chemotherapy or undergoing radiation may experience an increase in fatigue beyond initial presentation. Symptoms at the EOL are dependent on the type of cancer and the sites of metastases. NSCLC frequently goes to the bone, often causing excruciating pain. SCLC often progresses to the brain, causing headaches, nausea, and impaired mental status. These symptoms require aggressive palliative care intervention regardless of the point they occur in the disease trajectory (Kvale et al., 2007).

Chemotherapy and targeted agents used to treat lung cancer have the potential to cause side effects that negatively influence QOL. Body image, nausea and vomiting, and chemoinduced neuropathies require aggressive nursing management. However, it is important to note that for all individuals with NSCLC or SCLC, chemotherapy has been shown to relieve tumor-related symptoms such as pain, cough, and dyspnea, as well as offering survival benefit and many patients choose to continue treatment in advanced disease for palliation (Stinnett, Williams, & Johnson, 2007).

Chemotherapy-related toxicities are common, undertreated, and most likely underreported. The deleterious effect of chemotherapy and other anticancer treatments can alter the patient's QOL and inhibit further treatments if symptoms limit the patient's physical ability to make it to the next treatment appointment. Some of the most debilitating side effects from chemotherapy require hospitalization for stabilization and the patient's decreased function level most likely will cause a delay in the treatment series. Common causes of hospitalization due to chemotherapy toxicity include infection and fever; neutropenia or thrombocytopenia; electrolyte disorders like dehydration related to nausea, vomiting, or diarrhea; fatigue and vertigo; deep vein thrombosis or pulmonary embolism; and malnutrition. Other chemotherapy induced effects include anemia, constipation, oral mucositis, anxiety/depression, neurotoxicity, peripheral neuropathy, hand and foot syndrome, and cardiac toxicity (Moore, Johnson, Fortner, & Houts, 2008).

MANAGEMENT

Cancer care should be age appropriate and treatment should be easily accessed to insure successful treatment of physical, emotional, and spiritual symptoms. The family (or family of choice for some adults) should be considered within the unit of care throughout the lifespan for effective palliative management. From childhood to frail older adult, the responsibility of decision-making shifts from parental (or support group) with possible patient input, patient with support group input, and back to support group with possible patient input (Scullion, 2005). An interdisciplinary, sometimes referred to as an integrated approach, is the gold standard for cancer care regardless of age, life expectancy, and treatment choices.

Pediatric and Young Adult

Children. The life of a child who has been diagnosed with a life threatening illness is drastically altered with wide reaching and long lasting effects on the family as a unit. Palliative care health professionals working in the field of pediatrics have reported the parental need to provide every available therapy to their child, in order to feel confident they have given their child the best chance to defy death. Often, the attempt to defy death with anticancer treatment eliminated the chance of expert symptom management occurring simultaneously. Parental direction towards measures to defy death is now considered the reality of pediatric cancer care and healthcare professionals, palliative care

specialists included, can philosophically support parents when they maintain dual goals of hope for comfort and emotional support at the same time as hope for life extension. This is a healthier alternative not only for the patient and family, but also for the healthcare professionals since it is distressing for healthcare professionals when expert symptom management is delayed until all other options have been exhausted (De Graves & Aranda, 2004; Wolfe et al., 2002). Pediatric oncology nurses report moral distress when "good nursing" is impeded as curative needs of the patient overshadow the patient's physical and emotional needs. It is necessary that cure and palliation goals interface in cancer care allowing an overlap and the palliative needs of the child are not sacrificed for the hope of a cure.

Symptom management, communication, and shared decision making resemble adult care with few exceptions, while spiritual care often presents slightly different issues for children. Identification of meaningful activity will change from one development stage to another. Play and relational connection are two identified mainstays for children. School age children may desire to maintain a school-day schedule to support their need to remain similar to and receive acceptance by their peers. Routine and normalcy are also recognized as important goals for care of children with life altering illness, and religious ritual as in routine visits to a church, synagogue, or mosque maintains the family's meaningful spiritual routine (De Graves & Aranda, 2004; Wolfe et al., 2000). Location of care and the pediatric patient's preference continues to merit attention. Some suggest that family adjustment after the child's death is better if the child dies at home, yet others have contended that family relationships are enriched if death occurs during hospitalization. Outpatient clinics resembling daycare allow the pediatric cancer patient who is receiving chemotherapy to spend nights at home and receive treatment elsewhere. These daycare clinics also encourage play that children need for emotional development. Parents frequently identify the decrease in their child's activity level in play as a source of emotional distress. No matter what the location is for anticancer treatment and EOL care, it is worth noting that healthcare professionals specialized in symptom management and bereavement support make a difference in the family's memory of the illness regardless of the outcome (Houlston, 2006; De Graves & Aranda, 2004; Wolf et al., 2000).

High quality care for children living with cancer includes expert pain and symptom management and healthcare professionals have an opportunity to make a difference in the perceived and actual experience of the parents of dying children. Children dying of cancer experience many symptoms and parents who witness the child suffering may experience additional suffering during grief work long after the child's death (Pritchard et al., 2008). Wolfe et al. (2000) discovered that discordance between parents and physicians regarding symptom recognition is similar to that of adults and their healthcare providers.

Wolfe et al., also discovered that there was a direct correlation between a parent's report of the child's suffering and the level of involvement the physician displayed during the final phase of the child's life. In other words, a parent was more likely to report the child suffering when the parent also reported feeling that the physician was not actively involved in care at the end of the child's life. Wolfe also found that earlier discussions about hospice care were associated with a higher likelihood that the parent would report the child as calm and peaceful during the last month of life. These observations support the theory that active involvement by healthcare providers committed to palliation helps to alleviate the suffering of dying children (Pritchard et al., 2008).

Young adults. Uncertainty while living with cancer has been identified as a significant aspect of pediatric cancer and a major concern of adolescent and young adult cancer survivors. Long-lasting disease control and long-term survival during and after childhood is now common due to major advances in surgery, chemotherapy, and radiotherapy. However, treatment success can also have serious implications through each phase of the patient's life. Chemotherapy and radiation therapy can harm developing organs, and surgery can alter normal physical functioning or cause disfigurement. Previous studies have reported that as many as 69% of survivors of childhood cancer have physical, mental, or emotional limitations resulting from successful anticancer treatment (Decker, Haase, & Bell, 2007).

A study of 226 adult survivors of childhood cancer showed that 12% of those interviewed reported some level of suicidal symptoms. Risk factors found for a higher significance of suicidal symptoms included younger age at diagnosis, a greater time lapse since diagnosis, and radiation treatments to the head. Add those risk factors to feelings of depression and hopelessness, chronic pain, physical dysfunction, and appearance alterations due to treatment and the data suggest that healthcare professionals should perform a thorough psychosocial assessment upon long-term follow up of survivors (Carroll, 2007). Decker et al. (2007) conducted a cross-sectional, secondary analysis study to examine uncertainty in three "time-since-diagnosis" groups of adolescents and young adults. The most recent diagnozed survivors had significantly higher uncertainly for recurring pain, an unpredictable illness course, and self-care concerns. Interestingly, survivors with 5 or more years from diagnosis had higher uncertainty related to knowing what to expect for disease reoccurrence. All survivor groups exhibited a significantly high uncertainty about multiple meanings of communication from doctors leading the investigators to conclude that providers should direct communication to adolescent and young adulthood patients. Uncertainty should be considered a concern throughout cancer survivorship and long-term support of the young cancer survivor is warranted.

Adults and Older Adults

Critical assessment of the individual with cancer is important when determining life expectancy, treatment tolerance, and palliation. Physical reserve, psychosocial support, economic support, and comorbidity impact treatment outcomes (Repetto & Comandini, 2000). The Karnofsky Performance Status (KPS) is the most widely used assessment tool in the field of oncology (Repetto, Comandini, & Mammoliti, 2001). The KPS evaluates physical function, and draws a close parallel with mortality (Repetto et al., 2001). The Eastern Cooperative Oncology Group (ECOG) assessment scale has also been used widely in oncology care to determine functional status and eligibility for treatment.

The Palliative Performance Scale (PPS) is correlated with the KPS and has been used by palliative care specialists, most generally hospice professionals, to determine and monitor a patient's eligibility for hospice services. The PPS is a reliable, valid tool which correlates well with actual and median survival times for cancer patients (Anderson, Downing, & Hill, 1996).

Age itself is not the most useful factor to determine prognosis and consider treatment options for older adults; however, a standardized nomenclature is required for a large and growing population. The concept of senescence by the passing of biological time is most useful in predicting survival, chemotherapy toxicity, postoperative morbidity, and mortality as opposed to chronological age (Exterman & Hurria 2007; Audisio et al., 2004). Chronological age can be used as a functional status indicator for the older adults because it is assumed that adults living with cancer are more likely to need functional assistance than their same-age peers without cancer. For the sake of discussion and predicting functional needs of older adults, geriatric terminology categorizes elders as "young old" (70–74 years), "old-old" (75–84 years), and "oldest old" (85 years and older). These age-related categorizations should be considered with a complete functional assessment when developing a treatment plan, since aging involves a progression of organ systems decline, coexisting physical conditions, cognitive impairment, social isolation, functional dependence, and economic limitations (Audisio et al., 2004; Balducci & Extermann, 1999). Natural changes associated with age often leads to a greater susceptibility to chronic and acute disease, yet a comprehensive evaluation of the older adult's coexisting disease (comorbidities), cognition, functional status, nutritional status, social supports, psychological state, and personal resolve give a more accurate definition of age in relation to cancer treatment tolerance (Extermann & Hurria 2007).

Another commonly used geriatric classification of the older adult is the "frail elder." The use of the term elder is most generally reserved for patients exceeding the age of 65 and "frail" is a traditional term not well defined. The medical literature often refers to a frail individual as someone with poor physiological reserves and a high prevalence of repeated chronic illness requiring multiple hospital admissions. Additional characteristics of frailty include complex psychosocial problems and limited social support, which increases the risk of treatment-related complications and cancer-specific mortality (Audisio et al., 2004). In addition, the term is associated with more than one geriatric syndrome, a limited life expectancy not much beyond two years, the inability to maintain homeostasis in nonstressed conditions, and a greater risk of developing treatmentrelated toxicities with the loss of functional independence (Repetto & Comandini, 2000). Geriatric syndromes should also be included in a comprehensive assessment in order to determine accurately the elder's stage of life and functional capabilities. Geriatric syndromes that have been defined and used in treatment planning within the last 10 years include dementia, depression, abuse/neglect, incontinence, osteoporosis, failure to thrive, and risk for falls (Balducci & Extermann, 1999).

Since the evaluation of the older adult is obviously influenced by many factors, a geriatric assessment tool can equip healthcare providers to manage the complexity of geriatric oncology healthcare needs. The comprehensive geriatric assessment (CGA) is recommended to determine the medical, psychological, and functional capabilities of elderly cancer patients. The CGA focuses on frail elderly people with complex conditions, functional status relating to QOL, and incorporates an interdisciplinary team approach to assessment (Repetto et al., 2003). Activities of daily living (ADL) and instrumental activities of daily living (IADL) are useful tools for assessing functional ability and are incorporated into many comprehensive assessment tools (Repetto et al., 2003). Dependence in ADLs and IADLs closely parallel limited life expectancy and dependence in IADL correlates with treatment intolerance, while comorbidity, a normal process of age, is known to complicate cancer diagnosis, prognosis, and treatment (Lazzaro & Comandini, 2000; Balducci & Monfardini, 1999). Comorbidity is associated with decreased survival rates, and merits attention during a comprehensive assessment.

Family Support

In addition to the physical care of a loved one with advanced cancer, comprehensive care requires family support. Palliative care includes physical, emotional, and spiritual comfort of the patient and family. Spouses, adult children, extended relatives, and neighbors account for the 7 million Americans who consider themselves caregivers. Approximately 15% of those Americans care for individuals with serious illness and disability. Spouses represent roughly 62% of those caregivers, with women as 72% of those caregivers (Derby & O'Mahony, 2006). Often, primary caregivers

are spouses with their own healthcare needs that may make them susceptible to depression, fatigue, and frequent acute illness. Other caregiving relationships involve adult children as dual role caregivers to parents and their own children, or the staff at the elder's nursing facility or assisted living environment. Researching the use of home medical/social services by elders in the last 6 months of life, Kobayashi (2000) found that the focus of care needed by the patient and family is that of medical and psychosocial treatment. Symptom management is more intense and requires regular evaluation. A large part of the advanced stage of illness may require more physical symptom monitoring, however, the psychosocial needs of the patient and family is just as important. Utilization of the palliative care team is vital at the end of life (Kobayashi, 2000).

End-of-life decisions place additional burdens on the family. Those decisions include where the final days will be spent, what impact there will be on loved ones, and whether the family can afford the care involved. Family members often take a leave of absence from their jobs to care for a dying loved one; those that do not have that option may experience feelings of remorse for taking a more peripheral role in the care of the older adult. Many Americans report they would prefer to die in the comforts of their home; however, a majority die in an acute-care or long-term facility. Nurses can support a dying patient by providing a home-like environment and a familiar surrounding with the patient's personal items, aroma, music, and support people (Hsieh, Huang, Lai, & Lin, 2007; Tang, 2003; Beardsmore & Fitzmaurice, 2002; Higginson & Sen-Gupta, 2000).

When patients reach the terminal phase of cancer, conflict may occur among the patient, family members, and healthcare workers. Conflict at the EOL transpires due to the disparity of patient/family expectations with the patient's function and symptom status and the patient's attempt to maintain physical, emotional, and existential control. As the disease progresses, symptoms, and physical function are in flux. Family members attempt to adjust to the changes, however, in advanced cancer, the changes can occur quickly, which provokes conflict. Family concerns throughout the course of advanced illness are directed towards the physical comfort of the patient, the emotional impact on the family, and the desire for accurate information (Milberg et al., 2008; Griffin et al., 2007; Valdimarsdottir et al., 2007; Tang, 2003; Kristjanson & White, 2002). Vachon, Kristjanson, and Higginson (1995) report that most families feel that information concerning their loved ones' illness is difficult to obtain, and that support is inadequate. It is commonly perceived by family members that once the terminal prognosis is discussed, healthcare professionals do not feel the need to provide additional information. Due to the rapid change in physical and cognitive status, information updates are just as significant as before. Out of 22 terminally ill patients interviewed, Kutner, Steiner, Corbett, Jahnigen, and Barton, (1999) concluded that 98.2% requested information concerning changes in their disease status. It is interesting to note that even though most patients and families request the truth, they still want healthcare providers to be optimistic and maintain a sense of hope (Kutner et al., 1999). It is also worth noting that bereaved family members report higher satisfaction, fewer concerns, and fewer unmet needs pertaining to the care of a loved one when palliative care and hospice teams provide EOL care (Teno et al., 2004). Initially, the family's focus of hope is often on cure. It is also the hope and goal of the family to provide comfort and support to their loved one as death becomes imminent. The palliative care team assists caregivers to develop the physical, emotional, and mental reserves that are required to maintain hope; coupling that with the provision of timely, accurate, and honest information of the impending death. Nurses should respond to patient and family concerns with patience and assurance of nonabandonment and an increase in attention to aggressive symptom management (Valdimarsdottir et al., 2007; Borneman, Stahl, Ferrell, & Smith, 2002). Physicians often choose to limit or tailor prognostic information with the intention of maintaining a patient's hope. Mack et al. (2007) conducted a cross-sectional, questionnaire-based study of parents and physicians of children with cancer. The study evaluated relationships between parental recall of prognostic disclosure from the physician and how that disclosure affected hope, trust, and emotional distress. In this multivariable model, parents frequently reported that "high quality" physician communication (defined by parents as trusting a familiar physician to give honest information) involving more elements of prognostic disclosure made them feel more hopeful. The result of this study found that when the physician has established a compassionate, trusting relationship with the patient and family prognostic disclosure can support hope, even when the prognosis is poor. In fact, no data are available that show hope can be taken from patients and families despite the longstanding fear of clinicians (Harrington & Smith, 2008).

Parents of dying children often have an intellectual knowledge or emotional awareness of the child's impending death. Vladimarsdottir and colleagues (2007) discovered that healthcare providers can influence that awareness of parents encouraging a "preparatory phase" of care that fosters an environment of talking about the child's impending death and making a long lasting beneficial effect on bereavement. Emotional awareness enables parents to see the patient's weakening condition, obtain more information and assistance from healthcare providers, and discuss important issues on life and death. As the family's focus of hope shifts due to the patient's weakening physical condition, family members may strengthen the connection with their faith system, their relationship to the patient, and others. The connection made with healthcare providers prior to the death of the loved one is considered integral in the grieving process (Milberg et al., 2008; Griffin et al., 2007; Valdimarsdottir et al., 2007; Tang, 2003; Kristjanson & White, 2002).

Bereavement Support

Saying goodbye to a loved one is important to survivors. Those who lose a loved one unexpectedly often exhibit less resilience and more anger during the bereavement period. Anticipatory grief has not been shown to alter actual grief, but giving family members sufficient warning of an impending death will foster a shift of focus to meaningful discussions with the cancer patient. That meaningful time will have a lasting impact on the survivor, possibly alleviating any guilt the survivor may normally experience as a grieving caregiver. Since mourning is culture based, this is also a good time for the healthcare provider to inquire about and honor cultural and religious practices surrounding death. This display of respect for cultural and spiritual rituals surrounding the dying process and memorial can make the experience of death less traumatic.

Data from two small studies (Cohen et al., 1997) of terminally ill cancer patients show that scores of existential well being correlate with scores of physical well being. Even in the presence of physical pain, depression, and hopelessness are inversely related to spiritual well being. After the death, a caring call from a familiar healthcare provider allows the survivor to reconnect with someone who shared the death experience and to discuss concerns regarding emotional and physical responses to grief. The bereaved often report the need to talk about the death experience many times. These phone calls can lend an additional listening ear for that purpose (Griffin et al., 2007). Milberg et al. (2008) learned from bereaved family members that half of them requested bereavement follow up and many wanted to talk about the events occurring in the palliative phase of the decendent's care, their own response to loneliness, and the future. Follow-up contacts were preferred in person and respondents expressed appreciation to be recognized as a person with specific needs for contact.

PALLIATIVE CARE ISSUES

Palliative Chemotherapy

Goals and use of chemotherapy near the EOL. Since the 1970s, oncological trials have focused on chemotherapy response rates, disease-free intervals, and overall survival endpoints. At the same time, clinicians have observed and recorded the symptom improvement benefits during curative treatment efforts. As a result, the concept of "palliative chemotherapy" for the purpose of symptom improvement and slowing cancer growth became not only an acceptable practice, but also a desirable choice for patients whose cancer was impossible to eradicate (Archer et al., 1999). Chemotherapy is increasingly available and better tolerated, therefore patients with incurable cancer are frequently offered the option of palliative chemotherapy even though there is no certainty that symptom burden will be relieved or survival will be extended. Patients and families will put their hope in treatments offered with limited scientific evidence of benefit, therefore, chemotherapy use for patients with advanced disease requires sophisticated oncologic assessment, clarity of the patient's goals for care, and balanced shared decision-making between patient and oncologist. Like other treatment decisions, it requires a complete burden versus benefit analysis. Since solid data are not available to support the palliative benefits of chemotherapy, smaller community hospice agencies are not willing to take on the cost of such treatment. Community resources offering interdisciplinary support not linked to the hospice benefit provide valuable support to individuals receiving palliative chemotherapy. Cancer clinics may be linked to national and local programs and area hospices may have additional services for individuals ineligible to elect the hospice benefit.

Knowing what patients and families understand from diagnosis, treatment, and prognosis discussions with their oncologists is paramount. Many studies have shown that patients and families report not knowing that late-stage chemotherapy was not intended to cure. Within those studies reported by Harrington and Smith (2008), many patients did not recall such a discussion regarding prognosis and the goal to treat with palliative chemotherapeutic agents. In an effort to support a patient's hope for disease outcome, it has also been reported that many physicians will offer a wide range of outcomes to allow patients to assume for themselves the most favorable. Supporting a balanced exchange of information and shared decision-making between patients and their oncologists remains important. People living face to face with death will choose aggressive treatment with major adverse effects and a small chance of benefit. This is largely different from what their physicians and nurses who are not living with illness would choose. Individuals representing many socioeconomic levels and value systems are willing to place their hope in experimental drugs with 10% mortality rate for one last chance of benefit (Harrington & Smith, 2008).

A discussion of patient preference for quality and quantity of life with or without chemotherapy is a good start to a palliative treatment discussion. Before chemotherapy is recommended, a definable benefit must be indentified, and a straightforward discussion can be initiated by asking the patient how much they want to know about their current condition and prognosis. Define the words response and cure. Many patients will use these terms interchangeably. Provide printed resources listing benefits of and adverse reactions to chemotherapy, keeping in mind that there must be a

definable benefit to chemotherapy before treatment can be medically justified. Ask the patient about goals for treatment, their views on undesirable side effects, and plans for the future. Extending survival time for an upcoming special event may be the benefit that could justify treatment in the patient's mind. Also, initiate discussion, with the intent of revisiting the plan when the cancer is resistant to chemotherapy.

Upon evaluation of the palliative treatment, the nurse can facilitate a meeting with the treating and palliative care team to clearly report on how the cancer is responding to chemotherapy. Working within an interdisciplinary framework, the physician, a nurse specialist, clergy, patient, and family should be involved in this discussion. Continue a straightforward approach to communication by clearly defining the cancer's response to treatment. Provide hope if there is reason to be hopeful; however, avoid offering false hope. Many people are able to be hopeful about something even if the cancer is growing, yet some physicians believe that disclosing a poor prognosis will reduce a patient's hope. In a study of 194 parents of children living with cancer, Mack et al. (2007) discovered that clinician communication can foster hope even when the news is bad. In almost half of the parents receiving more prognostic, high quality information from their child's physician, a greater communication-related hope was reported (Mack et al., 2007). High quality was designated by clinician sensitivity and the clinician's active listening skills. Supporting previous research findings, Mack and associates suggest that meaningful experiences and relationships can serve as a foundation for hope, as opposed to a hope based on unrealistic expectations for treatment outcome. In fact, there are no data that supports the previous belief that hope can be taken away from patients and that patients are harmed by sensitive, compassionate information exchange regarding prognosis (Harrington & Smith, 2008).

Body image changes associated with targeted agents including facial and upper body rash and hair loss associated with many of the chemotherapeutic agents can be devastating for patients and families. The pathophysiology of nausea and vomiting is quite complex and requires strong assessment skills to identify appropriate pharmacologic and nonpharmacologic interventions. Neuropathies associated with thoracic surgical resection and with chemotherapeutic agents, especially the platinum drugs and taxotere, can be very burdensome and require aggressive management. Medications for neuropathic pain, such as gabapentin, pregabelin, duloxetine, or the tricyclic antidepressants, may improve QOL.

In addition to addressing physical symptoms associated with lung cancer, the nurse may be involved with palliative care to help the patient and family with complex decision making during the staging process, at the time of disease progression and end of life.

With the minimally toxic targeted agents now available, many are opting to choose treatment rather than supportive care alone. Hospice referral length of stay may decrease as more patients are continuing treatment late into the disease. The current hospice medicare regulations require patients to choose eitherhospice care or continued therapy. Until there is a change in the hospice benefit, many will not have access to needed hospice care until the last days of life (Temel et al., 2008). The role of the nurse as advocate is needed at this stage.

Palliative care can also improve psychological, social, and spiritual concerns that confront patients and families with cancer. Guilt, associated with a history of smoking or current tobacco use, may increase distress in patients throughout the disease trajectory. Counseling may be of help to address emotions, fears, and concerns. Changes in roles and relationships as a result of disease progression also may require intervention from the counselors and social workers on the palliative care team. Involving spiritual care is important as individuals face the reality of the end-of-life and the importance of life closure.

Over half of all patients with colorectal cancers are diagnosed in the advanced stages. Comfort measures to manage metastatic disease and side effects of treatment are essential for QOL. Tri-modality therapy is difficult with patients battling fatigue, nausea and vomiting, diarrhea, and pain. In late-stage disease, bowel obstruction, pain, ascites, and nausea and vomiting require aggressive palliative care. For bowel obstruction, pharmacologic management (octreotide) and nonpharmacologic interventions (percutaneous draining peg) may relieve pain and nausea/vomiting.

Along with managing physical symptoms, the nurse must address the psychological, social and spiritual issues that may be evident across the disease trajectory. Depression, frequently underdiagnozed and undertreated in patients with cancer should be managed with medication and counseling. Financial burdens associated with months of expensive treatment and inability to work requires help from social work. Spiritual care may alleviate the anxiety that comes from the uncertainty of disease progression in colorectal cancer and the challenges associated with treatment decisions. As hope and goals change from control of the disease to a comfortable death, the palliative care team in conjunction with the primary nurse can provide support to the patient and family.

Case Study conclusion: Mr. J. experienced the roller-coaster journey of advanced cancer. Throughout this journey, from diagnosis until death, he was supported by his primary treatment nurse and the cancer center's palliative care team. The best approach to patients with life-limiting illness is access to palliative care throughout the disease

trajectory (IOM, 2003). Interventions from the advanced practice nurse, social worker, counselor, and spiritual care coordinator on the palliative care team were a support to Mr. J. and his family.

For some months, Mr. J's CT scans demonstrated response to treatment or stable disease. During other times of restaging, the CT scans and clinical symptoms were evidence of progression. Over the course of the first 20 months, he received a variety of combinations of chemotherapy and targeted agents. Pain, nausea and vomiting, anxiety, and depression were managed with pharmacologic and nonpharmacologic interventions. Mr. and Mrs. J. participated in counseling. The spiritual care counselor provided listening and presence during each of his treatment sessions.

In March of 2008, Mr. J. had progressive disease in the abdomen and liver and new pulmonary metastases and he was enrolled in a Phase I clinical trial. At that time, he was experiencing right upper quadrant pain associated with liver metastases, nausea and vomiting related to the treatment, cough, lower extremity peripheral neuropathy, and depression. Current medications included oxycodone SR 10 mg p.o. b.i.d., oxycodone 5 mg p.o. every 2 hr as needed for pain, and dexamethasone 8 mg daily for abdominal pain, ondansetron 8 mg p.o. every 6 hr as needed for nausea and vomiting, lorazepam 1 mg p.o. every 8 hrs as needed for anxiety, benzonatate 100 mg p.o. every 4 hr for cough, gabapentin 300 mg p.o. b.i.d. for chemoinduced neuropathy, magnesium oxide 400 mg. p.o. b.i.d., and setraline 150 mg. p.o. daily for depression (which had been increased over time).

As his pulmonary metastases progressed, managing Mr. J.'s dyspnea became the major challenge. He was hoping to enroll in a second Phase I clinical trial but required hospitalization for shortness of breath. Since current recommendations for progressive colon cancer suggest chemotherapy for symptom management and increased survival, and since Mr. J.'s goal was quantity and QOL, continuing chemotherapy was appropriate. However, during this admission, it became evident that he was dying from his pulmonary metastases and would no longer be a candidate for more treatment.

The palliative care team worked with the nurses to manage his dyspnea with opioids and increase his intravenous lorazepam to alleviate his anxiety and restlessness. Mrs. J. met with the team in conjunction with the oncologists to review Mr. J.'s goals of care. Hospice was called in to help care for him at end of his life. Mrs. J. was very worried about caring for him at home with the children experiencing another loss, and Mr. J. preferred to stay in the hospital with the staff he had come to know over the 2 years of care. The decision was made to keep him in the hospital with hospice care.

The children were brought to the hospital to see their dad and had time to work with the hospital childlife workers and receive counseling. All the children participated in decorating squares on a premade quilt on Mr. J.'s bed, expressing their love for him. Time was set aside for Mr. J. and his wife to be alone in the room and their privacy was honored by the staff. Mr. J. died peacefully within 5 days of his sudden decline. The palliative care team, which had been with him throughout the cancer experience, supported him and his family at this difficult time, and hospice continued to provide bereavement support and counseling to the family.

EVIDENCE-BASED PRACTICE

Hilliard, R. E. (2003). The effects of therapy on the quality and length of life of people diagnozed with terminal cancer. *Journal of Music Therapy, 40*(2), 113–37.

Research problem. Researchers studied the effects of music therapy on QOL, survival benefit, physical well being, and relationship of death occurrence to the final music therapy interventions of hospice patients diagnozed with terminal cancer.

Design. Randomized control trial

Sample and setting. A total of 80 hospice patients participated in the study, randomly assigned to one of two groups: The experimental group received routine hospice services with clinical music therapy. The control group received routine hospice services without clinical music therapy. Both groups were matched on the basis of gender and age.

Methods. Quality of life (QOL) was measured with the Hospice Quality of Life Index-Revised (HQOLI-R) as a self report every visit. Functional status was assessed during weekly nursing visits. All subjects received a minimum of two visits. ANOVA used to analyze data.

Results. A significant difference was revealed between the two groups on scales used for visits one and two. QOL was higher for subjects receiving music therapy, and increased over time with more music therapy sessions. The control group reported lower QOL scores compared to the experimental group with QOL decreasing over time without music. There were no significant differences determined by age, gender, or condition of patient. There were also no significant differences between groups in functioning, survival benefit, or time of death in relation to the last music therapy session.

Commentary. Professionally trained, board certified music therapists (MT-BC) use live music to treat people living with advanced illnesses and people during the active dying phase. Music therapy includes making music, listening to music, writing songs that may include telling the story of the patient, and discussing the meaning of lyrics. It may also involve imagery and learning through music. The patient does not need to have any musical ability to benefit from music therapy. Music thanatology is the form of music therapy used at the end of a patient's life to ease the person's dying process. Music therapy can be provided in homes, hospices, or nursing homes.

Research provides support for music therapy to increase QOL, alleviate spiritual suffering, provide symptom (pain, dyspnea, anxiety) management, and promote relaxation in end-of-life care. Music therapy is an established allied health profession and is used with increasing frequency in the treatment of individuals living with a terminal illness and for those in the active phase of dying. Empirical research literature supporting the use of music therapy in EOL care is necessary to evaluate the effects of music therapy on QOL, longevity, symptom burden prior to and during the final phase of dying. There is some evidence that music therapy can help to reduce pain and relieve chemotherapy-induced nausea and vomiting, relieve stress, and provide a sense of well-being. Other studies have also found that music therapy can lower heart rate, blood pressure, and breathing rate.

This study conducted by Big Bend Hospice, in collaboration with Florida State University, showed that QOL was higher for those subjects receiving music therapy sessions. Conversely, those individuals in the control group receiving no music therapy exhibited a trend in decreasing QOL. This study did not show significant differences between the groups pertaining to longevity and physical function. Since QOL scales evaluate physical, emotional, and spiritual symptom burden, music therapy enhanced the recipient's physical comfort and overall well-being.

Music therapists can be found in many communities. The Centers for Music Therapy in end-of-life care provide training opportunities for professional and student music therapists, social workers, nurses, chaplains, and others. Participants who are board-certified music therapists can earn the hospice & palliative care music therapy certificate by completing required courses. In addition, The American Music Therapy Association represents over 5000 music therapists. An on-line search or calling a local hospice agency can be helpful to find state listings of board certified music therapists and services.

EVIDENCE-BASED PRACTICE

Given, C. et al. (2004). Effect of a cognitive behavioral intervention on reducing symptom severity during chemotherapy. *Journal of Clinical Oncology, 22*(3), 507–16.

Research problem. To test the efficacy of a behavioral intervention for reducing the severity of multiple symptoms among patients diagnozed with different solid tumor sites undergoing a first choice of chemotherapy.

Design. Randomized Control Trial.

Sample and setting. Patients ($n = 237$) were accrued from comprehensive and community cancer centers, interviewed, and randomly assigned to the experimental intervention ($n = 118$) or conventional care ($n = 119$) groups. Patients were older than 21 years of age, diagnozed with a wide range of solid tumors, undergoing first course of chemotherapy.

Methods. The control group received conventional care. The experimental group received a behavioral intervention based on the work of Bandura, using four approaches to developing self-efficacy: mastering skills through practice, observing others as they address problems, persuading oneself that the strategy will work, and convincing oneself that the strategy will reduce aversive symptoms. Fifteen symptoms (alopecia, constipation, cough, diarrhea, fatigue, fever, anorexia, coordination problems, nausea & vomiting, insomnia, dry mouth, pain, mouth sores, inability to concentrate, and shortness of breath), functional limitation, and emotional distress were evaluated at 10–20 weeks to assess the impact of intervention. Severity of symptoms was rated by patients on a 10 point scale ranging from 1 (barely noticeable) — 10 (worst possible). Nursing evaluation continued throughout the study to determine the appropriate intervention for the severity of symptom. Those evaluations were guided by computerized protocols. Intervention themes included self-care management; information, decision-making, and problem solving; communication with healthcare providers; and counseling and support. Data analysis through two-sample t tests for continuous variables and $x2$ tests for categoric variables was used.

Results. Two models were tested: 1) The additive effects of supportive medications, and 2) The possible interactions between group and numbers of supportive care medications on symptom severity at the 20-week observation. The behavioral intervention used a problem-solving approach designed to engage patients in specific intervention strategies to reduce total symptom burden. Baseline scores showed no statistically significant differences at entry. At 10 and 20-week evaluations, there was significant interaction between the experimental group receiving cognitive behavioral intervention and their baseline symptom severity. Patients in the experimental group who entered the trial with higher symptom burden reported significantly lower severity at 10 and 20 weeks. No evidence was found to indicate that supportive medicine confounded the effects of intervention.

Conclusion. The relationship between the presence and severity of symptoms reported by cancer patients undergoing chemotherapy and their impact of QOL has been demonstrated in prior studies. Those studies have represented large, vast final effect ranges. This study tested the efficacy of a behavioral intervention for reducing the severity of multiple symptoms among patients diagnozed with solid tumors undergoing a first course of chemotherapy.

This trial indicates that patients who entered the trial with higher symptom severity and undergoing a first course of chemotherapy, a 20-week, nurse administered cognitive-behavioral intervention resulted in significantly lower levels of symptom severity scores compared to patients receiving conventional care alone. The behavioral intervention was successful in engaging patients in specific intervention strategies designed to reduce total symptom burden. The intervention showed significant impact within 10 weeks with increasing impact evident at week 20. The intervention was integrated into the ongoing treatment plans equipping family caregivers and providing longstanding follow up via telephone. This is one of few trials contrasting the impact of behavioral intervention with supportive care medications to understand how these two approaches might work independently or complement one another. It is important to indentify interventions that can be directed toward a patient's high symptom burden while equipping the patient and family caregivers with tools to integrate behaviors learned into day-to-day life.

REFERENCES

Aebi, S., & Pagani, O. (2007). Treatment of premenopausal women with early breast cancer: Old challenges and new opportunities. *Drugs 67*(10), 1391–1401.

Albain, D., Swann, R., Rusch, V., Turrisi, A., Sheperd, F., Smith, C., et al. (2005). Phase III study of concurrent chemotherapy and radiotherapy (CT/RT) vs CT/RT followed by surgical resection for stage IIIA (pN2) nonsmall cell lung cancer (NSCLC): Outcomes update of North American Intergroup 0139 (RTOG 9309) [Abstract 7014]. *Journal of Clinical Oncology: ASCO Annual Meeting Proceedings*, Part I, *23*(165), 624s.

Aldridge, A., & Roesch, S. C. (2007). Coping and adjustment in children with cancer: A metaanalytic study. *Journal of Behavioral Medicine, 30*(2), 115–129.

American Cancer Society. (2008). *Cancer facts and figures 2002.* Atlanta, Georgia: ACS.

Anderson, F, Downing, G. M., & Hill, J. (1996). Palliative performance scale (PPS): A new tool. *Journal of Palliative Care, 12*(1), 5–11.

Archer, V. R., Billingham, L. J., & Cullen, M. H. (1999). Palliative chemotherapy: No longer a contradiction in terms. *The Oncologist, 4,* 470–77.

Armstrong, A. J., & Carducci, M. A. (2005). Chemotherapy for advance prostate cancer: Results of new clinical trials and future studies. *Current Oncology Reports, 7*(3), 220–227.

Aschele, C., & Lonardi, S. (2007). Multidisciplinary treatment of rectal cancer: Medical oncology. *Annals of Oncology, 18*(S9), 114–121.

Audisio, R. A., Bozzetti, F., Gennari, R., Jaklitsch, M. T., Koperna, T., Longo, W. E., et al. (2004). The surgical management of elderly cancer patents: Recommendations of the SIOG surgical task force. *European Journal of Cancer, 40,* 926–938.

Baker, D. (2001). Current surgical management of colorectal cancer. *Nursing Clinics of North America, 36*(3), 579–591.

Balducci, L., & Extermann, M. (1999). Management of cancer in the elderly. Home healthcare consultant oncology. *Clinical Geriatrics, 6*(3), 2–3, 7–10.

Balducci, L., & Monfardini, S. (1999). A comprehensive geriatric assessment (CGA) is necessary for the study and management of cancer in the elderly. *European Journal of Cancer, 53*(13), 1771–1772.

Beardsmore, S., & Fitzmaurice, N. (2002). Palliative care in paediatric oncology. *European Journal of Cancer, 38,* 1900–1907.

Becze, E. (2008). Put evidence into practice to manage dyspnea. *ONS Connect,* August, 2008, 18–19.

Besse, B., Ropert, S., & Soria, J. (2007). Targeted therapies in lung cancer. *Annals of Oncology, 18* (Suppl. 9), 135–142.

Borneman, T., Stahl, C., Ferrell, B., & Smith, D. (2002). The concept of hope in family caregivers of cancer patients at home. *Journal of Hospice and Palliative Nursing, 4,*(1). 21–33.

Bosset, J., Collette, L., Calais, G., Mineur, L., Maingon, P., Radosevic, J. et al. (2006). Chemotherapy with preoperative radiotherapy in rectal cancer. *The New England Journal of Medicine, 355,* 1114–11123.

Carbone, P. P. (2000). Advances in the systemic treatment of cancers in the elderly. *Critical Reviews in Oncology/Hematology, 35,* 201–218.

Carroll, S. (2007). Adult survivors of childhood cancer are at risk for suicide. *Oncology Nursing, 34*(2), 294.

Clinical Outcomes of Surgical Therapy Study Group. (2004). A comparison of laparoscopically assisted and open colectomy for colon cancer. *The New England Journal of Medicine, 35 0,* 2050–2059.

Cohen, S., Mount, B., Bruera E., Provost, M., Rowe, J., & Tong, K., et al. (1997). Validity of the McGill Quality of Life Questionnaire in the palliative care setting: A multicentre Canadian study demonstrating the importance of existential domain. *Palliative Medicine, 11*(1), 3–20.

Coyne, P., Lyckholm, L., & Smith, T. J. (2006). Clinical interventions, economic outcomes, and palliative care. In B. Ferrell & N. Coyle (Eds.), *Textbook of palliative nursing* (pp. 429–442). NY: Oxford University Press.

Curran, W., Scott, C., Langer, C., Kmaki, R., Lee, J., Hauser, B., et al. (2003). Long-term benefit is observed in a phase III comparison of sequential vs. concurrent chemo-radiation for patients with unresected stage III NSCLC: RTOG 9410 [Abstract 2499]. *Journal of Clinical Oncology, ASCO Annual Meeting Proccedings, Part I, 22,* 621.

Darmber, J., & Aus, G. (2008). Prostate cancer. *Lancet, 371,* 1710–1721.

De Graves, S., & Aranda, S. (2005). When a child cannot be cured-reflections of health professional. *European Journal of Cancer Care, 14,* 132–140.

Decker, C., Haase, J., & Bell, C. (2007). Uncertainty in adolescents and young adults with cancer. *Oncology Nursing Forum, 34*(3), 681–688.

Derby, S., & O'Mahony, S. (2006). Elderly patients. In B. Ferrell & N. Coyle (Eds.), *Textbook of palliative nursing* (pp. 635–660). NY: Oxford University Press.

DiSalvo, W., Joyce, M., Culkin, A., Tyson, L., & Mackay, K. (2008). Putting evidence into practice: Evidence-based interventions for cancer-related dyspnea. *Clinical Journal of Oncology Nursing, 12*(2), 341–352.

Djulbegovic, B., Kumar, A., Soares, H., Hozo, I., Bepler, G., Clarke, M., et al. (2008). Treatment success in cancer. *Archives of Intern Medicine, 168*(6), 632–642.

Dubey, S., & Powell, C. (2008). Update in lung cancer 2007. *American Journal of Respiratory and Critical Care Medicine, 177,* 941–946.

Engstrom, P., Arnoletti, J., Benson, A. Chen, Y., Choti, M., Cooper, H., et al. (2007). Colon cancer: Clinical practice guidelines in oncology. *Journal of the National Comprehensive Cancer Network, 5*(9), 884–925.

Engstrom, P., Arnoletti, J., Benson, A. Chen, Y., Choti, M., Cooper, H., et al. (2007). Rectal cancer: Clinicalpractice guidelines in oncology. *Journal of the National Comprehensive Cancer Network, 5*(9), 940–981.

Extermann, M., & Hurria, A. (2007). Comprehensive geriatric assessment for older patients with cancer. *Journal of Clinical Oncology, 25*(14), 1824–1831.

Foley, K., & Gelband, H. (2001). Background and recommendations. In K. Foley & H. Gelband (Eds.), *Improving palliative care for cancer* (pp. 9–61). Washington: National Academy Press.

Gelfman, L., Meier, D., & Morrison, S. (2008). Does palliative care improve quality? A survey of bereaved family members. *Journal of Pain and Symptom Management, 36*(1); 22–28.

Given, C., Given, B., Rahbar, M., Jeon, S., McCorkle, R., Cimprich, B., et al. (2004). Effect of cognitive behavioral intervention on reducing symptom severity during chemotherapy. *Journal of Clinical Oncology, 22*(3), 507–516

Griffin, J., Koch, K., Nelson, J., & Cooley, M. (2007). Palliative care consultation, quality of life measurements and bereavement for end-of-life care in patients with lung cancer: ACCP evidence -based clinical practice guidelines (2nd ed.). *Chest, 132,* 404–422.

Hampton, T. (2008a). New studies target lung cancer prevention, imaging, and treatment. *Journal of the American Medical Association, 300* (3), 267–268.

Hampton, T. (2008b). New treatment strategies provide more options for patients with breast cancer. *Journal of the American Medical Association, 300*(4), 381–382.

Harrington, S., & Smith, T. (2008). The role of chemotherapy at the end of life: "When is enough, enough?" *Journal of the American Medical Association, 299*(22), 2667–2678.

Harrington, S. E., & Smith, T. J. (2008). The role of chemotherapy at the end of life: Healthcare consultant oncology. *Clinical Geriatrics, 6*(3), 2–3, 7–10.

Higginson, I. J., & Sen-Gupta, G. J. A. (2000). Place of care in advanced cancer: A qualitative systemic literature review of patient preferences. *Journal of Palliative Medicine, 3*(3), 287–295.

Hilliard, R. E. (2003). The effects of therapy on the quality and length of life of people diagnosed with terminal cancer. *Journal of Music Therapy, 40*(2), 113–137.

Hoffman, A., Given, B., von Eye, A., Gift, A., & Given, C. (2007). Relationships among pain, fatigue, insomnia, and gender in persons with lung cancer. *Oncology Nursing Forum, 34*(4), 785–792.

Holcomb, S. S. (2006). Breast cancer therapy and treatment guidelines. *The Nurse Practitioner, 31*(10), 59–63.

Holland, J., & Chertkov, L. (2001). Clinical practice guidelines for the management of psychosocial and physical symptoms of cancer. In K. Foley & H. Gelband (Eds.), *Improving palliative care for cancer* (pp. 199–232). Washington: National Academy Press. http://www.nci.nih.gov/cancertopics/pdq/treatment/colon/healthprofessional/. Accessed 8/26/08.

Houlston, A. (2006). Hospital for the children. *Nursing Standard, 20*(25), 70–71.

Hsieh, M. C., Huang, M. C., Lai, Y. L., & Lin, C. C. (2007). Grief reactions in family caregivers of advanced patients in Taiwan. *Cancer Nursing, 30*(4), 278–84.

Hunter-Dorcas, R. (1991). Cancer and sexuality. In S. Baird, M. Donehower, V. Lindquist-Stalsbroten, T. Ades (Eds.), *A cancer source book for nurses* (6th ed., pp. 220–227). Atlanta, Georgia: ACS

Jassem, J. (2007). The role of radiotherapy in lung cancer: Where is the evidence? *Radiotherapy Oncology, 83*(2), 203–213.

Jemal, A., Siegel, R., Ward, E., Hao, Y., Xu, J., & Taylor, M., et al. (2008). Cancer statistics, *2008. CA: A Cancer Journal for Clinicians, 58*(1), 71–96.

Jonker, D., O'Callaghan, C., Karapetis, C., Zalcberg, J. T. D., Au, H., Berry, S., et al. (2007). Ceuximab for the treatment of colorectal cancer. *The New England Journal of Medicine, 357,* 2040–2048.

Kapiteijn, E., Marijnen, C., Nagtegall, I., et al. (2001). Preoperative radiotherapy combined with total mesorectal excision for resectable rectal cancer. *The New England Journal of Medicine, 345,* 638–646.

Kobayashi, N. (2000). Formal service utilization by the frail elderly at home during the last 6 months of life. *Nursing and Health Sciences, 2*(4), 201.

Kristjanson, L., & White, K. (2002). Clinical support for families in the palliative care phase of hematologic or oncologic illness. *Hematology Oncology Clinical North American, 16,* 745–762.

Kuebler, K., Lynn, J., & Von Rohen, J. (2005). Perspectives in palliative care. *Seminars in Oncology Nursing, 21*(1), 2–10.

Kutner, J. S., Steiner, J. F., Corbett, K. K., Jahnigen, D. W., & Barton, P. L. (1999). Information needs in terminal illness. *Social Science and Medicine, 48,* 1341–1352.

Kvale, P., Selecky, P., & Prakash, U. (2007). Palliative care in lung cancer: ACCP evidence-based clinical practice guidelines (2nd ed.), *Chest, 132* (Suppl. 3), 3685–4035.

Lally, R. M. (2007). Childhood cancer survivorship: A lifelong surveillance. *ONS Connect, 6,* 8–12.

Larson, S., & Wolk, A. (2007). Obesity and colon and rectal cancer risk: A meta-analysis of prospective studies. *American Journal of Clinical Nutrition, 86*(3), 556–565.

Lazzaro, R., & Comandini, D. (2000). Cancer in the elderly: Assessing patients for fitness. *Critical Reveiws in Oncology/Hematology, 35,* 155–160.

Lester, J., Macbeth, F., Toy, E., & Coles, B. (2006). Palliative radiotherapy regimens for non- small cell lung cancer. *Cochrane Database Systematic Review, 18*(4), CD002143.

Litsas, G. (2008). Sequential therapy with tamoxifen and aromatase inhibitors in early-stage postmenopausal breast cancer: A review of the evidence. *Oncology Nursing Forum, 35*(4), 714–720.

Mack, J., Wolfe, J., Cook, F., Grier, H. E., Cleary, P. D., & Weeks, J. C., et al. (2007). Hope and prognostic disclosure. *Journal of Clinical Oncology, 25*(35), 5636–5642.

Mackay, H. J. (2000). Metastatic and advanced breast cancer in the elderly. *Clinical Geriatrics.* Retrieved on 4/10/02 from http://www.mmhc.com/cg/articles/CG9912/mackay.html.

Matsuyama, R., Reddy, S., & Smith, T. J. (2006). Why do patients choose chemotherapy near the end of life? A review of the perspective of those facing death from cancer. *Journal of Clinical Oncology, 24*(21), 3490–3496.

Mauri, D., Pavlidis, N., Polyzos, N. P., & Ioannidis, J. P. (2006). Survival with aromatase inhibitors and inactivators versus standard hormonal therapy in advanced breast cancer: Meta analysis. *Journal International Cancer Institute, 98*(18), 1285–1291.

McBride, D. (2008). KRAS status predicts response to cetuximab for metastatic colorectal cancer. *ONS Connect, 8,* 25.

Merglen, A., Schmidlin, F., Fioretta, G., Verkooijen, H., Rapiti, E., Zanetti, R., et al. (2007). Short-and long-term mortality with localized prostate cancer. *Archives of Intern Medicine, 67*(18), 1944–1950.

Meyerhardt, J., & Mayer, R. (2005). Systemic therapy for colorectal cancer. Palliation of gastrointestinal obstructive disorders. *Nursing Clinics of North America, 36*(4), 761–778.

Milberg, A., Olsson, E. C., Jakobsson, M., Olsson, M., & Friedrichsen, M. (2008). Family members' perceived needs for bereavement follow-up. *Journal of Pain and Symptom Management, 35*(1), 58–69.

Molina, J., Yang, P., Cassivi, S., Schild, S., & Adjei, A. (2008). Non-small cell lung cancer: Epidemiology, risk factors, treatment, and survivorship. *Mayo Clinic Proceedings, 83*(5), 584–594.

Moore, K., Johnson, G., Fortner, B., & Houts, A. C. (2008). The AIM higher initiative: New procedures implemented for assessment, information, and management of chemotherapy toxicities in community oncology clinics. *Clinical Journal of Oncology Nursing, 12*(2), 229–238.

Murphy-Ende, K. (2001). Palliation of gastrointestinal obstructive disorders. *Nursing Clinics of North America, 36*(4), 761–778.

National Cancer Institute. (2007). Surveillance, epidemiology, and end results (SEER) cancer statistics review, 1975–2004. Retrieved August 22, 2008, from http://SEER.cancer.gov/CSR/1975_2004/results_merged/sect_15_lung_bronchus. pdf.

National Collaborating Centre for Cancer. (2005). Retrieved from http://www.wales.nhs.uk/sites3/page.cfm?orgid = 432&pid = 12500 on August 1, 2008.

National Comprehensive Cancer Network. (2008a). Practice Guidelines in oncology: Nonsmall cell lung cancer [v.2.2008]. Retrieved August 26, 2008, from http://www.nccn.org/professionals/physician_gls/PDF/palliative.pdf

National Comprehensive Cancer Network. (2008b). Practice guidelines in oncology: Palliative care [v.1.2008]. Retrieved August 26, 2008, from http://www.nccn.org/professionals/physician_gls/PDF/palliative.pdf.

Obasuju, C., Conkling, P., Richards, D., Fitzgibbons, J., Arceneau, K., & Boehm, L., et al. (2007). A randomized phase III trial of gemcitabine with or without carboplatin in performance status 2 (PS2) patients (pts) with advanced (stage IIIB with pleural effusion or stage IV) nonsmall cell lung cancer (NSCLC) [Abstract 7533]. *Journal of Clinical Oncology, ASCO Annual Meeting Proceedings, Part I, 25*(188), 392s.

Pawlik, T., Schulick, R., & Choti, M. (2008). Expanding criteria for resectability of colorectal liver metastases. *Oncology, 13,* 51–64.

Pignon, T., Horiot, J., Michel, B., van Poppel, H., Barelink, H., Roelofson, F., et al. (1997). Age is not a limiting factor for radical radiotherapy in pelvic malignancies. *Radiotherapy and Oncology, 42,* 107–120.

Pritchard, M., Burchen, E., Kumar Srivastava, D., Okuma, J., Anderson, L., Powell, B., et al. (2008). Cancer-related symptoms most concerning to parents during the last week and last day of their child's life. *Pediatrics, 121*(5), 1301–1309.

Repetto, L., & Comandini, D. (2000). Cancer in the elderly: Assessing patients for fitness. *Critical Reviews in Oncology/Hematology, 35,* 155–160.

Repetto, L., Comandini, D., & Mammolit, S. (2001). Life expectancy, comorbidity, and quality of life: The treatment equation in the older cancer patients. *Critical Reviews in Oncology/Hematology, 37,* 147–152

Repetto, L., Venturino, A., Fratino, L., Serraino, D., Troisi, G., Gianni, W., et al. (2003). Geriatric oncology: A clinical approach to the older patient with cancer. *European Journal of Cancer, 39,* 870–880.

Repetto, L., Comandini, D., & Mammolit, S. (2001). Life expectancy, comorbidity, and quality of life: The treatment equation in the older cancer patients. *Critical Reviews in Oncology/Hematology, 37,* 147–152.

Robinson, K.M., & Huether, S. (1998). Structure and function of the reproductive systems. In K.L. McCance, & S. L. Huether (Eds.), *Pathophysiology: The biologic basis for disease in adults and children* (3rd ed., pp. 788–790). St. Louis: Mosby.

Rosati, G., & Bilancia, D. (2008). Role of chemotherapy and novel biological agents in the treatment of elderly patients with colorectal cancer. *World Journal of Gastroenterology, 14*(12), 1812–1822.

Ryan, C., & Small, E. (2006). Prostate cancer update: 2005. *Current Opinion Oncology, 18,* 284–288.

Sandler, A., Gray, R., Brahmer, J., Dowlati, A., Schiller, J., Perry, M., et al. (2005). Randomized phase II/III trial of paclitaxel (p) plus carboplatin with or without bevacizumab (NSC#704865) in patients with advanced nonsquamous nonsmall cell lung cancer (NSCLC): An Eastern Cooperative Oncology Group (ECOG) Trial-E4599 [Abstract 4]. *Journal of Clinical Oncology, 2005, ASCO Annual Meeting Proccedings, Part I, 23*(16S), 2s.

Sauer, R., Becker, H., Hohenberger, W., Rodel, C., Wittekine, C., Fielkau, R. et al. (2004). Preoperative versus postoperative chemoradiotherapy for rectal cancer. *The New England Journal of Medicine, 351,* 1731–1740.

Scullion, F. (2005). An integrated model of care is needed for children and young people with cancer. *International Journal of Pallitive Nursing, 11*(9), 494–495.

Slotman, B., Faivre-Finn, C., Kramer, G., Rankin, E., Snee, M., Hatton, M., et al. (2007). Prophylactic cranial irradiation in extensive small-cell lung cancer, for the EORT Radiation Oncology Group and Lung Cancer Group. The *New England Journal of Medicine, 357* (7), 664–672.

Stinnett, S., Williams, L., & Johnson, D. 2007. Role of chemotherapy for palliation in the lung cancer patient. *Journal of Supportive Oncology, 5*(1), 19–24.

Surbone, A. (2008). Information to cancer patients: Ready for new challenges? *Support Care Cancer, 16,* 865–868.

Tang, S. T. (2003). When death Is imminent. *Cancer Nursing, 26*(3), 245–247.

Temel, S., McCannon, J., Greer, J., Jackson, V., Osteler, P., Pirl, W., et al. Aggressiveness of care in a prospective cohort of patients with advanced NSCLC. *Cancer, 113*(4), 826–833.

Teno J. M, Clarridge, B. R., Casey, V, & Welch, L. (2004). Family perspectives on end of life. *Journal of the American Medical Association, 291,* 88–93.

Terret, C., Zulian, G., Naiem, A., & Albrand, G. (2007). Multidisciplinary approach to the geriatric oncology patient. *Journal of Clinical Oncology, 25*(14), 1876–1881.

Vachon, M. L., Kristjanson, L., & Higginson, I. (1995). Psychosocial issues in palliative care: The patient, the family, and the process and outcome of care. *Journal of Pain and Symptom Management, 10*(2), 142–150.

Valdimarsdottir, U., Kreicbergs, U., Hauksdottir, A., Hunt, H., Onelov, E., Henter, J., et al. (2007). Parents intellectual and emotional awareness of their child's impending death to cancer: A population-based long-term follow-up study. *Lancet Oncology, 8,* 706–714.

Van Veldhuizen, P. J., Reed, G., Aggarwal, A., Baranda, J., Zulfiqar, M., & Williamson, S., et al. (2003). Docetaxel and Ketoconazole in advanced hormone-refractory prostate carcinoma. A phase I and pharmacokinetic study. *Cancer, 98*(9), 1855–1862.

Walker, S. (2003). Updates in nonsmall cell lung cancer. *Clinical Journal of Oncology Nursing, 127*(4), 587–596.

Willert, A., Semans, M. (2000). Knowledge and attitudes about later life sexuality: What clinicians need to know about helping the elderly. *Contemporary Family Therapy, 22*(4), 415–435.

Wolfe, J., Friebert, S., & Hilden, J. (2002). Caring for children with advanced cancer integrating palliative care. *Pediatric Clinical North America, 49,* 1043–1062.

Wolfe, J., Grier, H., Klar, N., Levin, S., Ellenbogen, J., Salem-Schatz, S., et al. (2000). Symptoms and suffering at the end of life in children with cancer. *The New Journal of Medicine, 342,* 326–33.

Wolfe, J., Klar, N., Grier, H., Duncan, J., Salem-Schatz, S., Emanuel, E., et al. (2000). Understanding of prognosis among parents of children who died of cancer: Impact on treatment goals and integration of palliative care. *Journal of the American Medical Association, 284*(19), 2469–2475.

Wolpin, B., Meyerhardt, J., Mamon, H., & Mayer, R. (2007). Adjuvant treatment of colorectal cancer. *CA: A Cancer Journal for Clinicians, 57,* 168–185.

Yamamoto, K., Padilla, A., Calvo, M., Garcia-Zarza, A., Pastor, G., Armengood, B., et al. (2003). Surgical results of stage I nonsmall cell lung cancer: Comparison between elderly and younger patients. *European Journal of Cardio-Thoracic Surgery, 23*(1), 21–25.

13

End-Stage Heart Disease

Judith B. Dyne

Key Points

- Heart failure (HF) is a terminal disease.
- Ten million patients will have HF by 2037.
- Direct/indirect cost in 2008 was $34.8 billion.
- Large-scale clinical trials give evidence-based guidelines as to the treatment.
- Palliative Care of HF is better recognized as an option.
- Predicting the illness trajectory is much harder in HF than in cancer.
- Communication of wishes continues to be a problem.
- Nursing has a key role in the management and outcomes of patients with heart failure.
- Patients often turn to nurses for information on their disease especially in the end stages of the disease.
- A coordinated effort by nursing has now been developed as to how to help patients with not only the physical symptoms of heart failure but also the psychosocial aspects.

Case Study: Mrs. L. is an 85-year-old woman who has been seen by the cardiologist on a weekly basis for the past 6 weeks in order to have her progressive symptoms of heart failure followed. At this point, she appears cachexic and now needs a walker, as she gets dyspneic and exhausted even at rest. She has been on the maximal medical therapy as reflected by current evidence-based guidelines, and continues to fail. She refuses another hospitalization but does not know what other options she has.

Her son, who has been bringing her into the office, is confused about why his mom is failing so quickly and does not understand why Mrs. L. would not go into the hospital again, as she seems to be better there. She has been living with him since her last discharge; and it is taking more and more time to care for her at home.

Mrs. L. recognizes that the weekly visits and constant changes in her diuretic doses are making her feel weaker and weaker. Today on exam she can barely speak in full sentences and her resting SaO_2 is 88% on room air. She tells her healthcare provider that she is exhausted and does not know where to turn.

The nurse practitioner who is her provider today needs to address some of the above issues with Mrs. L. and her son.

1) What concerns should be addressed?
2) What are the treatment options in this case?
3) What other healthcare team members should be brought into this conversation?
4) What referrals would be appropriate and why?

Heart failure is considered a terminal disease, and patients and their families continue to live a life of frequent hospitalizations, office visits, and decreased quality of life despite optimal therapy. These clients suffer with intractable dyspnea, pain, profound fatigue, orthopnea, and psychological despair. The disease itself remains difficult to prognosticate when end-of-life discussions should occur, and many healthcare providers find it difficult to face the facts themselves. What can we as professional nurses and nurse practitioners do in intervening with these patients who have very little "life" in them? How can we help family members come to the realities that death is imminent? This chapter will explore all of these issues from an evidenced-based point of view.

Among all cardiovascular diseases, heart failure (HF), despite considerable improvement of evidenced-based therapies, continues to lead to worse prognosis and quality of life than most cancers (Jessep & Brozena, 2003). According to the American Heart Association (2005) update, 5 million persons in the United States have the diagnosis of heart failure and there are 600,000 new cases diagnosed each year. Almost 75% of those diagnosed with congestive heart failure are over 65 years of age. Heart failure is the number one hospitalization diagnosis for the elderly, and the number has increased 150% over the last 20 years (American Heart Association, 2005). Perhaps the biggest factor boosting HF prevalence and incidence will be the burgeoning growth in the elderly population as the baby boomers reach the age of 65 years. In the United States, the number of elderly (> 65 years of age) is expected to grow from 35 million in the year 2000 to 70.3 million in 2030 (U.S. Department of Health and Human Services, 2002).

At the age of 40 years, the lifetime risk of developing heart failure in both men and men is 1 in 5. This risk doubles with blood pressure greater than 160/90 mm Hg compared to that of less than 140/90 mm Hg (American Heart Association, 2005). Patients with refractory symptoms of heart failure (Stage D) (Table 13.1), despite maximal care, have an average survival rate of 1 year (Lloyd-Jones, Larson, & Leip, 2002). This epidemic of heart failure in the United States is largely due to the success in the treatment of other heart diseases, especially heart attacks, whose symptoms are now more widely recognized and treated and have improved survival rates (Kirkpatrick & Kim, 2006). These same patients, however, usually have some long-term effects from the event and often have decreased left ventricular function. New medications and interventional devices have prolonged life, but these patients eventually go on to having heart failure as they age and the medications or devices no longer give them benefit (Kirkpatrick & Kim, 2006).

Heart failure continues to pose heavy economic burden in the United States with a projected total cost of $34.8 billion in 2008. The physical and mental distress and suffering from dying of heart failure can often be worse than that of some cancers (Hinton, 1963). In a prospective study done in the United States with 9105 patients of whom 1401 had heart failure, the SUPPORT (Study to Understand Prognoses and Preferences for Outcomes and Risks of Treatment) study found a mortality rate of 50% in 6 months in patients who were refractory to treatment. In the same study, these patientsreportedly had not only increased breathlessness, but alos increased pain, especially those who ended up dying 3 days later (Gibbs, McCoy, Gibbs,

Rogers, & Addington-Hall, 2002). This study confirmed that severe pain was the most common reported sign, which is not fully understood. The supposition is that this pain is caused by liver engorgement that occurs in heart failure. In this same study, the median depression scores and functional disabilities were also increased. Elderly women made up the largest majority of the population, and 75% of them had a long-term history of hypertension. As a result of this important study, the American Heart Association along with the American College of Cardiology developed a stratified

risk classification for the development of heart failure, which is outlined in Table 13.1.

One of the difficult issues in regard to predicting end-of-life treatment, which has been recognized in multiple studies, is the fact that patients with heart failure often have periods of waxing and waning in their disease process. There are weeks or months when patients seem to favorably respond to the data-driven therapies, and other times the same treatments need uptitrating or rehospitalization. This inability to predict death presents barriers to appropriate treatments for this last phase of

13.1 | Stages in the Development of Heart Failure/Recommended Therapy by Stage

AT RISK FOR HEART FAILURE			HEART FAILURE
STAGE A	**STAGE B**	**STAGE C**	**STAGE D**
At high risk for HF but without structural heart disease or symptoms of HF e.g., patients with: ■ hypertension ■ atherosclerotic disease ■ diabetes ■ obesity ■ metabolic syndrome or ■ using cardiotoxins ■ with family history of cardiomyopathy	Structural heart disease but without signs or symptoms of HF e.g., patients with: ■ Previous MI ■ LV remodeling including LVH and low EF ■ asymptomatic valvular disease	Structural heart disease with prior or current symptoms of HF e.g., patients with: ■ known structural heart disease and ■ shortness of breath	Refractory HF requiring specialized interventions e.g., patients with: ■ marked symptoms at rest despite maximal medical therapy (e.g., those who are recurrently hospitalized or cannot be safely discharged from the hospital without specialized interventions)
Goals ■ Treat hypertension ■ Encourage smoking cessation ■ Treat lipid disorders ■ Encourage regular exercise ■ Discourage alcohol intake and illicit drug use ■ Control metabolic syndrome *Drugs* ACE-I or ARB in appropriate patients for vascular disease or diabetes	**Goals** All measures under Stage A *Drugs* ■ ACE-I or ARB in appropriate patients ■ Beta-blockers in appropriate patients *Devices in selected patients* ■ Implantable defibrillators	**Goals** All measures under Stages A & B ■ Dietary salt restriction *Drugs for routine use* ■ Diuretics for fluid retention ■ ACE-I ■ Beta-blocker *Drugs for Selected Patients* ■ Aldosterone antagonist ■ ARBs ■ Digitalis ■ Hydralazine/nitrates *Devices in selected patients* ■ Biventricular pacing ■ Implantable defibrillators	**Goals** Appropriate measures under Stages A, B & C ■ Decision regarding appropriate level of care *Options* ■ Compassionate end-of-life care/hospice ■ Extraordinary measures ■ Heart transplant ■ Chronic inotropes ■ Permanent mechanical support/experimental surgery or drugs

HR: Heart Failure
ACE-I: angiotensin converting enzyme inhibitor
ARB: angiotensin receptor blocker
Source: American College of Cardiology Foundation & American heart Association. (2005). Based on ACC/AHA 2005 Guideline Update: Diagnosis and management of chronic heart failure.

the disease. It also makes it difficult for patients to receive the information they need to make informed decisions on what treatment options are afforded and how helpful treatments will be. These patients can be so uninformed about their disease that they think an increase in symptoms of breathlessness is "just getting old" or a process of "deconditioning".

The Seattle Heart Failure Model (SHFM) can also be used to assign as risk score for prediction of survival of patients with heart failure and has been derived from multiple clinical trial populations. This model was risk-score-derived from clinical trials that may enable prediction of survival of heart failure patients. One study done by May et al. (2007) examined about 4,000 hospitalized patients and found that the SHFM predicted survival in patients with HF. This was similar to the original findings of the model, but adding B-type Natriuretic Peptide levels to the model achieved significant reliability in the predication of survival rates. Baseline characteristics such as age, gender, The New York Heart Association (NYHA) class, weight, ejection fraction, blood pressure, as well as interventions that the patient were receiving for treatment were added to the model. When populated with this data, the model gives survival and mortality rates at 1, 2, and 5 years, as well as mean life expectancy. It is interesting to note that Allen et al. (2008) found that there was a 40% overestimation of survival and life expectancy with patients who completed the model as compared to actuarial-predicted life expectancy. It was felt that this was due to in part to lack of information regarding their disease and its prognosis. The model can be accessed at: www.cvoutcomes.org

In the Épidémiolgie de I'Insuffusance Cardiaque Avancée en Lorraine study (EPICAL) (Alla et al., 2000), 28 available factors using a multivariate analysis were used to develop algorithms for predicting prognosis in patients with ischemia or dilated cardiomyopathy. In this study, it was found that those with ischemic cardiomyopathy had a 25% or less chance of surviving 1 year; i.e., these individuals had three of the four of these factors:

- Serum sodium level below 138 mmol/L
- Resting heart rate of greater than 100 bpm
- Serum creatinine level of greater then 2.0 mg/dl
- History of previous decompensation.

Those with dilated cardiomyopathy had the same mortality rates if they had four of these seven factors (Alla et al., 2000):

- Serious comordity (cirrhosis, cancer, cerebral vascular accident or bronchopneumopathy)
- Known cardiomyopathy
- Institutionalization or dependence on assistance
- Serum sodium level below 138 mmol/L
- Resting heart rate of greater than 100 bpm

- Serum creatinine level of greater then 2.0 mg/dl
- Age over 70 years.

In the SUPPORT study, 50% of patients received adequate information on their terminal condition; many came to the conclusion themselves. Roger et al. (2004), in their study "Trends in Heart Failure Incidence and Survival in a Community-Based Population," found that most patients would welcome timely and frank discussion of their prognosis; unfortunately, many did not receive the information in time.

The Framingham Study which began in 1948 with a cohort of over 5,000 male and female subjects was the first large-scale study that looked at heart disease and heart failure in the United States. On routine examinations of the subjects in this study, it was found that the rate of congestive heart failure (CHF) increased in men from 8 per 1000 at age 50–59 years to 66 per 1000 at age 80–89 years. In women, the prevalence estimates go from 8 per 1000 to 79 per 1000 in the same age categories. In part, these estimates are due to the fact that women live longer than men with heart disease. One in three women over the age of 65 have some form of cardiovascular disease, which accounts for a greater proportion of deaths from heart disease in this age group (McGynn et al., 2003). Considered to be the hallmark study in modern cardiology, the Framingham study provided the data from which many worldwide clinical trials on heart disease and failure are based. In 2007, the Framingham heart Study published its latest findings, which reported that the incidence of heart failure has declined somewhat in women, but not among men over the past 50 years; and that the survival rates in both genders have improved (Levy et al., 2002). These findings are somewhat encouraging, but prolonged survival and the aging population, as outlined above, still mean that large numbers of patients will need extended care of their symptoms with results that will affect quality of life.

PATHOPHYSIOLOGY OF HEART FAILURE

Heart failure is a syndrome that encompasses many disease processes. These processes relate to the overall left ventricular function (LVEF) and changes the heart undergoes as a result of decreases in the LVEF.

Normally, the senescent heart goes through structural changes. There is an increase in the left ventricular (LV) wall thickness, septal hypertrophy, and a reduction of diastolic compliance (Taylor, 2001). It is felt that the hypertrophy is caused by an increased afterload on the LV, which is caused by increased pressure in the aorta (the higher the blood pressure, the greater the pressure), and leads to decreased compliance of the ventricles. As one ages, there is also felt to be an increase in collagen accumulation in the left ventricle, which adds to the diastolic rigidity (Taylor, 2001).

The aging process also affects the valvular structure. Valvular malfunction, which contributes to both systolic and diastolic heart failure, also plays a part in CHF. This occurs because of either pressure overload or volume overload. With age, the heart valves become calcified, leading to stenosis or narrowing of the valve diameter. This most often exists in the aortic valve, which slowly progresses over time. Volume overload, which is present in valvular insufficiency or regurgitation, most often occurs in the mitral and aortic valves. This condition also progresses insidiously, unless there is an associated acute cause, such as endocarditis, papillary muscle or chordae tendineae rupture, or interventricular rupture following a myocardial infarction (Laurent-Bopp, 2001). There is also an increase incidence of atrial fibrillation in patients who have calcium deposition in the mitral valve. Idiopathic bundle branch fibrosis may also occur with increasing age, and may be a cause of increased risk of heart block in elders. The arterial walls also become less elastic and distensible, and systolic hypertension can occur (Taylor, 2001).

Heart failure can be described as a clinical syndrome characterized by pulmonary or systemic congestion or both, with diminished or limited cardiac output. This decrease in cardiac output causes the associated symptoms of dyspnea, fatigue, and peripheral edema. The heart is unable to pump sufficient amounts of blood to meet the metabolic demands of the body (Micheal & Frances, 2001). It is the decreased myocardial contractile state that leads to a decreased stroke volume (volume of blood ejected by the ventricle each heart beat), which triggers acute compensatory neurohormonal mechanisms. These neurohormonal responses include the innervation of the sympathetic nervous system (increases heart rate), increased inotropy (increased contractile state in viable myocardium), arteriolar constriction (to maintain organ perfusion), and activation of the renin–angiotensin system (which mediates arteriolar vasoconstriction and retention of sodium). These compensatory mechanisms in the acute phase attempt to maintain adequate cardiac output and vital organ perfusion. However, when heart failure occurs on a chronic basis, ventricular remodeling develops in response to these neurohormonal influences (Woods, Froelicher, & Motzer, 2000). The ventricle takes on a spherical instead of an oval shape in order to make the most of the Starling Law. This law maintains that if the myocardial fibers can be stretched by increased volume of blood within it, the force of contraction will be greater and the ventricle will more completely empty (Lamb, 1984). However, when this adaptation occurs chronically, the combination of the neurohormonal response and the ventricular remodeling causes myopathy, which is a response to the increased afterload and fluid retention. Ventricular filling pressures (preload) increase further,

the myocardial fibers overstretch, the mechanism of Starling's Law fails, cardiac output is compromised, and the increased pressure in the left ventricle backs up into the pulmonary vasculature. The heart can no longer meet the metabolic needs of the body for oxygen delivery to the tissues, and systolic hypoperfusion, severe vasoconstriction (increased afterload), and poor pump performance occur.

There has also been investigation of the inflammatory mediators and their effect on cardiac dysfunction. Mann (2001), in an introduction to an article in *Heart Failure Review*, believes that inflammatory mediators, such as tumor necrosis factor, interleukin-1, interleukin-6, and nitric oxide negatively affect tissues in the same way that others substances or mechanisms affect heart dysfunction, and mediator modulation may be an emerging class of therapeutic agents.

Other causes of heart failure can be due to heart muscle abnormalities, ventricular systolic dysfunction, dysrhythmias (especially atrial fibrillation and ventricular tachycardia), sinus node dysfunction, valve malfunction, and myocardial rupture (rare) (Wyse et al., 2002). These disorders of the cardiac rhythm contribute to heart failure because when there is loss of filling pressure or filling time, stroke volume is affected by 25–30% and cardiac output decreases. Muscle abnormalities include myocardial infarction, ventricular aneurysm, cardiomyopathy, or excessive hypertrophy from pulmonary hypertension, aortic stenosis, or systemic hypertension (Kirkpatrick & Kim, 2006).

Ventricular dysfunction can be due to either systolic dysfunction or diastolic dysfunction. Systolic dysfunction occurs when the contractility of the heart is compromised, which is measured by the left ventricular ejection fraction (LVEF). The normal LVEF is approximately 60%, but with systolic heart failure, the LVEF is below normal, usually less than 40%. In end-stage heart failure due to systolic dysfunction, the LVEF can be as low as 15–20%. Common causes of systolic dysfunction are ischemic heart disease, cardiomyopathy, volume overload (valvular insufficiency), or pressure overload (hypertension or valvular stenosis). In diastolic dysfunction, the LVEF is normal or hyperdynamic (> 40%), but the ability of the ventricle to relax and fill is compromised (poor compliance). Cardiac output, especially in exertion, is limited because of the abnormal filling capacity. As ventricular pressures elevate, there is backflow of blood into the pulmonary vasculature, which causes dyspnea and edema. This type of dysfunction accounts for approximately 20–50% of all cases of heart failure, and is commonly seen in elderly women who are usually obese with hypertension and diabetes (Jessup & Bronzena, 2003). Causes may include ischemic heart disease with aging, myocardial hypertrophy, and restrictive cardiomyopathy. It is important to note that in the aging process, the relaxation of the heart in diastole is sometimes delayed, which causes a decrease in the filling time (Micheal & Frances, 2001). A comparison of symptoms of systolic and diastolic heart failure is illustrated in Table 13.2.

Congestive heart failure is also commonly classified according to the side of the heart that is affected. It is important to understand that the right ventricle and the left ventricle are independent of each other, but are serially connected. To function effectively, both ventricles must maintain equal outputs. Unless the patient has a history of chronic lung disease, the left ventricle is usually the first to become dysfunctional, which is due to the fact that the left ventricle must generate higher pressures than the right ventricle in order to maintain adequate cardiac output. The left ventricle must generate a great deal of force to eject its contents in systole (which in turn requires adequate oxygen). If the systemic vascular resistance is high (blood pressure), it increases afterload, which ultimately decreases stroke volume. If the left ventricle fails, there is backward flow of blood into the pulmonary capillaries, which eventually transudates into the alveoli. The clinical symptoms are related to the elevated pulmonary pressures and decreased cardiac output. High blood pressure, myocardial ischemia (MI), aortic stenosis or insufficiency, and mitral stenosis/insufficiency can also cause left ventricular failure.

Right ventricular failure is caused by increased pulmonary pressure. This increased pressure is usually due to chronic lung disease, pulmonary emboli, or left-sided heart failure. The clinical signs are those associated with increased systemic venous pressure, which gives rise to the signs of dependent peripheral edema. Although initial heart failure may be either right- or left-sided, in end-stage heart failure it is both or biventricular.

Coexisting conditions also factor into congestive heart failure such as diabetes mellitus, renal disease, anemia, obesity, sleep apnea, and depression. Diabetes is considered a cardiac risk equivalent. This means that a diabetic patient is treated medically as if he/she has already had a cardiovascular event. Renal disease causes fluid retention and activation of the renin system which vasoconstricts and increases myocardial demand. Obstructive sleep apnea is now known to cause many cardiovascular affects if left untreated. Pulmonary hypertension and right heart failure are two of the effects that can be easily treated by treatment of sleep apnea with a proper device. Depression and anxiety are important as they relate to the pathophysiology of CHF. Lett and Blumenthal (2007) found that depression may independently worsen heart failure and increase risk of death. It is also known that cortisol levels are persistently high in patients with depression, which, over time, leads to hypertension (increased afterload), increase in heart rate (decreased ventricular filling time), immunodepression, increased gluconeogenesis, inhibition of growth and reproduction systems, shunting of blood to the central nervous system, as well as maladaptive neural and hormonal pathways. It has also been found that proinflammatory cytokines, which are activated in the stress response, have major effects on the serotonergic system by reducing the available serotonin, which leads to not only depression but also to increased platelet aggregation and ultimately coronary artery occlusion (Kubzansky & Ichiro, 2000). The biggest study in the United States on the link between depression and heart disease was done by the National Health and Nutrition Examination Survey (NHANES), which began in 1960. In the latest report of 2005–2006, it is reported that more than 1 in 20 Americans, 12 years and older had depression, and 1 in 7 were poorer Americans (Pratt & Brody, 2008). In this report, it was found that 80% of persons with depression reported some level of functional impairment and 27% had problems with work and home issues.

Heart failure is typically classified using the NYHA Functional Classification System (Exhibit 13.1). In the patient with end-stage heart disease, the severity of symptoms is classified as NYHA Class III or IV, with associated radical clinical dysfunction affecting the quality of life of the individual (Criteria Committee NYHA, 1964).

13.2 | Characteristics of Patients with Diastolic vs. Systolic Heart Failure (HF)

CHARACTERISTIC	DIASTOLIC HF	SYSTOLIC HF
Age	Elderly	All ages (50–70 years)
Sex	Frequently female	Often male
Left ventricular function	Normal or even higher than normal	Depressed, 40% are lower
Hypertension	Usually present	Often present
Diabetes mellitus	Usually present	Often present
Previous heart attack	Occasionally present	Usually present
Obesity	Usually present	Occasionally present
Chronic lung disease	Often present	Not present
Sleep pnea	Often present	Often present
Chronic renal disease	Often present	Not present
Atrial fibrillation	Occasionally present	Occasionally present

Source: Jessup, M., & Bronzena, S. (2003). Heart failure. *New England Journal of Medicine, 348,* 2207–2218.

Stages of Heart Failure
New York Heart Association (NYHA)
Classification Scale

Early-Stage Heart Failure

- **NYHA Class I**
  No symptoms at any level of exertion and no limitation in ordinary physical activity.

- **NYHA Class II**
  Mild symptoms and slight limitation during regular activity. Comfortable at rest.

Advanced-Stage Heart Failure

- **NYHA Class III**
  Noticeable limitation due to symptoms, even during minimal activity. Comfortable only at rest.

- **NYHA Class IV**
  Severe limitations. Experience symptoms even while at rest (sitting in a recliner or watching TV).

The NYHA classification scale is very useful for physicians and nurses who treat patients with heart failure. It helps them determine if the condition is improving, staying the same, or getting worse. It is also used in research studies to evaluate the effectiveness of new treatments.

CLINICAL SIGNS AND SYMPTOMS OF CONGESTIVE HEART FAILURE

It is important as nurses and nurse practitioners to evaluate the clinical signs by understanding the symptoms of both right and left heart failure. A patient may have typical right or left heart failure symptoms, but often in patients with end-stage heart disease biventricular heart failure and combined symptoms occur. In Table 13.3, the symptoms of both right ventricular and left ventricular failure are outlined. The severity and progression of the symptoms are dependent on the extent of the failure and the type of dysfunction. Early on in the disease when cardiac output decreases due to heart failure, compensatory mechanisms come into play to keep tissue perfusion intact. The sympathetic nervous system releases catecholamines, which cause increases in the heart rate, systemic vascular resistance increases (SVR), preload, afterload, and contractility. These same compensatory mechanisms eventually cause the symptoms of congestive heart failure as ventricles begin to fail, and LVEF declines.

Dyspnea is the initial manifestation in most patients. This occurs as hypoxemia due to low cardiac output ensues. At first this may be a subtle change, but as the disease progresses this is the most common presenting symptom, especially in left heart failure. As the left ventricle fails, blood backs up to the left atrium and the pulmonary veins. As pressure rises in the pulmonary vasculature, blood moves into the alveoli and pulmonary edema occurs. Orthopnea and paroxysmal nocturnal dyspnea increase, and often patients have to sleep in upright position to rest. Cough is also a common symptom. The cough of CHF is a dry cough and can often be attributed to another cause (post-nasal drip, cough from ace-inhibitor medication). When fulminate pulmonary edema occurs, there is pink frothy expectorant and a feeling of "suffocating."

Fatigue progresses as the disease state becomes end stage. What patients often report is the inability to "do what they used to do." Activity tolerance decreases, and the smallest of tasks can be overwhelming. Cachexia and malnutrition are seen also, and muscle mass diminishes. Patients are often too tired to eat; it takes too much energy (which it does as eating increases myocardial oxygen demand). These men and women become frail and often have a low albumin level which only adds to their overall peripheral edema. The cardiac output becomes so low that the gut does not get adequate perfusion and becomes hypoxic; and a oxygen-deprived gastrointestinal system does not function as it should, which again leads to more cachexia and weight loss. Blood flow to the kidneys decreases, which causes a decrease in urinary output. Renal insufficiency and eventually renal failure occurs as the creatinine rises and again contributes to loss of appetite and the decision as to whether renal replacement therapy should be initiated. When oliguria and anuria occurs, fluid retention increases and peripheral edema and pulmonary edema become more pronounced. Eventually, cardiogenic shock occurs which leads to marked hypoperfusion of poorly oxygenated blood to the tissues, an increase in lactic acid, which causes metabolic acidosis, and death. Heart failure should always be ruled out in patients who present with recurrent pulmonary infections, frequent exacerbations of COPD, and elders who experience acute confusion.

Measurement of brain natriuretic peptide (BnP) can be helpful in the assessment of heart failure. BNP is a naturally occurring cardiac neurohormone secreted by the ventricular membrane in response to volume expansion

13.3 | Signs and Symptoms of Left and Right Heart Failure

LEFT HEART FAILURE	RIGHT HEART FAILURE
■ Dyspnea, orthopnea, paroxysmal nocturnal dyspnea	■ Decreased hemoglobin
	■ Jugular vein distention
	■ Peripheral edema
■ Pulmonary edema	■ Hepatojugular reflex
■ Dry cough	■ Liver engorgement (increased LFTs)
■ S3, S4	
■ Fine crackles, wheezing	■ Splenomegaly
■ Hypoxemia	■ Weight gain of > 2 lbs/day

and pressure overload. Its other functions are to regulate vascular tone and extracellular volume status as well as to counteract the effects of the renin–angiotensin syndrome. Results are elevated in the failing heart when ventricular stretching occurs. Therefore, the BNP should be ordered when it is unclear as to the cause of the dyspnea. It can also be used to help differentiate between CHF and chronic fibrotic lung changes, or an exacerbation of chronic obstructive pulmonary disease (COPD), which can present very similarly. The negative value of BNP is under 100 pg/ml. The finding of a low level of BNP of less than 50 pg/ml is good evidence of the absence of heart failure as the cause for dyspnea (Maisel, 2002).

PHYSICAL ASSESSMENT OF CONGESTIVE HEART FAILURE

The goal of physical assessment is to assess the type of heart failure (right, left, biventricular) and the severity of the condition. Assessment of the older adult with heart failure includes cardiac, pulmonary, integumentary, gastrointestinal, and functional assessments.

Cardiac Assessment. Assessment of the heart rate and rhythm are essential to determine if there are any dysrhythmias that are compromising the function of the heart. The pulse is usually the initial response to decreased cardiac output. Pulsus alternans, or alternating pulse, may be present due to the altered function of the left ventricle. This is exhibited by strong beats, alternating with weak beats on palpation, and low-voltage QRS complexes on the electrocardiogram.

On palpation of the chest wall, the point of maximum impulse (PMI), which normally is at the fifth intercostal space, mid-clavicular line, will be displaced laterally to the left toward the axilla. This displacement is due to the enlarged hypertrophied left ventricle. In patients with heart failure, a third heart sound (S3) is often the first clinical sign of CHF and is a highly specific one. This is caused by the overfilling of the ventricle and reduced cardiac output. A fourth heart sound may also be heard, which indicates chronic ischemic disease and lack of ventricular compliance. It is also important to be alert for murmurs.

Jugular vein pulses can estimate the venous pressure, and should be examined while the patient is positioned at a 35°. If the jugular vein is distended, it indicates right ventricular failure. The hepatojugular reflex should also be elicited, and is done by pressing on the right upper quadrant of the abdomen. When there is an increased peripheral venous pressure, the compression of the abdomen causes increased blood flow to the right atrium, which causes the right atrial pressure to rise, in turn engorging the jugular vein and causing jugular vein distention (JVD). These are key findings of heart failure and usually indicate a need for additional diuretic therapy (Jessup & Brozena, 2003).

Pulmonary assessment. When pulmonary pressures are elevated, the hydrostatic pressure within the pulmonary capillaries surrounding the alveoli is elevated. This occurs as the left ventricle fails and causes backward flow. This increased pressure causes transudation of the fluid within the capillary into the alveoli. This accumulated fluid can be heard when the patient inspires as "crackles." These crackles do not clear with coughing and are initially heard in the dependent portions of the lung. As pulmonary pressures continue to rise with left heart failure, these breath sounds can be heard throughout both lung fields. Pleural effusions can also be present. Dyspnea increases as fluid accumulates in the alveoli, oxygen saturation decrease, and the patient feels as if they are drowning.

Integumentary assessment. Dependent edema is a hallmark sign of right heart failure and biventricular failure and is important to the nursing assessment. Palpation of edema is felt in the ankles, the feet, and in the sacral area for those who are bedridden. This edema may lead to stasis dermatitis, hyperpigmentation, and ulceration. The temperature of the skin is also very helpful in assessing cardiac output. Cool, clammy, diaphoretic skin is an indicator of peripheral vasoconstriction, which is a sign of increased sympathetic nervous system response, a compensation for decreased cardiac output.

Gastrointestinal assessment. As mentioned in Table 13.3, liver enlargement occurs with heart failure (right ventricular, or biventricular) due to venous congestion. The liver when engorged can be felt below the right costal margin of the ribs. In advanced heart failure, the spleen can also be palpated below the left costal margin.

Functional status. In end-stage heart disease, symptoms of biventricular failure such as dyspnea, weakness, fatigue, and pain are present. It is important as healthcare providers to evaluate the impact of these symptoms on daily function by doing patient interviews or questionnaires at every visit.

The short form 36 [SF-36] (Ware & Sherbourne, 1996) is a 36-item questionnaire which measures eight dimensions of health covering three areas of general concern to individuals regarding their health: functional status, well-being, and overall evaluation of health. This tool asks the client to evaluate the dimensions in the past year. The eight dimensions are scored and coded and range on a scale of 0–100, with 0 being the worst possible health status and 100 being the best possible status (O'Mahoney, 1998). Some of the parameters used in this questionnaire are physical functioning, bodily pain, general health, vitality, social functioning, role emotional, mental health, and health transition. O'Mahoney (1998) found that this tool is suitable for interview administration, but found it was not useful in postal administration in the older population.

Disease-specific questionnaires such as the Kansas City Cardiomyopathy Questionnaire (KCCQ) looks at social patterns, mood status, and acceptance of limitations and has been used to screen for depression and anxiety which are prevalent in the heart failure patient (Hermann et al., 2005). The KCCQ is a relatively new self-administered 23-item questionnaire developed to provide a better description of quality of life (QOL) in a heart failure patient. It attempts to quantify QOL in a disease-specific way, where most questionnaires are generic in nature. It looks at frequency severity and recent change over time. The KCCQ is an instrument that measures activities of daily living and physical limitations and independently quantifies symptoms, social limitations, patient's use of self-efficacy and QOL. In a cross-sectional study by Krousel-Wood, Abdoh and Mehra (2003) of patients attending a heart failure clinic, it was found that both surveys were positively correlated. This instrument can be completed in 4–6 minutes, uses a Likert scale, and is easy to understand. Its clinical focus is primarily on fluid retention or the patient's perception of fluid retention. It is more effective in using with patients with systolic dysfunction.

It was found in a study by Green, Porter, Bresnahan and Spertus (2000), that there were significant changes in patients who were recovering from a hospitalization for decompensated heart failure, and that not only was the KCCQ scale closely correlated with NYHA classification (test for linear trend $F = 153$ and $R2 = 0.55$; $p < 0.001$), but baseline scores were also associated with subsequent death or hospitalization during follow-up procedures. Over the course of the study, 11 patients died and 13 patients required hospitalization. The baseline KCCQ functional status score was significantly lower among patients dying or requiring re-hospitalization during the follow-up period than among those with event-free survival (35.1 vs. 55.3, $p < 0.001$)

DIAGNOSTIC STUDIES IN CHRONIC HEART FAILURE

According to the practice guidelines written on the evaluation and management of chronic heart failure by the American College of Cardiology/American Heart Association (ACC/AHA) (2005) looking into the cause of the HF is important. Some conditions that lead to LV dysfunction are treatable and can be reversed. This begins with a thorough history and physical, with the following areas or comorbidites being assessed: hypertension (number 1 cause of CHF), diabetes, dyslipidemia, valvular heart disease, coronary artery disease, peripheral vascular disease (PVD), myopathy, rheumatic fever, sleep-disordered breathing, exposure to cardiotoxic medication (chemotherapy regimens; especially anthracyclines, herceptin, cyclophosphamide), current or past alcohol consumption, smoking, collagen vascular

disease, thyroid disorder, obesity, pheochromocytoma, and exposure to sexually transmitted diseases.

Family history should also be gathered, especially premature coronary artery disease, in a first-degree relative, sudden cardiac death, conduction system problems, cardiomyopathy, and history of strokes or PVD.

According to the ACC/AHA (2005) update, patients usually present in three ways:

- Syndrome of decreased exercise tolerance: usually due to dyspnea or fatigue. In this case it is important for the provider to ascertain whether these symptoms represent HF or another condition such as pulmonary disease.
- Fluid retention: complaints of leg edema, abdominal bloating, or sudden weight gain of 2 pounds or more in a 24–48 hour time span.
- Symptoms of another cardiac or non-cardiac disorder: diabetes, arrhythmia, pulmonary emboli, or a chest x-ray that has evidence of cardiac enlargement.

The following diagnostic studies are indicated:

1) Complete blood count (CBC), urinalysis
2) Serum electrolytes, blood urea nitrogen (BUN), creatinine, glucose, phosphorus, magnesium, calcium, albumin
3) Fasting transferrin saturation (to rule out hemochromatosis, a cause of cardiomyopathy)
4) BNP
5) Chest X-ray and electrocardiogram (EKG)
6) Thyroid studies (especially in those with atrial fibrillation and unexplained heart failure)
7) Transthoracic doppler–two-dimensional echocardiography
8) Noninvasive stress testing (in patients with previous history of myocardial infarction)
9) Cardiac catheterization in patients with angina or large areas of ischemic myocardium

DISEASE MANAGEMENT OF CHF

The evidence in the literature is abundant regarding the management of HF patients. There are many evidenced-based trials as to the appropriate treatment of end-stage heart failure (Table 13.4).

In the IMPROVE-HF trial, a prospective study that is ongoing, is identifying the gaps in cardiology practices in using evidenced-based therapies. Seven of the proven therapies were examined in patients who were ideal candidates to receive the treatment and did not. Some of the evidenced-based therapies were used in 100% of patients who were appropriate candidates to receive the treatment or device, but there was a large gap in treatments found in those who should have received a life-saving device and did not, such as cardiac resynchronization therapy (CRT). One third of cardiology practices in this study had

13.4 | Heart Failure Clinical Trials

TRIAL	POPULATION STUDIES	OUTCOMES/RECOMMENDATIONS
Cooperative North Scandinavian Enalapril Survival Study (CONSENSUS)	256 NYHA class IV assigned randomly to the Enalapril (an ACE-I) or placebo	1 year mortality rate: 64% in placebo group 46% in enalapril group At 10 year follow-up five patients from enalapril group had survived
Carvedilol Prospective Randomized Cumulative Survival (COPERNICUS)	Beneficial effects of beta-blocker carvedilol on mortality in NYHA class IV patients with chronic heart failure vs. placebo	1 year mortality rate: 19.6 % in placebo 11% in carvedilol
Randomized Aldactone Evaluation Study (RALES)	1663 patients with severe heart failure and LVEF > 35%, randomized to receive Aldactone 25 mg/day vs. placebo	After a follow-up of 24 months: mortality rates: 35% in aldactone group 46% in placebo group
Valsartan Heart Failure Study (V-HeFT)	Angiotensin II type receptor blocker, valsartan, vs. placebo	Significantly reduced the end-point mortality and morbidity and clinical symptoms in patients with HF.
Survival Trial of Antiarrhythmic Therapy in Congestive Heart Failure (CHF-STAT)	674 patients with symptoms of CHF, cardiac enlargement, 10 or more premature ventricular contractions (PVCs), LVEF of > 40% amiodarone vs. placebo	No significant differences in overall mortality between groups.
Multisite Stimulation in Cardiomyopathies (MUSTIC) trail	67 patients with severe heart failure received transvenous atrial bi-ventricular pacemakers (allows for better ventricular synchrony)	At 3 months QOL improved by 22%, hospitalizations decreased by 2/3rds
The Comparison of Medical Therapy, Pacing, and Defibrillation in Chronic Heart Failure (COMPANION) trial	Patients with NYHA III or IV, LVEF > 35%, looked at whether optimal pharmacological therapy used with ventricular resynchromization alone or combined with cardioverter-defibrillator capability was superior	Ongoing trial
IMPROVE HF	40,000 patients treated at 160 cardiology practices in USA.	Quantified seven guideline/recommended EBP

Source: Jessup, M., & Bronzena, S. (2003). Heart failure. *New England Journal of Medicine, 348,* 2207–18.

patients that could have benefited from some of the above therapies, but none was prescribed (Fonarow, 2008). A comprehensive multidisciplinary approach is imperative and was found in multiple studies to be the most successful in the treatment of this disease. The Joint commission on Accreditation of Healthcare organizations (JCAHO) developed a core measure set in 2002 as part of the quality care hospitals delivered with heart failure patients. The four standardized core measure sets for these patients are: 1) documentation of discharge instructions in six areas including medication management, low-sodium diet, activity and exercise, signs and symptoms of worsening condition, weight monitoring, and when to contact the healthcare provider; 2) assessment of left ventricular function; 3) use of angiotensin-converting enzyme inhibitors (ACE-I) or angiotenin II blockers (ARBs) in patients with left ventricular dysfunction; and 4) smoking cessation advice and counseling. The ACC and the AHA went onto add a fifth measure: that is, use of an anticoagulant in atrial fibrillation patients. In the OPTIMIZE-HF trial, the suggestion of adding a beta-blocker before discharge was also recommended.

The management of patients with heart failure is now widely based on the latest ACC/AHA guidelines that are illustrated in Table 13.1. Each stage suggests the appropriate lifestyle changes and appropriate pharmacological therapy. These guidelines were developed after reviewing multiple, large-scale studies. Based on clinical trials, treatment of all heart failure patients in Stages B though D should include the following:

1) Diuretics, the mainstay of controlling the symptoms of fluid overload. Thiazide or loop diuretics are most often used.
2) ACE-I based on the CONSENSUS trial. ACE-I are ideal in the treatment of HF in that it antagonizes the rennin–angiotensin–aldosterone system and has been proven to have an influence on disease regression, symptom improvement, and decreased mortality.
3) ARBs based on the V-HEFT trial. ARBs reduce end-point mortality and morbidity and improve clinical signs and symptoms.
4) Spironolactone based on the RALES trial. A Aldosterone antagonist has been found to decrease mortality rate.
5) Beta-blockers based on the COPERNICUS trial. Beta-blockers affect mortality in NYHA IV patients with chronic heart failure.
6) Digoxin, a positive inotropic medication that improves pump function. There was no difference in mortality of those receiving Digoxin vs. placebo, but there was a decrease in worsening of the failure when used (Deng, Ascheim, Edwards, & Naka, 2002).
7) Antiarrhythmics based on the CHF-STAT trial. Amiodarone with beta-blockers are the only interventions that have not been shown to increase the risk for mortality in patient with CHF [Deng et al., (2002)].

Diuretics

Loop diuretics are the preferred class of drugs for use with older adult patients. They are recommended due to the fact they are efficacious in sodium and water excretion even when renal function is compromised. Loop diuretics provide immediate relief of symptoms associated with fluid overload, but should not be used as the only pharmacologic agent because they lose effect over an extended period. Diuretics used on a chronic basis can increase renin, which magnifies the activation of the renin–angiotensin system (RAS), so therefore should be combined with ace inhibitors (Goldstein, 2001). Common loop diuretics used in CHF are furosemide (Lasix), torsemide (Demadex), and bumetanide (Bumex). Because loop diuretics cause loss of essential electrolytes (hypokalemia, hypomagnesemia, hyponatremia, glucose intolerance, and hyperlipidemia), careful ongoing assessment of the elder patient is recommended. The determination of the proper initial dose and readjustment of doses requires an ongoing evaluation of symptoms, especially in the elderly population. As heart failure increases, the absorption of loop diuretics in the gastrointestinal tract decreases, and increased dosage may be necessary (Goldstein, 2001). In end-stage disease, the addition of metolazone (Zaroxolyn) may be necessary, especially in patients with renal insufficiency (Arling, 1997). For older patients with mild congestive heart failure, hydrochlorothiazide (a thiazide diuretic) is recommended, but with caution because these preparations can cause hyperkalemia when combined with ace inhibitors.

ACE Inhibitors (ACEIs)

ACE inhibitors have been studied extensively over the last 10 years in many large series studies. ACEIs were introduced initially as treatment for hypertension. It was felt that since these agents vasodialated the peripheral blood vessels by inhibiting the RAS, there might be an indication for use in CHF. Extensive studies found that not only did these agents decrease afterload and preload as expected, but more importantly had a significant effect on ventricular remodeling. Through the mechanisms of decreasing aldosterone secretion and response of the sympathetic nervous system, symptoms dramatically improved almost immediately. There continues to be concern with hypotension and the use of ACEI especially in the elderly, and further large-scale studies should be done with patients over 65 years. Enalapril, one of the earliest ACEIs studied, has been shown to benefit elderly patients. ACEIs are better tolerated if patients are hydrated and electrolytes are within normal limits. ACEIs should not be used in patients with a history of angioedema or anuria. Also cautious use of ACEI is warranted in those with high serum creatinine levels (> 3 mg/dl), bilateral renal stenosis, high serum potassium levels (> 5.5 mmol/L) and those with low systolic blood pressure (Makalinao, 2000). Many patients complain of an irritating dry cough, a common side effect, which is caused by ACEI's ability to increase bradykinin release and can be a major reason for treatment failure.

Angiotensin Receptor Blockers (ARBs)

These agents block angiotensin II and aldosterone at the receptor level. Hemodynamic effects are the same as with ACEI as far as reducing preload and afterload and increasing cardiac output, but these agents do not increase bradykinin levels, thus diminishing the side effect of cough Gillespie, Darbar, Struthers, & McMurdo 1998). The first of these agents, Losartan, was found to be well tolerated in elder patients. And today there are many more on the market some of which are combined with HCTZ (a diuretic).

Aldosterone Antagonists

An aldosterone antagonist, spironolactone, at low doses (12.5–25 mg/d) has been found to helpful in patients with NYHA Class IV disease, or severe heart failure. These agents block aldosterone which causes diureses, and preload decreases. Patients, however, should have normal serum potassium levels (< 5.0 mEq/L) and adequate renal function (creatinine < 2.5 mg/dl)

Beta-Adrenergic Blocking Agents

Beta blocker (BB) use in patients with chronic heart failure has been studied in 20 clinical trials with over 10,000 patients. These trials have shown that these agents reduce the risk of sudden death by 40–50% and the need for hospital admission, and improve the overall functional capacity (Lonn, 2000). The beneficial effects of BB in heart failure are related to the blocking of adrenergic stimulation of the heart, specifically norepinephrine, which in CHF is related to increased mortality (Goldstein, 2001). BBs do have a negative inotropic effect and were for many years contraindicated in heart failure patients. In clinical trials, it was shown that this decrease in cardiac output was transient, and, in fact, BBs were shown to increase left ejection fraction. These benefits were found in patients who were receiving therapeutic responses to diuretics and ACEI. Patients with NYHA class II-IV disease were studied in multiple trials; one trial was able to show the decrease in mortality of 35% (MERIT-HF Study Group, 1999). The studies looking at BB in heart failure examined three agents: carvedilol, bisoprolol, and metoprolol CR/XL. The CIBIS-I trial found that there was a 34% reduction in hospital admission rates for patients who were on bisoprolol, and many showed improvements in overall quality of life (CIBIS, 1994). In the second trial CIBIS-II, in patients with NYHA class III and IV disease, there was a 34% reduction in mortality and a 20% reduction in hospital admissions in those treated with Bisoprolol (CIBIS-II, 1999). In the MERIT-HF (1999) study, it was found that carvedilol not only had a vasodilatation affect (due to its alpha-adrenergic properties), but also had antioxidant effects. BBs are contraindicated in patients with bronchospastic disease, advance heart block, or symptomatic bradycardia, and should be used with caution in those with low systolic blood pressure. BBs generally are added once diuretics and ACEIs have been optimized, and the patient is clinical stabile and euvolemic.

Digitalis

Digitalis glycosides, positive inotropic agents, have been a part of the medical regime for patients in heart failure for over 200 years. These agents are still indicated for use in patients with symptomatic heart failure in combination with ACEI and diuretic therapy. In the Digitalis Intervention Group Study (1997), patients with mild to moderate heart failure on digoxin experienced a decrease in the progression of heart failure, had decreased hospital admissions (28%), but had no overall decrease in mortality. Digoxin is still indicated in patients with heart failure and in those with atrial fibrillation with uncontrolled ventricular response.

The suggested dosings of these medications are shown in Exhibit 13.2.

There can be many adverse reactions to cardiovascular medications when used in the older adult population. Physiologically, changes in the metabolism and excretion of drugs occur with age. It is well known that with age there is a decrease in the glomerular filtration and tubular secretion. Cardiac medications that are dependent upon the kidney for excretion should be titrated appropriately; digoxin and ace Inhibitors are those that fit into this category. The hepatic metabolism of drugs also decreases with age. The commonly used medications for relief of symptoms in CHF can therefore have a delayed absorption that can be variable in the older patient. Careful dosing and titration of these drugs on an individual basis is imperative.

The following recommendations should be considered when prescribing cardiac medications for older adults:

1) Always begin with the smallest effective dose; titrate up in small increments, keeping in mind the patient's comorbid conditions that could influence the pharmacokinetics of the drug(s).
2) As dose adjustment is made, clinical evaluation should occur.
3) Review each medication the patient is currently taking, even over-the-counter medications, and herbal remedies, and be aware of contraindications or adjustments needed.
4) Avoid empiric treatment of symptoms. Have a diagnosis before initiating drug therapy.
5) Keep it simple! Adherence decreases as the number of medications and frequency of dosing increases.
6) Make sure that the patient can read the labels; if not, a family member or homecare nurse should set up a weekly pill dispenser. Patients can also have large print labels on their prescription bottles.
7) Patient education is key. Make sure that each patient understands the adverse reactions to watch for and knows when to call for assistance.

Electrical Therapy

Because the pharmacologic agents have fallen short in improvement of QOL and prognosis, especially in those with chronic ventricular dysfunction, recent consideration has been given to interventional therapies in heart failure. These therapies include biventricular pacing and implantable cardioverter defibrillators (ICDs).

EXHIBIT 13.2

DRUG NAME	STARTING DOSE	TARGET DOSE
Vasodilators (ACE-I)		
Captopril	6.25 mg 3×/day	50 mg 3×/day
Enalapril	2.5 mg 2×/day	10 mg 2×/day
Lisinopril	2.5–5 mg/day	20 mg/day
Ramapril	2.5 mg/day	5 mg/day
Accupril	5 mg 2×/day	20 mg 2×/day
Hydralazine + Isosorbide (BiDil)	1 tab 3×/day	2 tabs 3×/day
ARBs		
Candesartan	16 mg/day	32 mg/day
Valsartan	20–40 mg 2×/day	80 mg 2×/day
Atacand	4 mg/day	32 mg/day
Avapro	75 mg/day	150-300 mg/day
Beta-blockers		
Carvedilol	3.12→6.25→12.5→	25 mg 2×/day
Metoprolol	25→50→100→150→	200 mg/day
Bisoprolol	1.25→2.5→5→	10 mg/day
Digoxin		
	0.125 mg/day	0.25 mg/day
Aldosterone inhibitors		
Spironolactone	12.5–25 mg/day	25 mg 2×/day
Inspra	25 mg/day × 4 weeks	50 mg/day
HF Diuretics		
Lasix	40 mg/day	Increase as needed
Bumex	0.5–2 mg/day	
HCTZ	12.5–25 mg/day	
Zaroxolyn	5–20 mg/day ½ hour prior to Lasix dose	

Source: Albert, N (2006). Evidenced-based nursing care for patients with heart failure. *Advanced Critical Care, 17*(2), 170–185.

Biventricular pacing. Since the early 1990s, there have been numerous approaches to improve left ventricular function in patients with CHF by means of cardiac pacing. In the last 10 years, the most promising of these approaches has been biventricular pacing, or ventricular resynchronization therapy (VRT).

Normally, electrical impulses arise in the sino-atrial node of the heart, travel down through the atrioventricular node, to the Bundle of His, through the left and the right bundle branches to the purkinge fibers, where simultaneous depolarization of the atrium and the ventricles occurs. This coordinated conduction enables stroke volume to be maximized. If one or more of these conduction pathways (left bundle or right bundle) is damaged or blocked, the impulse will reach one ventricle before the other, causing asynchrony of the ventricular contraction. When this occurs, it is called intraventricular conduction defect (IVCD). This can be seen in the QRS (measurement of time for ventricular depolarization) of the EKG, which becomes prolonged : more than 120 ms. This IVCD has been found in 30–50% of patients with CHF (Naccarelli, 2001). These conduction delays cause inefficient ventricular contraction, with segments of the ventricle contracting at different times. Short diastole occurs with overlapping of systole and diastole and cardiac output decreases. If the patient already has a failing left ventricle, this asynchrony with decrease in cardiac output leads to further dysfunction, and increased symptoms.

The biventricular pacemaker looks like other pacemakers, but it has three leads instead of two. Electrical leads are threaded into both the left and right ventricle, and the right atrium. This device provides electrical stimulation that is programmed precisely to synchronize and coordinate the right and left ventricular contraction.

Evidence of the use of biventricular pacing with CHF patients in large series clinical trials has been done in the COMPANION, MUSTIC trials, and efficacy of this treatment has been well documented. Most patients in these trials had NYHA Class II-IV disease, prolonged QRS duration (> 150 ms), and were on optimum medical therapy (Naccarelli, 2001). Primary endpoints for these trials were 6-minute walk tests, QOL, and O2 consumption at peak exercise (Cazeau, Frank, Leenhardt, Clementy, & Barnay, 2002). Consistently it was found that there was an almost immediate increase in cardiac output, a positive effect on left ventricular remodeling, and an improvement of diastolic function.

Implantable Cardiac Defibrillators (ICDs) and Ventricular Resynchronization Therapy (VRT) in Combination

Sudden death occurs in 30–59% of patients in NYHA Class IV (Cazeau, et al., 2002). Because of these alarming statistics, the role of combining ICD and ventricular resynchronization devices in chronic heart failure patients has been investigated. ICD implantation is a therapy that is a life-saving option for the patient who has a substrate for sudden cardiac death due to lethal ventricular arrhythmia. In the VENTAK CHF, Insync ICD, and COMPANION trials, both of these devices have been investigated (Dresing & Natale, 2001). The differences between the inclusion criteria with these patients as compared with the patients in the biventricular studies were that these subjects also had an indication for implantable cardioverter defibrillator implantation (ventricular tachycardia) (Dresing & Natale, 2001). The results of these studies in primary reports have indicated an improvement of symptoms, increased QOL, and decreased incidence of sudden death. The efficacy of biventricular pacing and ICDs in patients with CHF and intraventricular conduction defects in the general CHF population is now a proven therapy and a life-saving device in those patients who meet criteria for placement.

Left Ventricular Assist Devices (LVADs)

These mechanical devices are implanted into the abdomen of the recipient and are attached to a weakened heart to help it pump. Doctors first used heart pumps to help keep heart transplant candidates alive while they waited for a donor heart. LVADs are now being considered as an alternative to transplantation. Implanted heart pumps can significantly extend and improve the lives of some people with end-stage heart failure who are not eligible for or able to undergo heart transplantation or are waiting for a new heart. Randomized Evaluation of Mechanical Assistance for the Treatment of Congestive Heart Failure (REMATCH) trial evaluated the survival benefit of this implanted left heart pumping device after 1 year and found that there was significantly more improvement in QOL than in those patients who were receiving optimal medical therapy (52% vs. 25%) (Quaglietti, Pham, & Frolicher 2005). There are serious side effects of this device, which include infection, bleeding, and stroke. This device is generally not recommended for use in palliative care.

Enhanced External Counterpulsation (EECP)

This noninvasive technique has been used as a treatment for heart-related chest pain. Researchers have found that this treatment is beneficial for people with heart failure. Inflatable pressure cuffs are placed on the calves, thighs and buttocks. These cuffs are inflated and deflated in sync with the heartbeat. The theory is that EECP increases blood flow back to the heart, which helps in the development of collateral circulation and decreased angina.

Complementary Therapies

People are becoming increasingly interested in holistic modalities in prevention and treatment of disease. Natural treatments, use of vitamins, herbs, antioxidants, and other nontraditional therapies are used by many to complement or even replace drugs and other interventions. Adjunctive healing modalities can be a benefit to traditional medicine, and there are specific homeopathic remedies that have shown some efficacy for the older patient with congestive heart failure.

Antioxidant drugs. Oxygen-derived free radicals, the byproducts of oxygen metabolism, have been found to cause damage to cells and is considered among the causes of many chronic diseases including CHF (Mak & Newton 2001). Antioxidants have been shown to inhibit atherogenesis and thrombosis in the coronary arteries by interfering with the oxidation of low-density lipoprotein (LDL) which prevents the formation of foam cells, a major cause of atherosclerosis (Anderson & Kessenich, 2001). Antioxidants are found naturally in a wide variety of foods and plants, including many fruits and vegetables, and they are also available as nutritional supplements (vitamins C and E, and beta-carotene). The foods that contain the greatest sources of antioxidants are carrots, tomatoes, yams, leafy greens, blueberries, garlic, and green tea.

Vitamin E, along with vitamin C and selenium, has been found to promote cardiovascular health. It has been shown in animal models to decrease oxidant injury to cardiac membranes, which in part, leads to the pathologic changes that occur in cardiomyopathy (Weglicki, Dickens, Wagner, Chmielinska, & Phillips, 1996). It was also found that magnesium deficiency produced a proinflammatory condition, resulting in overproduction of free radicals, which caused cardiovascular cell injury. The recommended dose per U.S. Drug Administration (USDA) for vitamin E is 400–800 IU/d. However, more recently the recommendation is to avoid vitamin E if taking a statin, as it has been shown to decrease HDL (good cholesterol); thus vitamin E should not be used with patients with CAD.

Coenzyme-Q10 is a fat-soluble vitamin-like compound, or ubiquinone. It is an endogenous antioxidant that protects free radical damage in the mitochondria (Skidmore-Roth, 2001). Coenzyme Q10 is a nutrient needed for cells to produce energy. In a small study by Hofman-Bang, Rehnquist, Swedberg, Wiklund and Astrom (1995), it was found that Coenzyme Q10 reduced hospitalizations and serious complications in patients with heart failure. It is indicated for use in ischemic heart disease, angina, hypertension, and CHF. The recommended dose is 300 mg/d. It has been shown to reduce the myalgia, which can be a side effect of statin use.

Hawthorn, a herb, has also been indicated for use in heart failure patients. It is an extract made from dried leaves, flowers, and fruits of the hawthorn bush. According to Pitter, Guo, and Ernst (2008), although 14 double blinded trials were conducted because of the fact that the trials did not measure the same outcomes, they could not be used in a meta-analysis of the product. The results did suggest that this extract used in addition to conventional therapies did have some benefit with chronic heart failure patients. Hawthorn is rich in flavonoids, which have been shown to benefit patients with heart disease. The dose is 100–250 mg/d.

Shengmai is a traditional Chinese herbal medicine that has been used for the treatment of heart failure and ischemic heart disease. It is a mixture of *Panax ginseng, Ophiopogon japonicas,* and *Schisandra chinensis.* Ten controlled clinical trials looked at the use of shengmai, but the evidence of benefit was weak; however, no adverse effects were reported [Chen et al., (2007)].

An herbal medicinal substance, Crataegus Extract WS® 1442, in a trial with 2,681 patients with severe left ventricular failure, was found to safely extend the lives of congestive heart failure patients already receiving pharmacological treatment for the disease, according to a study presented at the American College of Cardiology's 56th Annual Scientific Session. Crataegus Extract WS®1442 is an extract of leaves of the Crataegus tree and is a natural antioxidant. The herb is currently approved for use in some European countries to treat early congestive heart failure. Holubarsch (2007) and his team saw a 20% reduction in cardiac-related deaths among patients on WS® 1442, extending patients' lives by 4 months during the first 18 months of the study. The safety of the compound was confirmed by a lower number of adverse events among the study group than those on placebo.

"WS 1442 is safe in patients with more severe congestive heart failure and left ventricular ejection fraction lower than 35 percent," said Dr. Holubarsch of Median Kliniken Hospitals in Bad Krozingen, Germany, and lead study author. "It postpones death of cardiac cause after 18 months and sudden cardiac death in an important subgroup of patients" (Holubarsch, 2007).

For more information on herbal medicines: National Institute of Medical Herbalists www.nimh.org.uk

Other complementary therapies for CHF may include slow breathing exercises, meditation, prayer, biofeedback, and yoga. Slow breathing, according to Bernardi et al. (2002), improves oxygen saturation and exercise tolerance in heart failure patients by increasing the arterial baroreflex sensitivity.

Stress reduction techniques also have shown promise in the prevention and treatment of CAD. Transcendental meditation is associated with decreased hypertension and atherosclerosis (King, Carr, & D'Cruz, 2002).

Spirituality influences the manner in which a patient adjusts to a chronic illness. Patients with end-stage heart disease often reflect on their past and attempt to nurture hopes for the future. Westlake and Dracup (2001) looked at how spirituality affected adjustment in end-stage heart failure. Eighty-seven patients were interviewed using a semistructured questionnaire, and a three-step process was identified in which they adjusted or came to terms with their illness. The three steps were development of regret regarding past behaviors and lifestyles, the search for meaning within the present experience of heart failure, and the search for hope and optimism.

Experimental Treatments

- **Cardiac wrap surgery.** Researchers are studying a technique that wraps a failing heart in a mesh bag. A surgeon pulls the mesh wrap over the base of the heart and attaches it with stitches. The goal is to prevent a weakened heart from enlarging (dilating) and failing further. Studies are ongoing.
- **Ventricular restoration surgery.** This surgery is being used experimentally to treat some people with heart failure caused by a heart attack. During the surgery, doctors remove scar tissue in the ventricular muscle caused by a heart attack and reshape the remaining healthy tissue to restore a more normal elliptical left ventricle shape. Reducing the size of and reshaping the left ventricle help restore normal function to the pumping mechanism.
- **Cardiovascular regeneration.** This procedure of regeneration of myocardial cells and activation of myocardial stem cells to replace infracted myocardial cells is certainly an area that would have a positive effect on the heart failure patient and is in the experimental stages. In a book by Annarosa Anversa, and Frishman (2007), the potential for this therapy is reviewed to include the biology of stem cells, the biology of endogenous cardiac progenitors in the heart, the clinical results thus far of stem cell therapies in the infracted myocytes, and the potential of stem cell therapy in cardiomyopathies.
- **Xenotransplantation.** This is a therapeutic option for the hundreds of thousands of people dying each year of heart, kidney, lung, and liver failure. Xenotransplantation involves the transplantation of nonhuman tissues or organs into human recipients. It could provide an unlimited supply of cells and tissues needed for repair or replacement of myocardial cells (Deng et al. 2002). Xenotransplantation between closely related species, such as baboons and humans, offers an alternative to allotransplantation as a source of human organ replacement, but problems with rejection remains a major concern.

So, as one can see, there are many therapeutic options for the patient with heart failure. These multiple options as stated are not always prescribed even when the patient may benefit from the therapy. So there remain gaps in treatment, even in specialist's practice. The other option, palliative care, will be discussed later on in this chapter.

Now as we look at the nursing care of patients with heart failure, there are also gaps between the evidence offered by evidenced-based therapies and performance measures. According to Albert (2006), there are no uniform nursing actions and practice guidelines available.

The science of HF treatment has been well documented, and the nurse who cares for these patients needs to know about the latest 2005 ACC/AHA guidelines. These guidelines can be the basis of the goal setting, measurement outcomes, and development of care in these clients. Disease management is a method of increasing the use of evidenced-based therapies to improve patient education and decrease the usage of resources. Post-discharge interventions have been identified by multiple studies as being imperative for heart failure patients. These interventions include clinic follow-up with a nurse practitioner with cardiology or primary care physician supervision, home nursing follow-up, or a telephone follow-up with a nurse practitioner or specialized registered nurses (Whellan, Hasselblad, Peterson, O'Connor, & Schulman, 2005).

Albert (2006) suggests that algorithms, tables, development of "pocket cards," HF pre-printed discharge sheets, and systematic use of guideline summaries be developed to help nurses to manage HF patients so that the practice is more uniform and effective. Two studies (Albert et al., 2002; Washburn, Hornberger, Klutman, & Skinner, 2005) which assessed whether nurses had the knowledge base in heart failure to adequately educate patients on the disease process and management found that nurses did not have the knowledge needed, yet neither study tested whether patients understood the above delivered education.

Nursing is certainly more active in the planning and management of care in the HF patients, and now is present in collaborative, often nurse-directed, multidisciplinary heart failure clinics. Some have been very successful in achieving this goal. In a British study done by Murray et al. (2002), the illness trajectory of cancer was found to be far easier to predict than that of heart failure. By interviewing patients and healthcare providers, they found that there was a reported consensus of poor coordination and inadequate continuity of care. In Britain, nurses who coordinated care in these heart failure patients have become the main healthcare providers. Interventions by these nurse-based CHF clinics included education of patient and family, prescribed diet, social service consultation, review of medications, and close follow-up with physician. There still is a lack of nursing leadership, however, in defining the nurse care giving role for HF patients throughout all settings.

The Cleveland Clinic, considered a leader in cardiac care, has developed many nursing protocols in order to help standardize EBP in the care of the heart failure patient. Some guidelines already in place are algorithms on aldosterone-antagonists, beta-blockers, digoxin, hypertension, oral anticoagulation, oral vasodilator therapies, device therapies, and palliative care.

The optimal treatment for patients with CHF involves considerably more than prescribing the right medicine. It requires the full support of the patient to work with the healthcare team in managing his or her heart failure. It has been well established that the main reason for re-hospitalization is the discontinuation of prescribed medications, dietary indiscretions, and the failure to identify early signs of worsening heart failure.

Care provided by specialist nurses in heart failure clinics have been shown to improve outcomes for patients with CHF, significantly reducing the number of unplanned readmissions. Gutafsson and Arnold (2004) looked at 18 randomized studies with a total of 24, 551 patients and compared heart failure clinics using nursing interventions versus conventional care. Interventions included patient education, monitoring of medications, follow-up telephone calls, self-care, emotional support, and when to call the cardiologist for changing of symptoms. The majority of these studies showed that there was a reduction in hospital readmissions or shortening of hospitalizations in the nurse-run clinics. Some of the trials used home visits as part of the intervention, and it was found to be more effective than programs that did not have this option.

The role of the advanced practice nurse (APN) with cardiology background who has experience with heart failure patient is certainly a logical choice to help take a leadership role in the nursing management of this disease. In a study by Crowther (2003), it was found that APNs in hospital-based heart failure clinics provided multidisciplinary care which led to positive outcomes. Patients had less readmissions and improved scores on functional status. These APNs provided symptom monitoring, medication adherence, dietary compliance, and telemonitoring. Readmissions to hospitals were decreased, as well as medical costs. Patients felt better and had the benefit of improved QOL.

As part of the interdisciplinary integrated team, nurses, dieticians, social workers, pastoral care, physical therapists, occupational therapists, case managers, pharmacists, and physicians must take part in a coordinated approach in counseling and educating patients with end- stage heart disease, and the plan should be maintained across all settings.

For the elderly, aggressive use of the non-pharmacologic measures are imperative. Drug therapy can often cause unpleasant side effects, which often lead to non-adherence, and are costly now that Medicare D plans are in place. General measures are recommended:

a) Decreasing more or new cardiac injury by risk factor reduction
b) Limiting alcohol use to two glasses/day
c) Maintaining fluid balance by restricted salt intake (2 g/d)
d) Improving physical conditioning
e) Avoiding calcium channel blockers (except amoldipine) and NSAIDS
f) Careful management of comorbid conditions
g) Patient education regarding self-care
h) Influenza vaccination every fall
i) Pneumococcal immunizations after diagnosis and revaccination every 5 years.

j) Care of patients with heart failure across settings and by interdisciplinary team

k) Careful monitoring of fluid status.

PALLIATIVE CARE FOR PATIENTS WITH END-STAGE HEART DISEASE

As illustrated above, the evidenced-based management of heart failure has improved considerably over the last 10 years, but those who will eventually die from this disease are in need of respectful and comprehensive palliative care. The ACC/AHA 2005 guidelines certainly helped to develop benchmarks for palliative care of the heart failure patient. ACC/AHA's end-of-life considerations are as follows:

1) Ongoing patient and family education should be on regarding prognosis for functional capacity and survival.

2) Patient and family education should include options for formulating and implementing advanced directives and the role of palliative and hospice care.

3) Discussion is recommended regarding the option of inactivating implantable assist devices.

4) Continuity of medical care between inpatient and outpatient settings should be ensured.

5) Components of hospice care should include opiate use, inotropes, and intravenous diuretics.

6) All professionals should examine current end-of-life processes and work toward improvement of approaches to palliative care.

7) Aggressive procedures performed in the final days of life are not appropriate.

The writing committee also recommended that all involved with HF care make is a priority to improve the recognition of end-stage disease and provide appropriate care (ACC/AHA 2005). Although the ACC/AHA recommends hospice care as an option, the number of who are referred to this modality of treatment is small. According to the National Hospice and Palliative Care Organization (2004), 49% of hospice patients had a diagnosis of cancer and only 11% had a primary diagnosis of heart failure.

Discussions early in the disease process must be forthcoming. It is too late to discuss palliative care and end-of-life wishes when the patient is near death. As with all patients in this stage of life, ongoing communication is the key in achieving the goal of dying well. Communication skills needed for the discussions necessary in this phase of life are often lacking in the education of healthcare providers. Most patients are aware they they are dying and welcome the discussion of their death. Many patients are not aware of the choices they have and can make. When patients reach the place where they want and need to discuss wishes for this stage of their life, they often depend on their healthcare provider to initiate the conversation. These discussions need to happen before the patients become too ill to participate, because these decisions impact not only their own lives, but also the lives of their loved ones. This continues to be one of the biggest issues in the care of these end-stage patients, one I will address in a commentary at the end of this chapter.

Healthcare providers rarely raise these issues for fear of "decreasing hope." In a qualitative study done in London, Selman et al. (2007) reported that there was a wide range of preferences to end-of-life care reported by patients and their caretakers. Some were ready for death and preferred to die at home; those with poorer mobility said that they did not want their lives prolonged; family members were hesitant to make decisions regarding palliative care; and none of the respondents had discussed their preferences with their healthcare provider. I recommend the following for clinicians: 1) Improved communication with sensitive discussion of issues regarding end stage HF to include preferences; 2) Mutual education of staff who will be interacting with end-stage patients to include communication skills, and signs and symptoms of the disease; 3) CHF referral and care pathways to clarify roles and when to refer (Selman et al., 2007).

When it is time for hospice care, there is criterion from the National Hospice Organization that is important to be aware of. Besides the general criteria, added criteria for heart disease patients had been added to include intractable or recurrent symptoms of HF; optimal medical treatment to be in place; presence of symptomatic arrhythmias, history of cardiac arrest and resuscitation or syncope, cardiogenic brain embolism, or concomitant HIV disease. To enroll, patients also must have a physician to manage care and be expected to survive 6 months or less.

The National Hospice and Palliative Care Organization has a great web site that has many helpful information for patients and providers at: http://files/public/communications/OutreachGuide08/Hospice_Article_4-Don't_Wait.doc

Some of their suggestions as to how patients can discuss end-of-life decisions are the following:

- Talking about treatments that may be confusing
- Pain and options that are available
- Talking about advanced directive wishes and making sure he/she understands what those wishes are
- Giving a copy of advanced directives to all healthcare providers

Inherent in all palliative care are some fundamental precepts:

- Promotion of physical, psychological, social, and spiritual well-being
- Good symptom control
- Whole person approach

- Including both patient and family in the care
- Respecting the patient's wishes even if the choices are not what the healthcare provider may feel is appropriate
- Giving the patient autonomy in the decision making if requested.

Medications discussed in this chapter should continue, as they are palliative in nature. Medications that often are discontinued are statins, digoxin (as digtoxicity increases as renal function decreases). Furthermore, if hypotensive, ACE-I, ARBs, and other antihypertensives should be stopped. If the patient is in fluid overload, the beta-blocker should be tapered. Depression is common and normal during this time and should be treated. Selective serotonin receptor inhibitors are usually well tolerated and improve QOL.

Implantable devices are often turned off during this period, but this should be addressed early in the disease process and agreed upon by patient, family, and healthcare provider. This also should be included in advanced directives.

Symptom management is at the forefront of this care. In order to provide comfort to the patient, doses of up to 600 mg of Lasix may be required, and combinations of diuretics may be necessary in order to control fluid overload. Morphine is also indicated at doses that provide rest and comfort and also relieve suffering in the patient with CHF, which helps in decreasing preload, decreases dyspnea, and relieves pain. As there is no ceiling dose for opioids, the appropriate dose is whatever is needed to relieve pain when dying from heart failure, and the patient's cardiac output eventually decreases to a point where he/she has multiple organ dysfunction with involvement of the liver, kidneys, and lungs. Because of biventricular failure, the right-sided failure causes liver engorgement, which leads to not only nausea and vomiting but also ascites and the inability to eat. Pulmonary edema from left ventricular failure causes respiratory acidosis, which cannot be compensated normally by the kidneys, so renal failure and azotemia also occur. As azotemia increases, metabolic acidosis develops and the patient dies from both respiratory and metabolic acidosis. Sleep-disordered breathing occurs in half of the patients with advanced HF, and therefore treatment with CPAP improves the function of the left ventricle and reverses the adverse neurohormonal activation that occurs (Kohnlein, Welte, Tan, & Elliot, 2002). Unfortunately it is rarely used according to a survey done by Goodlin et al. (2005).

Now that palliative care has been widely studied in the heart failure population, we as nurses need to take advantage of the findings of these studies and discuss with our patients this option. Oncology nurses are a great role model for those of us who care for the heart failure patients, and their comfort in discussing this modality of treatment should be emulated. Education of this disease is where our efforts need to begin, and

then looking at our own feelings of death and dying should be explored. We have a wealth of information now, and we just need to keep abreast of all the nursing interventions that are evidence-based so that our practice reflects these standards of care.

> **Case Study conclusion:** Now back to Mrs. L, the 85-year-old patient presented at the beginning of this chapter. The fact that she doesn't know her options now that she is very ill and most likely nearing the end of her life certainly isn't unusual. Her son is struggling with the fact that his mom is failing and yet she doesn't want the treatment that helped her in the past. In his own mind he thinks that maximal medical care and hospitalization should be planned for his mom, but this may be the opposite of what Mrs. L. wishes at this point.

In a quantitative study by Rogers et al. (2000) looked at whether patients understood chronic heart failure and the investigated the difficulty patients had with communication with their healthcare provider. In this study, patients had symptomatic NYHA III or above, and had been hospitalized within the past 20 months. Thirty patients were interviewed and they all had decreased left ventricular function. Many patients gave accounts of their recurrent symptoms and lacked a clear sense of why they developed heart failure and what the disease entailed. Some patients had a desire to plan their death; others did not want to openly acknowledge their prognosis. Patients believed that their physicians did not want to talk about death. Many felt they could not raise certain issues with their physician; others believed that their doctor knew best and they should not question their recommendations of treatment. Some felt that a frank discussion about their diagnosis and prognosis would be helpful and even welcome.

This study and many others tell us as healthcare providers the same story .why are we so hesitant to talk about the full spectrum of heart failure? Why can't we share the prognosis of heart disease with our patients? Why can't we make their fears and misunderstandings about how they feel a priority in their care? Rather, we listen to their lungs, heart, adjust their medication, and have them come back to the office in 6 months to do the same. Is it because we have trouble with the idea of death ourselves? Or is it because we are afraid that it would be somehow a failure on our part if patients like Mrs. L give up too soon. Are we that omnipotent in our minds that we think that we do not need to discuss these issues as we "will save them" somehow some way?

Wouldn't our patients be better served if we could be more open with our communication? Wouldn't it be much more helpful to our patients if we could discuss where they prefer death to occur as in the case with Mrs. L? After all, we know from multiple studies that patients need to talk about these issues, but often that does not occur. Discussion about the possibility of death is certainly good nursing and medical practice, especially when there is a terminal disease like heart failure. Communication of this nature takes time, and much more thought and planning is required than an office visit where a physical exam is scheduled. But in my opinion it is worth the time and effort. Discussions on symptoms, the burden of heart failure on both the patient and family, financial burden, and what specific treatments each patient wishes to explore are also important. We also need to take into account gender and cultural differences. There are many cultural norms about death and dying that need to be part of the discussion. We need to use language that is understood; and most importantly, we need to allow the patient and his/her family to express their feelings without judgment. The outcomes of certain treatments should be explained; often patients will not choose a certain therapy if it seems (to them) to be either costly or of little benefit. Often patients will want to know how a treatment may affect their QOL. Those therapies that may affect their function or may have an effect on their cognition are often seen as not worthwhile options.

We know from experience when death is near. For Mrs. L, this was the case. At this point, I would talk to her frankly about what her options are, or we will have missed the chance. These conversations need to be ongoing as her symptoms change and as the disease progresses. Coping mechanisms need to be explored as functional impairment becomes worse, as is the case with Mrs. L. Depression needs to assessed and treated if present. Anxiety can make patients more dyspneic, and anxiolytics are often prescribed at this stage. Exploring the role of spirituality is important to include in our treatment of Mrs. L. It often brings inner peace and comfort in these end stages. We need to know what a "good death" is to Mrs. L. Hospice care should be offered and referrals made if Mrs. L. is ready for this option. Her symptoms and prognosis certainly qualify for these services. Her son is an important part of Mrs. L.'s care and he needs to be brought into these discussions from the start. He may have different worries or questions, and they need to be validated and explained. Mrs. L. may feel more comfortable talking about her wish to stay out of the hospital with the healthcare provider being in the room. There are some additional adjustments to therapy that may help in relieving her symptoms. Maximizing her diuretics would help her dyspnea with dosing in the morning, so she can sleep at night. Her ACEI should be slowly titrated up to a dose that is more beneficial. Home oxygen therapy would also help even when oxygen saturation levels are within normal range. General measures that could help alleviate some of her breathlessness should be reviewed, and referrals to homecare regarding dietitian and physical therapy can be arranged. Advance directives and living wills should be explained, and forms available for her to complete if she so desires.

When her condition becomes such that she needs parenteral medication, she needs to know what that therapy involves, and how hospice or homecare can help. Goals need to be outlined, and she can be reassured that a peaceful death is achievable.

A list of support groups for those in heart failure may be helpful: she may want to see a psychologist or a social worker, and referrals should be made. Mrs. L. can be reassured that she does not have to be readmitted to the hospital. Explain to her that it is always an option and that she can change her mind on this or any other choice at any time.

The plan that Mrs. L. has decided upon should be detailed in her chart. All colleagues in the practice should be aware of the plan so that continuity of care can be maintained. Above all, empower her to make the decisions that feel right for her at this time in her life, and respect her decision. Let her know that she can depend on the healthcare team and that her QOL in death matters.

CONCLUSION

In caring for the heart failure, there are nursing and medical evidence-based practices (EBPs) that should drive our decisions of care. Hopefully, this chapter has helped the reader to understand the state of this disease and its treatment, how important disease management is, how nurse-based heart failure clinics can lead to positive outcomes, and, most importantly, how to communicate with patients and families regarding their treatment options and what is important to them in the last days of life.

EVIDENCE-BASED PRACTICE

Dougherty, C.M., Pyper, G. P., Au, D.H., Levy, W.C., & Sullivan, M.D. (2007). Drifting in a shrinking future: living with advanced heart failure. *Journal of Cardiovascular Nursing*, 6, 480–7.

Background. Patients with advanced *heart* failure (HF) have an uncertain prognosis and low rates of advance *care* planning and hospice use. The purpose of this study was to describe how patients view and plan for their future.

Methods. Twenty-four (N = 24) patients took part in a semistructured interview in which they were asked to describe their experiences in living with *heart* disease and their understanding and planning for their future. Interviews were transcribed and analyzed using the constant comparative method to generate a grounded theory.

Results. The core category, "Living with HF," encompassed the subcategories of "My Experience of HF," "Help with HF," and "My Future with HF." This article reports on "My Future with HF." Patients wanted to discuss how HF affected their future with their providers, but initiation of these discussions was difficult and the absence of discussion led to frustration. Patients did not find specific life expectancy estimates helpful in coping or planning their future *care*.

Conclusions. Patients with advanced HF do not plan well for end-of-life *care* and tend to drift along while vaguely hoping for the best. End-of-life *care* in advanced HF should address difficulties in decision making and provider communication.

REFERENCES

Abraham, W., & Krum, H. (2007). *Heart failure: A practical approach to treatmen* New York: McGraw-Hill.

ACC/AHA. (2005). Guideline update for the diagnosis and management of chronic heart failure in the adult: Summary article: A report of the American College of Cardiology/American Heart association Task Force on Practice Guidelines (Writing Committee to update the 2001 guidelines for the evaluation and management of heart failure). *Journal of American College Cardiology, 46*, 1116–1143.

Albert, N. (2006). Evidenced based nursing care in patients with heart failure. *Advanced Critical Care, 17*(2), 170–185.

Albert, N. M., Collier, S., Sumodi, V., Wilkinson, S., Hammel, J. P., Vopat, L., et al. (2002). Nurse's knowledge of heart failure education principles. *Heart and Lung, 31*(2), 102–112.

Alla, F., Briancon, S., Julliere, Y., Mertes, P. M., Villemont, J. P. & Zannand, F., et al. (2000).

Differential clinical prognostic classification in dilated or ischemic cardiomyopathy and advanced heart failure: The EPICAL study. *American Heart Journal, 139*, 895–904.

Allen, L. A., Yager, H. E., Funk, M. J., Levy, W. C., Tulsky, J. A., Bowers, M.T., et al. (2008). Discordance between patient-predicted and model-predicted life expectancy among ambulatory patients with heart failure. *Journal of the American Medical Association, 299*(21), 2533–2542.

American Heart Association. (2005). *Heart disease and stroke statistics*. 2005 update. http://www.americanheart.org/downloadable/heart/107296–9766940HSStats2004Update.pdf

American College of Cardiology. (2005). Clinical statements/guidelines. http://www.acc.org/clinical/statements.htlm.

Anderson, J., & Kessenich, C. (2001). Cardiovascular disease and micronutrients therapies. *Topics in Advanced Practice Nursing Journal, I*(2). Available: http://www.medscape.com/viewarticle/408410 Medscape Portals, Inc.

Annarosa, L., Anversa, P., & Frishman, W. H. (2007). *Cardiovascular regeneration and stem cell therapy*. Hoboken, NJ: Wiley-Blackwell Publishing.

Arling, M. (1997). Management of heart failure in nursing facility residents according to AAMDA guidelines. *Nursing Home Medicine, 5*(11) 374.

Bernardi, L., Porta, C., Scpicuzza, L., Bellwon, J., Giammario, S., Frey, A., et al. (2002). Slow breathing increases arterial baroreflex sensitivity in patients with chronic heart failure. *Circulation, 105*, 143–145.

Cazeau, S., Frank, R., Leenhardt, A., Clementy, J. & Barnay, C. (2002). *Arch Mal Coeur Vasiss, 95*, (5 Spec 4), 33–36.

Chen, J., Wu, G., Li, S., Yu, T., Xie, Y., Zhou, L., et al. (2007). Shengmai (A traditional Chinese herbal medicine) for heart failure. *Cochrane Database of Systematic Review, 4*, Art. No. CD005052. doi: 10. 1002/14651878. CD005052.pub2.

CIBIS Investigators and Committees. (1994). A randomized trial of beta blockade in heart failure: The cardiac insufficiency bisoprolol study (CIBIS). *Circulation, 90*, 1765–1773.

CIBIS Investigators and Committees. (1999). The cardiac insufficiency bisoprolol study II (CIBIS II): A randomized trial. *Lancet, 353*, 9–13.

Criteria Committee of the New York Heart Association. (1964). *Diseases of the heart and blood vessels: Nomenclature and criteria for diagnosis* (6th ed.). Boston: Little-Brown.

Crowther, M. (2003). Optimal management of outpatients with heart failure using advanced practice nurses in a hospital-based heart failure center. *Journal of American Academy of Nurse Practitioners, 15*(6), 260–66.

Deng, M. A., Ascheim, D. D., Edwards, N. M. & Naka, Y. (2002). End-stage heart failure: Which options? *European Heart Journal*, (Suppl. D), 122–130

Dresing, T. J., & Natale, A. (2001). Congestive heart failure treatment: The pacing approach. *Heart Failure Reviews, 6*, 15–25.

Fonarow, G. C. (2008). Improving evidenced-based care of heart failure patients. *Medscape Cardiology*. Retreived 10/19/08. wwwmedscape.com.viewarticle/576072.

Fonarow, G. C., & Yancy, C. W. (2008). Heart failure care in the outpatient cardiology practice setting: Findings from IMPROVE HF. *Circulation: Heart Failure* . Published online May 28, 2008. doi: 10.1161/CIRCHEARTFAILURE.108.772228.

Gibbs, J., McCoy, A. S. M., Gibbs, L. M. E., Rogers, A. E., & Addington-Hall, J. M. (2002). Living with and dying from heart failure: The role of palliative care. *Heart, 88* (Suppl. III), ii–36–39.

Gillespie, N. D., Darbar, D., Struthers, A. D., & McMurdo, M. E. (1998). Heart failure: A diagnostic and therapeutic dilemma in elderly patients. *Age and Ageing, 27*, 539–543.

Goldstein, S. (2001). Heart failure therapy at the turn of the century. *Heart Failure Review, 6*, 7–14.

Goodlin, S. J., Kutner, J. S, Connor, S. R., Ryndes, T., Houser, J. & Hauptman, P., et al. (2005). Hospice Care for heart failure patients. *Journal of Pain and Symptom Management, 29*(5), 525–528.

Green, C. P., Porter, C. B., Bresnahan, D., & Spertus, J. (2000). Development and evaluation of the Kansas City Cardiomyopathy Questionnaire: A new health status measure for heart failure. *Journal of American College of Cardiology, 35*(5), 1245–1255.

Gutafsson, F., & Arnold, M. O. (2004). Heart failure clinics and outpatient management: Review of the evidence and call for quality assurance. *European Society of Cardiology, 25*(18), 1596–1604.

Hauptman, P. (2005). Integrating palliative care into heart failure care. *Archives of Internal Medicine, 165*(4), 374–378.

Hermann, F., Steinbuchel, T., Schowalter, M., Spectus, J. A., Stefan, S., & Angermann, C. E., et al. (2005). The Kansas City Cardiomyopathy Questionnaire: A new disease specific quality of life measure for patients with heart failure. *Psychotherapy, 55*,(3–4), 200–208.

Hinton, J. M. (1963). The physical and mental stress of dying. *Quarterly Journal of Medicine, 32*, 1–21.

Holubarsch, C. (2007). Crateagus extract WS 1442 postpones cardiac death in patients with congestive heart failure. Class

NYHA III: Arandomized placebo-controlled double-blind study of 2,681. Presented at March 27, 2007 American College of Cardiology 56th Annual Scientific Session.

Hofman-Bang, C., Rehnquist, N., Swedberg, K., Wiklund, I., & Astrom, H. (1995). Coenzyme Q 10 as an adjunctive in the treatment of chronic congestive heart failure. The Q 10 Study Group. *Journal of Cardiac Failure, 1,* 101–107.

Jessup, M., & Brozena, S. (2003). Heart failure. *New England Journal Medicine, 348*(10), 2007–2018.

King, M. S., Carr, T., & D'Cruz, C. (2002). Transcendental meditation, hypertension and heart disease. *Australian Family Physician, 31*(2), 164–168.

Kirkpatrick, J., & Kim, A.Y. (2006). Ethical issues in heart failure: Overview of an emergency need. *Perspectives in Biology and Medicine, 49*(1), 1–9.

Kohnlein, T., Welte, T., Tan, L. B., & Elliot, M. W. (2002). Central sleep apnea syndrome in patients with chronic heart failure: A critical review of current literature. *Thorax, 57,* 547–554.

Krousel-Wood, M., Abdoh, A., & Mehra, M. (2003). Academy heart meeting. *Abstract: Academy Heart Meeting. 20,* No. 792.

Kubzansky, L., & Ichiro, K. (2000). Going to the heart of the matter: Do negative emotions cause coronary heart disease? *Journal of Psychosomatic Research, 48,* 323–337.

Lamb, D. R. (1984). *Physiology of exercise: Responses and adaptations.* New York: Macmillan.

Laurent-Bopp, D. (2001). Heart failure. In S. L. Woods, E. S. Froelicher & S. Motzer (Eds.), *Cardiac nursing* (pp. 560–570). Philadelphia: Lippincott Williams & Wilkins.

Levi, A., Anversa, P., & Frishman, W.H. (Eds.). (2007) *Cardiovascular regeneration and stem cell therapy.* New Jersey: Wiley-Blackwell Publishing.

Levy, D., Kenchiach, S., Larson, M. G., Benjamin, E. J., Kupka, M., Kalon, K. L., et al. (2002). Long-term trends in the incidence and survival with heart failure. *New England Journal of Medicine, 347*(18), 1397–1402.

Lonn, E. (2000). Drug treatment in heart failure. *British Medical Journal, 320,* 1188–1192.

Lloyd-Jones, D. M., Larson, M. G., & Leip, E. P. (2002). Life time risk for developing congestive heart failure: The Framingham Heart Study. *Circulation, 106,* 3068–3072.

Makalinao, J. (2000). Chronic heart failure: Examining consensus recommendations for patients management. *Geriatric, 55,* 53–8

Maisel, A. (2002). B-type natriuretic peptide levels: Diagnostic and prognostic in congestive heart failure, what's next? *Circulation,105,* 2328–2331.

Mak, S., & Newton, G. (2001). The oxidative stress hypothesis of congestive heart failure: Radical thoughts. *Chest, 120,* 2035–2046.

Mann, D. L. (2001). The role of inflammatory mediators in the failing heart. *Heart Failure Review, 6*(69), 385–348.

May, H. T., Horne, B. D., Levy, M. C., Kfoury, A. G., Rasmusson, K. D., Linker, D. T., et al. (2007). Validation of the seattle heart failure model in a community-based heart failure population and enhancement by ading B-type natrriuretic peptide. *American Journal Cardiology, 100*(4), 697–700.

McGynn, E., Asch, S., Adams, J., Keesy, J., Hicks, J., DeChristafaro, A., et al. (2003). The quality of health care delivered to adults in the United States. *The New England Journal of Medicine, 348* (26), 2635–2645.

McPherson, M. (2007). Palliative care and appropriate medication use in end-stage heart failure. *Medscape Nurses.* Available at http://www.medscape.com/viewarticle/556035.

MERIT-HF Study Group. (1999). The effect of Metoprolol CR/XL in chronic heart failure: Metoprolol CR/XL randomized intervention trial in congestive heart failure (MERIT-HF). *Lancet, 353,* 2001–2007.

Micheal, A., & Frances, C. (2001). *Saint Frances guide to cardiology.* Philadelphia: Lippincott Williams & Wilkins.

Murray, S. A., Boyd, K., Kendall, M., Worth, A., Benton, T. F., Clause, H., et al. (2002). Dying of lung cancer or cardiac failure. *British Medical Journal, 325,* 929–32.

Naccarelli, G. V. (2001). *Biventricular pacing in congestive heart failure: A post-ACC meeting perspective.* 50th Annual Scientific Session of the American College of Cardiology, Day 3, March 20, 2001.

National Hospice and Palliative Care Organization. (2004). *NPHCO facts and figures.* Available at http://www.nhpco.org/files/public/facts_amd figures. Accessed October 28, 2008.

O'Mahoney, P. G. (1998). Is the SF-36 suitable for assessing health status of older stroke patients? (form used for self-reporting on health status in the United Kingdom). *Age and Ageing, 27,* 19–22.

Pantilat, S.Z., &. Steimle, A. E. (2004). Palliative care for patients with heart failure. *Journal of the American Medical Association, 291*(20), 2476–2482.

Pitter, M. H., Guo, R., & Ernst, E. (2008). Hawthorn extract for treating chronic heart failure. *Cochrane Database of Systematic Reviews* 10.1002/14651858.CD005312.pub2.

Pratt, L. A., & Brody, D. J. (2008). Depression in the United States household population 2005–2006. *National Center Health Statistics,* Number 7, September 2008.

Quaglietti, S. C., Pham, M., & Frolicher, V. (2005). A palliative approach to the advanced heart failure patient. *Current Cardiology Reviews, 1,* 45–52.

Rick, M. V. (1997). Epidemiology, pathopphsyiology and etiology of congested heart failure in older adult. *Journal American Geriatric Society, 45*(9), 968–975.

Roger, V. L., Weston, S. A., Redfield, M. M., Hellermann-Homan, J. P., Killian, J., Yawn, B., et al. (2004). Trends in heart failure incidence and survival in a community-based populatiom. *Journal of the American Medical Association, 292,* 344–350.

Rogers, A. E., Addington-Hall, J. M., Abery, A. J., McCoy, A. S. M., Bulpitt, C., Coats, A. J. S., et al. (2000). Knowledge and communication difficulties for patients with chronic heart failure: Qualitative study. *British Medical Journal, 32,* 605–607

Rose, E. G. (2001). Long-term use of a left ventricular assist device for end-stage heart failure. *The New England Journal of Medicine, 345*(20), 1435–1443.

Sherwood, A., Blumenthal, J. A., Trivedi, R., Johnson, K. S., O'Connor, C. M., Adams, K. F., et al. (2007). Relationship of depression to death or hospitalization in patients with heart failure. *Archives of Internal Medicine, 167*(4), 367–373.

Skidmore-Roth, L. (2001). *Handbook of herbs & natural supplements.* St. Louis, Mo: Mosby.

Selman, L. H., Harding, R., Beynon, T., Hodson, T., Coady, E., Hazeldone, C., et al. (2007). Improving end-of-life care for patients with chronic heart failure: 'Let's hope it'll get better, when I know in my heart of hearts it won't". *Heart, 93,* 963–967.

Taylor, G. (2001). *Primary care management of heart failure.* St. Louis, Mo: Mosby.

The Digitalis Investigation Group. (1997). The effect of digoxin on mortality and morbidity in patients with heart failure. *New England Journal of Medicine, 336,* 525–533.

Vaccarino, V. K. (2003). Depressive symptoms are the strongest predictors of short-term declines in health status in patients with heart failure. *Journal of American Cardiology, 38*(1), 199–205.

Ware, J. E., & Sherbourne, C. D. (1994). The MOS 36-Item short-form health survey (SF-36): I: Conceptual framework and item selection. *Medical Care, 30,* 473–483.

Washburn, S. C., Hornberger, C. A., Klutman, A., & Skinner, L. (2005). Nurses knowledge of heart failure education topics as reported in a small midwestern community hospital. *The Journal of Cardiovascular Nursing, 20* (3), 215–220.

Westlake, C., & Dracup, K. (2001). Role of spirituality in adjustment of patients with advanced heart failure. *Progress in Cardiovascular Nursing, 16*, 119–125.

Weglicki W. B, Dickens, B. F., Wagner, T. L., Chmielinska, J. J., & Phillips, T. M. (1996). Immunoregulation by neuropeptides in magnesium deficiency ex-vivo effect of enhanced substance P-production on circulating T-lymphocytes from magnesium-deficient mice. *Magnesium Research, 9*(1), 3–11.

Whellan, D. H., Hasselblad, V., Peterson, E., O'Connor, C. M., & Schulman, K. A. (2005). Meta-analysis and review of heart failure disease management randomized controlled clinical trials. *American Heart Journal, 149*, 722–729.

Gogen, J. S. (1999). Neither prevention nor cure: Managed care for women with chronic conditions. Women's Health Issues, (Suppl. 1), 68s-78s.

Woods, S., Froelicher, E., S., & Motzer, S. (2000). *Cardiac nursing* (4th ed.). Philadelphia: Lippincott Williams & Wilkins.

Wyse, D. G., Waldo, A. L., DiMarco, J. P., Domanski, M. J., Rosenberg, Y., Schron, E. B., et al. (2002). Atrial fibrillation follow-up investigation of rhythm management (AFFIRM): A comparison of rate control and rhythm control in patients with heart failure. *New England Journal of Medcine, 347*(23), 1825–1833.

Yancy, C. (2008). Predicting life expectancy in heart failure. *Journal of the American Medical Association, 299*(21), 2566–2567.

Zambroski, C. (2008). Self-care at the end of life in patients with heart failure. *The Journal of Cardiovascular Nursing, 23*(3), 266.

HELPFUL RESOURCES AND WEBSITES REGARDING HEART FAILURE

1) American Heart Association:
   - Very helpful in assessing data regarding statistics, patient information, risk factor identification, publications/brochures for patient education.
2) National Guideline Clearinghouse:
   - Latest evidenced-based guidelines on the care of patients with heart disease.
3) National Heart, Lung and Blood Institute (http://nhlbi.nih.gov/index.html):
   - Health information on cardiac risk factors with guidelines for management.
4) Framingham Heart Study (http://framingham.com/ heart/):
   - Score sheet for estimating risk of development of heart disease, good patient educational materials.
5) Center to Advance Palliative Care (http://www.capmssm.org/):
   - Publications, resources, conferences on palliative care.
6) Geriatric Medicine (http://www.mayo.edu/geriatrics-rst/Card_ToC.html):
   - Website of Mayo clinic, helpful for patient and provider information on geriatrics.

14

Chronic Lung Disease

Mary M. Brennan

Key Points

To provide palliative care for patients at every stage of chronic obstructive pulmonary disease (COPD), from diagnosis to end-of-life (EOL), the nurse needs to consider the following questions and acquire the knowledge and skills for expert nursing care.

- What are the pathophysiological changes associated with COPD?
- What are the etiologies involved in the development of COPD?
- How is COPD diagnosed and what are the current medical treatment modalities?
- What interventions are effective for smoking cessation?
- Are there alternative/complementary therapies that can assist the older adult with COPD?
- What can nurses do to assist the client at the end-stage of COPD?
- What are the goals of palliative care for patients with mild COPD and patients with very severe COPD?

Introduction

Chronic lung disease, specifically COPD, is the fourth leading cause of death (American Lung Association Fact Sheet, 2009) and is the most common cause of death from respiratory disease in the United States (American Lung Association Fact Sheet, 2009). Clients with COPD experience pulmonary complications as well as a spectrum of extrapulmonary complications arising from the disease including malnutrition, pain, anxiety, and depression (Global Obstructive Lung Disease [GOLD], 2008). As COPD progresses, it is the 7th leading cause of disability and the 12th most common cause of morbidity (American Lung Association Fact Sheet, 2009). About 80%–90% of COPD cases are the result of smoking (American Lung Association Fact Sheet, January 2009). COPD is progressive and the course of the disease is characterized as a slow decline with intermittent episodes of exacerbations (Curtis, 2008). Due to the progressive nature of COPD, as well as the increased complications and disability, palliative care should be implemented at the point of diagnosis. However, due to the variable and often unpredictable course of the disease, fewer patients with COPD receive palliative care than patients with other chronic diseases (Yohannes, 2007; Curtis 2008). According to the National Consensus Project for Quality Palliative Care (2009), the objective of palliative care is "to prevent and relieve suffering and to support the best possible quality of life (QOL) for patients and their families, regardless of the stage of the disease or the need for other therapies" (p. 6). As part of an interdisciplinary, team-based approach, integrated palliative care needs to be initiated at the time of diagnosis, and tailored to the stage of COPD to promote QOL for clients throughout the continuum of the disease. Both Mr. H. and Mrs. S require palliative care, although the objectives of palliative care need to be customized to the stage of their disease.

COPD DEFINITION

COPD is defined as:

> "a preventable and treatable disease with some significant extrapulmonary effects that may contribute to the severity in individual patients. Its pulmonary component is characterized by airflow limitation that is not fully reversible. The airflow limitation is usually progressive and associated with an abnormal inflammatory response of the lung to noxious particles or gases" (GOLD, 2008, p. 6).

The pulmonary aspect of COPD (2008) reflects airflow limitation and may or may not include changes associated with a combination of both emphysema and/or bronchitis. Emphysema, the destruction of alveoli with subsequent dysfunction of gas exchange, is only one of the changes that may occur with COPD (GOLD, 2008). Bronchitis, associated with excessive sputum production, may or may not occur with COPD, but does not reflect the major airflow obstruction that is characteristic of COPD (GOLD, 2008). The symptoms of COPD include dyspnea on exertion, cough and sputum (GOLD, 2008). Cough and sputum production may be early signs and may portend the onset of airflow limitation (GOLD, 2008).

Causes

Smoking is a major precursor to the development of COPD. Individuals who have been smoking for 10 years begin to develop pulmonary changes associated with COPD (American Lung Association, 2009). However, only 15% of smokers go on to develop COPD (Brashers, 2002). Urban living and air pollution have also been implicated in the development and the exacerbation of COPD (Brashers, 2002). Alpha-antitrypsin is a glycoprotein that appears to protect the alveolar walls from destruction; congenital deficiency of alpha-antitrypsin has been implicated in the diagnosis of COPD in persons who are young and nonsmokers (Weinberger, 1998). In the 15% of nonsmokers who will develop COPD, a deficiency of alpha-antitrypsin is suspected (Weinberger, 1998).

Pathophysiology

Clients with COPD have a number of pathological changes in the bronchioles, lower airways, lung parenchyma, and pulmonary vessels. Exposure to cigarette smoke, toxic gases, air pollution, and noxious substances induce widespread tissue damage and inflammation. Smokers are thought to have increased levels of inflammatory cells including neutrophils, macrophages, and T-Lymphocytes (GOLD, 2008). These cells damage the airways and stimulate proteases which destroy connective tissue and overwhelm the number of protective antiproteases. As the pulmonary cells undergo repeated episodes of damage, and cell repair, structural changes occur in the normal epithelium of the airways. Fibrosis and inflammation replace normal epithelium and cause a narrowing of the airways. The resultant narrowing of the airways causes an obstruction to airflow, particularly expiratory flow. As airways weaken and collapse, air in the airways is unable to be expired and becomes trapped. The residual air causes a breakdown of the alveoli and further damages the structure of the lungs.

Airflow limitation and obstruction of airflow are the hallmark consequences of COPD.

Airflow limitation can be accentuated by three main processes: a) Loss of elastic recoil of the alveoli, b) Inflammation causing narrowing of the airways, c) Hypertrophy of the mucous-producing goblet cells causing obstruction of the lumen of the airways with thickened mucous. As COPD progresses, there is a decline in lung function that is 3–5 times more dramatic than in age-related matched groups without COPD (Hardin, Meyers, & Louie, 2008).

Diagnosis

The diagnosis of COPD is often considered when a client reports a chronic cough, sputum production or dyspnea (GOLD, 2008). A comprehensive history should be obtained including the duration and type of cough, whether dyspnea occurs at rest or with exercise, and the amount of sputum production. The baseline, functional status of the client should be established and monitored over the course of the disease. Information regarding smoking history, recent exposure to toxic substances, or exposure to occupational fumes is necessary in establishing a diagnosis.

Once the diagnosis of COPD is considered, pulmonary function tests are needed to confirm the diagnosis. Pulmonary function tests measure the degree of airway obstruction. The stages of COPD (GOLD, 2008) are classified according to the degree of airway obstruction. Stage I COPD indicates mild airway obstruction; Stage II COPD indicates moderate airway obstruction; Stage III COPD indicates severe airway obstruction; Stage IV reveals very severe airway obstruction. Pharmacotherapy and treatments are individualized according to the degree of airway obstruction and symptoms (GOLD, 2008).

Additional diagnostic tests may be necessary for further investigation including a chest X-Ray, arterial blood gases, bronchodilator reversibility testing. If a client is diagnosed with COPD before the age of 45, and has a family history, alpha-1 antitrypsin testing may be performed. The chest X-ray examination may demonstrate hyperinflation, a flat diaphragm, and the increased AP diameter (Weinberger, 1998). The ABGs will remain fairly normal until the later stages of the disease. Use of the modified Borg Scale (see Exhibit 14.1)

EXHIBIT 14.1: MODIFIED BORG SCALE

0) Nothing at all.
0.5) Very, very slight (just noticeable).
1) Very slight.
2) Slight (light).
3) Moderate.
4) Somewhat severe.
5) Severe.
6)
7) Very Severe.
8)
9) Very, very severe (almost maximal).
10) Worst imaginable.

From Spector, N., & Klein, D. (2001). Chronic critically ill dyspneic patients: Mechanisms and clinical measurement. *AACN Clinical Issues. Advanced Practice in Acute and Critical Care, 12*(2), 220–233.

and noninvasive technology, such as pulse oximetry, may also help to quantify the changes in respiratory status of the older adult (Hall, 1998).

REVIEW OF SYMPTOMS AND PHYSICAL EXAMINATION FINDINGS

The client may complain of dyspnea upon exertion as well as at rest. A decrease in appetite, or a loss of appetite, can occur as dyspneic symptoms worsen. As a result of decreased food intake, the older adult may report weight loss. Mental status changes, due to decreased oxygenation, may be reported by family members or significant others.

Upon physical examination, auscultation of the lungs may reveal wheezing, rhonchi, or diminished lung sounds. With disease exacerbation, accessory muscle use will become visible—the sternocleidomastoid and trapezius muscle groups with intercostals muscle retractions as examples (Weinberger, 1998). Due to an increased anteroposterior (AP) diameter, the heart sounds may be distant.

Complications of COPD

The systemic and extrapulmonary complications of COPD may include cardiac, pulmonary, and gastrointestinal dysfunction. Some of the complications associated with COPD include pulmonary vascular vasoconstriction, cor pulmonale, atrial arrythmias, pneumothorax, recurrent respiratory infections (such as pneumonia), respiratory failure, and malnutrition. Pulmonary vascular hypertension develops as the result of hypoxia which causes vasoconstriction of the pulmonary arterioles (Weinberger, 1998). As the vasoconstriction worsens, increased pressure is reflected to the right side of the heart. Cor pulmonale, or enlargement of the right ventricle, occurs in response to increased pulmonary pressures and is a common feature of severe COPD (Sommers & Johnson, 2002). Cor Pulmonale accounts for 25% of all types of heart failure and is more common in middle-aged and older males (Sommers & Johnson, 2002). Cor pulmonale is a late sign of COPD and there is a poor response to therapeutic interventions (Marini & Wheeler, 1997).

A pneumothorax, an accumulation of air within the pleural space, may occur due to rupture of emphysematous bullae. Bullae develop as the result of cell and alveolar damage associated with COPD.

Recurrent respiratory infections, commonly viral and bacterial in origin, can cause a transient worsening of COPD symptoms and are the most common cause of acute exacerbations (Sethi & Muphy, 2008). COPD patients are likely to experience one to two acute exacerbations per year (Sethi & Murphy, 2008). Haemophilus, and Streptococcus infections are the most common bacterial infections (Sethi & Murphy, 2008). The rhinovirus is responsible for approximately 25% of acute exacerba-

tions (Sethi & Murphy). Frequent infections are likely to decrease pulmonary function (Weinberger, 1998).

The development of malnutrition is multifactorial in the older adult and occurs in up to 25%–50% of COPD patients (Manaker & Burke, 1999). There is a 20%–50% increase in metabolic demands associated with COPD as the normal work of breathing becomes more difficult and requires more effort (Witta, 1997). Calorie expenditure may increase 10-fold to more than 700 calories per day (Manaker & Burke, 1999). Patients with COPD find it difficult to satisfy the excessive caloric requirements associated with breathing. Malnutrition may develop as a result of decreased food intake due to dyspnea, or the increased energy expenditure due to the disease process (Marini & Wheeler, 1997). Early satiety may develop due to the diaphragmatic changes associated with COPD. The lowering and flattening of the diaphragm can result in gastric compression (Marini & Wheeler, 1997). Fatigue and dyspnea can result in decreased oral intake. Depression due to chronic illness or changes in lifestyle and personal losses may decrease the client's interest in eating (Witta, 1997).

Changes that occur with normal aging may predispose the patient to COPD or may worsen COPD. There are changes in lung function that are associated with the aging process. As individual age, elastic recoil decreases and the chest wall stiffens. As a result of these changes, there is a decrease in compliance resulting in decreased lung pressures and volumes (Hall, 1998; Sheahan & Musialowski, 2001). The residual volume, or air remaining in the lungs after a maximal expiration, increases (Hall, 1998). This increase in residual volume reflects the changes in lung elasticity. Airway compression occurs earlier in the expiratory phase of ventilation resulting in air trapping and altered gas exchange (Sheahan & Musialowski, 2001). Mucociliary clearance in both upper and lower airways may be diminished (Hall, 1998). Coupled with the earlier airway compression, the older client is predisposed to lung infection.

The partial pressure of arterial oxygen (PaO2) also decreases with age due to the premature airway closure. According to Hall (1998) and Sheahan and Musialowski (2001), exercise capacity can be diminished as a result of decreased muscle mass, decreased cardiac function, and decreased level of conditioning that may occur in some older adults. A decrease in the function of lymphocytes and a decreased humoral response also predispose the older client to viral and bacterial infections (Hall, 1998).

Respiratory failure is a serious complication of COPD and could necessitate hospitalization, intubation, and mechanical ventilation. Patients with COPD are at an increased risk of developing respiratory failure since the inflammation and damage of the alveoli-capillary membrane is progressive. Respiratory failure is characterized as a failure of either oxygen exchange or carbon dioxide elimination. The clinical criteria of respiratory failure include a PaO_2 of less than 60 mmHg, PCO_2 of greater than 50 mmHg, or respiratory rate of greater than 30 breaths per min (Sharma, 2006). The complication of respiratory failure can be due to an acute insult (such as an infection), or progressive worsening of COPD (Weinberger, 1998).

TREATMENT

The goal of palliative care for patients with COPD is to promote QOL (Hardin et al., 2008). The principles that underlie the provision of palliative care include effective communication among providers, clients and their families, maintaining independence, and promoting psychosocial, spiritual, and emotional health (Hardin et al., 2008). Patient education is an important component of communication and may help clients adjust to their illness. Effective communication may assist clients with smoking cessation. Providers should educate clients about the causes of COPD as well as the progressive nature of the disease. Discussions about advanced directives and EOL care should be carried out throughout the early and late stages of the disease. Education about the nature of COPD, the course of the illness and advance directives has been shown to allay patients' anxiety (Knauft, Nielsen, Engelberg, Patrick, & Curtis, 2006).

Treatment Modalities for COPD: Management of Stable COPD

Palliative care for patients with COPD involves comprehensive care including both disease-directed treatment, promoting independence, and reducing symptoms. The treatment of patients often depends upon the stage of their diagnosis and their symptoms. In mild COPD, therapy is targeted toward prolonging life. In contrast, treatment of patients with very severe disease is aimed toward providing care, comfort, and helping patients and families cope with EOL decisions and issues.

Current treatment modalities for all patients with COPD include smoking cessation, prevention of infection, maximizing pulmonary function, and education (Gaine & Terry, 1997; Barnes, 2001; Witta, 1997). After the age of 65, smoking continues to be a major risk factor for death as well as a decreased QOL (Hall, 1998). Cessation of smoking is the most effective intervention to reduce the progression of COPD (GOLD, 2008). Smoking cessation in the older adult can improve their QOL, prevent the progression of COPD, and therefore, reduce the development of complications due to COPD (Hall, 1998). The risk for the development of influenza and pneumonia decreases as the result of smoking cessation in the older adult.

Counseling has been shown to be a very effective intervention to reduce smoking. The GOLD guidelines (2008) recommend that clients should receive counseling at every healthcare visit. Counseling can range from a brief, informal episode to longer, more structured interventions, however both are effective (Fiore et al., 2008a, 2008b). A recommended strategy for healthcare providers is to utilize at every visit the five A's approach (GOLD, 2008; Fiore et al., 2008a, 2008b).

1) Ask: Identify all smokers.
2) Advise: Advise smokers to quit smoking at every visit.
3) Assess: Assess a client's willingness to quit smoking.
4) Assist: Assist client to quit by encouraging use of counseling, and pharmacotherapies.
5) Arrange: Arrange for the client to receive follow-up care (adapted from the GOLD Guidelines, 2008).

A growing evidence base reveals that several therapies are effective in achieving and sustaining smoking cessation (Fiore et al., 2008a, 2008b). Guidelines advocate the use nicotine replacement therapies in the form of nicotine inhalers, lozenges, gum, nasal spray, and patches (Fiore et al., 2008a, 2008b). The goals of nicotine replacement therapy are to reduce the desire to smoke and to decrease the physical, psychological, and physiological signs and symptoms of nicotine withdrawal. In a systematic review (Stead, Perrara, Bullen, Mant, & Lancaster, 2008), all of the different nicotine replacement therapies increased the success of smoking cessation by 50%–70%. The most effective medical therapy to date is Verenicline, a partial agonist of nicotine receptors. Venernicline is thought to increase levels of dopamine in the brain and decrease satisfaction associated with smoking (Cahill, Stead, & Lancaster, 2009). A systematic review (Cahill et al.) found the use of Verenicline was 2–3 times more effective in achieving smoking cessation when compared with placebo and was superior to Bupropion in achieving abstinence from smoking at 24 weeks and 52 weeks. Side-effects associated with the use of Vernenicline include nausea, insomnia and bad dreams. Bupropion, an antidepressant thought to antagonize nicotinic receptors in the brain, has been found to be effective in increasing smoking cessation; a few studies have shown it to be superior to nicotine replacement therapies (Stead et al., 2008; Hughes, Stead, & Lancaster, 2007). The addition of nicotine replacement therapies (NRT) to Bupropion is more effective than nicotine replacement alone (Stead et al., 2008). Side effects associated with Bupropion include dry mouth, insomnia, and nausea. Seizures occur in 1 of 1000 patients treated with this medication. Additionally, all forms of nicotine replacement therapy have been successful in achieving smoking cessation. While each of the aforementioned therapies has been successful in achieving outcomes, the combination of counseling and medications greatly increases the rate of cessation (Fiore et al., 2008a, 2008b).

The prevention of infection is an important consideration in the older adult with COPD. Simple interventions, such as hand washing and avoidance of exposure to illness, can reduce the development of respiratory infections. Inoculation, in order to prevent the development of influenza and pneumonia, are also recommended to prevent disease exacerbation (Barnes, 2001).

Maximizing pulmonary function includes pharmacologic therapy, pulmonary rehabilitation, breathing retraining, and the prevention of malnutrition. Standard pharmacologic therapies include bronchodilators, steroids, and supplemental oxygen (Exhibit 14.2). If the older client has developed cor pulmonale or atrial arrythmias, pharmacologic therapy is directed toward reducing the adverse cardiovascular effects that occur.

EXHIBIT 14.2: PHARMACOLOGIC INTERVENTIONS FOR CHRONIC LUNG DISEASE

*Bronchodilators:	Routes:
Sympathomimetics	
Epinephrine	Inhaled, oral, parenteral
Isoproterenol	
Albuterol	
Xanthines	
Theophylline	Oral
Aminophylline	Parenteral
Anticholinergics	Parenteral
Ipratroprium	Inhaled
Supplemental O$_2$:	
Nasal cannula	Compressed gas, liquid, or concentrate
*Steroids:	
Corticosteroids	
Prednisone	Oral
Methylprednisolone	Parenteral
Beclomethasone	Inhaled

*Not an inclusive list of medications

Respiratory Pharmacologic Therapy of Stable COPD

Pharmacotherapeutic agents are recommended for the treatment of symptoms and prevention of acute exacerbations for clients with COPD. Bronchodilators are the cornerstone of therapy for patients with COPD (GOLD, 2008). They are associated with a reduction of dyspnea and an improvement in exercise capacity (Cayley, 2008). Bronchodilators can be administered via metered-dose inhalers, by nebulizer, or by oral administration. The bronchodilators most often prescribed for patients with COPD include beta agonists and anticholinergic agents. Beta-2 agonists stimulate the beta receptors in the lung and promote bronchodilation of the proximal airways and vasoconstriction of the pulmonary vessels. In mild cases of COPD, short-acting beta 2 agonists

(SABAs) are prescribed on an as-needed basis to reduce symptoms such as wheezing, shortness of breath, and chest tightness. As COPD increases in severity to moderate, and severe forms of the disease, long-acting beta 2 agonists (LABAs) are recommended. Long acting beta-2 agonists (LABAs) provide sustained bronchodilation with daily or twice daily dosing. Research suggests that long-acting beta 2 agonists may be associated with improved QOL, reduced symptoms, and a decreased in the frequency of acute exacerbations (GOLD, 2008).

Anticholinergic agents promote bronchodilation in patients with COPD and work by activating muscarinic receptors in the airways. Tiotropium, a long-acting anticholinergic agent, is recommended for daily use. A recent systematic review (Barr, Bourbeau, & Camago, 2008) compared ipratropium, administered twice daily, as a less selective agent with tiotropoium, an agent with greater selectivity. Tiotropium was shown to reduce exacerbations of COPD and reduce the number of hospitalizations (Barr et al., 2008). Patients with moderate to severe COPD, who were managed with tiotropium, had significant improvements in QOL , and reduction in symptom scores when compared with long-acting beta agonists (Barr et al., 2008).

As the severity of COPD increases, and patients are diagnosed with moderate to severe forms of the disease, the GOLD guidelines recommend the addition of an inhaled corticosteroid (2008). Inhaled corticosteroids have been shown to decrease the number and severity of exacerbations (Cayley, 2008; Yang, Fong, Sim, Black, & Lasserson, 2007). Additionally, treatment with inhaled corticosteroids is associated with an improvement in QOL despite the fact that therapy does not slow the decline of lung function (Yang et al., 2007). Adverse effects associated with inhaled corticosteroids include hoarseness and vocal cord myopathy. Rinsing after administration of the inhaled steroids helps to reduce the oropharyngeal complications. At this point, there is insufficient evidence to know whether systemic effects occur as a result of long term therapy.

Theophylline, as an example of a bronchodilator, can be an effective therapy in the setting of COPD. Theophylline can increase the strength and effectiveness of respiratory muscles and improves blood flow to the diaphragm (Gaine & Terry, 1997). However, changes in cardiac or liver function associated with aging can decrease the clearance of theophylline (Barnes, 2001). Cigarette smoking can also negatively influence the metabolism of theophylline.

Acute Exacerbations

Acute exacerbations may be triggered by both bacterial and viral infections. Infections may exacerbate inflammation, impairment of cilia, and hypersecretion of mucous goblet cells. Oral and intravenous steroids are administered to patients to treat acute exacerbations of chronic obstructive lung disease. The main advantage to glucocorticoid steroids is their anti-inflammatory effect.

Glucocorticoids decrease the inflammation associated with the exacerbation. Evidence (Wood-Baker, Gibson, Hannay, Walters, & Walters, 2007) revealed that the use of systemic glucocorticoids for acute exacerbations significantly decreased dyspnea, the risk of treatment failure, and decreased recurrent exacerbations within 30 days. There was a significant increase in the volume of expired air and an improvement in arterial blood gases within the first 72 h (Wood-Baker, Gibson, Hannay, Walters, & Walters). However, even short term use is associated with an increased incidence of adverse side effects including increased risk of infection. The most common side effects include hyperglycemia, weight gain, and insomnia. Nonsignificant increases in depression and anxiety were also noted. Long term complications include muscle breakdown, suppression of the hypothalamus-pituitary axis and osteoporosis. Treatment for acute exacerbations is usually short term to avoid complications associated with their use.

Oxygen therapy can decrease the potentially harmful effects on the pulmonary vasculature by hypoxemia. Oxygen is utilized during acute exacerbations (Brashers, 2002), to reduce the dyspnea associated with cor pulmonale (Marini & Wheeler, 1997), and in the long-term management of COPD (Barnes, 2001). Oxygen therapy is titrated to a PaO_2 of 55–60 mm Hg in order to avoid "turning off" the hypoxic drive in clients with COPD (Weinberger, 1998).

Small breaths and a decreased respiratory rate is a COPD client's response to exercise (Collins, Langbein, Fehr, & Maloney, 2001). As stated previously, the older adult will reduce their activity in order to reduce the occurrence of dyspnea. Pulmonary rehabilitation is focused on exercise and muscle reconditioning (Witta, 1997). Rehabilitation can take place in a community setting, as well as in the client's home. By increasing physical activity, muscle atrophy may be reduced and the efficiency of oxygen uptake will be improved (Collins et al., 2001).

Breathing retraining for clients with COPD includes the techniques of pursed-lip breathing and diaphragmatic/abdominal breathing (see Exhibit 14.3). Due to the pathophysiology of COPD, air becomes trapped in the terminal airways and adequate ventilation decreases. Lung changes associated with aging can result in air trapping without the presence of COPD (Sheahan & Musialowski, 2001). Pursed-lip breathing facilitates the expulsion of air from the lungs by the client controlling and lengthening the expiratory phase of respiration (Dunn, 2001; Collins et al., 2001).

Diaphragmatic/abdominal breathing serves a similar purpose as pursed-lip breathing. The client utilizes the diaphragmatic and abdominal muscles to control both inspiration and expiration (Dunn, 2001). Both techniques assist the client to reduce panic and anxiety associated with dyspneic episodes (Dunn, 2001). The older client can perform both of these exercises while seated comfortably in a chair. Utilizing a controlled-breathing technique can

---

EXHIBIT 14.3: BREATHING EXERCISES

Abdominal/Diaphragmatic	Pursed-Lip
■ Sit comfortably with feet on floor.	■ Breathe slowly through nose.
■ Press one hand to abdomen, rest the other hand on chest.	■ Hold your breath to a count of 3 seconds.
■ Inhale through nose slowly; use abdominal muscles.	■ Purse lips like you will be whistling; breathe out slowly through pursed lips.
■ Abdominal hand should rise with a count of 3 sec.	■ By exhaling through pursed lips, air is expelled from the lungs and breathing is slowed.
■ Hand on chest should stay still.	

From Sheahan, S.L., & Musialowski, R. (2001). Clinical implications of respiratory changes in aging. *Journal of Gerontological Nursing, 27*(5), 26–34.

---

improve ventilation at the alveolar-capillary membrane by the reduction of air trapped at the end of expiration.

Malnutrition negatively affects the pulmonary system (Witta, 1997; Gaine & Terry, 1997), as well as the immune system (Witta, 1997; Hall, 1998) in the older adult. Due to the physiologic changes associated with aging, immunity and pulmonary function can already be compromised (Sheahan & Musialowski, 2001). If an older adult is concurrently on diuretic therapy, losses of phosphorus and potassium can contribute to further muscle weakness (Gaine & Terry, 1997). Recommendations to improve nutrition include eating smaller, more frequent meals (Witta, 1997; Sommers & Johnson, 2002), increasing protein and calories (Witta, 1997; Berry & Baum, 2001; Collins et al., 2001; Sommers & Johnson, 2002), and limiting carbohydrates to 50% of the total caloric intake (Marini & Wheeler, 1997).

Administering bronchodilators prior to meals can also facilitate intake by decreasing dyspneic episodes. Oral care prior to meals can improve the eating experience for clients who mouth-breathe or have sputum production. Improving nutritional intake can increase lung response to hypoxemia, increase the lung response to hypercarbia, and maintain immune function (Witta, 1997), which can be decreased as a result of the physiologic changes associated with aging as well as the pathophysiologic process of COPD.

Education is incorporated in the care of the older client during each contact. Explanations should be given regarding smoking cessation, medication administration and potential side effects of these medications, breathing, retraining, and pulmonary rehabilitation, and if necessary, home oxygen therapy. Because significant others often function as caregivers in the home, they should be included in the education sessions.

Once the older adult is diagnosed with COPD, he or she and his/her significant other should be made aware of the prognosis (see Exhibit 14.4). Death generally occurs within 5 years of diagnosis of advanced disease (Weinberger, 1998). There is no cure for COPD

EXHIBIT 14.4: MEDICAL GUIDELINES FOR DETERMINING PROGNOSIS: PULMONARY DISEASE

Determining prognosis in end-stage lung disease is extremely difficult. There is marked variability in survival. Physician estimates of prognosis vary in accuracy, even in patients who appear end-stage. Even at the time of intubation and mechanical ventilation for respiratory failure from acute exacerbation of chronic obstructive pulmonary disease (COPD), 6-month survival cannot be predicted with certainty from simple data easily available to the clinician. Far less information than this is available to most hospice programs at the time of referral.

Patients who fit the following parameters can be expected to have the lowest survival rates. Although end stages of various forms of lung disease differ in some respects, most follow a final common pathway leading to progressive hypoxemia, cor pulmonale and recurrent infections. Thus, these guidelines refer to patients with many forms of advanced pulmonary disease. At the present time, it is uncertain what number or combination of these factors might predict 6-month mortality; clinical judgment is required.

I. Severity of chronic lung disease documented by:
   A. Disabling dyspnea at rest, poorly, or unresponsive to bronchodilators, resulting in decreased functional activity, e.g., bed-to-chair existence, often exacerbated by other debilitating symptoms such as fatigue and cough. Forced expiratory volume in one second (FEV1), after bronchodilator, less than 30% of predicted, is helpful supplemental objective evidence, but should not be required if not already available.
   B. Progressive pulmonary disease.
      1. Increasing visits to emergency department or hospitalizations for pulmonary infections and/or respiratory failure.
      2. Decrease in FEV1 on serial testing of greater than 40 ml per year is helpful supplemental objective evidence, but should not be required if not already available.
II. Presence of cor pulmonale or right heart failure (RHF).
   A. These should be due to advanced pulmonary disease, not primary or secondary to left heart disease or valvulopathy.
   B. Cor pulmonale may be documented by:
      1. Echocardiography.
      2. Electrocardiogram.
      3. Chest x-ray.
      4. Physical signs of RHF.

III. Hypoxemia at rest on supplemental oxygen.
   A. pO_2 less than or equal to 55 mm Hg on supplemental oxygen.
   B. Oxygen saturation less than or equal to 88% on supplemental oxygen.
IV. Hypercapnia.
   A. pCO_2 equal to or greater than 50 mm Hg.
V. Unintentional progressive weight loss of greater than 10% of body weight over the preceding 6 months.
VI. Resting tachycardia greater than 100/min in a patient with known severe chronic obstructive pulmonary disease.

Source: National Hospice Organization (1996). *Medical guidelines for determining prognosis in selected non-cancer diseases* (2nd ed.), Arlington, VA: National Hospice Organization.

(Witta, 1997), only treatment of symptoms, and prevention of complications and exacerbations. The endpoint of the disease is pulmonary hypertension and the development of cor pulmonale (Marini & Wheeler, 1997). All information regarding the diagnosis and prognosis should be delivered honestly to the elder client and significant others at their level of understanding (Meier, Morrison, & Ahronheim, 1998).

Once the diagnosis has been made, it is appropriate to begin discussions about advance directives. Discussion regarding advance directives should begin prior to the development of a life-threatening event (Meier et al., 1998). Predictors of a poor prognosis are listed in Exhibit 14.6. If a patient has two or more of these clinical signs, discussions regarding EOL care are necessary. Even though predicting the exact time of death is difficult, the client and significant others should be offered options in treatment. Information regarding palliative care can also be included in the treatment plan for clients with COPD (Meier et al., 1998).

Pain and Symptom Identification and Treatment

Symptom management is important in the palliative care of clients with COPD but does not alter the trajectory of the disease or the survival odds. Dyspnea and the resultant development of anxiety are commonly associated with end-stage COPD (Meier et al., 1998). Dyspnea may also be associated with cor pulmonale, which is a late sign and poor outcome indicator of COPD (Marini & Wheeler, 1997). However, in the older adult with COPD, dyspnea and complaints of breathlessness may be difficult to ascertain (Hall, 1998). Dyspnea is a subjective symptom of breathlessness, but the older adult may compensate for its development by decreasing their level of activity (Hall, 1998).

Once dyspnea has been diagnosed, the underlying cause needs to be identified. In the older adult with COPD, dyspnea can be the result of the disease process itself, the development of cor pulmonale, or a respiratory infection, such as pneumonia. Non-pharmacologic interventions for symptom relief of dyspnea include repositioning the client with their head up or to a position of comfort in a chair (LaDuke, 2001; Kazanowski, 2001). A cool environment can decrease the perception of dyspnea (Meier et al.; Kazanowski, 2001). Balancing rest and exercise as tolerated can also assist the client to breathe easier (LaDuke, 2001; Kazanowski, 2001). Frequent reassurance and providing a physical presence can assist in decreasing anxiety and therefore decrease dyspnea (Meier et al., 1998).

The pharmacologic interventions chosen to treat dyspnea depend upon the underlying etiology. Oxygen can be an initial adjunctive therapy for dyspnea (LaDuke, 2001; Kazanowski, 2001; Meier et al., 1998) and can be delivered via nasal cannula, face mask with cool mist, Bi-level positive airway pressure (BiPAP), or mechanical ventilation. Oxygen is the only therapy associated with increased survival (GOLD, 2008). The administration of oxygen has a number of salient effects including improvements in pulmonary hemodynamics, functional status and well-being (GOLD, 2008). Although BiPAP is used in the acute care setting to reverse respiratory failure, it may provide some relief from dyspnea (McGowan, 1998). BiPAP may also be desirable because it may be chosen as a less invasive alternative to mechanical ventilation (McGowan, 1998).

Opioids, such as morphine sulfate, can be administered to decrease the perception of dyspnea as well as decrease the sensation of dyspnea (Kazanowski, 2001; LaDuke, 2001; Meier et al., 1998). Morphine can be administered sublingually, orally, parenterally, and via nebulizer (see Exhibit 14.5). Anxiety is also reduced because of the mood-altering effects of morphine (LaDuke, 2001; Meier et al., 1998). Somnolence is the main side effect of morphine, however, no severe respiratory compromise is noted (Kazanowski, 2001). Steroids can be administered to the client with COPD to alleviate the inflammatory effects within the lungs (LaDuke, 2001; Kazanowski, 2001). Bronchodilators can also relieve the dyspnea associated with end-stage COPD (LaDuke, 2001; Kazanowski, 2001).

Dyspnea related to cor pulmonale may respond to the administration of diuretics. If the client has tenacious secretions associated with COPD or a respiratory infection, mucolytics may be administered (Kazanowski, 2001). If a respiratory infection, such as pneumonia, has been identified as the source of dyspnea (fever, congested cough), antibiotic therapy is appropriate (LaDuke, 2001; Kazanowski, 2001). Anxiolytics, such as benzodiazepines, barbiturates, and phenothiazines, may be prescribed to relieve the anxiety and fear associated with the feelings of breathlessness (LaDuke, 2001; Kazanowski, 2001; Meier et al., 1998).

EXHIBIT 14.5: PHARMACOLOGIC INTERVENTIONS FOR DYSPNEA

Opiates:
Morphine sulfate
   Nebulized (5 mg/2cc 0.9 NS q4h)
Parenteral (1–2 mg IV every 10–15 min; 2–5 mg SC initially)
   Orally or sublingually (5–10 mg, repeat as needed every 1 h prn)
   Rectally (10–20 mg every 4 h)

Anxiolytics:
Benzodiazepines
   Lorazepam (0.5 mg orally or sublingually every 4 h)
Phenothiazines
   Thorazine (25–100 mg orally tid or qid)

Diuretics:
Furosemide
   Administered orally, SC, IV, or IM for signs/symptoms of fluid volume excess
   20–80 mg orally (per dose)
   20–40 mg IV/IM (per dose)

From Kazanowski, M. K. (2001).

Depression and anxiety are common in patients with COPD and are related to the increased morbidity and mortality, declining functional status, decreased QOL and difficult breathing. The prevalence of anxiety ranges from 10%–96% of individuals (Putman-Casdorph & McCrone, 2008). Increases in anxiety are associated with increased difficulty breathing (Putman-Casdorph & McCrone, 2008).

The incidence of depression is higher in clients with COPD than in the general public (Putman-Casdorph & McCrone, 2008). In COPD, depression rates range from 20%–80% (Putman-Casdorph & McCrone, 2008). Individuals who are African American, elderly, and those of lower socioeconomic status, experience a disproportionate incidence of depression (Putman-Casdorph & McCrone.). Other studies reveal an increased incidence of depression in those patients younger than 55 years of age (Putman-Casdorph & McCrone). Depression in COPD interferes with the client's ability to participate in activities of daily living, pulmonary rehab and breathing exercises. Depression may also impede the individual's ability to quit smoking, which is an integral component of care.

Although limited, studies to date indicate that antidepressants and psychotherapy may reduce a client's feelings of depression (Putman-Casdorph & McCrone, 2008). Providers should encourage clients to discuss their feelings and proactively encourage communication throughout the continuum of care. Clients should be assessed for depression and offered both antidepressants and/or cognitive psychotherapy.

Many providers are unaware that pain is a common symptom in COPD (Hardin et al., 2008). Often pain occurs as a result of both anxiety and depression which are prevalent in this population. Due to the lack of knowledge, clients are not routinely assessed for pain, and their pain is often undertreated. Additionally, many providers are concerned that treating pain may depress the patient's respiratory drive, or hasten their deaths. Common misperceptions and lack of knowledge may prohibit treatment of both pain and depression.

Mechanical ventilation is an intervention, which involves the creation of an artificial airway in order to deliver oxygen. In the setting of end-stage COPD, it is not an option that offers many advantages. There is an increased risk of nosocomial infection in an already compromised host, such as the older adult with COPD (Philbeam, 1998). It is difficult to wean a client with COPD from the ventilator because of diaphragmatic muscle weakness and in the older adult, a decreased physiologic response to hypoxemia and hypercarbia (Phelan, Cooper, & Sangkachand, 2002). Mechanical ventilation also increases the risk of cardiac problems, aspiration, and barotrauma (Philbeam, 1998). All oxygen delivery options should be offered to the client and family, along with the risks and benefits associated with treatment. In the setting of palliative care, the least invasive and intrusive therapies will promote comfort (Meier et al., 1998).

PALLIATIVE CARE

Complementary Therapies

Complementary therapies, when incorporated into the practice of nursing, can increase the repertoire of interventions available to older adult clients (Frisch, 2002). For those clients who are receiving symptom relief at the EOL, complementary therapies can positively enhance what is already being done. Complementary therapies enable the nurse to create care that is client-centered and holistic (Frisch, 2002). There is increasing demand by consumers to receive care that is holistic, that takes into account the mind, body, and spirit (Kreitzer & Jensen, 2000). Complementary therapies are already available in the community. The use of complementary therapies can give clients and their families control over their care decisions (Kreitzer & Jensen, 2000); most complementary therapies can be utilized in the home. Examples of complementary therapies include guided imagery, relaxation, massage, and music therapy.

Rest is necessary in order to decrease the intensity of dyspnea and it can also decrease the work of breathing.

Promoting rest and sleep can also decrease anxiety. Assessment of the older adult's sleep habits can be a helpful starting point to the promotion of restful sleep (Tullmann & Dracup, 2000). Assisting the client into a position of comfort can promote sleep (Tullmann & Dracup, 2000), and in the case of the client with COPD, this generally means elevation of the head of the bed, which also facilitates diaphragmatic expansion.

Guided imagery is a technique that can be utilized to promote sleep in the client with COPD (Tusek & Cwynar, 2000). Guided imagery can also assist the client through a stressful experience (Tusek & Cwynar, 2000). The older adult can practice guided imagery with a partner or via audiotape. Clients focus on the present, and then are taken to a safe place in their mind.

Massage can also be explored as an option for sleep promotion (Richards, Gibson, & Overton-McCoy, 2000). Prior to initiating massage, the nurse must first determine that the elder is comfortable with being touched (Richards et al., 2000). In the client at the end-stage of COPD, there are no contraindications to massage being utilized for the promotion of rest and sleep.

Music can also be added to the therapeutic plan for the promotion of rest and sleep (Chlan, 2000; Richards, et al., 2000). Music therapy can be helpful in elders with COPD who tire easily, however, music should be selected to their personal preference (Chlan, 2000). Anxiety reduction can also be facilitated through the use of complementary therapies such as massage (Richards et al., 2000), guided imagery (Tusek & Cwynar, 2000) and music therapy (Chlan, 2000). Reducing anxiety can also result in the reduction of dyspnea in the client with COPD.

Clients or their significant others may ask the nurse about the utility of herbal remedies in the treatment of COPD. There are several herbs that are used in the treatment of respiratory ailments. Chaparral, cinnamon, horehound, and pansy have been used in the treatment of bronchitis although Chaparral can cause severe liver damage, and cinnamon can precipitate shortness of breath (Skidmore-Roth, 2001). Anise and astragalus have been used in the treatment of COPD. For general respiratory care and cough, lobelia and wild cherry have been used (Skidmore-Roth, 2001). Lobelia is contraindicated in a client who has congestive heart failure or dysrhythmias, and wild cherry is contraindicated in a client who has respiratory or cardiovascular depression (Skidmore-Roth, 2001). If the client is self-medicating with ginseng, tachycardia, and hypertension can result if they also ingest caffeinated beverages, such as coffee or tea (Kuhn, 2002). St. John's wart taken in combination with theophylline can decrease the serum level of theophylline, making it less effective as a bronchodilator (Kuhn, 2002). Theophylline should not be used concurrently with the herb guarana, as it also contains theophylline (Kuhn, 2002). The benefits of herbal interventions should be weighed against the harmful side effects that could exacerbate COPD or the complications of cor pulmonale and respiratory failure.

More research is needed regarding the benefits of complementary therapies in the treatment plan of end-stage COPD. These therapies include massage, to promote rest and sleep, music, to promote sleep and reduce anxiety, and the role that spirituality plays in fostering a positive attitude in the client and the maintenance of hope in family members. Palliative care of the older adult encompasses the physical, psychological, and social domains of care. Complementary therapies can be incorporated with other pharmacologic and nonpharmacologic modalities in the care of the older adult with end-stage of COPD.

Death of the Older Adult with COPD

The death of the elder client with COPD is commonly the result of respiratory failure (Weinberger, 1998). Prognostication guidelines for COPD are listed in Exhibit 14.6 (NHO, 1996). Respiratory failure can be due to the development of either hypoxemia or hypercapnia. The older adult may initially present with dyspnea, disorientation, or confusion. Vague symptoms such as tachypnea, tachycardia, and restlessness can occur. If respiratory failure is due to hypercapnia, the client may become stuporous or lapse into a coma (Weinberger, 1998). Cyanosis is a late sign of respiratory failure. Therapeutic interventions are based on the etiology of the respiratory failure. Supplemental oxygen may be delivered either noninvasively or via mechanical ventilation. Dyspneic symptoms are treated with opiates, bronchodilators, and anxiolytics.

EXHIBIT 14.6: PREDICTORS OF POOR PROGNOSIS IN PATIENTS WITH COPD

1) FEV1 < 30% of predicted.
2) Declining performance status, with increasing dependence on others for activities of daily living.
3) Uninterrupted walk distance limited to a few steps.
4) More than one urgent hospitalization within the past year.
5) Left-heart and/or other chronic comorbid dease.
6) Depression/anxiety.
7) BMI < 21 kg/m^2.
8) Poor QOL per patient.
9) Long-term oxygen therapy.
10) Intolerable dyspnea.
11) BODE Index score > 7.

From Hardin, K. A., Meyers, F., & Louis, S. (2008). Integrating palliative care in severe chronic obstructive lung disease. *COPD: Journal of Chronic Obstructive Pulmonary Disease, 5,* 207–220.

In order to support the family through the death of their loved one, an honest discussion about the dying process needs to occur (Meier et al., 1998). Dyspnea is a symptom, which is seen during the dying process of a client with COPD. Family members can panic when these dyspneic episodes occur (Tarzian, 2000). Due to the fact that the elder has no control over his or her breathlessness (Tarzian, 2000), management of dyspneic episodes can decrease the sense of panic and increase his/her sense of control.

Case Study conclusions:

Mr. H.
Upon diagnosis, Mr. H. was educated about COPD, the progressive nature of the disease, and the variable course of illness. At that time, Mr. H. expressed a need to focus on disease-directed therapy and life-sustaining treatments. The multidisciplinary team emphasized improvements in QOL. He was started on nicotine replacement therapy, and successfully stopped smoking two years ago. A Tiotropium inhaler was initiated and he reports decreased symptoms of SOB with exertion. Mr. H. now visits with his minister twice a month and enjoys their regular discussions. The multidisciplinary team has continued to work with Mr. H. to address his emotional, physical, psychosocial and spiritual needs. Recently, Mr. H. decided against cardiopulmonary resuscitation and intubation in the future and signed an advance directive.

Mrs. S.
The EOL discussions were initiated approximately 2 years ago when Mrs. S. started on home oxygen. Mrs. S. determined that she did not want intubation or cardiopulmonary resuscitation. An advanced directive was signed at that time. Recently, Mrs. S. developed increased episodes of lethargy, confusion, and dyspnea. Morphine was added to her treatment regimen to ease her breathing. Mrs. S. died at home with her family in attendance 4 months after entering the hospice program.

CONCLUSION

COPD is the fourth leading cause of death in the US and it is the leading cause of death due to a respiratory cause; development of this disease occurs as the result of cigarette smoking and exposure to environmental pollution. These factors place older clients at particular risk for developing COPD because they have been exposed to smoking and pollution for an extended period of time. In addition to this, the normal physiologic changes due to the aging process places the older adult at increased risk for the development of complications, such as cor pulmonale and pneumonia. In order to reduce the risk of developing the complications of COPD, smoking cessation is recommended to the older adult. Pharmacologic modalities focus on improving ventilation, reducing inflammation, and preventing complications. Non-pharmacologic interventions including exercise, rest, and improved nutrition can be valuable adjunctive therapies in the care of elder patients with COPD.

Palliative care, integrated throughout the continuum of the disease from diagnosis to EOL, may help to provide comprehensive care that improves QOL, reduces symptoms and eases suffering for both patients experiencing COPD and their family members.

EVIDENCE-BASED PRACTICE

Epstein, C. D., El-Mokadem, N., & Peerless, J. R. (2002). Weaning older patients from long-term mechanical ventilation: A pilot study. *American Journal of Critical Care, 11*(4), 369–377.

Research problem. Accuracy is needed to determine the readiness for weaning from ventilatory support. A description of temporal changes in pulmonary and systemic variables in older adults was being sought. This is a descriptive study of weaning from long-term (3 or more days) ventilation. The purpose of the study was to determine whether there are differences between patients who can be weaned and those who cannot be weaned.

Sample, setting, and methods. The setting was a 750-bed level-one trauma center in Cleveland, Ohio. The study participants were admitted to the surgical intensive care unit (SICU) and were aged 60 yrs. or older. The mean age of the participants was 72.6 years.; sample size was 10 participants. Selection was based on convenience sampling. Each patient was monitored for weaning progress. The attending physician determined weaning initiation. The study investigators defined active weaning a priori as progress in ventilatory weaning by changes in ventilator mode or decreases in rate, oxygen level, and pressure support. Patients were monitored daily until successfully weaned, remained extubated for 24 hours, or up to 14 days. The instrument utilized to assess readiness for weaning was the Burns Weaning Assessment Program (BWAP), a 26-item checklist. Oxygen cost of breathing was measured by metabolic monitoring prior to and after each ventilator change. Multidimensional variables were also collected daily for each participant. Patient differences in weaning were compared by the Mann-Whitney and Wilcoxin signed

rank tests. Six participants were successfully weaned. The mean age of those successfully weaned was 70 years; for those not successfully weaned, the mean age was 76 years.

Implications for nursing practice. Age can prolong the weaning process due to the normal physiological changes in the pulmonary system. Older patients, due to age-related changes in physiology, may not be able to correct acid-base imbalances, excrete sedatives and opiates, etc. Nurses can utilize this information to provide interventions to optimize all factors that can promote weaning from mechanical ventilation. Because chronic lung disease can prolong a patient's time being mechanically ventilated, this information can improve care for this population group.

Conclusion. Further research is needed in the older adult population. The sample size was small (10 participants) and this limits generalization to other populations. Through further studies with older adults, weaning strategies can be tailored for this population.

REFERENCES

American Lung Association. (2009). *Fact sheet: Chronic obstructive pulmonary disease* (COPD). [On-line]. Available: lungusa. org/diseases/copd_factsheet_html

Barnes, P. J. (2001). Modern management of COPD in the elderly. *The Annals of Long-Term Care, 9*(5), 51–56.

Barr, R. G., Bourbeau, J., & Camargo, C. A. (2008). Tiotropium for stable chronic obstructive pulmonary disease. *The Cochrane Collaboration, 4,* 1–78.

Berry, J. K., & Baum, C. L. (2001). Malnutrition in chronic obstructive pulmonary disease: Adding insult to injury. *AACN Clinical Issues. Advanced Practice in Acute and Critical Care, 12*(2), 210–219.

Brashers, V. L. (Ed.). (2002). Chronic obstructive pulmonary disease. *Clinical applications of pathophysiology: Assessment, diagnostic reasoning and management.* St. Louis, MO: Mosby.

Cahill, K., Stead, L. F., & Lancaster, T., (2009). Nicotine receptor partial agonists for smoking cessation. *Cochrane Database of Systematic Reviews,* 1, 1–59.

Cayley, W. E. (2008). Use of inhaled corticosteroids to treat stable copd. *American Family Physician, 77*(11), 1532–1533.

Chlan, L. L. (2000). Music therapy as a nursing intervention for patients supported by mechanical ventilation. *AACN Clinical Issues. Advanced Practice in Acute and Critical Care, 11*(1), 128–138.

Collins, E. G., Langbein, W. E., Fehr, L., & Maloney, C. (2001). Breathing pattern retraining and exercise in persons with chronic obstructive pulmonary disease. *AACN Clinical Issues. Advanced Practice in Acute and Critical Care, 12*(2), 202–209.

Curtis, J. R. (2008). Palliative and end-of-life care for patients with severe COPD. *European Respiratory Journal, 32,* 796–803

Dunn, N. A. (2001). Keeping COPD patients out of the ED. *Registered Nurses, 64*(2), 33–38.

Fiore, M. C., Jaen, C. R., Baker, T. B., Bailey, W. C., Benowitz, M., & Curry, S. J. et al. (2008a). A clinical practice guideline for treating tobacco use and dependence: 2008 update. *American Journal of Preventive Medicine, 35*(2), 158–176.

Fiore, M. C., Jaen, C. R., Baker, T. B., Bailey, W. C., Benowitz, M., & Curry, S. J. et al. (2008b). Treating tobacco use and dependence: 2008 update. Clinical practice guideline. Executive Summary. *Respiratory Care, 53*(9), 1217–1222.

Frisch, N. C. (2002). *Nursing as a context for alternative/complementary modalities.*[On-line]. Available: nsgworld.org/ojin/topic 15/tpc15_2.htm

Gaine, S. P., & Terry, P. (1997). Treatment modalities for COPD in the institutionalized elderly. *The Annals of Long-Term Care, 5*(11), 390–397.

Global Initiative for Chronic Obstructive Lung Disease. (2009, January). *Global Strategy for the Diagnosis, Management and Prevention of Chronic Obstructive Pulmonary Disease.* Retrieved February 1, 2009 from: http://www.goldcopd.com/GuidelinesResources.asp Hall, W. J. (1998). Pulmonary disorders. In E. H. Duthrie & P. R. Katz (Eds.), *Practice of geriatrics* (pp. 494–504). Philadelphia, PA: W. B. Saunders Co.

Hardin, K. A., Meyers, F., & Louis, S. (2008). Integrating palliative care in severe chronic obstructive lung disease. *COPD: Journal of Chronic Obstructive Pulmonary Disease, 5,* 207–220.

Hughes, J. R., Stead, L. F., & Lancaster, T. (2007). Antidepressants for smoking cessation. *Cochrane Database of Systematic Reviews,*1, 1–106.

Kazanowski, M. K. (2001). Symptom management in palliative care. In M. L. Matzo & D. W. Sherman (Eds.), *Palliative care nursing: Quality care to the end of life* (pp. 327–361). New York, NY: Springer Publishing Co.

Knauft, E., Nielsen, E., Engelberg, R., Patrick, D., & Curtis, J. R., (2005). Barriers and facilitators to end-of-life care communication for patients with COPD. *Chest, 127,* 2188–2196.

Kreitzer, M. J., & Jensen, D. (2000). Healing practices: Trends, challenges, and opportunities for nurses in acute and critical care. *AACN Clinical Issues. Advanced Practice in Acute and Critical Care, 11*(1), 7–16.

Kuhn, M. A. (2002). Herbal remedies: Drug-herb interactions. *Critical Care Nurse, 22*(2), 22–28, 30.

LaDuke, S. (2001). Terminal dyspnea and palliative care. *American Jounal of Nursing, 101*(11), 26–31.

Marini, J. J., & Wheeler, A. P. (Eds.). (1997). *Critical care medicine: The essentials.* Baltimore, MD: Williams & Wilkins.

Manaker, S., & Burke, F. (1999). Pulmonary disease. In G. Morrison and L. Hark (Eds.), *Medical nutrition & disease* (pp. 268–275). Malden, MA: Blackwell Science, Inc.

McGowan, C. M. (1998). Noninvasive ventilatory support: Use of bi-level positive airway pressure in respiratory failure. *Critical Care Nurse, 18*(6), 47–53.

Meier, D. E., Morrison, R. S., & Ahronheim, J. C. (1998). Palliative care. In E. H. Duthrie & P. R. Katz (Eds.), *Practice of geriatrics* (pp. 99–111). Philadelphia, PA: W. B. Saunders Co.

National Hospice Organization. (1996). *Medical guidelines for determining prognosis in selected non-cancer diseases* (2nd ed.). Arlington, VA: National Hospice Organization.

National Consensus Project for Quality Palliative Care. (2009). *Clinical practice guidelines for quality palliative care.* National Consensus Project: Pittsburgh retrieved from http://www.nationalconsensusproject.org/guideline.pdf

Phelan, B. A., Cooper, D. A., & Sangkachand, P. (2002). Prolonged mechanical ventilation and tracheostomy in the elderly. *AACN Clinical Issues. Advanced Practice in Acute and Critical Care, 13*(1), 84–93.

Philbeam, S. P. (Ed.). (1998). Mechanical ventilation. *Physiology and clinical applications.* St. Louis, MO: Mosby.

Putman-Casdorph, H., & McCrone, S. (2009). Chronic obstructive pulmonary disease, anxiety and depression: State of the science. *Heart and Lung, 38*(1), 34–47.

Richards, K. C., Gibson, R., & Overton-McCoy, A. L. (2000). Effects of massage in acute and critical care. *AACN Clinical Issues. Advanced Practice in Acute and Critical Care, 11*(1), 77–96.

Sethi, S., & Murphy, T. F. (2008). Infection in the pathogenesis and course of chronic obstructive pulmonary disease. *The New England Journal of Medicine, 359,* 2355–2365.

Sharma, S., (2006). Respiratory failure. *E-Medicine.* Retrieved Febuary 2, 2009, from http://emedicine.medscape.com/article/167981-print

Sheahan, S. L., & Musialowski, R. (2001). Clinical implications of respiratory system changes in aging. *Journal of Gerontological Nursing, 27*(5), 26–34.

Skidmore-Roth, L. (Ed.). (2001). *Handbook of herbs and natural supplements.* St. Louis, MO: Mosby.

Sommers, M. S., & Johnson, S. A. (Eds.). (2002). *Diseases and disorders: A nursing therapeutics manual.* Philadelphia, PA: F. A. Davis Co.

Stead, L. F., Perrara, R., Bullen, C., Mant, D., & Lancaster, T. (2008). Nicotine replacement therapy for smoking cessation (Review). *Cochrane Database of Systematic Reviews,* 1, 1–221

Tarzian, A. J. (2000). Caring for dying patients who have air hunger. *Journal of Nursing Scholarship, 32*(2), 137–143

Tullmann, D. F., & Dracup, K. (2000). Creating a healing environment for elders. *AACN Clinical Issues. Advanced Practice in Acute and Critical Care, 11*(1), 34–50.

Tusek, D. L., & Cwynar, R. E. (2000). Strategies for implementing a guided imagery program to enhance patient experience. *AACN Clinical Issues. Advanced Practice in Acute and Critical Care, 11*(1), 68–76.

Weinberger, S. E. (1998). *Principles of pulmonary medicine.* Philadelphia, PA: W. B. Saunders Co.

Witta, K. M. (1997). COPD in the elderly. Controlling symptoms and improving quality of life. *Advance for Nurse Practitioners, 5*(7), 18–20, 22–23, 27, 72.

Wood-Baker, R. R., Gibson, P. G., Hannay, M., Walters, E. H., & Walters, J. A. E. (2008). Systematic corticosteroids for acute exacerbations of chronic obstructive pulmonary disease. *The Cochrane Database of Systematic Reviews,*(1), 1–63.

Yang, I. A., Fong, K., Sim, E. A., Black, P. N., & Lasserson (2007). Inhaled corticosterids for stable chronic obstructive pulmonary disease. *Cochrane Database of Systematic Review,* 2, 1–191.

Yohannes, A. M., (2007). Palliative care provision for patients with chronic obstructive pulmonary disease. *Health and Quality of Life Outcomes, 5*(17), 1–6. Retrieved from http://www.hqlo.com/content/5/1/17.

15

Neurological Disorders

Christine R. Kovach
Sheila Reynolds

Key Points

- Patients and families who are dealing with the consequences of severe stroke or a chronic and progressive neurological disease face multiple burdens and these burdens can be lessened through palliative care.
- Patients with severe stroke or chronic neurological disorders display great heterogeneity in symptoms and trajectory of illness.
- Common problems faced by many patients with these disorders include impairments in cognition, communication, sleep, swallowing, and mobility as well as dyspnea, pain, and depression.

Case Study: Mrs. Cohen is an 84-year-old woman in the late stages of Alzheimer's disease. Her dementia has severely impaired her short- and long-term memory as well as her functional ability. She lives in a nursing home and spends most of her day in her bed repetitively grunting and tapping the sides of the bedrails. She verbalizes few intelligible words, continually picks at her clothes, grimaces, and rocks her body. When approached she yells, and when bathed she screams and exhibits aggressive behavior. Attempts to bring her to the dining room or to therapeutic activities are met with resistance and screaming. Staff has responded by leaving her alone in the room, providing stimulation by keeping the TV on in her room, and hanging a mobile of flowers in her line of vision.

Introduction

This chapter will focus on management of people with severe stroke, chronic neurological disorders (CNDs), coma and brain death. Severe stroke and CNDs, while unique and individualized in many respects, share a cluster of common symptoms and treatment needs. While some people who suffer a stroke recover completely or nearly completely from the event, people with CND often exhibit unresponsiveness or only slight or temporary responsiveness to curative treatments. Symptoms associated with severe stroke and CND are amenable to palliative treatment, and a growing body of evidence supports that quality of life is increased from an array of palliative care interventions.

This chapter presents a description of common symptoms experienced from stroke and CNDs including Alzheimer's disease (AD) and related disorders, Parkinson's disease (PD), multiple sclerosis (MS), and amyotrophic lateral sclerosis (ALS). Co-morbid conditions that frequently accompany the latter stages of these illnesses are described, as well as interventions aimed to provide symptom management. Due to the unique assessment and management issues that accompany pediatric neurodegenerative disorders, coma, and brain death, these problems and their management are presented in separate sections of the chapter. All disorders discussed in this chapter except multiple sclerosis and specific pediatric disorders are more likely to occur in older adulthood, and therefore gerontological issues are incorporated throughout the chapter.

PREVALENCE, DISEASE TRAJECTORY, AND PATHOGENESIS

Stroke

Stroke is the third leading cause of death and the leading cause of severe long-term disability in the United States. It is estimated that each year 780,000 people will experience either a new or recurrent stroke. Eighty seven percent of strokes are ischemic and 10% are hemorrhagic (Rosamond et al., 1999). Stroke incidence rate is higher in men than women at younger ages; however, this pattern switches at the older ages. Stroke in children is highest under the age of 1 year (Hirtz et al., 2007). Overall incidence of stroke in children under the age of 15 years is 6.4/100,000 (Kleindorfer et al., 2006). Deaths from stroke fell 24.2% from the year 1994 to 2004. As a result, there is an increased number of people surviving, and currently there are an estimated 5.8 million stroke survivors in the United States (Rosamond et al., 1999). Stroke accounted for approximately 150,000 deaths in United States in 2004 (Rosamond et al., 1999).

The term "stroke" refers to the sudden onset of a focal or global neurological deficit that lasts longer than 24-hours and is caused by disrupted cerebral vascular circulation. Signs of impairment may be perceptual, motor, and cognitive or speech related. Risk factors include hypertension, heart disease, hyperlipemia, diabetes, obesity, physical inactivity, family history, and tobacco and alcohol abuse (American Heart Association, 2008b). There are two types of stroke: ischemic and hemorrhagic. Both result in injury to the brain tissue, but the mechanism involved is different. In ischemic stroke, there is decreased or absent circulation to an area of the brain due to an occlusion of a cerebral artery. Majority of occlusions occur from the formation of a thrombus or emboli (Book, 2007). In a thrombic event, atherosclerotic blood vessels cause complete or partial blockage of blood flow to a local area in the brain; whereas in an embolic event, a clot forms elsewhere in the body, such as in the heart, breaks off and travels through the arterial system and lodges in a cerebral vessel blocking blood flow. Atherosclerotic plaques tend to occur at the arterial bifurcations. Common sites for plaques formation include the internal carotid and vertebral arteries and the junctions of the basilar and vertebral arteries (Book, 2007).

In contrast to an ischemic stroke, a hemorrhagic stroke is the result of a ruptured intracerebral vessel. Ruptured intracerebral vessels occur as a result of hypertension, aneurysm, trauma, erosion of vessels by tumors, arteriovenous malformations, blood coagulation disorders, vasculitis, or from drugs. The bleeding that occurs within the brain tissue causes increased pressure within the skull, resulting in brain cell death.

Hemorrhagic stroke can progress rapidly resulting in coma and frequently death (Book, 2007).

The effects from an acute stroke are dependent upon the extent of the brain damaged and where in the brain the stroke occurred. Each stroke patient is unique in presentation. The greater the initial damage, the longer and more difficult the recovery. Abilities that can be affected by a stroke are memory, motor function, and speech. After a stroke, neurologic function begins to improve within a few days, with the majority of recovery occurring within the first 3 months. Neurologic and functional gains will continue over 6–12 months, however more slowly, with minimal gains seen beyond 1–2 years (Hankey, 2005). The National Heart, Lung, and Blood Institute's Framingham Heart Study reported that among stroke survivors 65 years of age or older at 6 months after discharge, 50% had some hemiparesis, 35% were depressed, 30% were unable to walk without assistance, 26% were dependent in activities of daily living (ADL), 26% were institutionalized in a nursing home, and 19% were aphasic (Kelly-Hayes, 2003). The median survival time for first time stroke is 6.8 years for men and 7.4 for women aged 60–69 years, 5.4 years for men and 6.4 years for women aged 70–79 years, and 1.8 years for men and 3.1 years for women 80 years and older (American Heart Association, 2008a).

Chronic Neurological Disorders

Alzheimer's disease is the sixth leading cause of death in United States, accounting for 72,914 deaths in the year 2006 (Heron, Hoyert, Xu, Scott, & Tejada-Vera, 2006). Approximately 5.2 million people of all ages are living in United States with Alzheimer's disease and this number is expected to increase as the population ages (Alzheimer's Association, 2008) There are more women than men with Alzheimer's disease because women tend to live longer and the greatest risk factor for Alzheimer's disease is advancing age (Alzheimer's Association, 2008). It is estimated that dementia of the Alzheimer's type affects over 13% of adults over the age 65 or 1 out of 8 people (Alzheimer's Association, 2008). Experts predict that by 2010 there will be almost a half million new cases of Alzheimer's disease each year; and by 2050, there will be almost a million new cases each year (Herbert, Beckett, Sherr, & Evans, 2001).

The cause of AD remains unclear. Cortical atrophy and loss of neurons are typically found in patients with AD. Researchers have found a link between ventricle dilatation, brain volume, and the degree of cognitive impairment and Alzheimer disease (Nestor, 2008). Beta-amyloid containing neuritic plaques and neurofibrillary tangles are the hallmark microscopic feature of AD (Book, 2007). Neuritic plaques occur as a result of an abnormal clumping of the ß-amyloid protein. The ß-amyloid protein breaks down into

toxic fragments, which accumulate in the brain and is thought to be responsible for the cascade of events that lead to neuronal dysfunction and death (Yaari & Corey-Bloom, 2007). The other hallmark, the neurofibrillary tangles, forms when a different protein called "tau" twist around each other in a helical fashion inside of abnormal neurons. The neurofibrillary tangle development causes disruption inside the neuron and later neuronal death (Yaari & Corey-Bloom, 2007). Neuritic plaques and neurofibrillary tangles are found in the hippocampus and amygdale areas. The hippocampus area controls information processing, acquisition of new memories, and retrieval of old memories (Book, 2007). Other pathological abnormalities found in Alzheimer brain tissue include inflammation, oxidative damage, and a decrease level of choline acetyltransferase responsible for synthesis of acetylcholine, a neurotransmitter involved with memory (U.S. Department of Health and Human Services, 2005).

People with Alzheimer's disease die on average of 4–6 years after diagnosis; however, the disease can last for as many as 20 years (Larson, 2004). The progression of the disease and rate of decline vary from person to person. Initially, people experience problems with memory that progress to confusion, disorganized thinking, impaired judgment, trouble expressing themselves, and disorientation as to time, space, and location (Alzheimer's Association, 2008). As the disease progresses to the advanced stages, functional abilities deteriorate and people become dependent for ADL (i.e., bathing, feeding, and toileting). In the final stage of the disease, impairment is considerable. People lose their ability to communicate, respond to the environment, walk, and swallow, and become bed-bound or chair-bound (Alzheimer's Association, 2008).

Parkinson's disease (PD) affects approximately 1.5 million people in United States, with about 60,000 new cases appearing each year (Dorsey et al., 2007). These figures are projected to grow as the age of the population increases. The average age of onset of Parkinson's disease is 60 years; however, up to 15% of people are diagnosed under the age of 50 (Fact Sheet, 2008). Men are affected more often than women (Hirtz et al., 2007).

Like AD, the exact cause of PD is not known. The hallmark features found in PD are the loss of pigmented dopaminergic neurons in the substantia nigra and the presence of Lewy bodies. Current research says PD is multifactorial and involves the complex interplay between genetic and environmental factors (Siderowf, 2007). PD develops when brain cells in the substantia nigra begin to degenerate and die (Parkinson's Disease Foundation, 2008). This structure makes and stores dopamine; the degenerative process results in depletion of the neurotransmitter, dopamine. The loss of dopamine alters the balanced functioning of neurotransmitters in the basal ganglia and creates the classic triad of motor symptoms: bradykinesia (i.e., slow movement), rigidity, and tremor. Other areas of the brain can be involved, causing the non-motor complications such as depression (frontal lobe mediated by serotonin), memory loss temporo-hippocampal mediated by acetylcholine), dysexecutive function (frontal lobe), dysautonomia, dysphagia, and sleep problems (brain stem) (Chan, 2008).

The course of PD spans years to decades, which can result in a reduced life expectancy. PD has become the 14th leading cause of death in the United States (Liao, 2007). Currently, there are no curative treatments; however, treatments can markedly reduce symptoms and slow the progression of Parkinson's (Liao, 2007). The progression of PD symptoms manifests differently from person to person. In some people, the disease progresses more quickly and in others it may take 20 years or more (National Institute of Neurological Disorders and Stroke, 2008c). Symptoms usually begin on one side of the body, and eventually progress to both sides body, causing balance problems and severe disability. In the late stage of PD, people are bedbound and are commonly afflicted by complications such as choking, pneumonia, and falls that can be the contributing factor leading to death (National Institute of Neurological Disorders and Stroke, 2008c).

Multiple sclerosis (MS) affects approximately 400,000 people in the United States with 200 newly diagnosed every week (National Multiple Sclerosis Society, 2008). Multiple sclerosis occurs at younger ages than the other neurodegenerative diseases discussed, with onset commonly occurring between the ages of 20 and 50 years. Women are more commonly affected than men (Richert, 1999).

MS is thought to be caused by a disturbance in the function of the immune system of genetically susceptible people (Porth, 2007). Unknown triggers stimulate an immune-mediated inflammatory response that causes demyelination and scarring (gliosis) of nerves. This scar tissue forms hard sclerotic plaques in multiple regions of the central nervous system (CNS). Early in the illness, the myelin sheath is affected but the nerve fiber is not affected and nerve impulses are still transmitted. As the damage to nerves progresses, and nerve axons become destroyed and nerve impulses are totally blocked, resulting in permanent loss of function (Porth, 2007).

MS is an unpredictable disease of the CNS that has the most variable disease trajectory. There are four main patterns to the presentation of MS. Relapsing-remitting is the most common form of MS and is characterized by flare-ups that appear for several days to weeks followed by remissions during which not all symptoms resolve completely. Primary-progressive is a less common form, in which the disease manifestations gradually worsen overtime without periods of remission. Secondary-progressive is the relapsing-remitting form with relapses that are more severe and occur on top of a continuous deterioration pattern. Progressive-

relapsing is an uncommon form MS where the person will have sudden acute episodes of new symptoms or worsening of existing ones (National Institute of Neurological Disorders and Stroke, 2008b). Most people with MS have a normal life expectancy. However, a rare form of the illness can be fatal within weeks. The average life span with MS is 20–40 years after the onset of symptoms (Liao, 2007).

Amyotrophic lateral sclerosis (ALS) or Lou Gehrig disease is a rare but a progressive neurodegenerative disease that typically occurs between the ages of 40 and 60 and affects more men than women (ALS Association, 2004). Death often occurs within a few years after diagnosis. However, 10% can live more than 10 years (National Institute of Neurological Disorders and Stroke, 2008a). The yearly incidence rate is approximately 2 cases per 100,000 individuals. Roughly, 30,000 Americans are living with ALS at any given time (ALS Association, 2004; Logroscino, 2007).

The etiology and pathogenesis of ALS remains unclear and multifactorial. However, 5–10% of the cases are familial, with 20% of those resulting from a mutation of the superoxide dismutase 1 (SOD1) gene (Porth, 2007). ALS progressively affects the upper motor neuron of the cerebral cortex and the lower motor neurons of the anterior horn cells of the spinal cord and motor nuclei of the brain stem resulting in progressive muscle weakness and wasting (Porth, 2007). ALS is selective within the motor system, sparing ocular movements, such as blinking, and the bowel and bladder function. Intellectual and sensory functions are rarely affected (Dangond, 2006). ALS affects both the upper and lower motor neurons (Swierzewski, 2000). Although the early symptoms can vary from person to person, the disease always starts off with muscle weakness. The muscle weakness progresses to muscle wasting and paralysis of the limbs and trunk. Eventually, in the more advanced stage of the disease, muscles that control vital functions are impaired, causing speech, swallowing, and breathing difficulties. Respiratory failure is the cause of most deaths (ALS Association, 2004).

Pediatric Neurodegenerative Disorders

The neurodegenerative disorders of childhood are a diverse group of very rare diseases that are most often fatal. These diseases can result from genetic problems, biochemical defects, viral infections, or toxic substances. Symptoms include a progressive loss of speech, hearing, vision, and strength as well as seizures, feeding difficulties, and cognitive deficits. The genetic neurodegenerative disorders are grouped into four categories: sphingolipidoses, neuronal ceroid lipofuscinoses, adrenoleukodystrophy, and sialidosis. These may be distinguished from one another based on head computerized tomography (CT), head magnetic resonance imaging

(MRI), nerve conduction velocities, visual evoked potentials, auditory evoked potentials, and electroretinography. Skin, conjunctival, and nerve biopsies as well as DNA tests and specific enzyme assays and cultures may also be used to diagnose the condition. While treatment success is uncommon, bone marrow transplant has been successful in treating ceroid lipofuscinoses. Transplanting myelin-producing cells to treat some of these disorders is being studied, and stem cell research is also discussed for these disorders (Green, 2008; Lukong, et al., 2000; Santavuori et al., 2000).

Coma

To date, valid estimates of the incidence and prevalence of severe disorders of consciousness are not available (Giacino et al., 2002). The state of arousal and wakefulness is dependent upon functioning cerebral hemispheres and the brain stem's regulatory system called the reticular activating system (RAS) (Book, 2007). The RAS is located at the core of the brain stem. Damage to the either the RAS area or both cerebral hemispheres will result in an altered level of consciousness or coma. Coma etiology can be classified into one of three main categories: supratentorial lesions, infratentorial lesions, and metabolic encephalopathy (Davis, 2005). Supratentorial caused coma results from the formation of a mass (i.e., brain tumor, stroke, head trauma with brain swelling, brain abscess) that expands producing brain herniation through the tentorial opening into the tentorial compartment causing fatal brainstem hemorrhages and ischemia (Davis, 2005). Infratentorial type coma occurs when a tumor or ischemic stroke involving the brainstem or cerebellum damages or compresses the reticular formation. Metabolic encephalopathy-type coma results from a variety of sources that affect the brain chemistry (i.e., drugs, hypoxia, blood glucose abnormalities, organ diseases, vitamin B deficiencies, poor cerebral perfusion, toxins, etc). Metabolic coma develops acutely and is often reversible if the underlying disorder is treated (Davis, 2005). Many comatose patients progress to being brain-dead. Unfortunately, to date there is a wide variation in brain death guidelines (Greer, 2008). Brain death is defined as the irreversible loss of function of the brain, including the brainstem (American Academy of Neurology, 1994).

Coma is the result of injury to the brain and is characterized as a deep state of unconsciousness in which a person cannot be awakened and does not purposefully respond to stimuli (National Institute of Neurological Disorders and Stroke, 2007). Those in the deepest coma are not conscious of self or their environment; they show no sleep wake cycles, no auditory or visual responses and have reflex and postural responses only to external stimuli (Giacino et al., 2002). The differential diagnosis for coma includes a structural lesion (stroke, head trauma, tumor), meningeal irritation (infection or bleeding),

metabolic encephalopathy (organ failure, drugs), and seizure (Simon, 2000). Getting a history from witnesses or significant others is helpful in making a differential diagnosis. If the coma was preceded by a period of confusion or delirium, this is more consistent with infection or metabolic etiologies, whereas sudden loss of consciousness suggests an intracranial bleed or infarct.

Some of the causes are treatable and reversible but others are not. The prognosis depends upon the cause, the severity of damage, and site of neurological damage (National Institute of Neurological Disorders and Stroke, 2007). A coma usually lasts only a few days to a few weeks, and it is rare that a coma would last more than 2–4 weeks. However, some comas can last for years (National Institute of Neurological Disorders and Stroke, 2007). Determining prognosis is dependent upon the underlying cause of the coma. Poor prognostic signs are when the coma follows cardiac arrest or if the patient has not regained pupillary function or purposeful movement after 72 hours. Coma, due to traumatic head injury, has a worse prognosis in older patients, with patients over 60 years old being three times more likely to die than patients less than 20 years old (Simon, 2000). Most comatose stroke patients do not survive. Medical comorbidity, advanced age, and complications all negatively affect survival. Refer to Table 15.1 for the National Hospice Organization's criterion for determining prognosis in stroke and coma patients. The majority of coma patients will die in the acute-care setting, except those whose coma is persistent and are transferred to a long-term care facility for supportive nursing care. Similar to stroke patients, they may die from the initial damage to the brain that precipitated the coma, or from subsequent complications or comorbid conditions.

After the coma phase, some people gradually recover, some progress into a vegetative state, and others become brain-dead. People who do emerge from a coma may have problems with complex thinking, emotional stability, and physical difficulties. The most common cause of death for someone in a persistent vegetative state is infection, such as pneumonia.

The common causes of pediatric coma are injury, shock, metabolic disorders, ingestions, and CNS infections. Altered mental status in children covers a range of behaviors and irritability; lethargy, changes in feeding or sleeping habits, and other subtle behavioral changes can be indicative of impairments in the child's CNS. History from the caregiver is critical. One recent study suggests that studying reactive encephalographic patterns in comatose children may be useful in prognostication of morbidity and mortality outcomes (Ramachandran Nair, Sharma, Weiss, & Cortez, 2005).

Comorbidities

Many of the predisposing factors for stroke, AD, and vascular dementia overlap with cardiovascular disease

15.1

| Medical Guidelines for Determining Prognosis: Stroke and Coma

After stroke, patients who do not die during the acute hospitalization tend to stabilize with supportive care only. Continuous decline in clinical or functional status over time means that the patient's prognosis is poor.

Conversely, steady improvement in the patient's functional or physiologic status may indicate that the patient is not terminally ill. Care should be taken to distinguish true recovery of performance and physiologic function from the improvement in symptoms and subjective well-being that can accompany hospice intervention.

I. *During the acute phase immediately following a hemorrhagic or ischemic stroke,* any of the following are strong predictors of early mortality:
  A. Coma or persistent vegetative state secondary to stroke, beyond three days' duration;
  B. In post-anoxic stroke, coma or severe obtundation, accompanied by severe myoclonus, persisting beyond three days past the anoxic event;
  C. Comatose patients with any four of the following on day 3 of coma have had 97% mortality by two months:
    1) Abnormal brain stem response
    2) Absent verbal response
    3) Absent withdrawal response to pain
    4) Serum creatinine >1.5 mg/dl
    5) Age >70;
  D. Dysphagia severe enough to prevent the patient from receiving food and fluids necessary to sustain life, in a patient who declines, or is not a candidate for, artificial nutrition and hydration.
II. *Once the patient has entered the chronic phase:* the following clinical factors may correlate with poor survival in the setting of severe stroke, and should be documented:
  A. Age greater than 70.
  B. Poor functional status, as evidenced by Karnofsky score of <50%.
  C. Post-stroke dementia, as evidenced by a FAST score of greater than 7.
  D. Poor nutritional status, whether on artificial nutrition or not:
    1) Unintentional progressive weight loss of greater than 10% over past six months;
    2) Serum albumin less than 2.5 gm/dl, maybe a helpful prognostic indicator, but not to be used by itself.

Source: National Hospice Organization. (1996). *Medical guidelines for determining prognosis in selected non-cancer diseases.*(2nd ed.). Arlington, VA: National Hospice Organization.

and include hypertension, diabetes, cigarette smoking, high cholesterol and African-American ethnicity. This can lead to complications with unstable blood pressure, angina, congestive heart failure, myocardial infarction, and arrhythmias (Cechetto, Hachinski, & Whitehead, 2008; Ostwald, Wasserman, & Davis, 2006).

As previously stated, the risk of stroke and most CNDs increases with age and the older patient is also more likely to have coexisting chronic illnesses. People with MS are likely to be younger at age of onset and thus have fewer coexisting chronic problems. Any limitations associated with comorbid conditions can impede functional status and complicate management. Comorbid illnesses have consistently been shown to affect function, mortality, and utilization of services (Studenski, Lai, Duncan, & Rigler, 2004).

People with stroke and CND are susceptible to secondary complications including pressure sores, malnutrition, venous thrombosis, contractures, pneumonia, conjunctivitis, depression, and problems with bowel and bladder function. These complications are frequent enough that they should be anticipated and nursing care should be aimed at prevention and early recognition and treatment of problems.

In addition, antiparkinson drugs are associated with the development of dyskinesias including on-off phenomena of recurring sudden changes from dopamine-deficient akinesia to dopamine-induced dykinesea. Antiparkinson drugs may also cause impaired thinking, delusions, and hallucinations.

COMMON SYMPTOMS AND TREATMENTS

Symptoms vary greatly between people who have had a stroke or neurodegenerative illnesses, depending on the locations and severity of damage or pathology. Specific chapters in this book that cover management of symptoms such as delirium, skin alterations, and gastrointestinal symptoms should be consulted for an overview of treatment options. This section will focus on some of the palliative care issues and their management for individuals with stroke and chronic neurodegenerative diseases such as cognition and communication, affect and behavior, recognizing and treating pain, eating and swallowing, dyspnea, sleep, and infection.

Cognition

There is great heterogeneity in cognitive deficits following a stroke. The person can exhibit reduced level of consciousness, attention deficits, and an array of perceptual deficits commonly impact functional ability. For example, some patients develop neglect or a loss of awareness of their affected limbs. It is associated with right hemispheric strokes and, in the extreme, can result in patients being completely unaware of the left side of their body or to stimuli coming from the left side of their environment. Patient safety is compromised, as neglect can increase the risk of injury and falls.

Neurodegenerative illnesses are associated with the development of cognitive deficits, and symptoms worsen as the illness progresses. Early in Alzheimer's disease, short-term memory, judgment, and visuospatial problems are common. During later stages, the person has severe impairment of all cognitive functions and may no longer recognize family members. Attention, orientation, as well as short- and long-term memories are impaired. In Parkinson's disease, it is more common to have impairment of learning and free recall of new information while is relatively well-preserved (Demakis, 2007). Cognitive changes for people with MS occur in 40 to 60% of cases and mainly affect attention, information processing speed, and episodic memory (Houtchens et al., 2007; Minden, 2000). Executive dysfunctions are the most common areas affected in those with ALS (Wheaton et al., 2007).

There is evidence that memantine and cholinesterase inhibitors are modestly effective in decreasing the severity of cognitive deficits in AD. Cholinesterase inhibitors are used in mild to moderate dementia, and memantine alone or in combination with cholinesterase inhibitors is used in the late stages of the illness (Potyk, 2005). Reality orientation is not recommended for people with AD, but the use of environmental cues and decreasing visual clutter are recommended.

Communication

Impairments in communication are common with all disorders discussed in this chapter. Strokes occurring in the left hemisphere, in particular, can impair the ability to communicate. Impairments in neuromuscular function cause dysarthria in people with PD, MS and ALS.

Cognitive deficits are associated with receptive and expressive aphasia in CNDs. As Alzheimer's disease progresses to late stages, the number of words in the person's vocabulary is usually limited to 20 or less. Those individuals with expressive aphasia may comprehend spoken language, but are unable to express themselves verbally to varying degrees. Receptive aphasia is the result of deficits in receiving the message/auditory perception or retaining it. Due to difficulty expressing their needs or interpreting what is going on around them, aphasic patients may become noncompliant, angry, fearful, or withdrawn.

Difficulty communicating severely reduces quality of life for people with stroke and chronic neurodegenerative disorders. Speech therapy is used to recover as much as possible from the dysarthria, aphasia, and apraxia impacting communication post stroke. The nurse should develop a plan for providing meaningful communication and socialization that considers the wishes of the individual and the accommodations needed because of dysarthria, aphasia, or cognitive impairment.

People with dysarthria use a wide variety of augmentative communication devices. As the person's condition deteriorates, there may be less ability to use the device. A consistent caregiver or family member is often able to understand speech that others consider unintelligible. Supporting the remaining demonstrations of attempts to communicate enables the patient to feel connected and accepted; they may begin using many more nonverbal cues to communicate needs. Behaviors listed in Table 15.2 may be used by patients with cognitive impairment to communicate that there is an unmet need such as pain or hunger, or the need to eliminate or change positions. An effective evidence-based intervention for treating pain and other unmet needs in people with dementia who no longer clearly or consistently verbally communicate unmet needs is presented in the Evidence-Based Box.

Anticipating physical needs decreases frustration for the person who is unable to clearly or consistently verbalize needs. Nonverbal communication through touch, massage, and eye contact should be used. Gestures are a three-dimensional language of communication;

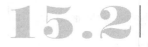

15.2 | Behavioral Symptoms of Unmet Needs in People with Impaired Communication and/or Cognition

- Any change in behavior
- Restless movement
- Moaning
- Tense muscles
- Facial grimace
- Agitation
- Combative/angry
- Pull away
- Changes in mobility
- Rubbing/holding or bracing of a body part
- Crying/tears in eyes
- Change in sleep
- Increased confusion
- Changes in appetite
- Verbal perseveration
- Withdrawal/quiet
- Increased pulse, respiration

waving hello, pointing, beckoning with outstretched hands, and hugging used judiciously by the caregiver may be effective communication tools. Presence of a family member or caregiver conveys to the individual that he/she is not alone and is respected.

When cognitive impairment is present, the strategies outlined in Table 15.3 may be useful to facilitate communication. A calm, gentle voice communicates safety and security. Listening to the person, even if the message is unclear, communicates respect. Compared to those with mild cognitive impairment, the individual who is severely impaired may require more focused stimulation to elicit a response. Making a compassionate and meaningful connection with a person who has severe dementia will often soothe a troubled anxious state.

Affect and Behavior

The development of depression, mood disorders, and anxiety associated with stroke and neurodegenerative illnesses are common. Frontal lobe pathology and disturbed neurotransmitter metabolism increase a person's

15.3 | Communication Strategies with the Cognitively Impaired

- Make sure the person knows you are present before communicating to avoid startling or frightening the person.
- Touching the person gently may be used to begin the communication. A conventional handshake may be well tolerated. Assess the person's reaction and gradually increase the use of appropriate touch, if tolerated.
- Keep voice, facial expression, and body movements calm, slow, clear, and positive.
- Use short, simple, adult sentences.
- Use the name of the person most familiar to him/her. Avoid the use of pronouns.
- Use visual cues to augment verbal message.
- Limit choices to two options to avoid overwhelming the person's cognitive ability.
- Avoid "why" questions, which may be perceived as threatening.
- Avoid negative feedback statements such as "don't."
- Avoid correcting the person or attempting to orient him/her. Since short-term memory is severely impaired, this is ineffective.
- Listen to the person's verbal message attentively and allow enough time for the person to communicate with you.
- Validate the feelings behind the words. For example, "I hear that you are upset and I am here to help" or "I'm glad you're okay."
- Tapes of family members may be used to provide simulated presence therapy.
- End all interactions with positive feedback such as "I appreciate this time with you," or "It was nice to visit with you today."

susceptibility to depression. Also, adapting to the loss of physical or cognitive abilities can be overwhelming, and the individual's premorbid personality, coping skills, and resources are all factors in making this adaptation. Medications can contribute to depressive and psychotic symptoms. In people with MS, frontal lobe symptoms of euphoria and pathological laughing and weeping are thought to result from demyelination of nerves (Minden, 2000). When cognitive impairment is present, the person may become increasingly frightened by a world that seems more and more unfamiliar.

The literature suggests that people with CND are both underdiagnosed and inadequately treated for mood and anxiety disorders (Minden, 2000). People with neuromuscular problems may appear less animated at baseline, so flat affect and decreased involvement in activity are not useful cues for depression or mood disorders. A recent systematic literature review using Cochrane methodology found a lack of evidence of an association between the severity of Alzheimer's disease and the prevalence of comorbid depressive symptoms or depression (Verkaik, Nuyen, Schellevis, & Francke, 2007). This review suggests that prevention and intervention strategies for depression should be aimed at all people with Alzheimer's disease regardless of their disease severity. Geropsychiatry consultations are often needed to competently assess and treat those with more complicated symptomatology. There are few systematic studies of psychotherapy and pharmacotherapy in individuals with CND. Evidence supports that selective serotonin re-uptake inhibitors are the drugs of choice for depressive disorders because of their safer drug profile, and anxiety disorders may be treated effectively with combined drug and non-pharmacological therapy (Chan, Cordato, & O'Rourke, 2008).

Behaviors listed in Table 15.2 are common in people with dementia and may indicate an underlying need such as pain or hunger. The person who has decreased competence, particularly cognitive competence, is more affected by stressors from the environment and has a decreased threshold for tolerating stressors from the environment (Kovach, 2000). Consideration of this environmental vulnerability creates the need for two foundational interventions:

- provide a positive environment with few environmental stressors;
- balance sensory stimulating and sensory calming activity throughout the day.

Health professionals should conduct a noise assessment by listening at various times of the day for sources of noxious or extraneous noise. Eliminate echo, background conversations, and television used for background sound. Provide brief periods of music listening with selections that are pleasing to the patient. The visually accessible environment may be quite circumscribed, so it is important that it be pleasant and as stress-free as possible. Avoid fluorescent lighting that often creates a glare. Keep some items that are familiar to the person in the immediate area; for example, pictures, afghans and pillows may convey home and familiarity. Spaces that are too big or too small and cluttered areas should be avoided. One or two plants or flower arrangements are preferred to an overwhelming clutter of flora. Avoid tactile stressors by keeping the room temperature comfortable. Avoid itchy skin by keeping the skin well lubricated and treating with medicated emollients; flannel sheets and silk pillowcases may provide some comfort.

In addition to decreasing environmental stress, there is a need to balance sensory stimulating and sensory calming activity. As the illness progresses, there may be a need for more sensory calming time, and the person will probably tolerate less than one hour of activity before needing a decrease in environmental stimulation. Often, only brief visits of 10 minutes or less will be tolerated. The person may need to engage in frequent inner retreat by withdrawing from others. This need should be explained to family, so they do not feel shunned; if the patient shuns socialization, allow him/her some solitary time and approach again later.

Agitated behaviors are associated with cognitive impairment and increase in frequency as dementia progresses (Chen, Ryden, Feldt, & Savik, 2000). Social contact and focused therapeutic stimulation have been associated with decreases in agitated behavior (Draper et al., 2000; McGonigal-Kenney, Schutte, Adams, & Titler, 2006). Stimulation of multiple senses may enhance engagement in the activity. Friendly visiting, hand massage, music listening, and pet therapy are just a few examples of therapeutic activities. Multiple activity therapy books provide suggestions for therapeutic activities that accommodate any level of cognitive or functional deficit and enhance quality of life.

Perseverant behavior, defined as repetitive movement or verbalization, may also occur in patients with CND. Perseverance may indicate boredom, discomfort, an unmet need, or it may be a simple tension-reduction mechanism. Calm repetitive movements or verbalizations may be a coping mechanism and not require treatment. It is important to determine if environmental stress needs to be decreased or, alternatively, if stimulating activity should be provided. Health professionals should assess for basic comfort needs: offer a drink, be certain elimination needs have been met, provide a warm blanket or sweater, check for pressure points, and good positioning. If pain is suspected, administer an analgesic.

Aggression and resisting care may also be present. Resisting care may indicate that pain control is inadequate. This behavior is often temporary, and so the caregiver should repeat the attempt to provide care following a short break. Paratonia is a primitive reflex that may be present, and is often mistaken for resisting care. Paratonia is involuntary resistance of an extremity in response to sudden passive movement. A caregiver who moves a patient's arm may evoke this movement that appears to be resistance to care. Slow and gentle touch decreases the likelihood of inducing paratonia.

Delusions and hallucinations, when present, are a real part of the person's mental life and can be very discomforting. These alterations in perception often respond well to psychotropic drugs. Caregivers should not agree or disagree with the false perception, but there is a need to provide comforting intervention. For example, saying, "I hear that you are afraid and I will keep you safe," validates feelings and provides reassurance. Distraction or provision of a comforting intervention such as friendly visiting will often soothe the person's troubled state. Also, check to be sure the person's glasses and hearing aid are in place and functioning properly. Many suspected delusions are actually mixed messages resulting from impaired hearing.

Eating and Swallowing

Dysphagia and aspiration are problematic in stroke and neurodegenerative illnesses. Dyspahagia resulting from stroke is temporary in 90% of cases but is a part of general progress of the illness for CNDs discussed in this chapter (Broadley et al., 2005). Dysphasia can occur in oropharyngeal or esophageal phases of swallowing. The oropharyngeal phase is voluntary and depends on motor and sensory pathways, triggering a series of movements that move food posteriorly to the oropharynx. Oropharyngeal dyspahagia has a neurological cause in 75% of cases (Ertekin & Aydogdu, 2003). Esophageal dysphagia is more likely caused by obstruction (White, O'Rouke, Ong, Cordato, & Chan, 2008). Patients with swallowing disorders are at risk for aspiration pneumonia. Drooling is common for those with PD because of a decrease in unconscious swallowing. Low food consumption, food pocketing, difficulty manipulating food on the plate and transporting it to the mouth, weight loss and nutritional impairments are common in PD (Westergren, Ohlsson, & Hallberg, 2002). All stroke patients should be evaluated by speech therapy, to determine if feeding by mouth is safe, and if aspiration precautions are needed. Techniques commonly used to assist individuals with dysphagia to swallow safely will be reviewed. Other options for managing eating problems will be discussed.

Prior to the meal, several interventions may be helpful. For example, oral hygiene is important in maintaining a normal viscosity to the saliva, and aggressive oral care may reduce the risk of pneumonia (Marik & Kaplan, 2003). If the person is taking medications that dry the mouth, artificial saliva products should be used. Safe swallowing methods include upright posture, chin-tucking, careful, slow swallowing, and specific maneuvers designed to improve swallowing (Marik & Kaplan, 2003). For the person with dementia, providing some cues that mealtime is coming is helpful. For example, in a long-term setting on units for individuals with late-stage CDN, in the late afternoon a tablecloth and vase of flowers are placed on each table to signal that it is the start of evening mealtime. The residents and staff enjoy a glass of nonalcoholic wine together while listening to relaxing music. It is important to reduce distractions during mealtime, so the focus is on eating and swallowing. If the person is in a long-term care facility, the dining room should optimally seat 16 or fewer residents to decrease the potential for overstimulation. Turning up lights, increasing visual contrasts, and improving acoustics have been suggested to enhance mealtimes in group dining rooms (Brush & Calkins, 2008). Be certain the person is comfortable and that the environment is comfortable and free from odors.

Provide verbal cueing to assist the person to eat; for example, say "the food is coming," and "swallow now." Do not rush the person to eat and swallow too quickly, but be aware that excessive time spent at the task may lead to fatigue and decrease eating. Provide positive encouragement during the meal. Plastic utensils should not be used because a biting reflex may occur, especially if the gums or teeth are touched with the utensil. Applying gentle pressure on the jaw and cheek muscles may break the biting reflex. The following feeder behaviors may help to sustain eating behaviors of the patient: talking and reorienting the person to the meal, offering drinks between bites, holding the spoon ready for a bite, and warmly touching the person.

There is a need for research on drugs used to stimulate appetite and promote weight gain in anorexic individuals with neurological illnesses. Dronabinol is a cannabis derivative which in one study of people with Alzheimer's disease was associated with a 0.5–1 kg greater weight gain than was placebo (Chapman, 2007).

The person with dysphagia will require alterations in diet. Dieticians can suggest foods that are easier to swallow. Calorie-dense pureed diets and thickened liquids may be used. One large randomized controlled trial found that honey-thick liquids were more effective than nectar-thick liquids, and chin-tucking was the least effective. All three interventions were more effective in people with PD than with AD (Logeman et al., 2008). Smaller, more frequent meals are used, and the person often takes in more food at meals earlier in the day. For some people, the stimulation of a soft bolus of food, such as mashed potatoes, may provide more stimuli for swallowing than liquids. The person should drink sufficient liquid to produce straw-colored urine. Consuming 20–35 g of fiber each day can help to manage constipation (Shagam, 2008).

For patients who have had a stroke, enteral feedings may be seen as a temporary intervention to allow time for rehabilitation and recovery or as a permanent intervention to prolong life. For those with CND, oral feeding may eventually become impossible and a person should never be force-fed. The decision to tube-feed is complex and controversial; the courts have recognized tube feeding as a medical treatment that can be refused.

Prior decision making by the patient relative to the desire to initiate assisted feeding is helpful.

There are no randomized clinical trials examining the outcomes of tube-feeding. In the case of ALS, percutaneous gastrostomy (PEG) tube placement is common, and evidence suggests survival is prolonged (Mitsumoto et al., 2003). There is no evidence that tube feedings reduce incidence of aspiration pneumonia, prolong life, or improve quality of life for people with advanced dementia (Gessert, Mosier, Brown, & Frey, 2000). Other possible problems associated with tube feeding include diarrhea, surgery risks, and burdens of hospitalization associated with tube placement, the need for physical restraints if tubes are pulled, wound infection, and skin breakdown.

Dyspnea

In people with chronic neurological disease involving motor systems, respiratory insufficiency is common late in the illness. Chronic nocturnal hypoventilation is also common. Weakness of the respiratory muscles produces a restrictive ventilatory defect with resulting atelectasis and a feeling of dyspnea or increased work of breathing. Expiratory weakness is generally more prominent than inspiratory and may contribute to impaired coughing, aspiration, and the development of pneumonia. Thick respiratory secretions may be difficult to manage and uncomfortable. Respiratory insufficiency is particularly severe in ALS and MS. People need to be given information regarding the mechanism of terminal hypercapnic coma and the resulting peaceful death, so that fear is decreased. Medications discussed in the chapter on dyspnea need to be administered skillfully to successfully prevent the feeling of "choking to death."

Noninvasive positive pressure ventilation (NPPV) is an option chosen by some patients, particularly those with ALS, to decrease feelings of dyspnea. In spite of recommendations that NPPV has beneficial effects on quality of life, it is utilized by only 36% of eligible patients (Jackson, Lovitt, Gowda, Anderson, & Miller, 2006; Miller, 2001). Refer to chapter 20 for further discussion of dyspnea.

Fatigue, Activity, and Sleep

Fatigue is a subjective feeling of early exhaustion that impacts an individual's ability to interact mentally or physically with his/her environment. It is a commonly reported symptom and can be overwhelmingly debilitating, especially for people with MS. Research is only beginning to investigate a possible correlation between fatigue and location of damage, such as brainstem and thalamic regions, that impact the reticular activating system (Staub & Bogousslavsky, 2001). An understanding of the relationship between fatigue and depression, sleep disturbances, and specific deficits is needed in order to better recognize and treat fatigue.

Sleep disruptions and insomnia are common in people with stroke, dementia, and other neurodegenerative illnesses (Subramanian & Surani, 2007). People with dementia show great alterations in the sleep-wake cycle with increased nighttime awakenings, decreased time spent awake versus time spent in bed, increased daytime napping, and changes in the amount of rapid eye movement and nonrapid eye movement sleep (Ancoli-Israel & Cooke, 2005; Subramanian & Surani, 2007). Sleep-disordered breathing has been reported in 33-70% of people with Alzheimer's disease, and obstructive sleep apnea is associated with agitation (Gehrman et al., 2003). Sundown syndrome, an increase in agitation in the late afternoon or evening, is often present (Volicer, Harper, Manning, Goldstein, & Satlin, 2001). Involuntary movements and muscle spasms for those with PD and MS and dyspnea during the night for those with ALS and MS can greatly impair sleep.

Patients should be carefully evaluated for factors that could be contributing to their fatigue, such as anemia, pain, occult infections, hypothyroidism, medications, malnutrition, and sleep apnea (Oken et al., 2006). Refer to chapter 23 for further discussion of fatigue. Adapting the environment to promote sleep, pacing activities, treating pain, and eliminating or reducing any offending medications, all should all be considered possible interventions for people with CND. Relaxation techniques such as breathing exercises, massage, imagery, or music may also promote sleep and reduce fatigue.

Light and fragmented sleep impairs quality of life. Nocturnal hypoventilation is discussed under dyspnea. It is important to keep a consistent schedule so that the diurnal rhythm is encouraged. Most people will need an afternoon nap, but keeping the person engaged in some activities during the daytime might help to improve nighttime sleep.

An increase in agitated behavior in the late afternoon or early evening is called sundown syndrome and occurs in some people with dementia. This often indicates there is a need to improve the balance between sensory stimulating and sensory calming activity earlier in the day (Kovach et al., 2004). Specifically, there may be a need for more physical activity early in the day, followed by an afternoon nap. Then, during the usual sundowning period, engage the person in a quiet one-on-one activity. Also, because of the severe sleep variations experienced by people with CND, try to keep diurnal rhythms intact by keeping lighting low during the night and up during the day. This may require increasing use of artificial light beginning in the late afternoon.

Movement

Stroke and neurodegenerative disease affect movement and these symptoms can severely impact functional ability and quality of life. People who suffer from a stroke display hemiparesis and a variety of symptoms, depending on location and severity of damage. People with neurodegenerative disease have slowed movement, and gait disturbances progress so that the person becomes more chair-bound or bed-bound. People with late-stage AD may display primitive reflexes such as hand grasping, and sucking reflexes and paratonia may be present. Paratonia is the involuntary resistance of an arm or leg to movement of the limb by another person. This may be misinterpreted by a caregiver as aggressive behavior, but is actually a reflexive process. Resting tremor is rarely present and muscles become rigid (Kurlan, Richard, Papka, & Marshall, 2000; Wilson et al., 2000).

PD is associated with a classic triad of motor symptoms: bradykinesia (i.e., slow movement), rigidity, and tremor. Late in the illness, motor problems occur, which may be a result from drug therapy, and include dyskinesias (involuntary movements), shorter duration of benefit or lack of benefit from medication, and end-of-dose deterioration. Severe muscle rigidity and bradykinesia contribute to the person becoming more bed- or chair-bound. When movement does occur, the person often needs physical help initiating the movement. Akinesia or freezing of movement becomes debilitating. Muscle rigidity moves from the cogwheel to pipe-like variety. Cogwheel rigidity is a "ratchety" catch of the limb when moved and is a manifestation of both rigidity and tremor. In severe Parkinson's disease, the resistance to passive movement of the limb is constant whether the limb is moved slowly or quickly (i.e., like bending a lead pipe) (Kurlan et al., 2000).

For people with MS, problems with walking, or gait, can arise from muscle weakness or stiffness, numbness, poor balance, spasticity, lack of ability to coordinate muscle movements, extreme fatigue, and visual disturbances. Depending upon the type of MS someone has, symptoms can become progressively worse or come and go over time. People with ALS experience weakness, particularly of the upper limbs, and progressive muscle wasting. The person loses muscle strength, muscle mass, and mobility, until becoming completely dependent.

Physical exercise is a cornerstone of rehabilitation following stroke. However, evidence is inconclusive regarding benefits of cardiovascular exercises on disability, activities of daily living, quality of life, and death (Meek, Pollock, Potter, & Langhorne, 2003). The goals of treatment of PD are to slow progression of the illness and to reduce disability without inducing long-term complications. Motor symptoms associated with PD are disabling. While levodopa/carbidopa is the cornerstone of treatment of motor symptoms of PD, optimal response only lasts 5–7 years. The classes of drugs approved for the treatment of PD includes dopamine agonists, catechol-O-methyl-ransferase (COMT) inhibitors, monoamine-oxidase type B (MAO-B) inhibitors, and anticholinergics. These drugs do not prevent neuronal degeneration but decrease motor symptoms (Lo, Leung, & Shek, 2007). Research is currently focused on developing neuroprotective drugs that will slow or halt progression of PD. Surgical options such as deep brain stimulation are options for some patients with PD who are not effectively managed through drug therapy.

Research on the effects of exercise for people with Alzheimer's disease and related disorders has shown maintenance of motor skills, decreased falls, reduced rate of cognitive decline, and improved mood (Teri et al., 2003). A systematic review and meta-analysis showed that strengthening and balance exercises in PD provide benefits to physical function, strength, balance, gait speed, and health-related quality of life (Goodwin, Richards, Taylor, Taylor, & Campbell, 2008). For people with ALS, exercise can help to maintain flexibility of the muscles, but will not strengthen muscles that have been weakened by ALS. For people with MS, exercise may decrease symptoms but must be done judiciously as overheating or overstressing the body can actually exacerbate symptoms. Occupational therapy may help patients to maintain independence for longer periods of time as the CNDs progress.

RECOGNIZING AND TREATING PAIN

Spasticity due to increased muscle tone is common, especially post stroke, with MS and PD and presents as resistance to passive range of motion. Brain lesions can interfere with the descending CNS pathways that regulate muscle tone (Gelber, 2002). For people with ALS, spasticity can actually be helpful in maintaining function, as the rigidity helps replace normal muscle strength, but it causes jerky, hard-to-control movements.

Shoulder pain after stroke is common, affecting from 16–72% of patients (Walsh, 2001). Both flaccidity and spasticity in the paretic arm can cause subluxation (partial separation), instability of the shoulder joint, pain, and increased risk of subacromial bursitis. Shoulder-hand syndrome or reflex sympathetic dystrophy is due to autonomic dysfunction in the affected upper extremity. Paresis in the shoulder and arm can lead to joint instability and trauma, which may trigger overstimulation of the sympathetic nervous system. It develops in stages and, typically, there is vasoconstriction in the affected arm with complaints of burning pain. If it progresses beyond three months, the limb may develop trophic changes with decreased hair, thin shiny skin, increased or decreased sweating, edema, and bone demineralization. Movement and touch usually cause pain and patients tend to guard the limb, leading to further dysfunction. After 9 months, atrophy and contractures may also occur. Central post-stroke pain (CPSP) is described as a neuropathic pain in all or part of the body affected by the stroke, which may develop immediately or up to 2 years after the initial stroke (Frese, Husstedt, Ringelstein, & Evers, 2006). It is associated with sensory deficits and tactile allodynia (pain elicited by a normally non-painful stimulus). This often prompts patients to lie perfectly still in order to avoid discomfort.

Pain in MS occurs both as a consequence of the disease process and the resulting disability. Prevalence of pain in patients with MS is nearly 50%, and approximately 75% of patients report having had pain within 1 month of assessment. The presence of pain in patients with MS is associated with increased age, duration of illness, depression, degree of functional impairment, and fatigue. Pain in MS may originate from trigeminal neuralgia, headache, facial pain, tonic seizures, and limb pain. The pain may indicate an underlying inflammatory process or demyelinating lesion affecting a pain pathway (O'Connor, Schwid, Herrmann, Markman, & Dworkin, 2008). Pain associated with optic neuritis is caused by traction of the meninges surrounding the swollen optic nerve (Maloni, 2000).

Dysesthetic extremity pain in people with MS is a result of demyelinating lesions and is described as persistent and burning. Most commonly affected are the legs and feet, but upper extremities and the trunk can also be affected. Pain is often worse at night and after exercise, and may be precipitated by changes in temperature, particularly the use of warm water. Joint pain and back pain are common, resulting from the disease process, steroid-induced osteoporosis, postural changes, immobility, and weakness with improper use of compensatory muscles (Maloni, 2000). Approximately 50% of patients in the late stage of ALS report pain as a result of immobility, ligament laxity, spasticity, fasciculations, muscle cramps, and associated problems (Miller, 2001).

Pain experienced by individuals with stroke and neurodegenerative illnesses may also arise from the medical conditions commonly prevalent in the older age group, or as a result of comorbid conditions such as pressure ulcers, urinary retention, constipation, and contractures. Older people more commonly suffer from arthritis, back problems, and other chronic conditions.

The consequences of untreated pain are far reaching, and assessing for pain and treating it early may help to improve psychosocial and functional outcomes. Early and continued range-of-motion exercises done at least twice daily and individualized splinting of affected areas may reduce the risk of contractures. Given the risk of sedation and mental status changes, particularly in the older adult, the decision to treat pharmacologically must be weighed carefully. Drugs such as baclofen, tizanidine, benzodiazepines, or dantrolene, each work slightly differently, but all patients using them must be closely monitored for side effects. Baclofen can also be administered intrathecally for spasticity. Nerve blocks with phenol or botulinum toxin to focal areas of spasticity can be effective for a number of weeks to months, but need to be repeated for sustained symptom relief. In order to restore a functional position or facilitate hygiene, surgical tendon release or lengthening can also be an option in extremities with no voluntary movement. Non-drug treatments that may be helpful include the application of heat or cold to areas of spasticity, but not if there is reduced sensation given the risk of injury. Gentle massage and relaxation techniques such as imagery or music may also promote comfort.

Establishing the underlying cause of the shoulder pain in patients with stroke is necessary to choose the appropriate intervention. The effect of electrical stimulation on shoulder pain is inconclusive (Price & Pandyan, 2001), but it may offer relief for some patients. Intra-articular steroid injections can be helpful, especially with bursitis. Shoulder pain due to spasticity has also responded to intramuscular botulinum toxin injections. Non-pharmacological treatments such as ice, heat, transcutaneous electrical nerve stimulation (TENS), and ultrasound may also relieve pain in some patients. Range of motion exercises, proper positioning, and techniques to manage edema should be initiated immediately post stroke in the affected limb.

Treatment options used for neuropathic pain can include anticonvulsants (e.g., gabapentin) and tricyclic antidepressants (e.g., amitriptyline and nortriptyline). The risk versus the benefit of a trial of a tricyclic antidepressant in an older adult must be carefully considered given the anti-cholinergic side-effect profile. Opiates play a relatively small role in the management of neuropathic pain. Vestergaard, Anderson, Gottrup, Kristensen, and Jensen (2002) tested the anticonvulsant lamotrigine on patients with central post-stroke pain (median age 59 years). Pain scores were reduced by 30%, and at 200 mg/day, the drug was well tolerated. Further study with older age groups and different doses may prove lamotrigine to be a promising new treatment alternative. Another study found gabapentin effective for paroxysmal pain experienced by people with MS (Yetimalar, Gurgor, & Basoglu, 2004). Adapting relaxation techniques to assist patients in coping with neuropathic pain may be helpful.

It may be difficult to recognize pain in people who have dementia and/or communication impairment. While self-report remains the gold standard for assessing pain, for those who cannot communicate pain verbally, it is important to be vigilant in assessing for potential causes of pain, to observe for changes in patient behavior that may be indicators of pain, to seek surrogate report from caregivers, and to attempt an analgesic trial if pain is suspected (Tsai & Chang, 2004). Refer to chapter 19 and the Evidence-Based Box for further discussion of pain management.

ADDITIONAL ILLNESS-SPECIFIC SYMPTOMS

Autonomic nervous system symptoms are most common in MS and PD and can include postural hypotension, constipation bowel dysfunction, urine retention, urgency, and incontinence. Bowel dysfunction may result from both a delay in colon transit time and

impaired muscle coordination in the anorectal area (Pfeiffer, 2000). Delayed gastric emptying, caused by reduced parasympathetic activity, can affect timing of drug response. Damage to the sensory system in MS can cause or contributes to a variety of problems including loss of sensation and sexual dysfunction. Visual dysfunction is common including diplopia, vision loss, and nystagmus.

Infection. Severe infection, commonly pneumonia and septicemia arising from the urinary tract, may be the cause of death in those with CND. Delayed diagnosis of infection may contribute to the severity of infection because of both altered clinical presentations for infection and inability to clearly report symptoms. Nurses should work to prevent infection through common practices such as good hand-washing, skin care, and

---

EXHIBIT 15.1: GLASGOW COMA SCALE

Eye Opening (E)
- spontaneous 4
- to speech 3
- to pain 2
- no response 1

Best Motor Response (M)
To Verbal Command:
- obeys 6
To Painful Stimulus:
- localizes pain 5
- flexion-withdrawal 4
- flexion-abnormal 3
- extension 2
- no response 1

Best Verbal Response (V)
- oriented and converses 5
- disoriented and converses 4
- inappropriate words 3
- incomprehensible sounds 2
- no response 1

E + M + V = 3 to 15
* 90% less than or equal to 8 are in coma
* Greater than or equal to 9 not in coma
* 8 is the critical score
* Less than or equal to 8 at 6 hours - 50% die
* 9–11 = moderate severity
* Greater than or equal to 12 = minor injury

Coma is defined as: (1) not opening eyes, (2) not obeying commands, and (3) not uttering understandable words.

Source: Teasdale, G., & Jennet, B. (1974). Assessment of coma and impaired consciousness: A practical scale. *Lancet*, 2, 81–84.

adequate hydration. As the illness progresses, the question of how vigorously to treat infection, or whether one should treat infection at all, is commonly raised. A comparison of nursing home residents with dementia in the Netherlands and Missouri found more aggressive treatment of lower respiratory tract infection and lower mortality rates in the Missouri homes (van der Steen, Mehr, Druse, Ribbe, & van der Wal, 2007). However, parenteral antibiotic treatment was not associated with better outcomes in residents with low to moderate risk of mortality (van der Steen et al., 2007).

Coma. Initial priority in the emergency management of comatose patients is to evaluate and maintain respiratory and circulatory functions and then to establish the underlying disease process. Timely diagnosis will improve the likelihood of reversing the coma, when this is possible, and reducing mortality. The Glasgow Coma Scale (Exhibit 15.1) is often used to assess and score the level of consciousness. Eye opening, verbal response, and motor response to stimuli are evaluated. The scores range from 3 to 15 and patients with scores between 3 and 8 are said to be "in a coma." A pediatric version of this scale is available (Reilly, Simpson, Sprod, & Thomas, 1988). The CHOP Infant Coma Scale or Infant Face Scale (IFS) may be more useful for children under 2 years of age. This scale relies on objective behavioral observations, assesses cortical as well as brainstem function, and is based on infant-appropriate behaviors. It can also be used with intubated patients and has better inter-rater reliability than the pediatric version of the Glasgow Coma Scale (Durham et al., 2000).

PALLIATIVE CARE ISSUES

The illness trajectory for patients with stroke and CNDs is often long and unpredictable. This prognostic uncertainty is associated with a host of patient, family, caregiving, and reimbursement challenges. Patients with CND have heavy physical and emotional care needs. Care in a hospice or long-term care facility may reduce the caregiving required of the family, but may lead to feelings of loss of control as well as feelings of isolation. Deciding on the preferred setting for end-of-life care is complex with many factors to consider; family members may disagree with each other or the individual him/herself. The nurse can serve as a nonjudgmental listener, can help to explore options, and facilitate working through the process of decision making with family members.

Regardless of the setting of care, people with stroke and CND do not receive enough palliative or hospice care even though overall quality of care is rated highly by family members of decedents (Mitchell et al., 2007). Approximately 11.3% of patients receiving hospice care

have a diagnosis of dementia (Mitchell et al., 2007).

Physicians and other healthcare providers often do not understand that hospice services are extremely helpful to those with non-cancer diseases, nor do they understand the criteria or mechanisms for establishing hospice services in their agencies or homes.

There are guidelines established by the National Hospice Organization (NHO) for determining prognosis in selected non-cancer diseases, including dementia, stroke, and coma. These guidelines (Tables 15.2 and 15.4) are designed to predict 6-month mortality, so that the person can be entered into Medicare/Medicaid reimbursed hospice services. The accuracy of these guidelines at predicting mortality is debated.

Family members should optimally be a part of a continued process of decision making throughout the illness trajectory. In the case of illnesses that are associated with dementia, early discussions and assignment of trusted family members to decision-making roles when capacity is compromised are essential. With these illnesses, there is a lot of anticipatory grieving that occurs, and family members need to be supported in accepting their feelings. Acknowledging conflicting feelings, particularly both the dread and desire for the death to occur, as common and natural can be helpful. Early discussions about the typical course of the illness that are honest but sensitive are needed.

Coping with the late stages of chronic neurodegenerative illness is both physically and emotionally demanding. The patient's stress should not be amplified by an awareness of the burden on family or professional caregivers. Discussions about the burdens or problems of care giving should be held away from the patient. The person should feel cared for and safe.

Brain Death

Improved medical technology capable of sustaining life and organ transplantation protocols has created circumstances in which the individual may have cardiopulmonary functions but are brain dead. With the need to define and determine brain death, the President's Commission developed the Uniform Determination of Death Act, which allowed brain death to be a legal definition of death (Guidelines for the determination of death, 1981).

Declaring persons dead requires that either their heart function has ceased or their brain no longer functions due to irreversible damage. There is continued controversy and ongoing research to improve accuracy in determining irreversible brain death, and a variety of confirming tests have been suggested. These include electroencephalogram, cerebral angiography, magnetic resonance imaging, and testing of cerebrospinal fluid. Major differences exist in the guidelines used to determine brain death in major neurological hospitals in the Unites States (Greer, Varelas, Haque, & Wijdicks, 2008).

15.4 | Medical Guidelines for Determining Prognosis: Dementia

The term "dementia" refers here to chronic, primary, and progressive cognitive impairment of either the Alzheimer or multi-infarct type. Although most research on prognosis in dementia is done with patients with Alzheimer's disease, the vascular (multi-infarct) dementias appear to progress to death more quickly. These guidelines do *not* refer to acute, potentially reversible, or secondary dementias, i.e., those due to drug intoxication, cancer, AIDS, major stroke, or heart, renal, or liver failure.

I. Functional Assessment Staging
  A. Even severely demented patients may have a prognosis of up to 2 years. Survival time depends on variables such as the incidence of comorbidities and the comprehensiveness of care.
  B. The patient should be at or beyond Stage 7 of the Functional Assessment Staging Scale (Sclan & Reisberg, 1992). The factors listed below should be understood explicitly, since many patients do not progress in an orderly fashion through the substages of 7.
  C. The patient should show *all* of the following characteristics:
    1) Unable to ambulate without assistance.
      This is a critical factor. Recent data indicate that patients who retain the ability to ambulate independently do not tend to die within 6 months, even if all other criteria for advanced dementia are present.
    2) Unable to dress without assistance.
    3) Unable to bathe properly.
    4) Urinary and fecal incontinence.
      a. Occasionally or more frequently, over the past weeks.
      b. Reported by knowledgeable informant or caregiver.
    5) Unable to speak or communicate meaningfully.
      a. Ability to speak is limited to approximately a half dozen or fewer intelligible and different words in the course of an average day or in the course of an intensive interview.
II. Presence of Medical Complications
  A. The presence of medical comorbid conditions of sufficient severity to warrant medical treatment, documented within the past year, *whether or not the decision was made to treat the condition,* decrease survival in advanced dementia.
  B. Comorbid conditions associated with dementia:
    1) Aspiration pneumonia.
    2) Pyelonephritis or other upper urinary tract infection.
    3) Septicemia.
    4) Decubitus ulcers, multiple, stage 3–4.
    5) Fever recurrent after antibiotics.
  C. Difficulty swallowing food or refusal to eat, sufficiently severe that patient cannot maintain sufficient fluid and calorie intake to sustain life, with patient or surrogate refusing tube feedings or parenteral nutrition.
    1. Patients who are receiving tube feedings must have documented impaired nutritional status as indicated by:
      a. Unintentional, progressive weight loss of greater than 10% over the prior 6 months.
      b. Serum albumin less than 2.5 gm/dl, which may be a helpful prognostic indicator, but should not be used by itself.

Source: National Hospice Organization. (1996). *Medical guidelines for determining prognosis in selected non-cancer diseases* (2nd ed.). Arlington, VA: National Hospice Organization.

Direct damage to the brain stem (head trauma, intracranial hemorrhage, infarcts, mass lesions) and diffuse damage to neuronal metabolism (drugs, renal failure, hypoglycemia) are the mechanisms by which irreversible brain death may occur. Patients who are being evaluated for brain death are most likely being treated in the intensive care unit or emergency room. Families need significant education and support throughout the diagnostic evaluation and the process of treatment withdrawal. If brain death has occurred as the result of a long illness with multiple organ failure, they may have had time to absorb information and

develop realistic expectations about their loved one's survival, as opposed to a sudden unpredictable trauma. It is important to have staff available who are comfortable discussing the implications of brain death, the need for withdrawal of treatment, and how to incorporate any previous wishes of the patient and requests by the family.

Truog et al. (2001) recommend that families be given a very straightforward but compassionate explanation that the patient died when his/her brain died and that treatment is being withdrawn from someone who is already dead. This may relieve feelings of guilt that withdrawal of treatment contributed to the patient's death. Due to the extent of the brain stem injury, brain-dead patients do not feel pain. Reassurance that they are not suffering and that measures to ensure patient dignity are in place is important, as well as incorporating any cultural or spiritual rituals. Nurses can help to establish an environment where the family feels supported and valued.

Before withdrawing life support, families should be offered adequate time to process and cope with the information they have been given and to spend time with the patient if requested. Discussion of any possible organ donation should be separate from the notification of brain death and should be done by those trained to have such discussions.

Pediatric Brain Death

The concept of brain death, particularly in children, remains difficult. The American Academy of Pediatrics has established guidelines for the determination of brain death in children (Guidelines for the Determination of Brain Death, 1987).These guidelines provide an algorithm for declaration of brain death in infants and children. The patient's history must provide a proximate cause of the irreversible coma, and potentially correctable conditions must be excluded. The guidelines include the need for the patient to have coma coexisting with apnea, absent brainstem function, absence of multiple reflexes, and flaccid tone without spontaneous or induced movements, excluding spinal cord reflexes. The recommended period of observation as well as ancillary testing recommendations vary by age of the patient (Crain & Boyle, 2002). Ancillary testing is particularly critical in infants and young children, as clinical examinations have been less reliable in these groups (Chang, McBride, & Ferguson, 2003).

In instances of brain death due to severe head trauma, one survey found that the majority of hospitals and neurosurgeons do not strictly adhere to these guidelines and that there is substantial variability in criteria for determining brain death (Chang et al., 2003). Waiting periods for establishing brain death, particularly of infants and young children, require further research. There has been no study of whether the recommended observation periods are effective in preventing the incorrect diagnosis of brain death in trauma patients (Chang et al., 2003). Also it is important to be aware of legal requirements specific to states as well as institutional policies regarding brain death and organ procurement.

Palliative Care Nursing for Comatose and Brain-Dead Patients

Assessing for signs and symptoms of discomfort is difficult because of the lack of response to stimuli from patients who are in a coma. It is possible that some comatose patients may feel painful stimulation, but be unable to respond in any meaningful way depending upon the depth of the coma. Physiological responses, such as changes in blood pressure, heart rate, respiratory rate and rhythm, diaphoresis, and decreased oxygen saturation levels, may be possible cues of pain sensation. Monitoring facial electromyography and electroencephalographic tracings have both been used, but they remain invalidated measures. Bispectral analysis using encephalographic signals to assess level of consciousness and comfort during withdrawal of life support has been attempted (Truog et al., 2001). This technology may assess the level of arousal, but is not able to quantify pain. The use of opiates to relieve potential pain in unresponsive patients with diagnoses consistent with pain or undergoing painful procedures should be initiated.

Although brain-dead patients, by definition, do not feel pain, they should be treated with the intent to maximize their physical integrity and minimize discomfort. Families may be comforted by touching and speaking to them and should be offered privacy to do so. Attention should be focused on the physical and emotional needs of the family members throughout these events.

Withdrawal of Life Support

By the time it is determined that any meaningful recovery is unlikely, healthcare providers may have had the opportunity to process the implications. Families, however, may require additional time and counseling to reconcile with the poor prognosis and the option of treatment withdrawal. It is always a difficult and emotionally charged issue to begin discussing the withdrawal of life support from a patient. Having consistent staff members communicating with families and ongoing opportunities to discuss diagnosis, prognosis, and quality of life issues should help to prepare them for potential outcomes.

Information regarding the actual process for withdrawal of treatment can be reviewed to the extent that the family requests, and input from all appropriate disciplines should be encouraged. The actual process of withdrawal needs to incorporate any preferences for timing, those who will be present, and religious and cultural rituals. This promotes the family's ability to infuse personal meaning into the experience. Ideally, this should occur in a calm environment with respect for privacy.

Protocols vary between institutions, and more evidence-based data is needed to determine the optimum management of patients during the withdrawal of life support. Prior to discontinuing mechanical ventilation, all other treatments that do not contribute to the patient's level of comfort and unnecessary electronic monitoring may be discontinued. An intravenous line may be maintained in order to administer medications. Rubenfeld and Crawford (2001) recommend that given the uncertainty regarding the potential for pain and suffering in comatose patients, clinicians administer an appropriate level of sedation. However, due to the extent of their neurological injuries, sedation is not required in brain-dead patients. Opioids and benzodiazepines are the primary drugs used for sedation and analgesia in comatose patients before and during the withdrawal of life support (von Gunten & Weissman, 2001) and these should be titrated up to effect or comfort.

After removing all other life-supportive equipment, ventilator withdrawal in comatose or brain-dead patients can be done by simply removing the endotracheal tube (extubation), or by gradually reducing the ventilator settings (terminal weaning). Terminal weaning may take several minutes or longer depending on the pace of the process that causes hypoxia and hypercarbia. For unconscious patients unlikely to experience discomfort, Truog et al. (2001) suggest rapidly withdrawing ventilator support by removing the artificial airway or disconnecting the ventilator rather than the process of terminal weaning. For any distress during or after extubation, Pendergast (2002) recommends midazolam (2–5 mg iv. every 7–10 min.) or diazepam (5–10 mg iv. every 3–5 min.) and/or morphine (5–10 mg iv. every 10 min.) or fentanyl (100–250 mcg iv. every 3–5 min.).

Following the withdrawal of supportive measures, the family may need time to share their feelings and have their decisions reaffirmed. Information on grief counseling should be offered to all that were involved in the person's care. Staff members should also have opportunities to debrief after withdrawing a patient from life support. Discussing reactions with coworkers can be therapeutic and lead to quality improvement initiatives.

Research Implications Regarding Care of Comatose and Brain-Dead Patients

Future research is needed to develop technology that could better assess pain perception in unconscious patients. This same technology might be applied to patients with impairments in cognition or communication as well. Currently, protocols for withdrawal of life support vary within and among institutions. Analysis of staff competencies, perceived patient comfort, and family acceptance to different protocols would support evidence-based clinical guidelines for the care of comatose and brain-dead patients. Putting the available resources of the healthcare system to the most appropriate use takes on added meaning with patients who require advanced technology for life support.

Case Study conclusion: Mrs. Cohen's case, introduced at the beginning of this chapter, is unfortunately not atypical for people with late-stage Alzheimer's disease. The physical assessment of Mrs. Cohen was unremarkable, except for stiff, inflexible muscles, arthritic changes, and the start of some contractures. Her history revealed arthritis of the hands and knees, though she currently was not taking any pain medication. Acetaminophen 500 mg was started on a twice-a-day schedule. The effect was a decrease in screaming and agitated behaviors but she still was resistant and agitated by physical contact. The television was turned off and the mobile was removed to decrease extraneous and potentially confusing environmental stimulation. Mrs. Cohen had a new activity plan that included two 10-minute sessions of friendly visiting, soft massage, and gentle range of motion, as well as music therapy for 15 minutes and pet therapy twice each week. She was also given a small silk pillow that she enjoyed feeling on her skin. Flannel sheets were applied to her bed to keep her joints warm. Mrs. Cohen was also transferred to a comfortable chair each day and ate at least one meal a day in the dining room. Though she did not participate, she watched the sing-a-long after lunch each day. Following these interventions, her appetite improved; verbalization was more coherent; her gaze often tracked events in the room; and she would smile in response to activities, such as pet therapy and massage. Her agitated behavior and repetitive vocalizations significantly decreased.

Mrs. Cohen had pain, social isolation, and boredom, and was receiving environmental stimulation that exceeded her stress threshold. All of these factors were compromising the quality of her life. Even though Mrs. Cohen was at the end of her life and would die soon, she could still engage in a range of positive activities and stay socially connected. While Mrs. Cohen did not have complex comorbid physical conditions, she clearly needed comprehensive nursing interventions to improve her comfort and quality of life.

CONCLUSION

Patients and their families who are dealing with the consequences of stroke, coma, CNDs or a diagnosis of brain death face enormous challenges and are ideal candidates for palliative care. Challenges may occur over a period of hours in the acute-care setting with immediate decisions to be made regarding prognosis and life support, or they may be experienced for years and require lifelong coping strategies. From a palliative care perspective, nurses in all settings need to combine knowledge of the disease, its trajectory, and related symptoms with appreciation of the values and goals of the patient and their family. Comfort and quality of life interventions have been found to greatly assist people to cope with an array of debilitating symptoms. While nursing spends a good deal of time focused on pain management and symptom control, nurses are also responsible for addressing the quality-of-life needs of patients who are at the end of their lives. Family members may need help learning how to avoid just sitting at the bedside in a "death watch" but rather share meaningful moments with their loved one. Family members and caregivers should still engage the person in activities designed to evoke feelings of pleasure, meaningfulness, and being socially connected. Warm conversation, music and pet therapy, massage, and activities designed to share beauty in the world and to maintain social connections should be a part of everyday life for the non-comatose patient. For families whose loved one is in a coma or determined brain-dead, palliative care nursing can provide information and support along the illness trajectory and into the bereavement period. Such support is central in assisting families to cope effectively with illness and to find strength in facing their loss.

Since patients with serious neurological problems are often not able to advocate for themselves, it is the nurses' responsibility to continue to work to improve the care delivered to this population who are nearing the end of their lives. There is a need for the profession of nursing to develop a host of evidence-based interventions to meet the palliative care needs of people with serious neurological disorders.

EVIDENCE-BASED PRACTICE

Kovach, C.R., Logan, B., Noonan, P.E., Schlidt, A.M., Smerz, J., Simpson, M., & Wells, T. (2006). Effects of the Serial Trial Intervention on discomfort and behavior in demented nursing home residents. *American Journal of Alzheimer's Disease, 21* (3), 147–155.

Research Problem. To address the problems of pain and other unmet needs in people with advanced dementia residing in nursing homes, an innovative clinical protocol, the Serial Trial Intervention (STI), was developed and tested for effectiveness. When behavior change is noted, the STI uses five sequential steps of assessment and treatment: (1) physical assessment followed by targeted treatment if indicated; (2) affective assessment followed by targeted non-pharmacological treatment if indicated; (3) non-pharmacological treatment trial; (4) analgesic treatment trial; and (5) consultation and possible trial of psychotropic medication. The STI

allows a standardized treatment to be customized to the individual's specific need.

Design. The study design was a double-blinded experiment with random assignment of matched nursing homes to treatment or control conditions.

Sample and setting. Fourteen long-term care facilities in one Midwestern state participated. There were 114 participants and all had advanced cognitive and functional impairment, had no chronic psychiatric diagnosis other than dementia associated diagnosis, and were at least 4 weeks post admission.

Methods. Discomfort and return of behavioral symptoms to baseline were assessed at pretest and 2–4 weeks post initiation of the STI. Discomfort was assessed using the observational visual analog scale called the Discomfort-Dementia of the Alzheimer's Type (Discomfort-DAT). Return of behavioral symptoms to baseline was assessed by nurse interventionists using a visual analog scale with demarcations from 0 to 100%. Nurse interventionists were staff nurses from the unit who received 7 hours of training in use of the STI. Regular protocol compliance testing was done to insure treatment fidelity.

Results. The treatment group had significantly less discomfort and agitation than the control group at post testing. The group of nurses using the STI also showed more persistence in assessing and treating participants than nurses in the control group. There was a statistically significant difference between the groups in the use of pharmacological, but not non-pharmacological, comfort treatments.

Implications for nursing practice. Results suggest that the STI is effective and that effective treatment of discomfort and agitation is possible for people with late-stage dementia. The finding that the STI increased nursing assessment, analgesic administration, and persistence of the nurse in intervening to resolve a person's troubled state is particularly encouraging given the overwhelming evidence that people with late-stage dementia are inadequately assessed and undertreated for discomfort.

Commentary. The use of an experimental design with random assignment and blinding of subject's and data collector's increases confidence in the validity of the findings. The STI intervention was completed by nurses who worked at the facility, and they were given no additional time to carry out the intervention, which may make this a feasible intervention for wide adoption in nursing homes. The STI has multiple assessment and treatment components, and this study does not allow conclusions about which parts of the STI, either separately or in combination, affected the outcomes.

Solaro, C., Brichetto, G., Battaglia, M.A., Uccelli, M.M., & Mancardi, G.L. (2005). Antiepileptic medication in multiple sclerosis: Adverse effects in a three-year follow-up study. *Neurological Sciences, 25,* 307–310.

Research problem. Neuropathic pain and paroxysmal symptoms are common in chronic neurological disorders. The purpose of this study was to evaluate prospectively the frequency of using antiepileptic medications and reported adverse events in a cohort of patients with multiple sclerosis.

Design. The study design was a longitudinal descriptive design in which data were collected for 3 years. There was a nonrandom allocation of patients to treatment arms.

Sample and setting. The study was conducted at a large neuroscience department in Genoa, Italy. During the study period, 735 patients were evaluated in 3,963 neurological evaluations.

Methods. For a period of 3 years, the rationale for prescribing antiepileptic medications, adverse events, treatment duration, and reasons for discontinuation were recorded in a database. Discontinuation due to neurological side effects was defined as a relapse presentation that included worsening of at least 1 point on the Expanded Disability Status Scale.

Results. Gabapentin was prescribed for 94 patients, with 16 experiencing adverse symptoms, of which 1 mimicked a relapse. Carbamazepine was prescribed for 36 patients, with 20 experiencing adverse symptoms, of which 12 mimicked a relapse. Lamotrigine was prescribed for 22 patients, with 4 experiencing adverse symptoms, and none mimicked a relapse.

Implications for nursing practice. In this study, carbamazepine had a significantly higher incidence of side effects, with a higher rate of discontinuation at lower dosages and episodes of worsening neurological functioning compared to gabapentin or lamotrigine. This study suggests that recognizing worsening neurological status due to medication and not disease course is important for maintaining optimal functional status.

Commentary. The use of a descriptive design without random assignment and blinding of subject's to drug conditions means that results must be interpreted cautiously. There is a need for a randomized double-blind study comparing effectiveness of drugs as well as side-effect profiles for treating neuropathic pain in people with chronic neurological disorders and stroke. The study does highlight that medication safety is a priority and that medication side effects should be considered as a potential source of deterioration in functional status for patients on these medications.

REFERENCES

ALS Association. (2004). *About ALS*. Retrieved August 6, 2008, from http://www.alsa.org/

Alzheimer's Association. (2008). *Alzheimer's disease facts and figures*. Retrieved August 14, 2008, from www.alz.org/national/documents/report alzfactsfigures2008.

American Heart Association. (2008a). *Heart disease and stroke statistics -2008 Update*. Dallas, TX: American Heart Association.

American Heart Association. (2008b). *Stroke risk factors* Retrieved August 25, 2008, from http://www.americanheart.org/presenter.jhtml?identifier = 4716.

American Academy of Neurology. (1994). *Practice parameters determining brain death in adults.*

Ancoli-Israel, S., & Cooke, J. R. (2005). Prevalence and comorbidity of insomnia and effect on functioning in elderly populations. *Journal of American Geriatrics Society, 53*(7), 264–271.

Book, D. (2007). Disorders of brain function. In C. M. Porth (Ed.), *Essentials of pathophysiology concepts of altered Health states* (pp. 823–854). Philadelphia: Lippincott Williams & Wilkens.

Broadley, S., Cheek, A., Salonikis, S., Whitham, E., Chong, V., Cardone, D., et al. (2005). Predicting prolonged dysphagia in acute stroke: The royal adelaide prognostic index for dysphagic stroke (RAPIDS). *Dysphagia, 20*(4), 303–310.

Brush, J. A., & Calkins, M. P. (2008). Environmental interventions and dementia: Enhancing mealtimes in group dining rooms. *The ASHA Leader, 13*(8), 24–25.

Cechetto, D. F., Hachinski, V., & Whitehead, S. (2008). Vascular risk factors and Alzheimer's disease. *Neurotherapeutics, 8*(5), 743–750.

Chan, D. C. (2008). Management for motor and non-motor complications in late Parkinson's disease. *Geriatrics, 63*(5), 22–27.

Chan, D., Cordato, D., & O'Rourke, F. (2008). Management for motor and non-motor complications in late Parkinson's disease. *Geriatrics, 63*(5), 22–27.

Chang, M. Y., McBride, L. A., & Ferguson, M. A. (2003). Variability in brain death determination practices in pediatric head trauma patients. *Pediatric Nerurosurgery, 39,* 7–9.

Chapman, I. M. (2007). The anorexia of aging. *Clinics In Geriatric Medicine, 23*(4), 735–756.

Chen, Y., Ryden, M. B., Feldt, K., & Savik, K. (2000). The relationship between social interaction and characteristics of aggressive, cognitive impaired nursing home residents. *American Journal of Alzheimer's Disease and Other Dementias, 15*(1), 10–17.

Crain, N. & Boyle, R. J. (2002). Pediatric brain death. *Pediatrics in Review, 23,* 222–223.

Dangond, F. (2006). *Amyotrophic lateral sclerosis*. Retrieved August 27, 2008, from http://www.emedicine.com/neuro/TOPIC14.HTM.

Davis, L. D. (2005). *Fundamentals of neurologic disease: An introductory text*. Demos Medical Publishing, LLC.

Demakis, G. J. (2007). The neuropsychology of Parkinson's disease. *Disease-A-Month, 53*(3), 152–155.

Dorsey, E. R., Constantinescu, R., Thompson, J. P., Thompson, K. M., Biglan, R. G., Holloway, K., et al. (2007). Projected number of people with Parkinson's disease in the most populous nations. *Neurology, 68*(5), 384–386.

Draper, B., Snowdon, J., Meares, S., Turner, J., Gonski, P., McMinn, B., et al. (2000). Case-controlled study of nursing home residents referred for treatment of vocally disruptive behavior. International *Psychogeriatrics, 12*(3), 333–344.

Durham, S. R., Clancy, R. R., Leuthardt, E., Sun, P., Kamerling, S., Dominguez, T., et al. (2000). CHOP Infant Coma Scale ("Infant Face Scale"): A novel coma scale for children less than two years of age. *Journal of Neurotrauma, 17*(9), 729–737.

Ertekin, C. & Aydogdu, I. (2003). Neurophysiology of swallowing. *Clinical Neurophysiology, 114*(12), 2226–2244.

Fact Sheet. (2008). Retrieved August 11, 2008, from www.parkinson.org/NETCOMMUNITY.

Frese, A., Husstedt, I. W., Ringelstein, E. B., & Evers, S. (2006). Pharmacologic treatment of central post-stroke pain. *The Clinical Journal of Pain, 22*(3), 252–260.

Gehrman, P. R., Martin, J. L., Shocat, T., Nolan, S., Corey-Bloom, J., & Ancoli-Israels., S. (2003). Sleep-disordered breathing and agitation in institutionalized adults with Alzheimer's disease. *American Journal of Geriatric Psychiatry, 11*(4), 426–433.

Gelber, D. (2002). Management of stroke-related spasticity in the long-term care setting. CNS/LTC, 1(1), 33–37.

Gessert, C. E., Mosier, M. C., Brown, E. F., & Frey, B. (2000). Tube feeding in nursing home residents with severe and irreversible cognitive impairment. *Journal of the American Geriatrics Society, 48*(12), 1593–1600.

Giacino, J. T., Ashwal, S., Childs, N., Cranford, R., Jennett, D., Katz, D. I., et al. (2002). The minimally conscious state: Definition and diagnostic criteria. *Neurology, 58*, 349–353.

Goodwin, V. A., Richards, S. H., Taylor, R. S., Taylor, A. H., & Campbell, J. L. (2008).The effectiveness of exercise interventions for people with Parkinson's disease: A systematic review and meta-analysis. *Movement Disorder, 23*(5), 631–640.

Green, A. (2008, October 24). *Neurodegenerative disorders.* Retrieved October 24, 2008 from http://www.drgreene.com/21_525.html

Greer, D. V. (2008). Variability of brain death determination guidelines in leading US neurologic institutions. *Neurology, 70*(4), 252–253.

Greer, D. M., Varelas, P. N., Haque, S., & Wijdicks, E. F. (2008). Variability of brain death determination guidelines in leading US neurologic institutions. *Neurology, 70*, 284–289.

Guidelines for the Determination of Death. (1981). Report of the medical consultants on the diagnosis of death to the President's Commission for the Study of Ethical Problems in Medicine and Biomedical and Behavioral Research. *Journal of the American Medical Association, 246*, 2184–2186.

Guidelines for the Determination of Brain Death. (1987). Pediatrics, 80(2), 298–300.

Hankey, G. J. (2005). *Stroke treatment and prevention: An evidence-based approach.* New York: Cambridge University Press.

Herbert, L., Beckett, L., Sherr, P., & Evans, D. (2001). Annual incident of Alzheimer's disease in the United States projected to the years 2000. *Alzheimer Disease and Associated Disorders, 56*, 49–56.

Heron, M. P., Hoyert, D. L., Xu, J., Scott, C., & Tejada-Vera, B. (2006). Deaths: Preliminary data for 2006. *National Vital Statistics Report, 56*(16), 1–52.

Hirtz, D., Thurman, D. J., Gwinn-Hardy, K., Mohamed, M., Chaudhuri, A. R., & Zalutsky, R., et al. (2007). How common are the "common" neurologic disorders? *Neurology, 68*(5), 326–337.

Houtchens, M. K., Benedict, R. H. B., Killiany, R., Sharma, J., Jaisani, Z., Singh, B., et al. (2007). Thalamic atrophy and cognition in multiple sclerosis. *Neurology, 69*, 1213–1223.

Hurley, A. C., Volicer, B. J., Hanrahan, P. A., Houde, S., & Volicer, L. (1992). Assessment of discomfort in advanced Alzheimer patients. *Research in Nursing and Health, 15*, 369–377.

Jackson, C. E., Lovitt, S., Gowda, N., Anderson, F., & Miller, R. (2006). Factors correlated with NPPV use in ALS. *Amyotrophic Lateral Sclerosis, 7*, 80–85.

Kelly-Hayes, M. B. (2003). The influence of gender and age on disability following ischemic stroke: The Framingham Study. *Journal of Stroke and Cerebrovascular Disease, 12*(3) 119–126.

Kleindorfer, D., Khoury, J., Kissela, B., Alwell, K., Woo D., Miller, R., et al. (2006). Temporal trends in the incidence and case fatality of stroke in children and adolescents. *Journal of Child Neurology, 21*(5), 415–418.

Kovach, C. R. (2000). Sensoristasis and imbalance in persons with dementia. *Journal of Nursing Scholarship, 32*(4), 379–384.

Kovach, C. R., Taneli, Y., Dohearty, P., Schlidt, A. M., Cashin, S., & Silva-Smith, A. (2004). Effect of the BACE (Balancing Activity Controls Excesses) Intervention on agitation of people with dementia. *The Gerontologist, 44*(6), 797–806.

Kovach, C. R., Logan, B., Noonan, P. E., Schlidt, A. M., Smerz, J., Simpson, M, et al. (2006). Effects of the serial trial intervention on discomfort and behavior in demented nursing home residents. *American Journal of Alzheimer's Disease, 21*(3), 147–155.

Kukull, W. A., LaCroix, A. Z., McCormick, W., & Larson, E. B. (2003). Exercise plus behavioral management in patients with Alzheimer disease. *Journal of the American Medical Association, 290*, 2015–2022.

Kurlan, R., Richard, I. H., Papka, M., & Marshall, F. (2000). Movement disorders in Alzheimer's disease: More rigidity of definition is needed. *Movement Disorders, 15*, 24–29.

Larson, E. B. (2004). Survival after initial diagnosis of Alzheimer disease. *Annuals of Internal Medicine, 140*(7), 501–509.

Liao, S. A. (2007). Attitudinal differences in neurodegenerative disorders. *Journal of Palliative Medicine, 10*(2), 430–432.

Lo, K., Leung, K., & Shek, A. (2007). Management of Parkinson disease: Current treatments, recent advances, and future development. *Formulary, 42*, 529–544.

Lou, J. S. (2008). Fatigue in Amyotrophic lateral sclerosis. *Physical Medicine and Rehabilitation Clinics of North America, 19*, 533–543.

Logeman, J. A., Gensler, G. Robbins, J., Lindblad, A. S., Brandt, D., Hind, J. A., et al. (2008). A randomized study of three interventions for aspiration of thin liquids in patients with dementia or Parkinson's disease. *Journal of Speech, Language, Hearing Research, 51*(1), 173–183.

Logroscino, G. A. (2007). Amyotrophic lateral sclerosis: A global threat with a possible difference in risk across ethnicities. Neurology, 68(13), E17.

Lukong, K. E., Elsliger, M., Chang, Y., Richard, C., Thomas, G., Carey, W., et al. (2000). Characterization of the sialidase molecular defects in sialidosis patients suggests the structural organization of the lysosomal multienzyme complex. *Human Molecular Genetics, 9*(7), 1075–1085.

Marik, P. E., & Kaplan, D. (2003). Aspiration pneumonia and dysphagia in the elderly. *Chest, 124*(1), 328–336.

Maloni, H. W. (2000). Pain in multiple sclerosis: An overview of its nature and management. *The Journal of Neuroscience Nursing, 32*(3), 139–144.

McGonigal-Kenney, M. L., Schutte, D. L., Adams, S., & Titler, M. G. (2006). Nonpharmacologic management of agitated behaviors in persons with Alzheimer Disease and other chronic dementing conditions. *Journal of Gerontological Nursing, 32*(2), 9–14.

McCormack, A. L., Thiruchelvam, M., Manning-Bog, A. B., Thiffault, C., Langston, J. W., Cory-Slechta, C., et al. (2002). Environmental risk factors and Parkinson's disease: Selective degeneration of Nigral Dopaminergic neurons caused by the herbicide Paraquat. *Neurobiology of Disease, 10*(2), 119–127.

Meek, C., Pollock, A., Potter, J., & Langhorne, P. (2003). A systematic review of exercise trials post stroke. *Clinical Rehabilitation, 7*(1), 6–13.

Miller, R. G. (2001). Examining the evidence about treatment in ALS/MND. *Amyotrophic Lateral Sclerosis and Other Motor Neuron Disorders, 2*, 3–7.

Minden, S. L. (2000). Mood disorders in multiple sclerosis: Diagnosis and treatment. *Journal of Neurology, 6* (Suppl. 2), S160–S167.

Mitchell, S. L., Kiely, D., Miller, S., Connor, S., Spence, C., Teno, J., et al. (2007). Hospice care for patients with dementia. *Journal of Pain and Symptom Management, 34*(1), 7–16.

Mitsumoto, H., Davidson, M. Moore, D., Gad, N., Brandis, M. Ringel, S., et al. (2003). Percutaneous endoscopic gastrostomy (PEG). In patients with ALS and bulbar dysfunction. *Amyotrophic Lateral Sclerosis and Other Motor Neuron Disorders, 4*(3), 177–185.

National Hospice Organization. (1996). *Medical guidelines for determining prognosis in selected non-cancer diseases* (2nd ed.). Arlington, VA: National Hospice Organization.

National Institute of Neurological Disorders and Stroke. (2007, February 12). *Coma and Persistent Vegetative State.* Retrieved August 17, 2008, from http://www.ninds.nih.gov/disorders/coma/coma.htm.

National Institute of Neurological Disorders and Stroke. (2008a, February 7). *Amyotrophic Lateral Sclerosis.* Retrieved August 17, 2008, from http://www.ninds.nih.gov/disorders/amyotrophiclateralsclerosis/amyotrophiclateralsclerosis.htm#What_is_the_prognosis.

National Institute of Neurological Disorders and Stroke. (2008b, August 13). *Multiple sclerosis: Hope through research.* Retrieved August 17, 2008, from http://www.ninds.nih.gov/disorders/multiple_sclerosis/detail_multiple_sclerosis.htm#126133215.

National Institute of Neurological Disorders and Stroke. (2008c, August 1). *Parkinson's Disease: Hope through research.* Retrieved August 15, 2008, from http://www.ninds.nih.gov/disorders/parkinsons_disease/detail_parkinsons_disease.htm#71273159.

National Multiple Sclerosis Society. (2008, August 1). *How many people have MS.* Retrieved August 1, 2008, from http://www.nationalmssociety.org/about-multiple-sclerosis/FAQs-about-MS/index.aspx#howmany.

Nestor, S. R. (2008). Ventricular enlargement as a possible measure of Alzheimer's disease progression validated using the Alzheimer's disease neuroimaging initiative database. *Brain, 131*(9), 2443–2454.

Oken, B. S., Flegal, K., Zajdel, D., Kishiyama, S. S., Lovera, J., Bagert, B., et al. (2006). Cognition and fatigue in multiple sclerosis: Potential effects of medications with central nervous system activity. *Journal of Rehabilitation Research and Development, 43*(1), 83–90.

O'Connor, A. B., Schwid, S. R., Herrmann, D. N., Markman, J. D., & Dworkin, R. H. (2008). Pain associated with multiple sclerosis: systematic review and proposed classification. *Pain, 137*(1), 96–111.

Ostwald, S. K., Wasserman, J., & Davis, S. (2006). Medications, Co-morbidities, and medical complications in stroke survivors: the CAReS study. *Rehabilitation Nursing, 13*(1), 10–14.

Parkinson's Disease Foundation. (2008). *Parkinson's disease: An overview.* Retrieved August 27, 2008, from http://www.pdf.org/AboutPD/.

Pendergast, T. (2002). Palliative care in the intensive care unit setting. In A. Berger, R., Portenoy, & D. Weissman (Eds.), *Principles and practice of palliative care and supportive oncology* (2nd ed., pp. 1086–1104). Philadelphia: Lippincott Williams & Wilkins.

Pfeiffer, R. F. (2000). Gastrointestinal dysfunction in Parkinson's disease. *Clinical Neuroscience, 5*, 136–146.

Porth, C. (2007). Disorders of neuromuscular function. In C. M. Porth (Ed.), *Essentials of pathophysiology concepts of altered health states* (pp. 787–821). Philadelphia: Lippincott Williams & Wilkins.

Potyk, D. (2005). Treatments for Alzheimer disease. *Southern Medical Journal, 98*(6), 628–635.

Price, C., & Pandyan, A. (2001). Electrical stimulation for preventing and treating post-stroke shoulder pain: A systematic Cochrane review. *Clinical Rehabilitation, 15*, 5–19.

RamachandranNair, R., Sharma, R., Weiss, S., & Cortez, M. (2005). Reactive EEG patterns in pediatric coma. *Pediatric Neurology, 33*(5),345–349.

Reilly, P., Simpson, O., Sprod, R., & Thomas L. (1988). Assessing the conscious level in infants and young children: A pediatric version of Glasgow Coma Scale. *Child's Nervous System, 4*, 30–33.

Richert, J. R. (1999). Demyelinating illness. In W. N. Kelly (Ed.), *Textbook of internal medicine* (pp. 2385–2388). Philadelphia: J.B. Lippincott.

Riise, T., Nortvedt, M. W., & Ascherio,A. (2003). Smoking is a risk factor for multiple sclerosis. *Neurology, 61*, 1122–1124.

Rosamond, W. D., Folsom, A. R., Chambless, L. E., Wang, C., McGovern, P. G., Howard, G., et al. (1999). Stroke incidence and survival among middle-aged adults 9-year follow-up of the atherosclerosis risk in communities (ARIC) cohort. *Stroke, 30*, 736–743.

Rubenfeld, G., & Crawford, S. (2001). Principles and practices of withdrawing life-sustaining treatment in the ICU. In J. Curtis & G. Rubenfeld (Eds.), *Managing death in the intensive care unit* (pp. 127–147). New York: Oxford University Press.

Santavuori, P., Lauronen, L., Kirveskari, E., Åberg, L., Sainio, K., & Autti, T., et al. (2000). Neuronal ceroid lipofuscinoses in childhood. *Neurological Sciences, 21*(Suppl.t 1), S35–S41.

Sclan, S. G. & Reisberg, B. R. (1992). Functional assessment staging (FAST) in Alzheimer's disease: Reliability, validity and ordinality. *International Psychogeriatrics, 4*, 55–69.

Shagam, J. Y. (2008). Unlocking the secrets of Parkinson disease. *Radiologic Technology, 79*(3), 227–239.

Shapiro, J., & Downe, L. (2003).The evaluation and management of swallowing disorders in the elderly, *Geriatric Times, 4*(6). Retrieved August 25, 2008, from www.cmellc.com/geriatrictimes/g031217.html.

Siderowf, A. D. (2007). *The emerging role of neuroprotection in Parkinson's disease.* Retrieved August 27, 2008, from http://www.medscape.com/viewprogram/8418.

Simon, R. (2000). Coma and disorders of arousal. In L. Goldman (Ed.), *Cecil textbook of medicine* (21st ed., pp. 2023–2026). Philadelphia: Saunders.

Solaro, C., Brichetto, G., Battaglia, M. A., Uccelli, M. M., & Mancardi, G. L. (2005). Antiepileptic medication in multiple sclerosis: Adverse effects in a three-year follow-up study. *Neurological Sciences, 25*, 307–310.

Staub, F., & Bogousslavsky, J. (2001) Fatigue after stroke: A major but neglected issue. *Cerebrovascular Diseases, 12*, 75–81.

Studenski, S., Lai, S. M., Duncan, P. W., & Rigler, S. K. (2004). The impact of self-reported cumulative comorbidity on stroke recovery. *Age and Aging, 33*(2), 195–198.

Subramanian, S., & Surani, S. (2007). Sleep disorders in the elderly. *Geriatrics, 62*(12), 10–16, 32.

Swierzewski, S. (2000). *Amyotrophic Lateral Sclerosis/Lou Gehrig's Disease.* Retrieved August 17, 2008, from http://www.neurologychannel.com/als/index.shtml.

Tsai, P. F., & Chang, J. Y. (2004). Assessment of pain in elders with dementia. *Medsurg Nursing, 13*(6), 364–370.

Teasdale, G., & Jennet, B. (1974). Assessment of coma and impaired consciousness: A practical scale. *Lancet, 2*, 81–84.

Teri, L., Gibbons, L. E., McCurry, S. M., Logsdon, R. G., Buchner, D. M., Barlow, W. E., Kukull, W. A., et al. (2003). Exercise plus behavioral management in patients with Alzheimer disease. *Journal of the American Medical Association, 290*, 2015–2022

Truog, R., Cist, A., Brackett, S., Burns, J., Curley, M., Danis, M., et al. (2001). Recommendations for end-of-life care in the intensive care unit: the Ethics Committee of the Society of Critical Care Medicine. *Critical Care Medicine, 29*, 2332–2348.

U.S. Department of Health and Human Services. (2005). Progress report on Alzheimer's disease 2004–2005. New discoveries, new insights. (NIH Publication No. 05-5724). Retrieved August 14, 2008, from www.ajnonline.com/pt/re/ajn/fulltext.00000446-200612000-00018.

van der Steen, J., Mehr, D. R., Druse, R. L., Ribbe, M. W., & Van Der Wal, G. (2007). Treatment strategy and risk of functional decline and mortality after nursing-home acquired lowered respiratory tract infection: Two prospective studies in residents with dementia. *International Journal of Geriatric Psychiatry, 22*, 1013–1019.

Verkaik, R., Nuyen, J., Schellevis, F., & Francke, A. (2007). The relationship between severity of Alzheimer's disease and prevalence of comorbid depressive symptoms and depression: A systematic review. *International Journal of Geriatric Psychiatry, 22*, 1063–1086.

Vestergaard, K., Anderson, G., Gottrup, H., Kristensen, B. T., & Jensen, T. S. (2002). Lamotrigine for central post stroke pain: A randomized controlled trial. *Neurology, 56*, 184–190.

Volicer, L., Harper, D. G., Manning, B. C., Goldstein, R., & Satlin, A. (2001). Sundowning and circadian rhythms in Alzheimer's disease. *American Journal of Psychiatry, 158*, 704–711.

von Gunten, C., & Weissman, D. (2001). *Fast facts and concepts #34: Symptom control for ventilator withdrawal in the dying patient.* Retrieved from ww.eperc.mcw.edu.

Walsh, K. (2001). Management of shoulder pain in patients with stroke. *Postgraduate Medical Journal, 77*, 645–649.

Westergren, A., Ohlsson, O., & Hallberg, I. R. (2002). Eating difficulties in relation to gender, length of stay, and discharge to institutional care, among patients in stroke rehabilitation. *Disability and Rehabilitation, 24*(10), 523–533.

White, G. N., O'Rouke, F., Ong, B. S., Cordato, D. J., & Chan, D. K. (2008). Dysphagia: Causes, assessment, treatment, and management. *Geriatrics, 63*(5), 15–20.

Wilson, R. S., Bennett, D. A., Gilley, D. W., Beckett, L. A., Schneider, J. A., & Evans, D. A., et al. (2000). Progression of Parkinsonian signs in Alzheimer's disease. *Neurology, 54*, 1284–1289.

Wheaton, M. W., Salamone, A. R., Mosnik, S. M., McDonald, R. P., Appel, S. H., Schmolck, H. H., et al. (2007). Cognitive impairment in familial ALS. *Neurology, 69*, 1411–1417.

Yaari, R., & Corey-Bloom, J. (2007). Alzheimer's disease. *Seminars in Neurology, 27*(1), 32–41.

Yetimalar, Y., Gurgor, N., & Basoglu, M. (2004). Clinical efficacy of gabapentin for paroxysmal symptoms in multiple sclerosis. *Acta Neurologica Scandinavica, 109*(6), 430–431.

16

End-Stage Renal Disease

Lynn Noland

Key Points

- The incidence and prevalence of end-stage renal disease (ESRD) is increasing as the population ages, the median age of occurrence being 65 years.
- Patients with ESRD have a high symptom burden and often have multiple comorbid conditions.
- Patients with ESRD have a shortened life expectancy with a 5-year survival probability of 38%—which is worse then that of most cancer diagnoses.
- The rate of palliative care and hospice use by patients with ESRD is around 10%, well below that of the general population.

Case Study: Gene lost his renal function from hypertensive nephrosclerosis. Years of poor blood pressure control caused irreversible scarring of the kidneys and finally end-stage renal disease (ESRD). He initially declined dialysis because he simply could not see how, at age 62, he could tolerate being tied to any sort of technologic life support, but later agreed to a trial of dialysis. He would ultimately spend 10 years on dialysis.

He and his family adjusted to the 4-hour treatments three times a week. His wife became an expert in managing the various aspects of therapy required to compensate for loss of renal function. Both were kind and supportive to the other patients undergoing dialysis at the same time. They were deeply religious people who brought a sense of grace and peace to the dialysis setting.

Late one August, Gene told his family and the dialysis staff that he could no longer tolerate dialysis. His feelings were understandable but emotionally difficult to accept. Because of progressive severe peripheral vascular disease, he had begun to experience constant pain. The cause of the increasingly intense pain seemed to have been related to a revision of his hemodialysis graft, which necessitated stopping the coumadin that he took to treat chronic deep venous thrombosis (DVT). As his prothrombin ratio (PR) and international normalized ratio (INR) drifted into a non-therapeutic range, he began having problems with thrombosis and leg pain that did not resolve even after the coumadin was resumed. Soon, he was no longer able to participate in church and family events, and this made his quality of life unacceptable to him. Each time he had to come in for dialysis, he experienced more pain

than was tolerable and he was now wheelchair-bound with leg and foot ulcerations from ischemia. It became clear from his lab values that he was not eating adequately (albumin 3.1 g/dl; BUN 30 mg/dl; PO_4 3.0 mg/dl—these values should be higher in patients undergoing dialysis).

After extensive discussion with Gene and his wife, the dialysis care team arranged for him to be seen by palliative car. Gene, his wife, and I went to the appointment. The doctor skillfully questioned him about what he found intolerable about his current situation. He determined that Gene was not amenable to amputation, which was the definitive treatment for intractable leg pain, and that his pain and subsequent inactivity were the reasons for his desire to withdraw support. He was offered a trial of several different types of pain control medications, including oxycontin and fentanyl lozenges for breakthrough pain. Gene agreed to try these therapies for 1 month. If there was no relief at the end of that period, he wanted to withdraw from treatment. He also said that he only wanted to dialyze twice weekly. All understood and sadly agreed.

Miraculously, by the end of the month, the pain, with the help of powerful analgesics, had lessened greatly. Circulation to his legs also improved sufficiently for the ulcers to begin to heal. Gene was able to resume some of his church and family activities. He even decided to dialyze three times weekly. A good prognostic indicator was that his appetite and his lab values improved. Unfortunately, in a short period of time Gene's medical problems would take a turn for the worse and withdrawal from dialysis with hospice care would become necessary.

Introduction

A diagnosis of end-stage renal disease (ESRD) is an ominous diagnosis, which means a patient has severe end organ kidney damage and failure. ESRD is the final renal outcome of stage-5 chronic kidney disease (CKD). Stage-5 CKD is defined as a glomerular filtration rate (GFR) of 0–15 ml/min, normal GFR being 60–90 ml/min depending on age and race. GFR is a measurement that is calculated from the serum creatinine level and is the accepted method of measuring kidney function. In ESRD, pathology is so extensive that the normally resilient kidneys finally reach a point where they no longer function well enough to remove fluid, balance electrolytes, stimulate red blood cell production, or accomplish the myriad other physical and chemical processes necessary to sustain life (Exhibit 16.1). ESRD requires renal replacement therapy in the form of dialysis or

transplantation, or death will occur within a relatively short time, usually 10–20 days.

The nursing care of ESRD patients is complex, as they typically have multiple disabling comorbidities that result in often serious complications. Most of the comorbidities such as the different forms that vascular disease can take, e.g., myocardial infarction (MI), stroke, hypertension, or the end organ complications of diabetes, can result in life-changing disability and premature death. Given that the mortality rate for patients with ESRD is high (23% per year) and death often does not occur before a spiral of worsening symptoms and chronic overall decline, the care challenges that family and staff face are substantial.

When confronted with the extensive list of medical and psychological problems of ESRD patients, the temptation for healthcare professionals is to focus primarily on correcting laboratory values or on the numerous

EXHIBIT 16.1: FUNCTIONS OF THE KIDNEYS

1) Maintenance of chemical and water equilibrium. The kidneys regulate the volume of fluid in the body and its osmolarity, electrolyte content, and acidity by varying urine excretion of ions and water. Electrolytes that are excreted or preserved by the kidneys include sodium, potassium, chloride, calcium, magnesium, and phosphate. Numerous functions in the body are dependent upon maintenance of optimal body fluid composition and volume such as
   i. Cardiac output
   ii. Blood pressure
   iii. Most enzymes in the body, which function best within a narrow range of pH
   iv. K+ concentration, which directly affects cell membrane potentials
   v. Membrane excitability, which depends on calcium concentration in the body fluid.
2) Excretion of metabolic end products and foreign substances. The kidneys excrete metabolic end products such as urea and creatinine as well as the end products of metabolized drugs and toxins.
3) Production and secretion of enzymes and hormones.
   a. Renin is a catalyst in the formation of angiotensin and is a potent vasoconstrictor that is involved in sodium balance and blood pressure regulation.
   b. Erythropoietin stimulates the maturation of erythrocytes in the bone marrow and when absent causes anemia of chronic renal disease.
   c. 1,25-Dihydroxyvitamin D3 is a steroid that is integral in parathyroid hormone function and in regulating calcium and phosphorus in the body (Schena, 2001).

physical manifestations of ESRD. Not surprisingly, this approach is too simplistic, resulting in less than satisfactory outcomes. The goal for patients with ESRD cannot be simply to preserve life but also to promote quality of life. These two goals can be in conflict and can certainly add to the complexity of care. The broader goal that incorporates quality of life necessitates a holistic team oriented with shared decision-making approach, the importance of which will be discussed later in the chapter. It is this approach that should prevail throughout the course of ESRD up to and including end-of-life care.

In this chapter, palliative care will be discussed in relation to two groups of patients: ESRD patients who are being treated with ongoing dialysis, and ESRD patients who are not being treated with dialysis either because they have decided not to have treatment or they want dialysis treatment withdrawn. Quality of life is crucial for both groups.

INCIDENCE AND PREVALENCE

The occurrence of ESRD has reached almost epidemic proportions. In the United States in 2007, the incidence rate was 106,000 new cases per year or 11/2 times the 1988 rate with a tripling of the prevalence rate to 341,000 combined peritoneal and hemodialysis patients. The median age of onset of adult ESRD was 64.6 years, and not surprisingly the highest rate of occurrence was in the 45–64 year age group (36.9%) with incidence rates increasing in all age groups. As expected, ESRD rates are being driven up proportionate to the overall rate of increase in kidney disease (USRDS, 2007). The scope of the problem is massive given that an estimated 15.5 million adults age 20 or greater (7.69% of adult population) have evidence of chronic kidney disease defined as moderate to severe reduction in GFR (Coresh, Stevens, & Levey, 2008) It is believed that a substantial number of these patients will progress to ESRD. The increase in ESRD is also of concern for economic reasons, as it is the only disease entity in the United States that is reimbursed primarily with public funds. Medicare pays for 80% of all costs of care for patients diagnosed with ESRD. This averages around 60,000 dollars per patient per year (USRDS, 2007).

The increase in ESRD is not simply a health problem of the United States. In 2001, it was estimated that the global maintenance dialysis population was just over 1 million, which is increasing at approximately 7% per year. One author states "If current trends in ESRD prevalence continue, as seems probable, the [world] ESRD population will exceed 2 million patients by the year 2010. The care of this group represents a major societal commitment: the aggregate cost of treating ESRD during the coming decade will exceed $1 trillion globally, a thought-provoking sum by any economic metric" (Lysaght, 2002).

Even though ESRD is an international health problem, dialysis is predominantly a phenomenon of highly industrialized societies, with the United States, Great Britain, and Japan accounting for almost 80% of all dialysis treatments worldwide. Developing nations cannot begin to afford the price tag attached to providing renal replacement therapy when access to basic food and shelter is a daily challenge (Iglehart, 1993).

To understand the societal scope of the problem, it is important to look at more than incidence and prevalence rates. Survival statistics for ESRD are informative as well. Although the lifespan of a particular individual with ESRD cannot be reliably known, survival data are eye-opening for the group as a whole. The 5-year survival rate for the ESRD dialysis population is 32% (USRDS, 2007), which is worse than the 5-year survival rate for many cancer diagnoses including breast cancer (90%), colon cancer (65%), and melanoma (90%). The death rate among ESRD patients is only slightly lower than the deadliest cancer killers (lung, liver, and pancreas) (SEER, 2007). Compared to the general population, ESRD patients live about one third as long as individuals without ESRD of the same age and gender (Henrich, 2004). In summary, statistics points to the reality that ESRD patients have a shortened life expectancy, thus solidifying the argument that palliative care should be a commonplace consideration for this patient population.

PATHOGENESIS

ESRD can be caused by any disease process that can damage the kidney; however, some diseases are more likely than others to cause irreversible damage and kidney failure. We know that glomerular diseases are the primary cause of ESRD but the reason why diseases cause glomerular destruction still remains unclear. The cause can be diseases that originate in the kidney, or they can be diseases in which kidney involvement is part of a systemic disorder that involves other organs and tissues (Brenner & Rector, 2007). The most common etiologies are diabetes, hypertension, glomerulernephritis, autoimmune diseases, lupus, and HIV. There are other causes, but they make up a fraction of the etiology of ESRD.

Almost 44% of all adult patients are on dialysis because of diabetes. Another 27% are being dialyzed because of uncontrolled hypertension. Sadly, in the case of both these diseases, i.e., diabetes and hypertension, if they had been treated aggressively in the early onset phase of the disease, most patients would not end up losing their kidney function. Given that diabetes accounts for almost 505 of the cases of ESRD, the really alarming statistic is that the incidence of diabetes is increasing exponentially worldwide. Recent statistics setsw the rate of diabetes at 578 per million population or slightly over 5% of the population (Center for Disease Control, 2007).

The underlying renal pathology of ESRD varies according to the etiology. For example, in the case of diabetic kidney disease, the renal lesion includes changes in the afferent and efferent arteries, tubular fibrosis, and thickening of the basement membrane with impingement on the filtration surfaces of the glomerulus. These changes progress as hyperglycemia persists and the resultant proteinuria contributes to hyperfiltration and high GFR and ultimately GFR decline (Johnson & Feehally, 2004). Each disorder that causes ESRD will have a different histopathologic look, but all will have one thing in common; i.e., sufficient destruction of the nephron in one form or another which, if left unchecked, will cause cellular death and ESRD.

In the pediatric population, the most common diagnoses that lead to ESRD differ from those of adults. They include, in order of frequency, glomerular nephritis (GN), vasculitis, and familial cystic disease, with GN having the best prognosis. The mortality rate for children regardless of cause is 55.3 per 1,000 patient years, which is better than that of adults (226 per 1,000 patient years); however, the most recent statistics demonstrate a lack of progress in the 5-year survival rate for children. As with adults, the most common cause of death for children with ESRD was cardiovascular disease, at 23.4% (USRDS, 2007).

DISEASE TRAJECTORY

We know, after 30 + years of caring for ESRD patients treated with renal replacement therapy, that the disease trajectory involves brief stable periods followed by intervals of steady decline, and death usually within 5 years of starting dialysis (Holley, 2007). The explanation for this compressed life span includes several speculative considerations and, truthfully, no concrete conclusions. There is simply not enough research available on patients undergoing dialysis at this time to pinpoint the reason for their high death rate.

What is clear is that ESRD patients commonly experience an acceleration of many disease processes found in the general population. For example, the most common cause of ESRD is diabetes, a disease wrought with complications and a prognosis of early disability and death. If ESRD is added to the diabetic milieu, the diabetic patient's life span is even more shortened. Additionally, ESRD patients most often die from atherosclerosis and myocardial infarction, which are present at a several fold higher rate of occurrence in patients with ESRD than in the age-matched non-ESRD population (Sarnak & Levey, 2000). The problem is illustrated by an early paper on the incidence of atherosclerotic cardiovascular disease (ASCVD) in dialysis patients. On postmortem examination of 106 consecutive dialysis patients, 86% had some degree of evidence of ASCVD regardless of age, 36% had acute cardiovascular events of some type as cause of death, with 15% dying of MI (Anasari, Kampke, Miller, & Barbari, 1993).

Other reasons exist as well for low survival rates in ESRD. It is well documented that patients on dialysis are immune-suppressed and therefore more prone to serious infection (Hauser et al., 2008), develop genitourinary tumors at a disproportionate rate (Mandyam & Shahinian, 2008), and are considered to be in a constant prothrombotic/pro-inflammatory state (Heinrich, 2004). ESRD patients also develop bone disease and complications such as calciphylaxis due to disorders in calcium, phosphorous, and parathyroid hormone levels, which result in disability and premature death. These are only a few examples of why the lives of patients with ESRD are shortened and wrought with disability.

If you are an ESRD provider, disability and death are seen as frequent and expected occurrences. Although a grim fact, this knowledge can serve the useful purpose of guiding the healthcare team and patients to make more appropriate therapy decisions that prioritize the desire to preserve quality of life and not simply extend life. In fact, the poor prognostic picture associated with ESRD adds to the justification for a conservative treatment approach for many patients. Excluding those patients who have the option of a living donor kidney transplant, the most realistic way for clinicians to think about ESRD is as a chronic disabling, if not terminal, disease for which palliative care may often be the most effective form of therapy. A palliative care approach places appropriate emphasis on symptom management, preservation of quality of life, as well as quality of the dying process. This should not preclude an aggressive treatment approach when it is warranted, however. Because ESRD is a chronic disease characterized by early disability and death, it is appropriate to describe the dying trajectory as well.

Dying Trajectory

As expected, the dying trajectory for ESRD patients is characterized by symptoms of uremia, a term that literally means urine in the blood. Toxins that the kidney normally eliminates, such as urea, excess phosphorous, potassium, acids, hormonal and protein by-prod ucts, sodium, and water, begin to accumulate. Symptoms from this abnormal systemic state cause discomfort as fluid and toxins build up. For example, if dying ESRD patients are volume-overloaded, dyspnea is almost certain. Knowing this, palliative care providers encourage fluid restriction and recommend that fluids be given only to provide comfort from thirst and dry mouth.

Uremic pruritus can become unbearable, and treatment should be used liberally. See palliative care issues section in this chapter on pruritus for specific treatment. Anorexia, nausea, vomiting, and diarrhea are common and should be treated symptomatically as described in other sections of the text. Hyperkalemia commonly occurs and can be the ultimate cause of death. Hyperkalemia first results in hyperreflexia and muscle fasciculation, eventually progressing to muscle weakness, paralysis, cardiotoxicity, and finally death as cells are no longer able to sustain normal electrical activity. One rare but significant symptom that can cause discomfort is hypothermia and should be treated symptomatically with warm blankets and heating pad (Henrich, 2004).

The final phase of the ESRD dying trajectory is due to the effect of uremic toxins on the brain causing mental and behavioral changes. Memory deficits including amnesia, accompanied by lethargy and drowsiness, are common early symptoms. Gait disturbances, paresthesias, organic psychosis, and finally coma can be seen in the later stages of dying. Families are benefited greatly by being informed prior to the occurrence of these symptoms of their possibility (Henrich, 2004).

COMMON SIGNS AND SYMPTOMS

Early in the course of chronic kidney disease (CKD), there may be few if any noticeable symptoms of disease much less evidence of failure. Patients adjust to the gradual onset of symptoms that occur as a result of an underlying chronic disease process such as diabetes or hypertension that can ultimately result in ESRD. In fact, progression to ESRD is often so insidious that patients do not realize that they have kidney disease until it is quite advanced. It is commonly revealed for the first time when patients have laboratory work done for other purposes. Even after diagnosis of CKD, the movement to ESRD can be so gradual that patients may be unaware of how badly they feel until they are dialyzed for several weeks and symptoms of uremia subside. Symptoms increase in severity as renal function (GFR) decreases. Different patients develop symptoms at varying GFRs. Amazingly, many patients do not develop life-limiting symptoms of chronic kidney disease until their GFR is around 10 ml/min or the point at which they have lost 90% of their kidney function. Patients who are under-dialyzed or who have opted to stop dialysis will develop the manifestations of uremia found in the second list below. Signs and symptoms include the following:

Early Signs and Symptoms
Hyperparathyroidism
Anemia
Hypertension
Leg cramps, joint pain, gout, arthritis, muscular pains, muscle weakness
Pitting edema
Gains in weight with fluid retention
Weakness and fatigue

Late Signs and Symptoms (Uremic Indicators)
Dry scaly skin and pruritus
Frequent headaches
Heat or cold intolerance
Ammonia or urine smell to breath
Metallic taste in mouth causing food to taste different
Poor healing of cuts, abrasions
Chest pain or palpitations
Dyspnea, orthopnea, paroxysmal nocturnal dyspnea
Pericardial friction rub
Easy bruising, purpura, bleeding
Loss or gain in weight
Anorexia
Nausea and vomiting
Fainting, seizures, peripheral neuropathy, decreased concentration and memory, mood swings and depression
Grayish-bronze skin color with underlying pallor, uremic frost
Coma, death (Henrich, 2004)

COMORBIDITIES AND COMPLICATIONS

This section combines comorbidities and complications of ESRD, as they are intimately connected. Proper management of both determines life expectancy and quality of life for ESRD patients. Comorbidities and complications associated with ESRD develop because as the kidneys are no longer able to fulfill their function, problems become compounded. Treatments of ESRD (including dialysis) are simply imperfect replacements for the kidneys, a point that is difficult for patients to grasp. Patients often think that dialysis can replace all of the kidney's function.

Most of the comorbidities of ESRD are present for years before the kidneys fail completely. This is important because early identification and treatment of comorbid conditions by a nephrology team can often delay ESRD and, when dialysis is required, help the patient arrive at that point in reasonably good health. Early referral can save kidneys and prolong lives as well as ward off or delay debilitating complications. Only 25% of adults and 40% of pediatric ESRD patients have pre-ESRD care by a nephrologist (USRDS, 2008). This is important because aggressive treatment of hyperglycemia, hypertension, anemia, bone disease, and lipid disorders, prior to the onset of ESRD improves survival statistics and nephrologists are aware of this and motivated to act accordingly.

The greater the number and severity of the comorbidities, the lower the survival rate; for example, diabetes mellitus effectively ages a dialysis patient by a decade (Henrich, 2004). Consider that an adult with CKD alone has a relative risk of dying of 2 1/2 as compared to an adult with CKD, diabetes, and congestive heart failure, who has a relative risk of dying 7, a greater than twofold higher probability (USRDS, 2008).

The age of the patient also plays a role in the type of complications and their outcomes. Both children and older patients with ESRD present special challenges because of the unique comorbid conditions and ESRD-related complications that are superimposed upon the normal anatomic and physiologic changes associated with those age groups. For example, patients with ESRD almost universally have growth failure, often necessitating the use of growth hormone, which has complications associated with it. Disease management for pediatric ESRD patients is also so specialized that adult nephrologists are often ill prepared to care for this age group. A distinct subspecialty has grown up for this reason. Elders often have age-related complications in addition to their ESRD complications as well; for example, they may have age-related osteoporosis as well as bone disease associated with ESRD or cognitive effects of aging that make following treatment regimens even more challenging than they already are.

Finally, one of the most controllable causes of complications in ESRD is adequacy of dialysis treatment. The care team typically has the capability to increase the quality of dialysis for almost every patient. Research has shown that dialysis adequacy can be estimated using a formula based on pre- and post-treatment blood urea and nitrogen (BUN) levels and that there is an optimal level of dialysis that should be achieved. If patients have inadequate dialysis, they are more prone to develop many of the complications associated with uremia such as infection, anemia, and overall poor quality of life. Dialysis adequacy is improved when patients have functional dialysis vascular access, receive their full treatment every time as scheduled, and are dialyzed with the correct size artificial kidney for the correct amount of time, just to name a few of the variables that need to be considered.

A brief review of the major comorbidities and complications associated with ESRD and their palliative treatment options follows. Treatment of these problems would be appropriate for patients who are continuing dialysis. If a decision is made to withhold or withdraw dialysis, then it would not be reasonable to treat most of the conditions discussed in this section. Treatment would then move into a hospice mode using appropriate palliative options to promote a compassionate death.

Disorders of Calcium, Phosphorous, and Bone

The calcium phosphorous imbalance associated with ESRD is responsible for many of the most discouraging and disabling complications that these patients have to face. The most common calcium-phosphorous disorder is a type of bone disease referred to as renal osteodystrophy (RO). RO is the result of the effects of secondary hyperparathyroidism or hyperparathyroidism that arises initially not from pathology of the glands themselves but as a result of another disease process. Hyperparathyroidism often begins to develop when the GFR is 50–70 ml/min, which is very early in the course of renal failure. Certain factors rev up the parathyroid glands which mostly exist to secrete parathyroid hormone (PTH) to maintain serum calcium levels in a tight range. The factors that cause this upregulation of the parathyroid glands in ESRD include hypocalcemia, diminished circulating levels of activated vitamin D (calcitriol), and phosphate retention.

Why does this triad of events occur? First, serum calcium levels fall as pathologic changes associated with kidney failure cause retention of phosphorous. The high levels of serum phosphorous cause calcium to complex with the phosphorous and become less available to the cells. This upregulates the parathyroid glands to secrete PTH, which stimulates calcium retention and normally reabsorption by the kidney. However, the diseased kidney cannot retain calcium, so the feedback system fails to accomplish the goal of raising serum calcium levels.

Another major cause of secondary hyperparathyroidism is that calcitriol or activated vitamin D decreases. Calcitriol is synthesized in the kidney and acts on cells in the parathyroid gland to reduce PTH synthesis when there is adequate calcium absorption. So the normal response to low serum calcium would be to upregulate calcitriol. Unfortunately, in uremia, calcitriol is less available (cannot be synthesized), and the calcitriol receptors in the parathyroid glands become reduced in number and less sensitive to calcitriol. The combination of low calcium levels and insufficient calcitriol then cause the parathyroids to produce more PTH.

Further, hyperphosphatemia, which occurs in late stage CKD and ESRD, directly stimulates PTH secretion. Without medical and dietary intervention, these events cause the glands to enlarge and continue to pour out PTH. The constant, high levels of PTH cause calcium to be leeched from the bone thereby causing the unique form of bone thinning and weakening seen in ESRD referred to as RO (Henrich, 2004). It is a complex cycle that requires aggressive intervention, or quality of life becomes drastically reduced as bone pain, fractures, and decreased mobility occur.

One of the most devastating complications of the calcium-phosphorous imbalance associated with ESRD is metastatic calcification or calciphylaxis. Prolonged elevation of PTH, as well as calcium-phosphorus complexing, leads to calcium-phosphorous being deposited in blood vessels, tissues, organs, and joints. In severe cases, the calcium deposits inflame the conjunctiva and produce palpable deposits under the skin that can become infected and cause tissue breakdown. This can be extraordinarily painful and is difficult to treat.

The best treatment for calciphylaxis is prevention, which involves maintaining calcium and phosphorus balance through diet and the use of phosphate binders (drugs like Tums and Renagel that are taken with food). Foods high in phosphorus include dairy products, meats, legumes, nuts, whole-grain breads and cereals, and many soft drinks. Parathyroid levels can also be maintained in goal ranges with the use of synthetic activated vitamin D (calcitriol). In severe cases where the glands are hypertrophied from continued stimulation because serum phosphorus levels have been high for a period of time and have become desensitized to synthetic calcitriol, parathyroidectomy becomes the treatment of choice. This is a last resort, however, because postoperative complication of parathyroidectomy, hypocalcemia, can be life-threatening and a treatment challenge for months after surgery (Henrich, 2004)

Anemia of Chronic Renal Disease

Insufficient production of the hormone erythropoietin by the kidneys is the most common cause of anemia in patients with renal disease. Without treatment, the hematocrit will often range from 18 to 24%. Before the advent of commercially manufactured erythropoietin, dialysis patients were frequently transfused with blood products, exposing them to bloodborne diseases, transfusion reactions, viral infections, iron overload, and immune sensitization. The development of injectable erythropoietin was obviously a tremendous breakthrough in the treatment of anemia of renal disease.

Treatment of anemia with erythropoietin should begin as soon as it is diagnosed, and almost all ESRD patients require it to maintain their hematocrit and to avoid complications associated with anemia. For example, adequate anemia management can help prevent left ventricular hypertrophy (LVH), the development of which increases morbidity and mortality for all patients. When the hemoglobin concentration drops below 10 g/dl, patients are particularly prone to develop LVH as well as congestive heart failure. So vigilance in diagnosing and aggressively treating anemia may be life preserving. Anemia may be present a year or more before dialysis is indicated and may not be reliably associated with creatinine levels (National Kidney Foundation, 1997).

Erythropoietin therapy is started in the pre-dialysis period and continued once patients start dialysis. Interestingly, the optimal hematocrit for a dialysis patient is not known, as studies have been inconclusive. The National Kidney Foundation's Dialysis Outcomes Quality Initiative (NKF, 1997) recommends a target range of 33 to 36%. Erythropoetin can be given subcutaneously or intravenously, and side effects include worsening of hypertension, seizures, and dialysis graft clotting.

Additionally, there are complicating factor associated with anemia of renal disease. One is that hemodialysis patients lose blood with each dialysis treatment. This necessitates careful monitoring of the hematocrit. Patients with advanced kidney disease and on dialysis also generally have low iron stores necessitating iron replacement intravenously, as oral iron is not absorbed well from the gastric mucosa. Finally, any inflammatory process such as infection or cancer creates erythropoietin resistance and impairs release of iron from storage sites. Hyperparathyroidism can also cause erythropoietin resistance, which is another reason to actively control this disorder.

Cardiovascular Disease

As previously mentioned, cardiac complications are the leading cause of death in the ESRD population, as the prevalence of cardiovascular disease is elevated in this group because of their increased risk of atherosclerosis. Risk factors for atherosclerosis include diabetes mellitus, hypertension, and factors associated with uremia such as hypertriglyceridemia, hyperparathyroidism, vascular calcification, abnormal calcium and phosphorus metabolism, and elevated levels of inflammatory mediators. As mentioned, LVH is also common in the dialysis population and is a strong risk factor for cardiovascular mortality.

Because the morbidity of cardiovascular disease influences the quality and ultimately the length of life in ESRD, prevention and treatment are crucial. Treatment includes screening for LVH and coronary artery disease (CAD), treating hypertension and hyperlipidemia using goals for patients who have preexisting CAD, low-sodium and low-fat diets, fluid restrictions, maintaining a calcium/phosphorus product below 55 (this is obtained by multiplying the serum calcium number by the serum phosphorous number), counseling for smoking cessation, exercise, and aggressive treatment of diabetes mellitus. For patients with CAD, attention to maintaining the hematocrit above 30 can help alleviate anginal symptoms. Dialysis patients also have increased risks for endocarditis, pericarditis, and arrhythmias, especially if they are inadequately dialyzed. Sudden death risk is increased and has been linked to hyperkalemia, usually related to dietary intake (Henrich, 2004).

Dialysis Access Problems

Dialysis access procedures and complications of dialysis access are a major cause of morbidity, hospitalization, and cost for dialysis patients. Access problems can significantly affect quality of life. Dialysis access is defined as the vascular entry point by which hemodialysis is accomplished or the abdominal catheter used for peritoneal dialysis. There are three types of access used for hemodialysis. They are in order of preference: 1) fistula: in which a native artery and vein are joined together to produce one large vessel; 2) graft: in which a synthetic material is used to create a large conduit between an artery and vein; and finally 3) catheter: in which a double lumen catheter is placed in a vein, usually the subclavian. In the case of peritoneal dialysis, a catheter is placed through the abdominal wall into the peritoneal space and dialysis fluid is infused into the peritoneal space and drained out through the catheter after an exchange of electrolytes and systemic toxins.

Arteriovenous fistulas are least likely to have complications associated with them. They are the safest type of access and have the lowest infection rate as compared to dialysis catheters or grafts. They are also less likely to cause arterial steal syndromes in which blood supply is routed away from the hand of the access arm causing ischemic pain. Infection rates are highest in patients who have dialysis catheters, but can also occur with grafts. Graft infections can be superficial or, worse, they may be deep-seated. Both catheter and graft infections can lead to sepsis and require surgical removal (Oreopoulos, Hazzard, & Luke 2000).

In the case of both the old and the young, successful access placement and maintenance for dialysis can be complicated by anatomy and physiology. Older patients frequently have peripheral vascular calcification or narrowing caused by diabetes, hyperlipidemia, high phosphorus levels, or hypertension. Placement of vascular access in calcified vessels increases the rate of ischemia and thrombosis. In children, blood vessels are often too small, necessitating the use of the peritoneal dialysis modality.

Intradialytic Hypotension

A combination of factors associated with the older, sick ESRD population may cause hypotension during dialysis. Factors such as low cardiac reserve and autonomic neuropathy can make removing fluid during the dialysis process difficult and uncomfortable for patients. If fluid is removed from the intravascular space too rapidly, it can exceed the plasma filling capacity. When combined with an inability to increase peripheral vascular resistance and the host of drugs that dialysis patients are prescribed, abrupt hypotension can occur. Postprandial hypotension is also common and occurs because of increased blood flow to the stomach and gut to digest food when patients eat during treatment. Dialysis often interferes with mealtimes for many patients and they must skip meals to avoid hypotension. Many dialysis units prohibit eating and drinking during dialysis treatment because of this. Complications of intradialytic hypotension include seizures, thrombotic events such as cerebrovascular accidents, myocardial ischemia and infarction, and thrombosis of the dialysis access (Henrich, 2004).

Treatment involves careful monitoring of patient weight and fluid intake in between dialysis sessions to prevent the necessity of having to take off too much fluid in one sitting. Patient education can be useful, but effectiveness is individual-specific and not well documented. This is an area for further research. Immediate treatment consists of volume replacement with normal saline and placing the patient in a recumbent position. Obviously, vigilance by the dialysis staff during treatment is required to identify hypotension as soon as there are detectable signs and to then treat it quickly. Older patients typically cannot tolerate as much fluid removal as younger patients. Ideally, no more than 500–1000 cc of fluid is removed per hour in older patients. Hypotensive episodes are avoided if at all possible due to reasons cited previously and because they can leave patients weak, contribute to falls outside of the dialysis center, cause cramping during and after treatment, and decrease quality of life (Henrich, 2004).

Some patients cannot take any antihypertensive medication before dialysis, even if their blood pressures are elevated, or they will have severe hypotension during treatment. Using shorter acting medications in the evening prior to dialysis can help the patient arrive at treatment with a more acceptable blood pressure without the risk of intradialytic hypotension (Schena, 2001).

Severe Hyperkalemia

The development of severe hyperkalemia by ESRD patients results from reduced or absent renal excretion of potassium in combination with normal or increased intake of potassium in the diet. ESRD patients may have no signs or symptoms of hyperkalemia, or they may have signs as severe as flaccid paralysis. ESRD patients tend to tolerate much higher serum potassium levels then the population at large, but even they have a upper limit before symptoms and death occur. Electrocardiogram changes parallel the degree of hyperkalemia. There can be initial tenting of the T wave, then P-wave flattening, widening of the QRS complex, and development of a deep S wave. Ventricular fibrillation is usually the cause of death when hyperkalemia is severe (Schena, 2001).

Emergency dialysis is the treatment of choice for patients who are already established on dialysis. IV calcium and insulin are also commonly used as mechanisms to drive potassium from the serum into the cell where the effects are neutralized.

Peritonitis

Peritonitis is a leading complication associated with peritoneal dialysis. It is best avoided by emphasizing to patients the need to use aseptic technique when they are working with the dialysis catheter connections. Patients who perform peritoneal dialysis are taught to visualize the fluid in each dialysate bag at exchanges for turbidity because it can be an indication of peritonitis. Other symptoms include abdominal pain, fever, or vomiting. The diagnosis is confirmed by the presence of 100 white blood cells/ml of dialysate and later by peritoneal fluid cultures. Catheter removal may be necessary if the infection cannot be cleared with it in place and the patient is then dialyzed using the hemodialysis modality. In an effort to prevent catheter site infection, in some facilities mupiricin is routinely applied to the nares of patients several times a week to avoid nose-to-catheter cross-contamination with gram-positive organisms.

Early diagnosis and treatment with antibiotics provide the best chance for cure and preserving the access. Repeated infections can cause scarring of the peritoneum, which may cause failure of this dialysis method.

Leaks of Peritoneal Fluid

Internal and external peritoneal dialysis fluid leaks can occur at any time. Common signs of internal leaks are edema of the labia, scrotum, or penis; of the soft tissue planes of the catheter insertion site; or of a preexisting hernia. Hydrothorax is a rare and life-threatening complication that can occur. External leaks are detected when fluid drains out around the catheter. In either case, peritoneal dialysis should be stopped and a work-up begun by the nephrology team. Prophylactic antibiotics, such as cephalexin, are commonly prescribed. Temporary hemodialysis may be necessary if the work-up or treatment is prolonged.

GENERAL MANAGEMENT—TREATMENT OPTIONS

The following section will address a general care management philosophy and broad treatment options for ESRD, as specific management strategies have been outlined in the preceding section. Adherence to this sound general management approach is the best way to palliate the disturbing symptoms of ESRD. At the end of the section, there is a discussion of the nontreatment option, withholding or withdrawing dialysis

Care management should be designed to give ESRD patients the best possible medical, psychological, and social outcomes. This is best accomplished using a shared decision-making approach as recommended by American Society of Nephrology and the Renal Physicians Association (Renal Physicians Association/ American Society Nephrology (RPA/ASN, 2000)). This approach is compatible with a palliative care philosophy that effectively utilizes all members of the health care team to achieve treatment goals. The main emphasis is on the alleviation of disabling symptoms and prevention of complications that affect longevity and quality of life. Ideally, with shared decision making, patients and providers understand and agree on diagnosis, prognosis, and treatment goals. Providers are also aware of personal data such as medical and social history and patient preferences including advance directive information. The intent of shared decision making is to mesh the patient and provider goals into a seamless treatment plan to accomplish desirable endpoints through mutual understanding. This is true whether the treatment goals are designed to preserve life or to allow it to end with care and dignity. The ASA/RPA group established a 10 step process for shared decision making to be used with ESRD patients by their providers during the initial discussion of treatment options for ESRD that focuses primarily on candid communication regarding diagnosis and prognosis and culminating in encouraging patients to explore end of life planning with family and friends (RPA/ASN, 2000).

Included in general palliative treatment strategies are the different dialysis modalities. How renal failure is treated is a significant factor in relief of symptoms and quality of life. As previously mentioned, treatment options for ESRD include peritoneal dialysis (PD), hemodialysis (HD), kidney transplant, or only supportive care with eventual death. The form of treatment or renal replacement therapy (RRT) to be used should be a major focus and lends itself particularly well to the shared decision-making approach. The type of RRT should be decided well in advance of the need to dialyze. In this chapter, transplantation will not be discussed in any depth, as it is a highly specialized field and transplant patients have very specific palliative care issues that overlap the discussion of ESRD only if the transplant fails. Once this occurs, then the palliative care needs are the same as those of ESRD patients.

When should dialysis begin? This is a common question asked by patients and their family. The most reliable answer is that the presence of uremic symptoms is the best indication for initiation of dialysis. Symptoms that indicate the need to begin dialysis in all age groups include confusion and lethargy, which would indicate uremic encephalopathy, pericarditis, gastritis as manifested by nausea and vomiting, fatigue, accumulation of fluid and dyspnea, anorexia, severe anemia, or hyperkalemia. Patients without symptoms are usually started at a GFR of 10 ml/min or 15 ml/min if they are diabetic (Henrich, 2004).

Indications for choosing one dialysis modality (HD vs. PD) over another include life-style choice by the patient, physician preferences, distance to the nearest dialysis center, as well as concurrent illnesses and their symptoms. Comorbidities, such as CHF or hypertension, contraindications to a specific dialysis modality, financial allocation of scarce resources, vascular access limitations, and provider and patient bias are also considerations. Either type of dialysis can generally be used; however, in the United States, hemodialysis is the most frequent form of renal replacement therapy for the adults. Peritoneal dialysis is the most common modality used in pediatrics due to limited vascular access. Internationally, hemodialysis and peritoneal dialysis are used in equal proportions (Henrich, 2004). All treatment options are replete with complications, especially for older and younger patients.

Older patients have more complications with hemodialysis than with peritoneal dialysis. They include arrhythmias, vascular-access-related infections, and gastrointestinal bleeding. Older peritoneal dialysis patients often have poor nutrition, and require back-up hemodialysis more often because peritoneal dialysis becomes ineffective more often in older patients. Older patients predictably are also hospitalized more frequently than younger patients. Interestingly, peritoneal dialysis access catheter infections are less frequent in elders than in the young (Oreopoulos, Hazzard, & Luke, 2000)

As the patients' physical and emotional health declines, or when patients decide or circumstances dictate that dialysis is not desirable, aggressive palliative and hospice care becomes crucial in order to manage symptoms and preserve comfort until death. This may be when patients decline dialysis altogether from the beginning, or dialysis may be withdrawn after a trial or at any time if it becomes overly burdensome. These are all morally valid options, especially for patients with a high symptom burden. Healthcare practitioners should

be prepared to accept these decisions as long as the patient has the mental capacity to make a decision of this magnitude, and the decision is not the result of overwhelming clinical depression.

A "trial" of dialysis can be suggested with clear stopping points established with the patient, such as time to feel well or finish family or personal business (RPA/ASN, 2000; Robert Wood Johnson Foundation, 2002). The patient who is not mentally competent places the provider in a more difficult situation. Finding the appropriate decision maker and involving the patient in a reasonable way is most important. Often the social worker and the ethics consult team can be helpful in wading through the legal and ethical implications of deciding for or against dialysis for patients who lack mental capacity. The primary question to ask is how would the patient decide if they were ever competent or if never competent, and how would a reasonable person decide given the same circumstances.

The healthcare team should view as ethically equivalent the stopping of dialysis for patients when it is overly burdensome or never starting dialysis when the risk or burden outweighs the benefit. Withdrawal from dialysis cannot be equated with killing the patient. In fact, if there is any difference, it is that a trial of dialysis is in many ways a more compassionate and life-honoring approach. According to government data, withdrawal of dialysis is actively utilized. In the older dialysis population, withdrawal is the second most common reason for death. In the younger dialysis population, death is usually caused by a secondary disease process (USRDS, 2007).

Interestingly, African-American patients are 50–66% less likely to stop dialysis than Caucasian patients (Oreopoulos et al., 2000). It is not known why there is such a discrepancy associated with race. The most likely patients to withdraw from dialysis are Caucasian female nursing home residents older than 65 years of age. Further, they are more likely to have other chronic diseases, such as dementia or malignancy. Patients who perform their own hemodialysis at home are more likely to withdraw from dialysis when compared to patients that have in-center hemodialysis. Patients elect withdrawal from dialysis most commonly in their third month of treatment (Leggat, Bloembergen, Levine, Hulbert-Shearon, & Port, 1997). Implications for caregivers and management of patients who opt to not start or to withdraw from dialysis are discussed in the next section.

PALLIATIVE CARE ISSUES

Modern palliative care has benefited from the efforts of professional groups that have promoted the establishment of clinical practice guidelines (CPGs) that are both general and specific to particular patient populations like ESRD. General palliative care guidelines include American Association of Colleges of Nursing Guidelines for End of Life Care; Hospice and Palliative Care Nursing Competencies; and National Quality Forum Guidelines and Preferred Practice for Quality Palliative care. Guidelines specific to care of ESRD patients include those from the American Society of Nephrology entitled "Shared Decision Making in the Appropriate Initiation and Withdrawal from Dialysis" (ASN/RPA, 2000). This guideline was designed to help nephrology professionals decide who will truly benefit from dialysis. A second guideline is the "End-stage Renal Disease Workgroup–Recommendations to the Field," which was developed in affiliation with the Robert Wood Johnson (RWJ) Foundation's national program of Promoting Excellence in End of Life Care (RWJ Foundation, 2002).

The RWJ workgroup in particular has been instrumental in moving forward to improve palliative care services for those with ESRD. This group identified the gaps, lack of consensus, and the absence of available research specific to ESRD palliative care and made recommendations to address these needs to all involved parties. Based on these recommendations, a demonstration project, the Renal Palliative Care Initiative (RPCI), was developed by eight dialysis clinics and Baystate Medical Center in Springfield, Massachusetts, with the cooperation of a large nephrology practice. Physicians, nurses, and social workers established a group that became educated in techniques of palliative care, developed programs to implement palliative care, and introduced them to the routines of dialysis patient care in the hospital and dialysis units. They also established survey instruments to ask family and patients about the quality of dying (Dialysis Quality of Dying Apgar) (Cohen, Poppel, Cohn, & Reiter, 2001) and programs to support bereaved families.

The RPCI developed initiatives to holistically address the needs of patients, families, and the care team as they grappled with the challenges of renal disease, dialysis, and transplantation. They incorporated strategies to help with confronting the inevitability of eventual early death in the ESRD population even while continuing with renal replacement therapies. The group found that the initiatives' measures enabled providers to become more likely to address palliative needs of ESRD patients and they became more proficient in doing so (Poppel, Cohen, & Germain, 2003). Gaps still exist but the RWJ ESRD workgroup provided a well-thought-out plan to improve the quality of life and dying for ESRD patients. It is a process that is still in infancy but is slowly changing the lives of ESRD patients for the better.

Never Starting or Withdrawing Dialysis

Although discussed above under general palliative care options, the non-treatment option is re-examined here in more detail to reiterate the need to consider it carefully when treatment possibilities are being developed. As stated above, the Renal Physicians Association and the American Society of Nephrology (RPA/ASN, 2000) responded to a request by the Institute of Medicine to issue guidelines for evaluating patients for whom the burdens of renal replacement therapy may substantially outweigh benefits. The report is intended to provide direction to providers who frequently find themselves confronting end-of-life issues in the ESRD population (Levine, 2001). At the core of the report is the belief that initiation of and withdrawal from dialysis should be a decision that the informed patient actively participates in (RPA/ASN, 2000). The discussion has to be broached in the context of shared decision making, or an interactive mutual relationship between patient and provider.

When discussing the option of never starting or stopping dialysis with patients and families, candor is a most prized professional trait. Candor associated with death is regrettably somewhat rare institutionally and culturally in the United States. This is partially because American patients and families have an idealized view of the capabilities of medicine. As ethicist Daniel Callahan writes, "We expect medicine to devise ever more ingenious ways to save our lives. That is why the NIH budget has always risen, budget crisis or not....Why should anyone be astonished...that the other message many are trying to deliver—the need to stop treatment—has such a hard time getting through?" (Callahan, 1987). If the illusion is allowed to remain that medicine has an unlimited ability to preserve life, patients suffer as inappropriate care is opted for. Candor regarding quality of life, prognosis, and life expectancy is crucial to patients who are considering either withdrawal of dialysis or not starting treatment in the first place.

Openness with patients and families who are considering the non-treatment option is a deeply important part of the holistic care and shared decision making that enables the best most well-informed decisions to be made by chronically ill ESRD patients. When the limits of medicine and technology are reached, patients are best served when they are accurately informed and all who are significant to them work towards agreement on a plan of care. This means that the team begins the important work of care and comfort both for the dying and for those who remain after the patient's death. The ability to adjust thinking from preservation of life to care of the dying is crucial for the provision of full spectrum therapy, especially when working with a high-risk population, such as ESRD patients. Any lag time in this transition of thought and deed can create both psychological and physical suffering for all involved. When patients indicate a readiness to think of and speak about their death, the proper approach at that point is discussion of hospice care when indicated, available general support, and recognition of the importance of therapeutic presence.

Management of Symptoms at the End of Life

Over 70,000 patients, or 22% of the total dialysis population, died in 2006 (USRDS 2007) and statistics suggest that less than 10% of ESRD patients are enrolled in hospice when dialysis is discontinued (Poppel et al., 2003). Once dialysis is stopped, death usually occurs in 6–8 days but can range over weeks if there is residual kidney function (Braveman, 2002). The work groups and organizations trying to address this gap in the use of hospice services and the need for better EOL care for ESRD patients all agree that a good death is a priority and that the only way this can be accomplished is through the provision of excellent palliative care. Cohen et al. (2001) surveyed ESRD patients and families who discontinued dialysis and asked what a good death would consist of for them. Their findings were that patients and families defined a good death as one that was pain-free, peaceful, and brief. The researchers developed a tool to evaluate the quality of dying in the ESRD group known as the "Dialysis Discontinuation quality of Dying" (DDQOD) tool as well as a second tool the "Dialysis Quality of Dying Apgar" (DQODA) which measures the quality of dying of ESRD patients who did not discontinue dialysis (Cohen et al., 2001). As is the case with other dying patients, families believed that the most distressing symptoms at the end of life were pain, weakness, and dyspnea (Cohen, Germain, Woods, Mirot, & Burleson, 2005). Several end-of-life symptoms and their treatment will be reviewed below.

Nausea and Vomiting

If dialysis is withdrawn (or never begun) or it becomes difficult to dialyze patients adequately, patients eventually revert to a uremic state where uremic toxins accumulate and can cause chemically induced nausea and vomiting. These two symptoms are reported as highly distressing by sufferers (Neely & Roxe, 2000). The mechanism of nausea associated with uremia is stimulation of the central nervous system center referred to as the chemoreceptor trigger zone (CTZ). Blocking receptors in this zone, located in the fourth ventricle of the brain, seems to be the most effective pharmacologic therapy for treatment of metabolically induced nausea and vomiting (Mannix, 2004). The tool recommended by the ESRD workgroup for assessment of the symptom of nausea is the Edmonton Symptom Assessment Scale (Breura, Kuehn, Miller, Selmser, & Macmillan, 1991).

Haloperidol and prochlorperazine are two agents that effectively block the CTZ. Haloperidol, which can also treat the confusion that may be present at the end of life, is given at 1.5–5 mg daily by mouth or subcutaneously but may cause extrapyramidal side effects such as dystonia, dyskinesia, and akathisia at higher doses. Promotilty agents such as metoclopramide or serotonergic antagonists like ondansetron may be useful to treat the nausea of uremia as well (Mannix, 2004). Even though treatment is available, further research is still needed to assess and treat uremic nausea and vomiting effectively, as the current treatments have side effects that make them less than desirable.

Pain

Pain can occur from any of several comorbidities of ESRD patients. Cancer and peripheral vascular disease are common causes of pain in this patient population and should be aggressively treated prior to but especially at the end of life. Pain is the symptom most frequently reported by dying ESRD patients (Cohen, Germain, Poppel, Woods, & Kjellstrand, 2000). It is more common when patients die in institutions versus at home and is viewed as being unnecessary and highly treatable.

There are a few important points to be made in the case of pain palliation in ESRD at the end of life. Analgesics should be used on a regular schedule using the WHO analgesic ladder as guidance for the management of pain in ESRD. There are some drugs that should not be used, and there are some drugs for which dosing should be monitored because their metabolites can accumulate in renal failure and cause unwanted side effects. Opioids are generally metabolized in the liver but some accumulate. For example, demerol should not be used for pain control in ESRD because the metabolite normeperidine accumulates and leads to seizures and neuro-excitation. Propoxyphene is another opioid narcotic that should not be used because of the accumulation of metabolites. Morphine has a distinct place in ESRD end-of-life care because of the analgesic effect and the positive effect on dyspnea, but it can accumulate and so side effects such as myoclonus should be carefully monitored (Cohen, Moss, Weisbord & Germain, 2006). If myoclonus occurs, it can be treated with benzodiazepines such as clonazepam which may help anxiety as well (Holley, 2008). There is anecdotal evidence that alternative strong opioids (hydromorphone, methadone, and fentanyl) are better tolerated but there is inadequate research to support this presently (Davison, 2007).

Dyspnea

With the addition of complicating illnesses, respiratory symptoms are not uncommon, and, as generalized systemic failure occurs at the end of life, they become more prevalent. Dyspnea, tachypnea, cough, and breathlessness may be common end-of-life symptoms experienced by patients with ESRD. These are typically the result of hypervolemia, congestive heart failure, and pleural effusion. Relief of these symptoms is crucial to providing comfort at the end of life. Prevention is highly desirable and is best accomplished by limiting fluid intake yet providing mouth care to prevent thirst and dry mouth.

One of the most potent causes of dyspnea is pleural effusion. It may be necessary to remove fluid from the chest by pleural aspiration to relieve air hunger and promote comfort regardless of the phase of the dying trajectory. This procedure can effectively improve symptoms and lessen air hunger, even if death is imminent. Management of respiratory symptoms involves acknowledging the goals of end-of-life care and providing comfort through symptom management (Ahmedzai, 1998).

Pruritus

Pruritus is one of the most bothersome symptoms of ESRD. It is a prominent symptom of uremia and is difficult if not impossible to control for some. One estimate is that 60% of ESRD patients experience it. Multiple reasons are proposed for it: hyperphosphatemia, hyperparathyroidism, calcium-phosphorous deposition in the skin, inadequate dialysis, anemia, allergy to the dialyzer materials (Cohen et al., 2006). Palliative treatment should be both preventative and symptomatic. Prevention includes adequate dialysis and lowering of the traditionally high phosphorous and parathyroid levels through a well-controlled diet. When necessary, phosphate binders such as calcium carbonate and renagel are added at meal times and activated vitamin D is used to control PTH levels. When prevention fails, symptomatic management for pruritus becomes necessary, with antihistamines, urea, and oatmeal-based creams being the most frequently used.

Since itching from renal failure is thought to be the result of uremic toxin accumulation, it makes sense that in the face of dialysis withdrawal, uremia increases and itching may worsen. Logically, in the hospice setting, continuing to give phosphate-binding drugs, such as calcium carbonate, may be useful to control this uncomfortable symptom; however, these drugs are notorious for their gastrointestinal side effects such as bloating and nausea and so may not be useful in many hospice cases. Other interventions include a 0.5 to 2% phenol solution, Sarna, or other menthol phenol creams topically, and systemic therapies such as antihistamines, thalidomide, and oral corticosteroids. It is imperative to find at least one intervention that will be effective, because pruritus is described as one of the more miserable of symptoms to endure (Oreopoulos et al., 2000).

Pediatric Palliative Care

Pediatric palliative care is offered as a summary section for this very rare but specialized population. In the United States, over 40,000 children die from trauma, lethal congenital conditions, or acquired illnesses every year. ESRD falls mostly into the latter category. Children account for only a fraction of the total dialysis patients in the United States. The U.S. Department of Vital Statistics indicate although pediatric ESRD mortality rates are lower than adult mortality rates, pediatric

rates have not improved in the last 5 years as compared to adult rates (USRDS, 2007). Given this, palliative care is an important intervention for children with ESRD, but as in the case of adult ESRD it is underutilized.

The issue of palliative care as it relates to children with ESRD is similar to the issue of palliative care in adult ESRD in that both children and adults with ESRD may need palliative care not only as treatment to promote a good death but to alleviate symptoms during life—or while a cure (transplantation) is being pursued. The American Academy of Pediatrics (American Academy Pediatrics, 2000) supports palliative care throughout the course of a wide range of illnesses and, due to the high symptom burden in ESRD, believes it to be appropriate whether cure is possible or not (AAP, 2000; (Himmelstein, Hilden, Boldt, & Weissman, 2004). Both curative treatments, which seek to reverse the illness and palliative treatments that are focused on relieving symptoms, have a place in the care of pediatric ESRD patients. According to the AAP, pediatric ESRD falls into a category of conditions for which palliative care is appropriate and requires intensive long-term treatment aimed at maintaining quality of life (Himmelstein et al., 2004). Unfortunately, there is little research available, however, on the quality-of-life outcomes of palliative care in this age group.

Incidence/Prevalence

Pediatric ESRD is devastating but rare. The most recent statistics from 2004 shows an incidence of 14 cases per million population with a prevalence of 80 cases per million. In 2000, the incidence was the same but the prevalence was 20 per million (USRDS, 2007).

Pathogenesis

The cause of ESRD and the primary cause of mortality in pediatrics differ from those of adults. Two congenital abnormalities, posterior urethral valves (PUVs) and hypoplastic/dysplastic kidneys, and a third disorder, focal segmental glomerulosclerosis (FSGS), are the primary causes of long-term kidney failure in children. PUV is the most common cause of obstruction of the lower urinary tract in males. This abnormality consists abnormal urethral folds that lead obstruction to the normal flow of urine. The incidence is 1 case for every 12,000 births, with nearly one third of children born with PUV progressing to ESRD.

Hypoplastic kidneys, the second most common cause of pediatric ESRD, are small kidneys that contain a reduced number of normal nephrons, while dysplastic kidneys contain a normal number of components but are abnormally developed. Children may have either or both disorders, although the two typically occur together. Children with one affected kidney generally do well; in contrast, those with bilateral hypoplasia/dysplasia characteristically progress to kidney failure.

FSGS is the third disorder that can lead to ERSD in children. This disorder causes primary nephrotic syndrome, which is characterized by the presence of heavy proteinuria, hypoproteinemia, hyperlipidemia, and edema. Other kidney diseases may cause nephritic syndrome; however, FSGS is most significant because of the tendency of the disorder to cause glomerular destruction (Warady, 2002).

Mortality rates for children are significantly lower than for adults: 41 per 1,000 patient years for patients 19 and younger as compared to 148 per 1,000 patient years for adults. As in adults, cardiovascular disease is still the most common cause of death in pediatric ESRD patients, with infection being the second most common cause of death in pediatric ESRD (USRDS, 2007).

Pediatric Palliative Care Issues

The use of palliative care and hospice services are relatively low in ESRD in general but especially so in children. The younger the patient, the less likely is he/she to be referred for palliation and hospice care. The presumed reason is that attempted curative care is ongoing in the case of pediatric patients, and providers and parents are less willing to move in the direction of withdrawing dialysis. Theses two goals do not have to be at odds. The AAP has a helpful position on this dilemma. They recommend the availability of palliative care to children with a broad range of illnesses even when cure remains a possibility. The components of palliative care should be offered at diagnosis and continued throughout the course of illness, whether the outcome ends in cure or death. One author describes it this way: "Pediatric palliative care should...intersect with the aims of curing and healing...improving the quality of life... maintaining dignity and ameliorating the suffering of seriously ill or dying children..." (AAP, 2004, p.1752). The main issue associated with pediatric palliative care is helping patient and family confront the reality of the illness with compassion and hope so that the treatment approach is appropriately (not overly) aggressive. With this approach the topic of palliation and hospice can be introduced.

Case Study conclusion: Gene's turnaround continued for approximately 3 months, until after Christmas. He then began to experience nosebleeds from the coumadin, deterioration in the perfusion to his legs as the coumadin dose was reduced, and a resumption of the pain.

Gene told his family that he was ready to stop dialysis; he was unwilling to tolerate the current symptoms; the pain and disability were just too great. He wanted to die at home and his family was committed to granting this last request.

The palliative care team engaged home hospice services to provide comfort and supportive care. The dialysis team agreed to provide dialysis for fluid removal and comfort purposes on an as-needed basis. This provision proved unnecessary because he never returned to the dialysis center. Those of us who had cared for him over the years stayed in touch with his wife during the 10-day process of his death; some nurses visited the home to say good-bye.

He remained committed to not having any more invasive therapy and never wavered from this final decision. Gene spent his last days with his family, his friends and pastors from his church, and the healthcare professionals who knew him best. As symptoms of uremia emerged, the hospice team treated them. His family faithfully followed directions to not overload him with fluids, as this would almost certainly add to his discomfort.

In the end, he died quietly in the night with his wife of almost 40 years at his side. He had assured her that day that he was ready to die, reliant to the last on his faith. He whispered to her that he would see her again. His dying was difficult for the family, but Gene's faith and conviction eased the pain. The dialysis staff loved him. He was a quiet, respectful man with a smile that illuminated the room. His family was devoted to him, as he was to them. He was 72 when he died. The funeral was a tribute to a life well-lived. As providers, we gathered with family and friends in the church one last time on his behalf.

Gene's case is paradigmatically significant, not only because of what happened and how events occurred, but what did not happen as well. Gene did not die in a hospital cared for by strangers; there were no intravenous drips, tube feedings, and futile attempts to preserve life when the body was clearly unable to sustain life. All talked, agreed, and were sad but comfortable with the decision. Essentially, this is an example of the beneficial effect of open dialogue and shared decision making around emotionally difficult topics such as death. Desirable outcomes occur when all involved are willing to speak candidly about prognosis and death with patients and their families and think about death as a part of the care continuum and not as failed therapy.

CONCLUSION

ESRD is a chronic disease that is characterized by steady functional decline, a 20% yearly mortality rate, and early death for most patients. It is increasing in incidence and prevalence in all age groups in the United States and globally. Significantly for our purposes, it is a disease with a high symptom burden that takes a toll on patient and family alike and for which palliative care is crucial to foster quality life and death.

A shared decision-making model facilitates preservation of patient values and preferences and effective care management across the life span for the patient, his/her family, and the healthcare team. Full integration of palliative care principles and standards provides support for ESRD patients to make difficult decisions concerning withdrawal of dialysis and can offer guidance during the process of ending life and seeking a good death. As nurses, we are often unable to deliver patients from illness and death for very long, but we can always stand with them in their struggle, and ease their suffering by promoting and utilizing effective palliative care practices.

EVIDENCE-BASED PRACTICE

Holley, J. L. (2002). A single center review of the death notification form: Discontinuing dialysis before death is not a surrogate for withdrawal from dialysis. *American Journal of Kidney Diseases*, *40*(3), p. 6.

Research problem. How do dialysis patients die? How many die because they no longer wish to be dialyzed? This should be a relatively simple question to answer. Renal replacement therapy for ESRD is 80% funded by the federal government through Medicare and, therefore, a death notification form must be filled out to notify the insurer when ESRD patients die. It is logical to think that review of these forms would provide answers to questions like the one above. This is not necessarily the case.

Methodology. Review of 212 of the federal death notification forms.

Finding. Few patients died because of an active decision to withdraw from dialysis, although discontinuation of dialysis was listed as the cause of death for 26% or 56 patients. Only 8 of the 56 patients were listed as having death attributed to uremia. Most died from cancer and cardiovascular disease in hospitals not in hospice (only two died in hospice care).

Conclusion. The authors concluded that use of the death notification forms might not provide an accurate answer to the question of how dialysis patients die, as there appears to be provider uncertainty about the meaning attributed to the phrase, "discontinuing dialysis." Discontinuing dialysis and active withdrawal from dialysis by patients do not have the same meaning, and substituting one for the other term does not allow accurate evaluation of events leading to death of dialysis patients. A secondary finding is the low number of ESRD patients referred for hospice care, which suggests that adequate end-of-life support may be lacking for dialysis patients.

EVIDENCE-BASED PRACTICE

Holley, J. L., Hines, S. C., Glover, J. J., Babrow, A. S., Badzek, L. A., & Moss, A. H. (1999). Failure of advance planning to elicit patients' preferences for withdrawal from dialysis. *American Journal of Kidney Disease, 33*(4), 688–693.

Research question. For patients with renal failure, who are doing advanced care planning, how many included consideration of dialysis withdrawal?

Methodology. A stratified random sample of 450 adult hemodialysis patients located in two geographic areas: six dialysis units within 75 miles of Morgantown, WV, and all nine dialysis units in Rochester, NY. Interviews were conducted by trained interviewers during a hemodialysis session with the patient and either face to face or by telephone with the patient's surrogate decision maker.

Findings. Fifty-one percent of the patients had advanced directives. Of these, 29% had a living will and health care proxy, and 22% had a living will or health care proxy. Only 18% of patients had discussed stopping dialysis. This was the least often discussed intervention compared, for example, to 69% who discussed mechanical ventilation, 55% who discussed tube feedings, and 43% who had discussed cardiopulmonary resuscitation. Thirty-one percent of the patients who had completed a living will and named a health care proxy had discussed withdrawal from dialysis with their surrogate decision makers compared to 8% of the patients who had not completed an advance directive.

Implications. Withdrawal from dialysis is very common and occurs before death in at least 19% of chronic dialysis patients, but it appears that patients do not routinely discuss it with their surrogate decision makers. Further, nephrologists and dialysis staff rarely discuss this issue with patients. Patients should be made aware of their options concerning withdrawal of dialysis. Staff should help patients consider conditions under which they might want to withdraw dialysis as part of their advance care planning and help them communicate their wishes to their surrogate decision makers.

REFERENCES

Ahmedzai, S. (1998). Palliation of respiratory symptoms.

Anasari, A., Kampke, C. J., Miller, R., & Barbari, A. (1993). Cardiac pathology in patients with end stage renal disease. *International Journal of Artificial Organs,16*(1), 31–36.

Breura, E., Kuehn, N., Miller, M. J., Selmser, P., & Macmillan, K. (1991). The Edmonton symptom assessment system: A simple method for assessment of palliative care. *Journal of Palliative Care, 7*(2), 6–9.

Brenner, B. M., & Rector, R., (2007) *The kidney* (8th ed.). Philadelphia: Saunders Elsevier.

Callahan, D. (1987). *Setting limits: Medical goals in an aging society.* New York: Simon and Schuster, p. 56.

Center for Disease Control-Online. (2007). National diabetes surveilance system.

Cohen, L. M., Moss, A. H., Weisbord, S. D., Germain, M. J. (2006). Renal palliative care. *Journal Palliative Medicine, 9*(4), 977–992.

Cohen, L. M., Germain, M. J., Woods A. C., Mirot, A., & Burleson, J. A. (2005). The family perspective of end stage renal disease deaths. *American Journal of Kidney Diseases, 45*(1), 154–161.

Cohen, L. M., Poppel, D. M., Cohn, G. M. & Reiter, G. S. (2001). A very good death: Measuring quality of dying in end stage renal disease. *Journal of Palliative Medicine, 4*(2), 167–172.

Cohen, L. M., Germain, M., Poppel, D. M., Woods, A., & Kjellstrand, C. M. (2000). Dialysis discontinuation and palliative care. *American Journal of Kidney Diseases, 36*(1), 140–144.

Cohen, L. M., McCue, J. D., Germain, M., & Kjellstrand, C. M. (1995). Dialysis discontinuation: A good death? *Archives of Internal Medicine, 155*, 42–47.

Davison, S. N. (2007). The prevalence and management of chronic pain in end stage renal disease. *Journal of Palliative Medicine, 10*(6), 1277–1287.

Hauser, A. B., Stenghen, A. E., Kato, S., Bucharles, S., Aita, C., Yuzawa, Y., et al. (2008). Characteristics and causes of immune dysfunction related to uremia and dialysis. *Peritoneal Dialysis International, 3*, S183–S187.

Henrich, W. L. (2004). *Principles and practice of dialysis.* (3rd ed.). Philadelphia: Lippincott Williams & Wilkins.

Himmelstein, B. P., Hilden, J. M., Boldt, M. S., & Weissman, D. (2004). Pediatric palliative care. *New England Journal of Medicine, 350*(17), 1752–1762.

Holley, J. L. (2008). Palliative care in end stage renal disease. *Uptodate.com* version 16.2, 1–5.

Holley, J. L. (2007). Palliative care in end stage renal disease: Illness trajectories, communication and hospice use. *Advances in Chronic Kidney Disease, 14*(4), 402–408.

Holley, J. L. (2002). A single center review of death notification forms: Discontinuing dialysis before death is not a surrogate for withdrawal of dialysis. *American Journal of Kidney Diseases, 40*(3), 525–30.

Holley, J. L., Hines, S. C., Glover, J. J., Babrow, A. S., Badzek, L. A., Moss, A. H., et al. (1999). Failure of advanced care planning to elicit patient preferences for withdrawal form dialysis. *American Journal of Kidney Diseases, 33*(4), 688–693.

Iglehart, J. K. (1993). The American health care system: The end stage renal disease program. *New England Journal of Medicine, 328*, 366–371.

Leggat J. R., Bloembergen, W. E., Levine, G., Hulbert-Shearon, T. E., & Port, F. K. (1997). An analysis of risk factors for withdrawal of dialysis before death. *Journal of the American Society of Nephrology, 8*(11), 1755–1763.

Levine, D. Z. (2001). Nephrology ethics forum. Shared decision making in dialysis: The new RPA/ASN guideline on the appropriate initiation and withdrawal of treatment. *American Journal of Kidney Diseases, 37*, 1081–1091.

Lysaught, M. J. (2002). Maintenance dialysis population dynamics: Current trends and long term implications. *Journal of the American Society of Nephrology, 13*(5), 37–40.

Mandyam, S., & Shahinian, V. B. (2008). Are chronic dialysis patients at increased risk for cancer? *Journal Nephrology, 21*(2), 166–174.

Mannix, K. A. (2004). Palliation of nausea and vomiting. In D. Doyle, G. W.C. Hanks, & N. MacDonald (Eds.), *Oxford textbook of palliative medicine* (3rd ed., pp. 459–468). Oxford, U.K.: Oxford University Press.

Murray, A. M., Arko, C., Chen, S. C., Gilbertson, D. T., & Moss, A. H. (2006). Use of hospice in the United States dialysis population. *Clinical Journal of the American Society of Nephrology, 1*(6), 1248–1255.

National Kidney Foundation. (NKF). (1997). *National Kidney Foundation dialysis outcomes quality initiative(DOQI): Clinical practice guidelines for the treatment of anemia of chronic renal failure.* New York: National Kidney Foundation.

Neely, K. J., & Roxe, D. M. (2000). Palliative care, hospice and withdrawal of dialysis. *Journal of Palliative Medicine, 3*(1), 57–67.

Oreopoulos, D. G., Hazzard, W. R., & Luke, R. (Eds.). (2000). *Nephrology and geriatrics integrated.* Dordrecht, The Netherlands: Kluwer Academic Publishers.

Poppel, D. M., Cohen, L. M., & Germain, M. D. (2003). The renal palliative care initiative. *Journal of Palliative Medicine, 6*(2), 321–326.

Renal Physicians Association and American Society of Nephrology. (RPA/ASN). (2000). Shared decision making in the appropriate initiation and withdrawal from dialysis. Clinical practice guide. #2. Washington DC, RPA/ASN.

Robert Wood Johnson Foundation. (2008). *Promoting excellence in end of life care: End stage renal disease workgroup-recommendations to the field.* Retrieved from www.promotingexcellence.org.

Sarnak, M. J., & Levey, A. S. (2000). Cardiovascular disease and chronic renal disease: a new paradigm. *American Journal of Kidney Diseases, 35* (S4), S117-S131.

Schena, F. P. (Ed.) (2001). *Nephrology.* Milan, Italy: McGraw-Hill International.

SEER. (2007). Surveillance research program, NCI. *Surveillance, Epidemiology and End Results Program (SEER).* Washington, DC: U.S. Government Publications.

U.S. Renal Data System. (USRDS). (2007). *Annual data report: Atlas of end stage renal disease in the United States.* Bethesda, MD: National Institutes of Health, National Institute of Diabetes and Digestive and Kidney Diseases.

Warady, A. M. (2002). End stage renal disease in children: What causes it? *Renal Life, 17,* (4), 1.

17

End-Stage Liver Disease

Robert B. Davis

Key Points

- Liver disease is the fourth leading cause of death in individuals aged 45–54 years.
- Nurses should have a proactive role in educating individuals about the prevention of liver disease.
- Nurses need to be aware of the pathophysiology and etiologies of liver disease.
- Hepatitis C has replaced alcohol cirrhosis as the leading cause of liver transplantation.
- Patients with end-stage liver disease (ELSD) present with malnutrition, muscle wasting, hyperlipidemia, electrolyte imbalances, fatigue, and jaundice.
- The only effective treatment for ESLD is liver transplantation.
- Patients with liver disease benefit from the physical, emotional, social, and spiritual interventions offered through palliative care.

Case Sudy: Shelia was brought into our urgent care clinic by her mother. Her problem was "itchiness" for the past three days. Shelia was in the ninth grade and was a "typical teenager" according to her mother. There had been an outbreak of head lice at some of the schools in the area and Shelia and her mother were concerned that this could be the culprit. Examination of her scalp and other areas of skin showed no rash, signs of lice, or discoloration. There were the marks from fingernails where Shelia had been "clawing at myself." Otherwise, her physical examination was normal. Environmental history was unremarkable with no new pets, changes in laundry products, or new clothes. Shelia did admit that school was very demanding for her that year and that she had broken up with a boyfriend a week before.

Lacking any obvious physical explanation for the itching, we drew a set of basic labs that included a comprehensive metabolic panel, a sedimentation rate, urine sample, drug screen, and a complete blood count. While we waited for the results our social worker met with Sheila and her mother. We were beginning to consider the itching to be the result of a stress reaction and that Shelia could benefit from counseling.

The returning labs showed all liver function tests to be six to eight times higher than normal. The drug screening and all other labs were within normal ranges. We interviewed Shelia again and concentrated on her use of alcohol as well as prescription, nonprescription, and illegal drugs. She told us that she occasionally drank with her friends and that a week before had been at a party where she and her then boyfriend had gotten into an argument. After that argument she had finished off an open bottle of acetaminophen with a wine cooler. She admitted that this was a "half-hearted" suicide attempt and really did not take the whole incident seriously. She had been sick to her stomach that night and ill the next day but attributed this to being "hung over."

INCIDENCE AND PREVALENCE

In the United States 27,257 people died in 2002 from chronic liver disease and cirrhosis. Death rates from chronic liver disease and cirrhosis are highest among Native-Americans (22.5 per 100,000) where it is more than double that of Whites (9.2) and African-Americans (7.2). The rate among women (5.8) of all ethnicities is half that of males (12.4). There has been a significant reduction in death rates among all persons from a peak in the 1970s and 1980s (Kung, Hoyert, Xu, & Murphy, 2008). Although this trend has been attributed to the World War II generation passing out of the population pool and the influx of "Baby Boomers," some believe that, in part, this change can be attributed to refinements in reporting the cause-of-death.

Deaths from liver disease as a whole peaks between the ages of 45–54 years where it is the fourth leading cause of death, behind neoplasms, heart disease, and accidents, respectively. Among those people 35–44 and those 55–64 years of age, liver disease is the seventh leading cause of death. After the age of 65, liver disease drops to 70th as diseases correlated to advancing age dominate (Jemal, et al., 2008).

Cancer of the liver and intrahepatic bile duct are expected to kill 18,410 Americans in 2008 with an alarming upward trend over the past decade (Jemal et al., 2008). The age distribution of new diagnoses of liver and bile duct cancers is displayed in Exhibit 17.1.

The percentage of people who go onto die from liver cancer increases with advancing age. Liver and bile duct cancer is the fifth leading cause of cancer deaths among men and accounts for 4% of cancer deaths. This form of cancer accounts for 2% of deaths

EXHIBIT 17.1: AGE DISTRIBUTION AND PERCENTAGES OF NEW DIAGNOSES AND DEATHS FROM LIVER AND BILE DUCT CANCER

AGE	PERCENTAGES OF NEW DIAGNOSES	PERCENTAGES OF DEATHS
Under 20	1.2%	0.5%
20 to 34	1.2%	0.8%
35 to 434	4.2%	3.2%
45 to 54	18.2%	13.0%
55 to 64	21.0%	17.4%
65 to 74	26.4%	26.8%
75 to 84	21.2%	27.4%
85 or Older	6.6%	10.9%

Source: Jemal, A., Siegel, R., Ward, E., Hao, Y., Xu, J., Murray, T., & Thun, M., (2008). Cancer Statistics, 2008. *CA: A Cancer Journal for Clinicians, 58,* 71–96.

from neoplasms among women and is the ninth leading cause of cancer death (National Center for Health Statistics, 2007).

Viral hepatitis is becoming a leading cause of liver failure in the United States and throughout the world. Vaccinations have led to a sharp decline in incidences of hepatitis A and B but no vaccination or treatment for hepatitis C has yet been developed. As a result, hepatitis C is now the leading cause of chronic liver disease affecting approximately 4.1 million people in the US and is the primary cause of liver transplantation. IV drug use, high-risk sexual behavior, administration of blood products, tattooing, hemodialysis, and needle stick injuries are some of the key methods of transmission for hepatitis C.

Hepatic toxicity is another cause of liver failure. Ingestion of acetaminophen (APAP) resulted in 168,093 calls to the American Association of Poison Control Center's National poison Data System in 2006 alone. This has provoked a nation-wide public education program warning that over-use or chronic use of APAP can result in irreversible liver damage. This is critical information for people who ingest two or more ounces of alcohol or its equivalent per day, people who use other medications metabolized by the liver, or parents who administer APAP to their children for pain and fever.

Perhaps the most disturbing, but under reported, trend in hepatic disease is the rise in hepatic steatosis or "fatty liver" disease. Fatty liver disease is most often found in patients with Type-2 diabetes. Health officials are using the term "epidemic" to describe the escalation in the prevalence of obesity in the United States. With this rise has come an increase in the frequency of a constellation of type-2 associated comorbidities. These include the following:

- Abdominal obesity (excessive fat tissue in and around the abdomen).
- Atherogenic dyslipidemia (blood fat disorders—high triglycerides, low HDL cholesterol and high LDL cholesterol—that foster plaque buildups in artery walls).
- Elevated blood pressure.
- Insulin resistance or glucose intolerance (the body can not properly use insulin or blood sugar).
- Prothrombotic state (e.g., high fibrinogen or plasminogen activator inhibitor-1 in the blood).
- Proinflammatory state (e.g., elevated C-reactive protein in the blood).

It is estimated that one in 10 adolescents in the United States meets the definition of metabolic syndrome. It is projected that by the year 2020, fatty liver disease will surpass hepatitis as the primary cause of liver transplantation in the United States (American Liver Foundation, 2008).

PHYSIOLOGY AND PHYSICAL ASSESSMENT

To understand liver disease we must first touch on some salient anatomy and physiology. The liver is the largest solid organ in the body and has two primary functions. First, as an essential organ of digestion producing chemicals that breakdown food. Secondly, as the primary organ for the recycling of red blood cells. The liver receives approximately 20% of its oxygen-rich blood flow from the hepatic artery. Critical to understanding end-stage liver disease (ESLD) is knowing that the remaining 80% of the flow is nutrient-rich blood from the stomach, intestines, and spleen via the portal vein (Keith, 1985).

The liver is responsible for (Ghany, & Hoofnagle, 2001):

- Synthesis of most serum proteins (albumin, carrier proteins, coagulation factors, many hormonal and growth factors);
- Production of bile and its carriers (bile acids, cholesterol, lecithin, phospholipids);
- Regulation of nutrients (glucose, glycogen, lipids, cholesterol, amino acids);
- Metabolism and conjugation of bilirubin, cations, as well as medications and excretion of these compounds in the bile or urine.

The assessment of the liver begins with a history that includes the past and present use of alcohol, IV drug use, acetaminophen, herbs, prescription drugs, as well as over the counter medications. Immunizations against hepatitis A and B, tattooing, and sexual history are important to note. Blood work needs to include a comprehensive liver function panel, comprehensive metabolic panel with close attention paid to glucose metabolism, and a hepatitis panel if indicated. Jaundiced skin tone is usually a late sign of liver failure, but a careful examination of the patient's sclera may reveal discoloration earlier. Sometimes skin ulceration on skin surfaces that have sun exposure can indicate liver disease.

The liver is the largest organ in the body and rests in the upper right quadrant of the abdomen and a portion of the inferior aspect can often be palpated just under the rib cage. Since it is solid, and when percussed delivers a flat or dull tone in comparison to bowel that is more tympanic. The healthy live is smooth and non-tender to palpation. Evaluating the size of a patient's liver via percussion is imprecise, but should generally be about 6–12 cm vertically at the right nipple or mid-clavicular line. Ascites can be crudely distinguished from adipose tissue by assessing a wave action to a patient's abdominal girth. To do this the patient or a helper firmly places the ulnar side of his hand along the umbilical line of the patient. This stabilizes adipose tissue and internal organs. The examiner then quickly presses and retracts finger tips on one side of the patient's abdomen while feeling for a fluid wave on the opposite side of the abdomen with the palm of the other hand. Having the patient lay on his side and percussing laterally across the abdomen can reveal dullness in the dependent areas where the fluid collects (Rushing, 2005). Abdominal ultrasound is a more precise assessment technique for determining liver size and the presence of ascites and is relatively inexpensive as well as being minimally invasive.

COMORBIDITY AND COMPLICATIONS

The liver is a resilient solid organ and withstands 80%–90% loss in function before symptoms occur (McGrew, 2001). Liver disease is usually divided into obstructive and hepatocellular. Obstructive liver disease is most often caused by stones blocking the bile duct. This is an acute problem corrected surgically. The causes of ESLD are hepatocellular and can be divided into (1) chemical, (2) infectious, and (3) neoplastic origins. The various forms of viral hepatitis are the primary infectious agents. Alcohol is the primary cause of cirrhosis followed by medications like acetaminophen, and industrial chemicals such as acetone. Fatigue and pruritus are often the first sign of a failing liver's inability to process bilirubin. The excess bilirubin accumulates in the skin, first causing an itch, then later jaundice.

For these reasons, the patient with ESLD may present with a number of problems that may include (Ghany & Hoofnagle, 2001):

- Malnutrition with serum albumin levels less than 3.0g/L.
- Muscle wasting with abdominal and peripheral edema.
- Disseminated intravascular coagulation (DIC) or extended bleeding time.
- Hyperlipidemia.
- Fluid, vitamin, and electrolyte imbalances.
- Fatigue and mental status changes.
- Chronic wounds on sun-exposed areas of the skin.
- Urticaria and later jaundice.
- Functional changes in the liver that last for longer than 6 months distinguish acute liver failure (ALF) from chronic liver failure (CLF) *(Fontana, 2008)*.

Chemical and alcoholic cirrhosis. Many prescribed, herbal, and over-the-counter medications stress the aging liver. Acetaminophen, considered a benign pain killer outside the medical community, can, if used in combination with prescription drugs assimilated in the liver, be a deadly combination for the older person. Presently acetaminophen overdose is the leading cause of acute

liver failure in the United States and its increasing incidence has been attributed to (1) intentional suicide gestures, (2) a shift away from the use of aspirin as an analgesic and antipyretic, as well as (3) the use APAP in more and more over-the-counter and prescription combination products (Fontana, 2008).

Physiological Changes with Chronic Liver Failure

- Jaundice.
- Ascites.
- Hepatic encephalopathy.
- Portal hypertension.
- Esophageal and gastric varices.
- Variceal hemorrhage.
- Spontaneous bacterial peritonitis.
- Hepato-renal syndrome.
- Porto- and hepato-pulmonary syndrome.
- Possible development of hepato-cellular carcinoma. (Arora & Keeffe, 2008)

In a 4-year study in the metropolitan Atlanta region, Bower, Johns, Margolis, Williams and Bell (2007) found that acetaminophen poisoning was the leading cause of admission to local ICUs for acute liver failure. Of those admissions, 48% of adults and 25% of children were due to acetaminophen with "undetermined etiology" being the next most prevalent cause listed. In this study, there was a 40% mortality rate, 42% surviving with supportive care and 12% rate of liver transplant. In a similar study, Gyamlani and Parikh (2002) reported that 86% of acetaminophen poisons in the Denver, Colorado area were suicide attempts and the remainder were accidental overdoses.

At least 70% of adults in the United States drink alcohol to some degree but drinking more than two drinks (22–30 g) per day in women and three drinks (33–45 g) increases the risk for liver disease. Most patients with alcoholic cirrhosis have a much higher daily intake and have drunk excessively for 10 years or more before onset of liver disease. Alcoholism is often intertwined with depression and may be described by the patient as "the blues," fatigue, social isolation, and decreased interest in social, as well as physical activities.

Alcohol is the leading cause of chemical cirrhosis in the United States and alcohol induced cirrhosis is the primary cause of portal hypertension in the portal venous system or vena cava. This pressure increase eventually will cause an expansion of the veins surrounding the esophagus creating hemorrhoid-like sacks that are susceptible to sudden rupture. Without intervention early in the development of esophageal varices, the rupture of varices is a life-threatening emergency. Intervention must include abstinence from alcohol and may include sclerosis of the varices.

Increased pressure in the mesenteric arms to the portal vein causes fluid to leak into the peritoneal cavity causing ascites. Likewise, because blood is not circulated completely through the liver, toxins build up causing encephalopathy. Ammonia is produced by the breakdown of protein during metabolism or by the breakdown of protein by bacteria in the gut.

The digestion of protein leads to the production of ammonia which the healthy liver can breakdown and excrete. In the late stages of liver disease, ammonia accumulates in the blood stream and leads to ammonia portal-systemic encephalopathy (PSE). Symptoms included progressive behavioral change, memory loss, and may eventually include hallucinations. Butterworth (1995) outlines a grading schema for PSE in Exhibit 17.2.

As encephalopathy develops and progresses the patient's ability to make informed decisions about interventions diminishes and the burden of that responsibility falls onto family members who may not be prepared. A frank discussion of the patient's wishes for interventions and end-of-life care needs to be initiated early and be made clear to the patient's circle of caregivers. Lack of preparation may be due to communication problems among the family members, a family member's beliefs being at odds with those of the patient, guilt, or other factors (Larson & Curtis, 2006).

Alcohol consumption patterns should be a part of the physical assessment. Less than 50% of primary care physicians include the diagnosis of alcohol dependence for patients who consumed four or more drinks per day and less than a third of healthcare professionals can effectively identify patients with substance abuse patterns (Gambert, 1997). Exacerbating the lack of consistent assessment is the reluctance of many individuals to openly discuss how much they drink. To decrease the likelihood of conflict, several questionnaires are available for patients to answer while filling out their health history. The most commonly used questionnaire is "CAGE" which asks, "Have you ever..."

- tried to **C**ut down on your drinking?
- been **A**nnoyed by anybody criticizing your drinking?
- felt **G**uilty about your drinking?
- had an "**E**ye opener" (drink) in the morning?

A "yes" answer to two or more of these questions indicates alcohol dependence. The CAGE tool may not be as valid in older adults who are retired or living alone (Fingerhood, 2000; Rigler, 2000).

Developed by the World Health Organization, the Alcohol Use Disorders Identification Test (AUDIT) in Exhibit 17.3 provides more detail than the CAGE questionnaire. A score of 8 or more indicates alcohol dependence. High scores on the first three items and lower scores on items 4 through 10 suggests hazardous alcohol use. Higher scores on questions 4, 5, and 6 point to the presence or emergence of alcohol dependence. High scores on 7 through 10 suggest harmful alcohol use (Trotto, 2000).

Infectious liver disease. The primary infectious agents of the liver are an expanding cluster of viral hepatitis agents. Hepatitis can be subdivided into acute and chronic diseases. Hepatitis-A (HAV) is the most common acute form of hepatitis and has no chronic state. It is passed through the feco-oral route and normally produces flu-like symptoms among a nonimmune compromised population. In the older adults, and subsequently immune compromised, population hepatitis-A can be deadly as it stresses the already damaged liver.

Hepatitis-B (HBV), hepatitis-C (HCV), and others in this expanding list have both acute and chronic stages. The major sources of chronic hepatitis are blood, blood products, tattoos with contaminated tools, IV drug use, and unprotected sexual activity. A review of transfusions and other medical procedures should therefore be a part of medical history. HBV infects over 1.25 million Americans and is presently the leading cause of hepatitis mortality. Infection is not restricted to the young or

EXHIBIT 17.2: GRADING OF PORTAL-SYSTEMIC ENCEPHALOPATHY (PSE) AND CHARACTERISTIC SIGNS

STAGE OF PSE	COGNITIVE SIGNS	NEUROMUSCULAR SIGNS
Sub-clinical	Abnormal psychometric test scores	None
Grade 1	Abnormal sleep patterns, shortened attention span, irritability, apathy	Tremor, incoordination
Grade 2	Personality changes, time disorientation, memory loss	Asterixis, dysarthia, abnormal muscle tone
Grade 3	Confusion, drowsiness, sleeplessness, paranoia, anger, stupor	Hyperactive reflexes, muscle rigidity
Grade 4	Coma	

Source: Butterworth, R. F. (1995). The role of liver disease in alcohol-induced cognitive defects. *Alcohol and Health Research World, 19,* 122–129.

EXHIBIT 17.3: ALCOHOL USE DISORDERS IDENTIFICATION TEST (AUDIT)

1) **How often do you have a drink containing alcohol?**
   (0) Never **(1)** Monthly or less **(2)** 2–4 times a month **(3)** 2–3 times a week **(4)** 4 or more times a week

2) **How many drinks do you have in a typical day when you are drinking?**
   (0) 1or 2 **(1)** 3 to 4 **(2)** 5 to 6 **(3)** 7 to 9 **(4)** 10 or more

3) **How often do you have 6 or more drinks on one occasion?**
   (0) Never **(1)** Less than monthly **(2)** Monthly **(3)** Weekly **(4)** daily or almost daily

4) **How often during the last year have you found that you were unable to stop drinking once you had started?**
   (0) Never **(1)** Less than monthly **(2)** Monthly **(3)** Weekly **(4)** Daily or almost daily

5) **How often during the last year have you failed to do what was normally expected from you because of drinking?**
   (0) Never **(1)** Less than monthly **(2)** Monthly **(3)** Weekly **(4)** Daily or almost daily

6) **How often within the last year have you needed a drink first thing in the morning to get yourself going after a heavy drinking session the night before?**
   (0) Never **(1)** Less than monthly **(2)** Monthly **(3)** Weekly **(4)** Daily or almost daily

7) **How often in the past year have you felt guilty or remorse after drinking?**
   (0) Never **(1)** Less than monthly **(2)** Monthly **(3)** Weekly **(4)** Daily or almost daily

8) **How often during the last year have you been unable to remember what happened the night before because you had been drinking?**
   (0) Never **(1)** Less than monthly **(2)** Monthly **(3)** Weekly **(4)** Daily or almost daily

9) **Have you, or has someone else, been injured as a result of your drinking?**
   (0) No **(1)** Yes, but not within the last year **(2)** Yes, during the last year

10) **Has a relative, friend, doctor, or other healthcare worker been concerned about your drinking or suggested that you cut down?**
   (0) No **(1)** Yes, but not within the last year **(2)** Yes, during the last year

Source: World Health Organization (1992). *Audit: The Alcohol Use Disorders Identification Test: Guideline for use in primary health care.* Geneva: WHO.

middle aged. As the overall American population ages, rates of all hepatitis infections will increase.

Never assume that an older patient is not sexually active. While the number of sexual partners and frequency of coitus may decrease with age, elderly does not mean abstinent. Older women are at greater risk of sexually acquired hepatitis, HIV, and other sexually transmitted diseases (STDs) than might be expected. Older women may not see themselves as vulnerable due to their age and in comparison to younger women,

quantifiably diminished sexual activity (Davis, Duncan, Turner, & Young, 2001). Up until the mid-1980s condoms were primarily used as a birth control device. The post-menopausal woman may not view condoms as an integral part of the sex act. In addition, the aging tissue of the genitalia is more susceptible to microscopic tears during coitus.

Screening for the increasing variety of hepatitides will be a challenge for medical and laboratory science. When writing this chapter the alphabet variations of hepatitis was passing the letter "E" and rising. Due to lack of long-term experience, the natural disease history of hepatitis-C and beyond is unknown, but appears deadly and increasingly widespread. Interferon alpha-2b and lamivudine (Epivir®) are the treatments recommended for Hepatitis B at the present time (Malik & Lee, 2000).

Liver cancer. Primary liver cancer is significantly lower in the United State than in foreign countries, especially those in Africa and Asia. In these regions, the primary cause of liver cancer is chronic viral hepatitis infections. The rate of liver cancer is declining in developing countries and increasing in developed nations. This trend is due to an increase in HCV among developed countries and an increasing use of HBV vaccines in underdeveloped areas. As the incidence of viral hepatitis increases in the United States, it is also likely that liver cancer due to this etiology will increase. However, for now, like so many other diseases of the liver, risk of hepatic carcinoma in America increases proportionally with alcohol consumption (El-Serag, 2001; McGlynn, Tsao, Hsing, Devesa, & Fraumeni, 2001). Some of the increase in the incidence of liver cancer in the United States is due to an overall aging of our population.

Primary cancer of the liver is often in an advanced state before symptoms appear. The first symptom is usually liver pain. The patient is usually tender over the liver and a mass may be palpable. A friction rub or bruit may be heard when the abdomen is auscultated. Alkaline phosphatase and alpha–fetoprotein (AFT) may be elevated, however, AFT is not elevated in 20%–30% of liver cancers (Stuart, Anand, & Jenkins, 1996). Although survival rates for liver and bile duct cancers has doubled over the past two decades, less than 11% of liver cancer patients will be alive 5 years after diagnosis (Jemal et al., 2008) The most likely long-term survivor of primary hepatic carcinoma is someone whose cancer is detected early enough for surgical resection. If the older patient presents symptomatically, the prognosis is poor with the average survival between 3–6 months. As a solid organ which is rich in blood, the liver's structure and function make it unsuitable for radiation therapy. If the tumor is caught early, surgery is the only definitive treatment. Surgical debulking of the tumor and chemotherapy at this time are only palliative (Lau, 2000).

Because the liver filters blood, many of the cancers that affect the liver have their origin somewhere else in the body. The liver is therefore second only to lymph nodes as the most common site of metastasis. Metastatic cancer in the liver is over 20 times more prevalent than primary liver carcinoma.

Other causes of liver disease. Hepatic steatosis and nonalcoholic fatty liver disease (NAFL) or nonalcoholic steatohepatitis is the gradual metamorphosis from a normal cell structure to one of fatty tissue. NAFL is more common in obese diabetic patients with hyperlipidemia (Marchesini et al., 2001) or those on long-term parenteral nutrition. Patients with fatty liver disease may show few signs of disease other than mild to moderate tenderness over the upper right abdominal quadrant. Without control of their diabetes and lipids as well as alcohol abstinence, these patients may progress to acute liver failure.

In a study by Ford, Giles, and Dietz (2002), slightly less than 7% of the sample below the age of 30-years old met the criteria for metabolic syndrome, however approximately 43% of those older than 60 did. As obesity continues on its trend to become more prevalent among children and adolescents, so too is the incidence of developing Type-2 diabetes and metabolic syndrome at increasingly younger ages. Duncan, Li, and Zhou (2004) found that the prevalence of metabolic syndrome among children and adolescents has increased from 4.2% (1988–1994) to 6.4% from 1999 through 2000. With this comes increased incidences of chronic liver and renal end-organ damage in these age groups (Ford, Li, Cook & Choi, 2007).

DYING TRAJECTORY

The life expectancy of a person with ESLD is difficult to predict. Fox et al. (1999) followed over 2600 patients who had been diagnosed with the advanced stages of either chronic obstructive pulmonary disease (COPD), congestive heart failure (CHF), or ESLD. In the Fox et al. study, ESLD was defined as patients with a diagnosis of cirrhosis and at least two of the following:

- Serum albumin of 30 g/L or less.
- Cachexia.
- A serum bilirubin level of 51 μmol/L (30 mg/dL) or more.
- Uncontrolled ascites.
- Hepatic encephalopathy.
- Massive gastrointestinal bleed requiring two or more units of blood transfused within a 24- hour period.
- Hematemesis or gross blood on endoscopic exam or nasogastric tube aspiration.

Of those meeting these criteria and predicted to die within 6 months by their physician, over 50% were still alive 6 months later. Roth, Lynn, Zhong, Borum,

and Dawson (2000) likewise found the 6-month projection of death in liver failure to be tenuous, but very predictable only in the last two weeks when symptoms, such as significant jaundice developed.

The average size of esophageal varices increase 5% each year the alcoholic continues to drink. If varices hemorrhage, 20%–30% of these patients die. If left untreated, 70% of patients with varices will die within a year (Hegab & Luketic, 2001). Over 50% of patients will die within 2 years of their diagnosis of ascites (Garcia & Sanyal, 2001).

The latest tool in assessing the severity of liver failure and estimating survival is the "Model of End-Stage Liver Disease" (MELD) introduced by Kamath et al. (2001). In a large prospective and retrospective study of the variables that predicted the survival of ESLD patients, these researchers found a formula that assessed international normalized ratio(INR) for prothrombin time (INR), serum bilirubin, and serum creatinine:

$$\begin{aligned} \text{MELD} = {} & 3.8 \, [\log_e \text{serum bilirubin (mg/dl)}] \\ & + 11.2 \, [\log_e \text{INR}] \\ & + 9.6 \, [\log_e \text{serum creatinine (mg/dl)}] \\ & + 6.4 \end{aligned}$$

This formula produces a score that is inversely related to the patient's likelihood of survival over time. MELD scores are used to rank patients awaiting liver transplantation. Several studies of the MELD formula over the intervening years have supported this tool's predictive value and validity. Some of these studies have attempted to determine if other variables should be included in the MELD formula. Dunn et al. (2005) tested MELD to determine if the presence of ascites or encephalopathy should be included as predictive variables, but found that MELD was able to stand alone as the best predictor (Exhibit 17.4).

EXHIBIT 17.4: ENCEPHALOPATHY AND ASCITES AS PREDICTORS OF 90-DAY MORTALITY

ENCEPHA-LOPATHY	ASCITES	90-DAY MORTALITY/ TOTAL # (%)	MEAN ± SD (RANGE OF MELD)
Yes	Yes	7/9 (78%)	29 ± 9 (17–38)
No	Yes	7/33 (21%)	17 ± 8 (6–36)
Yes	No	2/8 (25)	21 ± 8 (7–33)
No	No	0/23 (0%)	10 ± (0–18)

Source: Dunn, W., Jamil, L. H., Brown, L. S., Wiesner, R. H., Kim, W. R., Menon, K.V. N., et al. (2005). MELD accurately predicts mortality in patients with alcoholic hepatitis. *Hepatology, 41,* 353–358.

Emergency Situations

Emergencies in ESLD can result from one, but more likely a combination of factors, specifically: (1) bleeding; (2) mental status changes; (3) electrolyte imbalance; or (4) infections. The goal of palliative care is to have a plan in place that addresses what actions to take if a crisis occurs. This plan is a joint undertaking by the patient and his circle of caregivers. Nurses, family members, and other medical personnel must be willing to respect the wishes of the patient. What has changed in the medical community is the willingness to accept exacerbations or collateral diseases as a part of a natural process. Although healthcare professionals have the capability to intervene and stop the course of a collateral disease process, such as pneumonia, should we? This section will address the key emergency conditions that will likely result in the death of patients with ESLD. The interventions outlined range from the aggressive to comfort care only.

The most immediate life-threatening emergency in liver failure is hemorrhage from esophagal varices. A gradual decline in hemoglobin level or changes in stool towards a dark or tarry consistency heralds a slow low-grade hemorrhage. The differential diagnosis of these changes may be ulcerative or cancerous lesions in the upper GI tract. A careful history that includes a thorough assessment of alcohol use focuses the clinician to evaluate the liver and esophagus. If varices are discovered on endoscopy, they can be sclerosed surgically.

An alcoholic vomiting bright red blood is always an emergency. Even when this occurs in a hospital emergency room, the bleeding may be so severe and the patient so debilitated by the disease, that survival is doubtful. Aggressive intervention in hemorrhage includes intubation to protect the airway, the careful infusion of blood products and crystalloid, then endoscopy to sclerose the varices. Endoscopic sclerotherapy or banding is more effective than balloon tamponade and pharmacological treatment to increase survival in patients with varices. The primary surgical intervention used in patient rescue at this time is a transjugular intrahepatic portosystemic shunt (TIPS) in which a metal tube is placed connecting the portal and hepatic veins, reducing portal hypertension (Hegab & Luketic, 2001). Like many of the treatments for varices, TIPS does not improve survival rates.

The ESLD-induced dementia is usually a gradual process, but dramatic changes are possible. Rapid behavioral changes can be due to: (1) resumption of heavy drinking; (2) ingestion of other hepotoxic chemicals such as acetaminophen; (3) cerebral-vascular disease, (4) electrolyte imbalance; or (5) infection. Stopping the alcohol or other drugs is the first step and may return the patient's mental status back near base-line. If the change is due to acetaminophen overdose, the antidote, *N*-acetylcysteine, must be given within 10 h if it is to be effective.

Cerebral-vascular accident (CVA), stroke, or brain-attack can result in the abrupt onset of dementia in ESLD patients. Family members will report that these changes occurred "over night" or within a matter of hours. On examination, the patient may not show unilateral weakness or hemiparalysis. Unless it is a hemorrhagic stroke, CT of the head has little diagnostic utility. Care of the stroke patient is dealt with elsewhere in this book and comorbid ESLD does not significantly change those interventions. The patient with slow-progressing liver disease, however, may be more malnourished than the heretofore-healthy stroke patient.

Assuming that someone is providing daily care directly to the ESLD patient, infections and electrolyte changes lead to a more gradual change in behavior rather than the more abrupt changes of a stroke. Because the patient may not be able to reliably relate pain or other symptoms, aggressive evaluation of the patient includes: (1) complete blood count with differential; (2) blood cultures; (3) urine analysis; (4) blood chemistries; and (5) chest x-ray. Chemical imbalances in ESLD often result from low serum albumin levels due to malnutrition or fluid shifts. Aggressive intervention for electrolyte imbalances includes parenteral nutrition and hydration.

The site of the infection is more likely to be in the lungs, bladder, or perineum. Risk of peritonitis associated with ascites is the only infection that separates the ESLD patient from any other older person. Spontaneous bacterial peritonitis (SBP) is common in patients with ascites and presents with fever, chills, and generalized abdominal pain (rarely rebound tenderness). However, symptoms may be vague in the confused and debilitated patient. IV cefotaxime coupled with an aminoglycoside are initiated while waiting for the results of the ascites culture. Left untreated the patient with SBP will quickly slip into septic shock (Garcia & Sanyal, 2001).

Common Symptoms—Early to Late

Fatigue, itching, decreased appetite, and abdominal bloating singly or in combination may be the presenting symptoms of a patient with ESLD. The patient will usually complain of fatigue with activity or lack of stamina. They will feel best early in the morning and later need periods of rest between activities of daily living. Chronic nausea may be accompanied by alterations in taste and aversion to food and food preparation smells.

The itch of liver failure is not localized and is not associated with a rash. In some instances, the patient may have open superficial wounds on the sun-exposed areas of the skin that reoccur and are slow to heal. The patient may report increasing right upper quadrant abdominal pain as the sack inclosing the liver expands as the size of the liver increases.

Darkening of the urine as bilirubin is excreted occurs before the development of jaundice. Jaundice, or the accumulation of bilirubin in the skin, is usually a sign of advanced disease and may only present as death approaches. The development of jaundice may be so slow that family members do not recognize the change.

Ascites may be distinguished from gas by having the patient lie flat. The abdomen is round or distended and is dull to percussion. Gas bloating has a tympanic sound to percussion and the abdomen may not be uniform in its contour. With ascites a fluid wave motion can be bolotted by placing your hands on both sides of the patient's abdomen and pushing one side in quickly. A ripple of abdominal fluid will roll across the other hand.

Because of the resilient nature of the liver, blood tests may be normal despite advanced disease. Likewise, measurements of liver function may be elevated for problems that do not have their origin in this organ. Laboratory testing is five-fold. First is to assess if the liver is damaged through liver function tests (LFTs). Secondly, blood work is used to determine if the patient is malnourished and the degree of malnutrition. Albumin of less than 4 g per l of blood is considered malnourished. If the albumin drops below 2.1 the patient is extremely malnourished. Next, complete blood chemistry is used to determine the fluid and electrolyte balance of the patient. High mineral concentration indicates dehydration. Approximately half of the patients with chronic liver disease have macrocytosis and thrombocytopenia but the rest will have no significant change to their CBC.

Drawing an ammonia level requires special handling and is best drawn at the lab running the test. In the hospital, check the protocol for drawing this test. An elevated ammonia level indicatesportal-systemic encephalopathy (PSE). Lastly a hepatitis panel is used to identify if there is an infectious cause to the liver disease. Muscle wasting can also result in an elevated serum ammonia level and cannot be taken alone as a measure of PSE.

All LFTs are measurements of serum bilirubin, albumin, and prothrombin time. The serum bilirubin level is a measure of hepatic conjugation and excretion, and the serum albumin level and prothrombin time are measures of protein synthesis. Abnormalities of bilirubin, albumin, and prothrombin time are typical of hepatic dysfunction. Decreased intake and absorption of vitamin K is common in alcohol cirrhosis and prolonged bleeding times can make the rupture of varices deadly. Bilirubin found in the urine is conjugated bilirubin and its presence implies liver disease. A urine dipstick test can give the same information as the serum bilirubin and is almost 100% accurate.

While a thorough history, physical examination, and testing just described will provide enough information to make a diagnosis, liver biopsy is "gold standard" for grading and staging of the disease.

Complications of End-Stage Liver Disease

The onset of ascites or esophageal varices coupled with low albumin or any gastrointestinal bleeding are thought to be sentinel events in the decision to initiate palliative care in advanced liver disease (McGrew, 2001). Essential to any treatment is abstinence from alcohol.

Ascites. The patient, family, and even the clinician may misidentify ascites as the bloating of simple fluid retention or weight gain. This may be attributed to excess sodium in the diet or congestive heart failure. Without a thorough physical examination, the first reaction to a patient presenting with fluid "bloating" is to prescribe a diuretic. Diuretics can cause hypovolemia, therefore concentrating ammonia. This patient may quickly become disoriented, demented, and then comatose. Other causes of ascites besides liver failure include cancer, tuberculosis, renal failure, and pancreatic disease (Riley & Bahatti, 2001).

Progressive ascites push up on the diaphragm, making it difficult for patients to take a deep breath, exert themselves, or sleep lying down. As the degree of ascites increases the patient will feel increasing shortness of breath. All these factors raise the risk of pneumonia. With increased abdominal girth is a shift in the patient's center of gravity and this affects his ability to walk.

Bed rest is the first nonaggressive treatment for ascites and keeping the patient reclined for a few days reduces the activation of the renin-angiotension system. However, this is impractical for long-term treatment. Dietary sodium restriction is the mainstay of ascites treatment. The addition of the diuretic spironolactone (Aldactone) that reduces aldosterone-dependent sodium reabsorption is very effective in reducing ascites if used in conjunction with dietary sodium restriction. A daily dose of 100 mg spironolactone is given. Rapid diuresis can result in hyponatremia, azotemia, potassium imbalance, and onset of or increase encephalopathy.

One treatment for ascites is paracentesis which is the drainage of excess fluid in the abdominal cavity. The primary purpose of paracentesis is decompression of chest and abdominal cavity's organs. The patient will be able to breathe with less strain and they will feel less bloated and therefore able to eat. His gait may be improved. Paracentesis is not without risk of secondary infection and potential puncture of an abdominal organ. Overly aggressive paracentesis can result in extracellular fluid shifts and orthostatic hypotension. First, a sample of the fluid is examined for infection, blood, and tumor. One kilogram of fluid can be removed in an outpatient setting if the ascites is coupled with peripheral edema. Without comorbid peripheral edema, no more than 0.5 kg should be drained. More aggressive or "large-volume" paracentesis of up to 5 l of fluid requires hospitalization and parenteral albumin supplementation (Garcia & Sanyal, 2001). Fifty percent of patients with either ascites or encephalopathy will die within 2 years of onset (Sanchez & Talwalkar, 2006).

Portal-systemic encephalopathy (PSE). Ammonia is a byproduct of protein metabolism. Restricting protein in the diet is controversial. On one side are those who recommend initiation of a low protein diet once PSE has been confirmed by an elevated ammonia level in the arterial blood and mental status changes (McGrew, 2001). Pharmacological management includes 15–30 ml of lactulose given three times a day to reduce protein absorption in the gut. If lactulose alone is effective at reducing symptoms of encephalopathy, this regime is continued. If encephalopathy continues, neomycin can be added to reduce bacterial activity in the gut (Abiy-Assi & Vlahcevic, 2001). Patients have difficulty staying on a regimen of neomycin and lactulose due to stomach upset, cramping, and diarrhea. Ascites will likely return, requiring multiple procedures.

Other specialists in ESLD believe that long-term protein restriction is counter productive because of the advanced malnourished state that accompanies ESLD (Bashir & Lipman, 2001). Vitamin and mineral supplementation is a special need with alcoholic cirrhosis. Dietary restriction of sodium to no more than 800 mg or 2 g of salt per day may be helpful in reducing fluid retention. Diet in ESLD should employ a team approach consisting of the patient, family, healthcare provider, and dietician.

Esophageal varices. Treatment of esophageal varices is limited because the surgical interventions are invasive and have not been shown to improve the overall survival rate. A noninvasive approach is to reduce portal hypertension using nonselective beta-blockers such as propranolol (Inderal) or nadolol (Corgard). Higher doses that are normally used to treat hypertension will be required and dosage is adjusted upward until the resting heart rate is reduced by 25%, but not below 55 beats per min. The advantage of nadolol is that it can be given in a single daily dose of 40–320 mg. Propranolol at a dose between 10–480 mg may be divided over the course of the day. Use of beta-blockers has been shown to reduce the risk of bleeding by 45% and bleeding-related death by 50%. Surgical intervention using a laser to cauterize the varices is a recent innovation, but can result in fatal hemorrhage. Endoscopic sclerotherapy and banding are presently the first-line treatments for bleeding varices (Hegab & Luketic, 2001).

Pain management. Pain control and comfort are the primary patient and family concerns in patients with terminal diseases (Cleary & Carbone, 1997). Aggressive chemotherapy is costly, often has no effect on the course of the disease, and the therapy itself results in discomfort. Pain in the later stages of ESLD can be equivalent to that of late-stage lung or colon cancer (Roth et al.,

2000). Without appropriate medical pain control, the patient may turn to over-the-counter medications that may be hepatotoxic or resort to alcohol. Codeine or codeine analogs without acetaminophen and later morphine are the initial choices (Stravitz et al., 2007). As the patient has difficulty swallowing or retaining oral medications, the use of transdermal Fentanyl or a morphine pump may be used. Family members will likely be concerned that their loved one will become "addicted" to these pain medications or become "doped-up." The patient and family need to be repeatedly reassured that comfort is the priority and that addiction is extremely rare.

Diphenhydramine (Benadryl), hydroxyzine (Vistaril), or promethazine (Phenergan) often act synergistically with pain medications in addition to reducing nausea, decreasing the severity of itching skin, but their primary benefit for the ESLD patient is these medication's sedative properties (Larson & Curtis, 2006). Often with progressing ascites and shortness of breath, the patient becomes increasingly restless and anxious even though pain is adequately controlled. Family members may become frightened with a loved one who is struggling to breathe or who is confused. In these cases, they are more likely to call paramedics or take the patient to the emergency room. Antianxiety agents such as lorazepam (Ativan), alprazolam (Xanax), or diazepam (Valium) are essential in reducing these symptoms. Diazepam has the advantages of being cheap and coming in an IV or IM injectable forms. While finding the appropriate combination of medications to control pain, anxiety, urticaria, and nausea may require some trial and error, no patient should suffer in pain (Tremblay & Breitbart, 2001).

Hospice can be an effective source of information, family counseling, and pain control if this resource is initiated early in ESLD. As mentioned before in this chapter, prediction of life expectancy is problematic and clinicians often wait until death is certain and eminent before involving Hospice. Effective pain control is, therefore, inconsistent and pain appraisal is made difficult as the patient's level of consciousness diminishes. If Hospice is not involved, problems with pain control are confounded by withdrawal of contact with the healthcare community as the patient deteriorates. In a study of people who died at home, Desbiens and Wu (2000) found that half were conscious in the last 3 days of life and of the conscious patients, 40% reported severe uncontrolled pain.

CONCERNS AND IMPLICATIONS FOR NURSING PRACTICE

Proactive Role of Nursing in the Prevention of Liver Disease

- Early immunizations against hepatitis.
- Alcohol moderation.

- Acetaminophen safety.
- Weight management.
- Exercise.
- Safer sex practices.
- Dangers of needle contamination (tattooing and IV drug use).
- Regular primary care evaluation including glucose monitoring and liver function testing.

Patients with ESLD may first seek care due to increasing fatigue. This sense of fatigue will increase as the disease progresses. Community health nurses need to assess the patient's capabilities and the home environment to determine what support resources are needed. The patient must learn to self-pace his activities, to take frequent breaks and build naps into his day.

The goals of professional nursing care for the ESLD patient are the following:

- Maintain activities of daily living.
- Prepare the family and circle of caregivers for their roles.
- Help the patient avoid alcohol and other hepatotoxic chemicals.
- Maintain nutrition and hydration.
- Management of symptoms such as pain and itching. Larson & Curtis, 2006)

Nurses are in a pivotal position to assess the family for their capacity to give care (Groen, 1999). There may be unresolved issues of guilt and recrimination surrounding the patient's alcohol abuse. Spouse and children may need counseling to deal with these issues. The circle of caregivers must be willing to help the patient avoid alcohol. Likewise, the family needs to be informed of the natural course of the disease process and what changes should be expected. There should be a written plan of the steps to be taken in the event of an emergency or rapid deterioration so that the patient's wishes are addressed. At a minimum every family member should read and discuss this advanced directive.

Referral to palliative care is late for most terminally ill patients, not just those with ESLD (Medici et al., 2008). Because the only effective treatment for ESLD is liver transplantation, these patients can be on a transplant registry and receive hospice care at the same time. Unfortunately, many of those awaiting transplant will die and palliative care's role is to control symptoms as they occur.

The first step to alcohol abstinence may be detoxification in a specialized facility. With advanced disease the patient may be hemodynamically unstable with severe nutritional and mineral deficits. These will need to be stabilized before the patient can return to family or long-term care. Most detoxification facilities interface with Alcoholics Anonymous (AA) and arrangements for follow up with AA should be established before the patient is discharged. Older patients may have more severe alcohol withdrawal symptoms with increased hallucinations, sleep disturbance, and confusion.

Older alcoholics are often malnourished because alcohol has been a significant source of calories. A dietician is an essential part of the caregiver circle, especially if the decision is made to restrict protein. "Meals On Wheels" can deliver food to home-bound patients that conform to specialized diet. Vitamin and mineral supplementation is specialized to avoid chemicals that are hepatotoxic. Extra vitamin K may be needed to correct bleeding irregularities. Aspirin should be avoided and salt intake reduced.

Elderly alcoholic patients are at increased risk of falls. Due to increased prothrombin time, bleeding precautions such as the use of soft toothbrushes is a part of the lifestyle change. The patient needs to be weighed daily on the same scale and report any sudden gain of over 2 kg in a day. The patient needs to be assessed daily for pain, itching, fever, edema, increased shortness of breath, and mental status changes (Martin, 1992).

In cases of cerebral edema leading to encephalopathy, the palliative care nurse is a vital link in shaping the environment for the liver failure patient.

O'Neal, Olds, and Webster (2006) developed and described a protocol for the administration of mannitol when acute liver failure patients in an ICU develop signs of encephalopathy. Their protocol incorporate evidence-based practice interventions, a criteria for patient assessment, as well as a collaborative model of nursing and medicine.

EXHIBIT 17.5: NURSING INTERVENTIONS FOR PATIENTS WITH ENCEPHALOPATHY

STAGE	COGNITIVE SIGNS	INTERVENTIONS
Grade 1	Sleep disturbance, mild mood and speech changes.	Reassurance, nutritional and hydration support. Avoid hypnotics and sedatives.
Grade 2	Mild irritability, agitation, and somnolence.	All in Grade 1 plus quiet environment with minimal stimuli.
Grade 3	Confusion, arousable by painful stimuli only.	All in Grades 1 & 2 and elevate head of bed to 30° from horizontal. Give IV mannitol.
Grade 4	Coma	Life support. Give IV mannitol.

Source: Fontana, R. J. (2008). Acute liver failure including acetaminophen overdose. *Medical Clinics of North America, 92,* 761–794.

Family Concerns and Considerations—Caregiver Fears

The progression to death from liver disease is often a slow and tedious process. Roth et al. (2000) studied 575 patients with ESLD. Two thirds of these patients died within 2 years. Eighty-nine percent of the patients rated their quality of life as fair to poor with the inability to perform activities of daily living as the major source of dissatisfaction. Eighty-eight percent of the study's patients had a family caregiver in the home and two thirds required professional home-health services. One third of family's savings were devastated by the costs of healthcare for the dying patient.

The circle of caregivers needs to be supported by health professionals. Support of the family members is also extremely important particularly in certain cultures. Pain control and comfort measures are, however, universal goals. African Americans, Hispanics, and recent immigrants are less likely to utilize advance directives (Huff & Kline, 1999; Waters, 2001). This is primarily due to distrust or lack of familiarity with the medical system in the United States. In a study of palliative care choices, Phillips et al. (2000) found no differences between races with regard to decisions to withdraw or withhold life support for dying patients. Clergy should also be included as a part of the care-giving circle early in the disease process while the patient is oriented and can have meaningful interaction. In many ethnic, national, and religious groups, clergy can act as a bridge between the family and healthcare providers.

Alcohol cirrhosis and hepatitis from drug use or sexual contact will likely create issues of guilt and blame that will be difficult to resolve as the patient deteriorates rapidly. While alcoholic cirrhosis is the more common origin of ESLD today, hepatitis will likely result in the death of many older adults in the future. The caring circle, to include health professionals and family, needs to be rallied around the patient-present rather than dwelling on the patient's past actions.

Children of a dying alcoholic parent will likely harbor memories of neglect or even abuse. Spouses may also be the victims of neglect or abuse. The codependent model may be exceedingly difficult to maintain if the other partner is frail and unable to provide the increasingly demanding day-to-day care of his spouse. Family members need to be informed of the mental status changes that take place when death is imminent. In Roth's study less than 10% of the patients showed confusion 6 months before death, however, within the last month of life one third displayed serious mental status changes.

Case Study conclusion: The story of Shelia in the opening of this chapter is but one of over

450 Americans who die each year from acetaminophen overdose (Nourjah, Ahmad, & Karwoski, 2006).

Shelia was transferred to our adjacent emergency room and was admitted to our hospital. Over the next week her liver function continued to decline and she was put on the transplant list. She became jaundiced and was transferred to our medical intensive care unit. During her second week of hospitalization Shelia experienced increasing periods of delirium. She died during her third week at our facility.

Had Shelia been treated within 10 h of her acetaminophen ingestion, N-acteylcysteine (NAC) could have been given intravenously (IV) and possibly limited the damage done to her liver. IV NAC was approved for use in such cases in 2004 and has come to replace the less well-tolerated oral form of this drug. In a study by Doyon and Klein-Schwartz (2008) of 77 patients treated for acute acetaminophen poisoning within the time window outlined by the FDA, only 4 patients developed hepatotoxicity, with one death and one liver transplantation.

As a result of recent press coverage of the dangers associated with the chronic use of acetaminophen and its interaction with alcohol as well as other medications, the makers of Tylenol have televised a public information warning. Unfortunately, the public continues to view acetaminophen as a benign over-the-counter drug with few side effects, and it is the most commonly administered drug for children.

CONCLUSION

Today end-stage liver failure carries with it the stigma of alcohol cirrhosis and the risk-taking behavior associated with hepatitis C. With a growing number of children and older people suffering the effects of fatty liver disease they will likely be associated with the "shame" of obesity and the social perception that a person's lifestyle or lack of healthy behaviors lead to their disease state. Shelia's mother now carries the burden that her child committed suicide and that emotional trauma ripples through affected families. No matter what the cause of the liver failure, the treatment of the patient and family remains the same-reduction in the symptoms of the disease process and emotional support. Family members will likely feel guilty or want to assign blame, as they consider themselves or others as enablers who sat by while their loved one drank or become obese.

Over the next decade, it is hoped that the artificial or bio-artificial liver-support systems that are being tested will allow ELSD patients a means of survival until transplantation (Fontana, 2008; Kjaergard, Liu, Als-Nielsen, & Gluud, 2003; O'Grady, 2007). These devices would also have benefit for patients with acute liver failure as a bridge until some degree of spontaneous recovery of liver function occurs.

There is a changing face to ESLD as we progress through the first quarter of the 21stcentury. Hepatitis C has now surpassed alcoholic cirrhosis as the leading cause of liver transplantation. As the epidemic of obesity spreads through the US, by 2020, fatty liver disease will demand more transplantable livers than any other reason. The cost and public health burden is difficult to predict. As nurses we should be proactive in encouraging the public health initiatives of improving young people's diet and their access to exercise. Otherwise, as palliative care nurses, we will have to care for the aftermath.

EVIDENCE-BASED PRACTICE

Hofer, S., Oberholzer, C., Beck, S., Looser, C., & Ludwig C. (2008). Ultrasound-guided radiofrequency ablation (RFA) for inoperable gastrointestinal liver metastases. *Ultraschall in der Medizin, 29*(4), 388–92.

Background. Surgery is the most effective treatment for liver metastases. Some patients, however, cannot tolerate this procedure due to comorbidity, advanced age, site of the lesion or previous liver surgery. In our institution we have now increasing experience with radiofrequency ablation (RFA), a thermo-ablative modality. We compare our outcome and survival results to standard treatments for liver metastases.

Methods. From April 2000–June 2005, 30 consecutive patients with liver metastases from gastrointestinal primaries were treated with ultrasound guided RFA for their liver metastases (patients mean age 63.5 years, range 37–80. Size of lesions, range 0.4–6 cm). Main indications were nonoperable lesions due to site of the lesion or comorbidity. RFA was also applied as an additive to liver surgery and as a repetitive palliative treatment. 15 patients underwent one RFA-intervention, 8 patients two, 3 patients three, 1 patient four, 2 patients five and 1 patient six. RFA-interventions (n = 60) were performed either percutaneously (71.5%), in an open approach without liver surgery (22%) or in addition to liver surgery (6.5%).

Results. Mean observation time after first RFA was 23.5 months (range 3–63). Median survival in our patient cohort is 34 months, which compares favourably with results obtained by hepatic resection, the standard of care for liver metastases. Complication rate, attributed

to the RFA procedure, was small in our series (5.5%) with one pleural effusion and one abscess formation in the ablated lesion due to underlying bacteraemia.

Conclusion. RFA is an effective and low risk treatment modality in patients with liver metastases. The procedure is safe (complication rate < 6%) with low morbidity. RFA can be performed repeatedly on an outpatient basis with good palliative effects. Of note, surgery remains the treatment of choice in resectable liver metastases of colorectal origin.

REFERENCES

Abiy-Assi, S., & Vlahcevic, Z. R. (2001). Hepatic encephalopathy: Metabolic consequence of cirrhosis often is reversible. *Postgraduate Medicine, 109*(2), 52–70.

American Liver Foundation. (2008). Retrieved November 27, from http://www.liverfoundation.org/education/info/fattyliver/

Arora, G., & Keeffe, E. B. (2008). Management of chronic liver failure until liver transplantation. *Medical Clinics of North America, 92*, 239–860.

Bashir, S., & Lipman, T. O. (2001). Nutrition in gastroenterology and hepatology. In M. L. Borum (Ed.), *Primary care: Clinics in office practice—Gastroenterology* (pp. 629–645). Philadelphia, PA: W. B. Saunders Company.

Bower, W. A., Johns, M., Margolis, H. S., Williams, I. T., & Bell, B. P. (2007). Population-based surveillance for acute liver failure. *American Journal of Gastroenterology, 102*, 2459–2463.

Butterworth, R. F. (1995). The role of liver disease in alcohol-induced cognitive defects. *Alcohol and Health Research World, 19*, 122–129.

Cleary, J. F., & Carbone, P. P. (1997). Palliative medicine in the elderly, *Cancer, 80*, 1335–1347.

Davis, R. B., Duncan, L., Turner, L. W., Young, M. (2001). Perceptions of HIV and STD risk among low-income adults: A pilot study. *Applied Nursing Research, 14*(2), 105–109.

Desbiens, N. A., & Wu, A. W. (2000). Perspectives and reviews of support findings: Pain and suffering in seriously ill hospitalized patients. *Journal of the American Geriatrics Society, 48*(Suppl. 5), S176–S182.

Doyon, S., & Klein-Schwartz, W. (2008). Hepatotoxicity despite early administration of intravenous *N*-acetylcysteine for acute acetaminophen overdose. *Academic Emergency Medicine, 15*, 1–6.

Duncan, G. E., Li, S. M., & Zhou, X. H. (2004). Prevalence and trends of a metabolic syndrome phenotype among US adolescents. *Diabetes Care, 27*, 2438–2443.

Dunn, W., Jamil, L. H., Brown, L. S., Wiesner, R. H., Kim, W. R., Menon, K.V. N., et al. (2005). MELD accurately predicts mortality in patients with alcoholic hepatitis. *Hepatology, 41*, 353–358.

El-Serag, H. B. (2001). Liver tumors. *Clinics in Liver Disease, 5*, 87–107.

Fingerhood, M. (2000). Progress in geriatrics: Substance abuse in older people. *Journal of the American Geriatrics Society, 48*, 985–995.

Fontana, R. J. (2008). Acute liver failure including acetaminophen overdose. *Medical Clinics of North America, 92*, 761–794.

Ford, E. S., Li, C., Cook, S., & Choi, H. K. (2007). Serum concentrations of uric acid and the metabolic syndrome among US children and adolescents. *Circulation, 115*, 2526–2532.

Ford, E. S., Giles, W. H., & Dietz, W. H. (2002). Prevalence of the metabolic syndrome among US adults: Findings from the third National Health and Nutrition Examination Survey. *Journal of the American Medical Association, 287*, 356–359.

Fox, E., Landrum-McNiff, K., Zhong, Z., Dawson, N. V., Wu, A. W., Lynn, J., et al. (1999). Evaluation of prognostic criteria for determining Hospice eligibility in patients with advanced lung, heart, or liver disease. *Journal of the American Medical Association, 282*, 1638–1645.

Garcia, N., & Sanyal, A. J. (2001). Minimizing ascites: Complications of cirrhosis signals clinical deterioration. *Postgraduate Medicine, 109*(2), 91–103.

Ghany, M., & Hoofnagle, J. H. (2001). Liver and biliary tract disease. In E. Braunwald, S. L. Hauser, A. S. Fauci, D. L. Longo, D. L. Kasper, & J. L. Jameson (Eds.), *Harrison's principles of internal medicine* (pp. 1707–1711). New York, NY: McGraw-Hill Medical Publishing Division.

Groen, K. A. (1999). Primary and metastatic liver cancer. *Seminars on Oncology Nursing, 15*, 48–57.

Gyamlani, G. G., & Parikh, C. R. (2002) Acetaminophen toxicity: Suicidal vs. accidental. *Critical Care, 6*, 155–159.

Hegab, A. M., & Luketic, V. A. (2001). Bleeding esophageal varices: How to treat this dreaded complication of portal hypertension. *Postgraduate Medicine, 109*(2), 75–76, 81–86, 89.

Huff, R. M., & Kline, M. V. (1999). *Promoting health in multicultural populations: A handbook for clinicians.* Thousand Oaks, CA: Sage Publications, Inc.

Jemal, A., Siegel, R., Ward, E., Hao, Y., Xu, J., Murray, T., et al. (2008). Cancer statistics, 2008. *CA: A Cancer Journal for Clinicians, 58,*71–96.

Kamath, P. S., Wiesner, R. H., Malinchoc, M., Kremers, W. Therneau, T. M., Kosberg, C. L., et al. (2001). A model to predict survival in patients with end-stage liver disease. *Hepatology, 33*, 464–470.

Keith, J. S. (1985). Hepatic failure: Etiologies, manifestations, and management. *Critical Care Nurse, 5*, 60–86.

Kjaergard, L. L., Liu, J., Als-Nielsen, B., & Gluud, C. (2003). Artificial and bioartificial support systems for acute and acute-on-chronic liver failure: A systemic review. *Journal of the American Medical Association, 289*, 217–222.

Kung, H. C., Hoyert, D. L., Xu, J. Q., & Murphy, S. L. (2008). *Deaths: Final data for 2005. National Vital Statistics Reports*(Vol. 56, p. 10). Hyattsville, MD: National Center for Health Statistics.

Larson, A. M., & Curtis, J. R. (2006). Integrating palliative care for liver transplant candidates: "Too well for transplant, to sick for life." *Journal of the American Medical Association, 295*, 2168–2176.

Lau, W. Y. (2000). Primary liver tumors. *Seminars in Surgical Oncology, 19*, 135–144.

Malik, A. H., & Lee, W. M. (2000). Chronic hepatitis-B infection: Treatment strategies for the next millennium. *Annals of Internal Medicine, 132*, 723–731.

Marchesini, G., Brizi, M., Bianchi, G., Tomassetti, S., Bugianesi, E., Lenzi, M., et al. (2001). Nonalcoholic fatty liver disease: A feature of the metabolic syndrome. *Diabetes, 50*, 1844–1850.

Martin, F. L. (1992). When the liver breaks down. *Registered Nurses, 55* (8), 52–57

McGlynn, K. A., Tsao, L., Hsing, A. W., Devesa, S. S., & Fraumeni, J. F. (2001). International trends and patterns of primary liver disease. *International Journal of Cancer, 94*, 290–296.

McGrew, D. M. (2001). Chronic illness and the end of life. In M. L. Borum (Ed.), *Primary care: Clinics in office practice—Gastroenterology* (pp. 339–347). Philadelphia, PA: W. B. Saunders Company.

Medici, V., Rossaro, L., Wegelin, J. A., Kamboj, A., Nakai, J., Fisher, K., et al. (2008). The utility of the Model for End-Stage Liver Disease score: A reliable guide for liver transplant candidacy and, for select patients, simultaneous hospice referral. *Liver Transplantation, 14*, 1100–1106.

National Center for Health Statistics. (2007). *Health, United States, 2007--With chartbook on trends in the health of Americans.* Hyattsville, MD: US Department of Health and Human Services.

Nourjah, P., Ahmad, S. R., & Karwoski, C. (2006). Estimates of acetaminophen (Paracetamol)-associated overdoses in the United States. *Pharmacoepidemiology and Drug Safety, 15*, 398–405.

O'Grady, J. (2007). Modern management of acute liver failure. *Clinics in Liver Disease, 11*, 291–303.

O'Neal, H., Olds, J., & Webster, N. (2006). Managing patients with acute liver failure: Developing a tool for practitioners. *Nursing in Critical Care, 11*(2), 63–68.

Phillips, R., Hamel, M. B., Teno, J. M., Soukup, J., Lynn, J., Califf, R., et al. (2000). Patient race and decisions to withhold or withdraw life-sustaining treatments for seriously ill hospitalized adults. *American Journal of Medicine, 108*, 14–19.

Rigler, S. K. (2000). Alcoholism in the elderly. *American Family Physician, 61*, 1710–1716.

Riley, T. R., & Bahatti, A. M. (2001). Preventive strategies in chronic liver disease: Part II. Cirrhosis. *American Family Physician, 64*, 1555–15560.

Roth, K., Lynn, J., Zhong, Z., Borum, M., & Dawson, N. V. (2000). Dying with end stage liver disease with cirrhosis: Insights from SUPPORT. *Journal of the American Geriatric Society, 48* (Suppl.), S122–S130.

Rushing, J. (2005). Assessing for ascites. *Nursing, 34* (2). 68.

Sanchez, W., & Talwalkar, J. A. (2006). Palliative care for patients with end-stage liver disease ineligible for liver transplantation. *Gastroenterology Clinics of North America, 35*, 201–219.

Stuart, K. E., Anand, A. J., & Jenkins, R. L. (1996). Hepatocellular carcinoma in the United States: Prognostic features treatment outcome and survival. *Cancer, 77*, 2217–2222.

Stravitz, R., Kramer, H., Davern, T., Shaikh, O. S., Caldwell, S. H., Mehta, R. L., et al. (2007). Intensive care of patients with acute liver failure: Recommendations of the U.S. Acute Liver Failure Study Group. *Critical Care Medicine, 35*, 2498–2508.

Tremblay, A., & Breitbart, W. (2001). Palliative care: Psychiatric dimensions of palliative care. *Neurologic Clinics, 19*, 949–967.

Trotto, N. E., (2000). Meeting the challenge of alcoholic liver disease. *Patient Care, 110–113*, 116–123.

Waters, C. M. (2001). Understanding and supporting African Americans' perspectives of end-of-life care planning and decision making. *Qualitative Health Research, 11*, 385–398.

World Health Organization. (1992). *Audit: The alcohol use disorders identification test: Guideline for use in primary health care.* Geneva: WHO.

18

Palliative Care for Patients with HIV/AIDS

Deborah Witt Sherman

Key Points

■ In countries with advanced healthcare, HIV/AIDS is managed as a chronic illness, while in underdeveloped countries individuals without access to care are continuing to die from AIDS.

■ HIV and AIDS are not synonymous terms but, rather, refer to the natural history or progression of the infection, ranging from asymptomatic infection to life-threatening illness.

■ The components of high-quality HIV/AIDS palliative care include competent, skilled practitioners; confidential, nondiscriminatory, culturally sensitive care; flexible and responsive care; collaborative and coordinated care; and fair access to care.

■ The control of pain and symptoms associated with HIV/AIDS enables the patient and family to expend their energies on spiritual and emotional healing, and the possibility for personal growth and transcendence even as death approaches.

■ Knowledge regarding HIV disease enables nurses to offer effective and compassionate care to patients and families at all stages of HIV disease.

Case Study: Miriam, a 36-year-old woman with *Mycobacterium avium intracellulare* (MAC), began to have daily episodes of diarrhea. She was admitted to the hospital with fever, fatigue, anorexia, nausea and vomiting, and weight loss of 15 lbs over the last 3 weeks. Her significant other was diagnosed with HIV 5 years ago and she reported unprotected sex on several occassions. Miriam's CD4 count was 60 cells/mm^3 with a viral load (VL) of 130,000. Her laboratory work indicated anemia and an elevated alkaline phosphatase. MAC was confirmed by biopsy with AFB (acid fast bacterial) stain. She was also anemic and labs indicated an elevated alkaline phosphatase. On physical exam, she had an enlarged spleen, and lymph nodes were palpable in her inguinal area. The diagnosis was advanced-stage AIDS. Miriam was begun on a highly active antiretroviral (HAART) regimen consisting of a protease inhibitor plus two nonnucleoside reverse transcriptase inhibitors. She was treated for MAC with azithromycin and rifabutin. Miriam's mother and sister, although close by, had a poor relationship with Miriam's significant other, and so Miriam was not in close contact with her family. Miriam had a 5-year-old son from a previous relationship. She was working as a secretarial assistant until 4 months ago when her health severely declined.

Miriam responded well following MAC treatment and her diarrhea improved. She still remained weak and found it difficult to climb the stairs of her four story walk-up apartment. Her son needed to be walked to school every day, and arguments ensued as her boyfriend was unwilling to assume any child-care responsibilities. Although Miriam was Catholic, she found little comfort in her faith, believing that her illness was a punishment from God for an abortion she had 2 years ago. Miriam was becoming increasingly depressed. The home health aid who assisted her in the first few weeks after discharge was no longer available. It became clear to Miriam that her life was threatened by this disease and she might never see her child grow up.

Despite HAART therapy, there was little improvement in her CD4 counts or in the lowering of her viral load. Miriam began to stay in bed for long periods of time during the day. She feared that she was never going to recover and worried about who would care for her son. The infectious disease physician, whom she saw at the AIDS clinic, changed her HAART regimen. Miriam was also treated with an antidepressant and within weeks her mood improved, as well as her appetite.

Within 3 months, Miriam's quality of life improved because she was free of opportunistic infections. Although unemployed, she kept busy with household activities and the care of her son. Even though Miriam had two friends, who lived in her building, they had their own personal and health-related issues. Miriam understood the fragility of her condition and was adherent to her medication regimen. She needed ongoing management of symptoms related to the disease and its treatment, as well as emotional and spiritual support as she faced her own mortality. With support from her family, Miriam was assured that her son would be cared for in the event of her death.

Introduction

It has been 28 years since the beginning of the HIV/AIDS epidemic, yet there remains no cure for this disease which has affected global health. In countries with advanced healthcare, the development and accessibility of highly active antiretroviral therapy (HAART) has significantly reduced the mortality from human immunodeficiency virus (HIV) and has transformed AIDS into a manageable chronic illness. However, in developing countries, the majority of people are not "living with AIDS," but, rather continue to die from AIDS due to a lack of access to medications and appropriate health care (Watt & Burnouf, 2002). In clinical practice, AIDS has stimulated the need to evaluate the interface between curative and palliative care, as there has been a false dichotomy created between disease-specific, curative therapies and symptom-specific palliative therapies (Selwyn & Forstein, 2003). Palliative care begins at the time of diagnosis with a life-threatening illness and continues across the illness trajectory. In the care of HIV/AIDS, despite the benefits of an increased of life expectancy given current therapies, the disease as well as its treatments can result in significant symptom burden warranting palliative care. Palliative care for patients with HIV/AIDS is an approach to care not only in the advanced stage of the illness, but as an aspect of care that begins in the early stage of illness and continues as the disease progresses (National Consensus Project, 2009). Furthermore, palliative measures can be beneficial in ensuring tolerance of and adherence to difficult pharmacological regimens. Given that there is not yet a cure for AIDS, it is recognized that AIDS treatment is primarily palliative, as antiretroviral drugs interfere with the replication of the virus, protect and reconstitute immune system function, and medications are used to treat infections and neoplasms and their related symptoms. Palliative care offers physical, emotional, social, and spiritual support to promote the patient's quality of life and that of his/her families over many years of the illness (National Consensus Project, 2009).

INCIDENCE AND PREVALENCE

AIDS has been characterized as a volatile and dynamic epidemic, which has spread globally. This epidemic is complex due to the viruses' ability to mutate and cross all socioeconomic, cultural, political, and geographic boundries. As a worldwide epidemic, HIV/AIDS has affected more than 33 million people. In the United States, an estimated 2.5 million acquired HIV in 2007, with an estimated 2.1 million people dying from AIDS (UNAIDS/WHO, 2007). The Centers for Disease Control and Prevention (CDC) in 2008 reported that through December 2006, there were more than 1,014,797 reported cases of AIDS in the United States since the beginning of the epidemic. Of these cases, 783, 786 cases were men, 189,566 were women, and an estimated 9,144 cases were children under age 13 (CDC, 2008). In the United States, the estimated number of deaths of persons with AIDS is 565,927, including 540,436 adults and adolescents and 5,369 children under age 15 (CDC, 2008). Although, HIV is no longer a leading casue of death in the United States, in populations and nations without access to antiretorviral therapy and treatments for opportunistic infections, AIDS remains a life-threatening and progressive illness that marks the final stage of a chronic viral illness.

PATHOGENESIS OF HIV

The HIV virus survives by reproducing itself in a host cell, replacing the genetic machinery of that cell, and eventually destroying the cell. The HIV is a retrovirus whose life cycle consists of 1) attachment of the virus to the cell, which is affected by cofactors that influence the virus's ability to enter the host cell; 2) uncoating of the virus; 3) reverse transcription by an enzyme called reverse transcriptase, which converts two strands of viral RNA to DNA; 4) integration of newly synthesized proviral DNA into the cell nucleus, assisted by the viral enzyme integrase, which becomes the template for new viral components; 5) transcription of proviral DNA into messenger RNA; 6) movement of messenger RNA outside the cell nucleus, where it is translated into viral proteins and enzymes; and 7) assembly and release of mature virus particles out of the host cell (Orenstein, 2002).

These newly formed viruses have an affinity for any cell that has the CD4 molecule on their surface, such as T lymphocytes and macrophages, and become major viral targets. Because CD4 cells are the master coordinators of the immune system response, chronic destruction of these cells severely compromises individuals' immune status, leaving the host susceptible to opportunistic infections and eventual progression to AIDS.

Since the identification of the first case of HIV in 1984, there has been significant scientific advancements made in the diagnosis and treatment of the disease, specifically the virus has been identified; screening for HIV infection has been implemented; biological and behavioral cofactors have been identified related to infection and disease progression; prophylactic treatments are available to prevent opportunistic infections; HIV RNA quantitative assays have been developed to measure viral load (VL), combination antiretroviral therapies are available to treat the infection; and vaccines are being tested (Orenstein, 2002).

DISEASE TRAJECTORY

HIV and AIDS are not synonymous terms but, rather, refer to the natural history or progression of the infection, ranging from asymptomatic infection to life-threatening illness characterized by opportunistic infections and cancers. This continuum of illness is associated with a decrease in CD4 cell count and a rise in HIV-RNA VL (Melroe, Stawarz & Simpson, 1997). Although, low CD4 cell counts are generally correlated with high VLs, some patients with low CD4 counts have low VLs and vice versa. The most reliable current measurement of HIV disease progression is the viral load and the more consistent surrogate marker is the percentage of lymphocytes that are CD4 cells, rather than the absolute CD4 cell count (Guidelines for Prevention and Treatment of Opportunistic Infections, 2008).

The natural history of HIV infection begins with primary or acute infection in which the virus enters the body and replicates in large numbers in the blood. As a result, there is an initial decrease in the number of T cells and a rise in viral load during the first 2 weeks of the infection. The amount of virus present after the initial viremia and the immune response is called the viral set point. Within 5 to 30 days of infection, the individual experiences flulike symptoms such as fever, sore throat, skin rash, lymphadenopathy, and myalgia. Other symptoms of primary HIV infection include fatigue, splenomegaly, anorexia, nausea and vomiting, meningitis, retro-orbital pain, neuropathy, and mucocutaneous ulceration (Orenstein, 2002). Within 6 to 12 weeks of the initial infection, the production of HIV antibodies results in seroconversion as the patient now tests HIV positive.

Clinical latency refers to the chronic, clinically asymptomatic state in which there is a decreased VL and resolution of symptoms of the primary infection. Recent advances in the understanding of pathogenesis of the virus reveal that there is continuous viral replication in the lymph nodes at this time with more than 10 billion copies of the virus being made every day. Combination antiretroviral therapy is therefore recommended as an early intervention in non-acute HIV infection, as studies have shown that it may reverse immune-mediated damage (Al-Harthi et al., 2000).

After years of HIV infection, the individual enters the early symptomatic stage which is apparent by conditions indicative primarily of defects in cell-mediated immunity. Early symptomatic infection generally occurs when CD4 counts fall below 500 cells/mm³ and the HIV VL copy count increases above 10,000/ml up to 100,000/ml, which indicates a moderate risk of HIV progression and a median time to death of 6.8 years. Early symptoms of HIV infection include, oral candidiasis and hairy leukoplakia, as well as ulcerative lesions of the mucosa. Gynecological infections are common in women with HIV disease, as well as dermatological manifestations, which include bacterial, fungal, viral, neoplastic, and other conditions such exacerbation of psoriasis, severe pruritus, or the development of recurrent pruritic papules (Al-Harthi et al., 2000).

The late symptomatic stage begins when the CD4 count drops below 200 cells/mm³ and the VL generally increases above 100,000/ml. At this point, the CD4 count defines the progression from HIV to the classification of AIDS according to the CDS (2008). Patients experience opportunistic infections or cancers in the late stage of disease and their related symptoms. In addition to such illnesses as Kaposi Sarcoma (KS), *Pneumocystis jiroveci* pneumonia, HIV encephalopathy, and HIV wasting, diseases such as pulmonary tuberculosis, recurrent bacterial infections, and invasive cervical cancer may be seen.

Advanced HIV disease stage occurs when the CD4 cell count drops below 50 cells/mm³. At this point, the immune system is so impaired that death is likely within 1 year. Common conditions are central nervous system (CNS) non-Hodgkin's lymphoma, KS, cytomegalovirus (CMV) retinitis, or *Mycobacterium avium* complex (MAC) (UNAIDS/WHO, 2007). With advanced disease, most individuals have health problems such as pneumonia, oral candidiasis, depression, dementia, skin problems, anxiety, incontinence, fatigue, isolation, bed dependency, wasting syndrome, and significant pain (UNAIDS/WHO, 2007). Research regarding AIDS patients experiencing advanced disease confirms the multitude of patient symptoms and factors that contribute to mortality. In a study of 83 hospitalized AIDS patients, factors contributing to higher mortality include the type of opportunistic infections, serum albumin level, total lymphocyte count, weight, CD4 count, and neurological manifestations (Gerard et al., 1996). In the last month of life, a retrospective study of 50 men who died from AIDS indicated that the most distressing symptoms included pain, dyspnea, diarrhea, confusion, dementia, difficulty swallowing and eating, and loss of vision. Dehydration, malnutrition, and peripheral neuropathy are also important problems (Malcolm & Dobson, 1994).

Death from AIDS is usually due to multiple causes, including chronic infections, malignancies, neurological disease, malnutrition, and multisystem failure. However, even for patients with HIV/AIDS for whom death appears to be imminent, spontaneous recovery with survival of several more weeks or months is possible. The terminal stage is often marked by periods of increasing weight loss and deteriorating physical and cognitive functioning. The general rule related to mortality is that the greater the cumulative number of opportunistic infections, illnesses, complications, and/or deviance of serological or immunological markers in terms of norms, the less the survival time (Goldstone, Kuhl, Johnson, Le Clerc, & McCleod, 1995). Survival time is also decreased by psychosocial factors such as a decrease in physical and emotional support as demands increase for the caregivers, feelings of hopelessness by the patient, and older age (> 39 years). In the terminal stage of HIV disease, decisions related to prevention, diagnosis, and treatment pose ethical and clinical issues for both patients and their healthcare providers because they must decide on the value and frequency of laboratory monitoring, use of invasive procedures, use of antiretroviral and prophylactic measures, and patients' participation in clinical trails.

AIDS-Related Opportunitistic Infections and Comorbidities

Opportunistic infections are the greatest cause of morbidity and mortality in individuals with HIV disease. Given the compromised immune system of HIV-infected individuals, there is a wide spectrum of pathogens that can produce primary, life-threatening infections, particularly when the CD4 cell counts fall below 200 cells/mm³. Given the weakened immune systems of HIV-infected persons, even previously acquired infections can be reactivated. Most of these opportunistic infections are incurable and can at best be palliated to control the acute stage of infection and prevent recurrence through long-term suppressive therapy. In addition, patients with HIV/AIDS often experience concurrent or consecutive opportunistic infections that are severe and cause a great number of symptoms.

In addition to opportunistic infections, ethnically diverse populations are also diagnosed with other comorbidities such as hepatitis B and C, end-organ failure, and various malignancies which increase mortality rates (Selwyn & Rivard, 2003). Based on patients (n = 230) in a large urban New York Medical Center who had been referred to the HIV palliative care team, Shen, Blank, and Selwyn (2005) reported that close to half of all deaths for these patients were attributable to non-AIDS-specific causes, including cancer and end-organ failure. Age and markers of functional status were more predictive of mortality than traditional HIV prognostic variables. With the occurrence of opportunistic infections, specific cancers, and neurological manifestations, AIDS involves multiple symptoms not only from the disease processes but also from the side effects of medications and other therapies. Patients with AIDS present with complex care issues because they experience bouts of severe illness and debilitation alternating with periods of symptom stabilization (Bloomer, 1998).

HIV/AIDS AND PALLIATIVE CARE

Pallitive care is the comprehensive management of the physical, psychological, social, spiritual, and existential needs of patients with incurable progressive illness (National Consensus Project, 2009). Palliative care has become an increasingly important component of AIDS care from diagnosis to death involving ongoing prevention, health promotion, and health maintenance to promote the patient's quality of life throughout the illness trajectory. The components of high-quality HIV/AIDS palliative care, as identified by healthcare providers, include competent, skilled practitioners; confidential, nondiscriminatory, culturally sensitive care; flexible and responsive care; collaborative and coordinated care; and fair access to care. Resources aimed at prevention, health promotion and maintenance, symptom survillance and end-of-life care are essential (Higginson, 1993). Not only the treatment of chronic debilitating conditions but also the treatment of superimposed acute opportunistic infections and related symptoms is necessary to maintain quality of life. As one example, health prevention measures, such as ongoing IV therapies to prevent blindness from CMV retinitis, must be available to patients with AIDS to maintain their quality of life.

The precepts of palliative care include comprehensive care with respect for patient goals, preferences, and choices, and acknowledgment of caregivers' concerns (National Consensus Project, 2009). These precepts are fundamental in addressing the complex needs of patients and families with HIV/AIDS and require the coordinated care of an interdisciplinary palliative care team, involving physicians, advanced practice nurses, staff nurses, social workers, dietitians, physiotherapists, and clergy. The management decisions for patients with advanced AIDS must consider the benefits and burdens of the various diagnostic and treatment modalities, and the patient's expectations and goals, as well as anticipated problems (Sherman, 2001). Healthcare providers and patients must determine the balance between aggressive and supportive efforts, particularly when increasing debility, wasting, and deteriorating cognitive function are evident in the face of advanced disease. As the unit of care is the patient and family, the palliative care team offers support not only for patients to live as fully as possible until death but also for the family to help them to cope during the patient's illness and in their own bereavement (National Consensus Project, 2009).

Although, the hospice and palliative care movement developed as a community response to those who were dying, primarily of cancer, the advent of the AIDS epidemic made it necessary for hospices to begin admitting patients with AIDS. This meant applying the old model of cancer care to patients with a new infectious, progressive, and terminal disease. Unlike the course of cancer, which is relatively predictable once the disease progresses beyond cure, AIDS patients experience a series of life-threatening opportunistic infections. It is not until wasting becomes apparent that the course of AIDS achieves the predictability of cancer (Malcolm & Sutherland, 1992). Furthermore, while the underlying goal of AIDS care remains one of palliation, short-term aggressive therapies are still needed to treat opportunistic infections. Also, unlike cancer palliation, AIDS palliation deals with a fatal infectious disease of primarily younger people, which requires ongoing infection control and the management of symptoms. The neglect of the palliative care needs of patients with HIV disease relates to certain barriers to care, such as reimbursement issues. Specifically, public and private third-party payers have reimbursed end-of-life care only when physicians have verified a life expectancy of less than 6 months to live. Given the unpredictability of the illness trajectory, many patients with AIDS were formally denied access to hospice care. Currently, these policies are under review, and the 6-month limitation is being extended so that patients with AIDS are eligible for comprehensive care, with control of pain and other symptoms along with psychological and spiritual support offered by hospice/palliative care.

A second barrier to hospice/palliative care for patients with AIDS has been the cost of continuing the administration of antiretroviral therapies and other medications to prevent opportunistic infections. The estimated cost of treatment for AIDS patients in hospices could amount to twice the cost of treating patients with cancer, particularly when the costs of medications are included. Financing of such therapies for patients with AIDS is now being addressed by hospice/palliative care organizations.

The third barrier to palliative care is the patients themselves. Many patients with HIV/AIDS are young and continue to hope that a cure will be found even when in the advanced stage of the disease. There is a need to shift the perception of palliative care as only end-of-life care, and to promote palliative care as an aggressive approach to enhance quality of life throughout the course of the illness. Over the years, there have been public initiatives and media campaigns to improve the care of the seriously ill in the United States and to inform patients and families about the availability of palliative care across health care settings.

A review of the evidence of barriers and inequality in HIV care by Harding et al. (2005) found that there is increased complexity in the balance of providing concurrent curative and palliative therapies given the prolongation of lifespan as a result of HAART therapy. Harding and colleagues believe that palliative care should not soley be associated with terminal care and propose four recommendations: specifically, the need for multidimensional palliative care assessment for differing populations; basic palliative care skills training for all clinical staff in standard assessments; the development of referral criteria and systems for patients with complex palliative care needs; and the availability of specialist consultation across all settings.

When patients are in the advanced stage of AIDS, Grothe and Brody (1995) suggested that four criteria be considered regarding the admission to hospice: functional ability, statistical prognosis, CD4 count and VL, and history of opportunistic infections. These criteria give a better understanding of the patient's prognosis and needs. Hospices are continuing to review their policies to offer the necessary support to patients with AIDS at the end of life. Different models of palliative care are being developed including partnerships with community hospitals or agencies. Conducting cost–benefit analysis will be important in meeting the healthcare needs of patients with AIDS and their families in the future (Al-Harthi et al., 2000).

Assessment of Patients with HIV/AIDS

Throughout the course of their illness, individuals with HIV disease require primary care services to identify early signs of opportunistic infections and to minimize related symptoms and complications. This includes a complete health history, physical examination, and laboratory data including determination of immunological and viral status.

Health history. In the care of patients with HIV/AIDS, the health history should include the following (Sherman, 2006):

■ History of present illness, including a review of those factors that led to HIV testing.
■ Past medical history, particularly those conditions that may be exacerbated by HIV disease or its treatments, such as diabetes mellitus, hypertriglyceridemia, or chronic or active hepatitis B infection.
■ Childhood illnesses and vaccinations for preventing common infections such as polio, DPT, or measles.
■ Medication history, including the patient's knowledge of the types of medications, side effects, adverse reactions, drug interactions, and administration recommendations.
■ Sexual history, regarding sexual behaviors and preferences and history of sexually transmitted diseases, which can exacerbate HIV disease progression.
■ Lifestyle habits, such as the past and present use of recreational drugs, including alcohol, which may accelerate progression of disease; cigarette smoking, which may suppress appetite or be associated with opportunistic infections such as oral candidiasis, hairy leukoplakia, and bacterial pneumonia.

■ Dietary habits, including risks related to foodborne illnesses such as hepatitis A
■ Travel history, to countries in Asia, Africa, and South America, where the risk of opportunistic infections increase.
■ Complete systems review, to provide indications of clinical manifestations of new opportunistic infections or cancers, as well as AIDS-related complications both from the disease and its treatments.

Physical Examination. A physical exam should begin with a general assessment of vital signs and height and weight, as well as overall appearance and mood. A complete head-to-toe assessment is important and may reveal various findings common to individuals with HIV/AIDS such as (Sherman, 2006):

■ Oral cavity assessment may indicate candida, oral hairy leukoplakia, or KS.
■ Funduscopic assessment may reveal visual changes associated with CMV retinitis; glaucoma screening annually is also recommended.
■ Lymph node assessment may reveal adenopathy detected at any stage of disease.
■ Dermatological assessment may indicate various cutaneous manifestations that occur throughout the course of the illness such as HIV exanthema, KS, or infectious complications such as dermatomycosis.
■ Neuromuscular assessment may indicate various central, peripheral, or autonomic nervous systems disorders and signs and symptoms of conditions such as meningitis, encephalitis, dementia, or peripheral neuropathies.
■ Cardiovascular assessment may reveal cardiomyopathy.
■ Gastrointestinal assessment may indicate organomegaly, specifically splenomegaly or hepatomegaly, particularly in patients with a history of substance abuse, as well as signs related to parasitic intestinal infections. Annual stool of guaiac and rectal examination, as well as sigmoidoscopy every 5 years, is also parts of health maintenance.
■ Reproductive system assessment may reveal occult sexually transmitted diseases or malignancies, as well vaginal candidiasis, cervical dysplasia, pelvic inflammatory disease, or rectal lesions in women with HIV/AIDS, as well as urethral discharge and rectal lesions or malignancies in HIV-infected men. Health maintenance in individuals with HIV/AIDS also includes annual mammograms in women, as well as testicular exams in men and prostate-specific antigen (PSA) annually.

Laboratory data. CD4 counts, both the absolute numbers and the CD4 percentages, are the strongest predictor of disease progression and patient survival (U.S. Department of Health and Human Services (DHHS), 2008).

Evaluation of these laboratory data are important in assisting the health practitioner in therapeutic decision making about treatments of opportunistic infections and antiretroviral therapy. Although quantitative RNA level or VL is a useful marker of disease progression, it is primarily used as a measure of the effectiveness of antiretroviral therapy. The DHHS's Panel on Clinical Practices for the Treatment of HIV recommends that the CD4 count and the VL be measured upon entry into care and every 3–6 months subsequently (U.S. Department of Health and Human Services, 2008). Immediately before a patient is started on HAART, the patient's HIV-RNA (VL) should be measured, and again 2–8 weeks after treatment is initiated, to determine the effectiveness of the therapy. With adherence to the medication schedule, it is expected that the HIV-RNA will decrease to undetectable levels (< 50 copies/ml) in 16–24 weeks after the intitiation of therapy (U.S. Department of Health and Human Services, 2008). If a patient does not significantly respond to therapy, the clinician should evaluate adherence, repeat the test, perform a genotyping or phenotyping resistance assay, and rule out malabsorption or drug interactions.

The decision regarding laboratory testing is based on the stage of HIV disease, the medical processes warranting initial assessment or follow-up, and consideration of the patient benefit-to-burden ratio (Sherman, 2006). Complete blood counts are often measured with each VL determination or with a change of antiretroviral therapy, particularly with patients on drugs known to cause anemia. Chemistry profiles are done to assess liver function, lipid status, and glycemia every 3–6 months or with a change in therapy, and are determined by the patient's antiretroviral therapy, baseline determinations, and coinfections. Abnormalities in these profiles may occur as a result of antiretroviral therapy. Increasing hepatic dysfunction is evident by elevations in the serum transaminases (AST, ALT, ALP, LDH). Blood work should also include hepatitis C serology (antibody), hepatitis B serology, and *Toxoplasma* IgG serology (Murphy & Flaherty, 2003).

Urine analysis should be done annually unless the person is on antiretroviral therapy, which may require more frequent follow-up to check for toxicity. Syphilis studies should be done annually; however, patients with low positive titers should have follow-up testing at 3, 6, 9, 12, and 24 months. Gonorrhea and chlamydia tests are encouraged every 6–12 months if the patient is sexually active. Annual Papanicolaou (Pap) smears are also indicated, with recommendations for Pap smears every 3–6 months in HIV-infected women who are symptomatic. In addition, HIV-infected persons should be tested for IgG antibody to Toxoplasma soon after the diagnosis of HIV infection to detect latent infection with *T. gondii*. Toxoplasma-seronegative persons who are not taking a PCP prophylactic regimen known to be active against Toxoplasma enecephalitis (TE) should be retested for IgG antibody to Toxoplasma when their CD4 + counts decline to < 100 cells/μl to determine whether they have seroconverted and are therefore at risk of TE (Guidelines for the Prevention and Treatment of Opportunistic Infections, 2008).

Individuals should be tested for latent tuberculosis infection (LTBI) at the time of their HIV diagnosis, regardless of their TB risk category, and then annually if negative. LTBI diagnosis can be achieved with the use of a tuberculin skin test (TST) or by interferon-γ release assay using the patient's serum. A TST is considered positive in patients with induration of greater than or equal to 5 mm. An interferon-γ release assay is reported as postive or negative. Any positive test warrants a chest radiograph for active disease and consideration of antituberculosis therapy based on history, laboratory, physical and radiographic findings.

Management of HIV/AIDS

With no current cure, the health management of patients with HIV/AIDS is directed toward controlling HIV disease and prolonging survival, while maintaining quality of life (Burgoyne & Tan, 2008). Quality of life is associated with health maintenance for individuals with HIV/AIDS, particularly as it relates to physical and emotional symptoms and functioning in activities of daily living as well as social functioning (Nichel et al., 1996). Quality of life is based on the patient's perceptions of his or her ability to control the physical, emotional, social, cognitive, and spiritual aspects of the illness. In a study regarding the functional quality of life of 142 men and women with AIDS, Vosvick et al. (2003) concluded that maladaptive coping strategies were associated with lower levels of energy and social functioning and that severe pain interfered with daily living tasks and was associated with lower levels of functional quality of life (physical functioning, energy/fatigue, social functioning, and role functioning). Therefore, health promotion interventions should be aimed at developing adaptive coping strategies and improving pain management.

In the management of HIV/AIDS, it is important to prevent or decrease the occurrence of opportunistic infections and AIDS-indicator diseases. HIV management therefore involves health promotion and disease prevention. In addition to the treatment of AIDS-related diseases and related symptoms, palliative care involves prophylactic interventions and the prevention of behaviors that promote disease expression (Bolin, 2006).

Through all stages of HIV disease, health can be promoted and maintained through diet, micronutrients, exercise, reduction of stress and negative emotions, symptom surveillance, and the use of prophylactic therapies to prevent opportunistic infections or AIDS-related complications. A health-promoting diet is essential for optimal functioning of the immune system. Cell-mediated immunity, phagocytic function, and antibody response are impaired by deficiencies in diet, including low protein intake. Alteration in nutrition leads to secondary infections, disease progression, psychological distress, and fatigue. In patients with AIDS, common nutritional problems are weight loss, vitamin and mineral deficiencies, loss of muscle mass, and loss or redistribution of fat mass. With the administration of antiretroviral therapy, there is the possibility of redistribution of fat, characterized by increased abdominal girth, loss of fat from the face, and a "buffalo hump" on the back of the neck (Keithley, Swanson, Murphy, & Levin, 2000). Diseases of the mouth and oropharynx, such as oral candidiasis, anular cheilitis, gingivitis, herpes simplex, and hairy leukoplakia may limit oral intake. Diseases of the GI tract that can cause malabsorption include CMV, MAC, cryptosporidiosis, and KS. These diseases are experienced in individuals with CD4 counts of 50 or less, and may adversely affect their nutritional status (Rene & Roze, 1991). Metabolic alterations may be due to HIV infection or secondary infections, as well as abnormalities in carbohydrate, fat, and protein metabolism (Vosvick et al., 2003). A good diet is one of the simplest ways to delay HIV progression and will bolster immune system function and energy levels and help patients live longer and more productive lives (Hussein, 2003). It is recommended to have 2 or 3 servings daily from the protein and dairy groups, 7–12 servings from the starch and grain group, 2 servings of fruits and vegetables rich in vitamin C, as well as 3 servings of other fruits and vegetables (Aron, 1994).

Research has also indicated a linkage between vitamin A (beta carotene) deficiency and elevated disease progression and mortality (Semba, Graham, & Caiaffa, 1994). It has been hypothesized that correcting both vitamin A and B6 deficiencies restores cell-mediated immunity (Freeman & MacIntyre, 1999). Research findings also indicate that an increase in dietary intake of n-3 polyunsaturated fatty acids, arginine, and RNA increases body weight and reduces wasting due to malabsorption. Increase in concentrations of amino acids such as arginine has been found to preserve lean muscle mass (Freeman & MacIntyre, 1999).

Exercise is also important to health promotion in patients with HIV/AIDS, as it increases natural killer-cell activity (Freeman & MacIntyre, 1999). However, variable results are reported on the effects of exercise on neutrophil, macrophage, and T- and B-cell function and proliferation (Nieman, 1996). LaPerriere et al. (1997) conducted a review of exercise studies and reported a trend in CD4 cell count elevation in all but one study, with the greatest effect from aerobic exercise and weight training. The CDC (2008) recommend a physical exercise program of 30–45 minutes four or more times a week to increase lung capacity, endurance, energy, and flexibility, and to improve circulation.

Furthermore, stress and negative emotions are associated with immunosuppression and increases an individual's vulnerability to infections. For patients living with HIV/AIDS, there is stress related to the uncertainty regarding illness progression and prognosis, stigmatization, discrimination, financial concerns, and increased disability as the disease progresses. Individuals with AIDS frequently cite the avoidance of stress as a way of maintaining a sense of well-being (Sherman & Kirton, 1998). Based on a study of 96 HIV-infected homosexual men without symptoms or antiretroviral medication use, Leserman et al. (2002) reported that higher cumulative average stressful life events, higher anger scores, lower cumulative average social support, and depressive symptoms predicted a faster progression to both the CDC AIDS classification and a clinical AIDS condition. In a study of quality of life of women with AIDS, cognitive-behavioral interventions have been shown to improve cognitive functioning, health distress, and overall health perceptions, yet there were no changes in energy/fatigue, pain, or social functioning (Lechner et al. 2003). Massage has also been linked to natural killer-cell activity and overall immune regulation as reported in a research study of 29 HIV-infected men who received daily massages for 1 month (Ironson et al., 1996). A further consideration is the use of recreational drugs such as alcohol, chemical stimulants, tobacco, and marijuana, which increases physical and emotional stress. In patients with HIV/AIDS, physical and emotional stress is associated with these agents, as they have an immunosuppressant effect and may interfere with health-promoting behaviors. Substance use may also have a negative effect on interpersonal relationships and are associated with a relapse to unsafe sexual practices (Sherman & Kirton, 1999). Patients who have substance abuse problems are encouraged to participate in self-health groups and harm-reduction programs to promote their health and quality of life.

Research further suggests that the promotion of health involves positive emotional coping. In a study by Remien, Rabkin and Williams (1992), patients diagnosed with AIDS demonstrated that long-term survivors used numerous strategies to support their health. These included a strong will to live, positive attitudes, feeling in charge, a strong sense of self, expressing their needs, and a sense of humor. The relationship between the use of humor to cope with stress (coping humor) and perceived social support, depression, anxiety, self-esteem, and stress was examined, based on a sample of 103 HIV/AIDS patients (Cohen, 2001). Although, patients who used more coping humor were less depressed, expressed higher self-esteem, and perceived greater support from friends did not buffer stress, anxiety, or immune-system functioning. Other health-promotion strategies frequently used by these patients included remaining active, seeking medical information, talking to others, socializing and pursuing pleasurable activities, good medical care, and counseling. It is recognized that stress can also be associated with the financial issues experienced by patients with HIV/AIDS. Therefore, financial planning, identification of financial resources available through the community, and public assistance offered through Medicaid are important in reducing stress.

In addition, health promotion for patients with HIV/AIDS includes avoidance of exposure to organisims in the environment and thereby prevention of the development of opportunistic infections. The immune system can be supported and maintained through the administration of prophylactic and/or suppressive therapies, which decrease the frequency or severity of opportunistic infections (Guidelines for the Prevention of Opportunistic Infections, 2008). The administration of a pharmacological agent to prevent initial infection is known as primary prophylaxis, while the administration of a pharmacological agent to prevent future occurrences of infection is referred to as secondary prophylaxis (Guidelines for the Prevention of Opportunistic Infections, 2008). There has been a significant decrease in the incidence of opportunistic infections due to the effectiveness of HAART. Prophylaxis for life for HIV-related coinfections is no longer necessary in many cases (Murphy & Flaherty, 2003).

With restoration of immune-system function, as evident by a rise in CD4 counts, clinicians may consider discontinuation of primary prophylaxis under defined conditions (Murphy & Flaherty, 2003). Ending preventive prophylaxis for opportunistic infections in selected patients may result in a decrease in drug interactions and toxicities, lower cost of care, and greater adherence to HAART regimens. However, prophylaxis remains important to protect against opportunistic infections in the late symptomatic and advanced stages of HIV disease, when CD4 counts are low and VL may be high. Therefore, throughout the illness trajectory, and even in hospice settings, patients may be taking prophylactic medications, requiring sophisticated planning and monitoring. The recommendation is that prophylaxis and suppressive therapy continues in hospice/palliative care if the patient is clinically stable and wants to continue prophylaxis drug therapy (Von Gunten, Martinez, Neely, & VonRoenn, 1995). However, if side effects occur, and the patient continues to be otherwise stable, alternative regimens should be considered. Furthermore, if the patient is intolerant of prophylaxis and/or the regimens are burdensome, medications should be discontinued. Furthermore, HIV-infected individuals are at risk for severe diseases such as hepatitis B, tetanus, influenza, pneumococcal and measles, rubella, and mumps. Therefore, it is important to offer such vaccinations as a component of health promotion and disease prevention.

The Use of Antiretroviral Therapy

The goal of antiretroviral therapy is to slow disease progression and limit the occurrence of opportunistic infections. HAART is administered to maximize long-term suppression of HIV-RNA and restore or preserve immune system function, thereby reducing morbidity and mortality and promoting quality of life (Murphy & Flahety, 2003). Assessment of the CD4 cell count and VL are used to determine the initiation of antiretroviral therapy. Clinicans must determine the potential risks versus benefits of early or delayed initiation of therapy for asymptomatic patients. The risks of early therapy initiation include lower quality of life due to the adverse effects of therapy, problems with adherence to therapy, and subsequent drug resistance, with the potential limitation of future treatment options as a result of premature administration of available drugs. Consideration must also be givern to severe toxicities associated with certain antiretroviral medications, such as elevations in serum levels of triglycerides and cholesterol, alterations in fat distribution, or insulin resistance and diabetes mellitus. However, the benefits of early therapy include earlier suppression of viral replication, preservation of the immune system functioning, prolongation of disease-free survival, and a decrease in the risk of HIV transmission (U.S. Department of Health and Human Services, 2008).

Given the available data in terms of the relative risk for the progression to AIDS, the evidence supports the initiation of therapy for asymptomatic HIV-infected patients with a CD4 T-cell count of < 350 cell/mm^3 or with an AIDS defining history. Antriretroviral therapy should also be started, regardless of CD4, in patients who are pregnant, who have HIV-associated kidney disease and who are coinfected with hepatitis B when treatment is indicated (U.S. Department of Health and Human Services, 2008). If a patient has a CD4 count > 350 cells/mm^3, arguments can be made for both conservative and aggressive approaches to therapy. The decision to start therapy for the asymptomatic patient should begin with discussions of the patient's willingness, ability, and readiness to begin therapy, and the risk for disease progression given the VL as well as CD4 count. Studies indicate that early in the course of disease, suppression of plasma HIV-RNA is easier to maintain when CD4 counts are higher and VLs are lower (U.S. Department of Health and Human Services, 2008).

It is also recommended that all patients with symptomatic infection be treated with antiretrovirals regardless of CD4 count or plasma VLs. When a patient is acutely ill with an opportunistic infection or other complication of HIV disease, the timing of antiretroviral therapy initiation is based on drug toxicity, ability to adhere to the treatment regimen, drug interactions, and laboratory abnormalities. In this case, maximally suppressive regimens should be used. Patients with advanced AIDS should not discontinue therapy during an acute opportunistic infection or malignancy unless there is drug toxicity, intolerance, or drug interactions (U.S. Department of Health and Human Services, 2008).

Classifications of Antiretroviral Therapies and Recommendations

Antiretroviral drugs are broadly classified by the phase of the retrovirus life cycle that the drug inhibits. Specifically, they act in the following ways:

- Nucleoside reverse transcriptase inhibitors (NRTIs) interfere with the action of an HIV protein called reverse transcriptase, which the virus needs to make new copies of itself.
- Non-nucleoside reverse transcriptase inhibitors (nNRTIs) inhibit reverse transcriptase directly by binding to the enzyme and interfering with its function.
- Protease inhibitors (PIs) target viral assembly by inhibiting the activity of protease, which is an enzyme used by HIV to cleave nascent proteins for final assembly of new virons.
- Integrase inhibitors inhibit the enzyme integrase, which is responsible for integration of viral DNA into the DNA of the infected cell.
- Entry inhibitors (fusion inhibitors and CCR5 antagonists) interfere with binding, fusion, and entry of HIV-1 to the host cell by blocking one of several targets. Maraviroc and enfuvirtide are the two currently available agents in this class (U.S. Department of Health and Human Services, 2008).

When patients are naïve to antiretroviral therapy, it is recommended that they begin a combination regimen that consists of either one NNRTI plus two NRTIs or, as an alternative regimen, one PI (preferably boosted with ritonavir) plus two NRTIs. The prefered NRTIs to be used in combination are tenofovir + emtricitabine. The preferred NNRTI is Efavirenz and the preferred PI is either Atazanvir, Darunavir, Fosemprenavir, or Lopinavir. When alternatives to the preferred regimen are needed for treatment, the prescriber should consult the latest treatment recommendations (U.S. Department of Health and Human Services, 2008).

If there is insufficient viral suppression, which is evident by an increase in VL, inadequate increase in CD4 cell counts, evidence of disease progression, adverse clinical effects of therapy, or compromised adherence, caused by the inconvenience of difficult regimens, it is appropriate to consider a change of the medication regimen. The decision to change therapy involves consideration of whether other drug choices are available, and determination of whether another regimen may also be poorly tolerated or fail to result

in better viral suppression. Consideration must also be given to whether a change in regimen may limit future treatment options (Murphy & Flaherty, 2003). According to Murphy and Flaherty (2003), the criteria for considering changing a patient's antiretroviral regimen include the following:

- Incomplete virologic suppression: when the HIV VL is > 400 copies after 24 weeks or > 50 copies after 48 weeks of therapy or there is a virologic rebound after complete virologic supression;
- Persistent decline in CD4 cell or failure to achieve an adequate CD4 response despite virologic supression;
- The occurrence or recurence of HIV-related events after at least 3 months on an antiretroviral regimen.

A change in an antiretroviral regimen can also be guided by drug-resistance tests, such as genotyping and phenotyping assays. Consultation with an HIV specialist is often of value.

Considerations Relevant to Antiretroviral Therapy in Palliative Care

Clinicians must consider possible drug interactions with the administration of drugs in the treatment of HIV/AIDS and relief of symptoms. Pharmacokinetic interactions occur when administration of one agent changes the plasma concentration of another agent. Pharmacodynamic interactions also occur when a drug interacts with the biologically active sites and changes the pharmacological effect of the drug without altering the plasma concentration. In palliative care, drug interactions have been reported for patients who are receiving methadone for pain management and who begin therapy with an nNRTI, nevirapine. These individuals have reported symptoms of opioid withdrawal within 4–8 days of beginning nevirapine due to its effect on the cytochrome P-450 metabolic enzyme CYP3A4 and its induction of methadone metabolism (U.S. Department of Health and Human Services, 2008).

Furthermore, patients and healthcare providers should discuss the continuation of antiretroviral therapy in hospice or palliative settings. Such decisions are often contingent on the feelings of patients regarding the therapy. Patients may be asked such questions as "How do you feel when you take your antiretroviral medications?" Patients who enter hospice may have a greater acceptance of their mortality and wish to stop antiretrovirals because of the side effects. However, patients may wish to continue antiretroviral therapy because of its symptom relief and the prevention of future symptoms related to opportunistic infections. Von Gunten et al. (1995) have recommended that antiretrovirals be discontinued if the drugs cause burdensome symptoms, or the patient no longer wants to use the drug. However, if the patient is asymptomatic and wishes to continue with antiretroviral therapy, medications should be continued with close clinical assessment.

In the hospice and palliative care settings, it is important for clinicians to discuss with patients and families their goals of care to make important decisions regarding the appropriateness of curative, palliative, or both types of interventions. More specifically, examples of clinical decisions about palliative or disease-specific care include use of blood transfusions, psychostimulants, or corticosteroids to treat fatigue in patients with late-stage AIDS; aggressive antiemetic therapy for PI-induced nausea and vomiting; discontinuation of such antiretroviral therapies that give severe side effects; continued suppressive therapy for CMV retinitis to prevent blindness; use of amphotericin B for azole-resistant candidiasis for patients who wish to continue eating; prophylactic medications in dying patients; palliative treatment of disseminated MAC in patients with advanced disease who are unwilling to take anti-infectives; withdrawal of MAC or PCP prophylaxis in patients who are expected to die soon; use of HAART for short-term palliation of symptoms related to high VLs, or withdrawal of HAART after evident treatment failure, with assessment of medical risk-benefit and emotional value of therapy; as well as decisions to initiate HAART in newly diagnosed late-stage patients (Selwyn & Rivard, 2003).

Given changes in hepatic and renal function and the effects on drug elimination, the use of antiretrovirals must also be seriously considered in patients who have organ dysfunction or failure. Patients with renal impairment may be at greater risk for zidovudine-induced hematological toxicity due to lowered production of erythropoietin. Because of the markedly decreased clearance of ZVD and increased drug half-life, it is recommended that the daily dosage of ZVD be reduced by approximately 50% in patients with severe renal dysfunction (CrCL, 25 ml/min), for those receiving hemodialysis, and for those with hepatic dysfunction (Hilts & Fish, 1998). Due to reduced drug clearance, patients should be monitored for ZVD-related adverse effects. As many of the antiretroviral agents are metabolized by the liver and excreted by the kidney, knowledge of pharmacokinetic properties of antiretroviral drugs is recommended to monitor drug therapy for efficacy and safety. Decisions regarding the use of antiretrovirals and other medications need to be based on the specific goals of care, such as quality of life or life prolongation (Selwyn & Rivard, 2003).

Symptom Management in HIV Disease

Patients with HIV/AIDS require symptom management not only for chronic debilitating opportunistic infections and malignancies but also for the side effects of treatments and other therapies. Based on a sample of 1128 HIV-infected patients, Fantoni et al. (1997) reported

that the most commonly experienced symptoms were fatigue (65%), anorexia (34%), cough (32%), and fever (29%), while Holzemer and colleagues (Holzemer, Henry, & Reilly, 1998) found that 50% of the participants experienced shortness of breath, dry mouth, insomnia, weight loss, and headaches. The last stage of HIV infection is often marked by increasing pain, GI discomfort, and depression. Avis, Smith, and Mayer (1996) reported, based on a sample of 92 HIV-positive men, that quality of life was more related to symptoms as measured by the Whalen's HIV Symptom Index than CD4 counts or hemoglobin. Based on a longitudinal pilot study of patients with advanced AIDS ($n = 63$), Sherman et al. (2007) reported that the most prevalent symptoms for AIDS patients, based on the Memorial Symptom Assessment Scale (MSAS), were lack of energy (75%), pain (73%), worry (65%) dry mouth (64%), feeling sad (62%), shortness of breath (58%), and difficulty sleeping (57%), as well as cough (57%) and numbness/tingling (51%), which significantly affected quality of life. With the myriad of symptoms experienced by patients with HIV disease across the illness trajectory, healthcare practitioners need to understand the causes, presentations, and interventions of common symptoms.

The five broad principles fundamental to successful symptom management include 1) taking the symptoms seriously, 2) assessment, 3) diagnosis, 4) treatment, and 5) ongoing evaluation (Newshan & Sherman, 1999). Patient's self-report of symptoms should be taken seriously by the practitioner and acknowledged as a real experience of the patient. An important rule in symptom management is to anticipate the symptom and attempt to prevent it. Assessment and diagnosis of signs and symptoms of disease and treatment side effects require a thorough history and physical examination. Questions as to when the symptom began and its location, duration, severity, and quality, as well as factors that exacerbate or alleviate the symptom, are important to ask. Patients can also be asked to rate the severity of a symptom by using a numerical scale from 0 to 10, with 0 being "no symptom" to 10 being "extremely severe." Such scales can also be used to rate how much a symptom interferes with activities of daily life, with 0 meaning "no interference" and 10 meaning "extreme interference." When a patient seeks medical care for a specific symptom, the clinician should conduct a focused history, physical exam, and diagnostic testing. Assessment of current medications and complementary therapies, including vitamin therapy, past medical illness that may be exacerbated by HIV disease, and the administration regimen of chemotherapy and radiation therapy, should also be ascertained to determine the effects of treatment, side effects, adverse effects, and drug interactions. In the case of extremely advanced disease, practitioners must re-evaluate the benefits versus burden of diagnostic testing and treatments, particularly the need for daily blood draws or more invasive and uncomfortable procedures. When the decision of the practitioners, patient, and family is that all testing and aggressive treatments are futile, their discontinuation is warranted. Ongoing evaluation is key to symptom management and to determining the effectiveness of traditional, experimental, and complementary therapies. Changes in therapies are often necessary because concurrent or sequential illness or conditions occur (Newshan & Sherman, 1999).

In an article regarding the symptom experience of patients with HIV/AIDS, Holzemer (2002) emphasized a number of key tenets; specifically, 1) the patient is the gold standard for understanding the symptom experience; 2) patients should not be labeled "asymptomatic" early in the course of the infection because they often experience symptoms of anxiety, fear, and depression; 3) nurses are not necessarily good judges of patients' symptoms, as they frequently underestimate the frequency and intensity of HIV signs and symptoms; however, following assessment, they can answer specific questions about a symptom, such as location, intensity, duration, etc.; 4) nonadherence to treatment regimens is associated with greater frequency and intensity of symptoms; 5) greater frequency and intensity of symptoms leads to lower quality of life; 6) symptoms may or may not correspond with physiological markers; and 7) patients use few self-care symptom management strategies other than medication.

Pain and symptom assessment and management have been related to quality of life in patients with HIV/AIDS. Using data from a nationally representative cohort of HIV patients ($n = 2,267$), Lorenz, Cunningham, Spritzer, and Hays (2006) reported that symptoms are significantly related to health-related quality of life and that the functional status and well-being of patients with HIV are inextricably linked to their symptoms.

Pain In HIV/AIDS. Pain syndromes in patients with AIDS are diverse in nature and etiology. For patients with AIDS, pain can occur in more than one site, such as pain in the legs (peripheral neuropathy reported in 40% of AIDS patients), which is often associated with antiretroviral therapy such as AZT, as well as pain in the abdomen, oral cavity, esophagus, skin, perirectal area, chest, joints, muscles, and headache. In a study to identify the most common sites of pain in patients with advanced AIDS, Norval (2004) reported that lower limb pain was the most prevalent (66%), followed by mouth pain (51%), headache (42%), throat pain (40%), and chest pain (18%). Pain is also related to HIV/AIDS therapies such as antiretroviral therapies, antibacterials, chemotherapy such as vincristine, radiation, surgery, and procedures (Lorenz et al., 2006). Patients may be suffering from inflammatory or infiltrative processes and somatic and visceral pain. Neuropathic pain is commonly a result of the disease process or the side effect

of medications. The survival rate of patients without pain was significantly higher than those who report pain (Frich & Borgbjerg, 2000). Shofferman and Brody (1990) reported that more than half of the patients cared for in hospice with advanced AIDS experienced pain. Cleeland et al. (1994) also reported significant undermedication of pain in AIDS patients (85%), far exceeding the published reports of undertreated pain in cancer populations.

Following a complete assessment, including a history and physical examination, an individualized pain management plan should be developed to treat the underlying cause of the pain, often arising from underlying infections associated with HIV disease. The principles of pain management in the palliative care of patients with AIDS are the same as for patients with cancer, and include regularity of dosing, individualization of dosing, and the use of combinations of medications. The three-step guidelines for pain management as outlined by WHO should be used for patients with HIV disease. This approach advocates for the selection of analgesics based on the severity of pain. For mild to moderate pain, anti-inflammatory drugs such as NSAIDs or acetaminophen are recommended. However, the use of NSAIDs in patients with AIDS requires awareness of toxicity and adverse reactions because they are highly protein-bound, and the free fraction available is increased in AIDS patients who are cachetic or wasted. For moderate to severe pain that is persistent, opioids of increasing potency are recommended, beginning with opioids such as codeine, hydrocodone, or oxycodone (each available with or without aspirin or acetaminophen), and advancing to more potent opioids such as morphine, hydromorphone (Dilaudid), methadone (Dolophine), or fentanyl either intravenously or transdermally. In conjunction with NSAIDs and opioids, adjuvant therapies also recommended (Trescot et al., 2008), such as the following:

- Tricyclic antidepressants, heterocyclic and noncyclic antidepressants, and serotonin reuptake inhibitors for neuropathic pain
- Psychostimulants to improve opioid analgesia and decrease sedation
- Phenothiazine to relieve anxiety or agitation
- Butyrophenones to relieve anxiety and delirium
- Antihistamines to improve opioid analgesia and relieve anxiety, insomnia, and nausea
- Corticosteroids to decrease pain associated with an inflammatory component or with bone pain
- Benzodiazepines for neuropathic pain, anxiety, and insomnia.

Caution is noted, however, with use of PIs because they may interact with some analgesics. For example, Ritonavir has been associated with potentially lethal interactions with meperidine, propoxyphene, and piroxicam. PIs must also be used with caution in patients receiving codeine, tricyclic antidepressants, sulindac, and indomethacin to avoid toxicity. Furthermore, for patients with HIV disease who have high fevers, the increase in body temperature may lead to increased absorption of transdermally administered fentanyl.

To ensure appropriate dosing when changing the route of administration of opioids or changing from one opioid to another, the use of an equianalgesic conversion chart is suggested. As with all patients, oral medications should be used if possible, with round-the-clock dosing at regular intervals, and the use of rescue doses for breakthrough pain. Often, controlled-release morphine or oxycodone are effective drugs for patients with chronic pain from HIV/AIDS. In the case of neuropathic pain, often experienced with HIV/AIDS, tricyclic antidepressants such as amitriptyline, or anticonvulsants such as Neurontin can be very effective (Trescot et al., 2008). However, the use of neuroleptics must be weighed against an increased sensitivity of AIDS patients to the extrapyramidal side effects of these drugs. If the cause of pain is increasing tumor size, radiation therapy can also be very effective in pain management by reducing tumor size, as well as the perception of pain. In cases of refractory pain, nerve blocks and cordotomy are available neurosurgical procedures for pain management. Increasingly, epidural analgesia is an additional option that provides continuous pain relief.

Nonpharmacological and Complementary Interventions for Pain and Symptom Management

In addition to pharmacologic management of pain and other symptoms, clinicians may consider the value of nonpharmacological interventions such as bed rest, simple exercise, heat or cold packs to affected sites, massage, transcutaneous electrical stimulation (TENS), and acupuncture. Psychological interventions to reduce pain perception and interpretation include hypnosis, relaxation, imagery, biofeedback, distraction, and patient education.

Patients with HIV disease seek complementary therapies to treat symptoms, slow the progression of the disease, and enhance their general well-being. Milan et al. (2008) found that more than 90% of inner-city, middle-aged, heterosexual women and men (n = 93) who were at risk for or who had HIV infection reported use of complementary and alternative medicine in the prior 6 months.

The 10 most commonly used complementary therapies and activities reported by 1,106 participants in the Alternative Medical Care Outcomes in AIDS study were aerobic exercise (64%), prayer (56%), massage (54%), needle acupuncture (48%), meditation (46%), support groups (42%), visualization and imagery (34%), breathing exercises (33%), spiritual activities (33%),

and other exercise (33%) (Milan et al., 2008). Nurses' knowledge, evaluation, and recommendations regarding complementary therapies are important aspects of holistic care.

PSYCHOSOCIAL ISSUES FOR PATIENTS WITH HIV/AIDS AND THEIR FAMILIES

Many practitioners focus on patient's physical functioning and performance status as the main indicators of quality of life, rather than on the symptoms of psychological distress such as anxiety and depression. Based on a sample of 203 patients with HIV/AIDS, Farber and colleagues (Farber, Mirsalimi, Williams, & McDaniel, 2003) reported that positive meaning of the illness was associated with a higher level of psychological well-being and lower depressed mood, and contributed more than problem-focused coping and social support to predicting both psychological well-being and depressed mood. Sherman et al. (2006), in a two-year longitudinal pilot study regarding quality of life for patients with advanced cancer and AIDS, found that while patients with advanced AIDS (n = 63) reported a total lower quality of life as compared to patients with advanced cancer (n = 38), AIDS caregivers (n = 43) reported greater overall quality of life, psychological well-being, and spiritual well-being than did cancer caregivers (n = 38). Sherman and colleagues posited that even as death approaches, health professionals can identify changes in quality of life and appropriate interventions to improve quality-of-life outcomes for HIV/AIDS patients.

Uncertainty is also a source of psychological distress for persons living with HIV disease, particularly as it relates to ambiguous symptom patterns, exacerbation and remissions of symptoms, selection of optimal treatment regimens, the complexity of treatments, and the fear of stigma and ostracism. Uncertainty is linked with negative perceptions of quality of life and poor psychological adjustment (Brashers, Neidig, Reynolds, & Haas, 1998). Friedland and colleagues (Friedland, Renwick, & McColl, 1996) identified the determinants of quality of life in a sample of 120 individuals with HIV/AIDS as emotional support, and problem-oriented and perception-oriented coping, while tangible support and emotion-focused coping were negatively related. The prevalence of depression in patients diagnosed with HIV/AIDS has been estimated at 10%–25% and is characterized by depressed mood, low energy, sleep disturbance, anhedonia, inability to concentrate, loss of libido, weight changes, and possible menstrual irregularities (McEnany, Hughes, & Lee, 1996). In patients experiencing depression, clinicians should assess also their use of alcohol, drugs, and opioids.

The psychosocial issues experienced by patients with HIV/AIDS include multiple losses, complicated grief, substance abuse, stigmatization, and homophobia, which contribute to patients' sense of alienation, isolation, hopelessness, loneliness, and depression (Sherman, 2006). Such emotional distress often extends to the patient's family caregivers as they attempt to provide support and lessen the patient's suffering, yet experience suffering themselves. Palliative care is therefore of great value as the focus of care in both the patient and his/her family (Sherman, 1998).

Psychosocial assessment of patients with HIV disease is important throughout the illness trajectory, particularly as the disease progresses and there is increased vulnerability to psychological distress. Psychosocial assessment includes the following (Sherman, 2006):

- Past social, behavioral, and psychiatric history, which includes the history of interpersonal relationships, education, job stability, career plans, substance use, preexisting mental illness, and individual identity;
- Crisis points related to the course of the disease as anxiety, fear, and depression intensify, creating a risk of suicide;
- Life-cycle phase of individuals and families, which influences goals, financial resources, skills, social roles, and the ability to confront personal mortality;
- Influence of culture and ethnicity, including knowledge and beliefs associated with health, illness, dying, and death, as well as attitudes and values toward sexual behaviors, substance use, health promotion and maintenance, and healthcare decision making;
- Past and present patterns of coping, including problem-focused and/or emotion- focused coping;
- Social support, including sources of support, types of supports perceived as needed by the patient/family, and perceived benefits and burdens of support;
- Financial resources, including healthcare benefits, disability allowances, and the eligibility for Medicaid/Medicare.

Patients diagnosed with depression should be treated with antidepressants to control their symptoms (Repetto & Petitto, 2008). Selective serotonin reuptake inhibitors (SSRIs) are as effective as tricyclic antidepressants but are better tolerated because of their more benign side-effect profile. SSRIs may interact with such antiretroviral medications as PIs and nNRTIs; therefore, initial SSRI dosage should be lowered with careful upward titration and close monitoring for toxic reactions (Repetto & Petitto, 2008). Serotonin and norepinephrine reuptake inhibitors (SNRIs), such as venlafaxine and duloxetine, are newer antidepressants which also are useful in treating chronic pain. Tricyclic antidepressants are indicated for treating depression only in patients who do not respond to newer medications. It is noted that monoamine oxidase inhibitors (MAOIs) may interact with multiple medications used to treat HIV disease and, therefore, should be avoided. Medication interaction and liver function profiles should be considered before antidepressant therapy is initiated.

Another pyschological symptom experienced by persons with HIV/AIDS is anxiety. Anxiety may also result from the medications used to treat HIV disease, such as anticonvulsants, sulfonamides, NSAIDs, and corticosteroids. Manifestations of generalized anxiety disorder include worry, trouble falling asleep, impaired concentration, psychomotor agitation, hypersensitivity, hyperarousal, and fatigue (Arriendel, 2003). The treatment for patients with anxiety is based on the nature and severity of the symptoms and the coexistence of other mood disorders or substance abuse. Short-acting anxiolytics, such as lorazepam (Ativan) and alprazolam (Xanax), are beneficial for intermittent symptoms, while buspirone (BuSpar) and clonazepam (Klonopin) are beneficial for chronic anxiety (Repetto & Petitto, 2008).

Significant stress is also associated with sharing information, related to the diagnosis, and particularly when such disclosures occur during the stage of advanced disease. The need for therapeutic communication and support from all health professionals caring for the patient and his/her family exists throughout the illness continuum. For many patients experiencing psychological distress associated with HIV disease, therapeutic interventions such as skills building, support groups, individual counseling, and group interventions using meditation techniques can provide a sense of psychological growth and a meaningful way of living with the disease (Chesney, Folkman, & Chambers, 1996; Kinara, 1996). Fear of disclosure of the AIDS diagnosis and stigmatization in the community often raise concern in the family about the diagnosis stated on death certificates. Practitioners may therefore write a nonspecific diagnosis on the main death certificate and sign section B on the reverse side to signify to the registrar general that further information will be provided at a later date.

Spiritual Issues in HIV/AIDS

Assessment of patients' spiritual needs is an important aspect of holistic care. Nurses must assess patients' spiritual values, needs, and religious perspectives, which are important in understanding their perspectives regarding their illness and their perception and meaning of life. Patients living with and dying from HIV disease have the spiritual needs of meaning, value, hope, purpose, love, acceptance, reconciliation, ritual, and affirmation of a relationship with a higher being (Kylma, Vehvilainen-Julkunen, & Lahdevirta, 2001). Assisting patients to find meaning and value in their lives, despite adversity, often involves a recognition of past successes and their internal strengths. Encouraging open communication between the patient and family is important to work toward reconciliation and the completion of unfinished business.

As with many life-threatening illnesses, patients with AIDS may express anger with God. Some may view their illness as a punishment or are angry that God is not answering their prayers. Expression of feelings can be a source of spiritual healing. Clergy can also serve as valuable members of the palliative care team in offering spiritual support and alleviating spiritual distress. The use of meditation, music, imagery, poetry, and drawing may offer outlets for spiritual expression and promote a sense of harmony and peace.

For all patients with chronic life-threatening illness, hope often shifts from hope that a cure will soon be found to hope for a peaceful death with dignity, including the alleviation of pain and suffering, determining one's own choices, being in the company of family and significant others, and knowing that their end-of-life wishes will be honored. Often, the greatest spiritual comfort offered by caregivers or family for patients comes from active listening and meaningful presence by sitting and holding their hands and knowing that they are not abandoned and alone.

Spiritual healing may also come from life review, as patients are offered an opportunity to reminisce about their lives, reflect on their accomplishments, reflect on their misgivings, and forgive themselves and others for their imperfections. Indeed, such spiritual care conveys that even in the shadow of death, there can be discovery, insight, the completion of relationships, the experience of love of self and others, and the transcendence of emotional and spiritual pain. Often, patients with AIDS, by their example, teach nurses, family, and others how to transcend suffering and how to die with grace and dignity.

Advanced Care Planning

Advanced planning is another important issue related to end-of-life care for patients with HIV/AIDS. It is important to understand the concept of competency, which is a "state in which the person is capable of taking legal acts, consenting or refusing treatment, writing a will or power of attorney" (Ferris et al., 1995). In assessing the patient's competency, the health provider must question whether the decision maker knows the nature and effect of the decision to be made and understands the consequences of his or her actions, and determine if the decision is consistent with an individual's life history, lifestyle, previous actions, and best interests. When an individual is competent, and in anticipation of the future loss of competency, he or she may initiate advance directives such as a living will and/or the designation of a healthcare proxy who will carry out the patient's healthcare wishes or make healthcare decisions in the event that the patient becomes incompetent. The patient may also give an individual the power of attorney regarding financial matters and care or treatment issues (Ferris et al., 1995). Advance directives include the patient's

decisions regarding such life-sustaining treatments as cardiopulmonary resuscitation, use of vasoactive drips to sustain blood pressure and heart rate, dialysis, artificial nutrition and hydration, and the initiation or withdrawal of ventilatory support. The signing of advance directives must be witnessed by two individuals who are not related to the patient or involved in the patient's treatment. Individuals who are mentally competent can revoke at any time their advance directives. If a patient is deemed mentally incompetent, state statutes may allow the court to designate a surrogate decision maker for the patient.

Most patients with AIDS have not discussed with their physicians the kind of care they want at the end of life, although more gay men have executed an advance directive than injection-drug users or women (Curtis, Patrick, Caldwell, & Collier, 2000a, 2000b). White patients were more likely to believe that their doctor was an HIV/AIDS expert and good at talking about end-of-life care, and recognize they have been very sick in the past, and that such discussions are important By contrast, nonwhite patients with AIDS report that they do not like to talk about the care they would want if they were very sick, and are more likely to feel that if they talk about death it will bring death closer (Curtis et al., 2000a, 2000b).

In addition to the discussion of goals of care and the completion of advance directives, healthcare providers can also assist patients and families by discussing the benefits of social support programs, unemployment insurance, worker's compensation, pension plans, insurance, and union or association benefits. In addition, they may emphasize the importance of organizing information and documents so that they are easily located and accessible, and suggest that financial matters be in order, such as power of attorney or bank accounts, credit cards, property, legal claims, and income tax preparation. Health professionals may also discuss matters related to the chosen setting for dying and the patient's wishes regarding their death.

Care of the Dying

The dying process for patients with advanced AIDS is commonly marked by increasingly severe physical deterioration, with patients becoming dependent on others for their care. Patients often are bedbound, and experience wasting as their appetite decreases as well as their energy. At the end of life, common symptoms include pain, dypsnea, and pressure ulcers. Febrile states and changes in mental status often occur as death becomes more imminent. Maintaining the comfort and dignity of the patients becomes a nursing priority. Symptomatic treatments, including pain management, should be continued throughout the dying process, since even obtunded patients may feel pain and other symptoms.

Because palliative care also addresses the needs of family, it is important to consider the vulnerability of family members to patients' health problems at the end of life. As illness progresses and death approaches, health professionals can encourage patients and family members to express their fears and end-of-life wishes. Encouraging patients and families to express such feelings as, "I love you," "I forgive you," "Forgive me—I am sorry," "Thank you," and "Good-bye," is important to the completion of relationships (Byock, 1997). Peaceful death can also occur when families give patients permission to die and assure them that they will be remembered.

Loss, Grief, and Bereavement for Persons with HIV/AIDS and Their Survivors

Patients with HIV disease experience many losses across the illness trajectory including a sense of loss of identity as they assume the identity of a patient with AIDS; loss of control over health and function; loss of roles as the illness progresses; loss of body image due to skin lesions, changes in weight and wasting; loss of sexual freedom because of the need to change sexual behaviors to maintain health and prevent transmission to others; loss of financial security through possible discrimination and increasing physical disability; and loss of relationships through possible abandonment, self-induced isolation, and the multiple deaths of others from the disease (Sikkema, Kochman, DiFranceisco, Kelly, & Hoffman, 2003). Each occurrence of illness may pose new losses and heighten the patient's awareness of mortality. Illness experiences are opportunities for health professionals to respond to cues of the patients in addressing their concerns and approaching the subject of loss, dying, and death. Given that grief is the emotional response to loss, patients dying from AIDS may also manifest the signs of grief, which include feelings of sadness, anger, self-reproach, anxiety, loneliness, fatigue, shock, yearning, relief, and numbness; physical sensations such as hollowness in the stomach, tightness in the chest, oversensitivity to noise, dry mouth, muscle weakness, and loss of coordination; cognitions of disbelief, confusion; and behavior disturbances in appetite, sleep, social withdrawal, loss of interest in activities, and restless overactivity (Rando, 1984).

The patient's family and significant others enter a state of bereavement upon the death of their loved one. Bereavement is a state of having suffered a loss, which is often a long-term process of adapting to life without the deceased (Rando, 1984). Family and significant others may experience signs of grief, including a sense of presence of the deceased, paranormal experiences or hallucinations, dreams of the deceased, a desire to have cherished objects of the deceased, and to visit places frequented by the deceased. Grief work is a dynamic process that is not time-limited and predictable (Mallinson,

1999). Those left behind never "get over" the loss but, rather, find a place for it in their life and create through memory a new relationship with their loved one.

Families and partners of patients with AIDS may experience disenfranchised grief, defined as the grief that persons experience when they incur a loss that is not openly acknowledged, publicly mourned, or socially supported (Doka, 1989). Support is not only important in assisting families in the tasks of grieving, but is also important for nurses who have established valued relationships with their patients. Disenfranchised grief may also be experienced by nurses who do not allow themselves to acknowledge their patient's death as a personal loss, or who are not acknowledged by others, such as the patient's family or even professional colleagues, for having suffered a loss.

Worden (1991) has identified the tasks of grieving as accepting the reality of the death; experiencing the pain of grief; adjusting to a changed physical, emotional, and social environment in which the deceased is missing; and finding an appropriate emotional place for the person who died in the emotional life of the bereaved. Mallinson (1999) recommends the following nursing interventions to facilitate grief work:

- Accept the reality of death by speaking of the loss and facilitating emotional expression.
- Work through the pain of grief by exploring the meaning of the grief experience.
- Adjust to the environment without the deceased by acknowledging anniversaries and the experience of loss during holidays and birthdays; help the bereaved to solve problems and recognize their own abilities to conduct their daily lives.
- Emotionally relocate the deceased and move on with life by encouraging socialization through formal and informal avenues.

The complications of AIDS-related grief often come from the secrecy and social stigma associated with the disease. Reluctance to contact family and friends can restrict the normal support systems available for the bereaved. The death of patients with AIDS may therefore result in complicated grief for the bereaved. Complicated grief may also occur when death occurs after lengthy illness, and the relationship has been ambivalent. Culturally sensitive and truthful communication is important as health professionals offer support to families in their grief.

Case Study conclusion: Within six months, Miriam experienced night sweats, fever, and diarrhea due to an exacerbation of MAC. This resulted in severe dehydration. The palliative care team was asked for a consultation by the AIDS specialist. The advanced practice nurse developed a very supportive relationship with Miriam and her significant other. She listened attentively and offered a comforting presence. The palliative care nurse provided effective symptom management and lessened their anxiety by working out a plan of care based on Miriam's wishes and preferences. They discussed her relationship with her mother and sister. Miriam decided to reach out and call her sister to tell her about her hospitalization. Her sister came to the hospital to visit. Over the next few weeks, a closeness was reestablished and her sister told her that she would be the guardian of her little boy. This conversation was faciliated by the advanced practice nurse. Miriam was coming to terms with her diagnosis and confided that she wanted to speak to a priest for confession. An intimate conversation with the nurse was of comfort and a visit by the chaplain was arranged.

Miriam never left the hospital as her fever began to rise and she became delirious. Several tests were conducted to identify other potential sources of the infection and other possible reasons for the delirium. Her symptoms were treated with Haldol and antipyretics. However, within a day, Miriam slipped into a coma. Her breathing was labored and she was given low doses of morphine to increase her comfort. With support from the advanced practice nurse, Miriam's little boy visited his mother. He kissed her hand and hung a picture he drew from the bedrail. With her mother, sister, and significant other at the bedside, tears flowed. In the nightstand, a letter from Miriam was left for her family. She reminded her son of her strong love for him and promised to watch over him from above. Miriam thanked her mother and sister for their promise to protect and care for her child. To her partner, she expressed a love and a wish that things were different. She asked the palliative care nurse to offer ongoing support to her family and to thank her for her loving and supportive care.

CONCLUSION

Palliative care offers a comprehensive approach to address the physical, emotional, social, and spiritual needs of individuals with incurable progressive illness throughout the illness trajectory until death. For patients with HIV/AIDS, palliative care offers a combination of disease-modifying and supportive interventions throughout the disease trajectory to relieve the suffering associated with opportunistic infections and

malignancies. Knowledge regarding HIV disease is important so that nurses can offer effective and compassionate care to patients, alleviating physical, emotional, social, and spiritual suffering at all stages of HIV disease. By establishing a partnership with their healthcare professionals in planning and implementing their healthcare, patients can maintain a sense of control during the illness experience. Through advanced care planning, patients can ensure that their end-of-life preferences and wishes are honored. The control of pain and symptoms associated with HIV/AIDS enables the patient and family to expend their energies on spiritual and emotional healing, and the possibility for personal growth and transcendence even as death approaches (Sherman, 2006). Palliative care preserves patients' quality of life by protecting their self-integrity, reducing a perceived helplessness, and lessening the threat of exhaustion of coping resources. Through effective and compassionate nursing care, patients with AIDS can achieve a sense of inner well-being even at death, with the potential to make the transition from life as profound, intimate, and precious an experience as their birth (Byock, 1997).

EVIDENCE-BASED PRACTICE

Sherman, D.W., Ye, X.Y., McSherry, C., Parkas, V., Calabrese, M., Gatto, M. (2006). Quality of life of patients with advanced cancer and acquired immune deficiency syndrome and their family caregivers. *Journal of Palliative Medicine*, 9(4) 948–63.

Background. Although definitions of palliative care include quality of life as a central concern, little research has been published about both the quality of life of patients with advanced illness and their family members, and particularly the changes in their quality of life over time.

Objectives. The aims of this prospective longitudinal pilot study were to: 1) establish the reliability of multidimensional quality of life instruments based on AIDS and cancer patients and caregivers; 2) identify differences in quality of life between patients with advanced AIDS and cancer, and their family caregivers with consideration of mortality, attrition, and compliance rates; and 3) examine differences in demographic variables and their potential confounding effect when measuring quality of life.

Methods. The sample included 101 patients with advanced illness (63 patients with advanced AIDS and 38 with advanced cancer) and 81 family caregivers (43 AIDS patients' caregivers and 38 cancer patients' caregivers). Data collection involved the monthly completion of the McGill Quality of Life Questionnaire (MQOL) for patients, and the Quality of Life Scale (QLS) for family caregivers.

Results. Reliability of the MQOL and QLS were established for AIDS and cancer patients and caregivers. Based on the MQOL, patients with advanced AIDS reported a lower total quality of life, and lower psychological quality of life, and a higher physical quality of life compared to patients with advanced cancer. There were no significant differences between patient groups on the one-item physical well-being subscale, or the existential well-being, and support subscales. Based on the QLS, AIDS caregivers reported greater overall quality of life, greater psychological well-being, and greater spiritual well-being than cancer caregivers. There were no significant differences between AIDS and cancer caregivers with respect to physical or social well-being. From baseline entry into the study to third month of participation, there were no significant changes in total quality of life scores for patient or caregiver groups, though trends indicated a moderately high total quality of life over time for all patient and caregiver groups. Fourteen out of 63 (22 %) of AIDS patients died, while 19 out of 38 (50%) of patients with advanced cancer died following enrollment. Forty-six out of 63 (73%) patients with advanced AIDS withdrew for various reasons other than death at some point during the 12 month time frame of the study, while 15 out of 38 (39%) patients with advanced cancer withdrew. There were significant differences on all demographic variables for patients with advanced cancer and AIDS. Only religious affiliation was significantly related to quality of life for patients with AIDS, while gender was the only variable associated with quality of life for cancer patients. There were significant differences on all demographic variables between caregivers with the exception of gender and living arrangements. Only the relationship between patients and caregivers and marital status were significantly associated with quality of life for cancer caregivers.

Conclusions. In palliative care research, the challenge is to design studies that will capture changes in the domains of quality of life over time, yet will minimize participant burden and subsequent attrition rates. By measuring quality of life as an outcome variable in palliative care, health professionals can identify changes in the domains of quality of life over time for various patient populations and their family caregivers, and respond with appropriate interventions, which promote or maintain their quality of life even as death approaches.

REFERENCES

Al-Harthi, L., Siegel, J, Spritzler, J., Pottage, J., Agnoli, M., & Landay, A., et al. (2000).
Maximum suppression of HIV replication leads to the restoration of HIV-specific responses in early HIV disease. *AIDS*, 14, 761–770.

Aron, J. (1994). Optimization of nutritional support in HIV disease. Nutrition and AIDS. In R. R. Watson. (Ed.). (pp. 215–233). Boca Raton, FL: CRC Press.

Avis, N., Smith, K., & Mayer, K. (1996). The relationship among CD4, hemoglobin, symptoms, and quality of life domains in a cohort of HIV-positive men. *International Conference on AIDS*, 11, 116 [Abstract].

Arriendel, J. (2003). Differential coping strategies, anxiety, depression, and symptomatology among African–American women with HIV/AIDS. Dissertationabstracts International. Section B: The Sciences & Engineering. 64:1481. US: UnivMicroFilms International.

Bloomer, S. (1998). Palliative care. *Journal of the Association of Nurses in AIDS Care*, 9, 45–47.

Bolin, J. (2006). Pernicious encroachment into end-of-life decision making: Federal intervention in palliative pain treatment. *American Journal of Bioethics*, 6, 34–36.

Brashers, D. E., Neidig, J. L., Reynolds, N. R., & Haas, S. M. (1998). Uncertainty in illness across the HIV/AIDS trajectory. *Journal of the Association of Nurses in AIDS Care*, 9, 66–77.

Burgoyne, R. W., & Tan, D. H. (2008). Prolongation and quality of life for HIV-infected adults treated with highly active antiretroviral therapy (HAART): A balancing act. *Journal of Antimicrobial Chemotherapy*, 61, 69–473.

Byock, I. (1997). *Dying well: The prospect for growth at the end of life*. New York: Riverhead Books.

Centers for Disease Control and Prevention. National Center for HIV, STD, and TB prevention: HIV/AIDS Survelliance report (2008). Available at http://www.cdc.gov/hiv/topics/surveillance/resources/reports/2006report/default.htm   Accessed, November 22, 2008.

Chesney, M. A., Folkman, S., & Chambers, D. (1996). Coping effectiveness training decreases distress in men living with HIV/AIDS. *International Conference on AIDS*, Vancouver, 11, 50.

Cleeland, C. S, Gonin, R., Hatfield, A. K., Edmonson, J. H., Blum, R. H., Stewart, J. A., et al. (1994). Pain and its treatment in outpatients with metastatic cancer: The eastern co-operative group's cooperative study. *New England Journal of Medicine*, 300, 592–596.

Cohen, M. (2001). The use of coping humor in an HIV/AIDS population. *Dissertation Abstracts International*, 61, 4976.

Curtis, R., Patrick, D., Caldwell, E., & Collier, A.(2000a). Why don't patients and physicians talk about end of life care?: barriers to communication for patients with acquired immunodeficiency syndrome and their primary care clinicians. *Archives in Internal Medicine*, 160, 1690–1696.

Curtis, R., Patrick, D., Caldwell, E., & Collier, A. (2000b). The attitudes of patients with advanced AIDS toward use of the medical futility rationale in decisions to forgo mechanical ventilation. *Archives in Internal Medicine*, 60, 1597–1601.

Doka, K.(1989). *Disenfranchised grief: Recognizing the hidden orrow*. Lexington, MA: Lexington Books.

Fantoni, M., Ricci, F., Del Borgo, C., Izzi I., Damiano, F., Moscati, A., et al. (1997). Multicentre study on the prevalence of symptoms and somatic treatment in HIV infection. Central Italy PRESINT Group. *Journal of Palliative Care*, 13, 9–13.

Farber, E., Mirsalimi, H., Williams, K., & McDaniel, J. (2003). Meaning of illness and psychological adjustment to HIV/AIDS. *Psychosomatics*, 44, 485–491.

Ferris, F., Flannery, J., McNeal, H., Morissette, M., Cameron, R., Bally, G., et al. (1995). *Palliative care: A comprehensive guide for the care of persons with HIV disease*. Toronto, Ontario: Mount Sinai Hospital/Casey House Hospice.

Freeman, E.M., & MacIntyre, R.C. (1999). Evaluating alternative treatments for HIV infection. *Nursing Clinics of North America*, 147–162.

Frich, L. M., & Borgbjerg, F. M. (2000). Pain and pain treatment in AIDS patients: A longitudinal study. *Journal of Pain and Symptom Management, 19*, 339–347.

Friedland, J., Renwick, R., & McColl, M. (1996). Coping and social support as determinants of quality of life in HIV/AIDS. *AIDS Care, 8,*15–31.

Gerard, L., Flandre, P., Raguin, G., Le Gall, J. R., Vilde, J. L., Leport, C., et al. (1996). Life expectancy in hospitalized patients with AIDS: Prognostic factors on admission. *Journal of Palliative Care, 12*, 26–30.

Goldstone, I., Kuhl, D., Johnson, A., Le Clerc, A., McCleod, A. (1995). Patterns of care in advanced HIV disease in a tertiary treatment centre. *AIDS Care, 7*, 47–56.

Grothe, T. M., & Brody, R. V. (1995). Palliative care for HIV disease. *Journal of Palliative Care, 11*, 48–49.

Guidelines for Prevention and Treatment of Opportunistic Infections in HIV-Infected Adults and Adolescents. (2008, June 18). Accessed December 15, 2008, http://aidsinfo.nih.gov/contentfiles/Adult_OI.pdf.

Harding, R., Easterbrook, P., Higginson, I. J., Karus, D., Raveis, V. H., Marconi, K., et al. (2005). Access and equity in HIV/AIDS palliative care: Review of the evidence and responses. *Palliative Medicine, 19*, 251–258.

Higginson, I. (1993). A review of past changes and future trends. *Journal of Public Health Medicine, 15*, 3–8.

Hilts, A. E., & Fish, D. N. (1998). Antiretroviral dosing in patients with organ dysfunction. *AIDS Reader, 8*, 179–184.

Holzemer, W., Henry, S., & Reilly, C.(1998). Assessing and managing pain in AIDS care: The patient perspective. *Journal of the Association of Nurses in AIDS Care, 9*, 22–30.

Holzemer, W. (2002). The symptom experience: What cell counts and viral loads won't tell you. *The American Journal of Nursing, 102*, 48–52.

Hussein, R. (2003). Current issues and forthcoming events. *Journal of Advanced Nursing, 44*, 235–237.

Ironson, G., Field, T., Scafidi, F., et al. (1996). Massage therapy is associated with enhancement of the immune system's cytotoxic capacity. *International Journal of Neurosciences, 84*, 205–217.

Keithley, J., Swanson, B., Murphy, M., & Levin, D. (2000). HIV/AIDS and nutrition implications for disease management. *Nursing Case Management, 5*, 52–62.

Kinara, M. (1996). Transcendental meditation: A coping mechanism for HIV-positive people. *International Conference on AIDS, 11*, 421.

Kylma, J., Vehvilainen-Julkunen, K., & Lahdevirta, J. (2001). Hope, despair and hopelessness in living with HIV/AIDS: A grounded theory study. *Journal of Advanced Nursing, 33*, 764–775.

LaPerriere, A., Klimas, N., Fletcher, M., et al. (1997). Change in CD4 cell enumeration following aerobic exercise training in HIV-1 disease: Possible mechanisms and practical applications. *International Journal of Sports Medicine, 18*, 56–61.

Lechner, S., Antoni, M., Lydston, D., LaPerriere, A., Ishii, M., Devieux, J., et al. (2003). Cognitive-behavioral interventions improve quality of life in women with AIDS. *Journal of Psychosomatuic Research, 54*, 252–261.

Leserman, J., Petitto, J., Gaynes, B., Barroso, J., Golden, R., Perkins, D., et al. (2002). Progression to AIDS, a clinical AIDS condition and mortality: Psychosocial and physiological predictors. *Psychological Medicine, 32*, 1059–1073.

Lorenz, K. A., Cunningham, W. E., Spritzer, L. K., & Hays, R. D. (2006). Changes in symptoms and health-related quality of life in a nationally representative sample of adults in treatment for HIV. *Quality of Life Research, 15*, 951–958.

Malcolm, J. A., & Sutherland, D. C. (1992). AIDS palliative care demands a new model. *Medical Journal of Australia, 157*, 572–573.

Mallinson, R. K. (1999). Grief work of HIV-positive persons and their survivors. In: D. W. Sherman (Ed.). HIV/AIDS Update. *Nursing Clinics of North America* (pp. 163–177). Philadelphia: W.B. Saunders.

McEnany, G. W., Hughes, A. M., & Lee, K. A. (1996). Depression and HIV. *Nursing Clinics of North America, 31*, 57–80.

Melroe, N. H., Stawarz, K. E., & Simpson, J. (1997). HIV RNA quantitation: Marker of HIV infection. *Journal of the Association of Nurses in AIDS Care, 8*, 31–38

Milan, F. B., Arnsten, J. H., Klein, S., Schoenbaum, E. E., Moskaleva, G., Buono, D., et al. (2008). Use of complementary and alternative medicine (CAM) in inner-city persons with or at risk for HIV infection. *AIDS Patient Care STDs, 22*, 811–816.

Murphy, R., & Flaherty, J. (2003). *Contemporary diagnosis and management of HIV/AIDS infections.* Newtown, PA: Handbooks in Health Care.

National Consensus Project. (2009). National consensus project for quality palliative care: Clinical practice guidelines for quality palliative care. [http://www.nationalconsensusproject.org].

Newshan, G., & Sherman, D. W. (1999). Palliative care: Pain and symptom management in persons with HIV/AIDS. *Nursing Clinics of North America, 34*(1),131–145.

Nieman, D. (1996). Exercise immunology: Practical applications. *International Journal of Sports Medicine, 18*, 91–100.

Nichel, J., Salsberry, P., Caswell, R., Keller, M., Long, T., & O'Connell, M., et al. (1996). Quality of life in nurse case management of persons with AIDS receiving home care. *Research in Nursing and Health, 19*, 91–99.

Norval, D. A. (2004). Symptoms and sites of pain experienced by AIDS patients. *South African Medical Journal, 94*, 450–454.

Orenstein, R.(2002). Presenting syndromes of human immunodeficiency virus. *Mayo Clinic Proceedings, 77*, 1097–1102.

Rando T.(1984). *Grief, dying, and death: Clinical interventions for caregivers.* Champaign, IL: Research Press Co.

Remien, R. H., Rabkin, J. G., & Williams, J. B. W. (1992). Coping strategies and health beliefs of AIDS longterm survivors. *Psychologial Health, 6*, 335–345.

Rene, E., & Roze, C. (1991). Diagnosis and treatment of gastrointestinal infections in AIDS. In D. Kotler (Ed.), *Gastrointestinal and nutritional manifestations of AIDS* (pp. 65–92). New York: Raven Press.

Repetto, M. J., & Petitto, J. M. (2008). Psychopharmacology in HIV-infected patients. *Psychosomatic Medicine, 70*, 585–592.

Selwyn, P., & Forstein, M. (2003). Overcoming the false dichotomy of curative vs palliative care for late-stage HIV/AIDS: "Let me live the way I want to live, until I can't." *Journal of the American Medical Association, 90*, 806–814.

Selwyn, P., & Rivard, M. (2003). Palliative care for AIDS: Challenges and opportunities in the era of highly active anti-retroviral therapy. *Journal of Palliative Medicine, 6*, 475–487.

Semba, R., Graham, P., & Caiaffa, J. (1994). Maternal vitamin A deficiency and mother-to-child transmission of HIV-1. *Lancet, 343*, 1593–1597.

Shen, J. M., Blank, A., & Selwyn, P. A. (2005). Predictors of mortality for patients with advanced disease in an HIV palliative care program. *Journal of Acquired Immune Deficiency Syndrome, 40*, 445–447.

Sherman, D. W., & Kirton, C. (1998). Hazardous terrain and over the edge: The survival of HIV-positive heterosexual minority men. *Journal of the Association of Nurses in AIDS Care, 9*, 23–34.

Sherman, D. W. (1998). Reciprocal suffering: The need to improve family caregiver's quality of life through palliative care. *Journal of Palliative Medicine, 1*, 357–366.

Sherman, D. W., & Kirton, C. A. (1992). Relapse to unsafe sex among HIV-positive heterosexual men. *Applied Nursing Research, 12*, 91–100.

Sherman, D. W. (2006). Patients with acquired immunodeficiency syndrome. In B.

Ferrel, B., & N. Coyle (Eds.), *Textbook of palliative nursing* (2nd ed., pp. 671–712). New York: Oxford University Press.

Sherman, D. W., Ye, X., McSherry, C., Calabrese, M., Parkas, V., Gatto, M., et al. (2007).

Symptom assessment of patients with advanced cancer and AIDS and their family caregivers: The results of a quality of life pilot study. *American Journal of Hospice & Palliative Medicine, 24*(5), 350–365.

Sherman, D. W. (2001). Palliative care. In C. Kirton, D.Talotta & K. Zwolski (Ed.), *Handbook of HIV/AIDS nursing* (pp. 173–194). Philadelphia: W.B. Saunders.

Sherman , D. W., Ye, X. Y., McSherry, C., Parkas, V., Calabrese, M., Gatto, M., et al. (2006). Quality of life of patients with advanced cancer and acquired immune deficiency syndrome and their family caregivers. *Journal of Palliative Medicine, 9*, 948–963.

Sikkema, K., Kochman, A., DiFranceisco, W., Kelly, J., & Hoffman, R. (2003). AIDS-related grief and coping with loss among HIV-positive men and women. *Journal of Behavioral Medicine, 26*, 165–181.

Trescot, A. M., Standiford, H., Hansen, H., Benyamin, R., Glaser, S. E., Adlaka, R., et al. (2008). Opioids in the management of chronic non-cancer pain: An update of American Society of the Interventional Pain Physicians' (ASIPP) Guidelines. *Pain Physician, 11*, S5–S62.

UNAIDS/WHO. (2007). AIDS epidemic update: December 2007. UNAIDS. Geneva 2007. ISBN 978 92 9 173621 86.

U.S. Department of Health and Human Services. Guidelines for using antiretroviral agents among HIV-infected adults and adolescents. (November 3, 2008). Accessed December 15, 2008 http://aidsinfo.nih.gov/contentfiles/AdultandAdolescent GL.pdf.

Von Gunten, C. F., Martinez, J., Neely, K. J., & Von Roenn, J. H. (1995). AIDS and palliative medicine: Medical treatment issues. *Journal of Palliative Care, 11*, 5–9.

Vosvick, M., Koopman, C., Gore-Felton, C., Thoresen, C., Krumboltz, J., Spiegal D., et al. (2003). Relationship of functional quality of life to strategies for coping with the stress of living with HIV/AIDS. *Psychosomatics, 44*, 51–58.

Watt, G., & Burnouf, T. (2002). AIDS: Past and future. *New England Journal of Medicine, 346* ,710–711.

Worden, J. (1991). *Grief counseling and grief therapy: A handbook for the mental health practitioner.* New York: Springer.

19

Pain Assessment and Pharmacological/ Nonpharmacological Interventions

Nessa Coyle
Mary Layman-Goldstein

Key Points

- Poorly controlled pain will be experienced by many patients at the end of life.
- This results in unnecessary suffering to both patients and their families.
- We have the knowledge and the art to control the pain and ameliorate the suffering and yet patients continue to die in pain.
- Pain is multidimensional and multifactorial and rarely occurs in isolation from other symptoms.
- Comprehensive assessment of pain is a necessary first step in management.
- A sound knowledge of clinical pharmacology of analgesic drugs is also essential.
- Nondrug pain interventions attempt to address aspects of a patient's pain that have not responded to pharmacological interventions. Or, when an individual is experiencing significant side effects from analgesic medications they may be considered a better option with less likelihood of adverse experiences.
- Consider whether a particular intervention will need high or low levels of patient or caregiver involvement at a time when both may be unable to participate at the level necessitated for success of the intervention.
- Evidence for the use of nondrug pain interventions at the end of life is frequently limited because of the lack of large, well-designed, rigorous studies. Evidence based literature continues to evolve.
- The nurse is a key figure in bringing a comprehensive pain management approach to the bedside.
- Ensuring that a dying patient has relief from pain is a moral obligation.

Case Study: Mr. J is a 68-year old gentleman with non-small cell lung cancer with widely metastatic disease to the bones. He was diagnosed 6-months earlier after a workup for a persistent cough and low back pain. He is married with two grown sons and recently retired from his job in the bank. His plans on retirement were to travel with his wife and to "enjoy life." He was, however, a pragmatist and "took life as it came."

His low back pain was described as dull, aching, persistent, worse with movement and better at rest—5/10 at its worse and 1/10 at its best. He was initially treated with palliative chemotherapy for his underlying disease and radiation therapy to his back for pain control. Residual pain was initially well managed with combination oxycodone/acetaminophen. He slept well at night and he moved his bowels on a regular basis. However, Mr. J. decided against further chemotherapy.

Over several weeks his back pain increased in severity—4/10 at rest and 7/10 on movement. He was using approximately 40 mg of oxycodone and 2,600 mg acetaminophen a day. Constipation had become a problem but there were no other side effects. He was started on controlled-release oxycodone—30 mg every 12 h (50% increase in oxycodone) and this was gradually increased to 120 mg every 12 h. Mr. J continued on acetaminophen as he found this gave him added pain relief. The rescue dose of oxycodone was 20 mg (approximately 10% of his 24/hr opioid dose) every 3 h as needed. He was also started on an effective bowel regimen of a laxative and stool softener. His back pain was now under adequate control with on average 3/10 on movement and he continued to enjoy life.

Unfortunately a change in his drug coverage mandated that he be given a trial of morphine therapy and that his controlled release oxycodone would not be covered. He was rotated to extended release morphine 100 mg every 12 h (based on his daily oxycodone intake of 300 mg: 240 mg around-the-clock + 60 mg prn—the oral equianalgesic dose of morphine = 450 mg). Because his pain control was good and because cross-tolerance is not complete, this dose was decreased by 25%. His final dose of extended release morphine was 200 mg per day. He was also prescribed immediate release morphine sulfate 30 mg every 3 h prn for breakthrough pain (15% of his 24 h dose).

Mr. J's pain remained well controlled on this regimen although he had some initial nausea after the opioid rotation to morphine and some increased sedation. Around the clock metoclopramide was added for 2 days with nausea resolving. It was then continued on a prn basis. His daytime sleepiness had not resolved after a week so he was started on a psychostimulant, methylphenidate 5 mg each morning and at 12 noon with good effect. He continued to move his bowels daily.

Mr. J well for several months and then had a sudden and severe exacerbation of his back pain 10/10 requiring hospitalization in a pain crisis. He was initially given 10 mg of intravenous dexamethasone and his oral morphine regimen was switched to the parenteral route for rapid pain control. Using a 3:1 ratio for the change form oral to parenteral route Mr. J's 300 mg of oral morphine/24 h was converted to 100 mg of parenteral morphine/day via PCA. This translated to his receiving 4 mg of morphine/h via PCA with 2 mg IV every 15 min as needed for breakthrough pain. Mr. J's pain returned to his base line of 3/10 and within 72 -h he was rotated back to his previous oral morphine regimen. He continued on dexamethasone. The cause of his pain exacerbation was identified as tumor impinging on the spinal cord but he decided against further treatment except for continued steroids.

Two weeks later Mr. J developed a burning, shooting pain in his right chest wall. Previous imaging studies revealed impingement of the brachial plexus by tumor. Neurontin was added to his current regimen with dose titrated up to an effective tolerated dose.

Hospice continued to work with this man and his family. He required no further hospitalizations and his pain remained under control. His opioids and coanalgesic/adjuvant drugs were adjusted as needed.

Questions

1) What types of pain was this man experiencing?
2) What principles of opioid and coanalgesic management were demonstrated in this case?
3) What would you add, if anything, to his analgesic regimen?

Introduction

Few things are of more concern to patients at end of life and to their families than that pain will be well controlled (Ferrell & Whiteman, 2003; Foley, 1991; Ng & von Gunten, 1998). In the words of one patient, "I can't emphasize enough that pain blinds you to all that is positive—I mean the real bad pain. It just closes you down." Unrelieved pain can consume the attention and energy of those who are dying, and create an atmosphere of impotency and despair in their families and caretakers (Chang, Hwang, Feuerman, & Kasimis, 2000; Coyle, 2004; Hwang, Chang, & Kasimis, 2002; van den Beuken-vanet al., 2007). The fear of unrelieved pain expressed by patients and their families is sadly often reflective of what they have or will experience (American Geriatrics Society, 2006; Coyle, 2004; Ehde et al., 2003; Kraft, 2003; Kutner, Bryant, Beaty, & Fairclough, 2007; SUPPORT 1995; Swica & Breitbart, 2002; Teno, Kabumoto, Wetle, Roy, & Mor, 2004). And yet, with the knowledge and art that is now available, we have the ability to relieve the majority of pain including pain at the end of life (Miaskowski et al., 2005).

The intent of this chapter is to provide nurses with a basic overview of the principles of pain assessment and pharmacological management at end of life. The needs of special populations who have been identified as "at risk" for inadequate pain control are highlighted including those who are elderly, children, those who are communication impaired, and those with a history of substance abuse. These tend to be patients "without a voice" or whose voice is not heard, not respected, or not believed. Sometimes there is a mismatch between the normative values of the patient and the healthcare provider. A discussion of the integration of nonpharmacological interventions into a comprehensive pain management plan occurs later in the chapter. The importance of these nonpharmacologic interventions cannot be overstressed but will not be reviewed in this chapter.

PAIN ASSESSMENT AND PHARMACOLOGICAL INTERVENTION

The prevalence of pain in those with advanced illness varies by diagnosis and other factors. Pain in the cancer population is highly prevalent, has been widely studied, and is therefore a useful model from which to review pain assessment and management at the end of life (Chang et al., 2000; Meuser et al., 2001; Morita, Ichiki, Tsunoda, Inoue, & Chihara, 1998). The assessment and management of cancer pain will be used as the framework for this chapter. It is recognized that pain associated with a terminal disease may be superimposed on many other chronic pain syndromes, including musculoskeletal pain such as osteoarthritis and low back pain. The principles outlined in this chapter can be applied to any pain situation.

Barriers to Pain Relief

Numerous clinician-related, institutional-related, and patient- and family-related barriers have been identified that consistently interfere with adequate pain management even at the end of life. In addition there is a growing research on the influence of sex and gender on the experience of pain and response to treatment (Hurley & Adams, 2009).

Clinician-related barriers include inadequate knowledge of pain management, incomplete assessment of pain, concern about regulation of controlled substances,

fear of causing patient addiction, concern about analgesic side effects, and concern that if strong opioids are used "too early" they will be ineffective later when the need is greatest. In addition, a failure of clinicians to evaluate or appreciate the severity of the pain problem and to appreciate the impact of pain on the patient's day-to-day existence is likely to be a major predictor of inadequacy of relief (Cleeland et al., 1994; Jones, Fink, & Clarke, 2005; Lasch et al., 2002; O'Brien, Dalton, Konsler, & Carlson, 1996; von Roenn, Cleeland, Gonin, Hatfied, & Portenoy 1993; Passik, Byers, & Kirsh, 2007; Weinstein et al., 2000).

Health care setting–related barriers include lack of visibility of pain, lack of a common language to describe pain, lack of commitment to pain management as a priority, and failure to use validated pain measurement tools in clinical practice (Bookbinder et al., 1995; Chih-Yi Sun et al., 2007; Goldberg & Morrison, 2007; Foley, 1998; Tarzian & Hoffman, 2004). Economic factors and drug availability are further impediments to adequate pain treatment, especially in underserved and minority communities and when pain is to be managed in the home (Anderson et al., 2002; Foley, 1998; Morrison, Wallenstein, Natale, Senzel, & Huang, 2000).

Patient-related barriers have many similarities to clinician-related barriers and include reluctance to report pain, reluctance to follow treatment recommendations, fears of tolerance and addiction, concern about treatment-related side effects, fears regarding disease progression, and belief that pain is an inevitable part of cancer and must be accepted (Coyle, 2004; Gunnarsdottir, Donovan, Serlin, Voge, & Ward, 2002; Jones et al., 2005; Potter, Wiseman, Dunn & Boyle, 2003; Ward et al., 1993).

It is extremely important to understand family-related barriers to pain management at the end of life (Berry & Ward, 1995; Keefe et al., 2003; Vallerand, Collins-Bohler, Templin & Hasenau, 2007; Ward, Berry & Misiewicz, 1996). Frequently, it is a family member who is the primary care provider in the home and it is a family member who will be assessing pain and administering the pain medications. An early small descriptive study investigated the experience of managing pain at home from the perspectives of the patient, the primary family care-giver, and the home-care nurse, and it encapsulated many of the important areas that still affect pain management in the home (Taylor, Ferrell, Grant, & Cheyney, 1993). Areas of decision making and conflict mainly centered around the use of medications. Patients were preoccupied with decisions about which pain medication to take and how much of it to take. Negative side effects and meaning in regard to these medications contributed to conflicts in the patient's mind as to whether they were doing the "right thing" in taking the pain medication. Nearly all the patients assumed their pain would increase with impending death.

Patient decisions about how to live with and cope with their pain included considerations of how what they did and said affected their healthcare professionals and family members. Sometimes these factors continue to lead the patients to deny the pain (Coyle, 2004; Taylor et al., 1993). Similarly, the decisions and conflicts that arose most frequently for family caregivers also related to pain medication and having to make decisions about which pill to give and when. Compounding these decisions were the concerns related to overdosing, adverse side effects, and addiction.

A variety of approaches and specific programs have been developed to address these barriers, for example, making pain visible within an institution by incorporating a pain measurement tool into institutional daily clinical practice and introducing broad educational efforts to change attitudes, behaviors, and knowledge deficits in patients, clinicians, and institutions (Bookbinder et al., 1995; Chih-Yi Sun et al., 2007). The Joint Commission on Accreditation of Healthcare Organizations (JCAHO) standards on pain management has been helpful in making institutions accountable for assessment and management of pain across care settings (JCAHO, 2006). In addition a variety of professional organizations have developed and regularly update clinical practice guidelines for the assessment and management of pain. These include: the American Pain Society, the National Comprehensive Cancer Network, the American Geriatric Society, and the National Consensus Guidelines for Quality Palliative Care. Clinical practice guidelines, as well as major national professional educational efforts on end-of-life care (End of Life Nursing Education Consortium [ELNEC] and Education for Physicians on End of Life Care [EPEC]) are ongoing efforts to improve care of the dying and address the problem of inadequate control of pain (Gordon et al., 2005; Herr et al., 2006; Idell, Grant & Kirk, 2007; Max et al., 1997; Oncology Nursing Society, 2006).

Basic Principles of Pain Assessment at the End of Life

Pain assessment is the underpinning of pain management. The goals of pain assessment are to prevent pain if possible and to identify pain immediately should it occur. This can be facilitated by standardized screening of all patients for pain, on a routine basis and across care settings (JCAHO, 2006). Standardized screening for pain can be as simple as asking the patient "Do you have pain?" A comprehensive assessment of pain follows if a patient reports pain that is not being addressed or adequately managed.

Pain is always subjective and is defined by the international association for the study of pain (IASP, 1979) as "an unpleasant sensory and emotional experience associated with actual or potential tissue damage

or described in terms of such damage." This definition clarifies the multidimensionality of pain. McCaffery's definition of pain "Whatever the person says it is, existing whenever he or she say it does" (McCaffery & Pasero, 1999) describes the subjectivity of pain. The patient is acknowledged as the expert on the severity of his pain and of the adequacy of relief obtained. The interdisciplinary team's expertise is in identifying the different etiologies of the pain and arriving at effective management strategies with the patient and/or family. Although verbal report of pain and adequacy of pain relief is considered the gold standard, some individuals at end of life are unable to communicate verbally (APS, 2003; Twycross & LIchter, 1998). Other behavioral measures for assessing pain are therefore required (Herr, Bjoro, & Decker, 2006; Taylor & Herr, 2003). For example, patients who are semiconscious or in a coma may moan or cry out or exhibit other signs of distress when moved. Although these behaviors are not necessarily associated with pain, the likelihood of pain should be strongly considered. If the decision is made to medicate the patient for pain, subsequent signs of diminished distress on movement would indicate that pain had been present. If such a patient had been on an analgesic regimen prior to diminution of consciousness, analgesics should be continued or increased until the patient shows signs of comfort.

Assessment of pain at end of life is often complicated by the presence of multiple other symptoms that are common in the last few days of life, including cognitive impairment (Coyle, Adelhardt, Foley & Portenoy, 1990; Miaskowski, 2002; National Institute of Health, 2002). Refer to Table 19.1.

In addition, the suffering that patients experience at the end of life is not necessarily related to the severity of the symptom. Mild symptoms may cause considerable distress to the individual sometimes because of the meaning of that symptom to the person, and sometimes because the individual has not yet come to terms with dying (Twycross & Lichter, 1998). Unrelieved pain and

19.1 | Challenges When Assessing Pain in the Far-Advanced Cancer Patient

- Multiple concurrent medical problems.
- Multiple symptoms and symptom clusters.
- Hepatic and renal failure and susceptibility to drug accumulation and adverse side effects.
- Prevalence of delirium when close to death.
- Requires more time than with patients who are less ill.
- Patients become easily fatigued and may be short of breath.
- May be in "too much pain" or bothered by other symptoms to answer questions.
- Possible tendency of family members to answer questions on patient's behalf.

suffering can deprive patients and their families of interaction at the end of life around anything other than pain. A time of potential growth, communication, and reconciliation can be lost. Nurses have an extraordinary responsibility to be patient advocates in the assessment and management of pain throughout the course of a disease process, but especially at the end of life (American Nurses Association 1990). Because of its complexity, the assessment of pain is enhanced by a multidimensional and interdisciplinary approach (Ingham & Coyle, 1997; Institute of Medicine Report, 2008; National Quality Forum, 2006). The tissue damage response leading to the complaint of pain, the suffering component of the pain, and the meaning of the pain to the individuals and their families all need to be addressed. Although this comprehensive pain assessment is usually interdisciplinary, it is the nurse who brings that assessment and plan to the bedside. The assessment of pain is carried out within the framework of goals of care, patient and family values, knowledge of the disease process, and nearness of the individual to death.

Types of Pain—Neurophysiological Mechanisms of Pain

Two major types of pain, *nociceptive pain* (which includes somatic and visceral pain) and *neuropathic pain,* have been described in the cancer patient (Payne & Gonzales, 2004). *Somatic* pain occurs as a result of activating pain sensitive structures, or nociceptors, in the cutaneous and deep musculoskeletal tissues. This pain is typically well localized and may be felt in the superficial cutaneous or deeper musculoskeletal structures. Examples of somatic pain include bone metastases, postsurgical incisional pain, and pain accompanying myofascial or musculoskeletal inflammation or spasm (Payne & Gonzales, 2004). Somatic pain is responsive to the nonsteroidal anti-inflammatory drugs, the opioid drugs, and steroids.

Visceral pain results from infiltration, compression, distention, or stretching of thoracic or abdominal viscera (e.g., liver metastases or pancreatic cancer). This type of pain is poorly localized, often described as deep, squeezing, pressure, and may be associated with nausea, vomiting, and diaphoresis (especially when acute). Visceral pain is often referred to cutaneous sites that may be remote from the site of the lesion, for example, shoulder pain associated with diaphragmatic irritation. Tenderness and pain on touching the referral cutaneous site may occur. Visceral pain is responsive to the nonsteroidal anti-inflammatory drugs, the opioid drugs and steroids (Payne & Gonzales, 2004).

Neuropathic pain results from injury to the peripheral or central nervous systems. In the cancer patient, neuropathic pain most commonly occurs as a consequence of the tumor compressing or infiltrating peripheral nerves, nerve roots, or the spinal cord. In addition, this type of pain may result from surgical trauma and chemical or radiation-induced injury to peripheral nerves or the spinal cord from cancer therapies. Examples of common neuropathic pain syndromes include metastatic or radiation-induced brachial or lumbosacral plexopathies, epidural spinal cord or cauda-equina compression, postherpetic neuralgia, and painful chemotherapy-induced neuropathies. Neuropathic pain is often described as having sharp, shooting, electric-shocklike qualities that are unfamiliar to the patient. It can also be described as a constant dull ache, sometimes with a pressure or viselike quality with episodic paroxysms of burning or electric-shocklike sensations. Neuropathic pain is often severe, very distressing to the patient, and sometimes difficult to control. Although partially responsive to the opioid drugs, neuropathic pain is also responsive to adjuvant drugs or coanalgesics such as antidepressants, anticonvulsants, steroids, local anesthetics and N-methyl-D-receptor antagonists (NMDA) such as ketamine (Elliot & Foley, 1998; Fine, 1999; Payne & Gonzales, 2004).

Temporal Pattern of Pain

Pain can also be defined on a temporal basis, for example, acute pain and chronic pain. Patients at the end of life frequently have a combination of both acute and chronic pain (Foley, 1998; Merskey, 1986).

Acute pain is characterized by a well-defined pattern of onset. Generally the cause of the pain can be identified and the pain may be accompanied by physiological signs of hyperactivity of the central nervous system such as a rapid pulse and elevated blood pressure. Acute pain usually has a precipitating cause, for example, small bowel obstruction, a painful dressing change, or a pathological fracture. The pain tends to be time-limited and responds to analgesic drug therapy, and where possible, treatment of the precipitating cause. Acute pain can be further subdivided into subacute pain and intermittent or episodic types (Foley, 2004). Subacute pain describes pain that comes on over several days, often with increasing intensity, and may be associated with a variety of causes such as a progressive pathological process or an analgesic regimen that has not been titrated upward to accommodate for a progressive painful disease process. Episodic pain refers to pain that occurs during defined periods of time, on a regular or irregular basis (Foley, 2004). Intermittent pain is an alternative way to describe episodic pain. Such pain may be associated with movement, dressing changes, or other activities. Because the trigger for intermittent pain often can be identified, the nurse, through appropriate use of analgesics prior to the pain-provoking event, can have a significant impact on decreasing these painful episodes for the patient. The fear of pain associated with these activities is therefore lessened for the patient.

Chronic pain differs from acute pain in its presentation. These differences are essential for the nurse to understand because patients with chronic pain are at risk to have their pain unrecognized, untreated, or undertreated. Chronic pain is defined as pain that persists for more than 3 months (Foley, 2004). Adaptation of the autonomic system occurs and the patient does not exhibit the objective signs of pain found so frequently in those with acute pain (e.g., there is no rapid pulse or elevated blood pressure). Poorly relieved chronic pain at the end of life can contribute to fatigue, depression, insomnia, general despair, withdrawal from interaction with others, and desire for death (Cherny & Coyle, 1994; Coyle, 2004; Ferrell, Rhiner, Cohen & Grant, 1991; Foley, 1991).

Breakthrough pain is defined as a transient increase in pain to greater than moderate intensity, occurring on a baseline pain of moderate intensity or less (APS, 2003; Foley, 2004; Portenoy & Hagen, 1990). Breakthrough pain has a diversity of characteristics. In some patients, for example, it is characterized by marked worsening of pain at the end of the dosing interval of regularly scheduled analgesics. In other patients, it occurs by the action of the patient or the nurse, for example, when turning or having a dressing change, and is referred to as incident pain. Patients frequently have a combination of these different types of pain; noting the patterns of pain in a particular individual is an essential component of pain assessment. Attention to such details is the essence of symptom control at the end of life. A pain diary or log, kept by the patient or family, can help identify the pattern of pain. The log can indicate, over the course of the day, the patient's rating of pain, medication taken, activity level, and any other pain relief measures tried.

Clinical Assessment of Pain

The previously described mechanisms of pain and types of pain that can be experienced by patients with advanced progressive disease are a useful background from which to start a clinical pain assessment. The clinical assessment is based on a process of both observation and interview. The basic principles of a pain assessment are outlined in Table 19.2.

It is based on the premise that the person experiencing the pain is the expert on his pain. The clinician's role is to sort out the etiology of the pain complaint and arrive at a targeted management approach with the patient and family. If the patient is too ill or cognitively impaired to respond to the questions, a family member or care provider is asked to give the pain history as best they can. A variety of validated pain assessment tools are available for use in the hospital or home setting. Ideally any pain assessment tool includes intensity of pain, relief of pain, psychological distress, and functional impairment. Examples of these tools are

19.2 | Clinical Assessment of Pain: Basic Principles

- Believe the patient's complaint of pain. The patient is the expert on the pain being experienced. The multidisciplinary staff are the experts in determining the etiology of the pain.
- Take a careful history of the pain complaint and place it within the context of the patient's medical history and goals of care. If the patient is unable to communicate verbally, obtain a history from those most involved in the patient's care, both family and formal health care providers.
- Observe the patient for nonverbal communication regarding pain, for example, guarding, wincing, and moaning, or crying out when turned or moved.
- Recognize that the patient near the end of life may have multiple symptoms complicating pain assessment.
- Assess the characteristics of each pain, including the site, pattern of referral, what makes it better and what makes it worse, and the impact of the pain on the individual's activity of daily living and quality of life; for example, mood, sleep, movement, and interaction with others.
- Clarify the temporal aspects and pattern of the patient's pain; for example, acute, chronic, baseline, intermittent, breakthrough, or incident.
- Assess the psychological state of the patient and the meaning of the pain to the patient and his or her family.
- Examine the site of the pain.
- Facilitate an appropriate diagnostic work-up making sure that the patient's pain is adequately managed during the work-up.
- Provide continuity of care for the patient and family during ongoing pain assessment and management.
- Assess and reassess the effectiveness of the pain management regimen both for baseline pain and breakthrough pain.
- Give a time frame where you would expect to see evidence of patient comfort after the start or adjustment of a pain management approach. If this is not evident, reassess the patient. Ongoing reassessment is essential in the setting of a complex patient with multiple symptoms.
- Assess and reassess for the presence of adverse side effects from the pain management regimen. Three categories of analgesic drugs are included in the three-step analgesic ladder: nonsteroidal anti-inflammatory drugs (NSAIDs), opioids, and adjuvant analgesics. With a focus on end-of-life care, discussion around these groups of drugs will include rationale for selection, dose titration, and routes of administration.

the memorial pain assessment card (Fishman, Pasternak, & Wallenstein, 1987), Wisconsin Brief Pain Inventory (Daut, Cleeland, & Flanery, 1983), the McGill Pain Questionnaire and the McGill Home Recording Chart (Melzack, 1993). Simpler scales that measure pain intensity only include numerical rating scales. Examples are, Visual Analog scales, Likert or Verbal Rating Scales (Ahles, Blanchard, & Rockdeschel, 1983; Serlin, Mendoza, Nakamura, Edwards, & Cleeland, 1995; Wallenstein, Rogers, Kaiko, & Houde, 1986), and Happy/Sad faces (Wong & Baker, 1995; Wong, Hockenberry-Eaton,

Wilson, Sinkelstein, & Schwartz, 2001). For the patient with severe cognitive impairment, various assessment tools are also available (Herr et al., 2006). In the terminally ill patient when multiple symptoms are common (Miaskowski, 2002; Portenoy et al., 1994). it can be useful to follow the intensity of pain and other symptoms in graph form longitudinally. With this approach the interrelatedness among symptoms may become clearer (Bruera, Kuehn, Miller, Selmser, & Macmillan, 1991).

Taking a focused pain history involves assessing the following parameters:

Onset. Have the patient describe when the pain first began. Was it associated with a particular activity or known medical event? Did other symptoms accompany the onset of pain such as nausea or vomiting?

Site(s). Ask the patient to point to the site or sites of pain. Frequently, individuals with pain have multiple sites of pain. Each site needs to be assessed as the management approach may differ depending on the etiology of the pain.

Quality of the pain. Have the patient describe the quality of each pain. Word descriptors used by patients to describe their pain help the clinician to arrive at an inferred pain mechanism. This in turn influences the choice of pharmacotherapy. For example, sharp, shooting, electric-shock-like descriptions of pain, often described by the patient as "unfamiliar," suggests a neuropathic component to the pain (Elliot & Foley, 1998). Such pain may be responsive to the coanalgesic/adjuvant drugs as well as to opioid analgesics.

Severity of the pain. Have the patient describe the severity of each pain. It is particularly important that the nurse recognize the significance of escalating pain within the context of that particular patient's disease process, value system, goals of care, and nearness to death. Treatment decisions take all of these factors into account. As previously described, a variety of tools for measuring pain are available for use in the hospital or home setting. Ask the patient the amount of distress caused by each site of pain. In this way each pain can be prioritized.

Although numerical estimates are the most frequently used method of assessing severity of pain and adequacy of pain relief, some patients cannot use a numerical estimate. In these cases one of the other tools may be more appropriate. Consistency in using a particular assessment tool with an individual patient is likely to enhance communication among team members regarding the efficacy of a pain management approach. Some patients will underreport their pain. The reasons are varied but include a patient's appraisal of the consequences of reporting pain (Coyle, 2004). For example, having an opioid dosage increased may lead to fear of increased constipation. This potential outcome may not be acceptable to the patient and therefore they chose not to report the pain. Other patients do not report escalating pain because previous reports of pain have led to ineffective management. In other words they "give up" trying.

Assess pain severity at times of different activity. Pain intensity should be assessed at rest, on movement, and in relation to daily activity and the patient's analgesic schedule. Asking certain questions helps establish if the appropriate drug has been selected, dose efficacy, and if the time interval between doses for this patient is correct: "How much pain is relieved when you take the pain medication?" "How long does the relief last?" and "Are side effects present?" A more global 24-hour assessment of the adequacy of pain management in general includes asking the patient his pain scores—"right now," "at its best," "at its worst," and "on average" (Daut et al., 1983).

Exacerbating and relieving factors. Identifying factors that increase or relieve the patient's pain can be helpful in arriving at a pain diagnosis and in giving the nurse the opportunity to reinforce techniques that the patient has found useful in the past to relieve pain. A patient with cancer who reports rapidly escalating back pain with a bandlike quality that is worse when lying in bed and better when standing is considered to have cord compression until proved otherwise (Posner, 1995). Early recognition of cord compression and treatment, frequently by steroids, radiation therapy, or both, may prevent paraplegia in the last few weeks or months of a patient's life. Escalating back pain may be the only sign of the impending cord compression. It is critical that the nurse who is caring for a patient at the end of life recognizes the significance of escalating pain within the construct of that particular patient's disease process and goals of care.

Impact of the pain on the patient's psychological state. The interface between pain and suffering has been well described (Cherney & Coyle, 1994; Cherney & Portenoy, 1994; Coyle, 2004; Foley, 1991; Saunders, 1967). In clinical situations, when patients are asked, "What does this pain mean to you?" and "What do you think is causing the pain?" a flood of suffering and fear is often expressed. Patients are fearful of what their dying will be like, of uncontrolled and excruciating pain, of being a burden on their family, and of being "drugged out." The same questions may be asked by the patient and family time and time again, and need to be responded to in a sensitive, accurate, and reassuring manner. Some clinicians, when meeting a patient in severe pain for the first time, ask if the pain has ever been so bad that the individual has thought of harming himself or herself. Again, the response may indicate that suicide has been considered as an option if the pain is not controlled or if things get "too bad." These are important questions for an experienced clinician to ask, so that the patient's vulnerabilities and anxieties are verbalized, suicide vulnerability factors identified, and education and support from other members of the interdisciplinary pain team including psychiatrists, psychologists, social workers, and chaplains mobilized (Coyle, 2004; Institute of Medicine Report, 2008; National Quality Forum, 2006). All of the patient's worries and fears need be addressed if the pain is to be adequately controlled. This is an ongoing process.

Pain Treatment History and Responses to Previous and Current Analgesic Regimens

The patient needs to be asked very specifically about what approaches have been used to manage pain in the past—both pharmacological (including over-the-counter medication) and nonpharmacological—and how effective those approaches have been. Included should be analgesics that have been previously prescribed, dosages, time intervals, routes of administration, effects, side effects, and the reasons why a particular approach was discontinued. Fear of recurrence of previously experienced side effects (e.g., sedation, nausea, mental haziness, and constipation) may make a patient reluctant to start a new analgesic regimen. Focusing attention on their concerns and a clear explanation of how side effects will be managed if they do occur can do much to allay these fears. This is a commitment that will require close monitoring of the patient's response to therapy and a rapid response to the management of any adverse side effects should they occur.

Examine the patient and the site of the pain. Examining the site of the pain and possible referral sites may help identify the source of the pain (Foley, 2004). This is always done within knowledge of the patient's disease process, extent of disease, possible referral sites of pain, and goals of care. The source of the pain may be obvious, for example, a distended abdomen associated with a full bladder, bowel obstruction or liver distention, a prior skin eruption with postherpetic neuralgia, a bony deformity or inability to use a limb due to a pathological fracture, or an open fungating infected wound. In the advanced cancer patient and others with advanced illness and co-morbidities, the cause of pain is frequently multifactorial requiring a multimodal approach (Ahles, Blanchard & Ruckdeschel, 1983; Bates, 1987; Foley, 2004; McGuire, 1995). Whenever possible, within the constraints of nearness to death and goals of care, an attempt is made to treat the cause of the pain as well as the pain itself. The extent of the diagnostic workup depends on the goals of care and the likely impact of the results of the diagnostic workup on the patient's treatment plan

and overall quality of life. The benefit-to-burden ratio to the patient is of uppermost concern and needs to be discussed fully with the patient and family or the patient's health care agent (Latimer, 1991). Although most pain can be adequately controlled to the patient's satisfaction, and that is always the goal, the complete absence of pain is not possible for some patients. Realistic goal setting with the patient, and establishing what level of pain would be acceptable and would not interfere with quality of life and function, is part of the assessment. The balance is to achieve maximum pain relief and minimal adverse effects of treatment. Realistic goal setting is likely to diminish later frustration and loss of trust in the clinician's competence.

Components of Pain Management

Pain is a multidimensional experience that involves sensory, affective, cognitive, behavioral, and sociocultural components (Ahles et al., 1983; Bates, 1987; McGuire, 1995). Although pharmacotherapy is the foundation of pain management, pharmacotherapy alone will not be an effective approach to pain management at the end of life. A multimodal approach is usually required including attention to the suffering and spiritual or existential component to the patient's pain (Byock, 1997; Cherny & Coyle, 1994; Saunders, 1967; Twycross & Lichter, 1998; Twycross & Wilcock, 2001). In addition, the needs of the family must be addressed (Ferrell, Grant, Chan, Ahn, & Ferrel, 1995; Herbert, Schulz, Copeland, Arnold, 2008; Rhodes, Mitchell, Miller, Connor, & Teno, 2008). Table 19.3 illustrates factors that contribute to the concept of "total pain" at end of life and its multidimensional nature.

PHARMACOLOGICAL THERAPY

Inadequate knowledge of analgesic pharmacotherapy is one of the most commonly cited reasons for undertreatment of pain. Developing expertise in the use of analgesic drugs is an integral part of nursing care at the end of life.

Over two decades ago, an expert committee convened by the cancer unit of the World Health Organization (WHO) developed a three-step "analgesic ladder" approach to the selection of drugs for the treatment of cancer pain (WHO, 1986). The basic principles of analgesic selection developed by this committee apply to pain management at the end of life. Three categories of analgesic drugs are included in the three-step analgesic ladder: nonsteroidal anti-inflammatory drugs (NSAIDs), opioids, and co-analgesics or adjuvant drugs. With a focus on end-of-life care, discussion around these groups of drugs will include rationale for selection, dose titration, routes of administration, and side-effect management.

19.3 | Factors Contributing to a Patient's "Total Pain" or "Existential Distress" at End-of-Life.

These factors are interrelated. Their interrelatedness is dynamic and non-linear. When one factor changes it influences other factors. The impact of each factor varies from patient-to-patient and within one patient at any given time. This list is not all-inclusive:

TISSUE DAMAGE RESPONSE ASSOCIATED WITH THE DISEASE OR ITS TREATMENT CAUSING PAIN:	■ Nociceptive pain ■ Neuropathic pain ■ Mixed pain syndrome
MULTIPLE OTHER DISEASE-RELATED OR TREATMENT-RELATED DISTRESSING SYMPTOMS:	■ Psychological, spiritual and social distress ■ Anxiety, fear and spiritual distress ■ Uncontrolled pain ■ Perceived loss of dignity ■ Loss of bodily control ■ Uncertainty about the future ■ Uncertainty about God ■ Fear of death ■ Fear of abandonment (by God, family, friends, the medical team) ■ Worry about exhausting and burdening the family, friends, and medical team ■ Worry about how will be remembered ■ Worry about finances and financially depleting the family
DEPRESSION ASSOCIATED WITH:	■ Loss of sense of "self" ■ Loss of social position and role in the family ■ Loss of control ■ Sense of helplessness and demoralization ■ Perceived loss of dignity ■ Loss of meaning and purpose in continued life ■ Loss of hope
ANGER ASSOCIATED WITH:	■ Delays in diagnosis resulting in late diagnosis and diminished hope for a cure ■ Bureaucratic bungling ■ Therapeutic failures ■ Insensitive communication ■ Friends who do not visit

Acetaminophen and Nonsteroidal Anti-Inflammatory Drugs

Acetaminophen although lacking in significant anti-inflammatory effects is a useful analgesic in the management of mild pain or in combination with an opioid for the management of more intense pain syndromes. Acetaminophen has fewer adverse effects than the NSAIDs. Gastrointestinal toxicity is rare, and there are no adverse effects on platelet function or cross-reactivity in patients with aspirin hypersensitivity (APS, 2003). Hepatic toxicity can occur, however, and patients with chronic alcoholism and liver disease can develop severe hepatotoxicity even when the drug is taken in usual therapeutic doses (Schiodt, Rochling, Casey, & Lee, 1997; Tanaka, Yamazaki, & Misawa, 2000). Reduced doses or avoidance of acetaminophen is recommended in the face of renal insufficiency or severe liver compromise.

The *NSAIDs* include many subclasses, are frequently used in all steps of the "analgesic ladder" (McQuay & Moore, 2004), and are analgesic, antipyretic, and anti-inflammatory. Table 19.4 shows guidelines for selection and use of NSAIDs. Aspirin is the prototype of the NSAIDs. Nonsteroidal anti-inflammatory drugs are most effective in treating mild to moderate pain when there is an inflammatory component present and are used in step 1 of the analgesic ladder. When greater relief is needed, they are continued along with the opioid drugs in steps 2 and 3 of the analgesic ladder. The NSAIDs can be extremely effective when combined with an opioid drug in treating bone pain in cancer patients; prostaglandins, which are rich in the periosteum of the bone, are implicated in pain modulation. Unlike the opioid drugs, NSAIDs have a ceiling effect, that is, a dose beyond which added analgesia is not obtained (APS, 2003). These drugs do not produce tolerance or physical dependence, and are not associated with psychological dependence (addiction) (APS, 2003). This class of drugs may also have an opioid sparing effect in some patients.

Mechanism of Action

The NSAIDs mainly affect analgesia by reducing the biosynthesis of prostaglandins, inhibiting the cascade of inflammatory events that lead to nociception (Jenkins & Bruera, 1998; Vane & Botting, 2008).

Adverse Effects and Their Management

Patients, particularly at end of life, are very susceptible to adverse side effects of pharmacotherapy. A careful balance is needed between achieving the desired effect of the selected drug for the patient and the potential for adverse effects. This is particularly important with NSAIDs. Unlike the opioids where the adverse effects are usually dose-dependent and controllable, NSAIDs have a largely "hidden" side-effects profile (Jenkins & Bruera, 1998). Although they occur in a minority of patients, these adverse effects are often "silent," not producing symptoms until a major event occurs such as gastrointestinal bleeding without prior warning. The nurse is an active participant in assessing this risk/benefit ratio for the patient and needs to become familiar with the relative side-effect profile for each of the drugs within this category. The potential adverse effects of the NSAIDs include those affecting the hematologic, gastrointestinal, renal, and central nervous systems (Hoppmann, Peden, & Ober, 1991; Mercadante, 2001; Perez, Rodriquez, Raiford, Duque, & Ris, 1996). The selective COX-2 inhibitors differ in their side-effect profile from other NSAIDs in relation to potential for less gastric irritation (at least with short term use) and interference with platelet aggregation. However, renal adverse effects are similar and concern about cardiovascular risks suggest that they should be used with caution in "at risk" patients (Juni, Rutjes, & Dieppe, 2002; Peterson & Cryer, 2002; Wright, Mather, & Smith, 2001).

Principles of Administration of the NSAIDs

Drug selection. A careful medical and pain history provides the nurse with information about potential benefits and risks for a patient about to receive a NSAID. An analgesic history should illuminate the patient's prior exposure to the NSAIDs, including frequency of administration, analgesic effects, and side effects. Information regarding the timing interval of other analgesics is important so that a prescribed NSAID regimen fits in with the patient's total analgesic plan. For example, if a patient is on an 8- or 12-h dosing regimen of a controlled release morphine preparation, an NSAID with a similar dosing profile would be appropriate. This may aid patient compliance and cut down on the feeling of having to take medication constantly.

Choice of a starting dose and dose titration. An NSAID is combined with an opioid drug in step 2 and 3 of the analgesic ladder. Doses are often started at the lower end of the recommended scale in these medically fragile individuals who are coming to the end of their lives and are increased as needed. Refer to Table 19.5. Although several weeks are needed to evaluate the efficacy of a dose, when NSAIDs are used in the treatment of grossly inflammatory conditions such as arthritis, clinical observation suggests that a shorter time period, usually a week, is adequate for pain relief in a patient with cancer pain. Pain and other symptoms should be monitored before and after starting the NSAIDs to document any improvement or adverse effects. If no benefit is seen or if adverse effects are noted, consideration should be given to discontinuing the drug or switching to an alternate NSAID, as marked variability has been noted in patients' response to different NSAIDs. Indicators of an effective response would be either a significant improvement in pain, or a significant decrease in the opioid use with a subsequent reduction in opioid-related side effects. The degree of monitoring for adverse effects from the NSAIDs should be individualized to the patient. Tables 19.4 and 19.5 provide guidelines to the nurse for the selection and use of NSAIDs in the management of pain.

The Opioid Drugs

A clear understanding of the clinical significance of tolerance, physical dependence, and psychological dependence, as these terms relate to the use of opioid drugs, is essential if nurses are to break down the pervasive barriers that surround the use of opioid analgesics and

19.4 | Key Points in the Selection and Use of NSAIDs and Acetaminophen

- The older adult with chronic heart failure, renal insufficiency, cirrhosis with ascites, significant atherosclerotic disease, or multiple myeloma is at risk for NSAID-induced renal failure.
- Unlike with opioids, the adverse side effects of NSAIDs often do no produce obvious symptoms until a major event such as a gastrointestinal bleed occurs.
- Selective Cox-2 inhibitors differ in their side effect profile from non-selective NSAIDs in relation to potential for gastric irritation and interference with platelet aggregation. However, selective Cox-2 inhibitors have adverse effects (e.g., sodium retention, edema, hypertension) similar to those of the nonselective NSAIDs.
- Avoid NSAIDs if possible in patient with gastroduodenopathy, bleeding diathesis, renal insufficiency, hypertension, severe encephalopathy, and cardiac failure.
- NSAIDs should not be used concomitantly with other drugs that have the potential to cause gastric erosion (e.g., corticosteroids).
- Avoid acetaminophen in patients with severe liver disease.

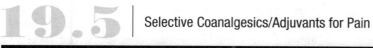

19.5 | Selective Coanalgesics/Adjuvants for Pain

DRUG CLASS	INDICATIONS	DRUG EXAMPLES OF DRUGS STARTING DOSE (RANGE)	ADVERSE EFFECTS
Antidepressants (PO)	Neuropathic pain (burning quality). Added benefit for insomnia or depression	Amitriptyline 10–25 mg/qhs Nortriptyline 10 –25 mg/qhs Desipramine 10–25 mg/qhs Venlafaxine 37.5 mg BID Duloxetine 30 mg BID	Anticholinergic effects Most prominent with amitriptyline Nausea; dizziness
Anticonvulsants (PO)	Neuropathic pain (sharp, shooting, electric shock-like quality)	Clonazepam 0.5–1mg/qhs, BID or TID Gabapentin 100 mg TID Pregabalin 50 mg TID	Sedation Dizziness; LE edema — elderly and frail more at risk
Corticosteroids (PO, IV, SC)	Cord compression, bone pain, neuropathic pain, visceral pain, pain crisis	Dexamethasone 2–20 mg/day Give up to 100mg IV for pain crisis. Prednisone 1530 mg TID or QID	"Steroid psychosis" — delirium Dyspepsia
Local anesthetics (PO) (IV, SC infusion) Transdermal	Neuropathic pain	Mexiletine 150 mg TID Lidocaine 1–5 mg/kg hourly Lidocaine patch 5% 12 h on 12 h off	Lightheadedness, tremor, paresthesias arrhythmias
N-methyl-D-aspartate (NMDA) Receptor antagonists (IV, SC) (PO)	Neuropathic pain	Ketamine 0.1–0.2 mg/kg per h 5 mg PO	Confusion, frightening dreams
Alpha-2 adrenergic agonists (PO, ED, transdermal)	Refractory pain. Can be used in combination with an opioid ED	Clonidine	
Bisphosphonates (IV)	Osteolytic bone pain	Pamidronate 60–90 mg	Pain flair over 2 h q 2–4 weeks
Antispasmodic (PO, IT)	Muscle spasms	Baclofen 10 mg (PO) qd or QID	Muscle weakness, cognitive changes
Botox (SC)	Dystonia Muscle spasms		
Calcitonin (SC, nasal)	Neuropathic pain, bone pain	25 IU/day	Hypersensitivity reaction nausea
Baclofen	Muscle spasm associated pain	10 mg PO daily or 3 times day	Muscle weakness; cognitive changes
Calcium channel blockers	Ischemic pain, neuropathic pain, smooth muscle spasms with pain	Nifedipine 10 mg PO TID	Bradycardia; hypotension

Note: This table should be used as a guide only and not replace a more in-depth review. Individual dosing depends on each patient's particular situation and comprehensive assessment.

q = ever; h = hour; PO = by mouth; IV = intravenous; SC = subcutaneous; ED = epidural; qhs = at bedtime; qd = daily; BID = morning and night; TID = three times a day; IU = international units

References cited in the section of text that discusses use of coanalgesics/adjuvants.

result in inadequate pain relief and much unnecessary suffering to patients and families. Refer to Table 19.6.

Tolerance is the phenomenon characterized by the need for increasing dose to maintain the same drug effect (APS, 2003). Usually the reason for dose escalation at the end of life occurs in the setting of increasing pain associated with progressive disease (Foley, 1993). Patients with stable disease do not usually require increasing opioid doses (Foley, 1993). This observation, integrated with the knowledge that there is no "ceiling" effect to the opioid drugs, implies the following: (1) concern about tolerance to analgesic effects should not impede the use of opioids early in the course of the disease, and (2) worsening pain in a patient on a stable dose of opioids is assumed to be evidence of disease progression until proven otherwise.

Physical dependence is an altered physiologic state that occurs in patients who use opioids on a long-term basis. If the drug is stopped abruptly or an antagonist is given, the patient exhibits signs of withdrawal. Signs of opioid withdrawal include anxiety, alternating hot flashes and cold chills, salivation, rhinorrhea, diaphoresis, piloerection, nausea, vomiting, abdominal cramping, and insomnia (APS, 2003). The time frame of the withdrawal syndrome depends on the half-life of the drug. For example, abstinence from drugs with a short half-life such as morphine and hydromorphone may occur within 6 to 12 h of stopping the drug and be most severe after 24–72 h. After withdrawal of drugs with a long half-life such as methadone, the symptoms may not occur for a day or longer (Hanks, Cherny, & Fallon, 2004). Gradual reduction of the opioid dose in the physically dependent patient who no longer has pain will

prevent the withdrawal syndrome (APS, 2003). Clinical experience suggests that administering 25% of the previous analgesic dose will prevent the withdrawal syndrome in most patients (Hanks et al., 2004). However, patients must be closely monitored during the tapering process to be sure they are not experiencing symptoms of withdrawal. A small proportion of patients require an extremely slow opioid taper because of persistent withdrawal symptoms.

The use of an antagonist such as naloxone in the physically dependent patient will precipitate acute withdrawal symptoms unless carefully titrated (Manfredi, Ribeiro, & Payne, 1996). If a drug overdose is suspected in a patient who has received opioids for more than a few days, a dilute solution of naloxone can be used (0.4 mg in 10 ml of normal saline solution) (APS, 2003). This may be administered in 1 ml bolus injections every 1–3 min until the patient becomes responsive. It is reiterated that the need to use naloxone to reverse opioid-induced respiratory depression at end of life is exceedingly rare (Fins, 1999).

Psychological dependence (addiction) is defined as a pattern of compulsive drug use characterized by a continued craving for an opioid, loss of control, and continued use despite harm. Clinical experience with cancer patients and limited studies suggest that addiction is extremely uncommon in patients without a history of drug abuse who are receiving opioids for pain (Passik & Portenoy, 1998; Porter & Jick, 1980; Schug et al., 1992). In patients who do have a history of drug abuse, the data is scant. Concerns about this outcome, however, continue to be a reason for undertreatment of pain (Cleeland, 1989; Hanks et al., 2004). In the setting of poorly relieved pain, "aberrant" drug-seeking behavior such as clock-watching requires careful nursing assessment. The term "pseudoaddiction" has been used to describe drug-seeking behavior reminiscent of addiction that occurs in the setting of inadequate pain relief and is eliminated by improved analgesia (Weissman, Burchman, Dinndorf, & Dahl, 1990). For the most part, this behavior signifies inadequate pain relief. Patients and their families need to be reassured that use of opioid drugs in the amount that is needed to control pain regardless of what that amount is, is unlikely to cause addiction if an individual does not have a history of drug abuse. In a patient who does have a history of previous drug abuse, there is minimal data in this respect; however, pain can still be well managed using this class of drug. The management of pain in patients with a history of drug abuse will be discussed in the section on special populations.

Opioids and the 3-Step Analgesic Ladder

Opioid analgesics are the mainstay of pain treatment at the end of life. These drugs are used for moderate to severe pain in steps 2 and 3 of the analgesic ladder.

19.6 | Clarification of Terms

- **Addiction** is a primary, chronic, neurobiological disease, with genetic, psychosocial, and environmental factors influencing its development and manifestations. It is characterized by behaviors that include one or more of the following: impaired control over drug use, compulsive use, continued use despite harm, and craving.
- **Physical Dependence** is a state of adaptation that is manifested by a drug-class-specific withdrawal syndrome that can be produced by abrupt cessation, rapid dose reduction, decreasing blood level of the drug, and/or administration of an antagonist.
- **Tolerance** is a state of adaptation in which exposure to a drug induces changes that result in diminution of one or more of the drug's effects over time. **Note** — need for opioid escalation in a patient with cancer is usually associated with progressive disease rather than tolerance per se.
- **Pseudo-addiction** is the mistaken assumption of addiction in a patient seeking pain relief.

Note: References cited in the section of text that discusses use of opioid drugs

They are frequently used in combination with an NSAID (APS, 2003). When formulated in combination with a NSAID drug, dose escalation is limited by reaching the maximum recommended daily dose of the NSAID. When formulated as a single agent, however, there appears to be no ceiling effect (Hanks et al., 2004). Dose escalation may be limited by adverse effects such as sedation, confusion, nausea and vomiting, myoclonus, and (rarely) respiratory depression (Hanks et al., 2004). Dose escalation is governed by the balance between pain relief and intolerable and unmanageable side effects (Hanks et al., 2004). This balance can be determined only by ongoing assessment and documentation of the effects and side effects produced by the opioid.

Mechanism of Action

Opioids produce their effects through binding to receptors in the brain and spinal cord to prevent the release of neurotransmitters involved in pain transmission (Inturrisi, 2003). Opioids also can have a peripheral site of action in the presence of inflammation (Stein, 1995). In addition, opioid receptors are present in immunocompetent cells that migrate to inflamed tissue (APS, 2003; Sibinger & Goldstein, 1988). The opioids can be divided into agonists, agonist-antagonists, and antagonists classes based on their interactions with the receptor types. Pure opioid agonists, for example, morphine, hydromorphone, OxyContin, fentanyl, and methadone bind primarily to the mu receptors.

Partial agonists and mixed agonist-antagonists either block or remain neutral at the mu opioid receptors while activating kappa opioid receptors (Jaffe & Martin, 1990). Partial agonists, for example, butorphanol and pentazocine, have limited use in palliative care. Their pharmacology is characterized by a ceiling effect to analgesia and the ability to precipitate withdrawal symptoms in patients who are physically dependent on pure agonist drugs (e.g., morphine) (Hanks et al., 2004). The incidence of psychomimetic effects (agitation, dysphoria, confusion) from the mixed agonist-antagonist is greater than that of pure agonists (morphine-like drugs) (Hanks et al., 2004). The opioid antagonist drugs include naloxone and naltrexone. These drugs bind to opioid receptors and block the effect of morphine-like agonists. Opioid side effects and their management are described below. This is followed by a brief review of the most commonly used opioids in palliative care and end of life care.

Opioid Side-Effects and Their Management

Constipation. Constipation in the palliative care setting is common and usually multifactorial (Kyle, 2007; Sykes, 2004; Thomas, Cooney, & Slatkin, 2008). It is the most frequently encountered side effect experienced during opioid therapy and the one to which patients rarely develop tolerance. Opioid binding to peripheral receptors in the gut prolongs colon transit time by increasing or decreasing segmental contractions and decreasing propulsive peristalsis (Sykes, 2004). Because the likelihood of constipation is so great in palliative care patients who are receiving opioid therapy, laxative medications should be prescribed in a preemptive manner (Walsh, 1990). Most clinicians recommend a laxative/softner. Bulking agents (e.g, psyllium) should be avoided as they tend to cause a large bulkier stool. In addition, debilitated patients are rarely able to take in sufficient fluid to facilitate the action of bulking agents. A new parenteral compound, methylnaltrexone, has been shown to be effective in relieving opioid-induced constipation when given subcutaneously at doses of 0.15 mg/kg (Becker, Galandi, & Blum, 2007; Holzer, 2008; Shaiova, Rim, Friedman, & Jahdi, 2007).

Sedation. Some level of sedation is experienced by many patients at the initiation of opioid therapy and during significant dose escalation. Patients usually develop tolerance to this effect in days to weeks (Hanks et al., 2004; Ripamonti, 2003). Should sedation persist, at a level that is unacceptable to the patient, a careful assessment by the nurse is needed. Confounding factors such as other sedating drugs, metabolic disturbances, sleep deprivation, and the somnolence that may occur at end of life must be identified. Management steps include elimination of nonessential drugs with central nervous system depressant effects, reduction of the opioid dose if feasible, changing to an alternate opioid drug, and if necessary adding a psychostimulant such as modafinil or methylphenidate (Breitbart, & Alici-Evcimen, 2007; Breitbart & Alici, 2008; Breitbart, Rosenfeld, Kaim, & Funesti-Esch, 2002; Bruera et al., 2003; Webster, Andrews, & Stoddard, 2003).

Confusion and/or delirium. Like sedation, mild cognitive impairment is common after initiation of opioid therapy. Patients may express this as feeling "mentally hazy" or "not as sharp as before." Patients should be reassured that these effects are transient in most individuals and last from a few days to a week or two (Ripamonti, 2003). Persistent confusion attributable to opioids alone is uncommon. More commonly, confusion or delirium in patients at the end of life is multifactorial including electrolyte disorders, neoplastic involvement of the CNS, sepsis, vital organ failure, and hypoxia (Breitbart & Alici, 2008; McNicol et al., 2003; Portenoy, 1994). If confusion or delirium persist opioid rotation may be warrented especially if the current opioid has active metabolites which may be contributing to the delirium. A common example of this would be an elderly patient with renal impairment who is receiving escalating doses of morphine to manage his pain.

Nausea and vomiting. Nausea and vomiting are not uncommon at the start of opioid therapy (Hanks et al.,

2004; Portenoy, 1994). Tolerance to this effect typically develops within days to weeks (Ripamonti, 2003). Both peripheral and central mechanisms are thought to be involved. Opioids stimulate the medullary chemoreceptor trigger zone and increase vestibular sensitivity. Direct effects on the gastrointestinal tract include increased gastric antral tone, diminished motility, and delayed gastric emptying (Hanks et al., 2004; Portenoy, 1994). Constipation may also be a contributing factor. Establishing the pattern of nausea may clarify the etiology of the symptom and guide management approaches. Frequently, a combination of cognitive and pharmacological approaches are used, depending on the pattern of the nausea and assumed underlying mechanism (Mannix, 2004; McNicol et al., 2003). Cognitive techniques might include relaxation training with focused breathing, guided imagery, and distraction. These are referenced and described in detail later in this chapter. For nausea associated with early satiation and bloating, metoclopramide is often the initial pharmacologic approach. If vertigo or movement-induced nausea are the predominant features, the patient may benefit from an antivertiginous drug such as scopolamine (transdermal) or meclazine. Scopolamine may cause confusion in the patient who is elderly or frail and so must be watched. Other options include trials of alternative opioids, treatment with an antihistamine (e.g., hydroxyzine or diphenhydramine), neuroleptic (e.g., haloperidol or chlorpromazine), benzodiazepine (e.g., lorazepam), or a steroid (e.g., dexamethasone) (Mannix, 2004; McNicol et al., 2003). The role of serotonin antagonists (e.g., ondansetron) has not been established in opioid-induced nausea and vomiting.

Multifocal myoclonus. Mild and infrequent multifocal myoclonus can occur with all opioids (Hanks et al., 2004). The effect is usually dose-related and the mechanism is unclear. Pronounced myoclonus is extremely distressing to the patient. The uncontrolled, abrupt, jerking movements of the patient's limbs or torso can increase already existing pain. Myoclonus can be a sign of opioid toxicity and is a reason to switch to an alternate opioid (Smith, 2000; Wright et al., 2001; Lee, Leng, & Tiernan. 2001; Klepstad et al., 2003). In addition, a benzodiazepine, for example, clonazepam, can be used to treat the symptom (Twycross & Lichter, 1998).

Urinary retention. Urinary retention can occur in patients receiving opioid drugs, especially in those who require rapid escalation of the drug, and are receiving other drugs with anticholinergic effects such as tricyclic antidepressants, or have compromised bladder function. Older men with an enlarged prostate are particularly at risk. Opioids increase smooth muscle tone and infrequently cause bladder spasm or an increase in sphincter tone, which may lead to urinary retention (Hanks et al., 2004).

Pruritus. Pruritus can occur with any opioid, is associated with histamine release, and is most commonly seen with morphine use. Fentanyl and oxymorphone may be associated with less histamine release (APS, 2003). Ondansetron has been reported to relieve opioid related pruritus (Larijani, Goldberg, & Rogers, 1996).

Respiratory depression. Respiratory depression is rarely a clinically significant problem in an opioid tolerant patient (APS, 2003; Sykes & Thorns, 2003a, 2003b). However, fear of respiratory depression is a frequently cited concern among medical and nursing staff when initiating opioid therapy or when rapidly increasing opioid drugs to control pain or dyspnea in a debilitated patient at the end of life. Clinically significant respiratory depression is always accompanied by other signs of central nervous system (CNS) depression, such as sedation and mental clouding, and is unusual in the patient receiving chronic opioid therapy unless other contributing factors are present. Pain antagonizes CNS depression, and respiratory effects are unlikely to occur in the presence of severe pain. With repeated administration of an opioid, tolerance develops rapidly to the respiratory depressant effects of the drug (Foley, 1991). Unwarranted fears of respiratory depression should not interfere with appropriate upward titration of opioid drugs to relieve pain (APS, 2003; Brescia, Portenoy, Ryan, Drasnoff, & Gray, 1992; Lipman & Gauthier, 1997). The onset or exacerbation of existing sleep apnea in patients taking opioids for pain has been reported (APS, 2003). Risk factors appear to be the use of methadone, concomitant use of benzodiazepines or other sedative agents, respiratory infections and obesity.

Occasionally staff unfamiliar with the dying process and altered breathing pattern that so frequently occurs at this time become concerned that continued use of opioids will hasten death, especially in the higher doses sometimes required to control pain at the end of life. The input and mentoring by a nurse who is knowledgeable in pain and palliative care will help refocus the more inexperienced staff on appropriate dosing strategies in the symptomatic dying patient.

Commonly Used Opioids in Palliative Care

Morphine is the prototype opioid agonist. The WHO placed morphine on the essential drug list and requested that it be made available throughout the world for cancer pain relief (WHO, 1986). Morphine is available in tablet, elixir, suppository, and parenteral form. Various oral controlled-relief preparations provide analgesia with a duration of from 8–12–24 h. Alternate routes of drug administration are available for patients who are unable to use the oral or rectal route.

Patients with severe pain are initially titrated with immediate-release morphine tablets, or if in a hospital setting with parenteral opioids, and once stabilized are converted to a controlled-release preparation. To manage breakthrough pain or incident pain, immediate-release morphine should be made available to all patients receiving controlled-release preparations. Absorption of morphine after oral administration occurs mostly in the upper small bowel. The average bioavailability for oral morphine is 20%–30% (Gourlay, Plummer, Cherry, & Purser, 2001). This explains why there is a need to increase the patient's opioid dose when changing from the parenteral to the oral route of drug administration. In patients with normal renal function, the average plasma half-life is 2–3 h, whereas the average duration of analgesia is about 4 h (Hanks et al., 2004). Morphine-3-glucoronide (M-3-G), an active metabolite of morphine, may accumulate in patients with impaired renal function. This accumulation may contribute to myoclonus, seizures, and hyperalgesia (increasing pain). in a dying patient with marked renal impairment (Anderson, Jensen, Christup, Hansen, & Sjogren, 2002; Smith, 2000). Because of these and other factors, the nurse must take note of the patient's renal status when administering morphine and monitor accordingly for signs of opioid toxicity. If adverse effects exceed the analgesic benefit of the drug, the patient should be rotated to a different opioid.

Hydromorphone is a synthetic, short half-life opioid that is a useful alternative to patients who tolerate morphine poorly. Hydromorphone is more potent than morphine and can be administered by the oral, rectal, parenteral, and intraspinal routes. The half-life of hydromorphone of ½–3 h is slightly shorter than that of morphine, and it has an oral bioavailability of 30–40% (Houde, 1986). The comparative potency of the opioid drugs and bioavailability dependent on route of administration underscore the need for nurses to be competent in the use of equianalgesic tables. Refer to Table 19.7. The main metabolite of hydromorphone, H-3-glucoronide, may lead to central nervous system (CNS) toxicity, including myoclonus, hyperalgesia, and seizure, especially in the setting of renal failure (Lee, Leng,& Tieernan, 2001; Fainsinger, Schooeller, Boiskin, & Bruera, 1993; Smith, 2000; Wright et al., 2001). Personal clinical experience suggests that these adverse effects usually occur in the setting of high parenteral doses being administered by continuous infusion. Hydromorphone is not presently available in a controlled-release formulation in the United States but is available in Canada and elsewhere.

Oxycodone is a synthetic opioid. The equianalgesic ratio to that of morphine is approximately 20–30:30. It has a half-life of 2–4 h and is mainly excreted by the kidneys. Oxycodone is available in combination with aspirin (Percodan) or acetaminophen (Percocet) or as a single immediate-release or controlled-release tablet. The controlled-release tablet (OxyContin) provides the patient with analgesia for 8–12 h. Both hydromorphone and oxycodone are used in steps 2 and 3 of the analgesic ladder. Oxycodone is not available in parenteral form.

Fentanyl is a lipid soluble, potent opioid that is being used with increasing frequency in palliative care, especially in the transdermal form. Because of its potency, fentanyl dosing is usually in micrograms. Clinical experience with cancer patients suggests that a 100 mcg fentanyl patch is equianalgesic to 2–4 mg of parenteral morphine per h (Hanks et al., 2004). Although most patients maintain satisfactory pain control with a patch change every 72 h, some patients require the patch to be changed after 48 h. Careful monitoring of adequacy of pain relief and evidence of end-of-dose failure will guide the nurse in the needs of the particular patient. It is important that the nurse also realize there is a lag in absorbing fentanyl through the skin. It takes 12–16 h for the patient to see a substantial therapeutic effect (Hanks et al., 2004; Payne, Chandler, & Einhaus 1995). Availability of a different route of drug administration is therefore necessary during the 12–16 h following initial patch placement. An alternate route of drug administration is also required for breakthrough pain medication. Significant concentrations of fentanyl remain in the plasma for about 24 h after removal of the patch because of delayed release from the tissues and subcutaneous depots. Drug side effects (if present) may persist for that length of time. Fever, cachexia, obesity, edema, and ascites may all have significant effect on absorption and clinical effect (Menten, Desmedt, Lossignol, & Mullie, 2002; Radbruch et al., 2001). Strength of patches range from 12.5 mcg to 100 mcg.

Oral transmucosal fentanyl (OTFC) provides a useful mode of delivering a potent, short half-life opioid to a patient who requires a potent drug with a rapid onset of action and short duration of effect for severe breakthrough pain (APS, 2003; Egan et al., 2000; Payne et al., 2001). Oral transmucosal fentanyl citrate is recommended only to be used in patients who are opioid tolerant and who are receiving the equivalent of no less than 60 mg of oral morphine a day or transdermal fentanyl 50 mcg every 3 days. Oral transmucosal fentanyl differs from other breakthrough pain medication in that there is no relationship between the baseline dose of the patient's pain medication, and the microgram dose of OTFC required to relieve breakthrough pain (APS, 2003; Streisand et al., 1998). In all other opioid drugs there is a relation between the two. With OTFC, the smallest available dose is initially chosen (200 mcg) and titrated up depending on the patient's response (available strengths range from 200–1,600 mcg per unit). Pain relief can usually be expected in about 5 min after beginning use (Payne et al., 2001). Patients should use OTFC over a period of 15 min because too rapid use will result in more of the agent being swallowed than absorbed transmucosally.

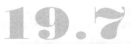

19.7 | Equianalgesic Dose Table: Relative Potencies of Commonly Used Opioid Analgesics*

DRUG	EQUIANALGESIC PARENTERAL DOSE (mg)**	PARENTERAL ORAL POTENCY	COMMENT
Morphine	10	3	Standard of comparison for opioid analgesics. Multiple routes of administration. Controlled-release available. M-3-G accumulation in patients with renal failure. Lower doses for the elderly.
Oxymorphone	1	10	Available in suppository form as Numorphan
Hydromorphone	1.5	5	Useful alternative for morphine. H-3-G accumulation in patients with renal failure. Multiple routes available.
Methadone	SEE TEXT AND TABLE		Long half-life
Levorphanol	2	2	Long half-life.
Fentanyl	—	—	Short half-life when used acutely. Parenteral use via infusion. Clinical experience suggests 4 mg IV morphine sulfate/hr = 100ug transdermal patch. Patches available to deliver 12.5, 25, 50, 75,100 ug/hr. Transmucosal delivery systems available
Oxycodone	Not available	2	Available in liquid or tablet preparation. Also in combination with a non-opioid. Controlled-release not available.
Codeine	130	1.5	Used orally for less severe pain. Usually combined with a nonopioid.
Hydrocodone	Not available		Usually combined with a nonopioid.

Note: This table should be used as a guide only and not replace a more in-depth review. Individual dosing and drug selection depends on each patients particular situation and comprehensive assessment.

** Dose that provides analgesia equivalent to 10 mg IM morphine. These ratios are useful guides when switching drugs or routes of administration (see text). In clinical practice, the potency of the i.m. route is considered to be identical to the IV and subcutaneous routes.

References cited in the section of text that discusses use of opioid drugs

Source: Reprinted from Lee. M. A., Leng, M. E., Tiernan, E. J. (2001). Retrospective study of the use of hydromorphone in palliative care patients with normal and abnormal urea and creatinine. *Palliative Medicine, 15,* 26-34

Buccal fentanyl—when compared with OTFC, fentanyl buccal tablets may provide more rapid onset of pain relief and greater extent of absorption (Darwish, Kirby, Robertson, Tracewell & Jiang, 2007). The adverse effects are similar to those of other opioids. A small group of patients cannot tolerate the sensation of the tablet effervescing in the buccal space. For patients who are unable to place the tablet buccally (between the gum and cheek pouch), sublingual (under the tongue) absorption appears to be comparable (Darwish, Kirby, Jiang, Tracewell & Robertson, 2008).

Methadone is another useful synthetic opioid for the management of pain, including pain at the end of life. It is especially useful for patients who have not done well on other opioids (Shaiova, Sperber, & Hord, 2002; Bruera, & Sweeney, 2002; Bruera et al., 2004). Patients, however, may be reluctant to use methadone for pain because of its association with addiction. Methadone is primarily metabolized by CYP enzymes. Drugs that induce CYP enzymes, for example, dexamethasone, carbamazepine, phenytoin, and barbiturates may accelerate the metabolism of methadone resulting in decreased plasma levels of the drug and decreased pain relief. On the other hand, drugs that inhibit CYP enzymes, for example, ketoconazole, omeprazole, and SSRI antidepressants, may potentially slow down the metabolism of methadone leading to sedation and the possibility of respirator depression (Bruera, & Sweeney, 2002). Awareness by the nurse of any changes in the patient's medication regimen and the potential effect on the patient's pain relief or development of adverse effects is an integral aspect of pain management. Methadone in inexperienced hands is a potentially dangerous drug because of its variable, long half-life (range 13 h—over 100 hours) (Hanks et al., 2004) and a discrepancy between drug half-life and the duration of analgesic effect (4–8 h). Patients are at increased risk for drug accumulation and subsequent toxicity when treatment is initiated, the dose is increased, or multiple organ failure develops. Warning signs of drug accumulation are, for example, a patient who becomes confused and increasingly sedated during the titration phase. Because of this risk, methadone should only be prescribed by experienced clinicians (Hanks et al., 2001).

The equianalgesic dose ratio of morphine to methadone has been a matter of controversy and confusing lack of clarity for clinicians (Mercadante et al., 2001). Available data indicate that the ratio correlates with the total opioid dose administered before switching to methadone. (Moryl et al., 2002; Watanabe, Tarumi, Oneschuk, & Lawlor, 2002). For example, when rotating a patient from morphine to methadone, the higher the current 24-h dose of morphine the patient has been re-ceiving, the larger the conversion ratio needs to provide pain relief. For example, if a patient is receiving from 30–90 mg morphine in 24 h the morphine to methadone ration is 4:1. If the patient has been receiving 91–300 mg of morphine in 24-h hours the morphine to methadone ratio is 9:1, and if the patient has been receiving greater than 300 mg of morphine in 24 h the morphine to methadone ratio is 12:1 or higher (Manfredi & Houde, 2003; Mercadanti et al., 2001). Refer to Table 19.8. Recently questions have been raised regarding the effect of methadone on cardiac conduction. Prolonged QTc intervals have been reported in patients receiving both oral and parenteral methadone (Cruiciani, 2008).

Other opioids. Oxymorphone a semisynthetic opioid is available in parenteral and more recently oral immediate release and controlled release formulations. Its safety and efficacy profile is similar to other opioids. Codeine, hydrocodone, levorphanol, and tramadol are other opioids available in the United States for pain.

Meperidine is rarely indicated for the management of chronic pain either at the end of life or earlier in the disease process. Meperidine has an active metabolite, normeperidine, that is twice as potent as a convulsant and half as potent as an analgesic as its parent compound (Kaiko, 1983). The half-life of normeperidine is 3–4 times that of meperidine, and accumulation of the metabolite with repetitive dosing can result in central nervous system excitability characterized by tremor, myoclonus, agitated delirium, and seizures (Szeto et al., 1977). Naloxone does not reverse meperidine-induced seizures and potentially could precipitate seizures by blocking the depressant effects of meperidine and allowing the convulsant effects of normeperidine to become manifest (Kaiko, 1983; Umans & Inturrisi, 1982).

Principles of Opioid Selection and Administration

Numerous factors, both patient-related and drug-related, must be considered in the selection of an appropriate opioid for a patient (Hanks et al., 2004). The opioid should be compatible with the patient's pain severity, age, dosing and route requirements, underlying illness, and metabolic state. Selection of an opioid that is available as a controlled-release formulation, such as morphine or oxycodone, may be an important consideration for some patients. In addition cost may be a factor for patients being cared for at home. For the older adult or those who have major organ dysfunction, an opioid without known active metabolites and with a short half-life, such as fentanyl, hydromorphone, or oxycodone, may be preferable. Patients with marked renal insufficiency must be monitored closely for signs of opioid toxicity.

The potential for additive side effects and serious toxicities from drug combinations must be recognized

---

19.8 | Guide for Rotation to Methadone from Morphine

- If oral morphine < 100mg/24 h, change to methadone 5mg every 8 h and discontinue previous opioid
- If oral morphine < 100 mg/24 h, use 3-day rotation period
  - ☐ Day 1—Reduce oral morphine dose by 30%–50% and replace with methadone using a 10:1 ratio. Administer methadone every 8 h
  - ☐ Day 2—Reduce oral morphine by another 30–50% of original dose and increase methadone if pain is moderate to severe.
  - ☐ Supplement with short-acting opioids.
  - ☐ Day 3—Discontinue oral methadone and titrate methadone dose daily

Alternate approach when rotating morphine to methadone. Conversion can be accomplished in one step using the following morphine to methadone ratios:
- Morphine 30–90 mg/24 h, use 4:1 ratio
- Morphine 91–300 mg/24 hours, use 8:1 ratio
- Morphine > 300 mg/24 h, use 12:1 ratio

(Higher doses requires higher ratios)

Note: References cited in the section of text that discusses opioid rotation.

by the nurse each time a new drug is added to a patient's regimen (Portenoy, 1994). Patients frequently have many distressing symptoms and are receiving multiple drugs. The impact of each new drug added to the patient's regimen must be carefully weighed for benefit versus burden.

Opioid rotation. Sequential trials of opioid drugs may be needed to find the most favorable balance for the patient between pain relief and adverse effects (Galer, Coyle, & Pasternak, 1992). The patient and family should be warned that this is a possibility so that they do not become discouraged during the process. Usually if one or two side effects are present and pain control is good, an attempt is made to treat the side effects and maintain the current opioid. If more than two side effects are present (excluding constipation), opioid rotation is probably warranted. Refer to Table 19.9.

The steps followed when rotating opioids are based on the following assessment:

1) Is the pain control good but significant side effects present? If so reduce the equianalgesic dose of the new opioid by 50% (to accommodate for cross-tolerance) and continue to monitor the patient for resolution of adverse side effects and adequacy of pain control. Frequent rescue doses should be available to the patient.

2) Is the pain control poor and are significant side effects present? If so reduce the equianalgesic dose by 25–50% and continue to monitor the patient closely for resolution of adverse side effects and improvement in pain control. Frequent rescue doses should be available to the patient.

3) Is the plan to convert the patient to methadone? If so, the around-the-clock equianalgesic dose of methadone should be decreased by 90%, with provision for frequent rescue doses and careful monitoring of the patient for signs of drug accumulation and toxicity, especially sedation. Refer to Table 19.8. Because of the large inter-patient variability, in all instances when an opioid dose is decreased or the drug is changed the patient must be closely monitored for adequacy of pain relief or presence of adverse side effects (Hanks et al., 2004).

This monitoring is a critical nursing function.

Choice of a Starting Dose and Dose Titration

A patient who is relatively opioid-naive should generally begin treatment at an opioid dose equivalent to 5–10 mg of parenteral morphine every 4 h (APS, 2003, National Cooperative Cancer Network [NCCN], 2008). Titration of the opioid dose is usually necessary at the start of pain therapy and at different points during the disease course. At all times inadequate relief should be addressed with dose escalation until relief is reported or until intolerable and unmanageable side effects occur. Integration of around-the-clock (ATC) dosing with supplemental rescue doses provides a rational stepwise approach to dose escalation and is appropriate to all routes of drug administration. Patients who require more than four to six rescue doses per day should generally undergo escalation of the baseline dose. In all cases, escalation of the baseline dose should be accompanied by a proportional increase in the rescue dose so that the size of the supplemental dose remains a constant percentage of the fixed dose. Refer to Table 19.10.

Nursing assessment of the patient's pattern of pain, rescue use, and level of pain relief is essential for appropriate dose titration. Table 19.11 summarizes the basic principles in the use of opioid drugs to manage pain.

Selecting a route. Opioids should be administered by the least invasive and safest route capable of producing adequate analgesia. Clinical experience indicates that the majority of patients can use the oral route of drug administration throughout the course of most of their disease. However, at times some patients become unable to use this route and require an alternate approach (Coyle et al., 1990; Foley, 2004). Nurses need to be skilled in selecting alternate routes to meet the

19.9 | Guidelines When Switching from One Opioid to Another—Opioid Rotation

- If one or two side effects are present and pain control is good, treat the side effects and maintain the present opioid.
- If more than two side effects are present, refer to the equianalgesic dose table (Table 19.7) prior to switching the opioid.
- In a minority of patients, two to three different opioids will need to be tried before a balance is reached between adequate pain relief and manageable side effects.
- A large interpatient variability is present in the way opioids are metabolized.
- If the pain control is good but significant side effects are present, reduce the equianalgesic dose of the new opioid by 25%–50% (accommodates for cross tolerance). Continue to monitor the patient for reduction in adverse side effects and adequacy of pain relief. Provide for rescue doses.
- If pain control is poor and significant side effects are present, rotate opioids without reduction in the equianalgesic dose. Continue to monitor the patient for reduction in adverse side effects and adequacy of pain relief. Provide for rescue doses.
- If converting to methadone refer to Table 19.8.
- In all situations of opioid rotation monitor the patient closely for adequacy of pain relief and gradual clearing of adverse effects.

Note: References cited in the section of text that discusses use of opioid analgesics and opioid rotation.

19.10 | Guidelines for Opioid Titration

Three choices are available when upward titration of an opioid dose is needed. The choice in approach is based on assessment of the patient's pain—both baseline pain and breakthrough pain:

- Increase the basal or around-the-clock (ATC) dose (oral, transdermal, subcutaneous, intravenous).
- Increase the rescue dose.
- Increase both the basal (ATC) dose and the rescue dose.

Most patients will require an increase in both the basal (ATC) dose and rescue dose:

- Calculate the number of rescue doses the patient has used in the past 24 h.
- Increase the basal (ATC) dose by that amount or increase by 25% or 50% for moderate to severe pain.
- Also increase the rescue dose by 10–15% of the new 24h dose

Monitor closely for the effectiveness of the new dose and presence of adverse effects such as sedation and or confusion.

Source: Information based on American Pain Society Guidelines (2003); National Comprehensive Cancer Network, Clinical Guidelines—*Pain, 2008;* and the clinical experience of the authors.

needs of a particular patient. The most commonly used alternate routes include rectal, sublingual, transmucosal, transdermal, subcutaneous, intravenous, epidural, and intrathecal.

A switch in route of opioid administration requires that the nurse have knowledge of relative potencies, to avoid overdosing or underdosing. Refer to Table 19.7. These times of transition from one drug or route to another place patients at risk for pain escalation or the development of adverse effects. Frequent assessment is therefore required during the transition period. The equianalgesic dose table provides a guide to dose selection when these changes are made. The calculated equianalgesic dose is usually reduced 25–50% when switching drugs to account for incomplete cross-tolerance (APS, 2003; Hanks, et al., 2004; NCCN, 2008). As noted previously, a much larger reduction (sometimes as much as 80%–90%) is necessary when switching to methadone.

Dosing interval. Patients with continuous or frequently occurring pain generally benefit from scheduled around-the-clock (ATC) dosing. This provides a more stable plasma level of the drug and helps prevent pain from recurring. A rescue dose is offered on a PRN basis and provides a means to treat pain that breaks through the fixed analgesic schedule. The drug used for

19.11 | Principles of Opioid Use in the Management of Pain

- Select analgesic(s) from Steps 1, 2 and/or 3 of the analgesic ladder appropriate to the patient's inferred pain mechanism(s), analgesic history, and severity of the pain.
- Take into consideration patient's age, metabolic state, presence of major organ failure (renal, hepatic, lung), and presence of coexisting disease.
- Consider pharmacologic issues (e.g., potential accumulation of active metabolites, effects of concurrent drugs, and possible drug interactions).
- Know the drug class (e.g., agonist, agonist/antagonist), duration of analgesic effects, and pharmacokinetic properties.
- Be aware of the various drug formulations available for the opioid selected (e.g., immediate release, controlled release, liquid, transmucosal).
- Be aware of the available routes of administration for the opioid selected (e.g., oral, rectal, transdermal, transmucosal, subcutaneous, intravenous, epidural, intrathecal).
- Select the least invasive route to meet the patient's needs.
- Consider issues that may affect patient ability to follow the prescribed regimen (e.g., convenience, ease for home management, cost).
- Administer the analgesic on a regular basis for persistent pain. Make sure that "rescue" doses are available for breakthrough or incident pain.
- Titrate to achieve a favorable balance between good pain relief and minimal adverse effects.
- Use drug combinations where appropriate to provide added analgesia (e.g., NSAIDs and coanalgesics).
- Avoid drug combinations that increase sedation without enhancing analgesia.
- Anticipate and treat distressing side effects (e.g., constipation).
- If one or two distressing side effects are present, treat the side effects and continue on the current opioid. If more than two side effects are present (excluding constipation), consider opioid rotation.
- Prevent precipitation of an acute withdrawal syndrome through abruptly discontinuing an opioid in the patient who has been on an around-the-clock regimen of an opioid for greater than one-week. Taper the opioids if they are to be discontinued.
- Systematically evaluate effectiveness of analgesic regimen (e.g., amount of pain relief, duration of relief, frequency of breakthrough pain, frequency and pattern of "rescue" dose use, presence of adverse side effects, and satisfaction with mode of therapy).
- Teach the patient and family the principles of analgesic therapy. Address the frequently held misconceptions regarding addiction and tolerance.

breakthrough pain is usually the same as that administered on a regular basis. An alternative short half-life drug is recommended when using methadone or transdermal fentanyl (Hanks et al., 2004). However, some clinicians prefer to use methadone as the rescue drug if a patient is already on methadone. For patients on parenteral opioids, the rescue dose should be calculated as about 25–50% of the hourly dose. For patients on an oral regimen, the rescue dose should be 5%–15% of the 24-h baseline dose (Hanks et al., 2004; Jacox et al., 1994). For example, a patient receiving 60 mg of a controlled-release oral morphine preparation every 12 h should have a rescue or supplemental dose of 10–15 mg of immediate-release morphine available on a 1- to 2-h basis as needed. The number of rescue doses used by the patient in a 24-h period, are a guide to titration of their around-the-clock dosage.

Patient-controlled analgesia. Patient-controlled analgesia (PCA) in the palliative care arena is a method that refers to parenteral drug administration in which the patient controls a pump that delivers analgesics according to parameters set by the nurse practitioner or physician. These parameters include concentration of the drug, basal infusion rate, and bolus dose with permitted intervals between doses for breakthrough pain (Coyle, Cherny, & Portenoy, 1994). Use of a PCA device is fairly common in palliative care patients who require a parenteral route of drug administration or severe pain to be brought rapidly under control. This technique can be managed safely at home by most patients, providing a system of education, monitoring, and support is in place.

Coanalgesics or Adjuvant Analgesics

Coanalgesics or adjuvant analgesics are those drugs that have a primary indication other than pain but are analgesic in certain pain states (Walsh, 1990). They can be used at any step of the analgesic ladder. As with the institution of any analgesic regimen, their use is based on a careful assessment of the pain, inferred pain mechanism(s), and analgesic history. Coanalgesics or adjuvant drugs in the palliative care setting are typically used to enhance the effects of the opioid drugs, or to allow for dose reduction because of adverse opioid side effects (Lussier & Portenoy, 2004). In the palliative care setting, it is useful to classify the adjuvant analgesics into three broad groups: multipurpose adjuvant analgesics, adjuvant analgesics used primarily for neuropathic pain, and adjuvant analgesics used for bone pain. Table 19.5 provides a guide to the commonly used coanalgesic/adjuvant drugs. As a general principle, low initial doses are suggested with dose titration until symptom relief is achieved.

Multipurpose coanalgesics. *Corticosteroids* are used to treat various types of neuropathic pain resulting from tumor infiltration or compression of neural structures such as nerve, plexus, root, or spinal cord. Corticosteroids can be extremely useful in the acute management of a pain crisis when neural structures or bone are involved. Dexamethasone (16–24 mg/day), in combination with an opioid, may be used to treat bone pain, neuropathic pain, back pain associated with cord compression, headaches associated with brain tumors, and pain associated with liver capsule distension (APS, 2003). Pain relief is assumed to be associated with anti-inflammatory and antiedema effects (Mercadante, Fulfara, & Casuccio, 2001; Wooldridge, Anderson, & Perry, 2001). Adverse effects of corticosteroids include hyperglycemia, gastric irritation, dysphoria, delirium, and myopathy. Lower dose corticosteroids (2–4 mg dexamethasone) can improve mood and appetite. These drugs should not be used concurrently with a NSAID and their use should be combined with gastroprotective therapy. Be aware that a patient who is on steroids for reasons other than pain, may experience increased pain or analgesic requirements if these steroids are tapered down.

Antidepressants are nonspecific analgesics that are used predominantly for the continuous dysesthesia component of neuropathic pain. Analgesia can occur in the absence of mood change, and the effective analgesic dose in the palliative care population is usually lower than that required to treat depression (Luisser & Portenoy, 2004). Their analgesic effect appears to be related to inhibition of norepinephrine and serotonin (Max et al., 1992). Common dose-related side effects include sedation, orthostatic hypotension, constipation, dry mouth, and dizziness. Tricyclic antidepressants are relatively contraindicated in patients with coronary disease in whom they can worsen ventricular arrthymias (McDonald & Portenoy, 2006). Amitriptyline has the best documented analgesic effect, but is less well-tolerated in frail seriously ill patients because of the anticholinergic effects (e.g., dry mouth, urinary retention, constipation, and delirium). Other tricyclic antidepressants have less potent anticholinergic effects and therefore may be better tolerated especially in the elderly (e.g., nortriptyline or desipramine) (McDonald & Portenoy, 2006).

Anticonvulsants are used to control the sharp, shooting, stabbing quality of neuropathic pain. Carbamazepine, phenytoin, valproate, and gabapentin and pregabalin have all been used in the management of neuropathic pain. Carbamazepine reduces pain by blocking sodium channels (Farrar & Portenoy, 2001). Gabapentin and pregabalin, a newer anticonvulsant, have been found to be useful in the management of both the dysesthetic and electric shock-like components of neuropathic pain and have a more favorable side-effect profile than other anticonvulsants (Backonja, 2002). Pregabalin like gabapentin is hepatically metabolized. It is distinguished from gabapentin in that it is more efficiently absorbed through the gastrointestinal track and the extent of absorption is proportional to the dose. Titration to the analgesic dose is likely to require just two or three steps rather than the multiple steps typically required with gabapentin (McDonald & Portenoy, 2006).

The *GABA-B agonists* include Baclofen, an agonist at the GABA-B receptor. Baclofen is primarily used for spasticity but is potentially analgesic for lancinating or paroxysmal pains associated with neural injury of any kind (Luissier, & Portenoy, 2003). Baclofen may interfere with mechanisms involved in neuropathic pain. The starting dose is 5 mg two to three times per day, and the dose can be titrated upwards to a range of 30–60 mg per day. The side-effect profile includes dizziness, somnolence, feelings of confusion and hallucinations. Slow upward dose titration is suggested in the palliative care setting. Abrupt discontinuation following prolonged use can result in a withdrawal syndrome including delirium and seizures. Doses should therefore always be tapered before discontinuation.

Alpha 2-adrenergic antagonists include Clonidine, the most commonly used alpha 2-adrenergic antagonist for neuropathic pain refractory to opioids and other coanalgesics or adjuvants. Systemic administration of clonidine via the oral or transdermal route or via intraspinal infusions have been used (Luisser & Portenoy, 2004).

Local anesthetics are generally considered second line drugs in the management of neuropathic pain. They can be given orally, topically, intravenously, subcutaneously, or spinally (Mao & Chen, 2000). A brief intravenous infusion of lidocaine or procaine has been used to relieve severe neuropathic pain that has not responded promptly to an opioid and adjuvant drugs and requires immediate relief (Luisser & Portenoy, 2004). Oral local anesthetics used in neuropathic pain include tocainide, mexiletine, and flecainide. The analgesic effects of local anesthetics is thought to derive from suppression of aberrant electrical activity or hypersensitivity in neural structures involved in the pathogenesis of neuropathic pain (Mao & Chen, 2000). Local anesthetics produce dose-dependent adverse effects that involve the central nervous system and cardiovascular system including dizziness, tremor, unsteadiness, paresthesias, nausea, bradycardia, and other arrhythmias (Luisser & Portenoy, 2004). Their use should be avoided in patients with a history of cardiac arrhythmias or cardiac insufficiency.

Topical local anesthetics, for example, the eutectic mixture of local anesthetics (EMLA) cream, when applied locally, produces a dense cutaneous local anesthesia that can be very soothing to patients with postherpetic neuralgia. Lidocaine patches (5%) to the site of the pain—12 h on and 12 h off—can also provide relief in some patients (Galer, Rowbotham, Perander, & Friedman, 1999). Topical lidocaine in the

form of a 5% lidocaine gel can also be effective in patients with postherpetic neuralgia. The risk of toxicity from systemic absorption of a topical local anesthetic appears small.

Topical capsaicin may be useful to control the constant, burning, local, dysesthetic pain of post herpetic neuralgia, for some patients. An unpleasant burning sensation, however, may follow topical application, making its use intolerable for some patients. This burning sensation may lessen or disappear after days or weeks of continued use. Capsaicin is thought to lessen pain by reducing the concentration of small peptides (including substance P) in primary afferent neurons, which activate nociceptive systems in the dorsal horn of the spinal cord (Luisser & Portenoy, 2004).

N-methyl-D-aspartate (NMDA) receptor antagonists are believed to block the binding of excitatory amino acids in the spinal cord. These antagonists in combination with the opioids are being increasingly used in the management of difficult to control neuropathic pain or when opioid dose reduction is the goal. Neuropathic pain includes a large number of diverse pain syndromes, some of which are thought to be mediated by NMDA receptors in the spinal cord (Chizh & Headley, 2005; Wilson et al., 2005).

Ketamine, a potent analgesic at low dose and a dissociative anesthetic at higher doses, is included in this class of drugs (Bell, Eccleston, & Kalso, 2003; Hocking & Cousins, 2003). Ketamine can produce psychomimetic effects (delirium, nightmares, hallucinations, and dysphoria). Assessment for these symptoms prior to initiating the infusion and on an ongoing basis is necessary. Haloperidol can be used to treat the hallucinations and scopolamine may be needed to reduce the excess salivation sometimes seen with this drug (Bell et al., 2003; Fine, 1999). As with an infusion of local anesthetics, anesthesia members of the pain and palliative care team are usually involved in decisions surrounding a ketamine infusion in palliative care. A ketamine trial can be initiated at low doses of 0.1–0.15 mg/kg for a brief infusion or 0.1–0.15 mg/kg/hr for a continuous infusion (Moryl, Coyle, & Foley, 2008). Case reports suggest that intravenous or oral ketamine can be used in children and adolescents (Finkel, Pestieau, & Quezado, 2007).

Adjuvant Analgesics for Bone Pain

Bone pain can be an extremely troublesome problem for cancer patients, especially those with advanced disease and multiple bone metastasis. As previously described, NSAIDs can be helpful in combination with the opioid drugs (Steps 2 and 3 of the analgesic ladder). Parenteral NSAIDs or corticosteroids can produce dramatic relief in difficult cases as previously reviewed, for example, the patient with bone pain who presents in a pain crisis. A concentrated course of radiation should also be considered for patients with focal bone pain (Janjan, 2001; Jeremic, 2001).

Bisphosphonates inhibit osteoclast-mediated bone resorption and can reduce pain related to metastatic bone disease and multiple myeloma. Pamidronate disodium has been shown to reduce pain, hypercalcemia, and skeletal morbidity associated with breast cancer and multiple myeloma. Dosing is generally repeated every 4 weeks with the analgesic effects occurring after 2 to 4 weeks. Zoledronic acid can relieve pain due to metastatic bone disease and be infused over a shorter period of time (Walker, Medhurst, Kidd, Glatt, Bowes, & Patel et al., 2002; Wong & Wiffen, 2002).

Radiopharmaceuticals such as strontium-89 and samarium-153 have been shown to be effective in reducing metastatic bone pain (Sciuto et al., 2001; Serafani, 2000). Thrombocytopenia and leukopenia are relative contraindications to the use of strontium-89 (Serafini, 2001). Because of the lag in response time to treatment from two to three weeks to beneficial effects, this approach is not appropriate for patients who are very close to death. Patients should be advised that a transient pain flair may occur following treatment and additional analgesia should be available in case of need.

Calcitonin is also an inhibitor of osteoclast-induced bone resorption and may be considered for patients with refractory bone pain or neuropathic pain, although results are inconclusive (Martinez et al., 2003). It can be administered via the subcutaneous or nasal route.

Managing a Pain Crisis

A pain crisis can be defined as pain that is severe, uncontrolled, and distressing to the patient (Moryl et al., 2008). It may be acute in onset or may have progressed gradually in severity. A pain crisis is considered a medical and nursing care emergency for those at the end of life. At the same time the pain is being managed, the probable etiology of the pain is assessed within the framework of the previous pattern of pain, probable cause of present pain crisis, goals of care, and the most effective long-term management approaches (Moryl, Coyle, & Foley).

In patients who do not respond to opioid titration, or who develop intolerable side-effects, the following adjuvants should be considered: (1) A parenteral NSAID, for example, ketorolac, for no longer than 5 days. During this period other longer-term approaches for pain relief should be considered; (2) Parenteral steroids, for example, dexamethasone, with the dose being gradually tapered down to the lowest effective dose for the patient. Anecdotal experience has shown the use of parenteral NSAIDs or steroids to be effective in a pain crisis associated with bone pain

and neuropathic pain; (3) If the pain is predominantly neuropathic, intravenous lidocaine or ketamine can be helpful for some patients (Ferrini, & Paice, 2004). The efficacy of a nerve block or spinal delivery system of drug administration for this particular clinical situation should be considered (Swarm, Karanikolas & Cousins, 2004).

Sedation at the End of Life

A proportion of patients at the end of life will experience refractory symptoms, including pain that is not possible to control in the absence of sedation, despite the use of state-of-the-art techniques. The number of patients involved is not clear. Palliative sedation at end of life is always an option for these individuals (Braun, Hagen, & Clark, 2003; Fainsinger et al., 2000; Wein, 2000). Clear documentation and communication among the team members and with the family is essential when the plan is to provide palliative sedation at end of life to ease intractable symptoms. It should reflect the goals of care, clearly stated in unambiguous terms with resuscitation status established; discussion with the patient or health care proxy with informed consent; symptom being treated and management approach selected; and end point to be achieved and monitoring parameters. Opioid or sedative drug dose escalation without clear indications should not occur. In this way, the integrity of the process is maintained.

Pain Management in Special Populations

The principles discussed concerning the assessment of the patient in pain, and the use of pharmacologic interventions in the comprehensive pain management plan, can be applied to all patients. However, there are issues specific to special populations that play a role in their pain assessment and pain management plan at end of life. The purpose of this section is to highlight briefly end-of-life pain-related issues in four populations as an example of some of the concerns in special populations and is not intended as a comprehensive approach. The following section will look at issues specific to the following four groups: those with a history of substance abuse, those with impaired communication, older adults, and pediatrics. These four groups were chosen because they are frequently encountered. Cultural factors and religious factors play a role in the pain management of certain groups. Sometimes there is a mismatch between the normative values of the patient and the health-care provider. It is the practice setting that frequently determines which populations a nurse cares for. It is the responsibility of the nurse to know the needs and special concerns of the populations that he or she cares for most often.

Special Considerations in Those with a History of Substance Abuse

The prevalence of substance abuse (or chemical dependency) in the United States and the association between drug abuse and life-threatening diseases such as AIDS, hepatitis C, and some types of cancer make it likely that nurses caring for patients at the end of life will work with some individuals who have a history of substance abuse (Passik & Portenoy, 1998). As a group, it is very heterogeneous with very diverse clinical problems. It will include individuals who are living drug-free lives, those in methadone maintenance programs, and those who are currently abusing drugs. It is not uncommon to find individuals with addictive disease who also have a concurrent psychiatric illness such as anxiety, depression, bipolar disorder, or schizophrenia (Compton, 1999). Changes in comorbid physical and psychosocial factors, which drugs an individual has abused, and with what frequency, can further complicate issues that clinicians face.

The challenge is to provide humane, high-quality care to people at the end of life who have a history of drug abuse in a society context that often views addiction from a moral or criminal perspective (Compton, 1999). The field of addiction medicine is a developing science that is based upon recent neuroscience advances that include identification of the brain mechanisms involved with addiction vulnerability and nociception. Despite this developing scientific understanding of the disease of addiction, individuals with a substance addiction are rarely cared for in an approach that draws upon this knowledge and their pain is frequently undertreated (Compton, 1999). This is true even in the area of palliative care. Formal involvements by experts from the fields of pain management and chemical dependency are working to remedy this problem.

The following points are helpful to keep in mind when working with palliative care patients who have a history of substance abuse (Gonzales & Coyle, 1992; Kirsh, Jass, Bennett, Hagen, & Passik, 2007; Kirsh & Passik, 2006; Passik & Kirsh, 2008; Passik, Byers, & Kirsh, 2007; Passik, Kirsh, Donaghy, & Portenoy; 2006; Passik & Kirsh, 2004; Savage, Kirsh & Passik, 2008).

- In order to maintain an objective, nonjudgmental approach, be aware of one's own reaction when asked to administer an opioid to a patient with a history of substance abuse.
- Individuals with a history of substance abuse, past or present, will be tolerant to opioids and will require higher doses of opioid to effectively treat pain than those with no history of drug abuse.
- Staff who may be reluctant to administer opioids in adequate amounts to relieve pain because of concerns of worsening addiction or "re-addicting" contribute to the problem of undermedication.

- Identify whether the individual has a far distant history of drug abuse, is in a methadone maintenance program (MMP), or is actively abusing substances.
- Patients who have a far distant history of drug abuse or who are in MMP may be reluctant to take opioids because of fear of readdiction.
- Patients who are actively abusing substances are the most challenging of the three groups to work with. An interdisciplinary team that emphasizes clear communication is most effective in addressing the multiple medical, psychosocial, and administrative problems present.
- If a patient is currently in MMP, permission must be obtained to contact the program and coordinate therapy. Some MMP providers wish to remain actively involved at the end of life, and others do not.
- Many MMP patients at the end of life frequently keep the methadone dose taken for addiction separate from whatever medication they take for pain control. For others, however, it may be useful to incorporate the equianalgesic daily methadone dose into their analgesic regimen, especially for those who are unable to swallow.
- Although sometimes time-consuming, support of the patient in managing his or her addictions can help support the integrity of the individual patient and in turn help reduce their suffering.
- Methadone may be stigmatized as an analgesic in patients who have a history of substance abuse. Patients and their families and friends may need education about the effectiveness of methadone as an analgesic.
- Providers need to be aware of the need for more frequent dosing of methadone when given for analgesia, usually at least every 6–8 hour. Some patients require a q-4-h schedule for adequate pain control.
- One nurse practitioner or physician should be identified to write all analgesic orders or prescriptions. This needs to be communicated to all caring for the patient.
- Consistent documentation that shows the assessment of the four domains of functioning-pain relief, patient functioning, adverse effects, and drug-related behaviors is important in the care of all patients receiving chronic opioid therapy including those who have a history of substance abuse.
- Individuals with a history of substance abuse frequently have difficulties handling stress and will need extra support at the end of life. Psychiatric symptoms and comorbidities such as anxiety, depression, and bipolar disorders are frequently encountered and are to be treated.
- Nondrug methods can be employed, as appropriate, in any pain management plan for dying patients, but these methods should not be used as substitutes for medications to treat pain, depression, anxiety, or other symptoms.

■ Individuals with a history of substance abuse who want to die at home need a careful assessment of their home environment to ensure adequate pain management and safety at home.

Special Considerations in Those with Impaired Communication

Impaired communication can be caused by a language barrier where the patient's primary language is not that spoken by the nurse or caregivers. The impaired communication can also be from an organic or functional etiology. This can include sensory impairment, cognitive impairment, aphasia, and others. This impairment may or may not be a result of the life-threatening illness the patient is experiencing. Because of the difficulties that these patients have with communication, they may not report their pain in an accurate or timely fashion. This may cause their pain to be undertreated. Other factors that can impede the communication of pain is the religious or cultural background of a patient. Cultural or linguistic differences may impair adequate assessment of pain and also may inhibit the patient's willingness to accept treatment for pain.

The American Pain Society (APS, 2003) recommends that patients who are unable to communicate and who undergo a procedure that would be painful for others are to be treated presumptively for pain. The Acute Pain Management Guidelines Panel (1992) recommends that if pain is suspected, an analgesic trial can be made to diagnose pain as well as to treat it. Terminally ill patients with pain who are unable to speak and who are known to have pain are likely to continue to have pain and should have continuing pain treatment.

In caring for dying individuals with impaired communication, the following are useful:

■ Identify the communication deficit that is impeding the patient's ability to report pain and pain relief and to comply with the pain management plan.
■ Obtain the appropriate pain assessment tools and place at the patient's bedside.
■ If the patient and his or her caretakers do not speak the same language, identify the patient's language and identify available translators. Obtain a pain scale in the patient's language and review it with the patient and translator. It is helpful to write key words or phrases in both the patient's language and the corresponding translations in the caregiver's language.
■ Provide more frequent pain assessments if a patient is unable to ask for pain medication or does not reliably ask for pain medication.
■ If the patient cannot communicate, it is useful to collaborate with the patient's family and caregivers to determine what behavioral activities may indicate

pain for this patient. These may be grimacing, pacing, restlessness, moaning, lying still, or guarding (Herr).
■ Document possible pain behaviors and any tools needed for pain assessment in the patient's record to assist other care-givers in providing continuity of care.
■ If the patient is to die at home, issues related to impaired communication need to be addressed in the home setting. Family members and other caregivers may need extra education and support. In some communities, it may be possible to obtain nurses or home health aides who speak the patient's language if language barrier is an issue.

Special Considerations for Older Adults

The probability is high that the older patient will experience pain at the end of life. Pain prevalence increases significantly with age and is due to both malignant and nonmalignant causes. Aggressive pain management is as necessary for those who are elderly as it is for younger individuals. In elderly patients, pain is frequently undertreated across all practice settings. The dying older patient may be cared for at home, in a nursing home, or in a hospital. In any setting, untreated pain can lead to loss of function and psychological complications in this vulnerable population.

Misconceptions regarding pain in the older adult can interfere with good pain management. Ferrell & Ferrell (1995) reported that common misconceptions may include the following: (a) pain is a normal or expected part of aging; (b) if individuals do not complain of pain, they must not have much pain; and (c) the side effects from opioids make them too dangerous to use with elderly people. Nurses need to reinforce that pain is not an inevitable part of aging. Pain in the older patient is to be evaluated and treated.

In treating pain in the older adult, it is important to be aware of the effects of age on the pharmacokinetic and pharmacodynamic responses to analgesic medications including risk of drug accumulation. The general rule for using medications with the older adult is to "start low and go slow." Those caring for dying older adult patients with pain need to be aware of the following (Bjoro & Herr, 2008; Dahl, 1996; Etzioni, Chodosh, Ferrell, & MacLean, 2007; Ferrell & Ferrell, 1995; Ferrell, Levy, & Paice, 2008; Goldstein & Morrison, 2005; Hadjistavropoulos et al., 2007; Herr et al., 2006; Kirsh, & Smith; 2008; Taylor, Harris, Epps, & Herr, 2005; Morrison, & Morrison, 2006).

■ Pain assessment can be disproportionately confounded by cognitive impairment or dysfunction, memory difficulties, depression, and abuse of alcohol.
■ The presence of polypharmacy, multiple diagnosis, and complex symptoms from comorbid conditions may further complicate the pain experience.

- The patient's ability to self-medicate independently and participate in the pain management plan may be affected by functional factors, such as impaired vision, impaired fine motor skills of hands, memory problems, and cognitive impairments.
- Identify the caregiver. The caregiver may be an older person, or the patient may live alone with the caregiver living elsewhere. Evaluate the ability, availability, and desire of the caregiver and of other family and friends to assist with care, administer pain medications, and participate in the pain management plan.
- Assess the role of the dying older patient within his family and community. Because of pain or disease, they may no longer be able to function in roles they had previously performed, such as care of a spouse or family member. The nurse may wish to facilitate discussion of the redistribution of roles and responsibilities

Special Considerations in Pediatric Patients

Until recently, the dying child with pain was not viewed as a significant problem. Children were not considered to feel pain as intensely as adults and were therefore considered not to need aggressive pain management. Fortunately, the literature on pediatric pain has expanded significantly since the 1970s and pediatric pain is viewed as a specialty in its own right. Nurses have played a significant role in this development (Eland, 1990). The nurse caring for the dying child needs to be well versed in how to manage pain in children, using a multidimensional approach with an awareness of issues specific to the pediatric population.

The following pointers are helpful in working with children with pain at the end of life (Berde & Sethna, 2003; Eland, 1990; Field & Behrman, 2003; Friebert, 2008; Hockenberry, Wilson, Winkelstein, & Klein, 2003; Gregoire & Frager, 2006; Hooke et al., 2007; Houlahan, Branowicki, Mack, Dinning, & McCabe, 2006; Schechter, Berde, & Yaster, 2003; Wolfe et al. 2008).

- The child and family is the unit of care.
- Parents and caregivers must be incorporated into the pain management plan as part of the therapeutic alliance, which also includes the child and the healthcare providers.
- Address family concerns regarding the risk of addiction in the medically ill child.
- Pain assessment is dependent upon the child's age and cognitive development stage.
- A child's self-report of pain is considered the most reliable and valid indicator for estimate of pain location and intensity.
- It is helpful to initiate discussions about pain and to learn the individual child's word for pain.
- Developmentally appropriate tools exist to evaluate the child in pain.

- Behavioral observation is the primary assessment measure for preverbal or nonverbal children. Observed pain behaviors may include vocalizations, facial expressions, body movements, autonomic responses, or changes in daily activities, usual behaviors, appetite, or sleep.
- The goal of pain management in children is to prevent as much pain as possible and to treat procedural pain aggressively.
- It is important to consider the child's age, developmental level, verbal capabilities, past experiences, cultural factors, type of pain, and context when developing a pain management plan.
- The pharmacologic management principles-by the ladder, by the clock, by the appropriate route, and by the child-are similar to those used with adults with the exception that the starting doses are determined by chronological age and body weight (milligrams or micrograms per kilogram). The child is frequently assessed and doses are titrated to effect.
- The oral route is the desired route whenever possible.
- Avoid IM injections and utilize the intravenous or subcutaneous route when parenteral administration is necessary.

Case Study conclusion: The case described earlier illustrates a man with advanced cancer who had a variety of pain syndromes—somatic pain, neuropathic pain, incident pain, and breakthrough pain. It also illustrated the need of many patients for opioid rotation and a switch in route of drug administration. The use of radiation therapy and coanalgesics in pain control are also seen, as well as the management of opioid side effects. The need to know a patient's insurance outpatient drug coverage is also shown, and the problems that it can create for patient.

Nondrug Pain Interventions

Case Study: Mr. R, a 74-year-old married Hispanic man, recently diagnosed with pancreatic cancer, was sent home on an analgesic regimen of around-the-clock sustained release oxycodone with immediate release oxycodone for breakthrough pain. At the time of his discharge his pain was well managed.

Two weeks later, he comes for an ambulatory oncology clinic visit and is found to be in significant pain. Evaluation by the ambulatory nurse revealed that his wife had not been consistently giving him his around-the-clock sustained release oxycodone. Discussion with his wife revealed that although she spoke English, she was unable to read the English patient-education materials that had been given to her when her husband was in the hospital and did not understand the pain management plan of care. She also reported being afraid that her husband "might become addicted" if he took this medicine on a regular basis. At that time the nurse addressed Mrs. R's concerns and reviewed the pain management plan and gave her appropriate educational materials written in Spanish. Mr and Mrs. R were encouraged to try using the pain diary that was included as part of the materials.

Three weeks later, they both return to the oncology clinic. Mr R's pain is better managed. Review of his pain diary by a nurse literate in Spanish revealed that to be comfortable, Mr R was taking PRN oxycodone 6–7 times a day. This was brought to the attention of the oncologist seeing Mr R. and his around-the-clock sustained release oxycodone dose was increased.

NONDRUG AND NONPHARMACOLOGICAL INTERVENTIONS

In addition to the pharmacological approach to pain management at the end of life, there are other approaches that may be useful. These nondrug or nonpharmacological interventions or techniques can complement the treatment of the underlying pain etiology and the mainstay pharmacological approach to pain management. Nondrug interventions cover a broad spectrum of approaches. These types of interventions can modify the pain experience and give individuals an increased sense of control, decrease anxiety, improve mood, and improve sleep.

Some of the nondrug approaches that will be discussed are considered mainstream, traditional Western medicine. Other nonconventional therapies fall under the heading of complementary or alternative. Although complementary and alternative therapies are often grouped together under the heading of complementary and alternative medicine (CAM), they are very different. Complementary therapies are used in addition to conventional therapies and in some settings are labeled "integrative." Alternative therapies are used in place of traditional, mainstream treatment (Berenson, 2005; Cassileth & Gubili, 2009). The National Center for Complementary and Alternative Medicine groups the CAM modalities into five main areas: 1. Alternative medical systems, 2. Mind-body interventions, 3. Biologically based therapies, 4. Manipulative and body-based therapies, and 5. Energy-based therapies. The nondrug interventions that will be discussed in this chapter, either

traditional or complementary/integrative, are considered a part of the overall pain management plan.

There are a variety of factors that promote and inhibit the use of nondrug techniques. On their own, patients often initiate nondrug interventions such as application of heat or use of vibration. The different methods chosen by patients are often based on previous use of a particular intervention or on home remedies and may or may not be an optimal method to relieve a particular type of pain. The National Center for Complementary and Alternative Medicine (NCCAM, 2002) released a study that showed that six of the top nine reasons that people use complimentary medicine are pain related. Although the inclusion of pharmacologic interventions are usually a well-thought-out part of the plan, the use of nondrug interventions often is not. There may be little input from an individual's doctor or nurse in initiating an intervention (Rhiner, Ferrell, Ferrell, & Grant, 1993). Many insurance plans do not currently cover nondrug methods even when prescribed by a licensed provider as part of a well-thought-out pain management plan.

Patients using nondrug methods may report reduced distress, a sense of control, improved mood, or more bearable pain. Some patients strongly believe that nondrug interventions should be used instead of analgesics or to increase the time between doses of analgesics. For most patients, the maximum benefit from nondrug interventions is obtained when they are used in addition to analgesics (Layman-Goldstein & Altilio, 1993).

Compared to the extensive studies that support the use of pharmacologic techniques, the strong scientific evidence supporting the use of many of these techniques is just being established (Deng, Cassileth, & Simon Yeung, 2004; Lorenz et al., 2008). Much of the work that has been done in this area explores the use on nondrug interventions in cancer populations although people dying from non-malignant disease can also have significant pain (Hall & Sykes, 2004). In 1999, the Center of Complementary and Alternative Medicine was established under the auspices of the National Institutes of Health to establish an information clearinghouse and to establish data for evaluating the clinical usefulness of various nontraditional interventions (Decker, 2000). It is hoped that as more money and energy goes into the rigorous evaluation of integrative techniques, it will be easier to appropriately add these interventions into an individual's plan of care. In 2009, the Cochrane Pain, Palliative and Supportive Care groups concluded that despite 10 years of solid achievement, many important questions in palliative care have not yet been answered because the relevant, rigorous studies have not yet been done (Wiffen & Eccleston, 2009). Yet, despite the current situation, patients express benefit from these methods and there are reasons to pursue their use (Berenson, 2005; Deng et al., 2004; Jacox et al., 1994).

The five main categories of nondrug approaches to pain management are (1) psychological interventions; (2) physiatric interventions; (3) neurostimulatory interventions; (4) invasive interventions; and (5) integrative interventions. In the following discussion, various techniques will be placed in the context of these categories. However, there is no common taxonomy and no uniformly accepted classification system for non-pharmacologic interventions (Devine, 2003). Often, an intervention may fall into more than one category or subcategory.

When reviewing the nondrug techniques for use in palliative care, it is useful to consider whether a specific intervention will need high or low levels of patient and caregiver involvement, and whether it is noninvasive or invasive. Some of the interventions, such as acupuncture, are invasive and should only be done by skilled practitioners. Because of this and other factors, it may or may not be possible to facilitate use of some of the nondrug techniques in individuals with advanced disease. The Clinical Practice Guidelines for the Management of Cancer Pain Panel Consensus stated that "with rare exceptions, noninvasive approaches should precede invasive palliative approaches" (Jacox et al., 1994, p. 89).

Psychological Interventions

A palliative care patient needs a biopsychosocial approach to pain management, one that includes the body, mind, and emotions. Incorporation of these elements into a patient's plan of care can lead to more effective pain management. Psychological interventions can help to do this. These interventions can primarily be classified as psychoeducational, cognitive, behavioral, or psychotherapeutic. They can include such things as patient and family education, distraction, self-statements, relaxation techniques, guided imagery and hypnosis, patient pain diaries, and cognitive-behavioral therapy (CBT). Devine's (2003) meta-analysis of the effects on pain of nonpharmacologic interventions, such as educational, psychosocial, and cognitive behavioral interventions in adults with cancer supported the use of the use of these interventions as an adjuvant to analgesic therapy. The Clinical Practice Guidelines for the Management of Cancer Pain Panel (Jacox et al., 1994) and the National Comprehensive Cancer Network (NCCN) Cancer Pain Guidelines for both adults (2009) and pediatrics (2007) encourage the use of psychosocial interventions for pain management early in the course of disease, as part of a multimodal approach. The nurse who is caring for an individual with life-threatening illness may find that this person is well versed in using specific psychological approaches and is open to using these techniques to aid in coping with pain and other symptoms. On the other hand, the person whom

the nurse may be caring for may be too weak, debilitated, and cognitively impaired to be taught or even to use a simple, previously utilized, relaxation technique. Assessment is key to developing a realistic plan. The intervention must match the specific problem with an appreciation for the patient's abilities and motivations.

Psychoeducational

Patient and family education regarding pain management is an intervention that can increase an individual's sense of control. Ideally, at the end of life, patients, their families, and their caregivers will be well informed about pain management. However, the nurse working with these individuals often will find that this is not the case, especially in individuals who initially present with advanced disease. Whatever the circumstances, it is necessary to maintain ongoing assessment and reinforcement of educational information as the clinical situation and patient's needs change. Lack of knowledge regarding pain management is a well-established barrier to good pain control (McCaffery & Pasero, 1999a). A 2009 systematic review and meta-analysis of the effectiveness of patient-based educational interventions in the management of cancer pain showed modest but significant benefits and suggested that his intervention is likely underutilized (Bennett, Bagnall, & Closs, 2009).

In the palliative care setting, especially for end-of-life pain management, the inclusion of family, supportive friends, and caregivers is essential. They too have important educational needs and their role in successful pain management cannot be underestimated. A study by Ferrell, Grant, Chan, Ahn, and Ferrell (1995) showed that a structured pain education program improved quality of life outcomes for both elderly patients and their family caregivers. The case for community-based interventions for cancer pain management utilizing care givers, community nurses, and pharmacists was further supported by Bourbonniere and Kagan (2004).

Knowledge regarding pain management (reviewed in chapter 12) should include pain and its etiology, the principles and methods of pain management, types of analgesics, potential side effects of analgesics and their management, equipment and devices used to deliver analgesics, the concepts of physical dependence, tolerance, and addiction, nonpharmacologic interventions, and expected participation in pain management (Adelhardt et al., 1995). Recent work suggests that to implement a pain management regimen successfully at home, patients, and families will also need other knowledge to assist them in problem solving to improve pain control. Challenges include obtaining and processing further information, obtaining prescribed analgesics, applying prescribed regimens to their very individual situation, managing new or changed pain, and managing side effects and other concurrently occurring symptoms

(Schumaker et al., 2002b). Knowledge of how to approach these challenges will enable individuals and their families to be active, informed participants in the plan of care. Knowledge deficits related to pain management encompass all dimensions of learning: cognitive, psychomotor, and affective. It is especially important to allay fears and concerns about opioid use, specifically addiction, tolerance, and physical dependence (refer to chapter 12 for a review of these concepts). Individuals who need equipment to relieve their pain will need special opportunities for their families and them to practice with that equipment management (Adelhardt et al., 1995).

There are several well-developed references that elaborate on teaching pain management information to patients, families, and care-givers which can be useful to nurses (Ferrell et al., 1995; Grant & Rivera, 1995; McCaffery & Pasero, 1999a). Readers are encouraged to review these references for more detailed information. An evaluation of all learners prior to any educational efforts will help to determine priorities and focus efforts. It is best to wait until pain is adequately controlled before giving patients and their families too much information. Teaching sessions may need to be brief with the most important information presented first and continually repeated. A wide variety of written, audio, CD, and DVD learning tools on pain management are available to reinforce information. All educational efforts are to be documented. This will improve continuity of care and provide a mechanism for identifying continuing education needs (Grant & Rivera, 1995).

Ideal outcomes of a successful pain management educational intervention will include the patient, family, or caregivers being able to notify the physician, nurse practitioner, physician's assistant, or registered nurse of any new or unrelieved pain; change in pain location, quality, or intensity, and any side effects experienced; identify the cause of pain; state the rationale of the prescribed analgesic regimen; identify the medications, doses, route, frequency, and potential side effects of an analgesic regimen; if indicated, use equipment related to pain management properly (such as PCA pump); comply with the analgesic regimen, using non-pharmacologic methods appropriately; and express understanding of the differences between tolerance, physical dependence, and addiction.

A small study by Oliver, Kravitz, Kaplan, and Meyers (2001) compared standard educational instruction on controlling cancer pain to an individualized education and coaching session in the outpatient setting, and showed an improvement in average pain outcomes for those in the individualized educational and coaching group.

In 2003, Devine performed a meta-analysis on the effect of nondrug interventions such as educational, psychosocial, and cognitive-behavioral interventions on adults with cancer-related pain by reviewing 25 interventional studies published from 1978 through 2001. Six of these studies tested the effect of education. A homogeneous small-to-moderate statistically significant beneficial effect on pain was found. In her discussion Devine pointed out that with the widely accepted strong mandate to educate patients about their pain and its management, there may not be much of a difference between experimental and control content (Devine, 2003).

A recent study of 64 patients with cancer-related pain and their primary caregivers was conducted to determine whether patients who were given access to continued information—either through a pain hot line or weekly provider-initiated follow-up calls for 1 month following the education program—had improved pain control during a 6-month follow-up period (Wells, Hepworth, Murphy, Wujcik, & Johnson, 2003). The basic pain management program that all study participants received included both structured and tailored components. Following this baseline education, all patient and caregiver study participants showed an improvement in knowledge and beliefs. The long-term outcomes of pain intensity, interference due to pain, analgesic adequacy, and relief from pain were not affected by continued access to pain information. It is important to note that the analgesic regimen of patients who had access to pain information was not adjusted by the nurse making the follow-up calls or by the hot-line respondent.

Education about pain and its management is an important component of any pain management plan. However, additional education without a systematic approach that addresses other barriers, such as inadequate analgesic titration or untreated side effects, may not enhance pain control (Wells et al., 2003). A recently developed program, the PRO-SELF pain control program "uses education along with repeated reinforcement, skill building, and ongoing nursing support to improve self-care pain management in patients with cancer and their family caregivers" (West et al., 2003). It has been successful in improving the management of cancer pain (Miaskowski et al., 2004).

A combination approach may be the wave of the future. The literature reveals four general categories that are useful in assisting patients with pain. These include (1) self-care management; (2) information, decision making, and problem solving; (3) communication with healthcare professionals; and (4) counseling and support (Given et al., 2004) Future work will evaluate whether this approach that combines education with ongoing nurse coaching and interactive nursing support may prove to be useful to patients and caregivers in other noncancer pain populations and how to best enhance outcomes for patients and their families.

Cognitive

Cognitive interventions are often discussed under the topic of mind-body therapies, which are techniques whose goal is to enhance a person's mental ability to reduce symptoms and enhance function (Deng et al., 2004; Given et al., 2004). This discussion will cover the areas of distraction, self-statements, relaxation, guided imagery, and hypnosis, which can be useful to individuals with pain at the end of their lives.

Distraction is an intervention that focuses on the cognitive component of the pain experience, and is sometimes referred to as cognitive refocusing or attention diversion. This technique's goal is to divert attention "away from the sensation of pain to a neutral of pleasant stimulus" (Thomas & Weiss, 2000, p. 161). It is thought that because a person has a limited capacity for processing information, the individual who focuses on something other than the pain pays less attention to the pain and is distracted from the pain. This distraction can be passive or active (Fernandez, 1986). Passive distraction can include such things as listening to music, watching a ball game, or watching a movie. Listening to or watching tapes that are humorous to an individual should be considered. Rhiner et al. (1993) promote the use by patients of a library of various musical and humorous choices when utilizing distraction as a nondrug treatment. Active distraction can include such things as mental problem-solving, singing, playing an instrument, or playing a video game.

Often, for distraction to be effective, its focus must be of interest to the individual. The distraction strategy for a particular individual will depend upon the individual's ability to concentrate and his or her energy level. At the end of life, one's energy level is not predictable. For example, an individual could start listening to recorded music but decide to make it a more active diversion by tapping out the rhythm and singing along. McCaffery and Pasero (1999b) review in-depth ways to assist patients effectively in using distraction. They suggest that effective distraction strategies should stimulate the four major sensory modalities of sound, sight, touch, and movement.

The use of distraction for short periods of time for such things as painful procedures, especially with children, is well established. Its use is thought to increase self-control and pain tolerance, and decrease pain intensity (Jacox et al., 1994; McCaffery & Pasero, 1999b; Rhiner, Ferrell, Ferrell, & Grant, 1993; Spross & Wolff Burke, 1995). It has been associated with positive mood and changes and decreases in pain intensity (McCaffery & Pasero, 1999). The use of distraction for chronic pain is more controversial. McCaffery and Pasero (1999), in their review of the literature, found that after using distraction, patients with chronic pain may experience more intense pain. It is uncertain why this occurs. It may be that distraction prevents the individual from recognizing that certain activities are causing more pain. Following the use of distraction, an individual may be fatigued, irritable, and more aware of the pain. Also, without education, family and caregivers may feel that the individual who is utilizing distraction does not have the pain or the degree of pain that he or she says. This can lead to a variety of negative situations, including a reluctance to administer analgesics.

Self-statements can be helpful in getting one through a painful experience. The use of self-statements is based on Bandura's theory of self-efficacy. This theory focuses on a person's beliefs regarding his or her ability to perform behaviors that will produce certain outcomes. It is hypothesized that a person's expectation of self-efficacy will determine "whether a person will initiate coping behavior, the amount of effort a person will put into it, and how long the person will persist in the face of obstacles" (Dunajcik, 1999, p. 501). Application of this theory involves teaching the patient methods the patient can use to lessen the severity of pain or improve the ability to cope with the pain. Practicing and reinforcement of these methods is important. A healthcare professional works in "coaching" the patient in the use of self- statements (Given et al., 2004).

All people carry on internal dialogues that both manifest and influence their belief systems. By becoming aware of the ongoing self-statements, one can gain insight into perceptions and appraisals. Once an appraisal is accessed, a determination is made concerning the helpfulness of the belief system. Clinicians can help patients to use cognitive coping statements to enhance adaptations and to counteract the maladaptive thought processes (Loscalzo, 1996).

Coping self-statements are devised to assist the patient in getting through a painful situation (Fernandez, 1986). For example, at the start of a pain flare, instead of focusing on the fear of the pain, a person is taught to say to himself or herself, "I've had this kind of pain before, I can keep it under control. I will do this and this. . . ." Another version of this technique is reframing or cognitive reappraisal. To use this, individuals are taught to be alert to negative thoughts they might be having and to replace them with more positive thoughts and images. Use of reframing can increase a person's sense of control. For example, instead of thinking, "I've had this kind of pain before and it was awful," an individual could say to himself or herself, "I've had this kind of pain before and it has gone away" (Jacox et al., 1994, p. 82).

Through the use of *relaxation techniques,* a person can be taught behaviors to independently release skeletal muscle tension and reduce the emotional stress that can make pain worse. The effects of relaxation and guided imagery can vary from patient to patient. (Kwekkeboon, Hau, Wanta, & Bumpus, 2008) These techniques are helpful for people whose pain experience causes them to feel out of control, those who will be experiencing procedures or activities that may be stressful or uncomfortable, and those who have successfully used relaxation techniques in the past, including meditation, yoga, and Lamaze.

There are a few relative contraindications to the use of relaxation techniques. These include individuals with a history of posttraumatic stress disorder, or thought disorders such as dementia, delirium, or schizophrenia; heavily sedated individuals or those experiencing respiratory compromise; and individuals who are experiencing a pain emergency (Layman-Goldstein & Altilio, 1993; Schaffer & Yucha, 2004). Only experts who are very experienced and well-trained in the use of these techniques should work with individuals with respiratory compromise. The unavailability of these experts or the presence of contraindicated conditions may be a barrier to the use of relaxation techniques at the end of life for some patients. Also, bear in mind that individuals who never have incorporated relaxation into their lives may find trying to do so during a period of increased stress to be countertherapeutic (Rhiner et al., 1993). During a pain crisis, relaxation will not be effective and the patient will associate the technique with severe pain instead of the desired outcome, pain relief. It is important not to set up a situation where the patient makes the paired association of severe pain and relaxation techniques. To optimize the patient's learning and effective use of this technique, it is better to wait until the pain is under better control. If you are able to stay with a patient during a pain crisis, you could consider having the patient breathe with you (Layman-Goldstein & Altilio, 1993). Also of concern is the use of relaxation techniques in individuals with bradycardia or heart block because of the physiological effects of relaxation. These effects can include decreased pulse, blood pressure, respiratory rate, oxygen consumption, carbon dioxide production, and basal metabolism (Spross & Wolff Burke, 1995). These effects may interact synergistically to cause adverse physiological effects. Spross and Wolff Burke (1995) suggest that in the acute care setting clinicians do a pre and postrelaxation exercise check on pulse and blood pressure when assisting patients with relaxation techniques.

The National Institutes of Health (NIH) Technology Panel evaluated the effects of relaxation on pain and sleep and provided strong evidence for the use of relaxation techniques to reduce pain. In its review, the panel divided relaxation techniques into brief and deep methods. In general, the brief methods take less time to acquire or practice. Very often brief methods are abbreviated forms of a corresponding deep method. The brief methods include deep breathing, focused breathing, paced respiration, and self-control. Deep methods include such techniques as progressive muscle relaxation (PMR), autogenic training, and meditation. To use autogenic training, one is taught to imagine a peaceful environment and focus on a "heaviness in the limbs, warmth in the limbs, cardiac regulation, centering on breathing, warmth in the upper abdomen, and coolness in the forehead" (NIH Technology Assessment Panel, 1996, p. 314). The use of PMR involves the tensing and then relaxing in sequence of each of the 15 major muscle groups.

Health professionals may benefit from practicing relaxation techniques on themselves before attempting to assist patients in its use. It is useful to have beginning practitioners practice with each other to gain experience and to provide each other with feedback. In learning the technique, consider taping oneself. An exercise that a beginning practitioner can use with patients teaches focused breathing and can be taped so that the patient can use it whenever he or she wants (Layman-Goldstein & Altilio, 1993). In this way, patients and their families also may be conditioned to associate the clinician's voice with support, comfort, and emotional connection in future interactions (Loscalzo, 1996). The reader is referred to several references that teach in detail the use of relaxation techniques (Benson, 1975; Copley Cobb, 1984; Loscalzo, 1996; Mast, Meyers, & Urbanski, 1987a, 1987b, 1987c; McCaffery & Pasero, 1999; Schaffer & Yucha, 2004, and chapter 2 of this text).

It is important to set the right tone before instructing individuals in relaxation techniques. Ideally, the environment should be as quiet and as calm as possible. This is often challenging, if not impossible, in hospital environments. How one enters the room, what one says, and how one communicates one's sense of competence is important. One may be able to influence a patient's sense of control and ability to cope. It is important when working with patients' families to calm them, increase their confidence, and engage them as collaborators.

Most relaxation techniques necessitate active patient involvement. However, McCaffery and Pasero (1999) describe specific techniques that utilize the patient as a passive recipient. These include superficial massage for relaxation, listening to music pleasing to the patient, and animal companion visits. These latter techniques may be effective when individuals are fatigued or are lacking the mental or physical ability to actively participate in relaxation techniques.

Guided imagery and *hypnosis* are related cognitive techniques used to manage pain. Guided imagery can be used to distract one's attention away from one's pain or to change or transform the pain sensations (Kwekkeboom, Hau, Wanta, & Bumpus, 2008). Patients can also use imagery to regain control of negative thoughts, to cope with limitations (such as immobility), and anticipate the future (Spross & Wolff Burk, 1995).

Although imagery can be a very useful technique, it may not be helpful for all individuals. Individuals who are not candidates for imagery include those with a history of mental illness such as psychosis or those with dementia or delirium (a common problem at the end of life). Unstructured, free-flowing imagery can bring to the surface "intense, latent feelings, and unconscious conflicts" (Stephens, 1993, p. 240). It is imperative to monitor an individual for distress, restlessness, or agitation during the use of imagery. Individuals need to be taught that they are in complete control of the situation at all times. If, for any reason, the imagery is unpleasant or distressing, they can simply open their eyes to stop the situation (Stephens, 1993).

A debriefing after the use of imagery can be helpful to identify what did or did not work and to determine how to proceed. Those who have positive experiences may wish to modify the original script to make it more effective. Some will want the therapist to create an audiotape for future use (Spross & Wolff Burke, 1995). Some clients who experience distress may be open to exploring the source of their feelings, some may not.

It is thought that the techniques of relaxation, imagery, and hypnosis do not differ empirically. For this reason, Syrjala, Donaldson, Davis, Kippes, and Carr (1995) relabeled hypnosis as "relaxation and imagery" in order to facilitate patient acceptance of their study entitled "Relaxation and imagery and cognitive-behavioral training reduce pain during cancer treatment: A controlled clinical trial." In this study, it was found that "relaxation and imagery," or hypnosis, reduced cancer treatment-related pain.

Hypnosis involves "achieving an intense state of relaxation, or trance" that enables one to receive suggestions to alter the individual's thoughts, feelings, sensations or behavior (Thomas & Weiss, 2000, p. 161). This state of being can be used "to manipulate the perception of pain" (Jacox et al., 1994, p. 186). Evidence supporting the use of hypnosis in adults and children is strongest for use in procedural pain (Montgomery, Bovbjerg, Schnur, et al, 2007; Richardson, Smith, McCall, & Pilkington, 2006). A Cochrane Database Systematic Review that looked at the use of psychological therapies for the management of chronic and recurrent pain in children and adolescents supported the use of psychological therapies in chronic headache but could find no evidence in nonheadache chronic/recurrent painful conditions (Eccleston, Yorke, Morley, Williams, & Mastroyannopoulou, 2003).

Historically, hypnosis is well established in the treatment of pain. It both induces deep relaxation and redirects the patient's attention away from his or her pain (Cleeland, 1987). Healthy, intact individuals vary in their ability to utilize hypnosis. Debilitated individuals who are at the end of life may have less than their usual ability to utilize hypnosis, making it suitable for even fewer. Hypnosis should only be done by specially trained professionals and will not be reviewed here in greater depth. It is important that entry into practice and advanced practice students are aware of the value of hypnosis and consider making a referral to a trained professional if hypnosis is something that a patient wishes to explore.

Behavioral

A *pain diary* is a tool that is especially useful for the ambulatory population of patients. Clinicians can review this diary with patients over the phone, at home, or on clinic visits.

Its use facilitates pain assessment, evaluation of pain management interventions, and need for further education (Grant & Rivera, 1995). It can be as simple or as sophisticated as the patient using it. The amount of information included often is a reflection of the patient's energy level. Essential information includes date and time of events, medication, dose of medication, and pain intensity before and after interventions. It is helpful if patients include their activities, periods of rest and sleep, pain quality, mood, and other symptoms, but this is up to the individual patient. Some prefer to use preprinted forms provided by pharmaceutical companies or other sources, whereas others prefer to use their computer or a Palm Pilot, or a simple spiral notebook. A pain diary can give a patient a sense of control and puts words to feelings that they can share with the family and others. These diaries have been shown to be helpful in heightening awareness of pain, facilitating communication, guiding pain management actions, and improving sense of control (Schumacher et al., 2002a). A recent randomized crossover study found that patients used an electronic diary more frequently than a paper pain diary. Patients in this study felt using the electronic pain diary led them to a more regular intake of their medicine. The reason for this may be related to the messages they received from the study manager that were generated by each log in, or from the built-in acoustic memory function (Gaertner, Elsner, Pollmann-Dahmen, Radbruch, & Sabatowski, 2004). The impact of technology on the use of patient pain diaries is evolving and merits further study.

Patients with advanced disease at some point may be unable to maintain a pain diary. Often their caregivers can be encouraged to record some of the basic information. Use of a pain diary can help patients or family members identify pain management barriers and successes. Use of this tool can assist some in gaining a sense of control in an overwhelming situation (Grant & Rivera, 1995) and promote communication (Schumacher et al., 2002b). Successful use of this tool requires patient and family education and reinforcement of its use and use of collaborative reviews.

Psychotherapeutic

Fishman (1992) writes of the experience of self-disintegration faced by individuals with advanced disease who are often dealing with the frustration of personal and interpersonal needs and aspirations while dealing with multiple symptoms and aggressive cancer treatments. The experience of total pain can add to an individual's sense of fear, anger, anxiety, hopelessness, and helplessness.

Cognitive behavior therapy (CBT) was originally developed by psychologists to treat anxiety, stress, and depression, using some of the psychoeducational, cognitive, and behavioral techniques previously described. Cognitive behavioral therapy has been used to treat individuals in a variety of situations with the goal of therapy based upon the situation. For the individual with cancer-related pain, the goal of CBT is to enhance the sense of self-efficacy or personal control (Fishman & Loscalzo, 1987).

CBT can be done in a variety of formats, including individual or group sessions (Thomas & Weiss, 2000). It works best in a series of structured sessions that are flexible and modifiable, according to the developing needs of the individual, no matter what the format. Fishman and Loscalzo (1987) suggest that there be clear and explicit goals for both the series of sessions and for each individual session. These goals are to be developed collaboratively by therapist and patient. Together, they will look at the range of problems present and prioritize them. This list will be reviewed on a regular basis and reprioritized as personal, social, and medical changes develop. Based on this list, appropriate interventions to address these problems will be determined. The purpose of the interventions is to resolve specifically defined current problems, not long-term personality and social-relations disturbances. Also, the interventions are to be made in a standard and systematic manner. The use of this flexible, adaptive collaboration is designed to enhance the patient's sense of self-control and sense of coherent purpose (Fishman & Loscalzo, 1987; Thomas & Weiss, 2000). Certain individuals and their families are more receptive to CBT than to traditional psychological approaches, which they may view as too intrusive (Loscalzo, 1996). CBT, a psychotherapeutic approach, provides a structure that some clinicians find useful, in which to collaborate with patients and their families to apply the nondrug psychological interventions to a pain management plan.

Ideally, work with CBT occurs early in the treatment phase of an illness. As disease progresses, an individual may experience cognitive impairment from a variety of causes that make it impossible to employ psychology. It may be necessary to focus more on the family and caregivers as the disease progresses. In this situation, the goal still would be to maximize their coping skills and increase their sense of control.

Cognitive behavioral therapy, a pragmatic psychological approach, and its techniques can be taught to interested clinicians who do not have specialized training in psychology or psychopathology. Nurses and social workers often obtain training in the use of some of these techniques. In an article aimed at the non-mental-health clinician, Fishman and Loscalzo (1987) review the principles and application of CBT. Realistically, the beginning staff nurse may be able to learn and apply the specific techniques of relaxation and distraction. More training would be needed for the use of CBT and the techniques of guided imagery and hypnosis and

structured support. Often the nurses who have expertise in using these techniques are advanced practice nurses, especially psychiatric clinical nurse specialists. The practice setting dictates what is possible. A busy, noisy inpatient unit may limit use of some techniques. Often the knowledge that a patient may benefit from CBT and a timely referral to a skilled practitioner are the most that can be achieved.

Techniques that tailor cognitive behavioral approaches to individual patients (Dalton & Coyne, 2003; Dalton, Keefe, Carlson, & Youngblood, 2004) and those that combine education with ongoing nurse coaching and interactive nursing support build upon the foundation of CBT. Research that evaluates the effectiveness of these approaches may lead to better assistance to individuals who choose to control their response to pain and suffering.

Physiatric Interventions

Physiatric interventions are another kind of nondrug intervention that can be helpful in the pain management plan. These interventions include positioning and movement, application of modalities such as heat, cold, vibration, and massage, and the use of supportive orthotic devices. Physical rehabilitation professionals are the experts in the use of physiatric interventions. The fact that pain is disabling is well established. Palliation and rehabilitation are not incompatible (Cheville, 1999). No matter what the goals of care are, the input from a physical rehabilitation expert may be useful to help the individual achieve his or her fullest physical, psychological, social, vocational, avocational, and educational potential (Dietz, 1982). The rehabilitation expert looks at an individual with cancer-related disability from four rehabilitation perspectives: (1) preventive, to minimize the effects of predictive disabilities; (2) adaptive, to assist the individual to adapt to definite changes; (3) maintenance, that is, maintaining the individual at the current level of functioning; and (4) palliative rehabilitation, keeping the individual functioning and involved in the environment. For nurses to set realistic, achievable goals with the patient with pain at the end of life, it is useful to consider these four possibilities as goals of care change and evolve.

Positioning and Movement

A debilitated individual with pain may be in static positions for extraordinary lengths of time. This in itself can exacerbate existing pain or produce new pain, including pressure sores and painful joint conditions. Healthy individuals are unconsciously and continuously initiating pain-relieving movements. A nurse can assist patients and their caregivers to promote positions or postures that maintain or facilitate normal physiologic function of the musculoskeletal system. When properly done, positioning places minimal stress on the joint capsule, tendons, and muscle structure (Spross & Wolff Burke, 1995). Basic nursing texts give thorough overviews of the basic principles of positioning and movement that are so essential to good nursing care at the end of life.

Patients who experience pain with movement may need to be premedicated prior to positioning. Care must be taken with patients who have bone disease and a high risk of pathologic fractures. An individual's pain or anxiety should not be increased with positioning. Although repositioning can be a helpful intervention to decrease pain, it may be appropriate to do it less often as death nears if the patient experiences significant discomfort from this activity.

For the palliative care patient who is not so close to death, range of motion (ROM), either active (AROM), active assisted (AAROM), or passive (PROM), can promote comfort and maintain or restore the integrity of muscles, ligaments, joints, bones, and nerves used in movement. It is hoped this will in turn prevent the development of additional complications. An individual who lacks the energy for AROM may attempt AAROM or PROM (for the patient who is neurologically impaired or unconscious). McCaffery and Wolff (1992) have written a useful review of the use of cutaneous modalities, positioning, and movement to facilitate pain relief in the hospice population.

Supportive Orthotic Devices

In attempting to decrease pain and increase functioning at the end of life, it may be helpful to consult with a physical therapist or rehabilitation-medicine physician to evaluate the possible use of a supportive orthotic device such as a splint, sling, brace, or corset. Their use can immobilize or provide support to painful tissues and maximize the use of weakened tissues to promote functioning. Appropriate use of such a device may decrease incident or mechanical-type pain for certain patients (Dunajcik, 1999; Tunkel & Lachmann, 1998). Also, the use of certain devices for patients with bone metastasis may immobilize areas of potential fractures to prevent this painful complication (Jacox et al., 1994).

Assistive devices such as canes, walkers, and wheelchairs when appropriately used can promote mobility, decrease pain, and prevent injury (Tunkel & Lachmann, 1998). Consulting with a rehabilitative specialist to obtain the correct assistive device for an individual patient and teaching the patient and the care-givers the proper use of such devices can be invaluable. Often, an evaluation of the home situation will be necessary to recommend the most appropriate device to maximize an individual's rehabilitation efforts.

Other modalities, such as the application of heat, cold, vibration, and massage, also fall under the heading of physiatric methods. Some would argue

that these techniques actually are neurostimulatory because of their activation of the large diameter nerve fibers. The gate control theory proposed that activation of the large diameter fibers inhibited the smaller "pain" fibers and closed the gate to the transmission of stimuli by smaller nerve fibers. These techniques frequently are referred to as cutaneous stimulation. As more information about the underlying mechanisms of pain has become known, the gate control theory gradually has been replaced. However, the actual mechanisms that affect pain relief from cutaneous stimulation are unclear. Most of the cutaneous interventions are thought to counteract the effects of decreased oxygen and accumulated metabolites associated with musculoskeletal pain and to promote superficial increases in circulation (Spross & Wolff Burke, 1995). These methods are thought possibly to reduce pain, inflammation, and muscle spasm. They are noninvasive, relatively low cost, easy to use, and often can be done by the patients themselves or by their caregivers (Jacox et al., 1994). To provide pain relief, these modalities can be applied directly over the site of pain, proximally to the site of pain, distally to the site of pain, or contralaterally to the site of pain (McCaffery & Pasero, 1999).

Superficial heating or cooling can cause a decrease in sensitivity to pain. There is a lack of well-controlled studies concerning the use of heat and cold. Most of the information discussed is based on clinical experiences presented in the literature. Despite the lack of firm evidence, the Management of Cancer Pain Guideline Panel recommends the offering of cutaneous stimulation techniques, such as applications of superficial heat and cold, to alleviate pain (Jacox et al., 1994). Patients with aching muscles, muscle spasm, joint stiffness, low back pain, or itching may benefit from the use of superficial heating or cooling. Their use seems to be most effective for well-localized pain (McCaffery & Passero, 1999). It is important to consider patient safety and comfort when using these interventions. This method should not be used with patients who have bleeding disorders, or pains such as causalgia (which are characterized by a hypersensitivity to touch); or in areas with recent injury, broken skin, open wounds, or skin where a patient is receiving radiation therapy (Jacox et al., 1994; McCaffery & Pasero, 1999; Spross & Wolff Burke, 1995). Sites proximal, distal, or contralateral should be considered if the area of pain is contraindicated. When using cold, care should be taken to not use cold for sustained periods of time to prevent peripheral nerve injury or local frostbite (Nadler, 2004). Cold should not be used if an individual has a history of peripheral vascular disease (such as Raynaud's disease), connective tissue disease, or reports an "allergy" to cold. Often, those who report an allergy to cold may experience an asthma attack upon exposure to cold air (Baily, 1999). Heat should not be used with topical menthol products because of the potential for tissue damage (Jacox et al., 1994; McCaffery & Pasero, 1999; Spross & Wolff Burke, 1995).

Most hospitalized individuals will need an order or institutional protocol before initiation of superficial heating or cooling. There are several convenient ways of utilizing these modalities for palliative patients. For example, cold application can be done safely using gel packs that are kept in the refrigerator, homemade cold packs (sealed plastic bags filled with 1/3 alcohol and 2/3 water placed in freezer), or 1-lb bags of frozen peas or corn (which have been hit gently to separate contents). Heat can be administered by heating pad, hot packs, immersion in water, or retention of body heat with plastic wraps. Care must be taken with both modalities to protect the skin with at least a layer of terry cloth or pillowcase. Moisture increases the intensity of the heat or cold. Patients are to be discouraged from lying on heat sources. The skin must be inspected at regular intervals for irritation, swelling, blistering, excessive redness that does not subside between treatments or bleeding. Some patients develop a "hunting reaction," in which the skin alternatively blanches and turns red after the application of cold. If this occurs, the use of cold should be immediately discontinued. Extreme vigilance is necessary for patients with impaired or decreased sensation, cognitive impairment, or who are unconscious and may be considered a relative contraindication. Treatment should be discontinued if the patient asks or if pain or any form of skin irritation occurs (Jacox et al., 1994; McCaffery & Pasero, 1999; Spross & Wolf Burke, 1995).

Research is lacking concerning the frequency and duration of such treatments. McCaffery and Pasero (1999) suggest a trial and error approach that is individualized to the patient. They suggest that a minimal effective duration for application of hot or cold is 5–10 min with the usual duration 20–30 min. The decision to use heat or cold will depend upon the patient's situation. When compared to heat, cold often relieves more pain and relieves it faster. Often, pain relief from cold will last longer. Cold can either relieve or exacerbate joint stiffness. Evaluation of each situation is necessary. It may be useful to alternate between heat and cold. The duration of application may be as short as 5–10 seconds or 3 min of heat, and then alternating to 1 min of cold for a period of 20–30 min (McCaffery & Pasero, 1999; Spross & Wolff Burke, 1995).

Individuals often will need education on the use of superficial heat and cold as a pain-relieving measure. Educational information that is useful in teaching patients and their family members and caregivers about the use of superficial heat and cold for pain relief can be found in several sources (McCaffery & Pasero, 1999; Rhiner et al., 1993).

Although helpful for some painful situations, methods of applying deep heat, diathermy, microwave diathermy, and ultrasound, will not be discussed in detail here. It is thought that they increase blood flow and metabolic rate even more than superficial heat does. Methods that deliver deep heat must be used with caution in patients with active cancer and are not to be used over areas of active tumor (Jacox et al., 1994; Tunkel & Lachmann, 1998). Also, methods that deliver deep heat may be fairly challenging to use with palliative care patients who have advanced disease. Consultation with a physiatrist would be necessary when considering the use of deep heat.

Massage, another form of cutaneous stimulation, uses touch in the various forms of pressure, friction, and vibration to muscle and connective tissue, potentially to reduce pain and tension, improve circulation, promote relaxation (Deng et al., 2004), and communicate care and concern, especially in patients who have a communication impairment or language barrier. Even children with pain can potentially benefit from massage. Pediatric nurses are key in implementing massage into a child's plan of care (Hughes, Ladas, Rooney, & Kelly, 2008). In a nondrug intervention program for pain relief, 63% of cancer patients selected massage/vibration as a nondrug intervention for pain relief (Rhiner et al., 1993). It is thought to decrease pain by increasing superficial circulation and, in some situations, by relaxing muscles.

Studies that utilized massage in ill populations showed that brief massages are tolerated and safe (Bauer & Dracup, 1987; Meek, 1993; Tyler, Winslow, Clark, & White, 1990). The National Center for Complementary and Alternative Medicine (NCCAM) recommends massage for refractory cancer pain (Berenson, 2005). The Integrative Oncology Practice Guidelines published in 2007 made a strong recommendation based on low or very low quality evidence that cancer patients who have pain have massage therapy given by an oncology trained massage therapist as the benefits clearly outweigh the risks and burdens (Deng, Cassileth, Cohen, Gubili, Johnstone, Kumar, Vickers; Society for Integrative Oncology Executive Committee, Abrams, Rosenthal, Sagar, & Tripathy). A 3-year study of 1,290 cancer patients receiving massage therapy showed a decrease in various symptom severity from pre- to postmassage symptom assessment, including a 40.2% improvement in pain (Cassileth & Vickers, 2004). A smaller massage study that utilized 41 hospitalized oncology patients also showed statistically significant outcomes for pain (Smith, Kemp, Hemphil, & Vojir, 2002). A meta-analysis of the effects of back-rub effleurage suggests that patient comfort and relaxation is enhanced by a simple 3-min back rub. Also, positive changes were demonstrated on heart rate, blood pressure, and respiratory rate. Some variables, such as gender, length of massage, and environmental conditions seem to play a role in effectiveness (Labyak & Metzger, 1997).

Massage is contraindicated over sites of tissue damage (such as open wounds or tissue undergoing irradiation), in patients with bleeding disorders or thrombophlebitis, patients uncomfortable with touch, or those who might misinterpret touch as sexual (although this might be acceptable if the massager was a spouse or close partner). In working with cancer patients, light pressure is best and deep or intense pressure is to be avoided (Berenson, 2005; Deng et al., 2004; Deng et al., 2007). When considering massage, it is important for the nurse to consider the patient's comfort with touch, previous experiences with massage, and preferred techniques (Spross & Wolff Burke, 1995).

Massage to the site of pain may or may not serve to decrease pain at that site. Palliative care patients may not be up to an extensive massage, but may find massage of limited sites beneficial and not requiring much effort on their part. For example, massage of the neck, back, or shoulders may be sufficient to promote comfort. Some may find this too strenuous. For these patients, the nurse could consider massage to the hands or feet. Massage movements can include rhythmic stroking, kneading or circular, distal-to-proximal movements. Effleurage, using slow, smooth, long strokes, is usually done to promote relaxation. The patient should be involved in choosing the sites and massage movements that provide the most comfort along with how long the massage should last. It may be helpful to try different types of strokes with varying degrees of pressure in an effort to find what is most effective for an individual (Jacox et al., 1994; McCaffery & Pasero, 1999; Spross & Wolff Burke, 1995). The patient may be sitting in a chair, or lying on his or her side, or prone on a bed or table. It is helpful to determine with the individual if the room will be quiet, if music will be played, or if conversation will take place during the massage (McCaffery & Wolff, 1992).

During the actual massage, ideally both the nurse and patient will be as relaxed as possible. The patient should be in a position that is supported and easy to maintain for the duration of the massage. The massager should be in a position that utilizes good body mechanics. Patient comfort and modesty are to be maintained with sheets, blankets, or towels. The use of a warmed, alcohol-free lotion will decrease friction. One hand should be on the patient at all times until the massage is over. For example, the right hand could begin its stroke as the left hand is completing its stroke. Removing both hands can communicate to the patient that the massage is over. Patients may fall asleep during massage (McCaffery & Pasero, 1999; McCaffery & Wolff, 1992). Feedback from the patient, if possible, is useful for future planning. If patients find massage helpful, it should be scheduled on a regular basis. Massage can be quite comforting to dying patients who are often deprived of human touch at the end of life. Family members and caregivers may wish to be instructed or included in this pain-relieving intervention. They should be taught to use the techniques that the patient found to be most

helpful (McCaffery & Pasero, 1999). Others who are overwhelmed may find this a burden, one more thing for them to do.

Vibration is a form of massage that passes fine tremors either electrically (using a vibrator) or manually (using one's hands) to the skin (Spross & Wolff Burke, 1995). It is thought to increase superficial circulation and stimulate large-diameter fibers (Jacox et al., 1994). It should not be used over sites overlying tumor, where skin has been injured, on areas of thrombophlebitis, with patients who bruise easily, or for migraine headache or headache that is worsened by sound or movement (McCaffery & Passero, 1999). Vibration can be used for itching, muscle spasm, neuropathic pain, phantom pain, and tension headache. It can be used as a substitute for TENS (McCaffery & Pasero, 1999; McCaffery & Wolff, 1992; Spross & Wolff Burke, 1995). One can vary the effect by varying the pressure of vibration. When applied with light pressure, its results are similar to massage. Moderate pressure vibration may act to relieve pain by causing numbness, paresthesia, or anesthesia to the stimulated area (McCaffery & Pasero, 1999).

Electric vibrators can be either hand-held or stationary. Some are battery powered and some are plugged into an electrical outlet. Many have at least two frequencies, high (100–200 Hz) and low (10–50 Hz); some have a heat-delivery option. Although the high setting is often the more effective frequency, it is advised to try the low frequency initially. Depending on the site of pain, some patients are able to administer the vibrator themselves. Use of the vibrator, like other cutaneous stimulation interventions, is often a trial and error situation with the site and duration of treatment up to the patient (McCaffery & Pasero, 1999; Spross & Wolff Burke, 1995). One study looked at the duration of poststimulatory pain relief resulting from brief (1–15 min) treatments and longer (30 min). The relief from the brief intervention was brief whereas the longer treatment resulted in prolonged relief (Lundeberg, Nordeman, & Ottoson, 1984). In most institutional settings, use of a vibrator will require an order from the healthcare provider (McCaffery & Pasero, 1999).

Further massage research may look at psychological, physiological, and molecular mechanisms that play a role in the central nervous pathways involved (Esch, Guarna, Bianchi, Zhu, & Stafano, 2004; Sagar, Dryden, & Myers, 2007). Ideally work with larger more homogenous populations will help determine which massage techniques are most beneficial to specific patient situations including those at end of life (Myers, Walton, & Small, 2008).

Neurostimulatory Interventions

Transcutaneous electrical nerve stimulation (TENS) has been defined as "a method of producing electroanalgesia through electrodes applied to the body" (Jacox et al., 1994, p. 188). The TENS system is a small battery-operated device that is attached by cables to electrodes taped to the skin overlying a nerve. Initiation requires an order from the healthcare provider. Patients with musculoskeletal, arthrogenic, or neurogenic pain may benefit from the use of TENS. It should not be used with patients who are unable to communicate its effects. It is contraindicated in individuals with demand-type pacemakers. Those who have a history of epilepsy, transient ischemia attacks, strokes, epilepsy, or myocardial disease should not have the TENS electrodes placed on the head, neck, or chest. The electrodes should not be placed over the site of tumors, near the carotid sinus, or directly on the eye. Specific patients at the end of life need to be carefully evaluated to determine if it is appropriate to use a TENS unit. For many, it will not be appropriate. The TENS unit should be started by a healthcare professional who is trained in its use and who will be able to take the time to instruct the patient in its use. Patients should be informed that it may take various adjustments to the TENS settings, electrode placements, and duration of treatment to find the most effective settings. The individual patient's feedback is essential in this process. A body chart can easily be used to document these trials (Spross & Wolff Burke, 1995). Thompson and Filshie (1998) describe the use of TENS in detail. Currently large multicenter randomized controlled studies evaluating the use of TENS for chronic pain, such as cancer-related pain, are lacking (Robb, Bennett, Johnson, Simpson, & Oxberry, 2008).

Use of a *spinal cord stimulator*, a more invasive technique that acts on sympathetic fibers, is usually not indicated in an actively dying patient. However, patients with neuropathic pain, such as postherpetic neuralgia pain or postthoracotomy pain, may benefit from this technique. Nurses caring for these individuals who are at the end of life and have permanently implanted spinal cord stimulators may need to become knowledgeable about this technique (Miguel, 2000).

Invasive Interventions

Invasive interventions can be considered for a small percentage of palliative patients whose pain cannot be adequately controlled by pharmacologic means. This population includes individuals whose pain is localized to one or two areas and is expected to persist, and who cannot achieve an acceptable balance between analgesia and intolerable, dose-limiting side effects from these analgesics.

In evaluating patients for invasive approaches, it is important to clarify that all feasible primary therapies that are likely to improve patient outcomes have been initiated, that the opioid dose has been titrated up to the maximal tolerated dose, that side effects have been treated with appropriate medication therapy or through

opioid rotation, that appropriate adjuvant analgesics have been considered or tried, and that the appropriate routes of drug administration have been instituted. Other patient-related factors to assess include presence of active infection, coagulopathy or use of anticoagulant drugs, coexisting medical conditions that increase risks (Cherny, Arbit, & Jain, 1996), functional status (Arbit & Bilsky, 1998), and the potential rapidity of tumor growth in areas unaffected by the neurodestructive intervention (Schroeder, 1986). Also to be considered is "the likelihood and duration of analgesic benefit, the immediate and long-term risks, the likely duration of survival, the availability of local expertise, and the anticipated length of hospitalization" (Cherney et al., 1996, p. 128). A procedure performed by an inexperienced surgeon or anesthesiologist on a medically ill patient may have a suboptimal ot unpredictable outcome (Hassenbush & Cherney, 2004).

Neurodestructive procedures should be considered irreversible with potentially irreversible side effects (Schroeder, 1986). A dying, bed-bound patient may be willing to accept the possible disabilities of motor weakness, loss of bowel or bladder functions, or loss of position sense as a reasonable exchange for adequate pain relief. However, hope for life, especially a "normal" one, frequently continues in those who are dying. An ambulatory patient is rarely receptive to the possibilities of these side effects (Swarm & Cousins, 1998).

Neural blockade is an anesthetic intervention for either temporary or permanent effect and is commonly called a nerve block. A local anesthetic (usually lidocaine or bupivacaine) is injected into or around a nerve. Nerve blocks can be considered diagnostic, prognostic, therapeutic, or preemptive/prophylactic. A diagnostic nerve block is done to determine the specific pain pathway and to aid in the differential diagnosis. A prognostic nerve block is one that is done to predict the efficacy of a permanent ablating procedure. A therapeutic nerve block is done to provide temporary pain relief in a pain crisis or to treat painful conditions that respond to these blocks (e.g., a celiac block for the relief of pain due to pancreatic cancer). A preemptive/prophylactic nerve block is done proactively to prevent the development of a chronic pain syndrome. Neurolysis is a permanent procedure that interferes with the transmission of a painful stimulus by injection of a chemical substance such as alcohol or phenol to destroy or ablate the nerve (Saberski, 1998).

A successful prognostic nerve block may not always mean a successful neurolysis. This may be due to such things as analgesic and sedating premedications, placebo response, spread of local anesthetic to adjacent neural structures, or systemic absorption of local anesthetics. Also, patients near the end of their lives may be unwilling or unable to undergo two blocking procedures, the prognostic followed by the neurolysis. In this situation, the anesthesiologist may decide on a neurolytic procedure without a preceding prognostic block (Swarm & Cousins, 1998). Contra-indications to an individual undergoing a nerve block includes infection, coagulopathies, ineffective prognostic block, inadequate patient and family preparation, patient refusal, inability to understand and sign informed consent, and inability to cooperate during the procedure. The use of ultrasound guidance—a more recent development that allows the anesthesiologist to position the needle more accurately and monitor the distribution of the local anesthetic medication—has improved both safety and efficacy of neural blockade (Marhofer, Greher, & Kapral, 2005; Marhofer & Chan, 2007).

General types of neural blockade are peripheral blocks (including brachial plexus, and cranial, intercostal, and sacral nerves), neuro-axial blocks (including epidural and intrathecal), and sympathetic nerve blocks (including celiac plexus block and superior hypogastric block) (Latifzai, Sites, & Koval, 2008). Specific nerve blocks are identified by the anatomical location where they are performed. Depending on the location of the block, some of the risks or complications include fatigue, oversedation (if analgesics are not decreased in relation to decreased pain), sensory loss, motor weakness, altered bowel and bladder function, altered sexual function, intravascular injection, hematoma, and new pain. If sufficient denervation occurs from a somatic block, for example, a deafferentation pain will result. It is estimated that 14–30% of individuals undergoing peripheral neurolytic blockade may develop neuropathic pain as a result (Swarm & Cousins, 1998). Side effects from nerve blocks can include Horner's syndrome, characterized by constricted pupil, ptosis, "and decreased sweating resulting from interruption of the sympathetic pathways to the eye" (Goldberg, 1983, p. 86); numbness, weakness, increased warmth, diarrhea, and lowered blood pressure. These effects are temporary if done with a local anesthetic, or long-lasting or permanent, if done with alcohol or phenol (as with a neurodestructive block). A recent systematic review of neurological complications after regional anesthesia found a neurological complication at 0.04% with permanent neurological injury rarely occurring (Brull, McCartney, Chan, & El-Beheiry, 2007). It is the responsibility of nurses caring for individuals undergoing these procedures to be knowledgeable about the side effects and alert to developing complications. Readers are encouraged to review the work of Latifzai, Sites, and Koval (2008), Michaels and Draganov (2007), De Tran, Clemente, and Finlayson (2007a), (2007b) and Datta et al. (2007) for more detailed information on neural blockade.

Cordotomy is a neuroablative, rarely done, neurosurgical procedure that involves making a lesion in the anterior spinothalamic tract, contralaterally to the pain site, either percutaneously or with an open surgical approach, to destroy the function of a portion of the particular spinothalamic tract that innervates the site of pain. The percutaneous approach is associated with less morbidity (Giller, 2003). The spinothalamic tract is important in several ways. Pain and temperature for the contralateral side of the body is mediated through the anterior spinothalamic tract. The area for superficial pain is found in the superficial area of this tract and the area for deep visceral pain and temperature is found in the deeper area (Arbit & Bilsky, 1998). Deliberate damage to the spinothalamic tract through a neuroablative procedure will affect the dermatomal area innervated by the selected level. Preservation of proprioception and power is often possible with cordotomy, but the level of analgesia may tend to decrease over time (Hassenbach & Cherney, 2004).

Cordotomy is most successful in patients with unilateral pain below C-5 (Arbit & Bilsky, 1998; Saberski, 1998). Cordotomy is indicated in pain that is unresponsive to other therapy in patients with a life expectancy of less than 1 year (Saberski, 1998; Hassenbach & Cherney, 2004). Because of a variety of factors, including progressive disease, it is difficult to ascertain its actual success rate. It is thought that in skilled hands, complete pain relief immediately after cordotomy is as high as 60%–80% (Saberski, 1998). As time progresses, pain relief drops, possibly due to progression of disease and the resulting development of new pain. Saberski (1998) and Sanders and Zuurmond (1995) discuss the possibility of developing a delayed postcordotomy dysesthesia, "a condition in which a disagreeable sensation is produced by ordinary stimuli" following a lesion in a peripheral or central pathway (Stedman, 1995, p. 531). Arbit and Bilsky (1998) estimate that 1% of patients can develop postcordotomy dysesthesia anytime after the cordotomy, even more than a year later. For this reason, it is advised to avoid this procedure in individuals with an extended life expectancy (Arbit & Bilsky, 1998).

Sometimes the relief of one pain by cordotomy unmasks a new or mirror pain in the ipsilateral side. Prior to the procedure, the patient may not be aware of this pain because of the overwhelming contralateral pain. Sometimes, the nociceptive components of a pain may be successfully relieved but not the neuropathic components (Arbit & Bilsky, 1998; Nagaro et al., 2001). A study by Sanders and Zuurmond (1995) demonstrated the effectiveness and safety of percutaneous cervical cordotomy in terminally ill cancer patients. Complications following cordotomy can include dysfunction of autonomic respiration, sleep apnea, Horner's syndrome, arterial hypotension, hemiparesis (usually transient), and bladder dysfunction (Arbit & Bilsky, 1998). As with neural blockade, the use of CT for guidance in percutaneous cordotomies can help to increase effectiveness and decrease complications of both unilateral and bilateral percutaneous cordotomies (Yegul & Erhan, 2003). The function of the ipsilateral diaphragm can be impaired by cordotomy (Saberski, 1998). Patients with pulmonary disease on the contralateral side of the cordotomy are at risk for respiratory decompensation. It is recommended that patients undergo preoperative pulmonary function tests to help identify individuals at increased risk. Bilateral cordotomy is associated with a higher risk of sleep apnea, respiratory compromise, and arterial orthostatic hypotension. These conditions may or may not be transient and self-limiting. Their presence is thought to be a major contributing factor to mortality following bilateral procedures. Because of this, the presence of a low ejection fraction or significant preexisting heart disease contraindicates the use of the bilateral procedure (Arbit & Bilsky, 1998). The unilateral percutaneous cordotomy is the preferred procedure. When bilateral lesions are necessary, the open approach may be indicated (Saberski, 1998). As a safety measure, Arbit and Bilsky (1998) suggest waiting at least 1 week between cordotomies to assess for the development of respiratory compromise from unilateral lesions. Sometimes, open cordotomy is done if the percutaneous procedure is not available, or if a patient is unable to lie supine for a percutaneous procedure (Saberski, 1998). An individual's ability to tolerate the actual procedure plays a role in what is done. Often, patients with advanced disease may be unable to tolerate multiple sessions to alleviate pain. Ideally, the neurosurgeon can make the most of a single opportunity to relieve the pain (Arbit & Bilsky, 1998). In recent years, invasive neurosurgical approaches have been used less frequently and replaced by neuromodulatory approaches; however, for select patients, neurosurgical approaches can be most useful (De Conno, Panzeri, Brunelli, Saita, & Ripamonti, 2003; Meyerson, 2001). A detailed review of other neurosurgical interventions for pain can be found in Giller (2003).

Integrative Interventions

In reviewing integrative interventions, it may be helpful to consider the five major classifications or domains used by the National Center for Complementary and Alternative Medicine (NCCAM). These are alternative medical systems, mind/body interventions, biologically based therapies, manipulative and body-based methods and energy therapies. The following review will include useful evidence-based techniques for pain management at the end of life from all of the NCCAM classifications except from the biologically based therapies. Acupuncture, mind-body therapy, and massage therapy are shown in studies to have the strongest evidence for their clinical use in pain control (Deng et al., 2004).

Alternative Medical Systems

Acupuncture, a treatment from traditional Chinese medicine (TCM), has been shown to treat pain, depression,

nausea, and other health problems effectively (Deng et al., 2004; NIH Consensus Conference, 1998). Despite even more evidence in the literature since 1998 supporting the use of acupuncture, it still is underutilized in end-of-life palliative care (Standish, Kozak, & Congdon, 2008). In this holistic, energy-based approach, thin, disposable needles, usually stainless steel, are placed in precise anatomical points (365 specific locations) to balance energy movement along the body's 12 meridians (Berenson, 2005; Decker, 2000). *Acupressure* is the application of finger pressure to the acupuncture points. *Moxibustion* is the stimulation of an acupuncture point by heat. This is done by burning a special compressed combustible substance near the acupuncture point. Other variations in acupuncture stimulation of sites include the use of electrical stimulators or lasers. The NIH Consensus Development Panel on Acupuncture (1998) found that the incidence of adverse effects from acupuncture is substantially lower than for many standard medical procedures or medications used for the same conditions. Adverse effects from acupuncture can include an occasional drop of blood or bruise at the needle insertion site, mild discomfort at site, infection, or, depending on insertion site, pneumothorax. The latter two effects are rare and depend on the experience and training of the acupuncturist (Berenson, 2005).

In TCM, it is thought that good health depends on the balance of energy in the body. Energy-called *chi*, or *qi*, is thought to be constantly circulating in the body. Acupuncture acts to promote circulation of chi or qi vital energy. Acupuncture is based on a holistic, energy-focused approach to individuals, not on a disease-oriented, diagnostic treatment approach. The fact that acupuncture causes a multitude of biological responses has been demonstrated clearly. Much work is currently underway to understand better the anatomy and physiology of the acupuncture points (NIH Consensus Conference, 1998). Western medicine considers the proposed mechanisms of action for pain relief by acupuncture to include endorphin release, mediation of pain-producing neurotransmitters, and stress-induced analgesia (Berenson, 2005; Spross & Wolff Burke, 1995).

In their review of the data, the NIH Consensus Development Panel on Acupuncture (1998) stated that at present the "data in support of acupuncture are as strong as those for many accepted Western medical therapies" (p. 1520). At present, there is fairly convincing data showing the effectiveness of acupuncture in postoperative dental pain, and in adult postoperative and chemotherapy nausea and vomiting. Some studies indicate that it may be helpful as an adjunct treatment in painful situations such as headache, menstrual cramps, fibromyalgia, myofascial pain, osteoarthritis, and low back pain. Its effectiveness in relieving musculoskeletal pain remains controversial (Deng et al., 2004). The Integrative Oncology Practice Guidelines published in

2007 recommended acupuncture as "a complementary therapy when pain is poorly controlled" as a strong recommendation based on high-quality evidence (Deng et al.). Controlled studies using acupuncture in palliative care patients are in the process of development. In this population, it may be both difficult and controversial to implement an acupuncture study comparing acupuncture to placebo or sham under controlled conditions, utilizing standardized outcomes. It is encouraging that a recent pilot study looked at using electrostimulation of acupuncture points in sedated, ventilated patients in an intensive care unit (Nayak et al., 2008). Ideally, as more research is done and acupuncture is further incorporated into the mainstream health care system, more informed decisions regarding the appropriateness of acupuncture for patients in varying situations will be made (NIH Consensus Panel, 1998). As healthcare professionals, it is important to guide patients from a perspective of evidence, not marketing.

More and more patients are seeking acupuncture treatments. It has been used to treat a variety of conditions (including pain) in children (Kundu, & Berman, 2007; Libonate, Evans, & Tsao, 2008). Acupuncture is gaining more practitioners with Western medicine backgrounds and more general support from Western practitioners. Along with others, some nurses are going through extensive training to become licensed practitioners of acupuncture. Issues of training, licensure, and accreditation are in the process of being clarified. In the United States, educational standards have been developed for the training of physician and nonphysician practitioners. An agency recognized by the U.S. Department of Education has accredited many of the acupuncture educational programs. Physician acupuncturists can sit for a nationally recognized exam. Nonphysician acupuncturists can sit for an entry-level competency exam that is offered by a national credentialing agency. Unfortunately, there is much variation from state to state. This includes differences in the requirements to obtain licensure and in the titles conferred. This variation leads to confusion and to less confidence in the qualifications of acupuncture practitioners. It is important that nurses be aware of the requirements and titles conferred in the states in which they practice, in order to guide patients who desire a TCM evaluation for acupuncture to the most qualified, safe practitioners (NIH Consensus Panel, 1998).

A more detailed discussion of acupressure and acupuncture is beyond the scope of this text. Nurse educators desiring to include more information of these techniques in the nursing curriculum are encouraged to seek out licensed practitioners of acupuncture for collaboration. Some schools of nursing have faculty who are also licensed acupuncturists. At this time, most insurance policies do not cover acupuncture or other integrative approaches, and most patients and families have to pay out of pocket for these interventions.

Mind-Body Interventions

Music has been shown to be an effective intervention for pain control through a variety of physiological and psychological effects. Affective, cognitive, and sensory processes can be engaged, activated, and altered by music. In palliative care, music therapy "strives to promote well being and quality of life for patients and caregivers (Magil, pg 37, 2009)." This is done by processes such as use of prior skills, relaxation, distraction, alteration of mood, and improved sense of control. Physical effects include increasing or decreasing pulse and blood pressure (Magill-Levreault, 1993; Tuls Hallstead & Tuls Roscoe, 2002). Music therapy, as defined by Spross and Wolff Burk (1995), is "the scientific and systematic use of music to effect beneficial changes in physiological and psychological processes that influence experiences of pain and illness" (p. 175). The use of music therapy in the medically ill can reduce mood disturbance (Cassileth, Vickers, & Magill, 2003) and affect the suffering and total pain that a sick individual experiences.

In using music with an individual, music therapists evaluate the patient's medical situation, the person's social and cultural history, and assess how emotions are affecting that person's pain. The music therapist can then utilize a variety of techniques to help ameliorate pain and suffering. Vocal techniques can include toning, chanting, singing precomposed songs, writing songs, and singing improvisations. Listening techniques and use of prerecorded or live instrumental music can provide opportunities for exploration and expression (Magill, 2001).

A patient's needs may change daily. Because of this, the music selection is best done with the individual on a day-to-day basis. "The aim is always to promote comfort, healing, and a decreased sense of pain. Working in collaboration with other pain modification approaches, music therapy can help soothe pain as well as heal the suffering" (Magill-Levreault, 1993, p. 45). Schroeder-Sheker (1994) explores the use of music in the actively dying. Tuls Halstead and Tuls Roscoe (2002) offer nurses many concrete examples of how to use music to assist patients as listeners and performers.

A recent Cochrane Review (Cepeda, Carr, Lau, & Alvarez, 2006) looked at the use of music for pain relief and concluded that music should not be considered the first line treatment for pain. Fifty one randomized controlled trials (RCTs) of adults or children met criteria to look at the effect of music on acute, chronic, or cancer pain. Despite the finding that music reduced pain and reduced requirements for morphine-like analgesics, the magnitude of the positive was small. Also of note, it may be that the types of pain included in studies that met criteria (acute postoperative pain, chronic, labor, procedural, or experimental pain with the majority involving procedural or postoperative pain) may not readily generalize to pain in individuals at the end-of-life. Clearly more rigorous, well designed studies looking at the use of music as part of a pain management plan for individuals at the end of life are needed.

The cognitive interventions discussed earlier under the umbrella of psychological interventions, such as relaxation, guided imagery and hypnosis, also fall under the NCCAM category of mind-body methods that may be helpful to the individual with pain.

Manipulative and Body-Based Methods

The use of massage, a manipulative mind-body technique, is covered under the physiatric intervention section as a cutaneous stimulation technique. However, readers desiring to learn more about the use of massage may also find information from integrative or complementary and alternative medicine sources (Berenson, 2005; Deng et al., 2004).

Energy Therapies

Therapeutic touch (TT) is a complementary technique based on systems theory of the multidimensional nature of the individual and the homeostatic concepts of balance and wholeness, which work with energy fields in promoting relaxation states, reducing pain, and promoting healing. It was developed by Dolores Krieger, a nurse physiologist, in conjunction with Dora Kunz, a healer (Owens & Ehrenreich, 1991a).

Despite its name, TT does not involve physical touching. It involves a conscious intention on the part of the healer to help the client (Spross & Wolff Burke, 1995). The practitioner of TT first centers himself or herself in the here and now. Then the practitioner does an assessment of the client's energy field for symmetry by placing his or her hands 4–6 inches from the body, starting at the head and moving towards the feet. The energy field is then "unruffled" by the practitioner's performing sweeping motions of the hands to smooth out the energy field. During the next phase, the treatment phase, the practitioner channels energy to areas of the field that the practitioner senses are imbalanced or void. Finally, in the last phase, reassessment, the energy field is reevaluated for repatterning of energy flow (Owens & Ehrenreich, 1991b).

Use of this technique for palliative patients who are interested may be useful because it involves no effort or expenditure of any energy on the part of the patient. Patients who are debilitated do not have to learn new skills at a time when they may be unable to do so. Also, there do not seem to be any adverse effects. It is thought to promote a profound relaxation response that alleviates the pain (Berenson, 2005). Anecdotal evidence suggests that TT can be a beneficial adjunct to traditional therapies (Kotora, 1997). A study that looked at the desire for serenity by persons nearing death and nursing interventions to facilitate this state found that pain control, TT, and assisting clients to

build trust were the three highest ranked interventions both in the frequency of use and in effectiveness (Messenger & Roberts, 1994).

The research base to support the use of TT in clinical practice is not solid. A recent meta-analysis of TT research found that there are many approaches to TT and that the TT practices vary from study to study. These factors may lead to less convincing conclusions when evaluating the effectiveness of TT as a modality. Although a number of studies had mixed or negative results, most studies supported the hypotheses regarding the efficacy of TT (Winstead-Fry & Kijek, 1999). One study (Giasson & Bouchard, 1998) looked at the effect of TT on the well-being of individuals with terminal cancer, and the results showed a positive increase in the sensations of well-being following three TT treatments. Well-being was measured using the Well-being scale, a visual analog scale that measures pain, nausea, depression, anxiety, shortness of breath, activity, appetite, relaxation, and inner peace (Giasson & Bouchard, 1998). Some of the proponents of TT feel that even if it is determined that TT is basically taking advantage of a placebo effect, this is still a beneficial adjuvant nursing intervention from a holistic nursing point of view. Meehan (1998) expresses the thought that "the potential of TT to enhance the placebo phenomenon requires further exploration but should not be discounted in seeking to relieve discomfort and distress and facilitate healing" (p. 117).

Therapeutic touch has been taught and researched since the 1970s. However, in recent years, its use has become more controversial. Mainstream American medicine is unconvinced about the value of TT. In 1998, one study was published in the very major mainstream *Journal of the American Medical Association*. It concluded that because 21 experienced practitioners of TT were unable to detect the investigator's "energy field" at a rate greater than chance, there was unrefuted evidence that the "claims of TT were groundless and that further professional use is unjustified" (Rosa, Rosa, Sarner, & Barrett, 1998, p. 1005). Some question the validity of this study and the biases inherent in the peer review. However, because this was published in a leading peer-reviewed medical journal, many in mainstream Western medicine are unsupportive of the use of TT. Eskinazi and Muehsam (1999) point out that conventional journals may have difficulty evaluating integrative techniques fairly because some of the concepts implicit in these techniques are outside the current biomedical framework. Often, information and opinions presented by mainstream medicine may be misinformed or based on a misunderstanding of an area of alternative medicine. It is important to explore knowledge outside the existing dogmas to promote real progress (Eskinazi & Muehsam, 1999).

Reiki, a Japanese term for universal life energy, is another energy therapy. This therapy is currently being studied to evaluate its role in symptom management, including that of pain. Reiki is defined as a vibrational or subtle energy most commonly facilitated by light touch whose use is thought to balance the biofield and strengthen the body's ability to heal itself. Reiki practitioners gently place their hands on a fully clothed individual's head, back, front, and the site of discomfort (if the person desires) to promote relaxation and decrease pain (Berenson, 2005; Vitale, 2007). A recent phase 2 study of Reiki in the management of pain in individuals with advanced cancer showed no overall reduction in opioid use, but did show improved pain control and improved quality of life using this safe, noninvasive intervention (Olson, Hanson, & Michaud, 2003).

A recent Cochrane Database Systematic review of touch therapies for pain relief in adults looked at the effectiveness of therapeutic touch, Reiki, and healing touch (developed by Janet Mentgen, RN, based on energy healing practices) (So, Jiang, & Qin, 2008). Only three studies met criteria for Reiki, five for Healing Touch, and seventeen for Therapeutic Touch. It found that these touch therapies may have a modest effect on pain relief. Of interest, it found that studies that utilized more experienced practitioners had greater reduction of pain. It concluded that more studies, especially those looking at the effect of touch therapies in children, are needed to provide sufficient evidence to promote the use of these interventions for pain relief.

Complementary services are being offered more frequently to patients at the end of life. A recent hospice survey found that 60% of 169 hospices offered complementary therapies to patients (Demmer, 2004). Massage therapy and music therapy, which are shown to have a positive effect on pain, were among the most popular. Barriers to providing integrative interventions were mostly limited to program constraints. These included lack of knowledge regarding these therapies, and how to offer them. Lack of qualified staff and funding problems also played a role.

SPECIAL POPULATIONS

Children

Children, like adults, experience pain at the end of life. Pain management for dying children is an important concern for both parents and clinicians. Although infants, children, and adolescents with many different life threatening conditions such as sickle cell disease or cystic fibrosis experience pain, most of the work documenting pain and its management has taken place in the field of oncology. Many of the principles of pain assessment and management reviewed in this chapter and the previous chapter can be applied to children. However, children should not be viewed as mini adults. Nurses caring for children need to be mindful of several important few points. (Layman-Goldstein & Sakae, 2010)

Pain assessment is dependant upon a child's chronological age and developmental state. A detailed review of pediatric pain assessment is beyond the scope of the chapter. Readers are directed to other resources when selecting age and population specific pediatric pain assessment tools which may be observational or self report depending upon the clinical situation and the infant or child's developmental stage and ability to verbalize. (Hockenberry & Wilson, 2007; Franck, Greenberg, & Stevens, 2000; Crellin et al., 2007; Ghai, Kaur Makkar, & Wig, 2008). Recently the Pediatric Initiative on Methods, Measurement, and Pain Assessment in Clinical Trials (www.immpact.org) commissioned a review of observational scales of pain for children ages 3 through 18. The goal was to identify particular scales that might be used as an outcome measure in clinical trials. This group found that no single observational measure can be recommended for pain assessment across all clinical contexts (von Baeyer & Spagrud, 2007). As established in the previous chapter, analgesic doses are initiated according to the child's chronological age and body weight.

Effective incorporations of nondrug pain interventions into a child's pain management plan is based upon the child's past experiences, developmental level, present response, and physical, emotional, and cultural factors. Like with adults, the nurse needs to consider what has worked well and what has not for a particular child. For some children there are there religious or cultural issues or concerns that would make certain interventions inappropriate for them or their families. A proposed intervention must be consistent with the developmental level of an individual child. The nurse also needs to keep in mind that just like with adults, the stress and fatigue from a prolonged illness may make it difficult for the child or family members to concentrate, follow directions, or learn new information.

It is important to keep in mind that the child and parent is the unit of care. Successful interventions can only happen when parents are included in the assessment and pain management plans. No one knows a child better than his or her parents. No one is better able to advocate for his or her child, than the parent of that child.

Over the last 20 years, the use of anesthetic techniques such as regional nerve blocks and use of intraspinal opioids has been established as safe and effective for children of all ages with specific needs who meet criteria for their use in acute, procedural, and chronic pain situations. Saroyan, Schechter, Tresgallo, and Granowetter (2005) described the use of an implanted infusion system in a 15 year-old girl dying of sarcoma to successfully manage what had been intractable pain that could not be managed with systemic therapy because of side effects. Through careful planning and education of all involved in her care, this girl was able to return home to die in her home country with her extended family present. In this situation and other less dramatic ones, special education and training for physicians and nurses using epidural analgesia in children is necessary. The nurse's role in setting institutional standards in using anesthetic techniques in children is important. Issues to be addressed include careful calculations and administration of medications, developmentally and situationally appropriate postprocedural assessment, and adequate nurse staffing are necessary to prevent serious complications. (Hockenberry & Wilson, 2007; Berde & Sethna, 2003; Marhofer, Sitzwohl, Greher, & Kapral, 2004; Tsue & Berde, 2005).

Use of nondrug pain interventions is well established in the pediatric population for procedural pain and acute pain (Evans & Tsao, 2008; Rheingans, 2007). There are many personal in the pediatric practice setting, such as childlife workers and pediatric social workers who are knowledgeable resources in the use of developmentally appropriate nondrug pain interventions. Perhaps as many as 30– 84% of children incorporate complimentary and alternative interventions into their care (Kudu & Berman, 2007). Many of the modalities, such as hypnosis, music therapy, and acupuncture appear promising. Yet, expert after expert is looking for large, well designed, rigorous studies in children to better establish these interventions as safe, effective, and acceptable. These studies could help establish more credible choices to help children and their families manage pain at the end of life (Evans & Tsao, 2008; Rheinans, 2007; Libonate et al., 2008).

Older Adults

Pain in the older adult, or pain in aging is emerging as a new subfield in pain research. Research indicates that pain in older adults has some differences from pain in younger adults. Some differences noted include increased difficulty using visual analogue pain scales, decreasing abilities to self report pain in individuals with dementing illness, increased risk to develop neuropathic pain, and prolonged hyperalgesia following tissue and nerve injury. The differences in psychosocial factors that influence how older adults adjust to pain compared younger adults may influence how psychological nondrug pain management interventions are implemented in geriatric patients. It is hoped that as more is known, age-tailored prevention, assessment and intervention protocols will lead to better quality of life for older adults (Gagliese, 2009).

At the moment, it is not clear how these and other factors play a role in the utilization of nondrug pain interventions for older adults. A recent study completed by Bennett, Closs, and Chatwin (2008) found that pain or pain management did not seem to be influenced by age. Much related to this topic is speculative. Obviously age-related changes in vision and hearing in the patient or caregiver play a role in educational strategies.

Bourbonniere and Kagan (2004) are among the many researchers that advocate for looking at interventions that result in more effective care for older adults. The evidence has yet to evolve.

HOW TO INTEGRATE NONDRUG INTERVENTIONS INTO A COMPREHENSIVE PAIN MANAGEMENT PLAN

A successful pain management plan is based on a comprehensive pain assessment and incorporates the components of treating underlying disease, pharmacologic interventions, psychological intervention, physiatric interventions, neurostimulatory interventions, invasive interventions, and integrative interventions. At the end of life, it may or may not be appropriate or feasible to treat underlying disease. Certainly, the patient with advanced disease may not be able to tolerate a surgery to remove a pain-producing tumor. Yet, some interventions aimed at treating underlying disease may be useful. For example, palliative radiation to areas of bony metastases may be well tolerated and decrease bone pain (Jacox et al., 1994). Pain caused by infection, such as pelvic abscess or occult infections from ulcerating tumors, may be relieved by treatment with appropriate antibiotics (Cherny & Portenoy, 1994a). The importance of pharmacological interventions, the mainstay of pain relief at the end of life, and how to integrate these interventions into the pain management plan have been well described in the previous chapter.

As part of the interdisciplinary team caring for a patient at the end of life, it is important for the nurse to understand how the nondrug interventions (psychological, physiatric, neurostimulatory, invasive, and integrative) are incorporated into the pain management plan. The availability of experienced consultants to perform certain interventions also plays a role. If no one is available to perform a specific intervention, it cannot be offered as an option in the pain management plan for that individual at that point in time. A palliative care team may need to work on system issues to improve access to specialists that may be helpful to their patients. Financial factors play a role in which resources are available to meet individual patient identified medical needs (Giordano & Schatman, 2008). Home health and hospice agencies have to keep financial and reimbursement issues in mind when incorporating integrative therapies into their programs. Ideas to consider include training current staff in techniques that could be incorporated into routine care while bearing in mind the scope of practice covered in each state or utilizing trained, certified volunteers (Johnson & O'Brien, 2009).

The use of any intervention is based upon the assessment of the patient. It is important to evaluate the individual carefully and apply what is appropriate for that individual in a particular situation. After the initiation of systemic analgesic therapy and treatment of underlying disease (if appropriate), the next step would be to consider the addition of psychological, physiatric, neurostimulatory, or integrative techniques to improve control and possibly improve the balance between analgesia and side effects (Cherny & Portenoy, 1994a; Rhiner et al., 1993). If these measures prove to be suboptimal, the consideration of the use of invasive techniques is appropriate (Miguel, 2000; Hassenbach & Cherney, 2004). Finally, if it is impossible to find the balance between pain relief and side effects, then sedation at the end of life (as described in chapter 12) must be considered.

THE ROLE OF NURSES IN IMPLEMENTING NONDRUG INTERVENTIONS

Nurses caring for patients at the end of life have both collaborative and independent functions in implementing nondrug interventions. First, nurses must be aware of which interventions they are able to perform. Factors to consider when making this determination include education in the use of particular techniques, comfort in teaching or implementing a particular technique, patient and family educational materials available, availability and affordability of specific necessary devices and materials, and time available to an individual nurse to initiate a particular intervention. Psychological interventions that an individual nurse must be comfortable initiating include patient and family education, and ideally cognitive interventions such as distraction, self-statements, brief-method relaxation techniques, and behavioral interventions such as a pain diary. Physiatric interventions that an individual nurse might initiate for an end- of-life patient's pain control could include positioning and movement, use of superficial heat or cooling, massage, or vibration. (Depending on the practice setting, the nurse may need to obtain orders for some of the physiatric interventions.) The use of music, an integrative technique, may also be initiated by an individual nurse. If the nurse has had additional training, he or she may consider the use of therapeutic touch, deep relaxation methods, or cognitive behavioral therapy. In addition, the nurse needs to know which members of the immediate primary team can perform nondrug interventions that may be useful as part of a comprehensive pain management plan. Also to be determined is the availability of special consultants, such as neurosurgeons, anesthesiologists, hypnotherapists, or acupuncturists, for consultation and intervention as necessary. The nurse may need to assist in making appropriate referrals to these consultants. Finally, as part of the team, it may be necessary to educate other team members about the efficacy of nondrug methods so that

these techniques can be integrated more efficiently into the pain management plan (Rhiner et al., 1993).

Only after it is determined who is capable and available to teach or perform a particular nondrug intervention can the nurse and his or her team realistically consider its use for an individual patient based upon the pain assessment. As with the pharmacological interventions, the nondrug interventions need to be directed at etiologic factors. For example, when applied with moderate pressure, vibration, a physiatric modality can help to relieve pain by decreasing sensation to a painful area and may act to decrease tension in muscles (Rhiner et al., 1993). This would make this approach a useful addition to the pharmacologic regimen already in place for an individual found to have pain from muscle spasm.

It is also important to consider whether a patient or the family has the physical, mental, or emotional energy necessary to participate in a particular intervention. Nondrug interventions that need a high level of patient involvement may not be possible when an individual is debilitated or when the caregiver is totally exhausted from the experience. Assessment needs to include a patient's ability to concentrate and follow directions, level of fatigue, and cognitive status (McCaffery & Pasero, 1999). Also include in the assessment an individual's previous experience and attitude towards nondrug interventions (McCaffery & Pasero, 1999; Rhiner et al., 1993). Determine which methods may be not useful because of religious or cultural issues or concerns or because they counter an individual's usual coping style (McCaffery & Pasero, 1999).

The next step is active collaboration by the nurse with the patient to choose a nondrug intervention that may be useful (Spross & Wolff Burke, 1995). As with CBT, it is useful to review with the patient the pain-related problems present, assign priorities to the problems, focus on the priority problems, set goals, and implement an intervention designed to address the priority problem (Fishman & Loscalzo, 1987). As part of this process, the nurse needs to be aware of what is realistically possible with the individual patient at that moment in time, given his or her medical condition (Loscalzo, 1996). Spross and Wolff Burke (1995) recommend focusing on only one or two nondrug interventions at a time. At this point, the patient's family, friends, and caregivers need to be asked if they wish to be involved in the nondrug intervention (McCaffery & Pasero, 1999; Spross & Wolff Burke, 1995). Some will want to be actively involved, and others will feel too overburdened (McCaffery & Pasero, 1999). Obstacles to the use of the selected nondrug intervention will need to be anticipated along with the development of strategies to overcome these obstacles (Spross & Wolff Burke, 1995).

Patient, family, and caregiver education follows. Even if the patient's family, friends, or caregivers are not actively involved, they will need information about the role of the nondrug intervention in the pain management plan (Spross & Wolff Burke, 1995). This helps to elicit their cooperation and promote successful use of the intervention (Rhiner et al., 1993). Written and audio materials that reinforce verbal information are useful (McCaffery & Pasero, 1999; Spross & Wolff Burke, 1995). It is important to emphasize that nondrug interventions are not a replacement for analgesics (McCaffery & Pasero, 1999). Patients and their families will need opportunities to develop skills using the nondrug intervention (Spross & Wolff Burke, 1995). Ideally, they actually will be able to use the intervention with the nurse present before utilizing it independently.

It is useful to debrief a patient and the caregiver following the use of a nondrug intervention. In this debriefing, the effect on pain and other outcomes and the need for more assistance should be assessed (Spross & Wolff Burke, 1995). If a nondrug intervention is assessed to be ineffective, then it should be modified or replaced (Spross & Wolff Burke, 1995).

Case Study conclusion: Mr R's pancreatic cancer progressed and he was readmitted to the hospital for uncontrolled pain several months after being successfully managed with oral systemic pain medications at home. Because there was an experienced anesthesiologist available, Mr R was evaluated for a celiac block. Imaging studies revealed that a successful block was possible. Mr. R underwent an ultrasound guided celiac plexus block with good results and a significant reduction in his analgesic requirements. This allowed him to return home to be successfully managed until his death 6 weeks later.

CONCLUSION

The assessment and pharmacologic management of pain in patients with life-threatening, progressive illness underscores the importance of integrating assessment and treatment strategies to address the needs of the individual patient. Nurses are expected to care for those who are seriously ill and dying from the moment the nurses' graduate. The delivery of optimal therapy depends on an understanding of the clinical pharmacology of the analgesic drugs and comprehensive assessment of the pain; the patient's medical condition, psychosocial state, and goals of care. Although the nurse will usually be part of an interdisciplinary team, he or she will often be the one responsible for assessing pain, administering analgesics, monitoring for adequacy of pain relief and presence of side effects, communicating with other members of the team, and

ensuring continuity of pain management across care settings. These responsibilities cannot be met unless the nurse is knowledgeable in the basic principles of pain assessment and pharmacological management, and in the recognition of patients who are at risk for inadequate pain assessment and control. In addition, recognition and respectful acknowledgment of the central role the family plays in managing pain in the home at end of life has major implications for nurses in their responsibility to educate and support families in this task. In few areas does the advanced practice nurse have a greater potential to impact on quality of life for those who are dying and their families than in facilitating effective pain management.

EVIDENCE-BASED PRACTICE

The Pain Management Indices—Cleeland (PMI) is a method of assessing the adequacy of clinician prescribing practices based on the World Health Organizations 3-Step analgesic ladder and other practice guidelines. (Cleeland et al., 1994)

Cleeland's PMI is based upon the patient's level of worst pain on the Brief Pain Inventory. Pain is categorized as: 0 = no pain; 1 = mild pain (1–3 on a 0–10 pain intensity rating scale); 2 = moderate pain (4–7 on a 0–10 pain intensity rating scale); or 3 = severe pain (8–10 on a 0–10 pain intensity scale). The patient's pain level is subtracted from the most potent level of analgesic drug therapies prescribed by the physician and is scored as 0 = no analgesic drug has been prescribed; 1 = a nonopioid has been prescribed; 2 = a weak opioid has been prescribed; and 3 = a strong opioid has been prescribed. The PMI can range from –3 (a patient with severe pain for whom no analgesic drug has been prescribed) to +3 (a patient for whom strong opioids have been prescribed and who is reporting no pain). Negative scores indicate inadequate orders for analgesic drugs, and score of 0 and higher are considered indicators of acceptable treatment.

Twenty-six national and international studies carried out between 1994 and 2007, in which the PMI was used to evaluate the adequacy of pain management in cancer patients, were reviewed. Analysis showed that a weighted mean of 43% of patients (8%–82%) had a negative PMI score indicating inadequate analgesic prescriptions for the level of pain experienced. Predictors of a negative PMI were publication before 2001, geographic location and socioeconomic variables, and setting. Although PMI is a rough estimate of how pain is treated in the population, it is a useful indicator of the clinicians' prescribing habits as compared to pain management practice guidelines (Deandear, Montanari, Moja & Apolone, 2008).

Cleeland CS, Gonin R, Hatfield AK, Edmonson JH, Blum RH, Stewart JA, Pandya KJ. (1994). Pain and its treatment in outpatients with metastatic cancer. *New England Journal of Medicine;* 330:592–596.

Deandear S, Montanari M, Moja L, Apolone G. (2008). *Annals of Oncology; 19:*1985–1991.

REFERENCES

Acute Pain management Guidelines Panel. (1992). Acute pain management: Operative medical procedures and trauma. *Clinical Practice Guideline.* AHCPR Pub. No. 92–0032. Rockvislle. MD: Agency for Health Care Policy and Research, Public Health Services, U.S. Department of Health and Human Services.

Adelhardt, J., Byrnes, M., Derby, S., Holritz, K., Layman-Goldstein, M., Racolin, A., et al. (1995). Care of the patient in pain: *Standard of oncology nursing practice.* New York: Memorial Sloan-Kettering Cancer Center.

Ahles, T. A., Blanchard, E. B., & Ruckdeschel J. C. (1983). The multidimensional nature of cancer-related pain. *Pain, 17,* 277–288.

American Geriatrics Society (AGS) Panel on Persistent Pain in Older Persons. (2006). Clinical practice guideline: The management of persistent pain in older persons. *Journal American Geriatric Society, 50*(Suppl. 6), S205–S224

American Nurses Association. (1990).*Position paper on the promotion of comfort and relief in dying patients.* Washington, DC: American Nurses Association. Revised December 5th, 2003.

American Pain Society. (2003). *Principles of analgesic use in the treatment of acute pain and cancer* (5th ed.). Glenview, IL: American Pain Society.

Anderson, K. O., Richman, S. P., Hurley, J., et al. (2002). Cancer pain management among underserved minority outpatients: Perceived needs and barriers to optimal control. *Cancer, 94,* 2295–2304.

Anderson, G., Jensen, N. H., Christup, L., Hansen, S. H., & Sjogren, P. (2002). Pain, sedation, and morphine metabolism in cancer patients during long-term treatment with sustained-release morphine. *Palliative Medicine, 16,* 107–114.

Arbit, E., Bilsky, M. H. (1998). Neurosurgical approaches in palliative care. In: D. Doyle, G. W. Hanks, & N. MacDonald (Eds.), *Oxford textbook of palliative medicine* (2nd ed., pp. 414–421). Oxford: Oxford Medical Publications.

Backonja, M. (2002). Use of anticonvulsants for treatment of neuropathic pain. *Neurology, 59* (5 Suppl. 2),S14–S17. [Review].

Baily, P. P.(1999). Asthma. In T. M. Buttaro, J. Trybulski, P. P. Bily, & J. SandbergCook (Eds.), *Primary care: A collaborative practice* (pp. 283–308). St Louis: Mosby.

Bates, M. S. (1987). Ethnicity and pain: A biocultural model. *Social Science Medicine, 24,* 47–50.

Bauer, W. C., & Dracup, K. A. (1987). Physiological effects of back massage in patients with acute myocardial infarctions. *Focus Critical Care, 14*(6), 42–46.

Becker, G., Galandi, D., & Blum, H. E. (2007). Peripherally acting opioid antagonists in the treatment of opioid-related constipation: a systematic review. *Journal Pain and Symptom Management, 34,* 547–565.

Berde, C. B., & Sethna, N. F. (2003). Analgesics for the treatment of pain in children. *New England Journal of Medicine, 347,* 1094–1103.

Bell, R. F., Eccleston, C. &, Kalso, E. (2003). Ketamine as adjuvant to opioid nonresponsive terminal cancer pain. *Journal Pain and Symptom Management, 26,* 867–875.

Bennett, M. I., Closs, S. J., & Chatwin, J. (2008). Cancer pain management at home (I): Do older patients experience less effective management than younger patients? *Support Cancer Care, 39*(3), 529–543.

Bennett, M. I., Bagnall, A. M., & Jose Closs, S. (2009). How effective are patient-based educational interventions in the management of cancer pain? Systematic review and meta-analysis. *Pain, 10*(3).

Benson, H. (1975). *The relaxation response.* New York: William Morrow.

Berde, C. B., Sethna, N. F. (2003). Analgesics for the treatment of pain in children. *New England Journal of Medicine, 347,* 1094–1103

Berenson, S. (2005). Complementary and alternative therapies in palliative care. In B. R. Ferrell & N. Coyle (Eds.), *Textbook of palliative care nursing.* New York: Mosby.

Bourbonniere, M., & Kagan, S. H. (2004). Nursing intervention and older adults who have cancer: Specific science and evidence-based practice. *Nursing Clinics of North America, 39*(3), 529–532.

Brull, R., McCartney, C. J., Chan, V. W., & El-Beheiry, H. (2007). Neurological complications after regional anesthesia: Contemporary estimates of risk. *Anesthesiology and Analgesia, 104*(4), 965–974.

Berry, P. E., & Ward, S. E. (1995). Barriers to pain management in hospice: A study of family caregivers. *Hospice Journal, 10,*19–33.

Bookbinder, M., Coyle, N., Kiss, M., Layman-Goldstein, M., Holritz, K., Thaler, H., et al. (1995). Implementing national standards for cancer pain management: Program model and evaluation. *Journal of Pain and Symptom Management, 12,* 334–347.

Bjoro, K., & Herr, K. (2008). Assessment of pain in the nonverbal or cognitively impaired older adult. *Clinical Geriatric Medicine, 24,* 237–362.

Braun, T. C., Hagen, N. S., & Clark, T. (2003). Development of a clinical practice guideline for palliative sedation. *Journal Palliative Medicine, 6,* 345–350.

Breitbart, W., Rosenfeld, B., Kaim, M., & Funesti-Esch, J. (2002). A randomized, double blind, placebo-controlled trial of psychostimulants for the management of fatigue in ambulatory patients with human immunodeficiency virus disease. *Archives Internal Medicine, 161,* 411–420.

Breitbart, W., & Alici-Evcimen, Y. (2007). Update on psychotropic medications for cancer-related fatigue. *Journal National Comprehensive Cancer Network, 5,* 1081–1091.

Breitbart, W., & Alici, Y. (2008). Agitation and delirium at the end of life: "We couldn't manage him." *Journal American Medical Association (JAMA), 300,* 2898–9100.

Brescia, F., Portenoy, R. K., Ryan, M., Drasnoff, J., & Gray, G. (1992). Pain, opioid use and survival in hospitalized patients with advanced cancer. *Journal of Clinical Oncology, 10,* 149–155.

Bruera, E., Kuehn, N., Miller, M. J., Selmser, P., & McMillan, K. (1991). The Edmonton Symptom Assessment System (ESAS): A simple method for the assessment of palliative care patients. *Journal Palliative Care, 7,* 6–9.

Bruera, E., & Sweeney, C. (2002). Methadone use in cancer patients with pain: A review. *Journal Palliative Medicine, 5,* 127–138.

Bruera, E., Driver, L., Barnes, E. A., Willey, J., Shen. L., Palmer, J. L., et al. (2003). Patient-controlled methylphenidate for the management of fatigue in patients with advanced cancer: A preliminary report. *Journal Clinical Oncology, 21,* 4439–4443.

Bruera, E., Palmer, J. L., Bosnjak, S., Rico, M. A., Moyano. J., Sweeney, C., et al. (2004). Methadone versus morphine as a first-line strong opioid for cancer pain: A randomized, double-blind study. *Journal Clinical Oncology, 22*, 185–192.

Byock, I. (1997). *Dying well: The prospect of growth at the end of life*. New York: Riverhead Books.

Cassileth, B. R., Vickers, A. J., & Magill, L. A. (2003). Music therapy for mood disturbance during hospitalization for autologous stem cell transplantation: A randomized controlled trial. *Cancer, 98*, 2723–2729.

Cassileth, B. R., & Vickers, A. J. (2004). Massage therapy for symptom control: Outcome study at a major cancer center. *Journal of Pain and Symptom Management, 28*, 244–249.

Cassileth, B. R., & Gubili, J. (2009). Integrative medicine: Complementary therapies. In D. Walsh, A. T. Caraceni, R. Fainsinger, K. Foley, P. Glare, C. Foh, M. Lloyd-Willimas, J. Nunex Olarte, & L. Radbruch (Eds.), *Palliative medicine*. Philadelphia: Saunders Elsevier.

Cepeda, M. S., Carr, D. B., Lau, J., & Alvarez, H. (2006). Music for pain relief. *Cochrane Database Systemic Reviews,*(2), CD 004843.

Cherny, N. I., Arbit, E., & Jain, S. (1996). Invasive techniques in the management of cancer pain. *Hematology/Oncology Clinics of North America, 10*, 121–137.

Chang, V. T., Hwang, S. S., Feuerman, M., & Kasimis, B. S. (2000). Symptom and quality of life survey of medical oncology patients at a veteran affairs medical center: A role for symptom assessment. *Cancer, 88*, 1175–1183.

Cherny, N., & Coyle, N. (1994). Suffering in the advanced cancer patient: A definition and taxonomy. *Journal of Palliative Care, 10*, 57–70.

Cherny, N., & Portenoy, R. K. (1994a). Sedation in the management of refractory symptoms: Guidelines for evaluation and treatment. *Journal of Palliative Care, 10*, 31–38.

Cheville, A. L. (1999). Cancer rehabilitation and palliative care. In R. Payne & A. L. Cheville (Eds.), *Conference course syllabus abstract of cancer rehabilitation in the new millennium: Opportunities and challenges* (pp. 125–128). New York: Memorial Sloan-Kettering Cancer Center.

Cleeland, C. S. (1987). Nonpharmacological management of cancer pain. *Journal of Pain and Symptom Management, 2*(2), S23–S28.

Copley Cobb, S. (1984). Teaching relaxation techniques to cancer patients. *Cancer Nursing, 7*, 157–161.

Crelin, D., Sullivan, T. P., Babl, F. E., O'Sullivan, R., & Hutchinson, A. (2007). Analysis of the validation of existing behavioral pain and distress scales for use in the procedural setting. *Pediatric Anesthesia, 17*, 720–733.

Chih-Yi Sun, V., Borneman, T., Ferrell, B. R., Piper B., Koczywas, M., Choi, K., et al. (2007). Overcoming barriers to cancer pain management: An institutional change model. *Journal of Pain and Symptom Management, 34*, 359–369.

Chizh, B. A., & Headley, P. M. (2005). NMDA antagonists and neuropathic pain: Multiple drug targets and multiple uses. *Current Pharmaceutical Design, 11*, 2977–2994.

Cleeland, C. E. (1989). Pain control: Public and physicians' attitudes. In C. S. Hill & W. S. Fields (Eds.), *Drug treatment of cancer pain in a drug oriented society. Advances in pain research and therapy* (pp. 81–89). New York: Raven Press.

Cleeland, C.S., Gonin, R., Hatfield, A.K., Edmonson, J. H., Blum, R. H., Stewart, J. A., et al. (1994). Pain and its treatment in outpatients with metastatic cancer. *New England Journal of Medicine, 330*, 592–596.

Compton, P. (1999). Substance abuse. In M. McCaffery & C. Pasero (Eds.), *Pain: Clinical manual* (2nd ed., pp. 428–466). St. Louis, MO: Mosby.

Coyle. N., Adelhardt, J., Foley, K. M., & Portenoy, R. K. (1990). Character of terminal illness in the advanced cancer patient: Pain and other symptoms in the last four weeks of life. *Journal of Pain and Symptom Management, 5*, 83–93.

Coyle, N., Cherny, N. I., & Portenoy, R. K. (1994). Subcutaneous infusions at home. *Oncology, 8*, 21–32.

Coyle, N. (2004). In their own words: Seven advanced cancer patients describe their experience with pain and use of opioid drugs. *Journal of Pain and Symptom Management, 27*, 300–309.

Cruiciani, R. A. (2008). Methadone: To EKG or not to EKG — that is still the question. *Journal Pain and Symptom Management. 36*, 545–552.

Darwish, M., Kirby, M., Robertson, P. Jr., Tracewell, W., & Jiang, J. G. (2007). Absolute and relative bioavailability of fentanyl buccal tablet and oral transmucosal fentanyl citrate. *Journal Clinical Pharmacology, 47*, 343–350.

Darwish, M., Kirby, M., Jiang, J. G, Tracewell, W., & Robertson, P., Jr. (2008). Bioequivalence following buccal and sublingual placement of fentanyl buccal tablet 400 mcg in healthy subjects. *Clinical Drug Investigation, 28*, 1–7.

Dahl, J. L. (1996). Effective pain management in terminal care. *Clinical Geriatric Medicine. 12*, 279–300.

Daut, R. L., Cleeland, C. S., & Flanery, R. C. (1983). Development of the Wisconsin brief pain questionnaire to assess pain in cancer patients and other diseases. *Pain, 1*, 197–210.

Dalton, J. A., & Coyne, P. (2003). Cognitive-behavioral therapy: Tailored to the individual. *Nursing Clinics of North America, 38*, 465–476.

Dalton, J. A., Keefe, F. J., Carlson, J., & Young-blood, R. (2004). Tailoring cognitive-behavioral treatment for cancer pain. *Pain Management Nursing, 5*(1), 3–18.

Datta, S., Everett, C. R., Trescot, A. M., Schultz, D. M., Adlaka, R., Abdi, S., et al. (2007). An updated systematic review of the diagnostic utility of selective nerve root blocks. *Pain Physician, 10*(1), 113–128.

De Conno, F., Panzeri, C., Brunelli, C., Saita, L., & Ripamonti, C. (2003). Palliative care in a national cancer center: Results in 1987 vs. 1993 vs.2000. *Journal of Pain and Symptom Management, 25*, 499–511.

de Leon-Casasola, O. A. (2000). Critical evaluation of chemical neurolysis of the sympathetic axis for cancer pain. *Cancer Control, 7*, 142–148.

De Tran, Q. H., Clemente, A., Doan, J., & Finlayson, R. J. (2007a). Brachial plexus blocks: A review of approaches and techniques. *Canadian Journal of Anesthesia, 54*(8), 662–674.

De Tran, Q. H., Clemente, A., Finlayson, R. J. (2007b). A review of approaches and techniques for lower extremity nerve blocks. *Canadian Journal of Anesthesia, 54* (11), 922–934.

Decker, G. M. (2000). An overview of complementary and alternative therapies. *Clinical Journal of Oncology Nursing, 4*(1), 49–52.

Demmer, C. (2004). A survey of complementary therapy services provided by hospices. *Journal of Palliative Medicine, 7*, 510–516.

Deng, G., Cassileth, B. R., & Simon Yeung, K. (2004). Complementary therapies for cancer-related symptoms. *Supportive Oncology 2*, 419–429.

Deng, G. E., Cassileth, B. R., Cohen, L., Gubilib, J., Johnstone, P. A., Kumar, N., et al. (2007). Society for intergarive oncology executive committee. In D. Abrams, D. Rosenthal, S. Sagar, & D. Tripathy (Eds.), Integrative oncology practice guidelines. *Journal of the Society for Integrative Oncology, 5*(2), 65–84.

Devine, E. C. (2003). Meta-analysis of the effect of psychoeducational interventions on pain in adults with cancer. *Oncology Nursing Forum 30*(1), 75–89.

Dietz, H. (1982). *Rehabilitation oncology*. New York: Wiley.

Dunajcik, L. (1999). Chronic nonmalignant pain. In M. McCaffery & C. Pasero (Eds.), *Pain: Clinical manual* (2nd ed., pp. 467- 521). St. Louis, MO: Mosby.

Eccleston, C., Yorke, S., Morley, S., Williams, A. C., & Mastroyannopoulou, K. (2003). Psychological therapies for the management of chronic and recurrent pain in children and adolescents. *Cochrane Database of Systematic Reviews, 1003* (1), CD003968.

Egan, T. D., Sharma, A., Ashburn, M. A., Kievit, J., Pace, N. L., Streisand, J. B., et al. (2000). Multiple dose pharmacokinetics of oral transmucosal fentanyl citrate in healthy volunteers. *Anesthesiology. 92*, 665–673.

Ehde, D. M., Gibbons, L. E, Chwastiak, L., Bombardier, C. H., Sullivan, M. D., Kraft, G. H., et al. (2003). Chronic pain in a large community sample of persons with multiple sclerosis. *Multiple Sclerosis, 9*, 605–611.

Eland, J. M. (1990). Pain in children. *Nursing Clinics North America, 25*, 469–475.

Elliot, K., & Foley, K. M. (1998). Neurologic pain syndromes in patients with cancer. *Neurologic Clinics, 7*, 333–360.

Etzioni, S., Chodosh, J., Ferrell, B. A., & MacLean, C. H. (2007). Quality indicators for pain management in vulnerable elders. *Journal American Geriatric Society, 55* (Suppl. 2), S403–S408.

Esch, T., Guarna, M., Bianchi, E., Zhu, W., & Stefano, G. B. (2004). Commonalities in the central nervous system's involvement with complementary medical therapies: Limbic morphinergic processes. *Medical Science Monitor, 10*(6), MS6-MS17.

Eskinazi, D., & Muehsam, D. (1999). Is the scientific publishing of complementary and alternative medicine objective? *Journal of Alternative and Complementary Medicine, 5*, 587–594.

Evans, S., & Tsao, J. C. I. (2008). Complementary and alternative medicine for acute procedural pain in children. *Alternative Therapies, 14*(5), 52–56.

Fanning, P. (1988). *Visualization for change.* Oakland, CA: New Harbinger.

Fainsinger, R., Schoeller, T., Boiskin, M., Bruera, E. (1993). Palliative care rounds: Cognitive failure and coma after renal failure in a patient receiving captopril and hydromorphone. *Journal Palliative Care, 9*, 53–55.

Fainsinger, R. L., Waller, A., Bercovici, M., Bengtson, K., Landman, W., Hosking, M., et al. (2000). A multicentre international study of sedation for uncontrolled symptoms in terminally ill patients. *Palliative Medicine, 14*, 257–265.

Farrar, J. T., & Portenoy, R. K. (2001). Neuropathic cancer pain: The role of adjuvant analgesics. *Oncology, 15*, 1435–1442.

Fernandez, E. (1986). A classification system of cognitive coping strategies for pain. *Pain, 26*, 141–151.

Ferrell, B. R., Rhiner, M., Cohen. M. Z., Grant, M. (1991). Pain as a metaphor for illness. Part 1: Impact of pain on family caregivers. *Oncology Nursing Forum, 18*, 1303–1309.

Ferrell, B. R., Grant, M., Chan, J., Ahn, C., & Ferrell, B. A. (1995). The impact of cancer pain education on family caregivers of elderly patients. *Oncology Nursing Forum, 22*, 1211–1218.

Ferrell, B. R., & Ferrell B. A. (1995). Pain in elderly persons. In D. B. McGuire, C. Henke Yarbro, & B. R. Ferrell (Eds.), *Cancer pain management* (2nd ed., pp.273–287). Boston: Jones and Bartlett.

Ferrell, B. A., & Whiteman, J. E. (2003). Pain. In R. S. Morrison & D. E. Mieier (Eds.). *Geriatric palliative care* (pp. 205–229). Oxford: Oxford University Press..

Ferrell, B., Levy, M. H., & Paice, J. (2008). Managing pain from advanced cancer in the palliative care setting. *Clinical Journal Oncology Nursing, 12*, 575–581.

Ferrini, R., & Paice, J. A. (2004). Infusional lidocaine for severe and/or neuropathic pain. *Journal Supportive Oncology, 2*, 90–94.

Field, M. J., & Behrman, R. (Eds.). (2003). When children die: Improving palliative and end of life care for children and their families. *Report of the institute of medicine task force.* Washington DC: National Academy Press.

Fine, P. G. (1999). Low dose ketamine in the management of opioid nonresponsive cancer pain. *Journal Pain and Symptom Management, 17*, 296–300.

Finkel, J. C., Pestieau, S. R., & Quezado, Z. M. (2007). Ketamine as an adjuvant for treatment of cancer pain in children and adolescents. *Pain, 8*, 515–521.

Finns, J. J. (1999). Acts of omission and commission in pain management: the ethics of naloxone use. *Journal of Pain and Symptom Management, 17*, 120–124.

Fishman, B. (1992). The cognitive behavioral perspective of pain management in terminal illness. *Hospice Journal, 8*(1–2), 73–88.

Fishman, B., & Loscalzo, M. (1987). Cognitive-behavioral interventions in management of cancer pain: Principles and applications. *Medical Clinics of North America, 71*, 271–287.

Fishman, B., Pasternak, S., & Wallenstein, S. L. (1987). The memorial pain assessment card. A valid instrument for the evaluation of cancer pain. *Cancer 60*, 1151–1158.

Foley, K. M. (1991) The relationship of pain and symptom management to patients' requests for physician-assisted suicide. *Journal of Pain and Symptom Management, 6*, 289–297.

Foley, K. M. (1993). Changing concept of tolerance to opioids: What the cancer patient has taught us. In C. R. Chapman & K. M. Foley (Eds.). *Current and emerging issues in cancer pain: Research and practice* (pp. 331–350). New York: Raven Press.

Foley, K. M. (1998). Pain assessment and cancer pain syndromes. In D. Doyle, G. W. Hanks & N. MacDonald (Eds). *Oxford textbook of palliative medicine* (2nd ed., pp. 310–331). Oxford, UK: Oxford University Press.

Foley, K. M. (2004). Acute and chronic pain syndromes. In D. Doyle, G. W. Hanks, N. Cherny, & K. Calman (Eds.). *Oxford textbook of palliative medicine* (3rd ed., pp. 298–316). New York: Oxford University Press.

Friebert, S. (2008). Pain management for children with cancer at the end of life: Beginning steps towards a standard of care. *Pediatric Blood Cancer, Dec 5* (Epub ahead of print).

Franck, L. S., Greenberg, C.S., & Stevens, B. (2000). Pain assessment in infants and children.

Gaertner, J., Elsner, F., Pollmann-Dahmen, K., Radbruch, L., & Sabatowski, R. (2004). Electronic pain diary: A randomized crossover study. *Journal of Pain and Symptom Management, 28*, 259–267.

Gagliese, L. (2009). Pain and aging: the emergence of a new subfield of pain research. *The Journal of Pain, 10*(4), 343–353.

Ghai, B., Kaur Makkar, J., & Wig, J. (2008). Postoperative pain assessment in preverbal children and children with cognitive impairmant. *Pediatric Anesthesia, 18*, 462–477.

Giasson, M., & Bouchard, L. (1998). Effect of therapeutic touch on the well-being of persons with terminal cancer. *Journal of Holistic Nursing, 16*, 383–398.

Giordano, J., & Schatman, M. E. (2008). A crisis in chronic pain care: An ethical analysis. Part three: Toward and intergrative, multidisciplinary pain medicine built around the needs of the patient. *Pain Physician, 11*(6), 775–784.

Giller, C. A. (2003). The neurosurgical treatment of pain. *Archives of Neurology, 60*, 1537–1540.

Given, C., Given, B., Rahbar, M., Jeon, S., McCorkle, R., Cimprich, B., et al. (2004). Effect of a cognitive behavioral intervention on reducing symptom severity during chemotherapy. *Journal of Clinical Oncology, 22*, 507–516.

Goldberg, S. (1983). *Clinical neurology made ridiculously simple.* Miami, FL: MedMaster.

Grant, M. M., & Rivera, L. M. (1995). Pain education for nurses, patients, and families. In D. B. McGuire, C. Henke Yarbro, & B. R. Ferrell (Eds.), *Cancer pain management* (2nd ed., pp. 289–319). Boston: Jones and Bartlett Publishers.

Galer, B. S., Coyle, N., & Pasternak, G. W. (1992). Individual variability in the response to different opioids: Report of five cases. *Pain, 49,* 87–91.

Galer, B. S., Rowbotham, M. C., Perander, J., & Friedman, E. (1999). Topical lidocaine patch relieves post herpetic neuralgia more effectively than a vehicle topical patch: Results of an enriched enrollment study. *Pain, 80,* 533–538.

Goldberg, G. R., & Morrison, R. S. (2007). Pain management in hospitalized cancer patients: A systematic review. *Journal of Clinical Oncology, 25,* 1792–1801.

Goldstein, N. E., & Morrison, R. S. (2005). Treatment of pain in older patients. *Critical Review: Oncology Hematology, 54,* 157–64.

Gonzales, G. R., Coyle, N. (1992). Treatment of cancer pain in a former opioid abuser: Fears of the patient and staff and their influence on care. *Journal of Pain and Symptom Management, 7,* 246–249.

Gordon, D. B., Dahl, J. L., Miaskowski, C. et al. (2005). American pain society recommendations for improving the quality of acute and cancer pain management. *Archives Internal Medicine, 165,* 1574–1580.

Gourlay, G. K., Plummer, J. L., Cherry, D. A., & Purser, T. (2001). The reproducibility of bioavailability of oral morphine under fed and fasting conditions. *Journal of Pain and Symptom Management, 6,* 431–436.

Gregoire, M. C., & Frager, G. (2006). Ensuring pain relief for children at the end of life. *Pain Research and Management, 11,* 163–171.

Gunnarsdottir, S., Donovan, H. S., Serlin, R. C., Voge, C., & Ward, S. (2002). Patient-related barriers to pain management: The Barriers Questionnaire 11 (BQ-11). *Pain, 99,* 385–396.

Hadjistavropoulos, T., Herr, K., Turk, D. C., Fine, P. G., Dworkin, R. H., Helme, R., et al. (2007). An interdisciplinary expert consensus statement on assessment of pain in older persons. *Clinical Journal Pain, 23*(Suppl. 1), S1–43.

Hall, E. J., & Sykes, N. P. (2004). Analgesia for patients with advanced disease: I. *Postgraduate Medicine, 80*(941), 148–154.

Hanks, G. W., Conno, F., Cherny, N., Hanna, M., Kalso, E., McQuay, H. J., et al. (2001). Morphine and alternative opioids in cancer pain: The EAPC recommendations. *British Journal Cancer, 84,* 587–593.

Hanks, G. W., Cherny, N. I, & Fallon, M. (2004). Opioid analgesic therapy. In D. Doyle, G. W. Hanks, N. Cherny, & K. Calman (Eds.). *Oxford textbook of palliative medicine* (3rd ed., pp. 316–341). Oxford: Oxford University Press.

Hassenbach, S. J., & Cherney, N. I. (2004). Neurosurgical approaches in palliative medicine. In D. Doyle, G. Hanks, N. Cherney, & K. Calman (Eds.), *Oxford textbook of palliative medicine* (3rd ed., pp. 396–405). New York: Oxford University Press, Inc.

Herman, P. M., Craig, B. M., & Caspi, O. (2005). Is complementary and alternative medicine (CAM) cost-effective? A systematic review. *BMC Complementary and Alternative Medicine, 5*(11), 1–15. Available from http://www.biomedicentral.com/1472–6882/5/11.

Hockenberry, M., & Wilson, D. (2007). *Wong's nursing care of infants and children* (8th ed.), St. Louis, MO: Mosby Elsevier.

Hughes, D., Ladas, E., Rooney, D., & Kelly, K. (2008). Massage therapy as a supportive care intervention for children with cancer. *Oncology Nursing Forum, 35*(3), 431–442.

Hearn, J., & Higginson, I. J. (2003). Cancer pain epidemiology: A systematic review. In E. D. Bruera & R. K. Portenoy (Eds.), *Cancer pain, assessment and management* (pp. 19–37). Cambridge, UK. Cambridge University Press.

Herbert, R. S., Schulz, R., Copeland, V., & Arnold, R. M. (2008). What questions do family caregivers want to discuss with health care providers in order to prepare for the death of a loved one? An ethnographic study of caregivers of patients at end of life. *Journal Palliative Medicine, 11,* 476–83.

Herr, K., Bjoro, K., & Decker, S. (2006). Tools for assessment of pain in non-verbal older adults with dementia: A state of the science review. *Journal Pain and Symptom Management 3,* 170–192.

Herr, K., Coyne, P. J., Key, T., Manworren, R., McCaffery, M., Merkel, S., et al. (2006). Pain assessment in the non-verbal patient: Position statement with clinical practice recommendations. *Pain Management Nursing, 7,* 44.

Hockenberry, M., Wilson, D., Winkelstein, M., & Kline, N. (2003). *Wong's nursing care of infants and children* (7th ed.). St Louis, MO: Mosby.

Hocking, G., & Cousins, M. J. (2003). Ketamine in chronic pain management: An evidence-based review. *Anesthesia Analgesia, 97,* 1730–1739.

Holzer, P. (2008). New approaches in the treatment of opioid-induced constipation. *European Medical review for Pharmacological Sciences,* Aug 12, 12 (Suppl. 1), 119–127.

Hooke, M. C., Grund, E., Quammen, H., Miller, B., McCormick, P., Bostrom, B., et al. (2007). Propofol use in pediatric patients with severe cancer pain at the end of life. *Journal Pediatric Oncology Nursing, 24,*29–34.

Hoppmann, R. A., Peden, J. G., & Ober, S. K. (1991). Central nervous system side effects of nonsteroidal anti- inflammatory drugs: Aseptic meningitis, psychosis, and cognitive dysfunction. *Archives Internal Medicine, 151,* 309–1313.

Houlahan, K. E., Branowicki, P. A., Mack, J. W., Dinning, C., & McCabe, M. (2006). Can end of life care for the pediatric patient suffering with intractable and escalating symptoms be improved? Journal *Pediatric Oncology Nursing, 23,* 45–51

Houde, R. W. (1986). Clinical analgesic studies of hydromorphone. In K. M. Foley & C. E. Inturresi (Eds.). *Advances in pain research and therapy,* Vol. 8 (pp. 129–136).

Hurley, R. W., & Adams, M. C. B. (2009). Sex, gender and pain: An overview of a complex field. *Anesthesia and Analgesia, 107,* 309–317.

Hwang, S. S., Chang, V. T., & Kasimis, B. (2002). Dynamic cancer pain management outcomes: The relationship between pain severity, pain relief, functional interference, satisfaction and global quality of life over time. *Journal Pain and Symptom Management, 23,* 190–200.

Idell, C. S., Grant, M., & Kirk, C. (2007). Alignment of pain reassessment practices and national comprehensive cancer network guidelines. *Oncology Nursing Forum, 34,* 661–671.

Ingham. J., & Coyle, N. (1997). Teamwork in end-of-life care: A nurse-physician perspective on introducing physicians to palliative care concepts. In D. Clarke, J. Hockley, & S. Ahmedzai, (Eds.), *New themes in palliative care* (pp. 255–274). Buckingham: Open University Press.

Institute of Medicine Report. (2008). *Cancer care for the whole person: Meeting psychosocial health needs.* Washington, DC: National Academy Press.

International Association for the Study of Pain. (1979). Pain terms: A list with definitions and usage. *Pain, 6,* 249.

Inturrisi, C. E. (2003). Pharmacology of analgesia: Basic principles. In E. Bruera, & R. K. Portenoy (Eds.), *Cancer pain: Assessment and management* (pp. 111–123). Cambridge: Cambridge University Press.

Jaffe, J. H., & Martin, W. R. (1990). Opioid analgesics and antagonists. In A. G. Gilman, T. W. Rall, A. S. Nies, & P. Taylor (Eds.),

The pharmacological basis of therapeutic (8th ed., pp. 485–521). New York: Permagon Press.

Jacox, A., Carr, D. B., Payne, R., Berde, C. B., Breithart, W., Cain, I. M., et al. (1994). *Management of cancer pain. Clinical Practice Guideline No. 9.* (AHCPR Publication No. 94–0592). Rockville, MD: Agency for HealthCare Policy and Research, U.S. Department of Health and Human Services, Public Health Services.

Janjan, N. (2001). Bone metastasis: Approaches to pain management. *Seminars in Oncology, 28*(4 Suppl. 11), 28–34.

Jenkins, C. A., & Bruera, E. (1998). Nonsteroidal anti-inflammatory drugs as adjuvant analgesics in cancer patients. *Palliative Medicine, 13*, 183–196.

Jeremic, B. (2001). Single fraction external beam radiation therapy in the treatment of localized bone pain. A review. *Journal of Pain and Symptom Management , 22*,1048–1058.

Johnson, E. L., & O'Brien, D. (2009). Integrative therapies in hospice and home health: introduction and adoption. *Home Healthcare Nurse, 27*(2), 75–82.

Joint Commission for Accreditation of Hospital Organizations (JCAHO). (2006). www.jcaho.org (accessed January 4th, 2009).

Jones, K., Fink, R., Hutt, E., Pepper, G., Voijir, C. P., Scott, J., et al. (2004). Improving nursing-home staff knowledge and attitudes about pain. *The Gerontologist, 44*, 469–478.

Jones, K., Fink, R., & Clark, L. (2005). Nursing home resident barriers to effective pain management: Why nursing home residents may not seek pain medication. *Journal of the American Medical Directors Association, 6*, 10–17.

Juni, P., Rutjes, A. W., & Diepp, P. A. (2002). Are selective COX 2 inhibitors superior to traditional nonsteroidal anti-inflammatory drugs? *British Medical Journal, 324*, 1287–1288.

Kaiko, R. F. (1983). Central nervous system excitatory effects of meperidine in cancer patients. *Annals of Neurology, 13*, 180–185.

Keefe, F. J., Ahles, T. A., Porter, L. S., Sutton, L. M., McBride, C. M., Pope, M. S. et al. (2003). The self-efficacy of family caregivers for helping cancer patients to manage pain at end-of-life. *Pain, 102*, 157–162.

Klepstad, P., Borchgrevink, P. C., Dale, O., Zahlsen, K., Aamo, T., Fayers, P, et al. (2003). Routine drug monitoring of serum concentrations of morphine, morphine- 3-glucoronide and morphine - 6-glucoronide do not predict clinical observations in cancer patients. *Palliative Medicine, 17*, 679–687.

Kirsh, K. L., & Passik, S. D. (2006). Palliative care of the terminally ill drug addict. *Cancer Investigation. 24*, 425–431.

Kirsh, K. L., Jass, C., Bennett, D. S., Hagen, J. E., & Passik, S. D. (2007). *Palliative Supportive Care, 5*, 219–26.

Kirsh, K. L., & Smith, H. S. (2008). Special issues for older adults who have pain. *Clinics Geriatric Medicine, 24*, 263–274.

Kotora, J.(1997). Therapeutic touch can augment traditional therapies. *Oncology Nursing Forum, 24*(8), 1329–1330.

Kundu, A., & Berman, B. (2007). Acupuncture for pediatric pain and symptom management. *Pediatric Clinics of North America, 54*, 885–899.

Kwekkeboom, K. L., Hau H., Wanta, B., & Bumpus, M. (2008). Patients' perceptions of the effectiveness of guided imagery and progressive muscle relaxation interventions used for cancer pain. *Complimentary Therapies in Clinical Practice, 14*, 85–194.

Kutner, J. S., Bryant L. L., Beaty L. L., & Fairclough D. L. (2007). Time course and characteristics of symptom distress of quality of life at the end of life. *Journal of Symptom Management, 34*, 227–236.

Kyle, G. (2007). Constipation and palliative care – where are we now? *International Journal Palliative Nursing, 13*, 6–16.

Lasch, K., Greenhill, A., Wilkes, G., Carr, D., Lee, M., & Blanchard, R., et al. (2002). Why study pain? A qualitative analysis of medical and nursing faculty and student's knowledge and attitudes to cancer pain management. *Journal of Palliative Medicine, 5*, 57–71.

Labyak, S. E., & Metzger, B. L. (1997). The effects of effleurage back rub on the physiological components of relaxation: A meta-analysis. *Nursing Research, 46*(1), 59–62.

Latifzai, K., Sites, B. D., & Koval, K. J. (2008). Orthopaedic anesthesia part 2. Common techniques of regional anesthesia in orthopaedics. *Bulletin of the NYU Hospital for Joint Diseases, 66*(4), 306–316.

Layman-Goldstein, M., & Altilio, T. (1993). *Cancer pain: Cognitive and behavioral approacheto cancer pain management-relaxation training* [video script]. New York: Memorial Sloan-Kettering Cancer Center.

Layman-Goldstein, M., & Sakae, M. (2010, in press). Knowing the child before you. In B. R. Ferrell & N. Coyle, (Eds.), *Textbook of palliative nursing* (3rd ed.). New York: Oxford University Press.

Libonate, J., Evans, S., & Tsao, J. C. I. (2008). Efficacy of acupuncture for health conditions in children: A review. *The Scientific World Journal, 8*, 670–682.

Lorenz, K. A., Lynn, J., Dy, S. M., Shugarman L. R., Wilkinson, A, Mularski R. A., et al. (2008). Evidence for improving palliative care at the end of life: A systematic review. *Annals of Internal Medicine, 148*(2), 147–159.

Loscalzo, M. (1996). Psychological approaches to the management of pain in patients with advanced cancer. *Hematology/ Oncology Clinics of North America, 10*, 139–155.

Lundeberg, T., Nordeman, R., & Ottoson, D. (1984). Pain alleviation by vibratory stimulation. *Pain, 20*(1), 25–44.

Larijani, G. E., Goldberg, M. E., Rogers, K. H. (1996). Treatment of opioid-induced pruritus with ondansetron: Report of four patients. *Pharmacotherapy, 16*, 958–960.

Lasch, K. E. (2000). Culture, pain and culturally sensitive pain care. *Pain Management Nurses, 1* (Suppl. 1), 16–22.

Latimer, E. J. (1991). Ethical decision-making in the care of the dying and its application to clinical practice. *Journal of Pain and Symptom Management, 6*, 329–336.

Lee. M. A., Leng, M. E., & Tiernan, E. J. (2001). Retrospective study of the use of hydromorphone in palliative care patients with normal and abnormal urea and creatinine. *Palliative Medicine, 15*, 26–34.

Lipman, A. G., Gauthier, M. E. (1997). Pharmacology of opioid drugs. In R. K. Portenoy & E. Bruera (Eds.), *Topics in palliative care*, Vol. 1 (Sch. 7). New York: Oxford University Press.

Luisser, D., & Portenoy, R. K. (2004). Adjuvant analgesics in pain management. In D. Doyle, G. W. Hanks, N. Cherny, & K. Calman (Eds.), *Oxford textbook of palliative medicine* (3rd ed., pp. 349–377). Oxford, UK: Oxford University Press.

Magil, L. (2001). The use of music to address the suffering in advanced cancer pain. *Journal of Palliative Care, 17*(3),167–172.

Magill, L. (2009). The meaning of the music in palliative care music therapy as perceived by bereaved caregivers of advanced cancer patients. *American Journal of Hospice and Palliative Care, 26*(1), 33–39.

Magill-Levreault, L. (1993). Music therapy in pain and symptom management. *Journal of Palliative Care, 9*(4), 42–48.

Manfredi, P. L., Ribeiro, S. W., & Payne, R. (1996). Inappropriate use of naloxone in cancer patients with pain. *Journal of Pain and Symptom Management, 11*, 131–134.

Manfredi, P. L., & Houde, R. W. (2003). Prescribing methadone, a unique analgesic. *Journal Supportive Oncology, 1*, 216–220.

Mannix, K. A. (2004). Palliation of nausea and vomiting. In D. Doyle, G. W. Hanks, N. Cherny, & K. Calman (Eds.), *Oxford textbook of palliative medicine* (3rd ed., pp. 459–468). Oxford: Oxford University Press.

Mao, J., & Chen, L. L. (2000). Systemic lidocaine for neuropathic pain relief. *Pain, 87,* 7–17.

Martinez, M. J., Roque, M., Alonso-Coelleo, P., Catala, E., Garcia, J. L., Ferrandiz, M., et al. (2003). Calcitonin for metastatic bone pain. *Cochrane Data Base Systematic Review.* CD003223.

Marhofer, P., Greher, M., & Kapral, S. (2005). Ultrasound guidance in regional anaesthesia. *British Journal of Anaesthesiology, 94*(1), 7–17.

Marhofer, P., Sitzwohl, C., Greher, M., & Kapral, S. (2004) Ultrasound guidance for infraclavicular brachial plexus anaesthesia in children. *Anaesthesia, 59*(7), 42–46.

Marhofer, P., & Chan, V. W. (2007). Ultrasound-guided regional anesthesia: Current concepts and future trends. *Anesthesia and Analgesia, 104*(5), 1265–1269.

Mast, D., Meyers, J., & Urbanski, A. (1987a). Relaxation techniques: A self-learning module for nurses: Unit I. *Cancer Nursing, 10,* 141–147.

Mast, D., Meyers, J., & Urbanski, A. (1987b). Relaxation techniques: A self-learning module for nurses: Unit II. *Cancer Nursing, 10,* 217–225.

Mast, D., Meyers, J., & Urbanski, A. (1987c). Relaxation techniques: A self-learning module for nurses: Unit III. *Cancer Nursing, 10,* 279–285.

McCaffery, M., & Wolff, M. (1992). Pain relief using cutaneous modalities, positioning, and movement. *Hospice Journal, 8,* 121–154.

McCaffery, M. (1999). Pain management: Problems and progress. In M. Caffery & C. Pasero (Eds.), *Pain: Clinical manual* (2nd ed., pp. 1–14). St. Louis, MO: Mosby.

McCaffery, M., & Pasero, C. (1999a). *Pain: Clinical manual.* (2nd ed.). St Loius, MO: Mosby.

McCaffery, M., & Pasero, C. (1999b). Practical nondrug approaches to pain. In M. McCaffery & C. Pasero (Eds.), *Pain: Clinical manual* (2nd ed., pp. 399–427). St. Louis, MO: Mosby.

Meehan, T. C. (1998). Therapeutic touch as a nursing intervention. *Journal of Advanced Nursing, 28,* 117–225.

Meek, S. S. (1993). Effects of slow stroke back massage on relaxation in hospice clients. *Image: Journal of Nursing Scholarship, 25*(1), 17–21.

Max, M. B., Lynch, S. A., Muir, J., Shoaf, S. E., Smoller, B., Dubner, R., et al. (1992). Effects of desipramine, amitriptyline, and fluoxetine on pain in diabetic neuropathy. *New England Journal Medicine, 326,* 1250–1256.

Max, M. B., Cleary, J., Ferrell, B. R., Foley, K. M., Payne, R., Shapiro, B., et al. (1997). Treatment of pain at the end of life: A position statement from the American Pain Society. *American Pain Society Bulletin, 7,* 1–3.

Messenger, T., & Roberts, K. T. (1994). The terminally ill: Serenity nursing interventions for hospice clients. *Journal of Gerontological Nursing, 20*(11), 17–22.

Meyerson, B. A. (2001). Neurosurgical approaches to pain treatment. *Acta Anaeshesiologica Scandinavica, 45,* 1108–1113.

Miaskowski, C., Dodd, M., West, C., Schumacher, K., Paul, S.M., Tripathy, D., et al. (2004). Randomized clinical trial of the effectiveness of a self-care intervention to improve cancer pain management. *Journal of Clinical Oncology, 22,* 1713–1720.

Michaels, A. J., & Draganov, P. T. (2007). Endoscopic ultrasonography guided celiac plexus neruolysis and celiac plexus block in the management of pain due to pancreatic cancer and chronic pancreatitis. *World Journal of Gastroenterology, 13*(26), 3575–3580.

Miguel, R. (2000). Interventional treatment of cancer pain: The fourth step in the World Health Organization analgesic ladder? *Cancer Control 7,* 149–156.

Montgomery G. H., Bovbjerg D. H., Schnue J. B., David, D., Goldfarb A., Weltz, C.R., et al. (2007). A randomized clinical trial of a brief hypnosis intervention to control side effects in breast surgery patients. *Journal of the National Cancer Institute, 99*(17), 1304–1312.

Myers, C. D., Walton, T., & Small, B. J. (2008). The value of massage therapy in cancer care. *Hematology/Oncology Clinics of North America, 22,* 649–660.

McCaffery, M., & Pasero, C. (1999). *Pain: Clinical manual* (2nd ed.). St Loius: MO: Mosby.

McDonald, A. A., & Portenoy, R. K. (2006). How to use antidepressants and anticonvulsants as adjuvant analgesics in the treatment of neuropathic pain. *Journal Supportive Oncology, 6,* 43–52

McGuire, D. B. (1995). The multiple dimensions of cancer pain: A framework for assessment and management. In D. B. McGuire, C. H. Yarbro, & B. F. Ferrell (Eds.), *Cancer Pain Management* (2nd ed., pp. 1–17). Boston: Jones and Bartlett.

McNicol, E., Horowicz-Mehler, N., Fisk, R. A., Bennet, K., Gialeli-Goudas, M., Chew, P. W., et al. (2003). Management of opioid side effects in cancer-related and chronic non-cancer pain: A systematic review. *Pain, 4,* 231–256.

McQuay, H. J., & Moore, A. (2004). Non-opioid analgesics. In D. Doyle, G. W. Hanks, N. Cherny, & K. Calman (Eds.), *Oxford textbook of palliative medicine* (3rd ed., pp. 342–349). Oxford, UK: Oxford University Press.

Melzack, R. (1993). The McGill Pain Questionnaire. In R. Melzack (Ed.), *Pain measurement and assessment* (pp. 41–48), New York: Raven Press.

Menten, J., Desmedt, M., Lossignol, D., & Mullie, A. (2002). Longitudinal follow-up of TTS-fentanyl use in patients with cancer-related pain: Results of a compassionate use study with special focus on elderly patients. *Current Medical Research Opinion, 18,* 488–498.

Merskey, H. (1986). Classification of chronic pain: Description of chronic pain syndromes and definition of pain terms. *Pain, 3*(Suppl. 3), S217.

Mercadante, S., Fulfaro, F., & Casuccio, A. (2001). The use of corticosteroids in home palliative care. *Supportive Care Cancer, 9,* 386–389.

Mercadante, S. (2001). The use of anti-inflammatory drugs in cancer pain. *Cancer Treatment Review, 27,* 51–61.

Mercadante, S., Casuccio, A., Fulfaro, F., Groff, L., Boffi, R., Villari, P., et al. (2001). Switching from morphine to methadone to improve analgesia and tolerability in cancer patients: A prospective study. *Journal Clinical Oncology, 19,* 2898–2904.

Meuser, T., Pietruck, C., Radbruch, L., Stute, P., Lehman, K. A., Grond, S., et al. (2001). Symptoms during cancer treatment following WHO guidelines: A longitudinal follow-up study of symptom prevalence, severity, and etiology. *Pain, 93,* 247–257.

Miaskowski, C. (2002). The need to assess multiple symptoms. *Pain Management Nursing, 3,* 115.

Miaskowski, C., Cleary, J., Burney, R., et al. (2005). Guidelines for the management of cancer pain in adults and children. *APS Clinical Practice Guidelines*, Series No. 3. Glenview, Ill.

Morita, T., Ichiki, T., Tsunoda, J., Inoue, S., & Chihara, S. (1998). A prospective study on the dying process in terminal ill cancer patients. *American Journal of Hospice and Palliative Care, 15,* 217–222.

Morrison, R. S., Wallenstein, S., Natale, D. K., Senzel, R. S., & Shuang, L. L. (2000). "We don't carry that" — failure of pharmacies in predominantly non-white neighborhoods to stock opioid analgesics (commentary). *New England Journal of Medicine, 342,* 1023–1026.

Morrison, L. J., Morrison, R. S. (2006). Palliative care and pain management. *Medical Clinics North America, 90,* 983–1004.

Moryl, N., Santiago-Palma, J., Kornick, C., Derby, S., Fishberg, D., Payne, R., et al. (2002). Pitfalls of opioid rotation: Substituting another opioid for methadone in patients with cancer pain. *Pain, 96,* 325–328.

Moryl, N., Coyle, N., & Foley, K. M. (2008). Managing an acute pain crisis in a patient with advanced cancer: "This is as much of a crisis as a code." *Journal of Ameican Medical Association, 26,* 1457–1467

Nagaro, T., Adachi, N., Tabo, E., Kimura, S., Arai, T., Dote, K., et al. (2001). New pain following cordotomy: Clinical features, mechanisms, and clinical importance. *Journal of Neurosurgery, 95,* 425–431.

Nadler, S. F. (2004). Nonpharmacologic management of pain. *The Journal of the American Osteopathic Association, 104*(11 Suppl. 8), S6–S12.

Nagaro, T., Adachi, N., Tabo, E., Kimura, S., Arai, T., Dote, K., et al. (2001). New pain following cordotomy: Clinical features, mechanisms, and clinical importance. *Journal of Neurosurgery, 95,* 425–431.

National Center for Complementary and Alternative Medicine. (2002). *The use of complementary and alternative medicine in the United States.* http://nccam.nih.gov/news/camsurvey fsl.htm.

National Comprehensive Cancer Network. (2009). NCCN clinical practice guidelines in oncology: Adult cancer pain, Version 1. 2009. Retrieved from http://www.nccn.org on April 22, 2009.

National Comprehensive Cancer Network. (2007). *NCCN Clinical practice guidelines in oncology: Pediatric cancer pain, Version 1.* Retrieved from http://www.nccn. org on April 22, 2009.

National Institutes of Health Technology Assessment Panel on Integration of Behavioral and Relaxation Approaches into the Treatment of Chronic Pain and Insomnia. (1996). Integration of behavioral and relaxation approaches into the treatment of chronic pain and insomnia. *Journal of the American Medical Association, 276,* 313- 318.

National Institutes of Health Consensus Conference. (1998). Acupuncture. *Journal of the American Medical Association, 280,* 1518–1524.

Nayak, S., Wenstone, R., Jones, A., Nolan, J., Strong, A., Carson, J., et al. (2008). Surface electrostimulation of acupuncture points for sedation of critically ill patients in the intensive care unit–a pilot study. *Acupuncture Medicine, 26*(1), 1–7.

National Cooperative Cancer Network. (2008). *NCCN clinical practice guidelines in oncology: Adult cancer pain, Version 2.* 2008.

National Quality Forum. (2006). *A national framework and preferred practices for palliative and hospice care quality.* www.qualityforum.org/publications/reports/palliative.asp

National Institute of Health. (2002). State-of-the-science statement on symptom management in cancer: Pain, depression, and fatigue. *NIH Consensus State-of-the: Science Statements,* 1–29.

Ng, K., & von Gunten, C. F. (1998). Symptoms and attitudes of 100 consecutive patients admitted to an acute hospital/palliative care unit. *Journal of Pain and Symptom Management, 16,* 307–316.

O'Brien, S., Dalton, J. A., Konsler, G., & Carlson, J. (1996). The knowledge and attitude of experienced oncology nurses regarding the management of cancer-related pain. *Oncology Nursing Forum, 23,* 515–521.

Oncology Nursing Society Position Paper on Cancer Pain Management -Revised. (2006). http://www.ons.org/publications/positions/Cancer.

Oliver, J. W., Kravitz, R. L., Kaplan, S. H., & Meyers, F. J. (2001). Individualized patient education and coaching to improve pain control among cancer patients. *Journal of Clinical Oncology, 19,* 2206–2212.

Olson, K., Hanson, J., & Michaud, M. (2003). A phase II trial of Reiki for the management of pain in advanced cancer patients. *Journal of Pain and Symptom Management,*(26), 990–997.

Owens, M. K., & Ehrenreich, D. (1991a). Literature review of nonphamacologic methods for the treatment of chronic pain. *Holistic Nursing Practice, 6*(1), 24–31.

Owens, M. K., & Ehrenreich, D. (1991b). Application of nonphamacologic methods of managing chronic pain. *Holistic Nursing Practice, 6*(1), 32–40.

Passik, S. D., & Portenoy, R. K. (1998). Substance abuse issues in palliative care. In A. Berger, , R. K. Portenoy, & D. E. Weisman (Eds.), *Principles and practice of supportive oncology* (2nd ed., pp. 513–529). Philadelphia: Lippincott-Raven.

Passik, S. D., & Kirsh, K. L. (2004). Opioid therapy in patients with a history of drug abuse. *CNS Drugs, 18*(1), 13–25.

Passik, S. D., Kirsh, K. L., Donaghy, K. B., & Portenoy, R. K. (2006). Pain and aberrant drug behaviors in medically ill patients with and without histories of substance abuse. *Clinical Journal of Pain, 22,* 173–178.

Passik, S. D., Byers, K., & Kirsh, K. L. (2007). Empathy and the failure to treat pain. *Palliative Supportive Care. 5,* 167–162.

Passik, S. D., & Kirsh, K. L. (2008). The interface between pain and drug abuse and the evolution of strategies to optimize pain management while minimizing drug abuse. *Experimental Clinical Psychopharmacology, 16,* 400–404

Payne, R., Chandler, S. W., & Einhaus, E. (1995). Guidelines for the clinical use of transdermal fentanyl. *Anti-Cancer Drugs, 6,* 50–53.

Payne, R., Coluzzi, P., Simmonds, M., Lyss, A., Rauk, R., et al. (2001). Long-term safety of oral transmucosal fentanyl citrate for breakthrough cancer pain. *Journal Pain Symptom Management, 22,* 575–583.

Payne, R., & Gonzales, R., G. (2004). Pathophysiology of pain in cancer and other terminal diseases, In D. Doyle, G. W. Hanks, & N. Cherny (Eds.), *Oxford textbook of palliative medicine* (3rd ed., pp. 288–298). Oxford: Oxford University Press.

Perez, S., Rodriguez, L. A., Raiford, D. S., Duque, A., & Ris, R. J. (1996). Nonsteroidal inflammatory drugs and the risk of hospitalization for acute renal failure. (comment). *Archives Internal Medicine, 156,* 2433–2439.

Peterson, W. L., & Cryer, B. (2002). COX-1-sparing NSAIDs: Is the enthusiasm justified? *Journal of American Medical Association, 282,* 1961–1963.

Portenoy, R. K., & Hagen, N. A. (1990). Breakthrough pain: Definition, prevalence and characteristics. *Pain, 41,* 273.

Portenoy, R. K., Thaler, H. T., Kornblith, A. B., Lepore, J. M., Friedlander, K. H., Coyle, N., et al. (1994). Symptom prevalence, characteristics and distress in a cancer population. *Quality of Life Research, 3,* 183–189.

Portenoy, R. K. (1994). Management of common opioid side effects during long term therapy for pain. *Annals of Academy of Medicine Singapore, 23,*160–170.

Porter, J., Jick, H. (1980). Addiction rare in patients treated with narcotics (letter to the editor). *New England Journal of Medicine, 302,* 123.

Posner, J. (1995). Neurological complications of cancer. Philadelphia:Davis

Potter, V. T., Wiseman, C. E., Dunn, S. M., & Boyle, F. M. (2003). Patient barriers to optimal pain control. *Psychooncology, 12,* 153–160.

Radbruch, L., Sabatowski, R., Petzke, F., Brunsch-Radbruch, A., Grond, S., Lehmann, K. A., et al. (2001). Transdermal fentanyl for the management of can pain: A survey of 1005 patients. *Palliative Medicine, 15,* 309–321.

Rhodes, R. L., Mitchell, S. L., Miller, S. C., Connor, S. R., & Teno, J. M. (2008). *Journal Pain and Symptom Management, 35,* 365–371.

Rheingans, J. I. (2007). A systematic review of nonpharmacologic adjunctive therapies for symptom management in children with cancer. *Journal of Pediatric Hematology/Oncology Nurses, 24*(2), 81–94.

Rhiner, M., Ferrell, B. R., Ferrell, B. A., & Grant, M. M. (1993). A structured non-drug intervention program for cancer pain. *Cancer Practice, 1,* 137–143.

Richardson, J., Smith, J. E., McCall, G., & Pilkington, K. (2006). Hypnosis for procedure-related pina and distress in pediatric cancer patients: A systematic review of effectiveness and methodology related to hypnosis interventions. *Journal of Pain and Symptom Management, 31*(1), 70–84.

Robb, K. A., Bennett, M. I., Johnson, M. I., Simpson, K. J., & Oxberry, S. G. (2008). Transcutaneous electrical nerve stimulation (TENS) for cancer-related pain in adults. *Cochrane Database of Systematic Reviews,* (3). Art. No.: CD006276. doi: 10.1002/12651858.CD006276.pub2.

Rosa, L., Rosa, E., Sarner, L., & Barrett, S. (1998). A close look at therapeutic touch. *Journal of the American Medical Association, 279,* 1005–1010.

Ripamonti, C. (2003). Pharmacology of opioid analgesia: Clinical principles. In E. Bruera, & R. K. Portenoy (Eds.), *Cancer pain: Assessment and management* (pp. 124–149). Cambridge: Cambridge University Press.

Saunders, C. M. (1967). *The management of terminal illness.* London: Hospital Medicine.

Saberski, L. R. (1998). Interventional approaches in oncologic pain management. In A. Berger, R. K. Portenoy, & D. E. Weissman (Eds.), *Principles and practice of supportive oncology* (pp. 93–107). Philadelphia: Lippincott-Raven.

Sagar, S. M., Dryden, R., & Myers, C. (2007). Research on therapeutic massage for cancer patients: Potential biologic mechanisms. *Journal of the Society for Integrative Oncology, 5*(4), 155–162.

Sanders, M., & Zuurmond, W. (1995). Safety of unilateral and bilateral percutaneous cervical cordotomy in 80 terminally ill cancer patients. *Journal of Clinical Oncology, 13,* 1509–1512.

Saroyan, J., Schechter, W., Tresgallo, M., & Granowetter, L. (2005). Role of intraspinal analgesia in terminal pediatric malignancy. *Journal of Clinical Oncology, 23*(6), 1318–1321

Savage, S. R., Kirsh, K. L., & Passik, S. D. (2008). Challenges in using opioids to treat pain in persons with substance abuse disorders. *Addiction Science and Clinical Practice, 4,* 4–25.

Schaffer, S. D., & Yucha, C. B. (2004). Relaxation and pain management: The relaxation response can play a role in managing chronic and acute pain. *American Journal of Nursing, 104*(8), 75–82.

Schroeder, M. E. (1986). Neurolytic nerve block for cancer pain. *Journal of Pain and Symptom Management, 1*(2), 91–94.

Schroeder-Sheker, T. (1994). Music for the dying: A personal account of the new field of music thanatology history, theories, and clinical narratives. *Journal of Holistic Nursing, 12*(1), 83–99.

Schumacher, K. L., Koresawa, S., West, C., Dodd, M., Paul, S. M., Tripathy, D., et al. (2002a). The usefulness of a daily pain management diary for outpatients with cancer-related pain. *Oncology Nursing Forum, 29,* 1304–1313.

Schumacher, K. L., Koresawa, S., West, C., Hawkins, C., Johnson, D., Wais, E., et al. (2002b). Putting cancer pain management regimens into practice at home. *Journal of Pain and Symptom Management, 23,* 369–382.

Schechter, N. L., Berde, C., & Yaster, M. (2003). *Pain in infants, children, and adolescents* (2nd ed.). Philadelphia: Lippincott, Williams & Wilkins.

Schiodt, F. V., Rochling, F. A., Casey, D. L., &, Lee, W. M. (1997). Acetaminophen toxicity in an urban country hospital. *New England Journal Medicine, 337,* 1112–1117

Schug, S. A., Zech, D., Grond, S., Jung, H., Meuser, T., Stobbe, B., et al. (1992). A long-term survey of morphine in cancer pain patients. *Journal of Pain and Symptom Management, 7,* 259–266.

Sciuto, R., Festa, A., Pasqualoni, R., Semprebene, A., Rea, S., Bergomi, S., et al. (2001). Metastatic bone pain palliation with 89-Sr and 186-Re-HEDP in breast cancer. *Breast Cancer Research, 66,* 101–109.

Serlin, R. C., Mendoza, T. R., Nakamura, Y., Edward, K. R., & Cleeland, C. S. (1995). When is cancer pain mild, moderate or severe? Grading pain severity by its interference with function. *Journal Pain, 61,* 277–284.

Serafani, A. N. (2000). Samarium Sm-153 lexidronam for the palliation of bone pain associated with metastasis. *Cancer, 88* (Suppl. 12), 2934–2939.

Shaiova, L., Sperber, K. T., & Hord, E. D. (2002). Methadone for refractory cancer pain. *Journal Pain and Symptom Management, 23,* 178–180.

Shaiova, L., Rim, F., Friedman, D., & Jahdi, M. (2007). A review of methylnaltrexone, a peripheral opioid receptor antagonist, and its role in opioid-induced constipation. *Palliative Supportive Care, 5,* 161–166.

Sibinger, N. E., & Goldstein, A. (1988). Opioid peptides and opioid receptors in cells of the immune system. *Annual review of Immunology, 6,* 219–249.

Smith, M. T. (2000). Neuroexcitatory effects of morphine and hydromorphone: Evidence implicating the 3-glucoronide metabolites. *Clinical and Experimental Pharmacology and Physiology, 27,* 524–528.

Smith, M. C., Kemp, J., Hemphil, L., & Vojir, C. P. (2002). Outcomes of therapeutic massage for hospitalized cancer patients. *Journal of Nursing Scholarship, 34,* 257–262.

So, P. S., Jiang, Y., & Qin, Y. (2008). Touch therapies for pain relief in adults. *Cochrane Database Systematic Reviews,* (4), CD006535.

Spross, J. A., & Wolff Burke, M. (1995). Nonpharmacological management of cancer pain. In D. B. McGuire, C. H. Yarbro, & B. R. Ferrell (Eds.), *Cancer pain management* (2nd ed., pp. 159–205). Boston: Jones and Bartlett.

Standish, L. J., Kozak, L., & Congdon, S. (2008). Acupuncture is underutilized in hospice and palliative medicine. *American Journal of Hospice and Palliative Medicine, 25*(4), 298–308.

Stedman, T. L. (1995). *Stedman's medical dictionary* (26th ed.). Baltimore: Williams & Wilkins.

Stephens, R. L. (1993). Imagery: A strategic intervention to empower clients part II—A practical guide. *Clinical Nurse Specialist, 7,* 235–240.

Swarm, R. A., & Cousins, M. J. (1998). An-aesthetic techniques for pain control. In D. Doyle, G. W. C. Hanks, & N. MacDonald (Eds.), *Oxford textbook of palliative medicine* (2nd ed., pp. 390–414). Oxford, UK: Oxford University Press.

Syrjala, K. L., Donaldson, G. W., Davis, M. W., Kippes, M. E., & Carr, J. E. (1995). Relaxation and imagery and cognitive-behavioral training reduce pain during cancer treatment: A controlled clinical trial. *Pain, 63,* 189–198.

Stein, C. (1995). The control of pain in peripheral tissues with opioids. *New England Journal of Medicine, 332,* 1685–1690.

Streisand, J., Busch, M. A., Egan, T. D., Gaylord Smith, B., Gay, M., Pace, N. L., et al. (1998). Dose proportionality and pharmacokinetics of oral transmucosal fentanyl citrate. *Anesthesiology, 88,* 305–309.

SUPPORT. (1995). A controlled trial to improve care for seriously ill hospitalized patients. *Journal of the American Medical Association, 274,* 1591–1598.

Swarm, R. A., Karanikolas, M., & Cousins M. J. (2004). Anesthetic techniques for pain control. In D. Doyle, G. W. Hanks, N. Cherny,

& K. Calman (Eds.), *Oxford textbook of palliative medicine.* (3rd ed., pp. 278–396). Oxford, UK: Oxford University Press.

Swica, Y., & Breitbart, W. (2002). Treating pain in patients with AIDS and a history of substance abuse. *Western Journal of Medicine, 176*, 33–39

Sykes, N., & Thorns, A. (2003a). Sedative use in the last week of life and the implications for end-of-life decision making. *Archives Internal Medicine, 163*, 341–344.

Sykes, N., & Thorns, A. (2003b). The use of opioids and sedatives at end-of-life. *Lancet Oncology, 4,*312–318.

Sykes, N. (2004). Constipation and diarrhea. In D. Doyle, G. W. Hanks, N. Cherny, & K. Calman (Eds.), *Oxford textbook of palliative medicine* (3rd ed., pp 483–490). Oxford, UK: Oxford University Press.

Szeto, H. H., Inturresi, C. E., Houde, R., Saal, R., Cheigh, J., Reidenberg, M. M., et al. (1977). Accumulation of normeperidine an active metabolite of meperidine, in patients with renal failure or cancer. *Annals of Internal Medicine, 86*, 738–741.

Tanaka, E., Yamazaki, K., & Misawa, S. (2000). Update: the clinical importance of acetaminophen hepatoxicity in non-alcoholic and alcoholic subjects. *Journal of Clinical Pharmacy and Therapeutics, 25*, 325–332

Tarzian, A., & Hoffmann, D. (2004). Barriers to managing pain in the nursing home: Findings from a statewide survey. *Journal of the American Medical Directors Association, 5*, 82–88.

Taylor, E. J., Ferrell, B. R., Grant, M., & Cheyney, L. (1993). Managing cancer pain in the home: The decisions and ethical conflicts of patients, family caregivers and homecare nurses. *Oncology Nursing Forum, 12*, 919–927.

Taylor, E. J., & Herr, K. (2003). Pain intensity assessment: A comparison of selected pain intensity scales for use in cognitively intact and cognitively impaired African American older adults. *Pain Management Nursing, 4*, 87–95.

Taylor, L. J., Harris, J., Epps, C. D., & Herr, K. (2005). Psychometric evaluation of selected pain intensity scales for use with cognitively impaired and cognitively intact older adults. *Rehabilitation Nursing, 30*, 55–61.

Teno, J. M., Kabumoto, G, Wetle, T., Roy J., & Mor, V. (2004). Daily pain that was excruciating at some time 8in the previous week: Prevalence, characteristic, and outcomes in nursing home residents. *Journal American Geriatric Society, 52*, 762–767

Thomas, J. R., Cooney, G. A., & Slatkin, N. E. (2008). Palliative care and pain: New strategies for managing opioid bowel dysfunction. *Journal Palliative Medicine, Sept 11*, (Suppl. 1), S1–S19– S21–S22.

Thomas, E. M., & Weiss, S. M. (2000). Nonpharmacological interventions with chronic cancer pain in adults. *Cancer Control, 7*, 157–164.

Thompson, J. W., & Filshie, J. (1998). Trans-cutaneous electrical nerve stimulation (TENS) and acupuncture. In D. Doyle, G. W. C. Hanks, & N. MacDonald (Eds.), *Oxford textbook of palliative medicine* (2nd ed., pp. 421–437). Oxford, UK: Oxford University Press.

Tsue, B., & Berde, C. (2005). Caudal analgesia and anesthesia techniques in children. *Current Opinions in Anesthesiology, 18*, 283–288.

Tuls Halstead, M., & Tuls Roscoe, S. (2002). Restoring the spirit at the end of life: Music as an intervention for oncology nurses. *Clinical Journal of Oncology Nursing, 6*, 332–336.

Tunkel, R. S., & Lachmann, E. A. (1998). Rehabilitative medicine. In A. Berger, R. K. Portenoy, & D. E. Weissman (Eds.), *Principles and practice of supportive oncology* (pp. 681–690). Philadelphia: Lippincott-Raven.

Tyler, D. O., Winslow, E. H., Clark, A. P., & White, K. M. (1990). Effects of a 1 minute back rub on mixed venous oxygen satu-ration and heart rate in critically ill patients. *Heart Lung, 19*, 562–565.

Twycross, R., & Lichter, I. (1998). The terminal phase. In D. Doyle, G. W. Hanks, & N. MacDonald (Eds.). *Oxford textbook of palliative medicine* (2nd ed., pp. 984–992). Oxford UK: Oxford University Press.

Twycross, R., & Wilcock, A. (2001). *Symptom management in advanced cancer* (3rd ed.). Oxford, UK: Radcliffe Medical Press.

Umans, J. G., & Inturresi, C. E. (1982). Antinociceptive activity and toxicity of meperidine and normeperidine in mice. *Journal of Pharmacology and Experimental Therapeutics, 223*, 203–206.

Vallerand, A. H., Collins-Bohler, D., Templin, T., & Hasenau, S. (2007). Knowledge of and barriers to pain management in caregivers of cancer patients receiving homecare. *Cancer Nursing, 30*, 31–37.

Van den Beuken-van, M. H., de Rijke, J. M., Kessels, A. G., Schouten, H. C., van Kleef, M., Patijn, J., et al. (2007). Prevalence of pain in patients with cancer. A systematic review of the past 40 years. *Annals of Oncology,18,*1437–1449.

Vane, J. R., Botting, R. M. (2008). Anti-inflammatory drugs and their mechanism of action. *Inflammation Research, 47* (Suppl. 2), S78–S87.

von Baeyer, C. L., & Spagrud, L. J. (2007). Systematic review of observational (behavioral) measures of pain for children and adloescents aged 3 to 18 years. *Pain, 127*, 140–150.

Vitale, A. (2007). An integrative review of Reiki touch therapy research. *Holistic Nursing Practice, 21*(4), 167–179.

Wells, N., Hepworth, J. T., Murphy, B. A., Wujcik, D., & Johnson, R. (2003). Improving cancer pain management through patient and family education. *Journal of Pain and Symptom Management, 25*, 344–356.

Von Roenn, J. H., Cleeland, C. S., Gonin, R., Hatfield, A. K., & Pandya, K. J. (1993). Physician attitude and practice in cancer pain management. A survey from the Eastern cooperative oncology group. *Annals of Internal Medicine, 119*, 121–126.

Walker, K., Medhurst, S. J., Kidd, B. L., Glatt, M., Bowes, M., Patel, S., et al., (2002). Disease modifying and antinociceptive effects of the bisphosphonate, zoledronic acid in a model of bone cancer pain. *Journal Pain, 100*, 219–229.

Wallenstein, S. L., Rogers, A. G., Kaiko, R. F., & Houde, R. W. (1986). Crossover trials in analgesic assays: studies of buprenorphine and morphine. *Pharmacotherapy, 6*, 228–235.

Walsh, T. D., (1990). Prevention of opioid side effects. *Journal of Pain and Symptom Management, 5*, 363–367.

Ward, S. E., Miller-McCauley, V., Mueller, C., Nolan, A., Pawlik-Plank, D., et al. (1993). Patient related barriers to management of cancer pain. *Pain, 52*, 319–324.

Ward, S. E., Berry, P. E., & Misiewicz, H. (1996). Concerns about analgesics among patients and family caregivers in a hospice setting. *Research Nursing Health, 19*, 205–211.

Ward, S. E., Wells, N. (2000). Pain intensity and pain interference in hospitalized patients with cancer. *Oncology Nursing Forum, 27*, 985–991

Watanabe, S., Tarumi, Y., Oneschuk, D., & Lawlor, P. (2002). Opioid rotation to methadone: Proceed with caution. *Journal Clinical Oncology, 20*, 2409–2410.

Webster, L., Andrews, M., & Stoddard, G. (2003). Modafinil treatment for opioid-induced sedation. *Pain Medicine, 4*, 135–140.

Weiner, D. K., & Rudy, T. E. (2002). Attitudinal barriers to effective treatment of persistent pain in nursing home residents. *Journal American Geriatric Society, 50*, 2035–2040.

West, C. M., Dodd, M. J., Paul, S. M., Schumacher, K., Tripathy, D., Koo, P., et al. (2003). The PRO-SELF©: pain control program: An effective approach for cancer pain management. *Oncology Nursing Forum, 30*(1), 65–73.

Wiffen, P. J., & Eccleston, C. (2009). The Cochrane pain, palliative and supportive care group: And update. *Palliative Medicine, 23*(2),179–180.

Winstead-Fry, P., & Kijek, J. (1999). An integrative review and meta-analysis of therapeutic touch research. *Alternative Therapies in Health Medicine, 5*(6), 58–67.

Wells, N., Hepworth, J. T., Murphy, B. A., Wujcik, D., & Johnson, R. (2003). Improving cancer pain management through patient and family education. *Journal of Pain and Symptom Management, 25,* 344–356.

Wein, S. (2000). Sedation in the imminently dying patient. *Oncology, 14,* 585–592.

Weinstein, S. M., Laux, L. F., Thornby, J. L., Lorimor, R. J., Hill, C. S., Thorpe, D. M. et al. (2000). Physicians' attitudes towards pain and the use of opioid analgesics: Results of a survey from the Texas cancer pain initiative. *Southern Medical Journal, 93,* 479–487.

Weissman, D. E., Burchman, S. L., Dinndorf, P., & Dahl, J. L. (1990). *Handbook of cancer pain management* (2nd ed.). Milwaukee: Wisconsin Pain Initiative.

Wilson, J. A., Garry, E. M., Anderson, H. A., Rosie, R., Colvin, L. A., Mitchell. R.,et al. (2005). NMDA receptor antagonist treatment at the time of nerve injury prevents injury-induced changes in the spinal NR1 and NR2B subunit expression and increases the sensitivity of residual pain behaviors to subsequently administered NMDA receptor antagonists. *Journal Pain, 117,* 421–432.

Wolfe, J., Hammel, J. F., Edwards, K. E., Duncan, J., Comeau, M., Breyer, J., et al. (2008). Easing of suffering in children with cancer at the end of life: is care changing? *Journal Clinical Oncololgy, 26,* 1717–1723.

Wong, D. L., & Baker, C. (1995). *Reference manual for the Wong-Baker FACES pain rating scale.* Tulsa, OK: Wong and Baker.

Wong, D. L, Hockenberry-Eaton, M., Wilson, D., Sinkelstein, M. L., & Schwartz, P. (2001).

Wong, R., & Wiffen, P. J. (2002). Bisphosphonates for the relief of pain secondary to bone metastasis. Cochrane Database Systematic Review, CD002068. *Wong's Essentials of Pediatric Nursing* (6th ed., p. 1301). St. Louis, MO: Mosby, Inc.

Wooldridge, J. E., Anderson, C. M., & Perry, M. C. (2001). Corticosteroids in advanced cancer. *Oncology, 15,* 225–1234; discussion 234–236.

World Health Organization (WHO). (1986). Cancer pain relief and palliative care. *Report of a World Health Organization (WHO). Expert Committee (WHO Technical Report Series, No 804).* Geneva, Switzerland: World Health Organization.

Wright, A. W., Mather, L. E., & Smith, M. T. (2001). Hydromorphone-3-glucoronide: A more potent neuro-excitant than its structural analogue, morphine – 3- glucoronide. *Life Science, 69,* 409–420.

Yegul, I., & Erhan, E. (2003). Bilateral CT-guided percutaneous cordotomy for cancer pain relief. *Clinical Radiology, 58,* 886–889.

20

Dyspnea

Cindy R. Balkstra

Key Points

- Dyspnea is a multidimensional symptom and assessment based on the patient's report.
- Assess dyspnea with an appropriate tool.
- Treatment should be aimed at the underlying cause(s) of the dyspnea when possible.
- Pharmacological mainstays in the management of dyspnea are opioids and anxiolytics.
- Complementary and behavioral therapies should be considered and offered to the patient in addition to pharmacological treatment.

Case Study: I first met Sam on the unit one Wednesday evening; he was 68 years old and retired from the military. He struggled with the symptoms of emphysema, a result of smoking 2 packs per day for nearly 50 years, although he had been smoke-free for the last 7 years. He also had severe rheumatoid arthritis that crippled his extremities and caused a condition known as rheumatoid lung that resulted in having both restrictive and obstructive lung disorders simultaneously. It was not surprising that Sam was huffing and puffing at rest. Initially, I assessed his level of understanding of his disease. He was fairly knowledgeable, but admitted he often denied the severity of his illness, causing him to avoid follow-up physician visits and to ignore his symptoms.

Finally, when he could not deny them any longer, he sought assistance, this hospitalization the result of such action. He spoke of how scary it was for him; he had been in intensive care for 2 weeks without much improvement. His poor condition upon arrival set the stage for a long uphill climb to recovery. He agreed that in the future early recognition and acknowledgment of his symptoms would be necessary to maintain his health. We reviewed the signs and symptoms of worsening chronic obstructive pulmonary disease (COPD) that would be a reason to consult with the doctor. Over the weeks that I continued to work with Sam and his wife a positive relationship developed. Sam typically welcomed me with a "play by play" account of his day. However, he grew depressed at his lack of progress on the sub-acute unit. He easily tired and remained extremely short of breath, rating his dyspnea an 8/10 with even slight activity. It varied between 6 at rest and 10 with physical exertion.

Muscle atrophy of his lower extremities caused weakness that made it even more difficult for him to meet the demands of physical therapy. Pursed lip breathing helped, but this was sometimes not enough. Energy conservation measures became essential; an occupational therapist worked with him daily to teach various techniques that allowed him to breathe more easily while performing activities of daily living. Anxiolytic agents and an antidepressant were added to combat the psychological effects of his illness, namely anxiety and depression. On the weekends, pet therapy was ordered to help lift his spirits. His wife, the primary support for him at home, was encouraged to make frequent visits.

DYSPNEA

According to the American Thoracic Society 1999 Consensus Statement, dyspnea is "a subjective experience of breathing discomfort that consists of qualitatively distinct sensations that vary in intensity (Author, 1999). The experience derives from interactions among multiple physiological, psychological, social, and environmental factors, and may induce secondary physiological and behavioral responses" (p. 1). In general, the definition of dyspnea is the sensation of difficulty breathing including the person's reaction to that sensation. Dyspnea can be acute, chronic, or terminal (Spector & Klein, 2002).

Acute dyspnea consists of high intensity, time-limited shortness of breath that occurs as an immediate response to an acute physiological or psychological event, seen in such conditions as myocardial infarction, pulmonary emboli, or with hyperventilation from an excitatory state. Chronic dyspnea is persistent shortness of breath of variable intensity, usually seen in chronic conditions, such as COPD or congestive heart failure (CHF). Terminal dyspnea occurs in people with end-stage diseases and is one of the most common symptoms reported in the last 48 h of life (Hall, Schroder, & Weaver, 2002). However, it is important to note that the etiology of dyspnea often changes over the course of an illness requiring different treatment approaches (Selecky et al., 2005). Common descriptions of dyspnea include air hunger, choking, congestion, tightness, and strangling as well as emotional responses such as panic, fear, worry, and frustration (Elia & Thomas, 2008; Schwartzstein, 1999).

Incidence

Dyspnea is a frequent and devastating symptom that occurs in as many as 94% of patients with advanced diseases, primarily those with lung cancer and end-stage heart or lung disease (Bruera, Macmillian, Pither, & MacDonald, 1990; Charles, Reymond, & Israel, 2008; Dudgeon, Kristjanson, Sloan, Lertzman, & Clement, 2001; Edmonds, Karlsen, Khan, & Addington-Hall, 2001). However, 24% of terminal patients participating in the National Hospice Study reported dyspnea despite the absence of pulmonary or cardiac disease (Reuben & Mor, 1986). In fact, dyspnea occurs in greater than 50% of individuals with breast, lymphoma, genitourinary and head/neck cancers (Dudgeon et al., 2001). Moreover, 41% of patients in palliative care experience dyspnea and 46% of those describe the severity as moderate to severe (Charles et al., 2008; Cleary & Carbone, 1997; Currow, 2008). Dyspnea can seriously affect the quality of life in those who experience it and may limit activity to the extent that even the slightest exertion may precipitate breathlessness. For example, eating may cause significant respiratory distress which will impact an individual's nutritional state as well as mobility and functional status.

In the terminal phase of the illness, fear of suffocation may be experienced. The frequency and severity of dyspnea often increases with progression of disease and/or when death is approaching. Other contributing factors include a history of or current smoking, environmental exposures, radiation treatment, Karnofsky < 40, anxiety, fatigue, and vital capacity or maximal inspiratory pressure < 80% predicted (Bruera, Schmitz, Pither, Neumann, & Hanson, 2000; Dudgeon et al., 2001). In advanced cancer patients dyspnea is considered a prognostic indicator of decreased survival time, whether alone or in association with other symptoms and/or performance status (Ben-Aharon, Gafter-Gvili, Paul, Leibovici, & Stemmer, 2008; Maltoni et al., 1995). Mercadante, Casuccio, and Fulfaro (2000) reported that advanced cancer patients treated at home experienced worsening dyspnea with advancing disease, peaking in the last week of life (Mercadante et al., 2000). This correlated with a reduction in performance status and a survival range of 4–6 days.

Mechanisms

Although the mechanisms of dyspnea are complex and not well understood, it may help to review the control of respiration. The respiratory center in the medulla activates the muscles that expand the chest wall, inflates the lungs, and produces ventilation. The process of breathing regulates the oxygen and carbon dioxide balance and hydrogen ion concentration in the blood and body tissues. The automatic regulation of breathing is controlled by chemoreceptor in the blood and brain. Changes in PCO_2 and PO_2 are sensed by central chemoreceptors in the medulla and peripheral chemoreceptors in the carotid and aortic bodies, which send feedback to the brainstem respiratory centers to adjust breathing to maintain blood-gas and acid–base homeostasis (Author, 1999). All the input returned to the brain from body sensors contributes in some fashion to the individual's perception of dyspnea.

While several physiologic mechanisms remain under investigation, three are recognized as dominant and interrelated in the creation of the dyspneic sensation. 1) A conscious awareness of the neuromotor command to the respiratory muscles, e.g., an increased sense of effort experienced with aging, malnutrition, deconditioning, and hypoxemia. 2) Stimulation of the receptors in the airways, lungs and chest wall, which detect changes in lung volume, stretch, and pressure. For example, the sensation of respiratory muscle abnormalities, such as those found in neuromuscular conditions and respiratory muscle fatigue, as well as diseases that inhibit normal airflow and ventilation, such as COPD, asthma, and pulmonary fibrosis. Lastly, is the stimulation of the chemoreceptors, e.g. the sensation of blood gas abnormalities, such as hypoxia and hypercapnia, that indirectly trigger ventilation, thereby causing dyspnea. Moreover, it is possible for more than one mechanism to be involved in any singular report of dyspnea (Spector & Klein, 2002).

These mechanisms support the idea that dyspnea is caused by a "mismatch" between central respiratory motor activity and feedback from receptors in the airways, lungs, and chest wall. However, psychological, social, spiritual, and environmental factors interact with the physiological ones to produce the subjective sensation of dyspnea. In other words, the sensation of dyspnea is produced by various physiological mechanisms (neural activation) but the perception of dyspnea is the reaction to the sensation as determined in the cortical and limbic areas of the brain (Author, 1999). Without recognizing all of the components contributing to the total suffering of dyspnea, successful management is difficult to achieve (Currow, 2008; Zepetella, 1998). Symptom control, therefore, is less frequently obtained than with other symptoms common in advanced disease (Williams, 2006).

Assessment

Dyspnea is a personal experience that accounts for a high proportion of disability, impaired quality of life, and suffering. The thorough interdisciplinary assessment includes a careful, comprehensive history to obtain a complete understanding of the patient's experience with dyspnea. Specific information about dyspnea, including its timing, precipitating factors, associated symptoms, alleviating factors, and quality of the symptom should be assessed. The influences of culture, race, age, and gender should also be taken into account.

Timing. Duration, frequency, and onset may provide insight into the etiology and management of dyspnea. For example, dyspnea that comes on suddenly may reflect bronchoconstriction, pulmonary embolism, cardiac ischemia or abrupt airway occlusion. Chronic dyspnea occurs gradually and is likely to be manifested in slow progressive disorders such as COPD, interstitial lung disease, or a slow growing tumor. If the dyspnea occurs more at night, then it may be secondary to the redistribution of fluid in the supine position from diseases such as CHF. Dyspnea can also result from an exacerbation of gastroesophageal reflux disease (GERD) that triggers bronchoconstriction. Assessing whether dyspnea is present with activity and/or at rest offers a better understanding of the severity of the condition.

Precipitating factors. Identification of precipitating factors assists in determining the underlying cause of the dyspnea (Hasson et al., 2008; Henoch, Bergman, & Danielson, 2008; Shumway, Wilson, Howard, Parker,

& Eliasson, 2008). Exercise or overexertion commonly precipitates dyspnea in most chronic cardiopulmonary conditions as does a change in position. Often patients with COPD or CHF feel dyspneic when supine while those with cirrhosis or pneumonectomy may feel the sensation when upright. Anticipation of stressful events is another typical precipitant. Inhalation of allergens (pollen, grass, and weeds), smoke, fumes, and other aerosolized substances may trigger bronchospasm in patients with COPD and asthma. Respiratory infections usually cause an exacerbation of symptoms.

Associated symptoms. Dyspnea is rarely an isolated problem. Concurrent symptoms can help clinicians identify the underlying pathophysiology. Clutching sternal chest pain is most likely indicative of myocardial ischemia, while brief, sharp lateral chest pain suggests pulmonary embolism, pneumothorax, or pleurisy. Wheezing is usually a sign of asthma, COPD, or CHF (Hasson et al., 2008). Coughing, if productive, may indicate the presence of an infection, especially if there is a change in color, consistency, or volume of sputum. Nonproductive coughing occurs with rhinitis, reactive airway disease, interstitial fibrosis, GERD, and others. Hemoptysis is most common with tuberculosis, lung cancer, and pulmonary embolism. Weight loss is another problem that occurs often in patients with cancer, cardiopulmonary diseases, and AIDS. Psychological symptoms are equally as important since anxiety has been found to correlate with the intensity of dyspnea in patients with cancer and lung disease (De Peuter et al., 2004; Smith et al., 2001). This requires tactful questioning and skilful observation as the patient may not admit to anxiety as a symptom. Often caregivers can assist with this component of the assessment.

Alleviating factors. Pharmacological and nonpharmacological strategies are necessary to relieve dyspnea and associated discomfort. Medications should be prescribed based on the identified etiology of dyspnea, such as cardiac or pulmonary problems (Lanken, Terry, Delisser, & Fahy, 2008). Bronchodilators relax bronchial smooth muscle and work well in diseases such as COPD and asthma (Williams, 2006). Nitroglycerin is the initial drug of choice for myocardial ischemia, which may cause dyspnea (Spector, Connolly, & Carlson, 2007). Benzodiazepines often provide relaxation by decreasing the anxiety that frequently accompanies shortness of breath (Elia & Thomas, 2008). Position changes can also offer clues as to etiology. Sitting up in a high Fowlers position or standing may relieve shortness of breath by allowing for better diaphragmatic expansion in the case of pulmonary disease or promoting redistribution of fluid in CHF (Spector et al., 2007).

Quality of dyspnea. Schwartzstein (1999) documented that dyspnea is composed of many distinct sensations

that are distinguishable by patients; patients' descriptive language of dyspnea can lead to a better understanding of etiology and management (Caroci & Lareau, 2004; Hasson et al., 2008; Hechler et al., 2008; Henoch et al., 2008; Mahler & Harver, 2000; Scano, Stendardi, & Grazzini, 2005; Schwartzstein, 1999; Wilcock et al., 2002). It is important to carefully question the patient about the quality and characteristics of the dyspnea experienced. For example, adults with more severe dyspnea may say they have an "urge to breathe," "need more air," or report a "sense of suffocation." Those with neuromuscular or chest wall disease may describe it as "heavy breathing." Still others, especially those with cardiac disease, may call it "chest tightness."

The assessment should include a thorough review of the patient's past medical history including all current and recent medications. Some medications become problematic related to drug-drug interactions that occurs secondary to multiple prescribers. Beta blockers, for example, antagonize beta-2 receptors and inhibit their potential bronchodilating effect (Henoch et al., 2008). An adequate nutritional history is valuable because malnutrition contributes to respiratory muscle fatigue and thus, promotes dyspnea. Information about exposure to chemicals, smoke, fumes and other environmental pollutants adds to the data obtained from the history.

Physical examination. A focused physical examination of the head, neck, and chest will yield specific information about the patient's condition and assist with identification of treatment options. Inspection should include the color of skin, nails, lips, nutritional state, sternal/spinal deformities, chest shape and movement, breathing rate and rhythm, capillary refill, the presence/absence of nasal flaring, tracheal deviation, jugular venous distention, costal retractions, accessory muscle use, and clubbing. Other clues include facial/oral expression and inspiration: expiration ratio. Palpation can yield information about tenderness, fremitus, masses, nodes, and crepitus. Percussion of the chest will indicate the degree of resonance, where dull is consolidation of tissue and tympanic is the presence of air. Auscultation of the lungs will detect adventitious or diminished breath sounds, voice sounds, or pleural friction rubs.

Diagnostic tests. Based on the need to determine the underlying cause(s) of dyspnea, several diagnostic tests may be of value. These include chest radiography, spirometry and/or pulmonary function tests, pulse oximetry (preferred) or arterial blood gas analysis, electrocardiogram, electrolyte profile, and complete blood count. Performance of any test should take into consideration the risk/benefit ratio, the patient and his/her family's wishes, the prognosis, and goals of care.

Measurement of Dyspnea

Dyspnea is a subjective, multidimensional symptom, therefore it is important that instruments used to measure it take into account the sensation, the impact of it on quality of life (patient and caregivers), and response to interventions. In 2007, a systematic review of tools to measure dyspnea in advanced disease was conducted by Bausewein and colleagues (Bausewein, Farquhar, Booth, Gysels, & Higginson, 2007). Seventy-three studies were identified from 1966 to August 2005 involving the development or validation of a tool to measure dyspnea. A total of 35 tools were reviewed but two were excluded due to the measurement of physical activity only. Of the 33 tools examined, 29 were multidimensional and 4 were unidimensional. Of the multidimensional instruments, 11 were dyspnea-specific and 18 were disease-specific. The majority of the latter have been validated primarily for chronic obstructive pulmonary disease (COPD), reducing the applicability for other conditions. No one tool assessed all dimensions (psychosocial, physical) of the symptom. This same conclusion was noted by other researchers (Dorman, Byrne, & Edwards, 2007). However, given the clinical diversity of patients experiencing dyspnea near the end-of-life, it is unlikely that one tool will ever be established as the gold standard. Therefore, clinicians, and researchers must choose the appropriate tool based on criteria such as the definition of dyspnea, setting, diagnostic group, disease stage, sensitivity required, and variables involved (Bausewein et al., 2007).

In general, the visual analogue scale (VAS), Numerical rating scale (NRS) or the Modified Borg scale provides useful assessment data. If there is a specific focus on quality of life, multidimensional tools such as the chronic respiratory questionnaire (CRQ) or lung cancer symptom scale (LCSS), would be best. If the focus is more on the sensation and its impact on function, then the cancer dyspnea scale (CDS) is most appropriate. Researchers should consider using both uni- and multidimensional instruments in order to understand the full impact on the patient and caregivers.

A visual analogue scale (VAS) is recommended due to its ease of use and availability. On either a 100 mm horizontal or vertical line, the anchors "not at all breathless" on the low end and "severely breathless" at the high end represent the extremes of dyspnea (Gift, 1989; Martinez et al., 2000). The VAS can measure even minute changes when used consistently. Another commonly used tool is the modified Borg scale, which has the numbers 0–10 listed horizontally with descriptors along the line. On both, the patient is asked only to rate the shortness of breath; no other dimensions are measured. While nonverbal adults can simply point to a number or position, some may find it difficult and need assistance to rate their symptom. For this reason, another choice would be a numerical rating scale (NRS)

as patients generally find it easier to verbally pick a number from a simple scale such as 0–5. Nevertheless, each of these uni-dimensional tools is reliable and valid and can be helpful when assessing dyspnea in a variety of settings. All are self-administered, quick, and can be used over the phone.

For patients with advanced disease, the cancer dyspnea scale (CDS), is a 12 question self-report of shortness of breath that includes aspects of dyspnea such as sense of effort, anxiety, and discomfort which continues to be validated and evaluated (Henoch, Bergman, & Gaston-Johansson, 2006; Tanaka, Akechi, Okuyama, Nishiwaki, & Uchitomi, 2000). The Chronic Respiratory Questionnaire (CRQ) has demonstrated validity, reliability, and responsiveness but only in the populations of chronic lung disease and heart failure. Further evaluation of these and other tools will benefit the patients, caregivers, and healthcare providers in dyspnea assessment.

Whichever instrument is used, the patient and family should feel comfortable and encouraged to utilize it in order to evaluate current therapeutic interventions. Consistency over time will maximize the relevance and usefulness of measurement. It is important to re-emphasize that physiological parameters may not always correlate with the degree of dyspnea reported. The patient must remain the singular authority on the symptom; if the patient is unable to communicate, objective indicators of dyspnea can be used, such as tachypnea, gasping, use of accessory muscles, anxiety, restlessness, agitation, grimacing, and tachycardia.

GERONTOLOGICAL CONSIDERATIONS

Three major factors contribute to the effects of aging on the pulmonary system: an increase in chest-wall stiffness; a decline in respiratory muscle strength; and a decrease in lung elasticity (Mahler, Rosiello, & Loke, 1986; Tan et al., 2009) [See Table 20.1].

Respiratory infections and inhalation of allergens, smoke, fumes, and other aerosolized substances are more likely to result in dyspnea in older adults as aging increases susceptibility to both infections and allergens due to a diminished immune system (Sheahan & Musialowski, 2001). Other effects of aging include a prevalence of silent GERD and sleep apnea secondary to discoordinated activity of the upper airway muscles and the diaphragm. Neurologically, age reduces chemoreceptor functioning causing an inadequate ventilatory response to hypercapnia and acute hypoxia (Thompson, 1996). This makes older adults more sensitive and vulnerable to adverse outcomes from conditions that produce lower oxygen levels, such as pneumonia and chronic obstructive pulmonary disease (COPD). Therefore, in the dyspneic elder, it is essential to take into consideration any underlying diseases and/or comorbidities, such as renal disease, congestive heart failure

20.1 | Effects of the Aging Process on the Pulmonary System

STRUCTURAL CHANGES (PEDIATRIC)	RESULT (PEDIATRIC)	STRUCTURAL CHANGES (GERIATRIC)	RESULT (GERIATRIC)
Upper Airways		**Upper airways**	
Infants = nasal breathers	Nasal congestion = airway obstruction	Nasal cartilage weakens causing obstruction	Difficulty in breathing through the nose
Large tongue	Easily occludes airway	Nasal blood flow decreases	Drying of secretions; nasal congestion
Narrowed cricoid cartilage	Potential for airway obstruction	Nasal turbinates shrink	Drying of secretions; nasal congestion
Cartilaginous larynx	Susceptible to edema, airway obstruction	Mucous increases in viscosity	Lodges in nasopharynx and stimulates coughing
Large Airways		**Large Airways**	
Trachea = diameter small finger of child	Easily obstructed	Trachea & large bronchi stiffen	Decreases air exchange
Small Airways		**Small Airways**	
Diameter increases over time		Diameter decreases	
		Alveolar ducts dilate	
Alveolar surface area increases		Alveolar surface area decreases	
		Combined changes	Increase residual volume
Thoracic Cage		**Thoracic Cage**	
Thin chest wall	Increases compliance (i.e., retractions)	Ribs decalcify	Affects posture
Cartilaginous ribs	Increases compliance (i.e., retractions)	Costal cartilages calcify	Affects posture
Cartilaginous sternum	Increases compliance (i.e., retractions)	Costal-vertebral joints stiffen (arthritic changes)	Decreases height
Flattened position of diaphragm	Any impedance affects work of breathing	Dorsal kyphosis occurs	Increases anterior-posterior diameter (barrel-shape)
		Combined changes	Decreases vital capacity, increases residual volume
Pulmonary Vasculature		**Pulmonary Vasculature**	
		Arteries enlarge and thicken (lose distensibility)	Decreases cardiac output during exercise/exertion

MECHANICAL CHANGES (PEDIATRIC)	RESULT (PEDIATRIC)	MECHANICAL CHANGES (GERIATRIC)	RESULT (GERIATRIC)
Small Airways		**Small Airways**	
Potential for premature closing	Grunting generates positive end-expiratory pressure (PEEP) and may prevent atelectasis	Premature closure	Air trapping/hyperinflation; impairs gas exchange & muco-ciliary clearance
Respiratory Musculature		**Respiratory Musculature**	
Immature	Easily fatigued	Strength decreases; oxygen needs increase	Muscle fatigue; less reserve
		Lung Volumes, Capacities, Flow Rates	
		Forced expiratory volume in 1 second decreases	Increases residual volume
		Forced vital capacity decreases	Increases residual volume
		Functional residual capacity increases	Increases work of breathing
		Diffusing capacity decreases	Impairs gas exchange

Source: McCaskey, 2007; Sheahan & Musialowski, 2001; Tan et al., 2009; Thompson, 1996.

or COPD, in order to formulate a successful treatment plan for dyspnea. For example, in the case of COPD, oxygen requirements need to be monitored more carefully for the possibility of carbon dioxide retention and subsequent acidosis (Ofir, Laveneziana, Webb, Lam, & O'Donnell, 2007). Renal or hepatic impairment will impact the dosages/frequencies of certain medications for elders with these conditions. Furthermore, nursing interventions similar to those offered in pulmonary rehabilitation have been found to help elders focus on attainable goals and learn techniques to enhance their quality of life (Booth, Farquhar, Gysels, Bausewein, & Higginson, 2006). Lastly, due to the thoracic changes attributable to aging, positioning, as described earlier, becomes a major factor in managing the symptom for the dyspneic elder.

PEDIATRIC CONSIDERATIONS

Twelve thousand children are diagnosed with cancer each year and 2,200 die from the disease (Houlihan, Branowicki, Mack, Dinning, & McCabe, 2006), making cancer the leading cause of non-accidental death in childhood (Wolfe et al., 2000). In addition, nearly 400,000 children live with chronic life-limiting conditions and approximately 25,000 die from their disease annually (Jennings, 2005). To this end, three fourths of pediatric deaths occur in hospitals, primarily in the intensive care unit (Davies et al., 2006). As many as 82% report dyspnea at the end-of-life, second only to loss of appetite (100%) (Teruaki et al., 2003) and fatigue (98%) (Wolfe et al., 2000). Wolfe et al. (2000) asked parents to rate the degree of suffering their child experienced in the last month of life. Approximately 50% reported "a lot" or "a great deal of" suffering due to dyspnea. According to the parents, 65% of those children were treated for dyspnea yet only 16% believed the treatment to be successful, even though the symptom is generally considered responsive to treatment.

The respiratory system in children continues to grow and develop long after birth. Because respiratory function is immature in younger patients, deterioration can occur rapidly when disease is present (McCaskey, 2007). Observation, assessment, and a medical history are the tools to evaluating respiratory distress as the pediatric patient is not always able to communicate how he or she feels, especially if very young. However, in those that can describe their symptom(s), it is important to use pediatric age-appropriate tools, such as the Wong-Baker faces. Once a baseline measurement has been obtained, the initial opioid dose is weight-based and may range from 2.1mg/kg/24 hr–4.4 mg/kg/24 hr (Hewitt, Goldman, Collins, Childs, & Hain, 2008). Children with solid tumors outside the central nervous system may need increased doses of opioids or multiple different opioids to successfully manage their symptoms (Hewitt et al., 2008). Complementary therapies may also assist with

dyspnea management but have not been evaluated in children (Ladas, Post-White, Hawks, & Taromina, 2006).

It is not surprising that one of the greatest fears parents have for their dying child is that he or she will be uncomfortable during the last days of life (Widger & Wilkins, 2004). Yet barriers to quality end-of-life care such as prognostic uncertainties and discrepancies in treatment goals between staff and family members prevent dying children from being kept as comfortable as possible (Davies et al., 2006). Fewer than 1% of children who need hospice care actually receive it (Mellichamp, 2007). Consequently, health professionals in both Canada and the United States have advocated to improve the quality of end-of-life care provided to dying infants, children, adolescents, and their families through identification of key components (i.e., pain and symptom management) and an integrated palliative care approach (Widger & Wilkins, 2004). Seeking positive outcomes such as an overall improvement in patient/family/staff satisfaction with care, a decreased number of emergency department visits and hospitalizations, and an increased ability of the patient/family to make informed decisions and set realistic goals is within reach but not yet seen often enough (Jennings, 2005).

TREATMENT AND INTERVENTIONS: NONPHARMACOLOGICAL

Cooling and vibration. When stimulated, temperature and mechanical receptors of the trigeminal nerve in the cheek and nasopharynx alter feedback to the brain and modify the perception of dyspnea. The use of a fan set on low speed and directed toward the face will stimulate this response (Booth, Moosavi, & Higginson, 2008; Elia & Thomas, 2008). Cooling the body may have a beneficial effect as well. Simple techniques include applying cool damp cloths to the forehead or chest, offering a cool water sponge bath, or providing a clean, fresh pillow. Altering the environment by circulating cool air with either an air conditioning unit, a ceiling fan, or placing the patient by an open window may add an element of comfort (Williams, 2006).

Stimulation of the mechanical receptors in the respiratory muscles can alter the sensation of dyspnea, too. This accounts for why chest wall vibration is helpful in some patients (Author, 1999). An electric massager can be purchased for this use, which also helps with relaxation and relief of pain. Another stimulatory modality, called acu-TENS, is showing promise using transcutaneous electrical nerve stimulation over acupoints. One randomized placebo-controlled study showed decreased dyspnea in ambulatory patients with COPD during a 45 minute acu-TENS session (Lau & Jones, 2008). Further investigation is warranted to evaluate the effects in a palliative care setting.

Breathing retraining. Diaphragmatic and pursed-lip breathing have been advocated to relieve dyspnea, especially in patients with COPD, however, relief is highly variable. Moreover, patients often resort to rapid, shallow breathing when unobserved. Despite these inconsistencies, both techniques offer an option that has no associated cost, is readily available, and can be easily learned. Families can play an active role in the patient's care by learning these techniques and coaching the patient during daily interactions.

Positioning. Patients should be assisted to find a position of comfort. The leaning forward position has been reported to improve overall inspiratory muscle strength, increase diaphragmatic excursion, and decrease abdominal paradoxical breathing as well as reduce dyspnea in patients with COPD (Author, 1999). While reducing participation of the chest wall and neck muscles overall, sitting and leaning forward with arms supported on a table facilitates a more focused effort on respiration rather than on maintenance of body posture and/or arm movement (Campbell, 1996; Spector et al., 2007).

Optimal comfort as well as ventilation and perfusion may be accomplished by placing the patient's good lung in a dependent position where gravity may assist in perfusing the healthiest area of lung tissue. In some patients, terminal dyspnea may only be relieved by an upright position where vital capacity is increased because of the lowered diaphragm. The clinician should accept the patient's position of choice, even if it belies traditional thinking.

Energy conservation. Activities of daily living strain the dyspneic patient, even if they are passive during the activity. Oxygen consumption is increased with any activity, so it is important to allow for an adequate recovery period. All care should be evaluated with regard to what the patient can tolerate and what is desired. In some cases, the activity or intervention can be modified to accommodate decreased tolerance. For example, a bath and linen change could be stretched out over the course of several hours, focused on face and hands only, or eliminated entirely. As noted earlier, a position of comfort is not only helpful, but also critical to accommodating the patient's wants/needs with any required activities. However, if the care is more burdensome than beneficial, it should be re-evaluated regarding the merit in continuing it (Ben-Aharon et al., 2008).

Cognitive-Behavioral Approaches/Complementary Therapies

Distraction and relaxation strategies are important and useful adjuncts in the treatment of dyspnea. Distraction helps to focus the patient on something other than breathing. Relaxation eases muscular tension thereby allowing breathing to be less strenuous and more effective. One method, guided imagery, uses mental images to promote relaxation. Other therapeutic activities include massage, music therapy, Reiki, therapeutic touch, and aromatherapy. However, a wide range of alternatives evaluated in a systematic review of eleven randomized controlled trials and two controlled clinical trials failed to provide enough evidence to yield specific recommendations (Pan, Morrison, Ness, Fugh-Berman, & Leipzig, 2000).

Acupuncture and acupressure have emerged as possible options for relief of dyspnea. Acupuncture has already been integrated into palliative care settings in the United Kingdom (Suzuki et al., 2008). A review of the literature found 27 randomized controlled clinical trials with 23 reporting statistically significant results for symptoms such as dyspnea, pain, nausea, and vomiting (Standish, Kozak, & Congdon, 2008). However, the evidence remains low to moderate and the results for dyspnea are mixed. More research is needed to evaluate the potential benefits of this modality.

A number of essential oils (highly concentrated plant constituents) are thought to enhance respiration (Cooksley, 1996). These oils possess certain qualities such as expectorant, mucolytic, anti-allergic, or immune stimulant; some also have anti-viral and anti-bacterial benefits. Most of the essential oils useful in respiratory conditions come from the bark, leaves, berries, and branches of certain trees. Once properly diluted, essential oils can be applied directly to the skin (check for sensitivity first), in the form of massage, placed on pulse points, or inhaled through the use of a diffuser, aroma lamp, vaporizer, humidifier, or an absorbent material, such as a cotton ball. Oils are non-habit forming and excreted via the kidneys, skin, or lungs. Some recommended essential oils that can be used for dyspnea include eucalyptus, peppermint, ginger, hyssop, lavender, bergamot, basil, pine, sandalwood, and cypress. Blends of various oils are commonly used to achieve the maximum effect.

Education of the patient and family on management techniques and the basic rationale for each empower them to take an active role in the treatment plan. Coaching both the patient and the family reinforces these interventions. Active listening and emotional support by the nurse encourages expression of thoughts and feelings and also helps with early identification of potential problems. Benefits have been achieved using a rehabilitative approach that combined breathing re-training, psychosocial support and help to develop adaptive strategies for breathlessness (Bredin et al., 1999; Corner, Plant, A'Hern, & Bailey, 1996; Hately, Laurence, Scott, Baker, & Thomas, 2003; Sola, Thompson, Subirana, Lopez, & Pascual, 2004). This was clearly found in a meta-analysis conducted by Salman, Mosier, Beasley, and Calkins (2003), where twenty randomized controlled trials showed strong evidence for pulmonary rehabilitation in the management of COPD (Salman et al., 2003). Focus groups specifically for caregivers of patients with dyspnea can be a helpful intervention both in terms of the caregiver as well as for evaluation of management techniques (Moody, Webb, Cheung, & Lowell, 2004).

Transfusion Therapy

For patients with advanced cancer, blood transfusions are commonly used to alleviate symptoms such as dyspnea, fatigue, weakness, and tachycardia (Ripamonti, 1999). There is scarce evidence documenting symptom relief and improvement of the subjective sense of well-being after blood transfusions in anemic adults. With the potential risks of a transfusion reaction and adverse responses to blood transfusions, a safer, effective non-transfusion form of therapy might be considered, such as recombinant human erythropoietin (Williams, 2006). Disadvantages to this therapy include cost and the significant length of time required for an improvement in hemoglobin concentration, which is normally 4–6 weeks (Author, 2009).

Noninvasive Positive Pressure Ventilation

Noninvasive positive pressure ventilation (NIPPV) represents a controversial alternative method to treat dyspnea. While it is widely accepted as a curative intervention, no studies have yet been done on NIPPV as a comfort measure at the end-of-life nor have any compared NIPPV with the use of pharmacological therapies such as morphine (Curtis et al., 2007). Nevertheless, NIPPV has found a place in palliative care for some patients with respiratory failure to either relieve symptoms or allow time for completion of life-closure tasks (Benditt, 2000).

For patients with advanced motor neuron diseases, NIPPV is considered the standard of care in the final phase of life (Tripodoro & De Vito, 2008). For patients who choose to forego endotracheal intubation in the presence of respiratory failure, the best candidates for NIPPV are patients with COPD and cardiogenic pulmonary edema (Schettino, Altobelli, & Kacmarek, 2005) with mixed results for patients with advanced cancer (Cuomo et al., 2004). Alternatively, some have suggested it is inappropriate to use NIPPV for patients who choose comfort over life support either because NIPPV is a form of life support itself, poor outcomes, or significant adverse events (Clarke, Vaughan, & Raffin, 1994; Delclaux, L'Her, & Alberti, 2000). Therefore, the Society of Critical Care Medicine Task Force on the Palliative Use of NIPPV developed a framework for using NIPPV in patients with acute respiratory failure, especially for those patients who decline endotracheal intubation or who are receiving palliative care (Curtis et al., 2007).

The proposed result is a categorical approach using an ethical framework based on the goals of care and informed patient and family preferences. Frequent, ongoing, interdisciplinary patient and family communication is inherent in choosing or continuing NIPPV as an intervention. Advantages include a lack of adverse effects when compared to medications, continued patient participation, maintenance of communication, as well as relief of dyspnea and other symptoms related to hypoxia or hypercarbia.

Disadvantages include the cost of equipment, hospice restrictions, lack of hypercarbic effect at the end-of-life (potential for increased suffering), the potential to decrease use of analgesics and anxiolytics prematurely, and the question of when/how to discontinue therapy (Booth et al., 2003; Williams, 2006). Adverse effects include facial irritation or discomfort, gastric distention, nasal/oral dryness or congestion, air leaks, failure to ventilate effectively, failure to tolerate and rarely, aspiration (Schettino et al., 2005). As yet, many questions remain about the role of NIPPV at the end-of-life. However, if used in conjunction with traditional therapies, it may evolve into an effective tool for relieving dyspnea and improving quality of life in terminal patients. At this point, surveys indicate that physicians and respiratory therapists are using NIPPV in patients with "do not resuscitate" orders but are less inclined to use it for patients choosing comfort measures only (Sinuff et al., 2008). Other technological advances that may be of value for the dyspneic patient include laser therapy and the placement of endobronchial or tracheal stents to facilitate airway dilation, especially with tumor encroachment.

Another advancement is a minimally invasive alternative to the treatment of malignant pleural effusion or non-hepatic abdominal ascites, both of which cause dyspnea. This is an indwelling, cuffed, tunneled catheter placed percutaneously in an outpatient setting that facilitates patient-controlled drainage of either pleural or ascetic fluid without requiring hospitalization or office visits (Haas, 2007). Not only has this device shown substantial relief of dyspnea in early studies (Gallo-Silver & Pollack, 2000) but it offers the patient a degree of control at the end of life.

PHARMACOLOGICAL THERAPIES

Oxygen. Supplemental oxygen depresses the hypoxic drive thereby reducing ventilation and subsequently relieving dyspnea. This physiologic response occurs at rest and during exertion in patients with a variety of lung diseases. Oxygen should be titrated to the individual's comfort level using the least restrictive device possible (e.g., nasal cannula does not interfere with eating and communication). Humidification is recommended for comfort and to prevent drying of mucous membranes at or above 4 l/min. Continuous oxygen has been proven to be beneficial, however, some may prefer to use oxygen intermittently, although assurance of the immediate availability of oxygen may be of greater importance (Currow, 2008; Elia & Thomas, 2008; Uronis & Abernethy, 2008).

High concentrations of oxygen can be problematic for those with COPD who are carbon dioxide retainers (i.e., their only drive to breathe is the hypoxic drive), but this should not be a major concern in the final hours of life because hypercarbia produces a sedating effect. Other potential adverse effects of oxygen include activity restriction, cumbersome apparatus, fire hazard, cost, psychological dependence, impaired communication, and difficult withdrawal.

It should be noted that the benefit of oxygen therapy for patients without hypoxemia remains controversial (Rousseau, 1997; Uronis & Abernethy, 2008; Zepetella, 1998). High quality evidence (20/22 RCTs) shows that oxygen improves dyspnea during short-term exercise in COPD while the evidence for patients with COPD at rest, heart failure, and cancer (3 small studies, 1 RCT) is weak (Brunnhuber, Nash, Meier, Weissman, & Woodcock, 2008). In fact, one review found oxygen equivalent to room air in patients with cancer (Booth et al., 2008). Clinical recommendations from the Association of Palliative Medicine emphasize tailored individual assessment and patient/family consultation with ongoing supervision to assure that the goals of care are met(Booth et al., 2003).

Recent reports of helium and oxygen (heliox) gas mixtures for the relief of dyspnea have stimulated interest in this modality. In patients with COPD, heliox reduces dynamic hyperinflation as well as decreases work of breathing, and improves exercise tolerance in patients with lung cancer (Laude & Ahmedzai, 2007). Further investigation is needed to determine best candidates and the potential for long-term benefits.

Opioids. Opioids reduce dyspnea through a number of mechanisms. They act on the respiratory center by decreasing the ventilatory response to hypercapnia and hypoxia, reducing metabolic rate and oxygen consumption, and altering the perception of breathlessness (Pinna, 2008). Furthermore, the cardiovascular effects of vasodilatation and decreased peripheral resistance help to improve oxygen supply and reduce lung congestion.

Despite concerns regarding the use of opioids, morphine therapy forms the basis for treatment of dyspnea at the end-of-life. One study found that improving the use of opioids is mostly a matter of improving communication and empathy between providers and patients (Bendiane et al., 2005). Opioids are very beneficial for many cardiopulmonary conditions, including lung cancer, CHF, COPD, interstitial lung disease, as well as neuromuscular problems and others. The strongest

evidence is for patients with COPD (12 RCTs) while the weakest is for patients with cancer (2 RCTs) (Ben-Aharon et al., 2008; Brunnhuber et al., 2008; Lorenz et al., 2008).

There is no ceiling dose with opioids, so it is appropriate to titrate morphine to the desired effect (limited only by intolerable side-effects). Commonly seen side effects include constipation, nausea & vomiting, urinary retention, altered mental status and drowsiness; tolerance to all of these side effects, except constipation, usually occurs within a week. A bowel regimen should always be established when opioids are prescribed to prevent constipation. While the most feared opioid-related side effect is respiratory depression, titration for symptoms has not been shown to cause it (Estfan et al., 2007).

The oral route of morphine is preferred at the end of life because it is better tolerated, least invasive, and less costly. Other routes can be utilized such as sublingual, rectal, intravenous, subcutaneous, or aerosolized. Furthermore, a recent pilot study demonstrated relief of dyspnea in patients with advanced emphysema using epidural methadone without adverse effects (Juan et al., 2005). Opioid-naïve adults start with the morphine equivalent of 5 mg orally every 4 h; increase dose 30%–50% daily or more frequently until dyspnea is relieved or sedation or other adverse effects become problematic (Elia & Thomas, 2008; Rousseau, 1997). For those already receiving morphine and experiencing dyspnea as a new symptom the dose should be increased by 25%–50% daily for mild to moderate dyspnea and 50%–100% for moderate to severe dyspnea then titrated accordingly (Elia & Thomas, 2008; Rousseau, 1997).

Since opioid receptors have been demonstrated to exist in the airways, nebulized morphine, hydromorphone, or fentanyl can be given in addition to systemic opioids or alone (Coyne, 2003; Shirk, Donahue, & Shirvani, 2006). Some patients experience relief of dyspnea with fewer side effects due to the lack of systemic concentration achieved by inhalation. However, morphine, and hydromorphone can cause histamine release leading to bronchoconstriction, thus the preference by some for fentanyl. Regardless, this method of delivery remains controversial as studies have been conflicting, with nine RCTs demonstrating no symptomatic improvement (Ben-Aharon et al., 2008; Jennings, Davies, Higgins, & Broadley, 2001). Nevertheless, commonly used initial doses of preservative-free injectable solution are morphine 2.5–10 mg, hydromorphone 0.25–1 mg, and fentanyl 25 mg diluted in 2 ml of normal saline (Charles et al., 2008; Ferraresi, 2005).

One protocol recommends nebulized morphine only when intolerable side effects have occurred from systemic administration (Spector, Klein, & Rice-Wiley, 2000). This protocol begins at a conservative dose of 5 mg and titrates up to a maximum of 40 mg every 4 h;

the protocol includes frequent re-evaluation of breathlessness. Dyspnea refractory to other routes of administration may justify a trial of nebulized opioids. However, further research is needed to determine which patients may achieve maximum benefit.

Anxiolytics. Although not supported by RCT evidence for frontline therapy, an anxiolytic may help relieve dyspnea when morphine is not completely effective; anxiety is often one of the dimensions of dyspnea (Navigante, Cerchietti, Castro, Lutteral, & Cabalar, 2006; Reddy, Parsons, Elsayem, Palmer, & Bruera, 2009). Anxiolytics should be considered in combination with opioids and nonpharmacologic anxiety-reduction measures (Elia & Thomas, 2008). Low dose benzodiazepines and phenothiazenes are the categories of anxiolytics most commonly used in the management of dyspnea (Elia & Thomas, 2008). These drugs have hypnotic, sedative, anxiolytic, anticonvulsant, and muscle-relaxant actions, therefore achieving control of dyspnea via multiple mechanisms of action (Author, 2009). Benzodiazepines depress the hypoxic/hypercapnic ventilatory response, as well as alter the emotional response to dyspnea (Author, 1999; Spector & Klein, 2002). Specifically, they bind to a site on the gamma-aminobutyric acid (GABA) receptor and potentiate the action of GABA, which acts as an inhibitory neurotransmitter in the central nervous system (Author, 2009).

Due to the long half-life of oral anxiolytics, some patients are unable to tolerate the side effects of prolonged sedation and cognitive impairment (Rousseau, 1997). Nevertheless, lorazepam 0.5–2.0 mg sublingual/oral every 4–6 hours as needed or around the clock is frequently used (Dahlin, 2006). To break a severe anxiety-dyspnea cycle, the medication can be given as often as hourly until the patient is comfortable (Dahlin, 2006). Side effects include drowsiness, ataxia, reduced psychomotor performance, loss of appetite, and perceptual disturbances (Author, 2009). Diazepam, alprazolam, clonazepam, buspirone, or chlorpromazine are considered alternative medications (Elia & Thomas, 2008; Spector et al., 2007). Subcutaneous midazolam (5 mg every 4 h) has been reported as a safe and effective adjunct to morphine in advanced cancer patients (Navigante et al., 2006). In this prospective, randomized, single-blind study, dyspneic cancer patients received either 1) around-the-clock morphine with midazolam for breakthrough dyspnea, 2) around-the-clock midazolam with morphine for breakthrough or 3) around-the-clock morphine plus midazolam with morphine for breakthrough. Dyspnea relief was achieved at the rates of 69%, 46%, and 92% respectively. Midazolam may be better tolerated than other benzodiazepines due to a shorter half-life (< 5 h) and lack of active metabolites.

Corticosteroids. Corticosteroids, while controversial in the treatment of dyspnea, may be of value because they reduce inflammation by suppressing the migration of polymorphonuclear leukocytes and reversing the increase in capillary permeability (Author, 2009). Euphoria in the form of an overall feeling of well-being, and an increase in appetite exhibit a secondary response. In the lungs, corticosteroids decrease airway inflammation that may be experienced with COPD and radiation pneumonitis, reduce edema associated with tracheal or lung tumors, and increase vital capacity in interstitial disease.

Corticosteroids can improve airway obstruction in cases of carcinomatous lymphangitis or superior vena cava syndrome (Ripamonti, 1999; Williams, 2006). Dose and duration of therapy for dexamethasone and prednisone, two commonly used drugs, depend on the patient's condition and response (Author, 2009). Starting doses are usually high, then reduced to a lower maintenance dose. Adverse reactions (such as insomnia, nervousness, dizziness, indigestion, and hyperglycemia) are not unusual; the nurse should monitor the patient closely for any untoward outcomes (Author, 2009). Corticosteroids can be given orally, subcutaneously, intramuscularly, intravenously, or by inhalation.

Bronchodilators. With substantial evidence from RCTs, a trial of bronchodilator therapy is warranted to relieve dyspnea, especially with COPD, asthma, or other problems associated with reactive airways (Author, 1999; Lorenz et al., 2008). Beta-2 agonists and anticholinergics cause smooth muscle dilation of the airways, thus removing any impedance to airflow (Spector & Klein, 2002). Specifically, bronchodilators exert synergistic action on cyclic 3–5-adenosine monophosphate (cyclic AMP) (Author, 2009). They also stabilize mast cells and stimulate the respiratory tract cilia to expel mucus. The preferred route is inhaled, either by metered dose inhaler or nebulizer, but the drug is also available in oral preparations (Ofir et al., 2007). Side effects, such as tremors, agitation, and anxiety that may heighten the dyspnea, are due to sympathetic stimulation. These potential systemic effects, however, are greater with the oral route. The patient's response should dictate the use of bronchodilators.

Diuretics. Dyspnea may be associated with fluid volume excess, which can be treated with diuretics, such as furosemide, to mobilize edema, normalize blood volume, reduce vascular congestion, and reduce the workload of the heart (Oxberry & Johnson, 2008; Spector et al., 2007). Furosemide inhibits reabsorption of sodium and chloride in the ascending loop of Henle and distal renal tubule, interfering with the chloride-binding cotransport system, thus causing increased excretion of water and electrolytes (Author, 2009). Normal doses can be administered orally, subcutaneously, intramuscularly, intravenously, and by inhalation. For conditions where diuresis is urgently needed (e.g., CHF or pulmonary edema), the intravenous form may be preferred (Kazanowski, 2001). Other disease states where diuretics may be helpful to relieve dyspnea include pulmonary hypertension and abdominal ascites (Selecky et al., 2005). For control of dyspnea refractory to standard treatments, inhaled furosemide has been tried. However, a few small trials in patients with COPD and advanced cancer thus far show mixed results and indicate a need for further investigation (Jensen, Amjadi, Harris-McAllister, Webb, & O'Donnell, 2008; Wilcock et al., 2008)

Antibiotics. Antibiotics may be indicated when dyspnea occurs secondary to a respiratory infection (Author, 1999; Ofir et al., 2007). Rather than pursue a traditional work-up for infection, an empiric trial of antibiotics is appropriate when the patient is near death (Kazanowski, 2001). Antibiotics can provide symptom relief and facilitate comfort in the presence of a respiratory infection characterized by an elevated temperature, abnormal breath sounds, acute cough, and nasal/chest congestion (Selecky et al., 2005).

Anticholinergics. The lack of ability to protect one's airway in the final hours of life contributes to the build-up of secretions that leads to what is commonly referred to as the "death rattle" (i.e., noisy breathing). While caregivers consider it to be a disturbing symptom for families and loved ones of the patient, recent studies have found this not necessarily the case (Wee, Coleman, Hillier, & Holgate, 2006). In contrast, it does have a negative impact on staff and volunteers working with dying patients, causing them to act without knowing which treatment is the most effective (Wee et al., 2006). The "death rattle" occurs in 25%–92% of dying patients, occurs more commonly in men and patients with brain and lung neoplasms, and predicts most will die within 48 h (Bennett, 1996; Plonk & Arnold, 2005; Wildiers & Menten, 2002). It is caused by the collection of secretions in the bronchi and posterior oropharynx, a decreased ability to swallow, an absent cough reflex, and in severe cases of cardiopulmonary failure, pulmonary edema (Bickel & Arnold, 2008; Picella, 1997).

Despite the lack of evidence-based guidelines, the standard of care has been to use anticholinergic drugs, namely scopolamine, hyoscyamine, glycopyrrolate, and atropine (Bickel & Arnold, 2008). The mechanism of action is the blockade of acetylcholine at parasympathetic sites in smooth muscle, secretory glands, and the CNS with the primary clinical effect of inhibition of salivary secretions (Author, 2009). Side effects are generally not reported as the patient is unresponsive but may include dry mouth, urinary retention, visual disturbances and less often confusion (Wee et al., 2006).

No controlled studies have determined if anticholinergics are the treatment of choice and if so, which drug/dosage/route is best. Only glycopyrrolate crosses the blood-brain-barrier, making it more potent but also

more erratically and poorly absorbed (Bickel & Arnold, 2008). The scopolamine patch is convenient with the dosage being 1–3 patches every 3 days (Bickel & Arnold, 2008). Hyoscyamine offers the most flexibility as it comes in short-acting, sustained-released oral tablets and solution (Bickel & Arnold, 2008). Anecdotal reports from hospice nurses suggest the use of atropine eye drops sublingually as a reasonable alternative, as long as side effects are monitored (e.g. tachycardia). Non-pharmacologic interventions have not been studied either but include positioning (side-lying or semi-prone), gentle oropharyngeal suctioning, postural drainage, and reduced fluid intake (Bickel & Arnold, 2008; Lawrey, 2005; Plonk & Arnold, 2005).

Anesthetics. Recent reports in the literature suggest that ketamine may have a place in treating intractable symptoms, namely pain, during a patient's final hours (Fine, 1999, 2003). Ketamine, an N-methyl-D-aspartate (NMDA) receptor antagonist, has strong analgesic, anxiolytic, and amnesiac properties that make it attractive as a treatment for uncontrollable dyspnea (Groover, 2009; Witte, 2002). Anecdotal reports on a small number of patients with severe dyspnea unresponsive to usual therapy suggest that a conservative induction of ketamine can be successful (Witte, 2002). Using trial and error, the following regime has safely facilitated control of severe dyspnea: initial intravenous bolus dose of 0.15 mg/kg (0.5 mg/kg SQ or IM); repeat every 10–15 min twice as needed (30–45 min for SQ or IM dosing) (Fine, 2003; Witte, 2002). If no effect is noted at this time, other options should be explored. If symptom(s) subside, a ketamine (IV or SQ) infusion can be started at a rate determined by dividing the relief-duration time into the total induction dose (Fine, 2003; Witte, 2002) (e.g. 50 kg person x 0.15 mg/kg = 7.5 mg IV bolus. Duration of relief is 3 h. 7.5 mg divided by 3 hrs = 2.5 mg/hr infusion.). The patient may need to be rebolused at the start of the infusion. Clinical signs and symptoms guide the number of boluses as well as the infusion rate of ketamine (Fine, 1999, 2003).

When using ketamine in sub-anesthetic doses, patients can respond and interact coherently and purposefully (Fine, 2003). Side effects such as vivid and disturbing dreams, hallucinations, and delirium common with anesthetic doses are rare but can be treated with a benzodiazepine or phenothiazine (Fine, 1999, 2003; Fitzgibbon & Viola, 2005). Opioids should be evaluated at the start of the ketamine infusion and reduced whenever possible to avoid opioid toxicity/tolerance (Fitzgibbon & Viola, 2005). Despite numerous reports of safety and efficacy, there may still be difficulty accessing this drug in palliative care due to lack of knowledge, professional bias, and financial constraints (Baumrucker, 2000). The success of using ketamine for pain control warrants further investigation regarding the role of ketamine in treating extreme dyspnea at the very end of life.

CONCLUSION

Dyspnea has long been recognized as a prevalent symptom near the end of life (Booth et al., 2003; Brunnhuber et al., 2008; Nauck, Klaschik, & Ostgathe, 2000; Williams, 2006). Similarly, noisy breathing (death rattle) is frequently observed in the last hours and days of life. Morita, Ichiki, and Tsunoda (1998) reported a mean of 57 h till death once noisy breathing began (Morita et al., 1998). A retrospective chart review of 185 residents who died in a long-term care facility indicated that dyspnea was the most commonly recorded symptom (62%) and noisy breathing was the third (39%) (Hall et al.,

2002). However, in nearly a quarter of the patients with dyspnea, symptoms were not treated. Of those who did receive treatment, oxygen was the therapy most often utilized. Opioids accounted for 27% of the treatment and nonpharmacological measures, 6%. About half of the cases with "noisy breathing" went untreated; those that did receive therapy were either suctioned or given hyoscine. The nurse was the only healthcare professional involved 40% of the time (Hall et al., 2002). Nearly a decade since the retrospective review done by Hall et al. (2002), 48% of patients in 230 long-term care centers across four states experienced dyspnea during the last 30 days of life (Hall et al., 2002; Hasson et al., 2008). Interviews with over 1000 staff and family caregivers rated the treatment very effective for only half. Furthermore dyspnea assessment remains primarily observational, even in hospice settings (Webb, Moody, & Mason, 2000). Lastly, while standard therapies have become more frequently employed, complementary alternatives are rarely utilized.

These and other similar findings continue to point to the tremendous need for end-of-life education and research, especially for dyspnea assessment and management. As the population ages and the symptoms of chronic diseases become even more prevalent, more people will suffer unnecessarily unless nurses advocate for quality end-of-life care.

EVIDENCE-BASED PRACTICE

Dorman, S., Byrne, A., & Edwards, A. (2007). Which measurement scales should we use to measure breathlessness in palliative care? A systematic review. *Palliative Medicine, 21,* 177–191.

Research problem. There are no universally accepted measurement scale to assess breathlessness in adult palliative care patients.

Design. Systematic search of electronic databases for patient-based scales with evaluations of at least two psychometric characteristics. Exercise based tests were excluded.

Sample. 29 scales: 6 to measure breathlessness severity, 4 to assess breathlessness descriptions, 19 to measure functional impact of breathlessness.

Methods. Scales were appraised with emphasis on construct validity and responsiveness.

Results. *Severity:* Numeric rating scale (NRS) and modified Borg Scale evaluated in COPD (NRS also in cancer). Both require further assessment of responsiveness and test–retest reliability over time intervals relevant to palliative care. Visual analogue scales (VAS) have also been evaluated but require larger sample sizes.

Descriptions. The Japanese Cancer Dyspnea Scale (CDS) evaluated in patients with cancer, requires further assessment of construct validity and responsiveness.

Functional impact. The Chronic Respiratory Questionnaire dyspnea subscale (CRQ-D) evaluated in chronic lung diseases and heart failure; the MND respiratory scale is similar. CRQ-D has face and construct validity, test–retest reliability, and responsiveness, and shows promise for palliative care.

Implications for nursing practice. Dyspnea needs to be assessed using a measurement tool, preferably one of the scales listed. Once used with a patient, the same tool should be continued.

Conclusion. The NRS, modified Borg, CRQ-D and CDS most suitable for use in palliative care; further evaluation required before adopting any scale as standard.

EVIDENCE-BASED PRACTICE

Lorenz, K. A., Lynn, J., Dy, S. M., et al. (2008). Evidence for improving palliative care at the end of life: a systematic review. *Annals of Internal Medicine, 148*, 147–159.

Research problem. What is the evidence for interventions aimed at the relief of dyspnea at the end of life?

Data sources. English language citations (January 1990–November 2005) from MEDLINE, the database of Abstracts of Reviews of Effects, the National Consensus Project for Quality Palliative Care bibliography, and November 2005–January 2007 updates from expert reviews and literature surveillance.

Study selection. Systematic reviews that addressed "end of life" including terminal illness and chronic, eventually fatal illness with ambiguous prognosis and intervention studies that addressed pain, dyspnea, depression, advance care planning, continuity, and caregiving.

Data extraction. Single reviewers screened 24,423 titles to find 6,381 relevant abstracts and reviewed 1,274 articles in detail to identify 33 high-quality systematic reviews and 90 relevant intervention studies. Related specifically to dyspnea, seven systematic reviews addressed this symptom, 3 for patients with COPD, 1 for patients with cancer, and 3 for patients with mixed diseases. Twelve additional reports of interventions included dyspnea evaluation, four focused on pharmacology and

one included several studies describing complementary and alternative medicines. The evidence was rated according to the GRADE standards (design, quality, consistency in results, and relevance of findings).

Outcomes. Quality palliative care focused on the relief of dyspnea at the end of life.

Main Results. Strong evidence supports treating dyspnea with B-agonists, opioids, pulmonary rehabilitation, and oxygen in COPD (the latter during short-term exercise). Weak evidence supports opioid use and oxygen for relieving dyspnea in cancer (the latter being just a few studies). Weak evidence supports care delivery interventions for dyspnea. No studies addressed dyspnea in heart failure.

Conclusion. Opioids and oxygen can be safely employed to treat dyspnea in the patient with COPD or cancer. B-agonists and pulmonary rehabilitation may be effective in patients with COPD alone. Care delivery interventions (e.g., nurse-led patient training in coping techniques, relaxation exercises) may also be helpful for patients with chronic lung disease, heart failure, and cancer.

Commentary. Dyspnea is a frequent and devastating symptom that occurs in as many as 94% of patients with advanced diseases, primarily those with lung cancer and end-stage heart or lung disease (Dudgeon et al., 2001, Edmonds et al., 2001). Consequently, many patients, and their families are burdened by this symptom at the end of life. The systematic review by Lorenz et al. (2008) synthesizes the available evidence for managing dyspnea primarily in COPD and cancer patients. Unfortunately, no research has been completed regarding the management of dyspnea in end-stage heart failure, for which it remains a significant problem. Two common therapies, opioids and oxygen, were supported by the evidence for patients with either disease.

However, dyspnea is a multidimensional symptom that simply cannot be successfully managed without taking co-morbidities into account, particularly anxiety. It is unclear whether anxiety was addressed in any of the trials evaluated. This would be helpful to address as co-management of anxiety could have a major impact on dyspnea. Also, while the benefits of pulmonary rehabilitation on dyspnea are well documented (12 RCTs), its use at the end of life may be limited due to the patient's functional decline.

This review cites 12 studies with 11 unique interventions that evaluated dyspnea as at least one of the endpoints. However, in the clinical arena there are numerous interventions attempted, some patient-driven, some clinician. It is unfortunate that so few of these are measured as the evidence base for dyspnea management could be strengthened if research was undertaken, even with initially small samples. Nevertheless, in addition to opioids and oxygen, studies involving acupuncture, exercise, and inspiratory muscle training measured dyspnea, thus meeting the criteria for inclusion. Cost effectiveness of interventions is yet another consideration to be examined.

REFERENCES

Author. (1999). American Thoracic Society. Dyspnea mechanisms, assessment, and management: A consensus statement. *American Journal of Respiratory and Critical Care Medicine, 159*, 321–340.

Author. (2009). *Physicians' Desk Reference.*

Baumrucker, S. J. (2000). Ketamine and problems with advanced palliative care in the community setting. *American Journal of Hospice and Palliative Medicine, 17*(6), 369–371.

Bausewein, C., Farquhar, M., Booth, S., Gysels, M., & Higginson, I. J. (2007). Measurement of breathlessness in advanced disease: a systematic review. *Respiratory Medicine, 101*(3), 399–410.

Ben-Aharon, I., Gafter-Gvili, A., Paul, M., Leibovici, L., & Stemmer, S. M. (2008). Interventions for alleviating cancer-related dyspnea: A systematic review. *Journal of Clinical Oncology, 26*(14), 2396–2404.

Bendiane, M. K., Peretti-Watel, P., Pegliasco, H., Favre, R., Galinier, A., Lapiana, J.-M., et al. (2005). Morphine prescription to terminally ill patients with lung cancer and dyspnea: French physicians' attitudes. *Journal of Opioid Management, 1*(1), 25–30.

Benditt, J. O. (2000). Noninvasive ventilation at the end of life. *Respiratory Care, 45*, 1376–1381.

Bennett, M. I. (1996). Death rattle: an audit of hyoscine (scopolamine) use and review of management. *Journal of Pain and Symptom Management, 12*, 229–233.

Bickel, K., & Arnold, R. M. (2008). Death rattle and oral secretions. *Journal of Palliative Medicine, 11*(7), 1040–1041.

Booth, S., Matukas, L. M., Tomlinson, G. A., Rachlis, A. R., Rose, D. B., Dwosh, H. A., et al. (2003). Clinical features and short-term outcomes of 144 patients with SARS in the greater Toronto area. *Journal of American Medical Association, 289*(21), 2801–2809.

Booth, S., Farquhar, M., Gysels, M., Bausewein, C., & Higginson, I. J. (2006). The impact of a breathlessness intervention service (BIS) on the lives of patients with intractable dyspnea: A qualitative phase 1 study. *Palliative and Supportive Care, 3*(4), 287–293.

Booth, S., Moosavi, S. H., & Higginson, I. J. (2008). The etiology and management of intractable breathlessness in patients with advanced cancer: A systematic review of pharmacological therapy. *Nature Clinical Practice Oncology, 5*(2), 90–100.

Bredin, M., Corner, J., Krishnasamy, M., Plant, H., Bailey, C., & A'Hern, R., et al. (1999). Multicentre randomised controlled trial of nursing intervention for breathlessness in patients with lung cancer. *British Medical Journal, 318*(7188), 901–904.

Bruera, E., Macmillian, K., Pither, T., & MacDonald, R. (1990). Effects of morphine on the dyspnea of terminal cancer patients. *Journal of Pain and Symptom Management, 5*, 341–344.

Bruera, E., Schmitz, B., Pither, J., Neumann, C. M., & Hanson, J. (2000). The frequency and correlates of dyspnea in patients with advanced cancer. *Journal of Pain and Symptom Management, 19*(5), 357–362.

Brunnhuber, K., Nash, S., Meier, D. E., Weissman, D. E., & Woodcock, J. (2008). *Putting evidence into practice: Palliative care.*

Campbell, M. (1996). Managing terminal dyspnea: Caring for the patient who refuses intubation or ventilation. *Dimensions in Critical Care Nursing, 15*(1), 4–13.

Caroci, A. D. S., & Lareau, S. C. (2004). Descriptors of dyspnea by patients with chronic obstructive pulmonary disease versus congestive heart failure. *Heart and Lung, 33*(2), 102–110.

Charles, M. A., Reymond, L., & Israel, F. (2008). Relief of incident dyspnea in palliative cancer patients: A pilot, randomized, controlled trial comparing nebulized hydromorphone, systemic hydromorphone, and nebulized saline. *Journal of Pain and Symptom Management, 36*(1), 29–38.

Clarke, D. E., Vaughan, L., & Raffin, T. A. (1994). Noninvasive positive pressure ventilation for patients with terminal respiratory failure: The ethical and economic costs of delaying the inevitable are too great [see comment][comment]. *American Journal of Critical Care, 3*(1), 4–5.

Cleary, J. F., & Carbone, P. P. (1997). Palliative medicine in the elderly. *Cancer Journal, 80*, 1335–1347.

Cooksley, V. G. (1996). Aromatherapy treatments for the respiratory system. In *Aromatherapy: A lifetime guide to healing with essential oils* (pp. 92–112). Paramus, NJ: Prentice Hall.

Corner, J., Plant, H., A'Hern, R., & Bailey, C. (1996). Non-pharmacological intervention for breathlessness in lung cancer. *Palliative Medicine, 10*, 299–305.

Coyne, P. J. (2003). The use of nebulized fentanyl for the management of dyspnea. *Clinical Journal of Oncology Nursing, 7*(3), 334–335.

Cuomo, A., Delmastro, M., Ceriana, P., Nava, S., Conti, G., Antonelli, M., et al. (2004). Noninvasive mechanical ventilation as a palliative treatment of acute respiratory failure in patients with end-stage solid cancer. *Palliative Medicine, 18*(7), 602–610.

Currow, D. C. (2008). Managing respiratory symptoms in everyday practice. *Current Opinion in Supportive and Palliative Care, 2*(2), 81–83.

Curtis, J. R., Cook, D. J., Sinuff, T., White, D. B., Hill, N., Keenan, S. P., et al. (2007). Noninvasive positive pressure ventilation in critical and palliative care settings: Understanding the goals of therapy.[see comment]. *Critical Care Medicine, 35*(3), 932–939.

Dahlin, C. (2006). It takes my breath away end-stage COPD. Part 1. *Home Healthcare Nurse, 24*, 148–155.

Davies, B., Sehring, S. A., Partridge, J. C., Cooper, B. A., Hughes, A., Philp, J. C., et al. (2006). Barriers to palliative care for children: perceptions of pediatric health care providers. *Pediatrics, 121*(2), 282–288.

De Peuter, S., Van Diest, I., Lemaigre, V., Verleden, G., Demedts, M., & Van den Bergh, O., et al. (2004). Dyspnea: The role of psychological processes. *Clinical Psychology Review, 24*(5), 557–581.

Delclaux, C., L'Her, E., & Alberti, C. (2000). Treatment of acute hypoxemic nonhypercapnic respiratory insufficiency with continuous positive airway pressure delivered by a face mask: A randomized controlled trial. *Journal of American Medical Association, 284*, 2352–2360.

Dorman, S., Byrne, A., & Edwards, A. (2007). Which measurement scales should we use to measure breathlessness in palliative care? A systematic review. *Palliative Medicine, 21*(3), 177–191.

Dudgeon, D. J., Kristjanson, L., Sloan, J. A., Lertzman, M., & Clement, K. (2001). Dyspnea in cancer patients: Prevalence and associated factors. *Journal of Pain and Symptom Management, 21*(2), 95–102.

Edmonds, P., Karlsen, S., Khan, S., & Addington-Hall, J. (2001). A comparison of the palliative care needs of patients dying from chronic respiratory diseases and lung cancer. *Palliative Medicine, 15*(4), 287–295.

Elia, G., & Thomas, J. (2008). The symptomatic relief of dyspnea. [Review]. *Current Oncology Reports, 10*(4), 319–325.

Estfan, B., Mahmoud, F., Shaheen, P., Davis, M. P., Lasheen, W., Rivera, N., et al. (2007). Respiratory function during parenteral opioid titration for cancer pain. *Palliative Medicine, 21*(2), 81–86.

Ferraresi, V. (2005). Inhaled opioids for the treatment of dyspnea. *American Journal of Health-System Pharmacy, 62*(3), 319–320.

Fine, P. G. (1999). Low-dose ketamine in the management of opioid, nonresponsive, terminal cancer pain. *Journal of Pain and Symptom Management, 17*, 296–300.

Fine, P. G. (2003). Ketamine: From anesthesia to palliative care. *American Academy of Hospice Palliative Medicine Bulletin, 3*(3), 1.

Fitzgibbon, E. J., & Viola, R. (2005). Parenteral ketamine as an analgesic adjuvant for severe pain: Development and retrospective audit of a protocol for a palliative care unit. *Journal of Palliative Medicine, 8*(1), 49–57.

Gallo-Silver, L., & Pollack, B. (2000). Behavioral interventions for lung cancer-related breathlessness. *Cancer Practice, 8*(6), 268–273.

Gift, A. G. (1989). Clinical measurement of dyspnea. *Dimensions of Critical Care Nursing, 8*(4), 210–216.

Groover. (2009). Ketamine.

Haas, A. R. (2007). Recent advances in the palliative management of respiratory symptoms in advanced-stage oncology patients. *American Journal of Hospice and Palliative Medicine, 24*(2), 144–151.

Hall, P., Schroder, C., & Weaver, L. (2002). The last 48 hours of life in long-term care: A focused chart audit. *Journal of the American Geriatric Society, 50*, 501–506.

Hasson, F., Spence, A., Waldron, M., Kernohan, G., McLaughlin, D., Watson, B., et al. (2008). I cannot get a breath: Experiences of living with advanced chronic obstructive pulmonary disease. *International Journal of Palliative Nursing, 14*(11), 526–531.

Hately, J., Laurence, V., Scott, A., Baker, R., & Thomas, P. (2003). Breathlessness clinics within specialist palliative care settings can improve the quality of life and functional capacity of patients with lung cancer. *Palliative Medicine, 17*(5), 410–417.

Hechler, T., Blankenburg, M., Friedrichsdorf, S. J., Garske, D., Hubner, B., Menke, A., et al. (2008). Parents' perspective on symptoms, quality of life, characteristics of death and end-of-life decisions for children dying from cancer. *Klinische Padiatrie, 220*(3), 166–174.

Henoch, I., Bergman, B., & Danielson, E. (2008). Dyspnea experience and management strategies in patients with lung cancer. [Research Support, Non-U.S. Gov't]. *Psycho-Oncology, 17*(7), 709–715.

Henoch, I., Bergman, B., & Gaston-Johansson, F. (2006). Validation of a Swedish version of the Cancer Dyspnea Scale. *Journal of Pain and Symptom Management, 31*(4), 353–361.

Hewitt, M., Goldman, A., Collins, G. S., Childs, M., & Hain, R. (2008). Opioid use in palliative care of children and young people with cancer.[see comment]. *Journal of Pediatrics, 152*(1), 39–44.

Jennings, A. L., Davies, A. N., Higgins, J. P., & Broadley, K. (2001). Opioids for the palliation of breathlessness in terminal illness. *Cochrane Database of Systematic Reviews*(4), CD002066.

Jennings, P. D. (2005). Providing pediatric palliative care through a pediatric supportive care team. *Pediatric Nursing, 30*(3), 195–200.

Jensen, D., Amjadi, K., Harris-McAllister, V., Webb, K. A., & O'Donnell, D. E. (2008). Mechanisms of dyspnoea relief and improved exercise endurance after furosemide inhalation in COPD. *Thorax, 63*(7), 606–613.

Juan, G., Ramon, M., Valia, J. C., Cortijo, J., Rubio, E., Morcillo, E., et al. (2005). Palliative treatment of dyspnea with epidural methadone in advanced emphysema. *Chest, 128*(5), 3322–3328.

Kazanowski, M. K. (2001). Symptom management in palliative care. In M. L. Matzo & D. W. Sherman (Eds.), *Palliative care nursing: Quality care to the end of life* (pp. 327–361). New York: Springer.

Ladas, E. J., Post-White, J., Hawks, R., & Taromina, K. (2006). Evidence for symptom management in the child with cancer. *Journal of Pediatric Hematology and Oncology, 28*(9), 601–615.

Lanken, P. N., Terry, P. B., Delisser, H. M., & Fahy, B. F. (2008). An official American Thoracic Society clinical policy statement: Palliative care for patients with respiratory diseases and critical illnesses. *American Journal of Respiratory and Critical Care Medicine, 177*, 912–927.

Lau, K. S. L., & Jones, A. Y. M. (2008). A single session of AcuTENS increases FEV1 and reduces dyspnoea in patients with chronic obstructive pulmonary disease: A randomised, placebo-controlled trial. *Australian Journal of Physiotherapy, 54*(3), 179–184.

Laude, E. A., & Ahmedzai, S. H. (2007). Oxygen and helium gas mixtures for dyspnoea. *Current Opinion in Supportive and Palliative Care, 1*(2), 91–95.

Lawrey, H. (2005). Hyoscine vs. glycopyrronium for drying respiratory secretions in dying patients. *British Journal of Community Nursing, 10*(9), 421–424.

Lorenz, K. A., Lynn, J., Dy, S. M., Shugarman, L. R., Wilkinson, A., Mularski, R. A., et al. (2008). Evidence for improving palliative care at the end of life: A systematic review.[see comment]. *Annals of Internal Medicine, 148*(2), 147–159.

Mahler, D. A., & Harver, A. (2000). Do you speak the language of dyspnea?[comment]. *Chest, 117*(4), 928–929.

Mahler, D. A., Rosiello, R. A., & Loke, J. (1986). The aging lung. *Geriatric Clinics of North American Journal of Health-System Pharmacy, 2*(2), 215–225.

Maltoni, M., Pirovan, M., Scarpi, E., Marinari, M., Indelli, M., Arnoldi, E., et al. (1995). Prediction of survival of patients terminally ill with cancer. *Cancer Journal, 75*, 2613–2622.

Martinez, J. A., Straccia, L., Sobrani, E., Silva, G. A., Vianna, E. O., & Filho, J. T., et al. (2000). Dyspnea scales in the assessment of illiterate patients with chronic obstructive pulmonary disease. *American Journal of the Medical Sciences, 320*(4), 240–243.

McCaskey, M. (2007). Pediatric assessment: The little differences. *Home Healthcare Nurse, 25*(1), 20–23.

Mellichamp, P. (2007). End-of-life care for infants. *Home Healthcare Nurse, 25*(1), 41–44.

Mercadante, S., Casuccio, A., & Fulfaro, F. (2000). The course of symptom frequency and intensity in advance cancer patients followed at home. *Journal of Pain and Symptom Management, 20*, 104–112.

Moody, L. E., Webb, M., Cheung, R., & Lowell, J. (2004). A focus group for caregivers of hospice patients with severe dyspnea. *American Journal of Hospice and Palliative Medicine, 21*(2), 121–130.

Morita, T., Ichiki, T., & Tsunoda, J. (1998). A prospective study on the dying process in terminally ill cancer patients. *American Journal of Hospice and Palliative Care, 15*, 217–222.

Nauck, F., Klaschik, E., & Ostgathe, C. (2000). Symptom control during the last three days of life. *European Journal of Palliative Care, 7*, 81–84.

Navigante, A. H., Cerchietti, L. C. A., Castro, M. A., Lutteral, M. A., & Cabalar, M. E. (2006). Midazolam as adjunct therapy to morphine in the alleviation of severe dyspnea perception in patients with advanced cancer [see comment]. *Journal of Pain and Symptom Management, 31*(1), 38–47.

Ofir, D., Laveneziana, P., Webb, K. A., Lam, Y., & O'Donnell, D. E. (2007). Mechanisms of dyspnea during cycle exercise in symptomatic patients with GOLD stage I chronic obstructive pulmonary disease. *American Journal of Respiratory and Critical Care Medicine, 177,* 622–629.

Oxberry, S. G., & Johnson, M. J. (2008). Review of the evidence for the management of dyspnoea in people with chronic heart failure. *Current Opinion in Supportive and Palliative Care, 2*(2), 84–88.

Pan, C. X., Morrison, R. S., Ness, J., Fugh-Berman, A., & Leipzig, R. M. (2000). Complementary and alternative medicine in the management of pain, dyspnea, and nausea and vomiting near the end of life. A systematic review. *Journal of Pain and Symptom Management, 20*(5), 374–387.

Picella, D. V. (1997). Palliative care for the patient with end stage respiratory illness. *Perspectives in Respiratory Nursing, 8*(4), 1–10.

Pinna, M. A. (2008). Re: Is there a higher risk of respiratory depression in opioid-naive palliative care patients during symptomatic therapy of dyspnea with strong opioids? *Journal of Palliative Medicine, 11*(6), 822.

Plonk, W. M., & Arnold, R. M. (2005). Terminally Ill. *Journal of Palliative Medicine, 5*(10), 1042–1054.

Reddy, S. K., Parsons, H. A., Elsayem, A., Palmer, J. L., & Bruera, B. (2009). Characteristics and correlates of dyspnea in patients with advanced cancer. *Journal of Palliative Medicine 12*(1), 29–36.

Reuben, D. B., & Mor, V. (1986). Dyspnea in terminally ill cancer patients. *Chest, 89,* 234–236.

Ripamonti, C. (1999). Management of dyspnea in advanced cancer patients. *Supportive Care for Cancer, 7,* 233–243.

Rousseau, P. (1997). Management of dyspnea in the dying elderly. *Clinical Geriatrics, 5*(6), 42–48.

Salman, G. F., Mosier, M. C., Beasley, B. W., & Calkins, D. R. (2003). Rehabilitation for patients with chronic obstructive pulmonary disease: Meta-analysis of randomized controlled trials. *Journal of General Internal Medicine, 18*(213–221).

Scano, G., Stendardi, L., & Grazzini, M. (2005). Understanding dyspnoea by its language. *European Respiratory Journal, 25*(2), 380–385.

Schettino, G., Altobelli, N., & Kacmarek, R. M. (2005). Noninvasive positive pressure ventilation reverses acute respiratory failure in select "do-not-intubate" patients [see comment]. *Critical Care Medicine, 33*(9), 1976–1982.

Schwartzstein, R. M. (1999). The language of dyspnea: Using verbal clues to the diagnosis. *Journal of Critical Illness, 14*(8), 435–441.

Selecky, P. A., Eliasson, C. A. H., Hall, R. I., Schneider, R. F., Varkey, B., McCaffree, D. R., et al. (2005). Palliative and end-of-life care for patients with cardiopulmonary diseases: American College of Chest Physicians position statement [see comment]. *Chest, 128*(5), 3599–3610.

Sheahan, S. L., & Musialowski, R. (2001). Clinical implications of respiratory system changes in aging. *Journal of Gerontological Nursing, 27*(5), 26–34.

Shirk, M. B., Donahue, K. R., & Shirvani, J. (2006). Unlabeled uses of nebulized medications. *American Journal of Health-System Pharmacy, 63*(18), 1704–1716.

Shumway, N. M., Wilson, R. L., Howard, R. S., Parker, J. M., & Eliasson, A. H. (2008). Presence and treatment of air hunger in severely ill patients. *Respiratory Medicine, 102*(1), 27–31.

Sinuff, T., Cook, D. J., Keenan, S. P., Burns, K. E. A., Adhikari, N. K. J., Rocker, G. M., et al. (2008). Noninvasive ventilation for acute respiratory failure near the end of life [see comment]. *Critical Care Medicine, 36*(3), 789–794.

Smith, E. L., Hann, D. M., Ahles, T. A., Furstenberg, C. T., Mitchell, T. A., Meyer, L., et al. (2001). Dyspnea, anxiety, body consciousness, and quality of life in patients with lung cancer. *Journal of Pain and Symptom Management, 21*(4), 323–329.

Sola, I., Thompson, E., Subirana, M., Lopez, C., & Pascual, A. (2004). Non-invasive interventions for improving well-being and quality of life in patients with lung cancer [see comment]. *Cochrane Database of Systematic Reviews* (4), CD004282.

Spector, N., Connolly, M. A., & Carlson, K. K. (2007). Dyspnea: applying research to bedside practice. *AACN Advanced Critical Care, 18*(1), 45–58.

Spector, N., & Klein, D. (2002). Assessing and managing dyspnea. *Nursing Profile,* 20–24.

Spector, N., Klein, D., & Rice-Wiley, L. (2000). Terminally ill patients breathe easier with nebulized morphine. *Nursing Spectrum,* 1–6.

Standish, L. J., Kozak, L., & Congdon, S. (2008). Acupuncture is underutilized in hospice and palliative medicine. *American Journal of Hospice and Palliative Medicine, 25*(4), 298–308.

Suzuki, M., Namura, K., Ohno, Y., Tanaka, H., Egawa, M., Yokoyama, Y., et al. (2008). The effect of acupuncture in the treatment of chronic obstructive pulmonary disease. *Journal of Alternative and Complementary Medicine, 14*(9), 1097–1105.

Tan, M. P., Wynn, N. N., Umerov, M., Henderson, A., Gillham, A., Junejo, S., et al. (2009). Arm span to height ratio is related to severity of dyspnea, reduced spirometry volumes, and right heart strain. *Chest, 135*(2), 448–454.

Tanaka, K., Akechi, T., Okuyama, T., Nishiwaki, Y., & Uchitomi, Y. (2000). Development and validation of the cancer dyspnoea scale: A multidimensional, brief, self-rating scale. *British Journal of Cancer, 82*(4), 800–805.

Teruaki, H., Watanabe, C., Okada, S., Shuhei, N. S., Fujii, Y., & Ohzeki, T., et al. (2003). Analysis of the circumstances at the end of life in children with cancer: Symptoms, suffering and acceptance. *Pediatrics International, 45*(1), 60–64.

Thompson, L. F. (1996). Failure to wean: Exploring the influence of age-related pulmonary changes. *Critical Care Nursing Clinics of North America, 8*(1), 7–16.

Tripodoro, V. A., & De Vito, E. L. (2008). Management of dyspnea in advanced motor neuron diseases. *Current Opinion in Supportive and Palliative Care, 2*(3), 173–179.

Uronis, H. E., & Abernethy, A. P. (2008). Oxygen for relief of dyspnea: What is the evidence? *Current Opinion in Supportive and Palliative Care, 2*(2), 89–94.

Webb, M., Moody, L. E., & Mason, L. A. (2000). Dyspnea assessment and management in hospice patients with pulmonary disorders. *American Journal of Hospice and Palliative Medicine, 17*(4), 259–264.

Wee, B. L., Coleman, P. G., Hillier, R., & Holgate, S. H. (2006). The sound of death rattle I: Are relatives distressed by hearing this sound? *Palliative Medicine, 20*(3), 171–175.

Widger, K., & Wilkins, K. L. (2004). What are the key components of quality pediatric end-of-life care? A literature review. *Journal of Palliative Care, 20*(2), 105–111.

Wilcock, A., Crosby, V., Hughes, A., Fielding, K., Corcoran, R., & Tattersfield, A. E., et al. (2002). Descriptors of breathlessness in patients with cancer and other cardiorespiratory diseases. *Journal of Pain and Symptom Management, 23*(3), 182–189.

Wilcock, A., Walton, A., Manderson, C., Feathers, L., El Khoury, B., Lewis, M., et al. (2008). Randomised, placebo controlled trial of nebulised furosemide for breathlessness in patients with cancer. *Thorax, 63*(10), 872–875.

Wildiers, H., & Menten, J. (2002). Death rattle: prevalence, prevention and treatment. *Journal of Pain Symptoms Management, 23*, 310–317.

Williams, C. M. (2006). Dyspnea. *Cancer Journal, 12*(5), 365–373.

Witte. (2002, July). *Terminal agitation and sedation.* Paper presented at the HOPE regional meeting, Tomah, Wisconsin.

Wolfe, J., Grier, H. E., Klar, N., Levin, S. B., Ellenbogen, J. M., Salem-Schatz, S., et al. (2000). Symptoms and suffering at the end of life in children with cancer. *New England Journal of Medicine, 342*(5), 326–333.

Zepetella, G. (1998). The palliation of dyspnea in terminal disease. *The American Journal of Hospice and Palliative Care(November/December)*, 322–330.

21

Anxiety, Depression, and Delirium

Constance M. Dahlin

Key Points

- Anxiety, depression, and delirium are common symptoms during the dying process.
- Anxiety manifests itself in four ways: physical symptoms, affective symptoms, behavioral responses, and cognitive responses.
- The patient and his/her family should be reassured that the symptoms of depression are effectively treated the majority of the time.
- Effective treatment of anxiety, depression, and delirium necessitates a collaborative effort between the patient, family, and the health team.

Case Study: Elizabeth is a 78-year-old retired university vice-president who has a history of depression, breast cancer, and low blood pressure. She lived alone in the house she and her husband had shared for 25 years, even after he died of cardiac disease 20 years ago. His death was a sudden event for the family. Until recently, Elizabeth insisted she didn't need much help. She was fiercely independent as she attended to her own shopping, errands, and church activities. Elizabeth's three daughters visit her periodically.

Everything changed 1 year ago. Elizabeth began to get forgetful and seemed to have a hard time caring for herself and her house. Her neighbors noticed her erratic behavior but did not say anything to her family. Elizabeth was then involved in several car accidents and her confusion worsened. She was found to have bilateral subdural hematomas and underwent surgery. However, since her surgery, she is more anxious, sometimes confused about events. She is now living in assisted living and able to participate in activities and walk to the dining room for meals, but she appears depressed. She has lost interest in her personal appearance, has stopped reading or swimming, and prefers to stay in her room.

She then developed several bouts of urinary tract infections and pneumonia within a 12-month period requiring multiple hospital admissions. After four admissions, Elizabeth was much weaker and unable to help in her self-care. She was admitted to the higher skilled area of the assisted living residence. She was subsequently diagnosed with depression and anxiety, and intermittent confusion.

Introduction

There is a strong correlation between the diagnosis of anxiety, depression, and delirium in patients receiving palliative care for a life-limiting illness (Gibson, Lichtenthal, Berg, & Breitbart, 2006; Cassem, & Brendel, 2004). Individuals cope in many ways; sometimes, patients may develop psychiatric symptoms including anxiety, depression, and delirium. As transient events, anxiety, depression, and delirium may not cause long-term issues. In severe forms, these psychiatric issues may inhibit the ability to have meaningful communication with family and friends as part of life closure, cause suffering, and affect quality of life.

Anxiety, depression, and delirium are common symptoms during the dying process. Patients and families have understandable fears about disease progression in terms of pain and symptoms, loss of independence, change of function, change in cognition, and being a burden on others (Gibson et al., 2006). Anxiety, confusion, or delirium may be the first sign of a medical problem, particularly in older adults. This makes it difficult to differentiate between these three disorders and other medical conditions (Cremens, 2004; Reichel & Gallo, 1999). Since these symptoms may be interwoven, diagnosis and treatment are even more challenging. Anxiety may precede depression in the diagnosis of certain medical conditions such as myocardial infarction or dementia. Often, anxiety and depression are seen together, for example with the shock of the diagnosis of a terminal illness. Delirium may cause anxiety stemming from the ensuing altered consciousness. This is particularly true if the delirium waxes and wanes and the patient has a sense of his or her loss of cognitive faculties. Depression may result if a patient understands his or her cognitive deficits (Lovejoy, Tabor, & Delaney, 2000; Reichel & Gallo, 1999).

The initial presentation of a medical condition may manifest itself as a psychiatric symptom, resulting in a misdiagnosis of anxiety, depression, or delirium. With the additional overlay of a life-threatening illness, diagnosis may be much subtle and more complex. Cardinal signs of a disease may be hidden or diminished, such as decreased pain in a myocardial infarction, or minimal fever in an infection. Other examples include the presentation of delirium of a patient with a neurological process, depression of a patient who has underlying pancreatic cancer, or anxiety for underlying cardiac ailments (Reichel & Gallo 1999). In children, it may be difficult to distinguish anxiety and depression from sadness or grief. Historically, it was thought that children experience less psychosocial effects. However, this has been found to be a great underestimation. In addition, there are fewer available mental health specialists to treat children and pediatrics (Tyler & Fisher, 2007).

Once a diagnosis is made, treatment issues related to a specific patient must be considered. In particular, a clinician must take into account the patient's age. Older adults and young children many have more pronounced and adverse effects from medications. Older adults may experience diminishing functional and physiologic processes or possible lack of social supports (Reichel & Gallo, 1999). The successful treatment of a patient includes pharmacological medications, complementary therapy, and mobilization of social support of the patient and family. This chapter addresses the holistic care necessary to effective diagnosis, assessment, and treatment of anxiety, depression, and delirium in the palliative care patient.

ANXIETY

Definition

Anxiety is defined as feelings of distress and tension that lack a known stimulus (Lehmann & Rabins, 1999). Generalized anxiety disorder (GAD) is described as chronic uncontrollable nervousness, fearfulness, and sense of worry that lasts for 6 months or longer (Pollack, Otto, Bersntein, & Rosenbaum, 2004). Patients may describe this as a sense of worry, fear, concern, or even foreboding. Although anxiety is a very subjective experience, it is often accompanied by somatic complaints such as tachycardia, fatigue, restlessness, difficulty concentrating, muscle tension, headaches, palpitations, sweating, abdominal discomfort, dizziness, urinary frequency, and sleep disturbances. Symptoms must be present for at least 6 months and cause impairment in social or occupational functioning. In the older adults, there may be a sense of phobia where they may stay at home because they are fearful to leave, stop activities, and become more isolated (Lantz, 2002).

Anxiety in pediatric patients is a common occurrence. The challenge is twofold: the anxiety of the child as well as anxiety related to the stress of family and caregivers around them (Kane & Himelstein, 2007; Hellsten & Kane, 2006). The symptoms that children experience are related to behavioral issues and the change in their functional abilities. Younger children may have worries related to separation, stranger, injury, and loud noises, while teens may have issues regarding personal appearance, self worth, and competence (Kersun & Shemesh, 2007).

Incidence

Anxiety symptoms may develop in any individual diagnosed with a life-limiting illness. Increased anxiety has been associated with female gender, young age, and low socioeconomic status. However, as a life-threatening disease progresses and a person's physical status declines, anxiety may increase (Tremblay & Breitbart, 2001). In one study, over half of cancer patients fit the International Classification of Disorders criteria for anxiety (Stark, Kiely, Smith, Velikova, & Selby, 2002). Cancer-related anxiety is a natural response to the crisis precipitated by such a diagnosis, the threat to life, and the future (Miller & Massie, 2007). Generalized anxiety is the most common anxiety disorder found in late life and at a rate of 10–20% with a prevalence rate of 7% in adults older than age 55 (Reichel & Gallo, 1999). Within the pediatric population, there are no prevalent studies related to anxiety at the end of life.

Etiology

Anxiety in patients with a life-limiting illness is common; and may have a multitude of causes. It may be a component of adjustment disorder, a panic disorder, a generalized anxiety disorder, phobia, or agitated depression (Gibsen et al., 2006; Breitbart, Chochinov & Passik, 2005). The etiology of anxiety includes a multitude of medical conditions such as poorly managed pain; endocrine disorders including hypo- and hyperglycemia, hypo- and hyperthyroidism, Cushing's disease, and carcinoid syndrome. Cardiovascular conditions include myocardial infarctions, angina, congestive heart failure, mitral valve prolapse, and hypovolemia; respiratory conditions include asthma, chronic obstructive pulmonary disease (COPD), pneumonia, pulmonary edema, dyspnea, and hypoxia. Neoplasms and neurological conditions such as akathisia, encephalopathy, seizure disorder, and post-concussion disorders can also contribute to or exacerbate anxiety disorders (Pasacreta, Minarik, & Neild-Anderson 2006; Pollack et al., 2004).

Stimulant substances may contribute to anxiety and include caffeine present in coffee, tea, chocolate, and soda. Ephedrine present in cold products and stimulant type drugs such as methylphenidate, and withdrawal from medications such as benzodiazepines, alcohol, and barbiturates may cause anxiety. Psychological distress such as worries about family relationships, family strife, and financial worries, may all cause anxiety for patients with a life-limiting illness. These may be exacerbated by concern of being a burden to other family members. Lastly, a family history may be a component of anxiety, which may become more pronounced in older patients as they lose physical functioning.

Cardinal Signs

Anxiety has four types of manifestations: physical symptoms, affective symptoms, behavioral responses, and cognitive responses (Pollack et al., 2004, Fisch, 2003) as outlined in Table 21.2. Generalized anxiety can be accompanied by symptoms of depression, panic, and phobias; however, in the elder patient, depression is the most common accompanying condition (Anxiety Fact Sheet, 2008). Patients may be observed with a tense posture and frequent sighing. Older adults are more likely to minimize emotions and feelings and report somatic complaints (Lantz, 2002). In addition, they have many attributes of suicide vulnerability, which include pain and suffering, poor prognosis, depression, delirium, loss of control, and lack of social support (Breitbart et al., 2005). In differentiating anxiety from fear, evaluation should explore the known presence of an external threat versus anxiety stemming from an unknown internal stimulus (Pollack et al., 2004).

Severity

Anxiety in its mildest form assists any person to participate in general life activities; it serves as an impetus to perform various functions in learning, working, and

21.1 | Medical Conditions Associated with Anxiety

CATEGORY/BASIS	EXAMPLES
CARDIOVASCULAR CONDITIONS	Angina, congestive heart failure, hypovolemia, mitral valve prolapse, myocardial infarction, paroxysmal atrial tachycardia
ENDOCRINE DISORDERS	Carcinoid syndrome, Cushing's disease, hyperglycemia, hypoglycemia, hyperthyroidism, and hypothyroidism
IMMUNE CONDITIONS	AIDS, infections
METABOLIC CONDITIONS	Anemia, hyperkalemia, hyperthermia, hypoglycemia, and hyponatremia
RESPIRATORY CONDITIONS	Asthma, chronic obstructive pulmonary disease, hypoxia, pneumonia, pulmonary edema, and pulmonary embolus
NEUROLOGICAL CONDITIONS	Akathisia, encephalopathy, brain lesion, seizure disorders, postconcussion syndrome, vertigo, cerebral vascular accident, and dementia
CANCER	Hormone-producing tumors, pheochromocytoma
MEDICATION AND SUBSTANCES	Withdrawal of alcohol, benzodiazepines, nicotine, or sedatives
UNCONTROLLED PAIN	Use of steroids, stimulants, and neuroleptics such as metoclopramide or prochlorperazine

Compiled from Breitbart et. al., 2005; Lantz, 2002; McCullough, 1992; Pasacreta et al., 2006; Wall & Caroline, 2000.

adapting to the ongoing changes in life. Levels of anxiety are mild (which is considered to be normal), moderate, severe, and panic (Pasacreta et al., 2006; Lehmann & Rabins, 1999). In its severest form, anxiety becomes panic, which prevents the patient from doing anything. The person may become paralyzed in fear and confined to his/her immediate surroundings, such as the home or room. Table 21.4 outlines the characteristics of mild anxiety to panic.

Assessment

Assessment requires vigilance for anxiety. A history and review of medical conditions for potential causes of anxiety is part of the initial evaluation. A thorough discussion of psychosocial situations including living conditions, recent changes in the patient's life, as well as anticipated changes, is warranted. This conversation is most revealing if it includes both the patient and family or friends. Moreover, there should be an assessment of

21.2 | Four Types of Anxiety Manifestation

CLASSIFICATION	MANIFESTATIONS
PHYSICAL SYMPTOMS	Autonomic responses such as tachycardia, tachypnea, diaphoresis, lightheadedness, tremors
AFFECTIVE SYMPTOMS	Nervous or restless behaviors such as pacing, picking, frequent movement
BEHAVIORAL RESPONSES	Avoidance, compulsions
COGNITIVE RESPONSES	Edginess, worry, panic, terror, apprehension, obsession, thoughts of self-injury

Source: Pollack et al., 2004; Fisch, 2003.

21.3 | Emergent Conditions Disguised as Anxiety in Patients with Life-Threatening Illness

Hypoxia
Sepsis
Uncontrolled pain
Pulmonary embolus
Impending cardiac or respiratory arrest
Electrolyte imbalance
Dehydration

Source: Gibson et al., 2006.

whether the anxiety is a secondary response to the following: an organic factor, a primary psychiatric disorder, or reactive or situationally related stress (Pollack et al., 2004). For children, a skilled assessment based on children's concerns and worries may help reveal both parent and child anxiety.

Physical exam. A physical exam may reveal tachycardia, tachypnea, skin changes, tongue changes, rapid speech, restlessness, and tremors. Further assessment includes ruling out associated conditions; for example, if the patient has tachycardia, a thyroid function panel can rule out hyperthyroidism. For patients feeling anxious, a glucose test can rule out hypoglycemia. If there is a sore tongue along with the anxiety, testing folate levels can rule out nutritional deficiencies. Pulmonary function tests and arterial blood gases can rule out hypoxia and pulmonary disease (McCullough, 1992).

Assessment tools. A tool for further assessing anxiety is the Anxiety Sensitivity Index (ASI) as seen in Table 21.5. This is a 16-item self-report index in which responses are rated from 0 to 4. A mean score of 20 and below indicates no anxiety. A mean score in the 20's is common for those with generalized anxiety disorders. A mean score of 35 and above indicates panic disorder (Candilis, 1998; Reiss, Peterson, Gursky, & McNally, 1986).

For children, there are several tools to assess anxiety in well children; however, none has been tested in chronically ill children, or terminally ill children. Two self-report measures are the Spence Children's Anxiety Scale and the Screen for Child Anxiety Related Emotional Disorders. One interview that may help is the Anxiety Disorders International Schedule for Children (Kersun & Shemesh, 2007).

Management

Pharmacological

In a younger, healthier population, benzodiazepines are the drug of choice, along with possible tricyclic antidepressants and beta-adrenergic agents. However, in the geriatric population, benzodiazepines are the drug of choice as tricyclics and beta-adrenergic agents are not well tolerated. Even so, in the older adult, one should not use longer acting benzodiazepines as they may cause more confusion; use of shorter acting agents such as lorazepam, oxazepam, or temazepam may be more appropriate. Suggested doses are 0.25–5.0 mg TID of lorazepam, or 10–15 mg TID of oxazepam. Selective serotonin reuptake inhibitors (SSRIs) may be worth a trial if benzodiazepines are not successful. This could include fluoxetine 20–80 mg a day or sertraline 50–200 mg per day (Pollack et al., 2004). If insomnia is also an issue, temazepam 15–30 mg at bedtime may be helpful. Drug-induced anxiety may be caused by neuroleptic medications such as haloperidol. For patients with generalized anxiety and history of substance abuse, buspirone may be useful. Patients with severe respiratory function, low-dose antihistamines may be helpful, as benzodiazepines may be too sedating and inhibit

21.4 | Mild to Severe Anxiety and Its Effects

MILD	– Reduced awareness, reduced attention for problem solving
MODERATE	– Perceptual field narrowed, decreased observation, and selective attention
SEVERE	– Reduced perceptual field, scattered, escalated anxiety with inability to attend
PANIC	– Feelings of awe, dread, fear, panic – Inability to focus – No perceptual field

Developed from Pasacreta et al., 2006.

21.5 | Anxiety Sensitivity Index

1) It scares me when my heart beats rapidly.
2) It scares me when I become short of breath.
3) It scares me when I am nauseous.
4) It scares me when I feel faint.
5) When I notice my heart is beating rapidly, I worry I might have a heart attack.
6) Unusual body sensations scare me.
7) It scares me when I feel "shaky."
8) It embarrasses me when my stomach growls.
9) When my stomach is upset, I worry that I might be seriously ill.
10) When I am nervous, I worry that I might be mentally ill.
11) When I cannot keep my mind on a task, I worry that I might be going crazy.
12) It scares me when I am unable to keep my mind on a task.
13) It scares me when I am nervous.
14) Other people notice when I feel shaky.
15) It is important to me to stay in control of my emotions.
16) It is important for me not to appear nervous.

Responses are rated from 0 (not true) to 4 (extremely true). A mean score of 20 and below indicates no anxiety. A mean score in the 20s is common for those with generalized anxiety disorders. A mean score of 35 and above indicates panic disorder.

Source: Reiss, S., Peterson, R.A., Gursky, D.M., & McNally, R.J. (1986). Anxiety sensitivity, anxiety frequency, and the prediction of fearfulness. *Behavioral Research Therapy, 24,* 1–8.

respiratory drive (Miller & Massie, 2007; Pasacreta et al., 2006). See Table 21.6 for drugs and dosages.

In children, short-acting benzodiazepines are the medication of choice. These include lorazepam or diazepam (Tyler & Fisher, 2007; Hellsten & Kane, 2006), and dosing is based on weight. Lorazepam is calculated at 0.05 mg/kg with a maximum of 2 mg per dose. Diazepam is calculated at 0.01–0.02 mg/kg with a maximum of dose of about 10 mg a day (Tyler & Fisher, 2007). SSRIs have not been studied for children with life-threatening illnesses, though they have been used in children with other anxiety disorders such as obsessive compulsive disorders.

21.6 | Medications to Treat Anxiety

ADULTS	
Benzodiazepines	
Short acting	
Lorazepam (Ativan)	0.25–5 mg TID-QID
Oxazepam (Serax)	10–15 mg TID-QID
Temazepam (Restoril)	15–30 mg at bedtime
Neuroleptics	
Haloperidol (Haldol)	0.5–5 mg q 2–12 hours
Olanzipine (Zyprexa, Zydis)	2.5–5 mg BID to TID
Chlorpromazine (Thorazine)	12.5–50 q 4–6
Antihistamines	
Diphenhydramine (Benadryl)	25–75 mg BID
Hydroxyzine (Vistaril)	10–50 mg QID–q 6 hours
Azapirones	
Buspirone (BuSpar)	5–20 mg TID

CHILDREN	
Benzodiazipines	
Lorazapan (Ativan)	Younger children
	0.05 mg/kg every 4–6 hrs
	Max dose 2 mg per dose
	Adolescents above 12 yrs.
	1–2 mg every 8 hrs
Diazepam (Valium)	Younger children
	0.01–0.02 mg/kg every
	8–12 hrs
	Adolescents above 12 yrs.
	5 mg every 8 hrs

Compiled from Breitbart et al., 2005; Lavretsky, 2001; Miller & Massie, 2007; Pasacreta et al., 2006; Kersun & Shemesh, 2007; & Tyler & Fisher, 2007.

Nonpharmacological

To help with anxiety, it is helpful to work with the patients to help them acknowledge their fears and anxiety about their disease, treatment, symptoms, and future care. In particular, patient may have fears and concerns about dying and the dying process. Inquiring about such fears and addressing them in terms of future possible care plans is helpful to patients and families and provides them with the knowledge that the healthcare provider is proactive. Providing structure and predictability can help to allay fears and can take place in the form of future appointments and symptom management (Bakitas, Dahlin, & Bishop, 2008). Offering summary information about progress and future events is helpful to help alleviate any surprises. Encouraging patient participation in care helps with a sense of control (Perley, 2007). In severe anxiety and panic, medications are usually necessary; nonpharmacological or complementary therapy may help in mild to moderate anxiety. Nonpharmacological treatment of anxiety includes modalities such as dietary intake, stress management, and psychotherapy. Dietary intake includes evaluating the diet for caffeine and alcohol (McCullough, 1992). Caffeine is an ingredient in tea, coffee, chocolate, and colas, as well as other products; sometimes, just decreasing the daily amount ingested is helpful. However, in many cases, the caffeine intake needs to be completely eliminated. If this is the case, weaning off the caffeine in a planned process helps to avoid headache, nausea, and general malaise. High alcohol intake is common in anxious patients, although it does not actually help the anxiety and it may worsen anxiety since it affects sleep and cognition. Alcohol may be commonly ingested as beer, wine, or hard liquors and can be present in cough medicines. Reduction or elimination of alcohol intake may be helpful in the management of anxiety.

Stress management can include exercise programs, breathing exercises, relaxation techniques, massage, touch, distraction, music therapy, and visualization. Guided imagery and hypnosis may offer the patient more control (Gibsen et al., 2006). Some hospitals, healthcare systems, and even insurances offer exercise programs. Many YWCAs/YMCAs offer gentle exercise programs or special programs directed at keeping people of various ages healthy. Shopping malls often offer ill patients the opportunity to walk in a safe, weather-friendly environment. For patients in assisted living or skilled nursing facilities, physical therapists can often help promote gentle exercise. For children, stress management may be developed into more structured programs. These may include activities such as sports, music, or, for younger children, play therapy activities with child-life specialists. Adherence to routines and schedules helps reduce stress and normalize their illness. Of particular importance may be attendance at school and related activities since this plays a major role in the context of their daily routine and social networks (Tyler & Fisher, 2007).

Massage therapy can be an effective method to help patients relax. However, as with any person, the patient must be assessed regarding his/her comfort of physical touch. Older adults may not have experience with formal massage and may be uncomfortable with such intimate touch. Often patients may receive modified massages from healthcare personnel in various settings, such as outpatient oncology setting, hospitals, skilled facilities, or day care centers.

Distraction occurs in many forms including having a television or radio or participating in arts and crafts, performing hobbies, and reading. It is important to assess how the patients spend their time and what activities are distracting for them and helpful. Various volunteer organizations in the community can help with these sorts of activities. Music therapy has been shown to be effective in anxiety, as it can reduce pain, promote physical comfort, and induce relaxation (Horne-Thompson & Grocke, 2008).

Environmental manipulation may be very important: sometimes patients are fearful of their living environment. Physical therapists (PTs) and occupational therapists (OTs) can assist with home safety evaluations, and social workers can assist with issues of personal safety. In the case of older adults, this may include situations of potential abuse and neglect, transportation, or nutrition. Helping the patient to maintain control of his/her daily schedule of activities may decrease anxiety. Too often, the patients lose control over the structure of their day, depending on their types of treatment. Facilitating their ability to schedule when appointments, meals, and other activities occur can help them feel less anxious and out of control.

Psychotherapy may include counseling, spiritual care, and cognitive behavioral therapy. Counseling should include an acknowledgment of fears and specific conversations about fears. Spiritual care should focus on existential fears around death and dying (Payne & Massie, 2000). Cognitive behavioral therapy focuses on restructuring the issues. Children will need specially trained clinicians to assist with these areas.

Dependent, Independent, and Collaborative Interventions

Treatment of anxiety for a patient with a life-threatening illness requires a collaborative approach by an interdisciplinary team. Specifically, the team needs to review the patient history and medications, and then determine symptom management together. Since treatment usually requires psychological support and medication management, clear delineation of roles should be clarified for the patient and his/her family. This provides consistent direction and support to the patient

and family without provoking further anxiety. Usually, a physician or an advanced practice nurse can diagnose and treat anxiety as well as provide medications and psychological support. A social worker can be quite effective in assessing the living conditions, the family dynamics that affect anxiety, as well as offering both counseling and stress management techniques. An OT or PT can assess in-home safety. The pharmacist can examine a medication regimen for polypharmacy. A common intervention for all disciplines working with patients who are anxious is to remind health clinicians to recognize their own anxiety and manage it so as not to transfer their anxiety to the patient and family (Miller & Massie, 2007). It is helpful to remind colleagues how to defuse a patient's anxiety when it begins to escalate.

Family Concerns and Considerations

Education for the family and caregiver is important regarding their understanding of anxiety and how it manifests itself. This enables early recognition and helping the patient utilize both medications and complementary strategies to manage symptoms. The patient and family should also understand that long-term use of medications to treat anxiety might be necessary. Moreover, these medications may cause some or all of the following side effects: daytime somnolence, confusion, unsteady stance or gait, paradoxical effects, memory disturbance, depression, withdrawal, abuse, dependence, and respiratory problems. Therefore, safety may be an issue, and how to prevent problems with medications should be discussed. The patient and family may need to discuss the risk-benefit ratio of interventions if medication side effects are debilitating and worse than the anxiety itself.

Medication information is imperative, including both prescription medications as well as over-the-counter medications that can cause anxiety. A careful review of each medication, its intent, and its dosage can help decrease confusion and help with compliance. A medication box prefilled by family or healthcare personnel with medications in the correct time slots can be tremendously helpful in ensuring correct medication dosage and timing. In addition, a patient or family member can keep a diary of medications, dosages, and time of administration. In creating medication schedules, it is best to work around previous rituals such as mealtime and activities of daily living, with particular attention to sleep schedules.

Stress management techniques that can be utilized by both the patient and family should be taught. These interventions include promoting control for the older adults over their environment (e.g., simple planning of daily activities, toileting, mealtimes, and visiting times), and review of the symptoms including recognition, management, and prevention of anxiety. Education is particularly important in terms of how to diffuse anxiety for the patient and suggestions for helpful behaviors or strategies that families can follow to de-escalate the patient's stress.

Care should be taken to simplify the day by not overbooking activities for the terminally ill patient. Encourage family or significant others to allow time for ventilation of feelings or concerns regarding their illness. In addition, preparing the patient for any treatment, change in plans, or visitation by other medical personnel can greatly help decrease anxiety because the patient knows what to expect. Finally, all persons involved with the anxious patient need be patient, speak calmly, and provide any direct care as gently as possible.

DEPRESSION

At the end of life, it is common for patients to experience psychological distress in response to their life-threatening diagnosis. For many years, it was thought that grief and depression were normal coping mechanisms to a terminal illness (Block, 2000; McDonald et al., 1999) and therefore it was unnecessary to treat depression. (The treatment would interfere with the natural dying process and the emotional work of dying.) In fact, not treating depression may interfere with a patient's ability to bring closure to his/her end-of-life issues and concerns. Identifying depression in some patients is complicated by possible numerous comorbidities. These include cardiovascular conditions, neurological conditions, autoimmune diseases, endocrine disorders, and other conditions (Pasacreta et al., 2006). Specifically in cancer, depressive symptoms mimic those caused the treatment including loss of appetite from chemotherapy, fatigue induced by the metabolic changes in cancer, and lack of sleep from compliance with continuous pain and symptom medication regimens (Gibson et al., 2006; Breitbart et al., 2005; Fisch, 2003).

Depression in children is complex to assess and manage due to the challenges of their developmental stage. Often their depression may stem from the social issues such as being different from their friends and losing connection with their communities within and around school. Children may understand their illness through their continued, repeated interactions within a healthcare system, rather than understanding the illness itself. They may also pick up signals from their parents, so it is important to assess the family system (Kersun & Shemesh, 2007; Tyler & Fisher, 2007). However, no specific studies have been done on depression in dying children.

Depression in the older adult may be masked by the normal aging processes. Age-related changes include changes in the sleep/wake cycles, appetite, and the ability to continue previous pursuits in life condi-

tions (Pasacreta et al., 2006; Finkel, 2004; Goy & Ganzini, 2003). In addition, the presence of fatigue may be perceived as age-related rather than disease-related (Brown and Von Roenn, 2004). McDonald et al. (1999) documented that depression was overlooked because healthcare focuses on physiologic treatment and management of side effects rather than emotional responses to an individual's changes in health.

Specific to the elder patient, it is difficult to recognize depression secondary to the misperception that all elders become depressed as part of the aging process. There is also a cohort characteristic in the current generation of older adults because they may be embarrassed to report psychological problems in general and depressive symptoms in particular because of the perceived stigma that depression represents weakness (Valente, Saunder, & Cohen, 1994).

Further complicating the diagnosis and treatment of depression in the terminally ill patient is inadequate healthcare provider knowledge regarding the treatment of depression (Kapo, Morrison, & Liao, 2007). A thorough assessment necessitates time to interview a patient more deeply than a cursory check in. Moreover, effective treatment and management requires a time commitment that involves working on psychological issues, prescribing psychotropic agents, and monitoring the potential side effects of such agents. Under the time constraints of various medical practices, time to perform a complete assessment may feel overwhelming to the novice clinician. Ageist attitudes on the part of the prescribing clinician can also affect treatment for elder and younger patients.

Some clinicians express feelings of hopelessness around a life-limiting illness and feel depression cannot be well treated (Block, 2000). Other clinicians, including nurses, may feel that by asking about depression they may add to the patient's psychological distress by further upsetting them (McDonald et al., 1999; Valente & Saunders, 1997). Furthermore, clinicians may feel overwhelmed by the responsibility of caring for patients with limited prognoses. They may feel pressure and urgency that once they have identified depression, they must attend to all the elements of the disease at once to cure the patient rather than understand that treatment is a process (Valente & Saunders, 1997).

Definition

Depression is defined as a mood disorder and contains both psychological and somatic symptoms that alter mood, affect, and personality. It is a compilation of signs and symptoms that are not usually a normal reaction to daily life occurrences. According to the Diagnostic and Statistical Manual of Mental Disorders (APA, 2000), it is defined as an episode of 2 weeks or longer where there is loss of interest or pleasure in nearly all activities (anhedonia). In addition, four or more symptoms are present from the following list: changes in appetite, sleep, weight or psychomotor activity; decreased energy, feelings of worthlessness, or guilt; difficulty thinking, concentrating, or making decisions; or recurrent thoughts of death, suicidal ideation, or attempts at such (APA, 2000).

Depression can be persistent and lasts for months if left untreated. There may be a family history of the disease. Symptoms could include inconsistent memory or complaints of memory loss, increased speech latency, and an irritable affect (Cassem, Papkostas, Fava, & Stern, 2004). There is lack of consensus regarding the criteria to define depression in older adults with cancer because their disease and treatment side effects alone may result in many of the criteria in the depression profile (NIH, 2002). Some authors suggest that a clinician assess cognitive mood symptoms rather than neurovegetative symptoms (Gibson et al., 2006).

Incidence

Depression is common in patients with cancer 10–25% of the time. This may increase with disease progression and particular types of cancer (e.g., pancreatic cancer) (Gibson et al., 2006). Depression is a major health problem and the most common psychiatric disorder secondary to the events that occur later in life (Kapo et al., 2007; Finkel, 2004; Fisch, 2003), but it may be overlooked and/or mistaken for dementia (Cremens, 2004). Most studies on depression look at prevalence rather than incidence. At the *National Institute of Health State of the Science Conference on Symptom Management in Cancer: Pain, Depression, and Fatigue,* the consensus was that there were no reliable incidence studies in cancer patients (NIH, 2002). Recent geriatric studies report a 1–2% prevalence of major depression; estimates are about 25% of patients with cancer and over 50% of patients with life threatening diseases (Lebowitz et al., 1997).

The incidence and prevalence of depression in children is less understood; there have been no large studies to evaluate these symptoms in children, since children have unique ways of coping depending on their age. More often than not, disruptions in routines, relationships, physical condition, and, for teenagers, loss of independence, can be risk factors for depression, along with the adult reports of low self-esteem, guilt, hopelessness, and suicidal ideation (Kerson & Shemesh, 2007; Hellsten & Kane, 2006).

Etiology

The etiology of depression is multifactorial and falls into four categories: physical, psychological, social, and biological (Kane, Ouslander, & Abrass, 1999). See Table 21.7. Physical factors encompass medical

conditions, specific diseases, medication effects, and sensory deprivation from loss of vision or hearing (Kane et al., 1999). Many medical conditions can cause depression, including cardiovascular conditions such as congestive heart failure, myocardial infarction, and cardiac arrhythmias; neurological conditions such as cerebral vascular accidents and cerebral anoxia; Huntington's, Parkinson's, and Alzheimer's disease; HIV; dementia; epilepsy; multiple sclerosis; post-concussion periods; myasthenia gravis; narcolepsy; subarachnoid hemorrhage; autoimmune diseases such a rheumatoid arthritis and polyarteritis nodosa; endocrine disorders such as hypothyroidism, hyperparathyroidism, diabetes mellitus, folate deficiency, hypoadrenalism, and Cushing's and Addison's disease; and other conditions such as anemia, alcoholism, anemia, systemic lupus, Epstein Barr virus, hepatitis, malignancies, malnutrition, sexually transmitted diseases (STDs), and encephalitis. Medications that may generate depression include propranolol, reserpine, and metoclopramide (Pasacreta et al., 2006: Pollack et al., 2004). See Table 21.8 for a list of medical conditions associated with depression.

Psychological issues that may precipitate depres-

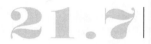 | Etiology of Depression for Adults and Children

CATEGORY	EXAMPLES
PHYSICAL	Medical conditions including cardiac disease; cerebrovascular disease; autoimmune disease; endocrine, liver, and renal failure; medication effects; symptom-related, such as pain or sleep disturbances; treatment effects; sensory deprivation
PSYCHOLOGICAL	Memory loss; unresolved conflict; loss of independence; change in living situation; financial consequences from illness; poor coping; substance abuse
SOCIAL	Changes in body image; loss of independence; loss of family and friends; loss of community, such as school-related activities; isolation; loss of employment; previous conflicted relationships
BIOLOGICAL	Family history; previous episodes of depression; neurotransmission deficiencies; central nervous effects of cytokines

Adapted from Edelstein et al., 1999; Kane et al., 1999. Tyler Fisher, 2007, Pasacreta, et al. 2006.

21.8 | Medical Conditions Associated with Depression

CATEGORY/BASIS	EXAMPLES
ENDOCRINE DISORDERS	Hypothyroidism, hyperparathyroidism, diabetes, Cushing's, Addison's
CARDIOVASCULAR CONDITIONS	Congestive heart failure, myocardial infarction, cardiac arrhythmias
NEUROLOGICAL CONDITIONS	Cerebral vascular accident, anoxia, Huntington's, Alzheimer's, dementia, multiple sclerosis, postconcussion syndrome, myasthenia gravis, narcolepsy, subarachnoid hemorrhage
IMMUNE DISORDERS	HIV, rheumatoid arthritis, polyarteritis nodosa
CANCER	Pancreatic, brain
OTHER	Pain, alcoholism, anemia, lupus

Compiled from Derby, 2007; Miller & Massie, 2007; Tyler & Fisher, 2007; Pasacreta et al., 2006; Breitbart et al., 2005; Cassem et al., 2004.

sion cover a wide spectrum, including unresolved conflicts, memory loss, loss of independence, change in living situations, and possible financial consequences incurred from a life-limiting illness (Pasacreta et al., 2006). For children and adolescents, the loss of independence and the loss of school and related community can be difficult (Tyler & Fisher, 2007). Coping with the debilitating physical aspects of having a life-limiting illness may also cause depression. Pain and exhaustion often trigger depression in some patients. Other triggers include loss of routines and, more importantly, changes in body image. Older children may retreat from the embarrassment of disease and treatment-related change in their physical appearance (Tyler & Fisher, 2007).

Social issues include loss of family or friends, isolation, loss of job, and previous conflicted relationships (Edelstein, Kalish, Drozdick, & McKee, 1999; Kane et al., 1999). Even without dealing with terminal illness, older adults face loss as a consequence of the aging process. Close friends and family members of similar age may predecease them, and retirement may result in multiple losses ranging from loss of social position as a working person, change in socioeconomic status, loss of friends and acquaintances, loss of routine, and a loss of purpose. Young children may have a loss of the school community including teachers, friends, sports, afterschool activities, and other social interactions.

Biological factors of depression include family history, prior episodes of depression, neurotransmission deficiencies, and central nervous effects of cytokines (Kane et al., 1999). Data suggests that deficiencies in serotonin, norepinephrine, and prolactin, as well as abnormal cortisol and dopamine levels, can cause depressive symptoms (Lovejoy et al., 2000). Family history may increase the risk of depression by a factor of 1.5–3, and 50% of people with depression have recurrence. Other mental disorders may accompany depression, including somataform disorders (Perley, 2007).

Cardinal Signs

Buckwalter and Piven (1999) describe a triad of depressive symptoms which include the following: 1) changes in mood; 2) perceptual disturbances of oneself, the environment, and the future; and 3) vegetative and behavioral signs. Depression may affect all aspects of a patient's life because of the possible element of depression in other conditions, such as aches and pains, confusion, agitation, anxiety, or irritability. Depression is not a symptom of normal aging but rather has a relatively discrete onset; the older adult may develop more physical symptoms rather than changes in emotional affect (Buckwalter & Piven 1999).

Patients may present with a dysphoric mood, or lack of pleasure. Signs in the older adult include poor personal hygiene and grooming; slow thought processes and speech; sadness, tearfulness, hopelessness, helplessness, worthlessness, and social withdrawal; changes in sleep patterns and appetite; fatigue; behavioral slowing; and complaints of diminished ability to think (Cremens, 2004; Kane et al., 1999; Costa et al., 1996). Signs of depression in children manifest as somatic complaints, periods of anger, and other behaviors. Patients of all ages may express recurrent thoughts of worthlessness, and excessive or inappropriate guilt (Derby, 2007). There may also be evidence of sadness or melancholy for children (Tyler & Fisher, 2007). For teenagers, it may be manifested by low self-esteem, guilt, and hopelessness (Kane & Himelstein, 2007).

The elder who has dementia does not manifest depression in the same way as the person whose cognitive function is intact. There may be more peripheral symptoms in the elder, with altered cognition, such as agitation, repetitive vocalization, apathy, insomnia, food refusal, or resisting care (Volicer, 2001). Depression in this population may lead to increased dependence in activities of daily living and decreased ability to engage in meaningful activities.

Most patients with a life-threatening illness fulfill several of the criteria for depression under DSM-IV (AMA, 2000). The challenge lies in differentiating depression from grief (Block, 2000). Grief is the normal response to a loss, injury, insult, illness deprivation, or disenfranchisement, which is usually proportionate to the disruption caused by the loss (Weissman, 1998). To differentiate between grief and depression in the patient with a terminal illness, one must perform a more thorough interview that examines how the patient has coped with past crises to assess resiliency. Evaluation of the somatic distress the patient is experiencing includes hopelessness or helplessness, whether they still the capacity for joy, and whether they look to the future. If they still have joy and can look forward to the future with joy and the symptoms come in wavelike fashion, the patient probably has grief rather than depression (Block, 2000).

Severity

Depression in its most severe form puts a person at a risk for suicide. The rate of suicide increases with age, with suicide being the third leading cause of death for older adults (Stern, Perlis, & Lagomasino, 2004; Depression Fact Sheet, 1998; Lehmann & Rabins, 1999). One out of five suicides involves a person 65 years or older (Stern et al., 2004; Edelstein et al., 1999). Suicidal behavior in the older adult differs from that of a younger person in that the elder is less likely to express suicidal ideation and more likely to utilize lethal methods. Older single men are at a higher risk for suicide than older single women (Edelstein et al., 1999).

In advanced illness, suicide has a higher incidence. Suicidal ideation should be considered a psychiatric emergency and assessed on an urgent basis. It is essential to assess for depression in any patient who verbalizes suicidal ideation because it plays a significant role. Lack of a previous suicide attempt may not be significant in assessing suicidal risk because the majority of older patients who commit suicide have no prior suicidal behaviors. Many elders who commit suicide have been found to have the most treatable types of depression; however, they have not received appropriate interventions (Edelstein et al., 1999; Depression Guideline Panel, 1993).

Risk for suicide in the general population includes prior psychiatric diagnosis including previous depression, family history of suicide, poor social support with isolation, delirium, fatigue, advanced illness with disfiguring disease or surgery, substance or alcohol abuse, poorly controlled pain, increasing age, and lack of control with hopelessness (Gibson et al., 2006; Depression Guideline Panel, 1993). The following issues are specific to the evaluation of the adult's potential for suicide: strong character, refusal of assistance, fear of becoming a burden, fear of dependence, fear of loss of control, fear of financial issues, retired or unemployed, severe pain that is unrelieved, poor functional status, poor health, poor/bad relationships with family, isolation, and previous psychiatric distress (Filiberti et al., 2001; Kane et al., 1999). Other factors include retirement, recent changes (such as a move), changes in health, history of poor

interpersonal relationships, and a terminal diagnosis (Kane et al., 1999). For teenagers, it can be a loss of social relationships with the school community, such as loss of relationships due to healthcare treatments and inability to attend school, activities, or sports.

Once a patient has been identified as a suicide risk, this must be taken seriously. Using a nonjudgmental approach, the clinician must develop a rapport with the patient in order to evaluate the intent. This includes evaluating the presence of suicidal thoughts, details of a suicide plan, the seriousness of the intent, the risk ratio, the precipitants of such intent, the patient's social supports, and the degree of the patient's impulsivity (Stern et al., 2004).

Suicidal ideation should be evaluated for its severity. There should be an examination of suicide plan, specifically looking at the risk rescue ratio and the level of planning. The patient's level of hopelessness should be examined. Further assessment of the possible precipitants should be determined as well as social supports. Specifically, a clinician should assess the history and determine the degree of intent and the existence and quality of internal and external controls (Gibson et al., 2006). Finally, the issue of suicide ideation should be discussed with family and friends (Stern et al., 2004).

Assessment

Assessment includes both cognitive and physical assessment. The Depression Guideline Panel (1993) outlines the steps in detecting and treating depression: 1) Be vigilant for depression and evaluate risk factors; 2) Perform clinical interview; and 3) Consider any mood disorders using clinical history, interview, and report by family, and evaluate other potential factors that may cause depression such as medications, medical conditions, previous psychiatric disorders, and substance abuse. In addition, the racial and ethnic culture of the older adult should be considered in assessment. This is particularly important since most of the depression literature, including description, presentation, and experience, focuses on that of the Caucasian culture (Edelstein et al., 1999). However, in many cultures the expression of depression may be in somatic complaints and certain affects. Therefore, it may be necessary to use interpreters when English is not the first language, as well as consult religious elders and community specific experts to assist with examining common practices within another culture.

Assessment focuses on the cognitive process of the patient, including a mental status examination. Depression assessment areas are reviewed in Table 21.9 (Block, 2000; Buckwalter & Piven, 1999; Lloyd-Williams, 2001).

Assessment of depression in children is more complicated. The age and developmental level must be taken into account. Like adults, they may experience

21.9 | Depression Assessment Areas

AREAS OF PSYCHOSOCIAL ASSESSMENT FOR THE PATIENT

ABILITY TO ENGAGE IN LIFE	Boredom vs. inability to be active
INTEREST IN WORLD AROUND THEM	Lack of interest vs. delight in shock, humor, etc.
ENGAGEMENT IN HOBBIES	Joy vs. lack or interest
PRESENCE OF ANHEDONIA	Inability to anticipate anything with pleasure
VIEW OF LIFE	Feelings of hopelessness vs. optimism and plans for the future
SELF WORTH	Worthfulness vs. worthlessness, any expressions of guilt or self-recrimination, expression of suicidal ideation

Compiled from Cassem & Brendel, 2004, Cassam et al., 2004; Block, 2000; Lloyd-Williams, 2001.

disease-related symptoms usually associated with depression, such as fatigue, anorexia, insomnia, and agitation (Hellston & Kane, 2006). Parents are often experts on their child's behavior and may notice signs such as persistent sadness, tearfulness, irritability, withdrawal from previously enjoyed activities, changes in school performance or activity level, and general feelings of unwellness. Also, parents must be evaluated for depression, as this may affect the child patient as well (Hellsten & Kane, 2006).

A thorough assessment of the patient would include laboratory tests to rule out other conditions, and may be appropriate if they do not present an undue burden on the patient and if there are plans to treat whatever deficiencies are found. Laboratory studies would include serum electrolytes to rule out dehydration; CBC and HCT to rule out anemia; thyroid profile to rule out hypothyroidism; a VDRL screen to rule out a sexually transmitted disease; B-12/folate levels to rule out vitamin deficiencies; liver function tests (LFTs) to rule out liver failure; renal function tests to rule out renal failure; a urinalysis to rule out infections; and an electrocardiogram (EKG) to rule out cardiac issues (Cassam et al., 2004; Cremens, 2004; Fisch, 2003).

Patients with pre-existing neurovegetative conditions such as Alzheimer's disease or Parkinson's may be unable to respond to questioning, so a cognitive assessment may be impossible or yield little helpful information. Volicer (1999) describes the high incidence

21.10 | Types of Conditions and Treatment of Related Depressions

CONDITION	CLASS OF MEDICATIONS
CARDIOVASCULAR DISEASE	SSRIs – Sertaline, Paroxetine, Fluosetine, Fluvoxamine, Citalopram Dopamine Reuptake Agents – Bupropion SNRIs – Venlafaxine 5-HT antagonists – Nefazodone, Trazadone
GASTROINTESTINAL DISEASE	Tricyclics Dopamine Reuptake Agents – Bupropion 5-HT antagonists – Nefazodone, Trazadone
RENAL DISEASE	Tricyclics SSRIs SNRIs – Venlafaxine Noradrenergic agonist – Mirtazapine
HEPATIC DISEASE	Tricyclics SSRIs SNRIs – Venlafaxine Noradrenergic agonist – Mirtazapine

Source: Pasacreta et al., 2006.

of depression in this population and stresses the importance to surveillance for behaviors that may indicate depression. These behaviors include food refusal, angry affect, labile mood, agitation, repetitive movements, or increased withdrawal. Treatment of possible depression with medications serves as a diagnostic tool (Volicer, 1999), and the current standard is to initiate treatment and see if there is a response. Even without any outward clues to the presence of depression, medications may improve behavior. Because this population is vulnerable to relapse, Volicer (1999) states that it is important to continue treatment for at least 1 year.

Physical assessment includes general examination of the following areas: cardiopulmonary, gastrointestinal, genitourinary, and neurological (Kane et al., 1999). If pain develops, radiological studies and gastrointestinal studies are indicated to rule our fractures, ulcers, and neoplasms. Complaints of chest pain should be evaluated with an EKG, and noninvasive cardiovascular studies to rule out myocardial infarctions, congestive heart failure, and arrhythmias. Shortness of breath justifies chest films, and pulmonary function test, pulse oximetry, and blood gases to rule out COPD, lung neoplasms, and other pulmonary conditions. The presence of constipation indicates occult blood test, barium enema, and thyroid function test to rule out neoplasms and ineffective thyroid. Neurological changes warrant an electroencephalogram with CT scan or MRI to rule out cerebrovascular accidents, tumors, or other brain conditions (Kane et al., 1999).

All too often, the symptom complaints of older adults are not taken seriously by their healthcare practitioners. The symptoms of depression can signal a medical condition, and a physical work-up may be necessary to find the cause of problems. However, it the older adult is already known to have a terminal illness, the extent of a work-up will depend on quality-of-life issues and how much a further work-up would change and inevitable outcome. However, if a condition is reversible and can have a positive effect on a patient, then at least a preliminary work-up may be appropriate. Evaluation of appropriate treatments needs to occur on an individual basis where the healthcare team can examine the totality of the patient's health condition and weigh the risks and benefit of work-up and treatment.

Assessment Tools. Assessment tools specific to screening for depression in the geriatric population include the Beck Depression Inventory (BDI) and the Geriatric Depression Scale (GDS). The BDI consists of 21 items with a 4-point scale, although there is a shorter 13-item version (Candilis, 1998). This self-report inventory investigates neurovegetative, cognitive, and mood symptoms. This scale is useful in examining psychological symptoms to develop a differential diagnosis of depression (Lloyd-Williams 2001). Candilis (1998) has a cut-off score of 10 (mild depression), 16 (mild to moderate depression), 20 (moderate to severe depression), and a score of 30 (severe depression). The GDS (Chapter 21 appendix, part A) was specifically developed for use with older adults. It is a 30-item questionnaire and takes approximately 10 minutes to complete. A score of 11 or more indicates depression. There is also a briefer 15-item GDS (Costa et al., 1996; Edelstein et al., 1999). A new scale, known as the Terminally Ill Grief or Depression Scale (TIGDS), is a self-report measure that contains preparatory grief and depression subscales (Periyakoil et al., 2005). See Table 21.11 for a review of tools.

Often asking, "Are you depressed?" as suggested by Block (2000) will result in an honest assessment by an adult patient. However, this may not be as appropriate in the older adult population because there is a generational attitude of denying mental health issues. Many older people are not comfortable expressing emotions or to directly answer a question. One study (Ohno et al., 2006) found that if a patient answers in the negative when asked "Are you depressed or not?" it signified further need for exploration. Rather than asking a single question, there is also a two-question screening assessment which includes the following questions: 1) Have you often been bothered by feeling down, depressed, or hopeless? 2) Have you often been bothered by having little pleasure or interest in doing things? (Fisch, 2003). Another measure of depression is the mood of the healthcare provider after an encounter. If a healthcare provider feels down, hopeless, and negative after an encounter, or has a desire to avoid the patient, there should be a high index of suspicion for depression and a rapid follow-up depressions assessment (Lee, Back, Block & Stewart, 2002). Of note, the U.S. Preventative Services Task Force (2005) found little evidence to sug-

21.11 | Depression Scales

BECK DEPRESSION INVENTORY (BDI)
  21-item questionnaire
  Multiple choice
  Scale of 11 or higher indicates depression
    11–19 mild depression
    20–30 moderate depression
    31 or higher severe depression

GERIATRIC DEPRESSION SCALE (GDS)
  30-item scale
  Yes/No format
  Scale of 11 or more is positive for depression

Complied from Edelstein et al., 1999.

gest that one assessment tool was more effective than another. Instead, they state a simple assessment may be just as effective. They offer two simple screening questions that relate to mood and anhedonia. They are:

1) Over the past 2 weeks, have you felt down, depressed, or hopeless?
2) Over the past 2 weeks, have you felt little interest or pleasure in doing things?"

Suicide assessment includes some specific questioning. One tool is the Suicidal Ideation Screening Questionnaire (SIS-Q) which is a 4-item screening tool that examines sleep disturbances, mood disturbances, guilt, and hopelessness with the following questions:

1) Have you ever had a period of 2 weeks or more when you had trouble falling asleep, staying asleep, and waking up too early, or sleeping too much?
2) Have you ever had 2 weeks or more during which you felt sad, blue, depressed, or when you lost interest and pleasure in things that you usually cared about or enjoyed?
3) Has there ever been a period of 2 weeks or more when you felt worthless, sinful, or guilty?
4) Has there been a period of time when you felt that life was hopeless?

A single positive response to a question correlates with 84% of patients with suicidal ideation, and necessitates further assessment (Candilis, 1998).

Kane et al. (1999) and Buckwalter and Piven (1999) suggest the following questions:

1) Do you feel life is not worth living?
2) Have you thought about harming yourself?
3) Are you thinking about suicide or taking your own life?
4) Do you have a plan? What is it?
5) Have you ever attempted suicide?

Any questions that receives a positive or "yes" answer warrants more further questioning, assessment, and intervention with the patient and family.

Management

Treatment of depression first includes management of pain and symptoms that will ensure that optimal comfort is achieved since physical pain and discomfort in itself increases depression (Block, 2000). Some of the major pain and symptoms areas include the use of medications: anti-emetics for nausea and vomiting; narcotics for cancer pain, chest pain, and dyspnea; nonsteroidal medications for bone pain, arthritis type pain, and various aches; and even low-dose antidepressant medications for nerve pain. In treating any one of these types of pain, the patient's mood may improve. However, in this last category of treating nerve pain, the use of low-dose tricyclics may simultaneously treat the depression and the pain.

For the older adult, it is judicious to use the lowest dose of antidepressants possible (Depression Fact Sheet 1996). This dose range may particularly vary in elders who have had a stroke, Parkinson's or Alzheimer's, or other comorbidities and may need longer treatment (Lavretsky, 2001). The underlying principle of medication management is to "start low and go slow." Practitioners should be careful not to stop therapy with a specific medication too soon because older patients may need a longer time to respond (Lavretsky, 2001).

For patients with a prognosis of 1 month or less, a psychostimulant, such as methylphenidate, may be very helpful. Psychostimulants typically work within 1–2 days. If the prognosis is longer than 1 month, one can start a psychostimulant to get an immediate effect and also start a longer acting antidepressant medication. The effect a patient gets from the psychostimulant can help with predicting how he/she will respond to a longer term medication; after a week on the psychostimulant, the dose can be decreased as the longer acting antidepressant dose is increased (Rozans, Dreisbach, Lertora, & Kahn, 2002).

In elder patients, tricyclic antidepressants (TCAs) and selective serotonin reuptake inhibitors (SSRIs) are roughly equivalent in efficacy (Lebowitz et al., 1997). However, the older adult tends to tolerate SSRIs better than TCAs. Side effects of TCAs include sedation, confusion, orthostatic hypotension, cardiac arrhythmias, dry mouth, constipation, ataxia, and confusion (Lavretsky, 2001; Lebowitz et al., 1997). SSRIs have fewer anticholinergic effects (Lebowitz et al., 1997) with other side effects of SSRIs including nausea, anorexia, diarrhea and insomnia (Lavretsky, 2001). In severe depression TCAs may be more efficacious (Depression Fact Sheet, 1998). Of note is that the use of herbal medications for treatment has shown no benefit over standard antidepressant therapy. More important is that these herbs (St. John's Wort, Kava, and Valerian) may interfere with other medications and foods, which may cause serious interactions (Miller & Massie, 2007). See Table 21.12 for a review of medications used in treating depression.

The treatment of children is difficult. The use of SSRIs in children is now not encouraged because of black box warnings from the Food and Drug Administration (FDA) that they could lead to suicide. Thus, until more research is done on SSRIs in children, their use in children is considered experimental (Kerson and Shemesh, 2007). Stimulants have been used in adults, but their use in children has been limited to ADHD. Their use in terminally ill children has not been well studied. Therefore, it is necessary to collaborate with child psychiatry to help with medication use and psychotherapy in children with depression.

One of the challenges in treating terminally ill patients with severe depression and potential suicidality is the question of psychiatric hospitalization. This is a difficult decision, but necessary in extreme cases. Sometimes a patient may require hospitalization to manage depression and maximize quality of life. However, focused attention and should be provided to the psychiatric unit to educate about symptoms seen at the end of life. Conversely, a patient may need to be on a medical floor with close psychiatric supervision to promote optimal management of other symptoms.

Nonpharmacological

The mainstay of nonpharmacological interventions is psychotherapy. Psychological counseling may be even more important in older patients since they may not physically tolerate medications (Cremens, 2004; Lavretsky, 2001). The ability to express emotions and feelings may be a novel process to the older adult and may take some adjustment, but psychotherapy allows the reduction of emotional distress and the improvement of morale and coping (Payne & Massie, 2000). Psychotherapy may focus on issues surrounding death and dying, including reminiscence and life review. In cognitive therapy, clinicians can help patients set realistic goals, provide compassionate listening, and validate the patient's feelings. In behavior therapy, clinicians can help patients develop structure for their day and activities (Pasacreta et al., 2006). This may allow a sense of making amends, identify accomplishments, improve interactions, and reduce fears of death.

21.12 | Medications to Treat Depression in Terminally Ill Patients

ADULTS

MEDICATION	STARTING DOSE	DAILY DOSE
Psychostimulants		
Dextroamphetamine	2.5–5 mg	10–20 mg 8a/noon
Methylphenidate	2.5–5 mg	5–10 mg 8a/noon
Selective serotonin reuptake inhibitors (SSRIs) less side effects		
Citalopram	10 mg q am	10–40 mg
Sertraline	12.5–25 mg	50–100 mg
Fluoxetine	5–10 mg	20–40 mg
Paroxetine	5–10 mg	20–40 mg
Nefazodone	100–500 mg	
Fluvoxamine	50–300 mg	
Serotonin noradrenaline reuptake inhibitors (SNRIs)		
Venlafaxine	37.5 mg	37.5–225 mg
Tricyclics		
Amitriptyline	25–50 mg	25–125 mg
Imipramine	25–50 mg	25–125 mg
Desipramine	25–50 mg	25–125 mg
Nortriptyline	25–50 mg	25–125 mg
Bupropion		200–450 mg

Compiled from Lavretsky 2001; Wilson, Chochinov, de Faye, & Breitbart, 2000; Block 2000; Breitbart et al., 2005; Fisch 2003.

CHILDREN

MEDICATION	STARTING DOSE
Methylphenidate	0.1 mg/kg twice a day – may need to give in afternoons to teens who want to stay up late
Antidepressants	SSRIs – but should consult child psychiatry

Source: Tyler and Fisher, 2007.

Cognitive therapy focuses on reframing and restructuring events.

Music therapy and movement therapy may be helpful in stimulating interaction, providing sensory input, and increased circulation. Other therapies may include pet therapy, group activities, and sensory stimulation. Music therapy allows a person to access his/her inner feelings because music can tap into emotions that words are unable to access. Pet therapy enhances self worth and fulfills a need to love and be loved in a safe environment while allowing tactile stimulation. Group activities and sensory stimulation increase contact and response to surroundings, stimulate thought and communication, and encourage interaction with other people (Buckwalter & Piven, 1999).

Dependent, Independent, and Collaborative Interventions

Team members may interact with the patient in different ways because of their different functions. In team conferences, vulnerable patients with a predisposition to depression can be identified. Reviewing specific patients in these team meetings can reveal subtle behavior changes that may indicate depression. Sometimes, certain behaviors alone may be difficult to evaluate, but putting into a more three-dimensional perspective may help to identify problems.

The effective management of depression requires a team approach. Physicians and advanced practice nurses may prescribe antidepressant medications. The social worker can provide counseling and assessment of social supports. In particular, family caregiver should be assessed for stress, and finances should be reviewed for potential burden. The chaplain can provide spiritual support (Block, 2000). Volunteers can add to the web of social support. If a patient has homecare, a psychiatric clinical nurse specialist can help with continuing care needs. Seeing the patient across the continuum and working within a collaborative approach may increase response to treatment.

Family Concerns and Considerations

Education is very important in depression. Families should understand that depression is neither a necessity of life nor a sign of weakness or failure, but rather it is a medical illness. Families should receive information on the factors that make patients vulnerable (e.g., multiple health problems, untreated pain, discomfort, and multiple losses). A review of depressive symptoms can help the family to recognize depression and may help the older adult to receive treatment sooner or alleviate suffering. In those patients with severe depression, clinicians can assist the family in reviewing patient safety issues for potential suicide including access to weapons, leftover medications, ability to drive, and extreme isolation.

Medical information is paramount. Patient and the family should understand that concurrent use of medications may cause depression or interfere with response to antidepressant medications. Discussion of treatment options comprises discussion of side effects of medication. The side effects include blurred vision, constipation, dry mouth, urinary retention, excessive perspiration, orthostatic hypotension, fatigue, weakness, drowsiness, tremors, twitching, and hallucinations. Family should understand these side effects further depress affect. With regard to medications and dosages, the family needs to understand that in the older adult population lower medication doses are prescribed because of slower metabolism (Buckwalter & Piven 1999; Depression Guideline Panel, 1993). The patient and family need to be reminded that it takes several weeks before the full effect of the medication is reached and may need encouragement to continue the medication for at least 6 weeks to receive the maximal effect of the medication. Medication education should also include continuing the medication when the patient feels better and thinks he/she can stop the medications.

Most important, the patient and his/her family should be reassured that the symptoms of depression are effectively treated most of the time (Waller & Caroline, 2000). They should be reassured that the patient will not be abandoned, and that a thoughtful treatment plan will be developed to improve quality of life. In the interim, education about severe depression should include information about support and obtaining emergency care if the depression worsens.

DELIRIUM

Delirium is defined as an acute disturbance of consciousness that affects cognition, arousal, and attention. It is also described as a confusional state resulting from a more global impairment in mental function (Waller & Caroline, 2000) and may also be referred to as confusion or agitation. This inconsistency in terminology makes management difficult. Alterations in thought processes are very common during the last weeks of life. Historically, this confusion has been thought to be a normal course of the dying process (Langhorne, 1999) and includes behaviors such as thrashing, agitation, muscle twitching, tossing or turning, moaning, and talking to the walls.

Delirium should be considered an emergency situation (Chan & Brennan, 1999). In the elder population, delirium may be associated with higher mortality rates, longer hospital admissions, increased costs of care, greater likelihood of being placed outside the home post hospitalization, and decreased functional ability (Cremens, 2004; Casarett and Inouye, 2001). Moreover, patients may be terrified of fluctuating cognitive deficits, hallucinations, misperceptions, paranoid and psychomotor agitation, and changes in sleep wake cycles (Casarett & Inouye 2001; Lawlor, Fainsinger, & Bruera, 2000). Families may become distressed by both the unusual behaviors and the sadness they feel from the premature loss of their loved one. If confusion is extreme, there is sadness and/or guilt if the patient falls and subsequent physical or chemical restraint is needed (Casarett & Inouye, 2001; Lawlor et al., 2000). Though delirium interferes with comfort and causes distress for family members, it was previously considered a stage of dying. Now state-of-the-art palliative care includes aggressive treatment of this symptom, allowing better quality of life for patients at the end of their lives.

Definition

According to the American Psychiatric Association, the essential feature of delirium is a disturbance of consciousness that is accompanied by a change in cognition that cannot be better accounted for by a pre-existing or evolving dementia (APA, 2000). The key elements which determine delirium, according to the Diagnostic and Statistical Manual of Mental Disorders-IV (APA, 2000), include changes in mental status in a short time, alternations in attention or consciousness, changes in cognition or memory, and a change in cognition from a direct physiologic consequence of a medical condition (APA, 2000).

Incidence

Estimates of delirium range from 20 to75% in cancer patients and up to 90% of all terminally ill patients (Casarett & Inouye, 2001; Tremblay & Breitbart, 2001). This symptom occurs frequently during perideath, particularly in the last days or hours, when estimates rise to 90–95% (Waller & Caroline, 2000). In hospitalized patients over age 70, delirium is very common and its treatment adds costly hospital days (Chan & Brennan, 1999).

Etiology

The precise pathophysiology of delirium is not well understood; however, it is thought to involve neurotransmitters in the cortical and subcortical areas of the brain. There are several neurotransmitters involved, and increased dopamine, serotonin, gamma-aminobutyric acid (GABA), beta-endorphins, and acetylcholine are thought to play the most important roles (Casarett & Inouye, 2001; Chan & Brennan, 1999). The etiology of delirium is multifactorial and includes medications, polypharmacy, brain metastases or other conditions, hypoxia,

sepsis, hypercalcemia, hepatic and renal dysfunction, electrolyte imbalances, bowel obstruction, urinary tract infection, past psych history, and medication withdrawal. Possible medications contributing to delirium include opioids, TCAs, diphenhydramine, antihistamines, H2 blockers, analgesics, sedatives, and cardiovascular drugs (Chan & Brennan, 1999; Langhorne, 1999).

Brain involvement may be secondary to metastases, primary cerebral disease, cancer, or cardiovascular accident. Systemic causes include organ failure, metabolic disturbances, infection, and toxic effects of an egonis substance (Lawlor et al., 2000). Other factors specific to the older adult include pre-existing dementia, a fracture, systemic infections, malnutrition, addition of three or more medications, simultaneous use of neuroleptics and narcotics, use of restraints, bladder catheters, and iatrogenic events (Chan & Brennan, 1999; Kane et al., 1999). Older adults are also susceptible due to their lack of resilience (Perley, 2007). Unfortunately, delirium may be misdiagnosed as dementia. See Table 21.13 for a summary of conditions that cause delirium.

Cardinal Signs

Delirium is a syndrome with many manifestations. Primarily, there are perceptual disturbances, which include misperceptions, illusions, and hallucinations (Lawlor, 2003). The cardinal signs of delirium include an acute onset, fluctuating course, presence of underlying organic cause, reduced sensorium, attention deficit, and cognitive or perceptual disturbances (Chan & Brennan, 1999; Lawlor et al., 2000; Costa et al., 1996). Specific symptoms include insomnia during the night and somnolence during the day, nightmares, restlessness, hypersensitivity to light or noise, and emotional lability (Breitbart & Cohen, 2000). Typical early signs of delirium include sundowning, withdrawal, irritability, new forgetfulness or befuddlement, and new onset of incontinence. Later signs include outbursts of anger, hostility, or abusive behavior (Waller & Caroline, 2000). Confusion, agitation, or restlessness is usually worse at night and when a patient becomes disoriented to person, place, date, and time.

Either increased activity (hyperactive delirium) or passivity (hypoactive delirium) may delineate delirium. Hyperactive delirium or agitated delirium is characterized by agitation and hallucinations and the delirium or confusion is readily apparent and more easily recognized. Hypoactive delirium often goes unrecognized because the patient may be quiet and lethargic and may be mistaken for sedation from opioids, an obtunded state in the last days of life, or comfort (if symptom management has been difficult) (Breitbart & Cohen, 2000; Casarett & Inouye, 2001; McElhaney, 2002). There may also be times when a patient experiences a mixed delirium, which means the patient alternates between a hypoactive and a hyperactive state.

Severity

Delirium usually becomes more severe in the hyperactive form. If a patient becomes more agitated and delusional, then she/he may become a safety risk (e.g., falls). Behaviors can be aggressive, combative, or physically threatening, resulting in a tendency placing the patients in physical restraints to keep them from injuring themselves. However, it is best to avoid restraints because this can further exacerbate the problem if the patient were to fall. Physical restraints can cause further agitation because the patient cannot move and feels frustrated by this. Delirium may include delusions, hallucinations, not understanding where they are, and a risk of suicide (Chan & Brennan, 1999; Langhorne, 1999; Costa et al., 1996).

The result of hypoactive delirium may be premature death. If pain and symptoms have been difficult to manage, the hypoactive patient will look sedated. The healthcare team may feel that they have finally managed the symptoms because the patient is very quiet. In particular, the patient may be lethargic and unable to communicate their confusion. Medications will continue and the vital functioning will be depressed; the result is premature death by weeks to months (Breitbart & Cohen, 2000; Casarett & Inouye, 2001; McElhaney, 2002).

Assessment

Evaluation of delirium includes several components: history, cognitive assessment, physical exam, and laboratory studies. Because it can be confused with dementia or depressions, the first step in diagnosing delirium is its identification as a potential symptom (Lawlor, 2003). Challenges of assessment include absence of uniform classification (as seen by its several names), lack of knowledge regarding early signs, staff tolerance of confused behavior, and the assumption that, with age, most people inevitably become confused (Boyle, Abernathy, Baker, & Wall, 1998).

Assessment DSM-IV (APA, 2000) defining characteristics includes disturbance in consciousness with impaired ability to focus or shift attention; changes in cognition or the development of perceptual disturbance that is not better accounted for by a pre-existing established or evolving dementia; fluctuating disturbance over a short period of time; and evidence from the history, physical exam, or lab findings that the disturbance is caused by psychological consequences of a general medical condition. Diagnostic studies should be ordered if they are likely to change patient management (Bakitas et al., 2008). Other assessment tools to screen for delirium include the Delirium Rating Scale or the Confusion Assessment Measure.

Assessment should first include a history and review of current medical conditions including the

21.13 | Causes of Delirium

CATEGORY/BASIS	EXAMPLES
DISEASE PROCESS	Primary brain tumor or secondary brain metastasis
SIDE EFFECTS OF TREATMENT	Chemotherapy Radiation to the brain
PAIN AND SYMPTOM MEDICATIONS	Corticosteroids Opioids Tricyclic antidepressants H_2 blockers – cimetidine, ranitidine Anticholinergics Antiemetics – thioridazine, amitryptyline, diphenhydramine OTC antihistamines Benzodiazepines Sedatives – triazolam Acyclovir Cardiovascular drugs – digitalis, nifedipine, quinidine, beta-blockers
MEDICATION WITHDRAWAL	Opioids Benzodiazepines Alcohol
PAIN	Uncontrolled pain syndrome Urinary retention Constipation/impaction Obstruction
METABOLIC FLUCTUATIONS	Glucose – hypoglycemia Sodium – hyponatremia Potassium Calcium
ORGAN FAILURE	Brain – stroke, seizure, CVA Kidney – uremia Lungs – hypoxia Heart – hypoxia, CO_2 retention, MI Thyroid or adrenal
INFECTION	CNS – meningitis Urinary tract - UTI Respiratory tract – pneumonia Generalized sepsis Steroid-induced immunocompromise
NUTRITIONAL DEFICIENCIES	Thiamine B-12/Folate
MISCELLANEOUS	Sleep deprivation Urinary retention Sensory deprivation Change in environment Immobilization
PAST PSYCHIATRIC HISTORY	Depression

Compiled from Casarett & Inouye 2001; Chan & Brennan, 1999; Langhorne, 1999; Waller & Caroline, 2000.

following: disease side effects, such as a tumor; side effects of treatment, such as chemotherapy or radiation to the head; medications used to treat symptoms, including corticosteroids, opioids, cimetidine, anticholinergics, antiemetics, benzodiazepines, and acyclovir; withdrawal of medications such as opioids, benzodiazepines, or alcohol; discomfort from uncontrolled pain, urinary retention, fecal impaction; metabolic fluctuations in glucose, sodium, potassium, or calcium; organ failure including the kidneys, liver, lungs, heart, brain, thyroid, or adrenal glands; infection from CNS, urinary tract, respiratory tract, generalized sepsis; and finally nutritional deficiencies from thiamine or folate/B-12 (Breitbart & Alici, 2008; Waller & Caroline, 2000). See Table 21.13. This is followed by a review of the patient's behavior and sleep cycles from the chart, followed by a review of the medication regimen.

A critical element of assessment includes the evaluation of mental status in order to develop a multidimensional clinical picture, functional performance status, and signs/symptoms. A mental status exam provides a baseline for monitoring the course of cognition and is a source of documentation for reference and repeat evaluations. The key aspects of mental status assessment include general state and appearance, orientation, state of consciousness, short- and long-term memory, language, visuospatial functions, cognitive functions (calculations, spelling), insight and judgment, thought control, and mood and affect (Kane et al., 1999; Costa et al., 1996).

Physical exam is important to rule out possible treatable causes. Vital signs can give information regarding infection, hypoxemia, and hypoglycemia. Integument inspection may reveal sepsis or cardiac failure from cold, clammy skin, or hot red skin from anticholinergic reactions. Head, eye, ears, neck, and throat exam may reveal signs of scleral icterus from liver failure, constricted pupils from opioids, or dilated from anticholinergic toxicity; oral exam reveals nutritional deficiencies; and chest exam will show rales of heart failure or dullness from pneumonia. The abdominal exam may reveal urinary retention, fecal slowing, extremities, Trousseau's sign, thiamine, and liver failure (Waller & Caroline, 2000). Helpful lab data may include glucose level, electrolytes, bilirubin, LDH, LFTs, urine culture, and oxygen saturation level. See Table 21.14 for a review of important elements to the physical exam for work-up of delirium.

Assessment Tools. There are several examinations available to assess mental status; the most frequently used is the Mini-Mental Status Examination (MMSE) (Folstein, Folstein, & McHugh, 2002). The MMSE is a brief tool that measures cognitive impairment, specifically examining immediate memory, short-term memory, aphasia, apraxia, agnosia, and construction ability along with concentration and spatial ability (Costa et al.,

21.14 | Physical Examination for Delirium

GENERAL	**Skin**	Cold clammy – cardiac failure, sepsis, hypoglycemia, hypocalcemia; warm, hot, red – anticholinergic
HEENT	**Head**	
	Face	Chostek's sign – hypocalcemia
	Eyes	
	Papilledema	Intracranial pressure
	Sclera	Icterus – liver failure
	Pupils	Constricted – opioid toxicity; dilated–anticholinergic toxicity
	Ears	
	Nose	
	Throat	
	Mouth	Smooth, shiny tongue – folate deficiency
CHEST	**Lungs**	Rales – heart failure Dullness – pneumonia
COR	S1 gallop	Heart failure
ABDOMINAL	Palpable feces	Constipation or impaction
	Palpable bladder	Urinary retention
EXTREMITY	Trousseau's sign	Hypocalcemia
	Tender, swollen calves	Thiamine deficiency
	Asterixis	Liver failure
NEURO	Mental status exam	Evaluation of cognitive functioning
	Hemiplegia/ hemiparesis	Stroke
	Proximal myopathy	Corticosteroid toxicity
	Ataxia, loss of vibration sense	Thiamine or B-12 deficiency
	Loss of position sense	

Compiled from Chan & Brennan, 1999; Waller and Caroline, 2000.

1996). The 30-item exam only requires approximately 10 minutes to complete. Out of a possible 30 points, scores below 20 indicate a possible organic brain disorders and a score of 23 is sensitive to thought disorders and mood (Candilis, 1998).

There are three tools used to assess confusion or delirium of patients with life-limiting illnesses. All have been used with the older adult and are outlined in Table 21.15. These are the Confusion Assessment Method diagnostic algorithm (CAM), the Delirium Rating Scale (DRS), and the Memorial Delirium Assessment Scale (MDAS).

The CAM assesses nine domains of cognitive functioning: acute changes in mental status w/ fluctuating course including, inattention (e.g., digit span, months backward), or observation; disorganized thinking (e.g., rambling, incoherent speech); and altered level of consciousness (e.g., sleepy, stuporous, hypervigilent) (Chan & Brennan, 1999). The presence of at least the

first three elements suggests a diagnosis of delirium (Flacker & Marcantonio, 1998).

The DRS (Chapter 21 appendix, part B) is a 10-item structured interview, each answer is rated on a 0–3 scale. It is the most widely assessment of delirium with the longest history of use in the psychiatric setting. It measures mood, onset of perceptual disturbances (including hallucinations and delusions), and behavior (Kuebler, Heidrich, Vena, & English, 2006). The MDAS (Chapter 21 appendix, part C) is a 10-item assessment tool measuring awareness and cognitive impairment with attention to memory, and psychomotor responses. Each response is rated from 0 to 3, and a score of 13 or higher is diagnostic of delirium (Breitbart & Strout, 2000).

Management

To treat the delirium, it is first necessary to decide on goals of care. Specifically, it must be determined if the patient is close to death and whether the delirium is reversible. A stepwise approach is taken regarding treatment (Boyle et al., 1998). Constipation and urinary retention should be treated, and any potential contributing factors should be removed.

For example, the clinician may initiate the discontinuation of problematic medications one by one to determine the causative drug. If complete discontinuation of the offending medication is not appropriate, then decreasing the dose may be helpful. Some patients may be sensitive to medications needed for pain and symptom management; therefore discussion is critical regarding the benefits and burdens of pain and symptom management. Alcohol or benzodiazapine withdrawal should be considered (Chan & Brennan, 1999).

Treatments should be provided with promotion of appropriate pacing and time for rest and sleep. Metabolic fluctuations should be corrected, including hydration (if appropriate), within the patient's entire clinical picture. Lastly, it may be appropriate to do further work-up with particular importance to discern delirium from dementia or possible depression. Table 21.16 compares the differences between depression, delirium, and dementia.

Bruera and Neumann (1998) suggest an algorithm approach in the patient with advanced disease. Their algorithm suggests determining whether it is a hypoactive or hyperactive delirium. If the delirium is hypoactive, then reversible causes should be ruled out. Assessment includes evaluating for causative factors, abnormal lab exams, metastatic processes, sepsis, and opioid review. Hydration and an opioid rotation may be necessary. Reassessment should occur to determine if the delirium is reversible. If the delirium is hyperactive, then the patient would be started on haloperidol. If delirium continues in spite of high doses of haloperidol, then the patient could

21.15 | Delirium Assessment Scales

DELIRIUM RATING SCALES

DELIRIUM RATING SCALE (DRS) (Chapter 21 appendix, part B)
  10-item scale
  4-point clinician rated scale
  Assesses
    Temporal onset
    Perceptual disturbance
    Delusions
    Psychomotor activity
    Cognitive status
    Sleep–wake disturbance
    Mood lability
    Symptom variability
Score of 12 or above from range of 0–32 indicates presence of delirium

MEMORIAL DELIRIUM ASSESSMENT SCALE (MDAS)
(Chapter 21 appendix, part C)
  10-item scale
  4-point clinician rated scale
  Assesses
    Disturbance in arousal
    Level of consciousness
    Cognitive functions
    Psychomotor activity
Score of 13 or above from range of 0–30 indicates presence of delirium

CONFUSION ASSESSMENT METHOD (CAM)
  10-item scale
  Clinician-rated scale
  Assesses nine domains from DSM-III-R
    Level of consciousness
    Thought clarity
    Perceptual disturbances
    Psychomotor activity
  Presence of first 3–4 items indicates presence of delirium

Compiled from Breitbart & Cohen, 2000; Casarett & Inouye, 2001; Kuebler et al., 2006.

receive a trial methotrimeprazine. If this medication had no effect, a benzodiazapine drip may be appropriate. Midazolam, diazepam, or lorazepam may be appropriate. Throughout the treatment of delirium, counseling and education would be offered to the patient, his/her family, and support staff, with continual reassessment focusing on determining any other causes of the delirium.

Pharmacological

Pharmacological interventions will depend upon the suspected problem. For undetermined causes, neuroleptics are the drug of choice. Haloperidol (a po-

tent dopamine blocker) and Olanzipine are the preferred medications (Chan & Brennen, 1999; Waller & Caroline, 2000). The initial dose of haloperidol is 1 mg three times a day and the dose of Olanzipine is 2.5–5 mg two to three times a day (Waller & Caroline, 2000). Historically, chlorpromazine has been used, but it is much more sedating. Risperidone has been suggested but the elder tends to experience more side effects (Zarate et al., 1997). Benzodiazepines may be helpful, particularly during medication withdrawal (Conn & Lieff, 2001), short-acting ones are better tolerated, making lorazepam the preferred drug. Doses can range 0.5–1 mg every 4 hours. For brain metastases, a trial of steroids may help. The dose

21.16 | Comparison of Depression, Delirium, and Dementia

	DEPRESSION	DELIRIUM	DEMENTIA
ONSET	Coincides w/ major life changes	Acute/abrupt	Insidious – chronic
COURSE	Diurnal effects – worse in AM usually, situational fluctuations	Short diurnal fluctuations, worse at night	Long – no diurnal effects, progressive
PROGRESSION	Variable – rapid or slow	Slow – uneven	Abrupt
DURATION	Persistent – at least 2 weeks	Days to hours – less than 1 month	Months to years
AWARENESS	Clear	Clear	Reduced
ALERTNESS	Normal	Fluctuates	Generally normal
ATTENTION	Minimal impairment	Impaired	Generally normal
ORIENTATION	Selective orientation	Generally impaired	Possibly impaired
MEMORY	Selective or patchy impairment	Recent and immediate impairment	Recent memory worse, remote impairment
THINKING	Intact w/ hopelessness, helplessness	Disorganized, distorted, fragmented, incoherent	Difficulty w/ abstraction, word finding
PERCEPTION	Intact except in severe cases	Distorted, illusions, hallucinations	Misperceptions usually absent
PSYCHOMOTOR BEHAVIOR	Variable – retardation or agitation	Variable – hypokinetic or hyperkinetic	Normal with apraxia
SLEEP/WAKE CYCLE	Disturbed early AM waking	Cycle reversed	Fragmented
AFFECT	Depressed/irritable	Labile	Variable
FAMILY HISTORY	May be positive	Noncontributory	May be positive for DAT

Compiled from Breitbart & Cohen, 2000; Chan and Brennan, 1999; Falk, 1998; Langhorne, 1999; Falk, Perlis, & Albert, 2004.

of dexamethasone ranges 16–36 mg every morning (Waller & Caroline, 2000). Patients who had Parkinson's disease may get relief from Risperidone (Chan &Brennan, 1999). If delirium is intractable and no treatment is successful, palliative sedation may be necessary (Wein, 2000). This may best be achieved through the use of propofol or midazolam (Casarett & Inouye, 2001; Waller & Caroline, 2000; Wein, 2000). Table 21.17 offers suggestions for medications and dosages in the treatment of delirium.

21.17 | Treatment of Delirium

ADULTS

NEUROLEPTICS	ORAL DOSE
Haloperidol	0.5–5 mg every 2–12 hours
Thioridazine	10–75 mg every 4–8 hours
Chlorpromazine	12.5–50 mg every 4 –12 hours
Methotrimeprazine	12.5–50 mg every 4–8 hours
Olanzipine	2.5–5 mg every 8–12 hours
BENZODIAZEPINES	
Lorazepam	0.5–2.0 mg every 1–4 hours
Midazolam	1.0–4.0 mg every 1–4 hours
ANESTHETICS	
Propofol	10 mg bolus w/ 10–20 mg/hr

Source: Breitbart & Alici, 2008; Breitbart et al., 2005; Casarett & Inouye 2001.

CHILDREN

BENZIDIAZIOPINES	ORAL DOSE
Midazolam	0.2–0.75 mg/kg every 6 hours
Lorazepam	0.02 mg/kg up to 2 mg every 4–6 hours
Diazepam	0.12–0.8 mg/kg every 6–12 hours
NEUROLEPTICS	
Haloperidol	0.01–0.03 mg/kg up to 6mg/day every 8 hours
Thioridazine	0.5–3 mg/kg every 8–12 hours
Chlorpromazine	0.5–1 mg/kg every 4–6 hours
Respiradone	0.25-1 mg every 6–12 hours
BARBITURIATES	
Phenobarbitol	2 mg/kg q 8 hours

Source: Wusthoff et al., 2007.

Nonpharmacological

Nonpharmacological treatments focus on the management of the environment, which includes creating a safe environment, reducing stimuli, and providing reassurance. A basic, but often ignored, intervention is to make sure patients have access to their hearing aids and vision correcting glasses. Other strategies focus on the patient's room and climate, such as soft lighting, that does not cause harsh images or shadows to prevent misinterpretation of the environment which can result in hallucinations. Cognitive devices (e.g., calendars or clocks) can cue orientation to time and date. Familiar sounds, smells, and touch may help promote calmness (Boyle et al., 1998). Personal effects (e.g., lotions, perfumes, foods) as well as family and friends can provide reorientation and reassurance.

Consistent nurses caring for the patient may also be of benefit. In order to avoid using restraints, family or healthcare providers may need to provide "sitters." Confused patients may unintentionally harm themselves trying to slip out of restraints (Conn & Lieff, 2001). Sitters can help with reorientation, respond to the patient's fear, and watch the patient to prevent falls. However, they may need to be reassured and coached about how much interaction to have with the patient, if interaction stimulates agitation.

Sleep deprivation may cause further confusion; therefore the elimination of both visual and sensory stimuli is paramount. Scheduling medications without constant interruption of sleep during the night can decrease sleep loss. Reduction and elimination of noise pollution such as from radios, television, or overhead announcements can also increase rest and promote sleep. Good nursing care such as gentle massage and warm drinks can promote sleep.

Family Concerns and Considerations

Education of the family is a cornerstone of management of the prevention and treatment of delirium. Families need to understand predisposing risk factors that can lead to delirium including pressure sores, poor nutrition, incontinence, sleep disturbances, and decreased functional ability including vision and hearing (Casarett & Inouye, 2001; Flacker & Marcantonio, 1998). Other preventative measures include judicious use of urinary catheters or removal of unnecessary tubes, avoiding restraints for confusion, prevention of skin ulcers, and maximal social support to the family caregivers (McElhaney, 2002). Teaching should be multifaceted; instructions regarding the use of cognitive assistive devices such as glasses and hearing aids can help maintain safety for the patient. Assessment of the home environment can be quite revealing, particularly whether the patient has the basic necessities such as food, finances, and medications. Family should be educated regarding the importance of skincare, the importance of a well-balanced diet, and hydration as long as these interventions are not a burden or source of distress to the patient.

When a patient becomes delirious at the end of life, ongoing support of the family is important. Delirium may be irreversible due to the various medical conditions the patient is experiencing as well as the dying process. In deciding treatment, an informed discussion of the realistic options should occur in the context of life expectancy and the risk versus benefit of any treatment. Families often welcome this clear discussion of all the current issues, including possible dying scenarios and what to expect so that they can become prepared for anticipated events.

Healthcare providers should role-model the art of "presence" or being with a patient. The patient's family should be encouraged to provide ongoing soothing communication, reassuring the elder patient he or she is safe, while not confronting the patient about what she or he sees or hears. Gentle reorientation should be provided and perhaps, if appropriate, gentle reassurance that the patient may be intermittently confused.

Often, in the search to find an explanation for delirium, the very fact that the patient is actively dying is overlooked. Therefore, families may need education that delirium may be a signal that their loved one is nearing the end of their life. The other signs and symptoms of the dying process should be reviewed in the larger context of the terminal illness (See chapter 25). Family should be encouraged to talk to the older adult even when death is imminent. They should also be reassured that pain and symptoms will be managed.

Gerontological Considerations

There are many developmental tasks of late adulthood include role changes related to retirement, widowhood, or caring for a spouse. In addition, there are normal biological changes in physical appearance and function that may result in loss of health and independence. Indeed, the older adult may have a keen sense of his or her mortality and limited life span (Buckwalter & Piven, 1999). In response to such events, individuals cope in many ways. Sometimes, individuals develop psychiatric symptoms including anxiety, depression, and delirium.

Older adults may be frail and have altered mental status and be unable to make decisions. Many patients experience delirium; in the older adult population, this confusion is even more prevalent. The aging process makes the elder more susceptible to delirium because of decreased kidney function causing inability to eliminate the body of toxic substances, decreased ability to metabolize medications, and decreased fluid balance

mechanisms. This is a serious prognostic marker for older adults (Kapo et al., 2007)

Depressive symptoms are more common in the elderly (Finkel, 2004) because of the effects from comorbidities, adjustment to loss of health, and independent living situations (Goy & Granzini, 2003). This includes grief and loss, fatigue, change in appetite that may cause metabolic imbalances, weight changes, changes in energy, and changes in sleep as well as changes in concentration. However, once the depression has been identified, treatment is usually effective (Cremens, 2004). Treatment focuses on the use of antidepressants within the SSRI class because TCAs may cause orthostatic hypotension and be too sedating (Finkel, 2004).

Anxiety is not well understood in the geriatric population due to lack of research. However, it can be stressed that loss of control and overall sense of vulnerability may increase the risk of anxiety. The challenge for treating anxiety in elders is that they may have a paradoxical effect to the use of benzodiazepines, which are commonly used in anxiety. Therefore, this class of medication should be used with caution. Mirtazepine may be helpful as it helps with sleep, appetite, and depression as well as Trazodone (Cremens, 2004).

Pediatric Considerations

Anxiety, depression, and delirium present differently in the younger population of patients. Indeed, it may be hard to differentiate between sadness, anxiety, depression, and panic. This is because these symptoms are typically unrecognized and underestimated, resulting in less research into these symptoms in the pediatric population.

Anxiety in terminally ill children may include separation anxiety. In older children and teens, anxiety may exhibit itself as post-traumatic distress disorder over treatment, social phobia over the results of treatment effects, and general anxiety in terms of the unknown future for living with a life-threatening illness (Ravitz, 2004). There are no specific tools for assessing pediatric anxiety; pediatric dosages of benzodiazepines are the first line of short-term therapy (Kersun & Shemesh, 2007).

Depression manifests itself in younger patients similar to that of older patients: changes in appetite and sleep, psychomotor retardation, with less energy. Grief in children is self-limited, and can be improved with reassurance. Depression can result from self-blaming and decreased self worth (Kersun & Shemesh, 2007). Similarly, there is limited experience in treating depression in children; SSRIs have been found to lead to a suicidal risk in the healthy child and no further research has been done in children with life-limiting illnesses. Optimal treatment is best achieved in consultation of a pediatric psychiatrist, who can also help with medication utilization and psychotherapy.

Delirium is difficult to determine in children. Like adults, it can be seen as agitation with loud, angry speech, irritability, crying, and nonpurposeful activity (Wusthoff, Shellhaas, and Licht, 2007). However, its frequency and prevalence, like many other issues in pediatrics, have not been studied. The usual diagnosis algorithm for delirium is followed in children. First, there is identification of symptoms and considerations of possible causes. Identification of symptoms includes changes in sleep, impaired attention, mood labiality, and confusion. An initial review of medications includes recent changes and side effects of medications. Further assessment includes pain, bladder fullness, positioning, and external stressors. The child should then be evaluated for medical issues such as increased intracranial pressure, hypoxia, and hypercapnia, along with kidney and liver failure. Additionally, infection should be considered (Wusthoff et al., 2007).

Treatment for agitation and delirium includes soothing touch and voice. Familiarity also provides calmness, so bringing objects from home such as pillows, pictures, and blankets may help by their touch and smell. It is important to limit television that is stimulating, and perhaps useful providing more calming music on radio, MP3 players, video players, and cell phones. Pharmacological treatment again focuses on sedatives and benzodiazepines, though there is a paucity of research in this area (Wusthoff et al., 2007). Neuroleptics are very controversial at this point due to their potent side effects. Specialist pediatric palliative care providers should be consulted for pediatric delirium.

Case Study conclusion: Elizabeth was a perfect candidate for palliative care. She was placed on a scheduled dose of a short-acting benzodiazepine, lorazepam 0.5 mg every 6 hours, for her anxiety. This lesser dose was chosen since Elizabeth weighed about 90 pounds. The lorazepam helped decrease her anxiety, which in turn helped with her confusion and her short-term memory. To treat her depression, she was started on sertraline 12.5 mg a day. In addition, a family meeting was held to determine her advanced care planning. It was decided that she would not be hospitalized for any further infections because this caused more confusion and agitation. Instead, she would be treated with oral antibiotics and antipyretics for fever control. A plan was made for the use of sublingual morphine elixir 0.5–1.0 mg every 6 hours to ease labored breathing. She will also receive hospice care at the assisted living facility where she lives.

Elizabeth was much less anxious and more engaged in her care. In fact, she felt so much better she thought she should stop her medica-

tions. However, with coaxing, she was made to understand the importance of the scheduled doses of these medications.

CONCLUSION

Previous life experiences can both positively and negatively affect coping. A life-threatening illness is an extreme crisis in life, and patients may develop psychiatric symptoms in response. Anxiety, depression, and delirium may be the first sign of an illness, or may be the response to an illness. Biological issues affect treatment considerations in the older and younger patient. For elders, these issues include slower metabolism, a higher side effect profile for many medications, and a lower threshold for any imbalances. For children, their small weight and developing organ systems must be considered. Moreover, there are many medications which are inappropriate for use in children because there is no research to support it or there are dangerous potential side effects.

Social issues such as isolation and lack of family supports may also have negative effects on treatment. Mobile families spread across the country and patients living alone in one town with families living in distant cities present challenges. Many patients may not want to burden relatives with their daily struggle (Reichel and Gallo, 1999).

Effective treatment of anxiety, depression, and delirium necessitates a collaborative effort between the patient, family, and the health team. The patient may perceive something is wrong but cannot articulate the problem; the family may perceive something is wrong but feels it is part of the aging process. The healthcare provider may not account for the biologic differences in the elder in evaluating the problem. These factors make communication and vigilance necessary components to care.

Anxiety, depression, and delirium can be difficult disorders to recognize and treat, and these conditions can cause suffering by reducing both daily functioning and quality of life. The result may be unnecessary placement in an institution outside the home and increased stress for family caregivers. Anxiety, depression, and delirium can be effectively treated; however, evaluation and treatment of patients require skill, time, and patience. The goal of palliative care is a holistic approach that improves physical, psychological, spiritual, and emotional well-being. It is incumbent upon clinicians to be vigilant for the presence of these disorders. A collaborative approach can provide a partnership in caring for the patient that supports his/her independence and dignity as long as possible.

EVIDENCE-BASED PRACTICE

Gagnon, Low, and Schreier (2005). Methylphenidte hydrochloride improves cognitive function in patients with advanced cancer and hypoactive delirium: a prospective clinical study. *Journal of Psychiatry Neuroscience. 30*(2)100–107.

Research Problem. Delirium is common on palliative care patients. However, little work had been done on hypoactive delirium. The purpose of this study was to evaluate the use of methylphenidate to improve cognitive function in patients with hypoactive delirium in the absence of an identifiable source

Methodology. To further evaluate this hypothesis, patients were prospectively screened at a tertiary palliative care day hospital by using a Mini-Mental Status Examination (MMSE). If it was reveled that the patients were delirious and did not manifest any signs of hyperactivity, the patients were categorized with hypoactive delirium. They were then treated for any metabolic, medication-induced, or opioid induced causes. Fourteen patients met these criteria and were treated with methylphenidate.

Findings. Thirteen patients had a positive effect to the methylphenidate in terms of alertness and resolution of psychomotor retardation and normalization of slurred speech. One died precipitously before a stable dose could be administered. Ten of these showed improvement in the MMSE, one improved in his activity level more that his cognition.

Limitations. This study is limited in its population of terminally ill cancer patients in a palliative care setting where clinicians are attuned to presence of all types of delirium.

Implications. Hypoactive delirium has often been neglected because these patients are quiet and cause little disturbance. Yet, their quality of life is impaired. This study offers a potential treatment when all other causes have been ruled out.

REFERENCES

Alexopoulos, G. S., Katz, I. R., Reynolds, C. F., Carpenter, D., & Docherty, J. P. (2001). *Postgraduate Medicine*, Special Report October.

American Psychiatric Association. (APA). (2000). *Diagnostic and statistical manual of mental disorders. Text Revision* (4th ed.).Washington, DC: American Psychiatric Association.

Bakitas, M., Dahlin, C., & Bishop, P. (2008). Palliative and end of life care. In T. Buttaro, J. Trybulski, P. Bailey, & J. Sandberg-Cook (Eds.), *Primary care: A collaborative approach* (3rd ed., pp 70–79). St. Louis, MI: Mosby Elsevier.

Barsevik, A. M., Sweeney, C., Haney, E., & Chung, E. (2002). A systemic qualitative analysis of psychoeducational interventions for depression in patients with cancer. *Oncology Nursing Forum, 29*(1), 73–87.

Block, S. D. (2000). Assessing and managing depression is the terminally ill patient. *Annals of Internal Medicine, 132*(2), 209–213.

Boyle, D. M., Abernathy, G., Baker, L., & Wall, A. C. (1998). End of life confusion in patients with cancer. *Oncology Nursing Forum,* 25(8), 1335–1343.

Breitbart, W., & Alici, Y. (2008). Agitation and delirium at the end of life. *Journal of the American Medical Association, 300*(24), 2898–2910.

Breitbart, W., Chochinov, H. M., & Passik, S. (2005). Psychiatric aspect of palliative care. In D. Doyle, W. C. Hanks, & N. MacDonald (Eds.), *Oxford textbook of palliative medicine* (3rd ed., pp. 740–771). New York: Oxford University Press.

Breitbart, W., & Cohen, K. (2000). Delirium in the terminally ill. In H. M. Chochinov & W. Breitbart (Eds.), *Handbook of psychiatry in palliative medicine.* New York: Oxford University Press.

Breitbart, W., Rosenfeld, B., Roth, A., Smith, M., Cohen, K., & Passik, S., et al. (1997). The memorial delirium assessment scale. *Journal of Pain and Symptom Management, 13*(3), 128–137.

Brown, J., & Von Roenn, J. (2004). Symptom management in the older adult. *Clinics in Geriatric Medicine, 20,* 621–640.

Bruera, E. D., & Neumann, C. M. (1998). The uses of psychotropics in symptom management of advanced cancer. *Psycho-Oncology, 7*(4), 346–358.

Buckwalter, K. C., & Piven, M. L. S. (1999). Depression. In J. T. Stone, J. F. Wyman & S. A. Salisbury (Eds.), *Clinical gerontological nursing—a guide to advanced practice.* Philadelphia: W.B. Saunders.

Caracine, A., & Grassi, L. (2003). Delirium: Acute *confusional states in palliative medicine.* New York: Oxford University Press.

Carmin, C. N., Pollard, C. A., & Gillock, K. L. (1999). Assessment of anxiety disorders in the elderly. In P. A. Lichtenberg (Ed.),. *Handbook of assessment in clinical gerontology.* New York: John Wiley.

Casarett, D. J., & Inouye, S. K. (2001). Diagnosis and delirium near the end of life. *Annals of Internal Medicine%, 135,* 32–40.

Cassem, N., & Brendel, R. (2004). End of life issues: Principles of care and ethics. In T. Stern, G. Fricchione, N. Cassem, M. Jellinek, & J. Rosenbaum (Eds.),. *The massachusetts general hospital handbook of general hospital psychiatry.* Philadelphia: Elsevier-Mosby.

Cassem, N., Papakostoas, G., Fava, M., & Stern, T. (2004). Mood-disordered patients. In T. Stern, G. Fricchione, N. Cassem, M. Jellinek, & J. Rosenbaum (Eds.), *The Massachusetts general hospital handbook of general hospital psychiatry.* Philadelphia: Elsevier-Mosby.

Chan, D., & Brennan, N. (1999). Delirium: Making the diagnosis, improving the prognosis. *Geriatrics, 54*(3), 28–42.

Costa, P. T., Williams, T. F., & Somerfield, M. S. et al., (1996). *Early identification of Alzheimer's disease and related dementia's. Clinical practice guideline 19.* U. S. Department of Health and Human Services. Rockville, New York: Agency for Health Care Policy and Research.

Conn, D. K., & Lieff, S. (2001). Diagnosing and managing delirium in the elderly. *Canadian Family Physician, 47,* 101–108.

Cremens, M. C. (2004). Care of the geriatric patient. In T. Stern, G. Fricchione, N. Cassem, M. Jellinek, & J. Rosenbaum. *The Massachusetts general hospital handbook of general hospital psychiatry.* Philadelphia: Elsevier-Mosby.

Derby, S. (2007). Geriatric populations. In M. J. Perley & and C. Dahlin (Eds.), *Core curriculum for the advanced practice hospice and palliative care nurse.* Hospice and Palliative Nurses Association.

Depression Guideline Panel. (1993). *Depression in primary care: Vol. 1 detection and diagnosis. Clinical practice guideline, 5.* U. S. Department of Health and Human Services. Rockville: Agency for Health Care Policy and Research.

Edelstein, B., Kalish, K. D., Drozdick, L. W. & McKee, D. R. (1999). Assessment of depression and bereavement in older adults. In P. A. Lichtenberg (Ed.), *Handbook of assessment in clinical gerontology.* New York: John Wiley.

Falk, W., Perlis, R., & Albert, M. (2004). Demented patients. In T. Stern, G. Fricchione, N. Cassem, M. Jellinek, & J. Rosenbaum (Eds.), *The Massachusetts general hospital handbook of general hospital psychiatry.* Philadelphia: Elsevier-Mosby.

Filiberti, A., Ripamonti, C., Totis, A., Ventafridda, V., De Conno, F., Contiero, P., et al.(2001). Characteristics of terminal cancer patients who committed suicide during a home palliative care program. *Journal of Pain and Symptom Management, 22*(1), 544–553.

Finkel, S. (2004). Geropsychiatry. In L. Goldman, T. Wise, & D. Brody (Eds.), *Psychiatry for primary care physicians* (2nd ed., pp. 375–384). American Medical Association Press.

Fisch, M. (2003). Depression and anxiety. In M. Fisch & E. Bruera (Eds.), *Handbook of advanced cancer* (pp. 382–389). Cambridge, England: Cambridge University Press.

Flacker, J. M., & Marcantonio E. R. (1998). Delirium in the elderly-optimal management. *Drugs and Aging, 13*(2), 119–130.

Folstein, M., Folstein, S., & McHugh, P. (2002). Mini-mental state: A practical method for grading the cognitive status of patients for the clinician. *Journal of Psychiatric Resident, 12,* 189.

Gagnon, B., Low, G., & Scheier, G. (2005). Methylphenidate hydrochloride improves cognitive function in patients with advanced cancer and hypoactive delirium: A prospective clinical study. *Review of Psychiatry Neuroscience, 30*(2), 100–107.

Gibson, C., Lichtenthal, W., Berg, A., & Breitbart, W. (2006). Psychologic issues on palliative care. *Anesthesiology Clinic of North America, 24,* 61–80.

Goy, E., & Granzini, L. (2003) End-of life in geriatric psychiatry. *Clinics in Geriatric Medicine, 19,* 841–856.

Hellsten, M., & Kane, J. (2006). Symptom management in pediatric palliative care. In B. Ferrell & N. Coyle (Eds.), *Textbook of palliative nursing* (2nd ed.). New York: Oxford University Press.

Horne-Thompson, A., & Grocke, D. (2008). The effect of music therapy on anxiety in patients who are terminally ill. *Journal of Palliative Medicine, 11*(4), 582–590.

Kane, J. L., & Himelstein, B. (2007). Palliative care in pediatrics. In A. Berger, J. Shuster, & J. Von Roenn (Eds.), *Principles and practice of palliative care and supportive oncology* (3rd ed.). Philadelphia: Lippincott William & Wilkins.

Kane, R. L., Ouslander, J. G., & Abrass, I. B. (1999). *Essentials of clinical geriatrics.* New York: McGraw-Hill.

Kapo, J., Morrison, L., & Liao, S. (2007). Palliative care for the older adult. *Journal of Palliative Medicine, 10*(1), 185–209.

Kersun, L., & Shemesh, E. (2007) Depression and anxiety in children. *Pediatric Clinics of North America, 54,* 691–708.

Kuebler, K. K., Heidrich, D. Vena, C., & English, N. (2006). Delirium, confusion, and agitation. In B. Ferrell & N. Coyle (Eds.), *Textbook of palliative nursing* (2nd ed., pp. 401–420). New York: Oxford University Press.

Langhorne, M. (1999). Confusion or delirium: Determining the difference. *Developments in Supportive Cancer Care, 3*(3), 82–87.

Lantz, M. (2002). Generalized anxiety in anxious times: helping older adults cope. *Clinical Geriatrics, 10*(1), 36–38.

Lawlor, P. G. (2003). Delirium. In M. Fisch & E. Bruera (Eds.). *Handbook of advanced cancer* (pp. 390–396). Cambridge, England: Cambridge University Press.

Lawlor, P. G., Fainsinger, R. L., & Bruera, E. D. (2000). Delirium at the end of life-critical issues in clinical practice and research. *Journal of the American Medical Association, 284*(19), 2427–2429.

Lavretsky, H. (2001). Choosing appropriate treatment for geriatric depression. *Clinical Geriatrics, 9*(5), 30–46.

Lebowitz, B. D., Pearson, J. L., Schneider, L. S., et al. (1997). Diagnosis and treatment of depression in late life-consensus statement update. *Journal of the American Medical Association, 248*(14), 1186–1190.

Lee, H. B., Ankrom, M., & Lyketsos, C. (2004). Cognitive disorders: Delirium, mild cognitive impairment and dementia. In L. Goldman, T. Wise, & D. Brody (Eds.), *Psychiatry for primary care physicians* (2nd ed., 197–223). American Medical Association Press.

Lee, S., Back, A., Block, S., & Stewart, S. (2002). Enhancing physician-patient communication. *Hematology, 1,* 464–478.

Lehmann, S. W., & Rabins, P. V. (1999). Clinical geropsychiatry. In J. J. Gallo, J. Busby-Whitehead, P. V. Rabins, R. A. Silliman, & J. B. Murphy (Eds.), *Reichels's care of the elderly-clinical aspects of aging.* Philadelphia: Lippincott Williams & Wilkins.

Lloyd-Williams, M. (2001). Screening for depression in palliative care patients: a review. *European Journal of Cancer Care, 10,* 31–35.

Lovejoy, N. C., Tabor, D. & Deloney, P. (2000). Cancer-related depression: Part II- Neurologic alterations and evolving approaches to psychopharmacology. *Oncology Nursing Forum, 27*(5), 795–808.

McCullough, P. K. (1992). Evaluation and management of anxiety in the older adult. *Geriatrics, 47*(4), 35–38.

McDonald, M. V., Passik, S. D., Dugan, W., Rosenfeld, B., Theobald, D. E., Edgerton, S., et al.(1999). Nurses' recognition of depression in their patients with cancer. *Oncology Nursing Forum, 26*(3), 593–599.

Medical Letter on Drugs and Therapeutics. (2002). Drugs that may cause psychiatric symptoms. *44,*59–62.

McElhaney, J. E. (2002). Delirium in elderly patients: How you can help. *Consultant, April 1,* 484–490.

Meagher, D. J. (2001). Delirium: Optimizing management. *British Medical Journal, 322,* 144–149.

Miller, K., & Massie, M. J. (2007). Depression and anxiety. In A. Berger, J. Shuster, J., & J. Von Roenn (Eds.), *Principles and practice of palliative care and supportive oncology.* Philadelphia: Lippincott William & Wilkins.

National Institute of Mental Health. (2008). *Anxiety fact sheet.* Retrieved 11/25/08 froam http://www.pueblo.gsa.gov/cic_text/health/factsabout-anxietydisorders/faxanxiety.htm.

Ohno, T., Noguchi, W., Nakayama, Y., Kato, S., Tsujii, H., & Suzuki, Y., et al. (2006). How do we interpret the answer "Neither" when physicians ask patients with cancer, "Are you depressed or not?" *Journal of Palliative Medicine, 9*(4), 861–865.

Pasacreta, J. V., Minarik, P. A., & Nield-Anderson, L. (2006). Anxiety and depression. In B. Ferrell & N. Coyle (Eds.), *Textbook of palliative nursing* (2nd ed., pp. 375–399). New York: Oxford University Press.

Payne, D. K., & Massie, M. J. (2000). Anxiety in palliative care. In H. M. Chochinov & W. Breitbart (Eds.), *Handbook of psychiatry in palliative medicine.* New York: Oxford University Press.

Periyakoil, V., Kraemer, H., Noda, A., Moos, R., Hallenback, J., Webster, M., et al. (2005). The Development and initial validation of the terminally ill grief or depression scale (TIFDS). *International Journal of Methods Psychiatry Resident, 14,* 202–222.

Perley, M. (2007). Psychiatric issues in palliative care. In M. J. Perley & C. Dahlin (Eds.), *Core curriculum for the advanced practice hospice and palliative nurse.* Dubuque, IA: Kendall Hunt, Hospice and Palliative Nurses Association.

Pollack, M. H., Otto, M., Bernstein, J. & Rosenbaum, J. (2004). Anxious patients. In T. Stern, G. Fricchione, N. Cassem, M. Jellinek, & J. Rosenbaum (Eds.), *The Massachusetts general hospital handbook of general hospital psychiatry.* Philadelphia: Elsevier-Mosby.

Ravitz, A. (2004). Child and adolescent disorders. In L. Goldman, T. Wise, & D. Brody (Eds.), *Psychiatry for primary care physicians* (2nd ed., pp. 69–93). American Medical Association Press.

Reichel, W., & Gallo, J. J. (1999). Essential principles in the care of the elderly. In J. J. Gallo, J. Busby-Whitehead, P. V. Rabins, R. A. Silliman , & J. B. Murphy (Eds.), *Reichels's care of the elderly–clinical aspects of aging.* Philadelphia: Lippincott Williams & Wilkins.

Reiss, S., Peterson, R. A., Gursky, D. M., & McNally, R. J. (1986). Anxiety sensitivity, anxiety frequency, and the prediction of fearfulness. *Behavioral Research Therapy, 24,* 1–8.

Roffman, J., & Stern, T. (2004). Diagnostic rating scales and laboratory test. In T. Stern, G.Fricchione, N. Cassem, M. Jellinek, & J. Rosenbaum (Eds.), *The Massachusetts general hospital handbook of general hospital psychiatry.* Philadelphia: Elsevier-Mosby.

Rozans, M., Dreisbach, A., Lertora, J., & Kahn, M. (2002). Palliative uses of methylphenidate in patients with cancer: A review. *Journal of Clinical Oncology. 20*(1), 335–339.

Shuster, J. (2007). Cognitive disorders: Delirium and dementia. In A. Berger, J. Shuster, & J. Von Roenn (Eds.),. *Principles and practice of palliative care and supportive oncology* (3rd ed.). Philadelphia: Lippincott, William, and Wilkins.

Simon, L., Jewell, N., & Brokel, J. (1997). Management of acute delirium in hospitalized elderly: A process improvement project. *Geriatric Nursing, 18,* 150–154.

Stark, D., Kiely, A., Smith, G., Velikova, A., & Selby, P. (2002). Anxiety disorders in cancer patients: Their nature, associations, and relations to quality of life. *Journal of Clinical Oncology, 20*(14), 3137–3148.

Stern, T., Perlis, R., & Lagomasino, I. L. (2004). Suicidal patients. In T. Stern, G. Fricchione, N. Cassem, M. Jellinek, & J. Rosenbaum (Eds.), *The Massachusetts general hospital handbook of general hospital psychiatry.* Philadelphia: Elsevier-Mosby.

Stevens, M. (2005). Psychological adaptation of the dying child. In D. Doyle, W. C. Hanks, & N. MacDonald (Eds.), *Oxford textbook of palliative medicine* (3rd ed.). New York: Oxford University Press.

Tremblay, A. & Breitbart, W. (2001). Psychiatric dimensions of palliative care. *Neurology Clinics, 19*(4), 949–967.

Tyler, M., & Fischer, D. (2007). Pediatric palliative care. In M. J. Perley & C. Dahlin (Eds.), *HPNA core curriculum for the advanced practice hospice and palliative care nurse.* Dubuque, IA: Kendall Hunt.

U.S. Preventive Services Task Forces. (2005). *Screening for depression: recommendations and rationale.* Rockville, MD: Agency for Healthcare Research and Quality.

Valente, S. M., & Saunders, J. M. (1997). Diagnosis and treatment of major depression among patients with cancer. *Cancer Nursing, 10*(3), 168–1777.

Valente, S. M., Saunders, J. M., & Cohen, M. Z. (1994). Evaluating depression among patients with cancer. *Cancer Practice, 2*(1), 65–71.

Volicer, L. (1999). Clinical guidelines for the treatment of Alzheimer's disease and other progressive dementia's. *Federal Practitioner Supplement,* May, 16–25.

Volicer, L. (2001). Management of severe Alzheimer's disease and end of life issues. *Clinics in Geriatric Medicine, 17*(2), 377–391.

Waller, A., & Caroline, N. L. (2000). *Handbook of palliative care in cancer.* (2nd ed.). Boston: Butterworth-Heinemann.

Wein, S. (2000). Sedation in the imminently dying patient. *Oncology, 14*(4), 585–592.

Weissman, A. (1998). The patient with acute grief. In T. A. Stern, J. B. Herman, & P. L. Slavin (Eds.), *The MGH guide to psychiatry in primary care.* New York: McGraw-Hill.

Well-Connected Fact Sheet. (1998). *Anxiety.* Report # 28, December 31,. Nidus Information Service, Inc.

Well-Connected Fact Sheet. (1998a). *Depression.* Report # 8, December 31,. Nidus Information Service, Inc.

Wilson, K. G., Chochinov, H. M., de Faye, B. J., & Breitbart. W. (2000). Diagnosis and management of depression in palliative care. In H. M. Chochinov & W. Breitbart (Eds.), *Handbook of psychiatry in palliative medicine.* New York: Oxford University Press.

Wusthoof, J., Shellhaas, R., & Licht, D. (2007) Management of common neurologic symptoms in pediatric palliative care: Seizures, agitation, and spasticity. *Pediatric Clinics of North America, 54,* 789–743.

Yesavage, J., Brink, T. L., Rose, T. L. (1983). Development and validation of a geriatric screening scale: A preliminary report. *Journal of Psychiatric Research, 17,* 37–49.

Zarate, C. A., Baldessarini, R. J., Siegel, A. J., Nakamura, A., McDonald, J., Muir-Hutchinson, L.A., et al. (1997). Risperidone in the elderly: A pharmacoepidemiologic study. *Journal of Clinical Psychiatry, 58,* 311–317.

A. Geriatric Depression Scale

Choose the best answer for how you felt over the past week.

1.	Are you basically satisfied with your life?	YES	NO
2.	Have you dropped many of your activities and interests?	YES	NO
3.	Do you feel that your life is empty?	YES	NO
4.	Do you often get board?	YES	NO
5.	Are you hopeful about the future?	YES	NO
6.	Are you bothered by thoughts you can't get out of your head?	YES	NO
7.	Are you in good spirits most of the time?	YES	NO
8.	Are you afraid that something bad is going to happen to you?	YES	NO
* 9.	Do you feel happy most of the time?	YES	NO
10.	Do you often feel helpless?	YES	NO
11.	Do you often get restless and fidgety?	YES	NO
12.	Do you prefer to stay at home, rather than going out and doing things?	YES	NO
13.	Do you frequently worry about the future?	YES	NO
14.	Do you feel you have more problems with memory than most?	YES	NO
*15.	Do you think it is wonderful to be alive now?	YES	NO
16.	Do you often feel downhearted and blue?	YES	NO
17.	Do you feel pretty worthless the way you are now?	YES	NO
18.	Do you worry a lot about the past?	YES	NO
*19.	Do you find life very exciting?	YES	NO
20.	Is it hard for you to get started on new projects?	YES	NO
*21.	Do you feel full of energy?	YES	NO
22.	Do you feel that your situation is helpless?	YES	NO
23.	Do you think that most people are better off than you are?	YES	NO
24.	Do you frequently get upset over little things?	YES	NO
25.	Do you frequently feel like crying?	YES	NO
26.	Do you have trouble concentrating?	YES	NO
*27.	Do you enjoy getting up in the morning?	YES	NO
28.	Do you prefer to avoid social gatherings?	YES	NO
*29.	Is it easy for you to make decisions?	YES	NO
*30.	Is your mind as clear as it used to be?	YES	NO

Score: ☐

*Non-depressed answers = yes, all others = no

Norms	
Normal	5 ± 4
Mildly depressed	15 ± 6
Very depressed	13 ±

Yesavage J., Brink, T.L., Rose, T.L. (1983). Development and validation of a geriatric screening scale: A preliminary report. *Journal of Psychiatric Research*, 17, 37–49. (Reprinted with permission from Pergamon Press PLC, Headington Hill Hall, Oxford OX3 OBW, UK.)

B. Delirium Rating Scale

Item 1: Temporal onset of symptoms

This item addresses the time course over which symptoms appear; the maximum rating is for the most abrupt onset of symptoms-a common pattern for delirium. Dementia is usually more gradual in onset. Other psychiatric disorders, such as affective disorders, might be scored with 1 or 2 points on this item. Sometimes delirium can be chronic (e.g., in geriatric nursing home patients), and unfortunately only 1 or 2 points would be assessed in that situation.

0) No significant change from long-standing behavior: essentially a chronic or chronic-recurrent disorder
1) Gradual onset of symptoms, occurring within a 6-month period
2) Acute change in behavior or personality occurring over a month
3) Abrupt change in behavior, usually occurring over a 1- to 3-day period

Item 2: Perceptual disturbances

This item rates most highly the extreme inability to perceive differences between internal and external reality, while intermittent misperceptions such as illusions are given 2 points. Depersonalization and derealization can be seen in other organic mental disorders like temporal lobe epilepsy, in severe depression, and in borderline personality disorder and thus are given only 1 point.

0) None evident by history or observation
1) Feelings of depersonalization or derealization
2) Visual illusions or misperceptions including macropsia, micropsia: e.g., mayurinate in wastebasket or mistake bedclothes for something else
3) Evidence that the patient is markedly confused about external reality: e.g., not discriminating between dreams and reality

Item 3: Hallucination type

The presence of any type of hallucination is rated auditory hallucinations alone are rated with less weight because of their common occurrence in primary psychiatric disorders. Visual hallucinations are generally associated with organic mental syndromes, although not

exclusively, and are given 2 points. Tactile hallucinations are classically described in delirium, particularly due to anticholinergic toxicity and are given the most points.

0) Hallucinations not present
1) Auditory hallucinations only
2) Visual hallucinations present by patient's history or inferred by observation, with or without auditory hallucinations
3) Tactile, olfactory, or gustatory hallucinations present with or without visual or auditory hallucinations

Item 4: Delusions

Delusions can be present in many different psychiatric disorders, but tend to be better organized and more fixed in nondelirious disorders and thus are given less weight. Chronic fixed delusions are probably most prevalent in schizophrenic disorders. New delusions may indicate affective and schizophrenic disorders, dementia, or substance intoxication, but should also alert the clinician to possible delirium and are given 2 points. Poorly formed delusions, often of a paranoid nature, are typical of delirium.

0) Not present
1) Delusions are systematized, i.e., well organized and persistent
2) Delusions are new and not part of a preexisting primary psychiatric disorder
3) Delusions are not w ∼ 11 circumscribed; are transient, poorly organized, and mostly in response misperceived environmental cues: e.g., are paranoid and involve persons who are in reality caregivers, loved ones, hospital staff, etc.

Item 5: Psychomotor behavior

This item describes degrees of severity of altered psychomotor behavior. Maximum points can be given for severe agitation or severe withdrawal to reflect either the hyperactive or the hypoactive variant in delirium

0) No significant retardation or agitation
1) Mild restlessness, tremulousness, or anxiety evident by observation and a change from patient's usual behavior

2) Moderate agitation with pacing, removing IV's, etc.

3) Severe agitation, needs to be restrained, may be combative: or has significant withdrawal from the environment, but not due to major depression or schizo phrenic catatonia

Item 6: Cognitive status during formal testing

Information from the cognitive portion of a routine mental status examination is needed to rate this item. The maximum rating of 4 points is given for severe cognitive deficits while only 1 point is given for mild inattention, which could be attributed to pain and fatigue seen in medically ill persons. Two points are given for a relatively isolated cognitive deficit, such as memory impairment, which could be due to dementia or organic amnestic syndrome as well as to early delirium.

0) No cognitive deficits, or deficits which can be alternatively explained by lack of education or prior mental retardation

1) Very mild cognitive deficits which might be attributed to inattention due to acute pain, fatigue, depression, or anxiety associated with having a medical illness

2) Cognitive deficit largely in one major area tested, e.g., memory, but otherwise intact

3) Significant cognitive deficits which are diffuse, i.e., affecting many different areas tested; most include periods of disorientation to time or place at least once each 24-hr period; registration and/or recall are abnormal; concentration is reduced.

4) Severe cognitive deficits, including motor or verbal perseveration, confabulations, disorientation to person, remote and recent memory deficits, and inability to cooperate with formal mental status testing

Item 7: Physical disorder

Maximum points are given when a specific lesion or physiological disturbance can be temporally associated with the altered behavior. Dementias are often not found to have a specific underlying medical cause, while delirium usually has at least one identifiable physical cause.

0) None present or active

1) Presence of any physical disorder which might affect mental state

2) Specific drug, infection, metabolic, central nervous system lesion, or other medical problem which can be temporally implicated in causing the altered behavior or mental status

Item 8: Sleep-wake cycle disturbance

Disruption of the sleep-wake cycle is typical in delirium, with demented persons generally having significant sleep disturbances much later in their course. Severe delirium is on a continuum with stupor and coma, and persons with a resolving coma are likely to be delirious temporarily.

0) Not present; awake and alert during the day, and sleeps without significant disruption at night

1) Occasional drowsiness during day and mild sleep continuity disturbance at night; may have nightmares, but can readily distinguish from reality

2) Frequent napping and unable to sleep at night, constituting a significant disruption of or a reversal of the usual sleep-wake cycle

3) Drowsiness prominent, difficulty staying alert during interview, loss of self control over alertness and somnolence

4) Drifts into stuporous or comatose periods

Item 9: Lability of mood

Rapid shifts in mood can occur in various organic mental syndromes, perhaps due to a disinhibition of one's normal control. The patient may be aware of this lack of emotional control and may behave inappropriately relative to the situation or to his/her thinking state, e.g., crying for no apparent reason. Delirious patients may score points on any of these items depending upon the severity of the delirium and upon how their underlying psychological state "colors" their delirious presentation. Patients with borderline personality disorder might score 1 or 2 points on this item.

0) Not present; mood stable

1) Affect/mood somewhat altered and changes over the course of hours; patient states that mood changes are not under self-control

2) Significant mood changes which are inappropriate to situation, including fear, anger, or tearfulness; rapid shifts of emotion, even over several minutes

3) Severe disinhibition of emotions, including temper outbursts, uncontrolled inappropriate laughter or crying

Item 10: Variability of symptoms

The hallmark of delirium is the waxing and waning of symptoms, which is given 4 points on this item. Demented as well as delirious patients who become more confused at night when environmental cues have decreased could score 2 points.

0) Symptoms stable and mostly present during daytime

2) Symptoms worsen at night

4) Fluctuating intensity of symptoms, such that they wax and wane during a 24-hr period

Total Score

From "A Symptom Rating Scale for Delirium," by P. T. Trzepacz, R. W. Baker, and J. Greenhouse, 1988, *Psychiatry Research*, 23, pp. 89–97. Copyright 1988. Reprinted with permission.

C. Memorial Delirium Assessment Scale

INSTRUCTIONS: Rate the severity of the following symptoms of delirium based on current interaction with subject or assessment of his/her behavior or experience over past several hours (as indicated in each time).

Item 1: Reduced Level of Consciousness (Awareness). Rate the patient's current awareness of an interaction with the environment (interviewer, other people/objects in the room, for example, ask patients to describe the surroundings).

0: none. Patient spontaneously fully aware of environment and interacts appropriately. Patient is unaware of some elements in the environment, or not spontaneously interacting appropriately with the interviewer: becomes fully aware and appropriately interactive when prodded strongly: interview is prolonged but not seriously disrupted.
2: moderate. Patient is unaware of some or all elements in the environment, or not spontaneously interacting with the interviewer: becomes incompletely aware and inappropriately interactive when prodded strongly; interview is prolonged but not seriously disrupted. Patient is unaware of all elements in the environment with no spontaneous interaction or awareness of the interviewer, so that the interview is difficult to impossible, even with maximal prodding.

Item 2: Disorientation. Rate current state by asking the following 10 orientation items: date, month, day, year, season, floor, name of hospital, city, state, and country.

0: none.
1: mild.
2: moderate.
3: severe.

Patient knows 9–10 items
Patient knows 7–8 items
Patient knows 5–6 items
Patient knows no more than four items

Item 3: Short-term memory impairment. Rate current state by using repetition and delayed recall of three words (patient must immediately repeat and recall words 5 minutes later after an intervening task. Use alternate sets of three words for successive evaluation (e.g., example, apple, table, tomorrow, sky, cigar, and justice).

0: none.	All three words repeated and recalled
1: mild.	All three repeated, patient fails to recall one
2: moderate.	All three repeated, patient fails to recall two
3: severe.	Patient fails to repeat one or more words

Item 4: lmpaired digit span. Rate current performance by asking subjects to repeat first three, four, then five digits forward and then three, then four backward: continue to the next step only if patient succeeds at the previous one.

0: none.	Patient can do at least five numbers forward and four backward
1: mild.	Patient can do at least five numbers forward, three backward
2: moderate.	Patient can do 4–5 numbers forward, cannot do three backward
3: severe.	Patient can do no more than three numbers forward

Item 5: Reduced ability to maintain and shift attention. As indicated during the interview by questions needing to be rephrased and/or repeated because patient's attention wanders, patient loses track, patient is distracted by outside stimuli or overabsorbed in a task.

0: none.	None of the above: patient maintains and shifts attention normally
1: mild.	Above attention problems occurs once or twice without prolonging the interview
2: moderate.	Above attentional problems occur often, prolonging the interview without seriously disrupting it

Above attentional problems occur constantly, disrupting and making the interview difficult to impossible

Item 6: Disorganized thinking as indicated during the interview by rambling, irrelevant, or incoherent speech, or by tangential, circumstantial, or faulty reasoning. Ask patient a somewhat complex question (e.g., "Describe your current medical condition.")

0: none.
1: mild.
3: severe.

Patient's speech is coherent and goal-directed.

Patient's speech is slightly difficult to follow; responses to questions are slightly off target but not so much as to prolong the interview. Disorganized thoughts or speech are clearly present, such that interview is prolonged but not disrupted.

Examination is very difficult or impossible due to disorganized thinking or speech.

Item 7: Perceptual disturbance. Misperceptions, illusions, hallucinations inferred from inappropriate behavior during the interview or admitted by subject as well as those elicited from nurse/family/chart accounts of the past several hours or of the time since last examination:

0: none.
1: mild.
2: moderate.
3: severe.

No misperceptions, illusions, or hallucinations.

Misperceptions or illusions related to sleep, fleeting hallucinations on 1–2 occasions without inappropriate behavior.

Hallucinations or frequent illusions on several occasions with minimal inappropriate behavior that does not disrupt the interview.

Frequent or intense illusions or hallucinations with persistent inappropriate behavior that disrupts the interview or interferes with medical care.

Item 8: Delusions. Rate delusions inferred from inappropriate behavior during the interview or admitted by the patient as well as delusions elicited from nurse/family/chart accounts of the past several hours or of the time since the previous examination.

0: none.	No evidence of misinterpretations or delusions
1: mild.	Misinterpretations or suspiciousness without clear delusional ideas or inappropriate behavior
2: moderate.	Delusions admitted by the patient or evidenced by his/her behavior that do

not or only marginally disrupt the interview or interfere with medical care

3: severe.	Persistent and/or intense delusions resulting in inappropriate behavior, disrupting the interview or seriously interfering with medical care.

Item 9: Decreased or increased psychomotor activity rate activity over past several hours as well as activity during interview by circling (a) hypoactive, (b) hyperactive, or (c) elements of both present

0: none. pormal psychomotor activity
a b c
1: mild.
a b c

Hypoactivity is barely noticeable, expressed as slightly slowing of movement. Hyperactivity is barely noticeable or appears as simple restlessness.

Hypoactivity is undeniable with marked reduction in the number of movements or marked slowness of movement: subject rarely spontaneously moves or speaks. Hyperactivity is undeniable, subject moves almost constantly, In both cases, exam is prolonged as a consequence.

Hypoactivity is severe, patient does not move or speak without prodding or is catatonic. Hyperactivity is severe; patient is constantly moving, overreacts to stimuli, and requires surveillance and/or restraint. Getting through the exam is difficult or impossible.

Item 10: Sleep-wake cycle disturbance (disorder of arousal). Rate patient's ability to either sleep or stay awake at the appropriate times. Utilize direct observation during the interview as well as reports from nurses, family, patient, or charts describing sleep-wake cycle disturbance over the past several hours or since last examination. Use observations of the previous night for morning evaluations only.

0: none.	At night, sleeps well. During the day, has no trouble staying awake.
1: mild.	Mild deviation from appropriate sleepfulness and wakefulness states at night, difficulty falling asleep or transient night awakenings, needs medication to sleep well: during the day, reports periods of drowsiness or during the interview is drowsy but can easily fully awaken him/herself.
2: moderate.	Moderate deviations form appropriate sleepfulness and wakefulness states at night; repeated and prolonged night awakening; during the day, reports of frequent and prolonged napping

or, during the interview, can only be roused to complete wakefulness by strong stimuli. Severe deviations from appropriate sleepfulness and wakefulness states at night, sleeplessness; during the day, patient spends most of the time sleeping, or, during the interview, cannot be roused to full wakefulness by any stimuli.

2: moderate. a b c

3: severe. a b c

From "The Memorial Delirium Assessment Scale," by W. Breitbart, B. Rosenfeld, A. Roth, M. J. Smith, K. Cohen, and S. Passlk. 1997. *Journal of Pain and Symptom Management,* 13(3). pp. 128–137. Copyright 1997 by the U. S. Cancer Pain Relief Committee. Reprinted with permission of Elsevier Science.

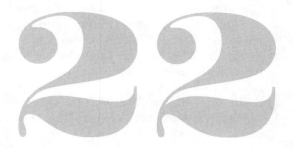

Gastrointestinal Symptoms

Pamala D. Larsen
Laura Mallett

Key Points

- Gastrointestinal (GI) symptomatology is very common in patients receiving palliative care; however, research to support evidence-based interventions is lacking.
- The evidence to support treatment of nausea and vomiting in palliative care is mostly drawn from chemotherapy-induced nausea and vomiting (CINV); however, the mechanisms and pathophysiology of CINV and the nausea and vomiting of the palliative care population are very different.
- The diagnosis and treatment of dysphagia is based on the patient's prognosis. With a longer prognosis, medically assisted feeding and hydration may be attempted. With a shorter prognosis, the treatment may be different.
- Medications, and primarily the opioids, are a primary cause of constipation in patients under palliative.
- Laxatives may be used as either a preventative measure for constipation or a treatment for the same.
- Signs and symptoms of bowel obstruction are based on the site of the obstruction.
- The most common cause of diarrhea in palliative care is inappropriate laxative therapy.

Case Study: Three months ago Mrs. Adams was diagnosed with pancreatic cancer with metastasis to her stomach, liver, and intestine, resulting in a poor prognosis. Mrs. Adams is 65 years of age with a history of smoking and drinking alcohol on a regular basis. There is no family history of cancer, and Mrs. Adams had no significant health history until this diagnosis. With the involvement of other organs, she made the decision not to have surgery. She is admitted to the medical unit today for severe abdominal pain, constipation, and nausea and vomiting.

She completed the admission assessment documents and finds that she is jaundiced and has a bruit located in the upper left quadrant. A nasogastric tube has been inserted and is connected to low suction. Breath sounds reveal fine crackles in the bases bilaterally. Mrs. Adams states that her appetite has been poor, and she has not been taking Viokase as ordered because of her vomiting. Her last stool was two days ago with diarrhea. She states that she has been taking morphine sulfate subcutaneously at home and an antiemetic that she cannot remember the name of. Mrs. Adams' daughter is with her and is concerned that her mother waited too long to come to the hospital. Lab results include total bilirubin of 4 mg/dl; amylase 2500 IU/dl; ASGOT 30 units/l; Hbg 4.0 g/dl and Hct 13%; Na 133; K + 3.45 mEq/l. Arterial blood gas results demonstrate pH at 7.33; $PaCO_2$ 34 and HCO_3 21. The chest X-ray shows bilateral pleural effusions.

Introduction

In most countries of the world, sharing meals with others is a social activity. The primary purpose of the meal may be consumption of food; however, the socialization with others while eating may be even more important. Communities, organizations, and churches often have potluck suppers where individuals gather to share a meal. If an individual is unable to share a meal with others due to gastrointestinal (GI) symptomatology, the effect on the emotional health of the individual from being socially isolated and unable to participate in such activities may be greater than the physical effects of the symptoms.

From an anecdotal perspective, adult patients at the end of life suffer from GI symptoms although there are limited data available to indicate the extent. For those with cancer, nausea and vomiting occurs in nearly 50% of cases (Dean, Harris, Regnard, & Hockley, 2006). Individuals with chronic kidney disease often suffer from numerous GI symptoms due to uremia (Germain & Cohen, 2005). GI symptomatology is also common in AIDS patients and end-stage heart failure (Dean et al., 2006). For patients suffering from continuous nausea, vomiting, or diarrhea, it precludes them from leaving their care setting, whether it is home, assisted living, or a long-term care facility, and affects their quality of life and the ability to function normally.

The incidence of GI symptoms in children who die of non-cancer-related illness is unknown; however, GI symptomatology in pediatric cancer patients at the end of life is significant (Santucci & Mack, 2007). Some symptoms may be the result of the disease process itself, complications of the disease, concurrent disorders, iatrogenic in nature, or from an unidentified cause. This chapter focuses on the cluster of GI symptoms that occur in the patient in palliative care.

There are multiple ways of assessing and diagnosing the symptomatology that a patient may develop from the side effects of treatment and/or comfort measures. A mnemonic, developed by Esper and Heidrich (2005, p. 20), gives the caregiver a resource in managing the multiple symptoms that are experienced by the patient.

R – Review the situation

E – Explore findings

S – Strategize a plan of action

C – Carry out the plan

U – Umbrella resources

E – Evaluate and modify as needed

NAUSEA AND VOMITING

Nausea and vomiting (N&V) are unpleasant GI symptoms and have been described by some patients as worse than pain and more disabling (Chilton & Faull, 2005). Although nausea may occur without vomiting on occasion, they commonly occur together and will be discussed together in this chapter. Nausea is a nonobservable subjective symptom involving an unpleasant sensation experienced in the back of the throat and the epigastrum, which may or may not result in vomiting (Rhodes & McDaniel, 2001). Vomiting is the forceful expulsion of gastric contents through the oral or nasal cavity (Rhodes & McDaniel, 2001).

Although N&V are typically associated with chemotherapy treatment in cancer, these symptoms occur in 40 to 70% of patients in palliative care settings (Dalal, Del Fabbro, & Bruera, 2006). Patients with AIDS, hepatic failure, and renal failure often have nausea during the disease process and at the end of life (Mannix, 2005).

Most of the management and treatment literature is derived from studying chemotherapy-induced nausea and vomiting (CINV). Because this type of N&V differs both in mechanism and pathophysiology from N&V due to advanced disease, those findings may not be applicable to palliative care (Tyler, 2000). Unfortunately, little progress has been made in understanding the mechanism and determining optimal treatment of multicausal N&V or non-chemotherapy-related N&V (King, 2006).

Etiology

Nausea and vomiting involve activity at multiple levels of the nervous system. Two distinct sites in the medulla are critical for the control of emesis: the vomiting center (VC) and the chemoreceptor trigger zone (CTZ) (Dalal et al., 2006). The VC is not a discrete anatomical structure but represents an interrelated neural network including the nucleus tractus solitarius (NTS) and the dorsal motor nucleus of the vagus (DMV) (p. 399). The NTS is where numerous afferent neuronal pathways from these sources converge. Once the NTS receives signals from the various afferent sources, the information is processed and the DMV emits an appropriate vasomotor response (respiratory, salivary, gut, diaphragm, and abdominal muscles) including nausea, retching, or vomiting depending on the intensity of the signals (Dalal et al.).

There are multiple pathways that stimulate the VC. Understanding the pathways is necessary to determine the cause and appropriate treatment (King, 2006). The various pathways include

- peripheral pathways of the
  - □ vagal afferents,
  - □ pharyngeal afferents,
  - □ vestibular system; and
- central pathways including
  - □ midbrain afferents and
  - □ CTZ.

Figure 22.1 demonstrates the various pathways and potential factors that may contribute to each.

Exhibit 22.1 lists potential causes and conditions associated with N&V that may occur in patients in palliative care. It must be emphasized that if comorbidities exist, the etiology of N&V may be difficult to ascertain. This is particularly an issue in the older adult who may have more than one disease process present. Without a clear indication of cause, successful treatment becomes even more difficult.

Signs and Symptoms

A sign is the objective evidence of what is occurring with the patient; the presence of vomitus in any amount is definitive objective evidence. Nausea, however, is a

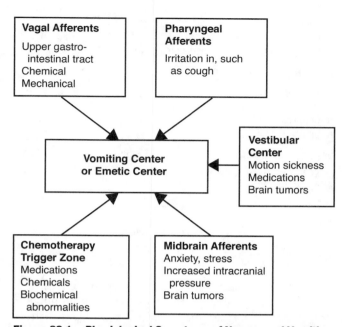

Figure 22.1   Physiological Symptoms of Nausea and Vomiting
Source: Reprinted from Dalal, S., Del Fabbro, E., & Bruera, E. (2006). Symptom control in palliative care – Part I: Oncology as a paradigmatic example. *Journal of Palliative Medicine,* 9(2), pp. 391-408.

EXHIBIT 22.1   CAUSES OF NAUSEA AND VOMITING IN PALLIATIVE CARE

CHEMORECEPTOR TRIGGER ZONE MEDIATED
- Medications
  - □ Opioids
  - □ Antibiotics
  - □ Chemotherapy
  - □ Corticosteroids
  - □ Digoxin
  - □ Nonsteroidal anti-inflammatory drugs
  - □ Iron

- Metabolic
  - □ Hypercalcemia
  - □ Hyponatremia
  - □ Uremia

MIDBRAIN AFFERENTS
- Emotional factors
  - □ Anxiety
  - □ Fear
  - □ Pain

- Increased intracranial pressure
- Primary or metastatic brain tumors
- Meningitis

VAGAL AFFERENTS
- Gastrointestinal distention, stasis, or obstruction

■ Constipation
■ Gastritis
■ External pressure ("squashed stomach syndrome")

PHARYNGEAL AFFERENTS

■ Thick sputum
■ Oral infection
■ Chronic cough
■ Unpleasant tastes

VESTIBULAR APPARATUS

■ Motion sickness
■ Brain tumors
■ Opioids

Source: Gullatte, Kaplow, & Heidrich (2005), p. 230.

subjective symptom that the patient experiences, and it is not measurable to the caregiver. Although it is not objective, nausea may produce significant distress for the patient and affect activities of daily living and quality of life.

N&V may have accompanying signs and symptoms. With nausea, there may be evidence of increased salivation and swallowing, perspiration, and tachycardia. In patients with N&V triggered by GI tract stasis, there may be accompanying epigastric pain, fullness, early satiety, flatulence, acid reflux, hiccup, and large volume vomitus (possibly projectile). In patients with N&V associated with increased intracranial pressure (ICP), headache and nausea, both diurnal in nature, may occur. Other neurological signs may or may not be present with increased ICP.

Assessment

There are a number of factors to consider when assessing the N&V of a patient. Some of the data will be obtained from self-report or report from family caregivers, while other data will be objective. Assessment includes frequency and duration, color, amount and consistency of vomitus, contributing factors to the N&V; pattern of the N&V; presence of pain; presence of other abdominal symptoms, and disruption to the patient (e.g., can the patient continue activities of daily living and other 'normal' activities with the N&V present?)

Patients should be questioned about the frequency of their bowel movements because in the palliative care population, chronic constipation is frequently present and may be contributing to the nausea. In patients with cancer, it is important to obtain details of the sites of the tumor involvement. As an example, in patients with intra-abdominal involvement, nausea with or without vomiting is often caused by liver metastasis, bowel obstruction by the tumor, or peritoneal carcinomatosis (Dalal et al., 2006). Another contributing factor to N&V could be unrelieved pain.

A large number of medications are associated with nausea; therefore a detailed medication history is necessary. Nausea often accompanies the use of opioids, nonsteroidal anti-inflammatories, anti-cholinergics, and antibiotics. Patients with HIV often have nausea, which is a side effect of all of the highly active anti-retroviral therapy (HAART) drugs. Medications that have been previously tolerated, e.g., digoxin, may become toxic and cause N&V because of reduced renal and hepatic function, particularly in the older adult (Gullatte, Kaplow, & Heidrich, 2005, p. 229). Assessing for hypercalcemia and syndrome of insufficient ant diuretic hormone (SIADH), particularly in cancer patients, is important. High levels of serum calcium and low sodium stimulate the CTZ and may cause N&V (Gullatte et al., 2005).

Assessing the young child may be more challenging. Although the above-mentioned assessment guide can be used, very young children may have difficulty differentiating between nausea and pain (Santucci & Mack, 2007). Even older children may view reflux as nausea.

Lastly, as part of the assessment, does the patient consider the N&V to affect his/her quality of life or is it seen merely as a nuisance? To have a clearer picture of the patient's N&V, an instrument with known reliability and validity should be used.

Instruments. Accurate assessment of signs and symptoms can better determine the pattern of occurrence, if there is one, and the effect of interventions. There are both self-report and observer-report tools, and there is a debate as to which type of tool is best (Saxby, Ackroyd, Callin, Mayland, & Kite, 2007). Some see self-report as essential to determine effective interventions, while others believe that the antiemetic medications given can cause sedation, mood alteration, disorientation, or memory loss and thus affect self-report (Saxby et al., 2007). Many of the specific tools have been validated in chemotherapy outpatient settings, and none has been extensively validated for assessment of emesis in a palliative care population (Saxby et al., 2007).

Rhodes (1997) recommends the following points when using an instrument to measure N&V: 1) use self-report tools; 2) determine and describe the symptoms; 3) consider the clarity, cultural sensitivity, and understandability of the tool; 4) reliability and validity of the tool; 5) use an instrument in an easy-to-read format; 6) consider the purpose of the tool and for what population of patients; and 7) consider the type of scoring and the ease of scoring.

The tools mentioned in this chapter have limited reliability and validity in a palliative care setting. The Index of Nausea, Vomiting and Retching-Revised (INV-R) instrument measures nausea, vomiting, retching, and the associated distress. The tool is an 8-item 5-point Likert type self-report tool with 'check the box inserts'. Although it was originally developed for the adult oncology population, it has been demonstrated to have use with other populations (Rhodes & McDaniel, 1997; Saxby et al., 2007).

A number of other instruments are more global in nature and include examining all symptomatology present. These include the Visual Analog Scale (VAS); Verbal Categorical Scale (VCS) and Adapted Symptom Distress Scale (SDS-2); and the Edmonton Symptom Assessment Scale (ESAS) (Saxby et al., 2007). The use of reliable and valid instruments is necessary to develop evidence-based interventions to assist patients with these symptoms.

Management

Interventions should take into account the symptoms and the central emetogenic pathways involved (Mannix, 2005). Unfortunately, there is a gap in the evidence regarding high-quality studies in the management of N&V in chronic advanced disease other than related to cancer treatment (Brunnhuber, Nash, Meier, Weissman, & Woodcock, 2008).

Pharmacological interventions. Although progress has been made in identifying antiemetic agents that alleviate CINV, little work has been accomplished to establish drugs that alleviate the N&V experienced at the end of life. As an example, in Lipman, Jackson and Tyler's book *Evidence Based Symptom Control in Palliative Care* published in 2000, there are a handful of descriptive studies listed, all with sample sizes of 5. All of these studies had a Level of Evidence of five case series without control groups. Similarly, in the newly published Putting Evidence into Practice: *Palliative Care*, a monograph by Brunnhuber et al. (2008), there are no studies listed that were conducted in a palliative care setting. Thus using the "evidence" in providing care for those with N&V in palliative care is difficult.

Different antiemetics act on different parts of the N&V process; therefore when antiemetics are not prescribed correctly, optimal results will not occur. For example, drugs that act on the CTZ would be given to patients with N&V stemming from uremia, chemotherapy, radiation, or opioid-inducted nausea.

Mannix (2005) recommends seven steps in choosing the appropriate antiemetic. Those steps include the following: 1) Identify the cause of the N&V; 2) Identify the pathway triggering the vomiting reflex; 3) Identify the neurotransmitter receptor involved in the pathway; 4) Choose the most potent antagonist to the receptor identified; 5) Choose a route of administration that ensures optimal action; 6) Titrate the dosage; 7) If symptoms persist, review the cause (pp. 459–460).

Table 22.1 lists examples of drugs, sites of action, receptors, and comments that may be useful in determining the appropriate antiemetic.

Some of the antiemetics are not well tolerated in older adults. For example, metoclopramide must be used with caution in older adults, as decreased hepatic function increases drug toxicity and increases the incidence of extrapyramidal effects such as tardive dyskinesia (Gridelli, 2004). Although typically the dosage guidelines between the most common 5-HT3 receptor antagonists do not differ, these drugs do differ in terms of receptor selectivity, duration of action and metabolism (Gridelli, 2004). These differences might have potential clinical implications in older adults. As an example, granisetron has duration of action of 24 hours, while ondansetron's action is 9 hours. Additionally, three of these drugs, dolasetron, palonosetron and tropisetron, have cardiovascular effects and should not be prescribed to patients of any age with a cardiovascular history (Gridelli, 2004).

Drugs from other classifications may be used in palliative care. These include corticosteroids, cannabinoids, and benzodiazapines. Corticosteroids have intrinsic antiemetic properties and have been known to enhance the effects of other antiemetics (Mannix, 2005). There is anecdotal evidence that cannabinoids may reduce N&V in CINV. However, studies assessing its use in individuals with advanced disease are lacking. Benzodiazepines have been used in combination with other antiemetics in chemotherapy. Although they have little antiemetic potency on their own, in drug combinations they reduce anxiety and akathisia (Mannix, 2005).

Medications appropriate for use in the pediatric client include ondansetron, lorazepam, promethazine, dexamethasone, metoclopramide, diphenhydramine, octreotide, meclizine, olanzapine, scopolamine, and hydroxyzine (Hellsten & Kane, 2006; Hinds, Oakes, Hicks & Anghelescu, 2005; Santucci & Mack, 2007). Ondanstetron is far less helpful in pediatric palliative care as opposed to children undergoing chemotherapy (Sibson, Craig, & Goldman, 2005).

Nonpharmacological and complementary interventions. Often there are adjunct interventions to accompany medications. Establishing a research basis for those interventions is more difficult, although much has been written using anecdotal data versus research data. Research studies in the literature are based on patients with CINV and on patients with N&V at the end of life.

Simple self-care strategies may be instituted to control N&V (Exhibit 22.2), which may consist of dietary and environmental changes. Encourage the patient to use interventions that have relieved N&V at other times in his/her life, such as during pregnancy, illness, or times of stress. A particular food associated with a positive past experience can be suggested (Enck, 2002). Dietary changes such as drinking clear liquids and eating bland foods may be helpful. Minimizing or even

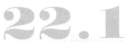

| | Receptor-Specific Antiemetics for Use in Palliative Care |

DRUG	SITE	RECEPTOR	COMMENTS
Haloperidol	CTZ	Dopamine antagonist	Use in opioid-induced nausea and chemical and mechanical nausea; use when anxiety symptoms aggravate N&V; may have additive effects with other CNS depressants
Metoclopramide cisapride	CTZ GIT	Metoclopramide is a dopamine antagonist at low doses; at doses greater than 120 mg/24 hour it becomes a 5-HT$_3$ antagonist	Use in gastric stasis, ileus, and chemotherapy; use diphenhydramine to decrease extrapyramidal symptoms; cisapride has potentially fatal cardiac arrhythmias
Phenothiazines (prochlorperazine, chlorpromazine, levomepromazine, thiethylperazine)	CTZ GIT VC	Predominantly as dopamine antagonists	Use in intestinal obstruction, peritoneal irritation, vestibular causes, raised ICP, and nausea of unknown etiology; extrapyramidal effects; not recommended for routine use
Scopolamine	VC	Anticholinergic	Use in intestinal obstruction, increased ICP, and peritoneal irritation; useful if N&V exists with colic
5-HT$_3$ receptor antagonists (ondanesetron, granisetron, tropisetron, palonosetron)	CTZ GIT VC	Serotonin antagonist	Use in chemotherapy, abdominal radiation and post-op N&V; safe for children and older adults; effectiveness increased by combining with dexamethasone
Antihistamines (cinnarizine, cyclizine, diphenhydramine, promethazine)	VC	H$_1$ receptor	Use in intestinal obstruction, increased ICP, vestibular causes and peritoneal irritation; cyclizine is the least sedative

CTZ = chemoreceptor trigger zone; VC = vomiting center; GIT = gastrointestinal tract; ICP = increased intracranial pressure.

Reprinted from Gullatte, M.M., Kaplow, R. & Heidrich, D.E. (2005). Oncology. In K.K. Kuebler, M.P. Davis & C.D. Moore (Eds.) *Palliative practices: An interdisciplinary approach* (pp. 197–245). St. Louis: Mosby Elsevier.

EXHIBIT 22.2 SELF-CARE ACTIVITIES FOR NAUSEA AND VOMITING

Oral hygiene after each emesis
Cool, damp washcloth to the forehead, neck, and wrists
Eat bland, cool foods
Have fresh air with a fan or open window
Limit environmental stimuli that precipitate N&V
Lie flat for 2 hours after eating
Eat small meals
Practice relaxation techniques and/or guided imagery
Provide distraction

Sources: Enck, 2002; Kemp, 1999; King, 2001; Rhodes & McDaniel, 2001.

eliminating liquids prior to a meal or during a meal may decrease nausea (Kemp, 1999). Patients with advanced disease often have decreased or altered taste (Tyler, 2000). When that occurs, they may prefer different foods than what they have previously enjoyed.

Patients and their family should be encouraged to keep a self-care log of symptoms, interventions, and responses. The log reinforces interventions that work for the patient and may demonstrate "good days" when the N&V was less. The log can also help the patient feel more in control of his/her life in addition to the providing the caregiver with information on which to base interventions.

Music therapy has shown some benefits as an adjunct therapy. Ezzone, Baker, Rosselet and Terepka (1998) demonstrated that music therapy was a statistically significant adjunct treatment during high-dose chemotherapy to reduce nausea and vomiting. Relaxation techniques and guided imagery are also adjuvant therapies that can be used to decrease N&V and reduce anxiety. However, the research basis of these nonpharmacological interventions (see Table 22.2) needs to be established to support evidence-based practice.

Acupuncture and ginger are two common complementary interventions used to manage nausea and vomiting (Thompson & Zollman, 2005). Acupuncture is an ancient healing art using insertion of fine-gauge needles to palliate symptoms. The needles are inserted into carefully chosen acupuncture points and left in place for up to 20 minutes. Vickers, in his review of acupuncture studies, found 11 high-quality, randomized, placebo-controlled trials that demonstrated positive results using acupuncture as an antiemetic intervention (Vickers, 1996).

Ginger has been used for centuries in folk medicine to decrease nausea (Langmead & Rampton, 2001; Wickham, 1999). Langmead and Rampton (2001) report four research studies that have been conducted using ginger in postoperative N&V, with two demonstrating statistically significant results.

Family concerns and considerations. N&V are visible signs of an unhealthy state, and, as such, family caregivers can be distressed and anxious about their loved one. It is important that the nurse addresses the family's anxiety associated with N&V. Family education is vital to facilitate functioning as a care team member and helping the loved one experience an optimal quality of life.

Families should be taught to systematically assess the patient's N&V. Use of a simple log of what activity the patient is engaging in when the episode of N&V

22.2 | Nonpharmacologic Interventions for Nausea and Vomiting

BEHAVIORAL INTERVENTION	DESCRIPTION	COMMENTS
Self-hypnosis	Evolution of physiologic state of altered consciousness and total body relaxation. This technique involves a state of intensified attention and receptiveness to an idea	Use to control anticipatory N&V; limited studies, mostly in children and adolescents; easily learned; no side effects; decreases intensity and duration of nausea; decreased frequency, severity, amount and duration of vomiting
Relaxation	Progressive contraction and relaxation of various muscle groups	Often used with imagery; can use for other stressful situations; easily learned; no side effects; decreases nausea during and after chemotherapy; decreases duration and severity of vomiting; not as effective with anticipatory nausea and vomiting
Biofeedback	Control of specific physiologic responses by receiving information about changes in response to induced state of relaxation	Two types of electromyographic and skin temperature; used alone or with relaxation; easily learned; no side effects; decreased nausea during and after chemotherapy; more effective with progressive muscle relaxation
Imagery	Mentally take self away by focusing on images of a relaxing place	Most effective when combined with another technique; increases self-control; decreases duration of nausea; decreases perceptions of degree of vomiting; feel more in control, relaxed and powerful
Distraction	Learn to divert attention from a threatening situation and to relaxing sensations	Can use videos, games, and puzzles; no side effects; decreases anticipatory N&V; decreases postchemotherapy distress; inexpensive
Desensitization	Three-step process involving relaxation and visualization to decrease sensitization to aversive situations	Inexpensive; easily learned; no side effects; decreases anticipatory N&V

Reprinted from King, C. (1997). Nonpharmacologic management of chemotherapy-induced nausea and vomiting. *Oncology Nursing Forum, 24* (Suppl), 41–48.

occurs provides evidence to the family and patient when the nausea increased or decreased and how and when the vomiting occurred as well. The family and healthcare professional can then assess the situation by viewing the log and determine what pharmacological or nonpharmacological intervention may work best for the patient.

DYSPHAGIA

Dysphagia is difficulty in transferring liquids or solids from the mouth to the stomach (Regnard, 2005, p. 468). Most of the data on incidence of dysphagia come from clients affected with head and neck cancer. These patients may suffer from dysphagia in the early, middle, and terminal stages of the disease. One source indicates that 79% of those patients have significant eating problems (Barbour, 1999). In the late stages of multiple sclerosis (MS), dysphagia is reported in 10–33% of clients (Dahlin & Goldsmith, 2006). In amyotrophic lateral sclerosis (ALS), 25% of patients present with dysphagia as their initial complaint at diagnosis (Dahlin & Goldsmith, 2006). Sixty-three percent of patients with Parkinson's disease have objective evidence of difficulty with swallowing (Regnard, 2005).

Etiology

Swallowing is a complex activity that requires intact anatomy; normal mucosa; normal functioning of six cranial nerves; the brainstem; the co-ordination of the cortex, limbic system, basal ganglia, and cerebellum; and brainstem centers involved in respiration, salivation, and motor function of 34 skeletal muscles (Regnard, 2005). Dysphagia may occur as a result of a disruption in any of the four stages of swallowing: oral preparatory stage, oral stage, pharyngeal stage, and the esophageal stage.

Both the oral preparatory and oral stages of swallowing are voluntary actions. In the oral preparatory phase, food is taken into the mouth and saliva helps form a paste bolus. During the oral phase, the bolus is centered and moved to the posterior oropharynx. The pharyngeal phase is not voluntary, but reflexive, as the swallowing reflex carries the food bolus through the pharynx. Peristaltic waves carry the food bolus to the stomach during the esophageal phase.

Each of the stages of swallowing is affected by aging, and dysphagia is a common complaint of the older adult. The skeletal muscles involved with swallowing may undergo age-related changes of atrophy and weakness that occur in all skeletal muscles (Plahuta & Hamrick-King, 2006). Similarly, there are aging changes that occur in the nerves that innervate the oral region. Each of the stages of swallowing is a precisely timed contraction/relaxation sequence and can be affected by the aging process. The sequence may become desynchronized, and the entire process of swallowing may become ineffective (Timiras, 1994).

Dahlin and Goldsmith (2006) list the causes of dysphagia commonly seen in palliative care: neoplasm (includes brain tumors, head and neck cancer, and esophageal tumors); progressive neuromuscular diseases such as ALS, Parkinson's disease, and multiple sclerosis (MS); dementia; systemic dysphagia as a result of inflammatory and infectious factors; and general deconditioning which may include multisystem disease and failure and the side effects of medications and/or polypharmacy. Each cause of dysphagia may occur for a different reason. For example, in Parkinson's disease there is disruption in the oral stage of swallowing because of rigidity of the lingual musculature (Dahlin & Goldsmith, 2006). As a result of this rigidity, pharyngeal swallow responses are delayed and aspiration may occur before or during the swallow. Regnard (2005) suggests there is a defect in the non-dopaminergic pathway from the medulla and a disturbance of the oral phase due to bradykinesia (p. 468). In head and neck cancers, dysphagia may occur because of the pressure and size of the tumor, or as a result of chemotherapy, radiation, or the surgery itself.

Common side effects of radiation, i.e., mucositis and xerostomia, may further exacerbate dysphagia (Rudd & Worlding, 2005), as well as pain on swallowing, dry mouth, anorexia, or anxiety (Baines, 1992). Dysphagia may not be a part of the terminal illness itself but be a result or symptom of a comorbidity. An example would be an older adult who is terminally ill with cancer and also has advanced Parkinson's disease or has suffered a previous cerebrovascular accident.

Signs and Symptoms

An initial indication of dysphagia is choking or coughing when eating or drinking. A patient may complain of having the feeling that something is caught in his/her throat. These signs of dysphagia are often accompanied by fear and anxiety on the part of the patients, fear that food may actually be trapped in their lungs, and the anxiety that they will be unable to breathe as a result of food "going down the wrong pipe." Some people exhibit no signs of choking, although food or liquids may be entering the trachea and lung; these patients are known as "silent aspirators." Noting the quality of the patient's voice and whether or not any expressive aphasia or dysphasia is present may provide clues to the nurse that the patient is aspirating (Easton, 1999).

Depending on the phase of swallowing that is affected, the signs of dysphagia may differ. Exhibit 22.3 delineates characteristics of dysphagia associated with the oral, pharyngeal, and esophageal phases. Each characteristic may have varying degrees of seriousness.

EXHIBIT 22.3 SIGNS AND SYMPTOMS OF DYSPHAGIA

Oral Phase	Drooling
	Pocketing of food
	Excessive chewing
	Facial asymmetry or weakness
	Tongue weakness
	Inability to close lips tightly or move lips
	Weakness or absence of gag reflex
	Weakness or absence of a swallowing reflex
	Nasal drainage due to nasal regurgitation
	Loss of internal or external sensation of the oral cavity or face
Pharyngeal Phase	Delayed or absence of swallowing
	Coughing while drinking or eating fluids
	History of aspiration pneumonia
	Wet, gurgling, moist or nasal voice
	Frequent clearing of throat
	Complaints of burning
Esophageal Phase	Burping or substernal distress due to esophageal reflux
	Coughing or wheezing

Source: J. Hickey (1997). Rehabilitation of neuroscience patients. In J. Hickey (Ed.) *The clinical practice of neurological and neurosurgical nursing* (4th ed.) (pp. 255). Philadelphia: Lippincott.

Assessment

In the terminal stages of illness, it is likely that dysphagia is not a new symptom but one that has been present for some time and is worsening. In assessment during palliative care, the goals of the swallowing evaluation should be clear. Dahlin and Goldsmith (2006, p. 202) list the following goals of assessment:

1) Identify the underlying physiological nature of the disorder;
2) Determine whether any short-range interventions can alleviate the dysphagia; and
3) Collaborate with the patient, family, and caregivers on the safest and most efficacious method of providing nutrition and hydration.

Difficulty with specific food consistencies provides the nurse with some assessment data, but may be misleading. Lesions and/or tumors that produce an obstruction generally produce dysphagia for solids first as opposed to liquids. However, patients with neuromuscular disorders may have dysphagia with both solids and liquids (Regnard, 2005).

Castell (1996) suggests that 80% of dysphagia can be diagnosed with a thorough history. Key questions

include the following: What type of food causes the symptom? Is the swallowing problem intermittent or progressive? Is heartburn present? (Cowely, Diebold, Coleman Gross & Hardin-Fanning, 2006).

The physical examination involves cognitive, neuromuscular, and respiratory assessment. Cognitive assessment includes interest in eating, ability to focus on and complete a meal, and ability to remember and follow directions for safe eating. Neuromuscular and respiratory assessment includes testing sensory and motor components of the cranial nerves, breath sounds, strength of cough, and ability to clear the throat (Cowely et al., 2006). Gag reflex is not a reflection of the patient's ability to swallow (Regnard, 2005). Evaluation of the patient's current medications is an important component of the assessment. Contributing medications to dysphagia are those that decrease saliva, decrease cognition, and decrease the strength of the muscles used in swallowing.

The prognosis of the patient will determine whether a professional swallowing evaluation merits consideration. If the patient's life expectancy is reasonably long and the patient is clearly in distress, a comprehensive evaluation performed by a speech-language pathologist with expertise in swallowing disorders may be indicated. A modified barium swallow is used to radiologically determine the phase of swallowing where the disturbance is occurring and thus identify potential interventions, as well as evaluating the compensatory mechanisms of the patient (Dahlin & Goldsmith, 2006).

Management

If the patient clearly has a very short prognosis (days), it may be determined by the patient, family, and caregivers that hydration and/or feeding are not warranted. If the patient has a longer prognosis, medically assisted feeding and hydration may be attempted. Regnard (2005) offers the following factors to help determine the appropriateness of interventions:

1) Rate of decline of the patient
2) Patient's opinion
3) Opinions of significant other and/or family
4) Opinions of formal caregivers
5) Feasibility/advantages/disadvantages of alternative feeding routes

Transnasal intubation, percutaneous endoscopic gastronomy or jejunostomy, or surgical gastrostomy or jejunostomy may be considered if the prognosis of the patient determines that these interventions will provide optimal palliation. Any surgical intervention is clearly undertaken with significant input from the patient and family and is determined by the goals of care.

Pharmacological interventions. If dry mouth and/or oral lesions are present and are exacerbating the dysphagia, pharmacological treatment is appropriate. The most common mucosal infection causing oral lesions is candidiasis. Antifungal medications such as nystatin, ketoconazole, miconazole, and fluconazole may be used in treatment (Dahlin & Goldsmith, 2006; Regnard, 2005).

Dry mouth (xerostomia) could be a result of prescribed medications, particularly anticholinergics and opiates. These medications may need to be continued if there are limited alternatives to treat other symptoms, making the dry mouth unavoidable. In that case, artificial saliva, such as Salagen or porcine mucin, may be used. Glycerin and lemon should be avoided because glycerin dehydrates the mucosa and the lemon affects the salivary glands (Regnard, 2005). A prokinetic agent such as ranitidine may be prescribed for poor esophageal motility. Prilosec and Zantac may be used in patients with gastroesophageal reflux disease.

Nonpharmacological interventions. After a thorough evaluation of the patient, and it has been determined that oral intake is "safe," the guiding principle of management is that a maximum amount of calories should be ingested for the least amount of effort (Dahlin & Goldsmith, 2001). If the degree of dysphagia is limited, simple positioning may be the primary intervention. Patients should be positioned in an upright, 90 degree angle, with the head tilted slightly forward and the chin tucked in to prevent food moving to the posterior oropharynx before it is properly chewed. If the patient is unable to hold his/her head independently, the caregiver can assist the patient in maintaining this position. If the older adult has had a past stroke, pocketing of food on the affected side of the mouth is a common problem. The patient, family, or caregiver can sweep the mouth with a finger after each bite to alleviate this problem.

In 2003, the American Dietetic Association published a monograph entitled the *National Dysphagia Diet: Standardization for Optimal Care (NDD)*. This diet aimed to establish standard terminology and practice applications of dietary texture modification in dysphagia management (McCullough, Pelletier, & Steele, 2003). Although the practice group that initiated this work consisted of speech-language pathologists (SLPs), dietitians, and a food scientist, there continues to be hesitation on the part of the American Speech-Language-Hearing Association to officially adopt this work. The hierarchy of the diet levels is provided here as an example of the different levels of semisolid/solid foods:

- Level I: Dysphagia-Pureed (homogenous, very cohesive, pudding-like, requiring very little chewing ability)
- Level II: Dysphagia-Mechanical Altered (cohesive, moist, semisolid foods, requiring some chewing)
- Level III: Dysphagia-Advanced (soft foods that require more chewing ability)
- Level IV: Regular (all foods allowed)

Liquid consistencies included spoon-thick, honey-like, nectar-like, and thin (McCullough et al., 2003). Viscosity ranges were prescribed for each level of liquid. Unfortunately there has not been research that validates the levels of foods or the liquid consistencies.

Simple dietary changes such as providing pureed or blenderized food may be appropriate. Patients with oropharyngeal dysphagia may require thickened liquids. There are a number of commercial products that are used in rehabilitation facilities (e.g., Thick-it) to address these issues; however, simple food starch can be used as effectively.

Family concerns and considerations. Positioning techniques that allow the patients to continue oral feeding can be easily explained and taught to the patients and/or their family. Dietary changes, such as using thickening agents, if appropriate, should be suggested to the family. Any interventions that can be taught to the family will increase their feeling of wanting to help the individual.

As described previously, eating is considered a social activity as much as it is a necessity of life. Society has conditioned us to believe that eating wholesome, healthy food will keep us well. As a family member sits by the bedside of their loved one and sees that oral intake is impossible due to dysphagia and potential aspiration, feelings of helplessness and anxiety may occur. Family may feel like they are neglecting their obligation to the person. For both the patient and the family, the act of eating is viewed as compatible with life; the inability to eat is a harbinger of death. Such factors influence decisions regarding feeding at the end of life.

Even if the decision to discontinue oral feeding and initiate alternate feeding methods is made, the decision is not easy. It is clearly difficult to make the initial decision to feed a patient or loved one "artificially," and more difficult if a decision is made to discontinue feedings. The patient and family must be fully aware of the risks and benefits of artificial nutrition and hydration. During this period, the support of the nurse to the patient and family is paramount. In addition to explaining what is occurring, the nurse must verbally support the decision of the patient and family even if he/she disagrees with it.

CONSTIPATION

Constipation is often seen in advanced disease related to bowel obstruction, adverse effects from medications, hypercalcemia, dehydration, and inadequate dietary intake (Esper & Heidrich, 2005). Similar to the concept of pain, constipation is often undertreated and is subjective (Economou, 2006). Dalal et al. (2006) define constipation as the infrequent and difficult passage of hard stool (p. 395). These authors also classify constipation as difficult to treat and to assess due to the wide variation in what is considered a normal stool. Typically, a normal stool is one that is passed three times a day to three times a week. Constipation is a common cause of morbidity in the palliative care setting and the numbers increase if the patient is treated with opioids. The incidence of constipation in older adults or ill persons may be 20 to 50% (Economou, 2006).

The "Rome criteria" offer other criteria to define constipation (Sykes, 2005). These criteria include the presence of two or more of the following symptoms for at least 3 months: straining at least 25% of the time; hard stools at least 25% of the time; incomplete evacuation at least 25% of the time; and two or fewer bowel movements per week (p. 483). However, it should be noted that these criteria may not be valid in a palliative care population.

Children are often symptomatic, and their symptoms increase with time, particularly within the terminal phase of illness (Collins, 2005). Constipation in children is distressing, but it often more distressing for the caregiver and not the child. Laxative use is generally not recommended in children. The research recommends a change in dietary intake, fluid intake, and mobility instead of laxative use (Collins, 2005). If these changes do not help in relieving the constipation, laxatives may be used, but the dosing is difficult to manage due to few resources for pediatric dosing.

Etiology

Bowel function includes three areas of control: small intestinal motility, colon motility, and defecation (Economou, 2006, p. 220). If any of these processes malfunction or is delayed, it can affect defecation. For example, the small intestine moves contents through in 1 to 2 hours, whereas the colon moves content much slower, in 2–3 days. Not eating properly or going without food, fluids, fiber, a decrease in activity, or even less privacy when using the bathroom, can all affect defecation and result in constipation. Other factors that affect bowel elimination are pain medications, cancer, obstructions, ascites, confusion, and diuretics (Economou, 2006). Dehydration is a common cause of constipation in the pediatric palliative care population (Dean et al., 2006). Figure 22.2 outlines some of the common causes of constipation.

Pharmacological-induced constipation may occur as a result of the use of opioids to control pain. Opioids affect the small bowel and the colon by binding with the receptors of the smooth muscle, thus affecting contractions and peristalsis of the bowel. Lengthening the time that the contents are in the colon causes more absorption of fluids and electrolytes, which in turn dries out and hardens the stool. However, there is some newer evidence, particularly associated with transdermal fentanyl use, indicating that constipation severity may differ among opioids (Economou, 2006).

Cimprich (cited in Economou, 2006, p. 220) describes three types of constipation:

1) Primary: generally caused by reduction of fluids and fiber intake, decrease in activity, and lack of privacy;

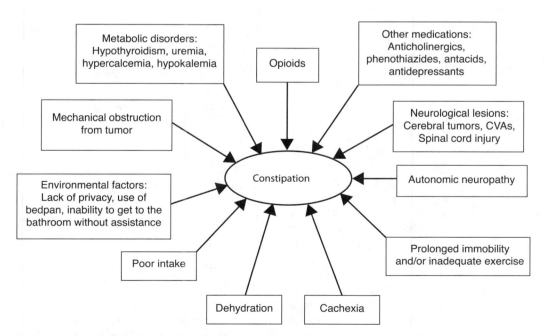

Figure 22.2 Common Causes of Constipation in Palliative Care
Reprinted from Dalal, S., Del Fabbro, E., & Bruera, E. (2006). Symptom control in palliative care – Part I: Oncology as a paradigmatic example. *Journal of Palliative Medicine*, 9(2), 391–408.

2) Secondary: related to the pathological changes the patient experiences; and

3) Iatrogenically induced: constipation related to pharmacological interventions.

Assessment

The patient receiving palliative care has multiple risk factors for constipation. The assessment begins with a history of bowel habits. Questions to ask include the following: Is the patient able to chew food? Does the patient wear dentures and do they fit properly? Is there a history of constipation prior to diagnosis? What has the patient's bowel pattern been prior to diagnosis? Has the patient been experiencing abdominal cramping, bloating, and nausea and vomiting? Does the bowel movement feel complete? Does the patient have an urge to defecate? Is the patient using laxatives and/or enemas? What pain medication does the patient take? Has there been a change in fluid intake or appetite?

Physical exam may reveal abdominal distention, diminished or hypoactive bowel sounds, and palpation of stool in the large intestine. Distention, however, may be associated with obesity, fluid, tumor, or gas. Percussion of the bowel may result in tympani over the abdomen, thus indicating gas in the bowel. Dullness is related to a solid mass, which could be intestinal fluid, tumor, or feces (Economou, 2006). Deep palpation may result in feeling a "sausage like" mass; however, determining if the mass is stool or a tumor is difficult with palpation alone. Sykes (2005) suggests that a fecal mass usually indents, if the patient can tolerate firm pressure, and may give a crepitus-like sensation because of entrapped gas. A fecal mass may also move over time. A digital rectal exam may reveal impaction, impaired sphincter tone, anal fissures, hemorrhoids, tumors, or even a rectocele (Economou, 2006).

Diagnostic tests. Diagnostic tests are used to confirm or determine the extent of bowel dysfunction due to constipation. The need for an extensive work-up in palliative care is rare, and should only be done when necessary to continue with comfort measures. If indicated, testing may include an upright and flat plate of the abdomen to determine air/fluid levels indicative of a partial or complete intestinal obstruction either due to tumor or secondary to fecal impaction. Radiographic examination, magnetic resonance imaging (MRI), or computerized tomography (CT), may also be appropriate to assess the abdomen. Laboratory data used to evaluate constipation may include blood urea nitrogen (BUN), as an elevation may signify dehydration, and blood glucose levels because elevation may indicate a diversion of fluids from the gastrointestinal tract to the kidneys with excess renal fluid loss (Bisanz, 1997).

Dalal and colleagues (2006) suggest the use of a constipation score based on findings from an abdominal X-ray. Scores from 0 to 3, based on the amount of feces, are obtained from each quadrant. "0" indicates no stool; 1 indicates less than 50%; a score of 2 indicates greater than 50%; and a score of 3 indicates full occupancy of the lumen with stool. Scores range from 0 to 12, and a score of 7 or greater indicates severe constipation.

Another tool developed in 1989, the Constipation Assessment Scale (CAS), has also proved to be useful in the assessment of constipation. The CAS has been tested for validity and reliability in measuring moderate to severe constipation (McMillan & Williams, 1989). The questionnaire is easy to complete.

Management

Prevention of constipation is an important strategy in providing palliative care. One method of prevention is the use of pharmacologic agents. Bulk-forming agents and stool-softening agents assist with normal peristaltic function (Beckwith, 2000). All patients beginning opioid therapy should be started on a laxative (Beckwith, 2000). Brunnhuber et al. (2008) suggest that senna and docusate be used, although they report that there is no supporting evidence for the use of docusate.

Each patient reacts differently to constipation and to the treatments used; thus individual assessments and interventions must be developed. Interventions that work for one patient may not work for the other. Increasing fluids is an initial intervention with a plan as simple as increasing fluids by as little as 100 ml. Care needs to be taken in increasing the fiber content. Fiber without increasing fluids absorbs what little fluid the patient may have available and contributes to more constipation (Economou, 2006).

Pharmacological interventions. Even with appropriate preventative strategies, most patients with advanced disease will require laxatives (Sykes, 2005). Laxatives are classified as follows by their action (Economou, 2006, pp. 224–225):

Bulk laxatives: provide bulk in the intestine, increase mass, and stimulate the bowel (usd in mild constipation);

Lubricant laxatives: lubricate the stool surface and soften the stool, leading to easier bowel movements;

Surfactant and/or detergent laxatives: increase absorption of water and fats which leads to a softer stool;

Osmotic laxatives: used more often in chronic constipation and in patients who have elevated ammonia levels, such as patients with hepatic failure. This form of laxatives has an osmotic effect not only on the small bowel but also the large intestine by increasing the colon volume in a short period of time;

Saline laxatives: increase gastric, pancreatic, and small intestine motility along with increasing the bowel secretions to form a stool;

Stimulant laxative: works on the colon increasing motility and inducing peristalsis.

Table 22.3 provides a listing of stool softeners and laxatives that may be used in palliative care.

Other approaches to management of constipation may include oral naloxone, an opioid antagonist, as a treatment for opioid-induced constipation. This treatment needs to be monitored closely because of inducing opioid withdrawal in the patient. Further work to classify its role is needed (Sykes, 2005).

Researchers are investigating the use of erythromycin in patients who do not respond to traditional treatments to relieve constipation. Erythromycin causes diarrhea in patients who use it as an antibiotic. Management of constipation with rhubarb or constituents of mulberry, which are similar to senna, can be used by patients who prefer not to use over-the-counter laxa-

tives. These patients need to be cautioned in purchasing herbal remedies and be aware of the side effects or the interaction with other medications they may be taking (Economou, 2006). Medications used in both the prevention and treatment in the pediatric palliative care population include docusate, lactulose, polyethylene glycol, and senna (Santucci & Mark, 2007).

It is a fine balance in managing the patient with constipation (Gullatte et al., 2005). The care provider does not want to have the stool so soft that it is leaking continuously. On the other hand, the patient should not suffer from cramping. The balance comes from adjusting the amount of stimulant and softener that the patient needs to have "normal" stools and not experience the side effects from the medication.

Family concerns and considerations. Family concerns regarding constipation can be addressed through education about the causes and methods of prevention and complications. Special attention should be given to the patient or family preferences with treatment modalities.

22.3 | Stool Softeners and Laxatives

TYPE	ACTION	COMMENTS
Lubricant softeners: ■ Mineral oil	Penetrates stool and prevents water absorption	Less palatable than some others
Bulk forming laxatives: ■ Methylcellulose ■ Psyllium ■ Polycarbophil	Resists bacterial breakdown, increasing bulk and shortening transit time	Must maintain fluid intake of 1½–2 L of fluid per day
Emollient/surfactant softeners: ■ Docusate sodium	Increases water penetration	Increased transit time caused by opioids negates action of these laxatives
Osmotic laxatives: ■ Lactulose ■ Sorbitol ■ Glycerin	Creates osmotic gradient in the intestine	Oral doses high enough to be effective may cause bloating, cramping, and diarrhea
Saline laxatives: ■ Magnesium citrate ■ Magnesium hydroxide ■ Sodium bisphosphate/sodium phosphate	Creates immediate osmotic gradient in the intestine	Oral forms are effective in ½–3 hours; enemas often effective within 15 minutes
Stimulant laxatives: ■ Senna ■ Cascara sagrada ■ Bisacodyl	Stimulates submucosal nerve plexus to increase motility	May cause cramping; often used in combination with a softener

Reprinted from Hickey, J. (1997). Rehabilitation of neuroscience patients. In J. Hickey (Ed.) The clinical practice of neurological and neurosurgical nursing (4th ed.) (pp. 255). Philadelphia: Lippincott.

Comfort level with routes of medication administration should be assessed, and if it is determined that rectal administration is not something the family is able to do, caregiver assistance should be provided.

Another concern includes dealing with patient privacy and the use of bedpan versus bedside commode. Privacy is a concern with patients in the hospital and in their homes. Often, if sharing a room in the hospital, using a bedside commode can be embarrassing to the patients and their families. The smell and noises during defecation make the patient unable to go. In the home or in the hospital, trying to use the bathroom in front of another person is generally not acceptable in the Western culture, which adds stress and anxiety to the patient. Typically, bedside commodes are more beneficial in constipation than bedpans.

BOWEL OBSTRUCTION

Bowel obstructions are common in patients with advanced abdominal or pelvic cancer, ovarian cancer, or primary bowel cancer (Chilton & Faull, 2005). An intestinal obstruction is occlusion of the lumen or absence of normal propulsion that produces elimination from the gastrointestinal tract (Economou, 2006; Sykes, 2005). Some disruption or dysfunction in motility leads to a mechanical obstruction but without occlusion of the intestinal lumen. This obstruction results in the accumulation of fluids and gas proximal to the obstruction (Economou, 2006). Abdominal distention occurs as a result of intestinal gas, ingested fluids, and digestive secretions. It then becomes a self-perpetuating phenomenon in that as distention increases, intestinal secretion of water and electrolytes increases (p. 233).

Etiology

Bowel obstructions can present in the clinical setting acutely or gradually and intermittently. Bowel obstructions can be due to constipation, adhesions, drugs, benign conditions, and/or progression of tumors in or around the intestine. A benign condition could be hypokalemia which can cause an ileus, or even hypercalcemia which can cause pseudo-obstructions (Chilton & Faull, 2005).

Signs and Symptoms

Signs and symptoms are based on the site of the obstruction (Ripamonti & Mercadante, 2005). If the obstruction is in the duodenum, the patient may experience severe vomiting with a large amount of undigested food. Pain or distention is not present, and the patient may have a succession splash present in the bowel soundsand there may be moderate to severe vomiting. Bowel sounds are hyperactive with borborygmi,

moderate distention is present, and there is pain in the upper and central abdomen that is colicky in nature. With an obstruction in the large intestine, vomiting is a late side effect, borborygmi bowel sounds and severe distention are present, and the colicky pain is in the central to lower abdomen (Economou, 2006). Diagnosis is suspected by clinical symptoms but is confirmed with abdominal radiography. Abdominal CT scan may be useful in evaluating the patient as well (Ripamonte & Mercadante, 2005).

Management

Lynch and Sarazine (2006) found that nurses can improve symptom management and quality of life for patients who are experiencing malignant bowel obstruction by frequent assessments and being aware that patients with intra-abdominal tumors are at the highest risk for bowel obstruction. Physical assessment that reveals dehydration, tachycardia, hypotension, and dry mucosa are all signs of impending bowel obstruction. Examination of the abdomen may reveal distention, pain, and varied bowel sounds. Malignant bowel obstruction is a pivotal point in the patient's illness, and nurses have an active role in helping the patient through the decisions that need to be made about aggressive treatment or a more palliative approach to the bowel obstruction.

In managing a bowel obstruction, it should be determined whether the obstruction is related to an underlying condition, such as a history of malignant bowel obstruction, a tumor, or an opioid-induced obstruction or opioid syndrome, which can occur with high doses of opioids. Medical management may offer good symptom control. Patients may live for surprisingly long periods, taking in small quantities of food and fluid, without the addition of nasogastric tubes or IV fluids (Chilton & Faull, 2005, p. 174).

Clearly, surgical intervention is the primary treatment for a complete bowel obstruction; however, in the palliative care population this is not typically an option. Self-expanding metallic stents may be used at the gastric outlet, proximal small bowel, and colon instead of surgery (Ripamonte & Mercadante, 2005). The use of continuous analgesics, antisecretory drugs, and/or antiemetics may be effective in controlling pain and N&V in patients who are not surgical candidates.

Octreotide may be an option in early management to prevent a full-blown obstruction. Its action slows the irregular and ineffective peristaltic movements of obstruction through reducing activity and balancing out the intestinal movement (Economou, 2006). Lynch and Sarazine (2006) note that once a bowel obstruction has occurred, the mean survival of the patient decreases to approximately 3 months in patients who are terminally ill. This sobering fact makes prevention of constipation and bowel obstruction important to not only the healthcare team but also to patients and their families.

DIARRHEA

Patients dealing with chronic and terminal illness may encounter bouts of diarrhea depending on the treatments they are receiving. Leakage of stool is common in bowel obstruction, and constipation can be overtreated causing the patient to experience diarrhea. Abrahm (1998) states that diarrhea may be associated with lactose intolerance post chemotherapy, bowel obstruction, fecal impaction, sphincter incompetence, chronic radiation enteritis, and infection.

Diarrhea is defined as the passage of frequent stools with urgency. Objectively, it is considered more than three unformed stools within a 24-hour period (Sykes, 2005). Although diarrhea occurs less frequently than constipation, patients report having acute episodes of diarrhea related to treatments, overeating of fruits and vegetables, and the use of antibiotics. Generally in episodes lasting a few days, the nurse needs to be aware of complications that can occur, along with the family being aware of the potential complications that could occur with diarrhea that is left untreated.

Etiology

There are four mechanisms of diarrhea: secretory, osmotic, hypermotile, and exudative (Economou, 2006). Secretory diarrhea persists with fasting and may be difficult to control because it occurs as a result of hypersecretion tumors, and endogenous mediators affecting electrolyte and water transport (Ratnaike, 1999). Enteral feedings, bleeding in the bowel, and lactose intolerance are all related to osmotic diarrhea. Increased intestinal motility in hypermotile diarrhea may result from overgrowth of bacteria, incomplete digestion of fat in the small intestine causing it to be expelled in

stool (steatorrhea), or due to chemotherapeutic agents. Prostaglandins are released secondary to inflammation of the intestinal mucosa in exudative diarrhea, which is commonly associated with radiation therapy (Economou, 2006).

Assessment

Initial assessment includes identification of the underlying cause of diarrhea. Specific description of previous bowel habits, along with current symptoms, may help to identify the etiology and appropriate management approaches. Fatty, pale yellow stool that is difficult to control may indicate an etiology of malabsorption. If diarrhea occurs after a period of constipation, fecal impaction should be suspected (Sykes, 2005). Diarrhea that persists beyond 2 to 3 days of fasting may be attributed to osmotic or secretory mechanisms (Economou, 2006).

Varying bowel habits make it difficult to assess diarrhea from the history alone. Typically, the complaint of loose, watery, or frequent stool is indicative of diarrhea. However, some patients describe diarrhea as frequent bowel movements even if consistency remains normal. The most accurate account of diarrhea is obtained from a 24–48-hour collection and measurement. Wadler (2001) states that this type of assessment in a clinical practice is rarely a reasonable method of assessment for diarrhea. Moreover, there is little need for this type of investigation in the palliative care setting. A more logical and objective approach to assessment would be the criteria for grading severity of diarrhea instituted by the National Cancer Institute (Table 22.4)

The most common cause of diarrhea in palliative care is an imbalance in laxative therapy (Sykes, 2005). It is also important to review all past, current, and new

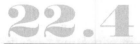 | National Cancer Institute Common Toxicity Criteria for Grading Severity of Diarrhea

	GRADE 1	GRADE 2	GRADE 3	GRADE 4
PATIENTS WITHOUT A COLOSTOMY	Increase of < 4 stools per day over pretreatment	Increase of 4 to 6 stools per day or nocturnal stools	Increase of ≥ 7 stools per day or incontinence or need for parenteral support for dehydration	Physiologic consequences requiring intensive care, or hemodynamic collapse
PATIENTS WITH A COLOSTOMY	Mild increase in loose, watery colostomy output compared with pretreatment	Moderate increase in loose, watery colostomy output compared with pretreatment, but not interfering with normal activity	Severe increase in loose, watery colostomy output compared to pretreatment and interfering with daily activity	Physiologic consequences requiring intensive care, or hemodynamic collapse

Adapted from Economou, D. C. (2006). Bowel management: Constipation, diarrhea, obstruction, and ascites. In B. R. Ferrell, & N. Coyle (Eds.), *Textbook of palliative nursing* (2nd ed.) (pp. 219–238). New York: Oxford University Press.

medications or treatment modalities. Metabolizing capabilities vary in older adults, but generally this population is more susceptible to medication side effects. Use of laxatives in conjunction with fiber intake should be explored. When antibiotics are in use or have been used recently and there is an onset of diarrhea, evaluation of stool culture for Clostridium difficile or other intestinal infections should be completed (Economou, 2006). Additionally, the patient who has abdominal or pelvic radiation may experience diarrhea up to 2–3 weeks after completion of treatment (Sykes, 2005).

Psychosocial effects of diarrhea, i.e., whether the diarrhea is acute or chronic in nature, must be evaluated. Physical activity may be limited due to dehydration and weakness if it has been an ongoing problem. The inability to control bowel movements can cause depression (Economou, 2006) and insecurity for the older adult. Diarrhea may prevent all patients from completing their activities of daily living and cause social isolation.

Management

Supportive care and medications are typically appropriate care for individuals in palliative care. The goal of treatment should be to eliminate the factors that led to the diarrhea, provide dietary intervention, and maintain fluid and electrolyte balance (Economou, 2006).

Pharmacological interventions. The antidiarrheal therapies of choice in palliative medicine are opioids, specifically loperamide (Imodium) (Benson et al., 2004). Initially 4 mg are given, followed by 2 mg after each loose stool up to a maximum of 16 mg per day. Codeine phosphate is also effective at a dose of 10–60 mg every 4 hours, and has the added benefit of being relatively inexpensive (Benson et al., 2004). Diphenoxylate (Lomotil) 2.5 mg may be given after each loose stool up to a maximum of 8 doses per day (Benson et al., 2004). However, if diarrhea is related to an infection, such as *Shigella* or C. *difficile*, the nonspecific diarrheal agents mentioned above will make it worse. Neither loperamide nor diphenoxylate is recommended in children under age 12 (Economou, 2006)

Secretory diarrhea, specifically with HIV patients, is often treated with octreotide (Sandostatin) 50–200 mg subcutaneously two to three times daily (Levy, 1991). Although costly, octreotide is a somatostatin analog with the ability to control even the most severe, intractable diarrhea (Doyle, 1994). Reduction of peristalsis and gastric secretions can also be accomplished using anticholinergics such as atropine and scopolamine (Economou, 2006).

Management of diarrhea also includes encouraging the patient and family to omit from the patient's dietary intake lactose-containing foods, spicy foods, and foods that contain high quantities of fat. Foods that can be added or that are tolerated well are potatoes, rice, and macaroni. Patients and families generally require instruction to not overuse the laxatives that they have been given to control constipation, which can lead to excessive diarrhea.

Nonpharmacological interventions. It is important to prevent dehydration and associated complications for patients who are at the end of their lives. Benson et al. (2004) recommend supportive care and rehydration by encouraging oral liquids rather than the parental route. A minimum of 2 quarts per day of un-carbonated fluids is suggested (Bisanz, 1997). Glucose and electrolyte concentrations (flat ginger ale; Pedialyte ½ strength) are most helpful in rehydration (Sykes, 2005). The adult patient and the family could also make their own electrolyte solution by mixing 1 tsp. salt, 1 tsp. baking soda, 1 tsp. corn syrup, 6 oz. of frozen orange juice concentrate, and 6 cups of water. This solution equals 47 kcal/cup with 515 mg Na+ and 164 mg K+ (Economou, 2006, p. 230)

Dietary modifications include clear liquids following the episodes of diarrhea, and then slowly adding simple or light carbohydrates such as toast or crackers in small amounts (Kemp, 1999). It is recommended to avoid milk until diarrhea subsides; then the patient can gradually add it back into the dietary intake (Economou, 2006). Dietary management is an important component in the management of diarrhea. As the episode resolves, proteins and fats can be added gradually into the diet (Economou, 2006).

Caregiver concerns. Incontinence of stool can be a disturbing problem for the older adult and the caregiver. Frequent checks and toileting should be made in cases where patients are confused or unable to express when they need to have a bowel movement. Nurses play a significant role in educating caregivers and family members regarding these issues. Care should be taken to prevent skin breakdown, perineal pain, and other complications with infection. Protective ointments and anesthetics can be applied for comfort measures, and should be initiated prior to skin problems developing (Kemp, 1999). It is also helpful to avoid toilet tissue after a few days of diarrhea; a spray bottle of warm-water washes or mild skin cleansers may be less painful.

If the etiology of diarrhea is infectious, appropriate contact precautions should be instituted. Patients, family members, and caregivers should be instructed on proper hand washing techniques to prevent the spread of infection. Disposable briefs should be discarded and tied in plastic bags to prevent contamination.

OTHER CONDITIONS

Hiccups

Hiccups, also referred to as singultus, are typically an intermittent phenomenon that is annoying, but benign. The exceptions are those termed persistent or protracted, lasting longer than 48 hours (Dahlin & Goldsmith, 2006). Chronic, reoccurring hiccups can negatively impact advanced conditions by causing dehydration, insomnia, or abdominal muscle pain (Kemp, 1999). Hiccups lasting longer than 1 month are considered intractable (Kolodzik & Eilers, 1991), and can produce exhaustion if sleep is disturbed for an extended period of time (Dahlin & Goldsmith, 2006). Intractable or persistent hiccups are more likely to be associated with anatomic or organic disorders, and may have complications including oxygen desaturation, ventilatory disturbances, and cardiac arrhythmias (Rousseau, 1995).

The characteristic sound of a hiccup is the result of a sudden, involuntary contraction of one or both sides of the diaphragm, causing a sudden inspiratory response and closure of the glottis (Regnard, 2005). The incidence of hiccups in patients with cancer is approximately 10–20% (Dahlin & Goldsmith, 2006). Protracted hiccups are 82% more common in men than women (Rousseau, 1995). Children are more at risk than adults.

Etiology. Although the exact pathophysiology is unknown, common causes of hiccups include esophagitis, gastric distension, diaphragmatic irritation, phrenic nerve irritation, uremia, infection, brain tumor, or possibly psychogenic in origin (Lewis, 1985). The numerous causes for hiccups are described with relationship to the type: benign, persistent (or chronic), or intractable. Some of the most common causes of benign hiccups are alcohol intake, emotional stress, sudden excitement, smoking, laughter, gastric distention from carbonated beverages, eating too fast, overeating, and indigestion. Gastric distention is thought to be the most common cause of hiccups in older adults with terminal cancer (Regnard, 2005).

Persistent and intractable hiccups can be classified according to causes from the central nervous system, diaphragmatic (phrenic nerve) irritation, vagal nerve irritation, drug or toxin induced, postoperative, infectious, metabolic, psychogenic, and idiopathic. Central nervous system causes of hiccups include structural lesions, neoplasms, hydrocephalus, encephalitis, epilepsy, vascular lesions, and head trauma (Kolodzik & Eilers, 1991). Diaphragmatic irritation may result from a hernia, organomegaly, esophageal neoplasms, pericarditis, intra-abdominal abscess, and gastroesophageal reflux disease. Irritation of any of the branches of the vagus nerve (auricular, meningeal, pharyngeal, laryngeal, thoracic, and abdominal) may cause intractable or persistent hiccups. Medications such as steroids, chemotherapy, dopamine antagonists, megesterol, methyldopa, nicotine, opioids, and muscle relaxants may contribute to hiccups (Dahlin & Goldsmith, 2006).

Recent evidence suggests that there is a correlation between partial pressure of carbon dioxide (pCO_2) and hiccups. A correlation was observed when there was an increase in pCO_2, resulting in a decrease in hiccups. It was also noted that a decrease in pCO_2 was related to increased frequency of hiccups (Dahlin & Goldsmith, 2006).

Assessment. In obtaining a thorough assessment of symptoms, it is necessary to enquire about duration, prior episodes, and the impact on activities of daily living. Interference with resting and sleeping may cause a patient to present with symptoms of exhaustion and fatigue. If the hiccups are so severe that eating habits are affected, and appetite is diminished, the patient may be dehydrated, thin, or weak, and even appear cachectic. The already predisposed terminally ill adult may exhibit signs of sepsis or metabolic dysfunction secondary to immunocompromised states. It may be necessary to perform lab work to determine whether metabolic dysfunction is the underlying cause of the hiccups (Dahlin & Goldsmith, 2006). These causes are often easily treated and may resolve persistent hiccups. In palliative care, a comprehensive work up to determine the etiology of persistent hiccups is appropriate only if the result assists in identifying an intervention. A chest X-ray may be necessary if mediastinal or pulmonary processes are suspected (Dahlin & Goldsmith, 2006).

Management: Pharmacological interventions. Pharmacological interventions are selected on the basis of the presumed etiology of hiccups. Hiccups are generally preventable or manageable by decreasing gastric distention and resolving esophageal irritation.

Gastric distention is likely to be the focus of an initial treatment approach in palliative care. Among the most effective medications for gastric distention are simethicone and metoclopramide (Reglan). Simethicone 15–30 ml is recommended before and after meals and at bedtime. Metoclopramide, 10–20 mg orally or intravenous, up to four times a day, can be used alone or in combination with simethicone. Metoclopramide works to decrease gastric distention by increasing overall gastric motility. This medication should be used with caution in older adults. Metoclopramide should not be used concurrently with peppermint water, another treatment, because of opposing effects on the lower esophageal sphincter (Regnard, 2005). Esophageal disorders or irritation can be treated with peppermint water, which decreases gastric distention that sometimes leads to esophageal irritation.

Chlorpromazine (Thorazine), 25–50 mg orally works by reticular formation and hiccup reflex suppression, and may be taken up to three times per day (Kolodzik & Eilers, 1991). It is an option for prophylactic treatment of intractable hiccups. However, due to side effects of CNS depression and postural hypotension, caution should be exercised in older adults (Regnard, 2005).

Haloperidol (Haldol) 3 mg orally at bedtime for acute treatment followed by regular dosing at bedtime for prophylactic management is successful in resistant cases of hiccups (Regnard, 2005). Anticonvulsants such as carbamazepine (Tegretol), phenytoin (Dilantin), and valproic acid (Depakote, Depakene), are most effective when the cause of hiccups is of a central origin (Kolodzik

EXHIBIT 22.4 NONPHARMACOLOGICAL INTERVENTIONS FOR HICCUPS

RESPIRATORY MEASURES
Breath holding
Rebreathing in a paper bag
Diaphragm compression
Ice application in mouth
Induction of sneeze or cough with spices or inhalants

NASAL AND PHARYNGEAL STIMULATION
Nose pressure
Stimulant inhalation
Tongue traction
Drinking from far side of glass
Swallowing sugar
Eating soft bread
Soft touch to palate with cotton-tipped applicator
Lemon wedge with bitters

MISCELLANEOUS VAGAL STIMULATION
Ocular compression
Digital rectal massage
Carotid massage

PSYCHIATRIC TREATMENTS
Behavioral techniques
Distraction

GASTRIC DISTENTION RELIEF
Fasting
Nasogastric tube to relieve abdominal distention
Lavage
Induction of vomiting

PHRENIC NERVE DISRUPTION
Anesthetic block

MISCELLANEOUS TREATMENTS
Bilateral radial artery compression
Peppermint water to relax lower esophagus
Acupuncture

Source: Economou, 2006, p. 214.

& Eilers, 1991). There has been an increase use of gabapentin in the treatment of hiccups as well (Dahlin & Goldsmith, 2006; Regnard, 2005). The skeletal muscle relaxant Baclofen 5–10 mg orally, twice a day, is also effective for treatment of hiccups (Regnard, 2005). In severe cases, phrenic nerve stimulation may be necessary to improve the patient's quality of life.

Nonpharmacological interventions. Determining the underlying cause of hiccups is the primary factor to consider when selecting treatment. This is not always possible, and, therefore, the healthcare provider should be most concerned with assessing the overall effect of persistent hiccups on the older adult's quality of life. The aggressiveness of treatment depends on how bothersome the hiccups are to the older adult.

Patients and family members often attempt nonpharmacological measures before they report hiccups to their healthcare provider. Pharyngeal stimulation by drinking a cold liquid or swallowing sugar granules or dry bread has been effective with acute attacks of hiccups (Baines, 1992). Increasing retention of carbon dioxide by re-breathing into a paper bag has also been suggested to relieve an acute attack (Baines, 1992).

Digital rectal massage and carotid massage can be used for vagal stimulation (Dahlin & Goldsmith, 2006). Gastric distention can be relieved by nasogastric tube insertion for decompression or lavage along with induction of vomiting (Lewis, 1985). Collaborative and complementary therapies that may be useful in the management of hiccups include chest physiotherapy to disrupt diaphragmatic spasms (Regnard, 2005).

Family concerns and considerations. Various treatment benefits, along with medication side effects, are necessary to make an informed decision regarding regimens they would like to pursue. When hiccups become overly disruptive to daily life, the patient may be willing to explore more aggressive therapies to obtain relief.

Ascites

Ascites can present either centrally, peripherally, or mixed. Central ascites is a condition which is related to a tumor that has invaded the hepatic parenchyma. This type of tumor generally compresses the portal venous and/or the lymphatic system (Economou, 2006). Peripheral ascites is associated with tumor cells from the parietal or visceral peritoneum. There is blockage within the peritoneal space resulting in a marked increase in macrophages causing ascites by increasing capillary permeability (Economou). The third type is called mixed-type and involves both central and peripheral ascites.

Etiology. In chronic liver disease, ascites initially begins as a result of portal hypertension that leads to increased

EXHIBIT 22.5 PHARMACOLOGICAL TREATMENT SUGGESTIONS FOR HICCUPS

AGENTS TO DECREASE GASTRIC DISTENTION
Simethicone 15–30 mL PO q 4h
Metoclopramide 10–20 mg PO/IV q 4–6 h (do not use with peppermint water)

MUSCLE RELAXANTS
Baclofen 5–10 mg PO q 6–12h up to 15–25 mg/d
Midazolam 5–10 mg

ANTICONVULSANTS
Gabapentin 300–600 mg PO TID
Carbamazepine 200 mg PO QD – TID, titrate up as needed
Valporic acid 5–15 mg/kg/d PO, then increase by 250 mg/week until hiccups stop

CORTICOSTERIODS
Dexamethazone 40 mg PO QD

DOPAMINE AGONISTS
Haloperidol 1–5 mg PO/SQ every 12 h
Chlorpromazine 5–50 mg PO/IM/IV q 6–8 h

CALCIUM CHANNEL BLOCKERS/ANTIARRYTHMICS
Phenytoin 200 mg IV, 300 mg PO QD
Nefopam 10 mg IV QD-QID
Lidocaine bolus 1 mg/kg/h IV, then 2 mg/min until hiccups terminated
Quinidine 200 mg PO
Nifedipine 10–80 mg PO QD

OTHER MEDICATIONS
Mephenesin 1000 mg PO QD
Amitriptyline 25–90 mg PO QD
Methyphenidate 5–20 mg IV, 5–20 mg QD
Sertaline 50 mg PO QD

Economou, 2006, p. 215.

levels of nitric oxide, vasodilatation, sodium retention, and decreased renal function (Runyon, 1998). Other disorders associated with the development of ascites due to increased hydrostatic pressure include congestive heart failure, constrictive pericarditis, and hepatic vein occlusion (Runyon et al., 1992). According to Runyon et al. (1992), tuberculosis, bacterial peritonitis, and malignant disease of the peritoneum may cause ascites, along with the decreased colloid osmotic pressure seen in malnutrition, nephritic syndrome with protein loss, and end-stage liver disease.

Signs and symptoms. Patients often complain of abdominal bloating and that their clothes no longer fit across their abdomen. Pain is often associated with the bloating and increase in abdominal girth. Some patients may have heartburn, nausea, and a decreased appetite. If the ascites is pronounced, dyspnea may be apparent (Economou, 2006).

Assessment. The most distressing physical symptom associated with ascites may be abdominal discomfort or pain caused by the distention. Additional complications, such as dehydration and electrolyte imbalances, should be assessed in the older adult. Depending on the extent of fluid present, scrotal edema may occur along with weakened hernial orifices (Heneghan & O'Grady, 2001). Physical mobility may be difficult, especially for patients who are weakened or fatigued secondary to the excess weight and pressure that occurs with ascites.

The most obvious sign of ascites is increased abdominal girth. Patients may complain of bloating, nausea, and decreased appetite. Secondary to increased abdominal pressure, there may be worsening of gastroesophageal reflux or heartburn (Economou, 2006), as well as dyspnea or orthopnea (Kichian & Bain, 2005). In the supine position, physical exam may reveal dullness on abdominal percussion in the dependent flank areas because ascitic fluid typically follows gravity. Tympany may be present towards the center of the abdomen. Shifting dullness can be assessed by turning the patient onto one side, noting the dullness of percussion shifts to the dependent side while tympany shifts to the top. There must be approximately 1500 ml of fluid present before dullness occurs with percussion of fluid alone (Cattau, Benjamin, Knuff, & Castell, 1982). A fluid wave test is performed by asking an assistant to press down firmly on the midline of the abdomen (to stop transmission of a wave through fat) while tapping on one flank of the abdomen. This causes an impulse to be transmitted through ascitic fluid that is felt on the other flank; if the impulse is easily palpable, it suggests the presence of ascites. Liver enlargement, tumor, or mass may also be palpable.

Management: Pharmacological interventions. The use of diuretics to decrease sodium reabsorption and urinary retention, along with increasing urinary excretion, are the primary interventions for ascites. As helpful as diuretic therapy may be, approximately 10–20% of patients will not respond to this intervention (Heneghan & O'Grady, 2001). The potassium-sparing agent spironolactone (100–400 mg per day) is the diuretic of choice for ascites; however, it may be necessary to initiate dieresis with a loop diuretic such as furosemide (40–80 mg per day) (Kichian & Bain, 2005). There is no theoretical reason to expect that sodium and fluid restriction or diuretics to be of use in peripheral ascites. A trial of diuretics and sodium restriction may be of use in individuals with mixed-type ascites (Kichian & Bain, 2005).

Ascitic fluid may be analyzed to determine whether albumin replacement is necessary, as well as bacterial infection of the fluid, which may require antibiotic therapy. Practitioner discretion and family requests will determine whether antibiotic therapy is appropriate, given the goals of care of older adults who are at the end of their lives. However, confusion and delirium are common when older adults have an infection, and may influence decisions regarding antibiotic therapy.

Administration of medications to help with dieresis and pain control is a primary intervention with ascites. Treatment for infection or albumin, and potassium replacement may also be warranted. Paracentesis or shunt placement and the prevention of infection may be important components of management. Nursing interventions include monitoring the client to promote symptomatic relief and educating the client and family about ascites and the interventions being performed.

If dieresis is accomplished with diuretic therapy, it is necessary to make elimination as easy as possible for the patient and caregivers. This may include urinary catheterization, if needed, to prevent injury if the patient has difficulty getting out of bed, or in patients who are confused and become agitated from urinary distention. Although it is important to monitor for signs and symptoms of urinary tract infection with catheterization, this intervention is usually considered a safe and effective treatment for patients at the end of life.

Nonpharmacological interventions. The goal of providing palliative care to a patient with ascites is to relieve discomfort. The poor prognosis related to ascites lends itself to palliation of symptoms without the expectation of altering patient survival rates. Management of ascites includes sodium restriction to prevent additional fluid retention. Ascites will be decreased from a dietary sodium restriction of 40–60 mcg/day, or 1–1.5 g of salt without the need for any further interventions (Heneghan & O'Grady, 2001). When there is marked sodium retention, restriction of sodium must be less than 20mcg per day, a goal that is not only difficult to achieve, but may so impair nutritional status (Heneghan & O'Grady, 2001).

Severe ascites requires therapeutic paracentesis alone or in combination with dietary sodium restriction. Symptomatic relief of malignant ascites may be accomplished with the removal of 5–10 L of fluid with each paracentesis (Kichian & Bain, 2005). Complete drainage of peritoneal fluid may actually cause an increase in pain (Doyle, 1994). Following removal of the ascitic fluid, diuretic therapy is often initiated to prevent re-accumulation. Heneghan and O'Grady (2001) cite conflicting data regarding albumin replacement to prevent electrolyte imbalance when large amounts of fluid are withdrawn. According to Doyle (1994), albumin replacement is rarely justified in palliative care and should be discussed with the patient and family.

Refractory ascites occurs when repeated attempts to restrict sodium and diuretic therapy are both unable to prevent reoccurrence of ascitic fluid. If drainage is frequently required or there is increased discomfort for the client, placement of a shunt may be warranted. Peritoneovenous shunting provides benefit for 3–4 weeks; however, insertion has high mortality rates (Doyle, 1994). Candidates for shunting include those with abdominal

scars preventing serial paracentesis, and limited access or distance from a physician able or willing to perform serial paracentesis (Heneghan & O'Grady, 2001).

Comprehensive nursing assessment is essential to identify any complications that may occur with ascitic fluid accumulation. The nurse should observe for signs and symptoms of infection or peritonitis. Monitor the patient for increased shortness of breath or dyspnea and notify the physician if positioning does not relieve dyspnea. With dieresis, older patients are also at increased risk of dehydration leading to poor nutritional status and skin breakdown. Frequent repositioning is necessary not only for comfort but also for prevention of pressure ulcers.

Collaborative care may include dietary consultation to aid with planning meals for sodium restriction, and it may also involve frequent discussions with the physician or palliative care team to accomplish symptom relief from refractory ascites

Family concerns and considerations. Caregiver(s) will need instruction on positioning. It may be difficult to achieve a comfortable position in which the pressure of ascitic fluid does not inhibit or make breathing more strenuous. Explain the importance of sodium restriction and provide education regarding how this may help to prevent fluid retention and the associated discomfort. If refractory ascites is present, the risks and benefits of paracentesis should be clearly discussed to ensure that informed decisions about management could be made. It is important that patients and caregivers understand the risks associated with re-accumulation of fluid.

Xerostomia

Xerostomia is a subjective feeling of dry mouth which may or may not be accompanied by decreased saliva flow (DeConno, Sbanotto, Ripamonti, & Ventabridda, 2005). Xerostomia receives little attention, so prevalence is unable to be estimated.

Etiology. A reduction in the salivary production by the parotid, submaxillary, and sublingual glands may occur as a result of radiotherapy, oral surgery, medication side effects, gland obstruction, brain neoplasms, and hypothyroidism. Typical saliva production a day is 1000–1500 ml (DeConno et al., 2005). Saliva functions as a protective mechanism against infection, dental caries, and extreme temperatures in food.

Medications may contribute to xerostomia either indirectly or directly. These may include anticholinergics, anticonvulsants, antidepressants, antihistamines, corticosteroids, opioid analgesics, nonsteroidal anti-inflammatory agents, calcium channel blockers, beta blockers, and diuretics. Indirect effects involve impairment of taste sensation, leading to a decreased secretion of saliva. Some polypharmacy is common for older adults, especially those that are terminally ill. It is likely that combinations of drugs increase the incidence of xerostomia. A study by Davies, Broadley, and Beighton (2001) revealed a positive correlation between the total number of drugs taken and the presence of xerostomia in older adults with cancer.

Oral cancer, chemotherapy or radiotherapy, stomatitis, and oral infections may cause actual erosion of buccal mucosa. Local causes of dehydration such as oxygen therapy or mouth breathing, may contribute to xerostomia, along with the systemic causes of diarrhea, vomiting, anorexia, and polyuria (Dahlin & Goldsmith, 2006).

Signs and symptoms. Xerostomia is generally considered a subjective sensation; the severity is related to the amount of discomfort or pain that the individual experiences. Symptoms that are most frequently voiced in relation to dry mouth include diminished taste (dysgeusia), difficulty chewing foods without fluids (dysmasesis), dysphagia, needing fluids during the night, and a burning sensation on the tongue (DeConno et al., 2005).

Assessment. When assessing the oral cavity, inspect the oral mucosa for dryness, cracking, fissures, pale color, ulcerations, and gingivitis (Cooke, Admedzel, & Mayberry, 1996). Remove the dentures to inspect for problems that may otherwise be hidden. Structures that should be evaluated on routine examination are the hard and soft palate, pharynx, buccal areas, floor of the mouth, gum and tooth or denture condition, as well as upper, lower, and sides of the tongue. Also evaluate the lips for dry, cracked areas or lesions along with the degree of mouth opening.

Xerostomia can be determined at the bedside utilizing a quick and easy test. Following inspection of the oral cavity, attempt to stick the tongue blade on the top surface of the tongue. If it remains in place, xerostomia is present (Cooke et al., 1996). Another test that can be attempted is the cracker/biscuit test. This involves asking the patient to eat a dry cracker or biscuit, and if they are unable to do so, xerostomia is present (Sreebny &

Valdini, 1987). It may difficult to perform this second type of test if patients are limited in their ability to tolerate oral intake. Caution should be used to prevent aspiration.

The Oncology Nursing Society has a documentation tool for xerostomia and nursing care that assists in making the assessment and documentation standardized. A zero is recorded for no evidence of dry mouth; 1 = mild dryness, slightly thickened saliva, minimal taste change; 2 = moderate dryness, thick and sticky saliva, markedly altered taste change; 3 = complete mouth dryness; and 4 = actual salivary necrosis (Oncology Nursing Society, 2002).

Management: Managing xerostomia is not based on prevention but on interventions intended to alleviate this complication from disease. A stepped approach is used in the management of xerostomia.

Pharmacological interventions. Implications for reversing symptoms accompanying xerostomia include discontinuing or changing medication regimens, when possible. In palliative care, this is rarely a viable option when the medications are utilized for pain and symptom management. There are more than 250 medications that can cause xerostomia (Jackson & Chambers, 2000). The healthcare team does have ways to increase secretions, increase salivation with medications, and the use of artificial saliva (see Table 22.5).

Nonharmacological interventions. Independent interventions for prevention of xerostomia include maintenance of good oral hygiene as frequently as every 2 hours, and humidifying the air especially when oxygen is being administered (Ventafridda et al., 1998). Gustatory stimulation can be enhanced using peppermint water or sugarless gum. Unfortunately, the results from these interventions tend to be short lived (Cooke et al., 1996). Vitamin C and citric acids may be helpful, but have been found to cause a burning sensation, and are not recommended if oral lesions are present (Davies, 1997). Acupuncture as been suggested to be effective in management of various types of xerostomia. Evidence demonstrated that that treatments of twice-a-week treatments for 6 weeks increased saliva for up to 1 year (Dahlin & Goldsmith, 2006). Another study cited in Chilton and Faull (2005) found that the key to mouth care was related to frequency of use and not so much the specific product that was used.

EXHIBIT 22.6 STEPWISE PROCESS FOR MANAGING XEROSTOMIA

- Treat underlying infections
- Review and alter current medications
- Stimulate salivary flow
- Replace lost secretions with saliva substitutes
- Protect teeth
- Rehydrate
- Modify diet

Source: Dahlin & Goldsmith, 2006, p. 210.

Case Study conclusion: Following a chest CT, Dr. Jameson requested the family to visit with him. Dr. Jameson informed Mrs. Adams and her family that the cancer had spread to the spleen. Before

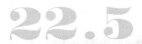

22.5 | Review of Interventions for Xerostomia

INTERVENTION	ROLE/EFFECT	BENEFIT	SIDE EFFECT
NONPHARMACOLOGICAL			
Peppermint water	Mucous saliva	Inexpensive	Interacts with metoclopramide
Vitamin C	Chemical reduction	Inexpensive, reduces viscosity	Can irritate mouth if sores present
Citric acid/sweets	Mucous saliva	Inexpensive	Can irritate like vitamin C, sweets can cause caries
Chewing gum, mints	Watery saliva	Inexpensive, more volume, only dentate	No side effects if sugarless, otherwise can promote caries
Acupuncture	Increased production	Noninvasive	Expensive
PHARMACOLOGICAL			
Pilocarpine	Nonselective muscarinic	Increases saliva production	Sweating, nausea, flushing, and cramping
Bethanechol	M-3 muscarinic	Relieves side effect of TCA	
Methacholine	Parasympathetic	Increases saliva	Hypotension
Cevimeline	M-1 & M-3 muscarinic agonist	Increases saliva	Fewer effects than pilocarpine
Yohimbine	Blocks alpha-2 adrenoreceptors	Increases saliva	Drowsiness, confusion, atrial fibrillation

Adapted from Nieuw Amerongen (2003).

the physician could say anything else, Mrs. Adams interrupted him and said, "I have lived a good life and I'm ready to go when God calls me home. What can be done to make me comfortable until that time comes?" Dr. Jameson explained to Mrs. Adams and her family the options of IV fluids, pain medications, and medications for nausea. Mrs. Adams requested time to be by herself. She called to speak with the physician 30 minutes later. She informed the physician that she wanted to be made comfortable, needed a DNR order in place, and to remove the nasogastric tube. The family called the remainder of her family and friends, and Mrs. Adams died 72 hours later in her sleep.

CONCLUSION

GI symptoms are a common symptom in terminal illness. Many patients have described the constant nausea, vomiting, and diarrhea as more disabling and disturbing than pain. GI symptoms affect patient's activities of daily living and influence their quality of life.

As in all palliative care, ongoing assessment of the patient is necessary to determine which interventions are working and which ones need modification. Interventions include pharmacological, nonpharmacological, and complementary therapies. Patient and family input remains the most important data to be considered in the assessment, planning, implementation, and evaluation of interventions in palliative care.

EVIDENCE-BASED PRACTICE

Miles, C. L., Fellowes, D., Goodman, M. L., & Wilkinson, S. (2006). Laxatives for the management of constipation in palliative care patients. Cochrane Database of Systematic Reviews 2006, Issue 4, Art. No.: CD0003448. DOI: 10.1002/14651858.

This Cochrane Systematic Review reviewed four randomized clinical trials (RCTs) involving 280 subjects to determine the effectiveness of laxative administration and the differential efficacy of the products used in the treatment of constipation in the palliative care population. Although a common symptom in palliative care, there were minimal RCTs to review on this subject. The four trials all included lactulose, senna, danthron combined with poloxamer, misrakasneham (an herbal preparation), and magnesium hydroxide combined with liquid paraffin (milpar). All four trials evaluated included number and frequency of bowel movements and relative ease of defecation in determining laxative efficacy.

Results indicated that all of the laxatives had limited efficacy, and a number of subjects required "rescue laxatives" in the studies. There was no evidence to support the use of one laxative over another one or a combination of laxatives being more effective. This review supported previous systematic reviews in their results

Nursing implications. Each patient in a palliative care setting is unique in their symptoms and the treatment of those symptoms. What treatment might be effective in the pharmacologically induced constipation of one patient (as an example) may not be effective in a similar patient. There continues to be a lack of evidence to support the treatment of constipation in the palliative care population.

REFERENCES

Abrahm, J. L., (1998). Promoting symptom control in palliative care. *Seminars in Oncology Nursing, 14*(2), 95–109.

Baines, M. J. (1992). Symptom management and palliative care. In J. G. Evans & T. F. Williams (Eds.). *Oxford textbook of geriatric medicine* (pp. 685–696). New York: Oxford University Press.

Barbour, L. (1999). Dysphagia. In C. Yarbro, M. Frogge, & M. Goodman (Eds.). *Cancer symptom management* (2nd ed.) (pp. 209–227) Sudbury, MA: Jones & Bartlett.

Beckwith, M. C. (2000). Constipation in palliative care patients. In A. G. Lipman, K. C. Jackson, & L. S. Tyler (Eds.), *Evidence based symptom control in palliative care* (pp. 147–158). New York: Haworth Press.

Benson, A. B., Ajani, J. A., Catalano, R. B., Engelking, C., Kornblau, S. M., Martenson, J. A., et al. (2004). Recommended guidelines for the treatment of cancer treatment-induced diarrhea. *Journal of Clinical Oncology, 22*(14), 2918–2926.

Bisanz, A. (1997). Managing bowel elimination problems in patients with cancer. *Oncology Nursing Forum, 24*(4), 679–686.

Brunnhuber, K., Nash, S. T., Meier, D. E., Weissman, D. E., & Woodcock, J. (2008). *Putting evidence into practice: Palliative care.* BMJ Publishing Group

Castell, D. O. (1996). The efficient dysphagia work-up. *Emergency Medicine,* 73–77.

Cattau, E. L., Benjamin, S. B., Knuff, T. E., & Castell, D. O. (1982). The accuracy of the physical exam in the diagnosis of suspected ascites. *The Journal of the American Medical Association, 247*(8), 1164–1167.

Chilton, A., & Faull, C. (2005). The management of gastrointestinal symptoms and advanced liver disease. In C. Faull, Y. Carter, & L. Daniels (Eds.), *Handbook of palliative care* (2nd ed., pp. 150–184). Malden, MA: Blackwell Publishing.

Collins, J. J. (2005). Symptom control in life-threatening illness. In D. Doyle, G. Hanks, N. Cherney & K. Calman (Eds.). *Oxford textbook of palliative medicine* (3rd ed., pp. 789–798). New York: Oxford University Press.

Cooke, C., Admedzel, S., & Mayberry, J. (1996). Xerostomia—A review. *Palliative Medicine, 10,* 284–292.

Cowely, J., Diebold, C., Coleman Gross, J., & Hardin-Fanning, F. (2006). Management of common problems. In K. L. Mauk (Ed.) *Gerontological nursing: Competencies for care* (pp. 475–560) Sudbury, MA: Jones & Bartlett.

Dahlin, C. M., & Goldsmith, T. (2006). Dysphagia, dry mouth, and hiccups. In B. R. Ferrell & N. Coyle (Eds.), *Textbook of palliative nursing* (2nd ed., pp. 195–218). Oxford, UK: Oxford University Press.

Dalal, S., Del Fabbro, E., & Bruera, E. (2006). Symptom control in palliative care – Part I: Oncology as a paradigmatic example. *Journal of Palliative Medicine, 9*(2), 391–408.

Davies, A. (1997). The management of xerostomia: A review. *European Journal of Cancer Care, 6,* 209–214.

Davies, A. N., Broadley, K., & Beighton, D. (2001). Xerostomia in patients with advanced cancer. *Journal of Pain and Symptom Management, 22*(4), 820–825.

Dean, M., Harris, J., Regnard, C., & Hockley, J. (2006). *Symptom relief in palliative care.* Oxford: Radcliffe Publishing.

DeConno, F., Sbanotto, A., Ripamonti, C., & Ventafridda, V. (2005). Mouth care. In D. Doyle, G. Hanks, N. Cherny, & K. Calman (Eds.) *Oxford textbook of palliative medicine* (3rd ed., pp. 673–87). Oxford: Oxford University Press.

Doyle, D. (1994). *Domiciliary palliative care: A handbook for family doctors and community nurses* (Oxford General Practice Series 27). New York: Oxford University Press.

Easton, K. (1999). *Gerontological rehabilitation nursing.* Philadelphia: Saunders

Economou, D. C. (2006). Bowel management: Constipation, diarrhea, obstruction, and ascites. In B. R. Ferrell & N. Coyle (Eds.). *Textbook of palliative nursing* (2nd ed.). (pp. 219–238). New York: Oxford University Press.

Enck, R. C. (2002). *The medical care of terminally ill patients* (2nd ed.). Baltimore: Johns Hopkins University Press.

Esper, P., & Heidrich, D. (2005). Symptom clusters in advanced illness. *Seminars in Oncology Nursing, 21*(1), 20–28.

Ezzone, S., Baker, C., Rosselet, R., & Terepka, E. (1998). Music as an adjunct to antiemetic therapy. *Oncology Nursing Forum, 10,* 27–35.

Germain, M., & Cohen, L. M. (2005). Nephrology. In K. K. Kuebler, M. P. Davis, & C. D. Moore (Eds.), *Palliative practices: An interdisciplinary approach* (pp. 181–196). St. Louis: Elsevier Mosby.

Gridelli, C., (2004). Same old story? Do we need to modify our supportive care treatment of elderly cancer patients? Focus on antiemetics. *Drugs and Aging, 21*(13), 825–832.

Gullatte, M. M., Kaplow, R. & Heidrich, D. E. (2005). Oncology. In K. K. Kuebler, M. P. Davis, & C. D. Moore (Eds.), *Palliative practices: An interdisciplinary approach* (pp. 197–245). St. Louis: Mosby Elsevier.

Hellsten, M., & Kane, J. (2006). Pediatric palliative care. In B. Ferrell & N. Coyle (Eds.), *Textbook of palliative nursing* (2nd ed., pp. 895–908). New York: Oxford University Press.

Heneghan, M. A., & O'Grady, J. G. (2001). Palliative care in liver disease. In J. M. Addington-Hall & I. J. Higginson (Eds.). *Palliative care for non-cancer patients* (pp. 82–103). New York: Oxford University Press.

Hickey, J. (1997). Rehabilitation of neuroscience patients. In J. Hickey (Ed.). *The clinical practice of neurological and neurosurgical nursing* (4th ed., pp. 255). Philadelphia: Lippincott.

Hinds, P. S., Oakes, L. L., Hicks, J., & Anghelescu, D. L. (2005). End-of-life care for children and adolescents. *Seminars in Oncology Nursing, 21*(1), 53–62.

Jackson, K. C., & Chambers, M. S. (2000). Oral mucosal problems in palliative care populations. In A. G. Lipman, K. C. Jackson & L. S. Tyler (Eds.), *Evidence based symptom control in palliative care* (pp. 143–161). *New York: Haworth Press.*

Kemp, C. (1999). *Terminal illness: A guide to nursing care* (2nd ed.). New York: Lippincott.

Kichian, K., & Bain, V. G. (2005). Jaundice, ascites, and hepatic encephalopathy. In D. Doyle, G. Hanks, N. Cherny, & K. Calman (Eds.), *Oxford textbook of palliative medicine* (3rd ed., pp. 507–520). Oxford: Oxford University Press.

King, C. (2006). Nausea and vomiting. In B. Ferrell & N. Coyle (Eds.), *Textbook of palliative nursing* (pp. 177–194). Oxford, UK: Oxford University Press.

King, C. (1997). Nonpharmacologic management of chemotherapy-induced nausea and vomiting. *Oncology Nursing Forum, 24* (Suppl.), 41–48.

Kolodzik, P. W., & Eilers, M. A. (1991). Hiccups (singultus): Review and approach to management. *Annals of Emergency Medicine, 20*(5), pp. 565–573.

Langmead, L., & Rampton, D. S. (2001). Review article: Herbal treatment in gastrointestinal and liver disease – benefits and dangers. *Alimentary Pharmacology Therapy, 15*, 1239–1252.

Levy, M. H. (1991). Constipation and diarrhea in cancer patients. *Cancer Bulletin, 43*, 412–422.

Lewis, J. H. (1985). Hiccups: Causes and cures. *Journal of Clinical Gastroenterology, 12*(6), 539–552.

Lynch, B., & Sarazine, J., (2006). A guide to understanding malignant bowel obstruction. *International Journal of Palliative Nursing, 12*(4), 164–166, 168–171.

Mannix, K. (2005). Palliation of nausea and vomiting. In D. Doyle, G. Hanks, N. Cherny, & K. Calman (Eds.), *Oxford textbook of palliative medicine* (3rd ed., pp. 459–468). Oxford UK: Oxford University Press.

McCullough, G., Pelletier, C., & Steele, C. (2003). National dysphagia diet: What to swallow? *The ASHA Leader* (November), 16, 27.

McMillan, S. C., & Williams, F. A. (1989). Validity and reliability of the constipation assessment scale. *Cancer Nursing, 12*(3), 183–188.

Nieuw Amerongen, A.V., & Veerman, E.C. Current therapies for xerostomia and salivary gland hypofunction associated with cancer therapies. *Support Care Cancer*, 11, 226–231.

Oncology Nursing Society. (2002). *Radiation therapy patient care record: A tool for documenting nursing care*. Pittsburgh, PA: Oncology Nursing Society Press.

Plahuta, J. M., & Hamrick-King, J. (2006). Review of the aging of the physiological systems. In K. L. Mauk (Ed.), *Gerontological nursing: Competencies for care* (pp. 143–264). Sudbury, MA: Jones & Bartlett.

Ratnaike, R. N. (1999). *Diarrhoea and constipation in geriatric practice*. New York: Cambridge University Press.

Regnard, C. (2005). Dysphagia, dyspepsia, and hiccup. In D. Doyle. G. Hanks, N. Cherny & K. Calman (Eds.), *Oxford textbook of palliative medicine* (3rd ed., pp. 468–483). Oxford UK: Oxford University Press.

Rhodes, V. (1997). Criteria for assessment of nausea, vomiting and retching. *Oncology Nursing Forum, 24*, 13–19.

Rhodes, V., & McDaniel, R. (2001). Nausea, vomiting and retching: Complex problems in palliative care. *CA—A Cancer Journal for Clinicians, 51*(4), 232–248.

Rhodes, V., & McDaniel, R. (1997). Measuring nausea, vomiting and retching. In M. Frank-Stromberg & S. Olsen (Eds.), *Instruments for clinical health-care research* (2nd ed., pp. 507–517). Sudbury, MA: Jones & Bartlett.

Ripamonti, C., & Mercadante, S. (2005). Pathophysiology and management of malignant bowel obstruction. In D. Doyle, G. Hanks, N. Cherny & K. Calman (Eds.), *Oxford textbook of palliative medicine* (3rd ed., pp. 496–507). Oxford: Oxford University Press.

Rousseau, P. (1995). Hiccups. *Southern Medical Journal, 88*, 175–181.

Rudd, N., & Worlding, J. (2005). The management of people with advanced head and neck cancers. In C. Faull, Y. Carter, & R. Woof (Eds.), *Handbook of palliative care* (2nd ed., pp. 240–255). Malden, MA: Blackwell Science

Runyon, B. A. (1998). Ascites and spontaneous bacterial peritonitis. In M. Feldman, B. F. Scharschmidt, & M. H. Sleisenger (Eds.), *Sleisenger and Fordtran's gastrointestinal and liver disease: Pathophysiology, diagnosis, management*, Vol. 2 (6th ed., pp. 1310–1333). Philadelphia: Saunders.

Runyon, B. A., Montano, A. A., Akrivadis, E. A., Antillon, M. R., Irving, M. A., & McHutchison, J. G., et al. (1992). The serum-ascites gradient is superior to the exudate-transudate concept in the differential diagnosis of ascites. *Annals of Internal Medicine, 117*(3), 215.

Santucci, G., & Mack, J. W. (2007). Common gastrointestinal symptoms in pediatric palliative care: Nausea, vomiting, constipation, anorexia and cachexia. *Pediatric Clinics of North America, 545*, 673–689.

Saxby, C., Ackroyd, R., Callin, S., Mayland, C., & Kite, S. (2007). How should we measure emesis in palliative care? *Palliative Medicine, 21*, 369–383.

Sibson,K., Craig, F., & Goldman, A. (2005). Palliative care for children. In C. Faull, Y. Carter, & L. Daniels (Eds.). *Handbook of palliative care* (2nd ed., pp. 295–316). Malden, MA: Blackwell Publishing.

Sreebny, L. M., & Valdini, A. (1987). Xerostomia: A neglected symptom. *Archives of Internal Medicine, 147*, 1333–1337.

Sykes, N. P. (2005). Constipation and diarrhoea. In D. Doyle, G. W. Hanks, N. Cherney, & K. Calman (Eds.). *Oxford textbook of palliative medicine* (3rd ed., pp. 483–496). Oxford, UK: Oxford University Press.

Thompson, E., & Zollman, C. (2005). Complementary approaches to palliative care. In C. Faull, Y. Carter, & L. Daniels (Eds.), *Handbook of palliative care* (2nd ed., pp. 437–461) Malden, MA: Blackwell Publishing.

Timiras, P. (1994). Aging of the gastrointestinal tract and liver. In P. Timiras (Ed.). *Physiological basis of aging and geriatrics* (pp. 247–257). Boca Raton, FL: CRC Press

Tyler, L. S. (2000). Nausea and vomiting in palliative care. In A. G. Lipman, K. C. Jackson, & L. S. Tyler (Eds.). *Evidence based symptom control in palliative care* (pp. 163–181). New York: Haworth Press.

Vickers, A. J. (1996). Can acupuncture have specific effects on health? A systematic literature review of acupuncture anti-emesis trials. *Journal of the Royal Society of Medicine, 89*(6), 303–311.

Wadler, S. (2001). Treatment guidelines for chemotherapy-induced diarrhea. *Oncology Special Edition, 4,* 81–84.

Wickham, R. (1999). Nausea and vomiting. In C. Yarbro, M. Frogge, & M. Goodman (Eds.) *Cancer symptom management* (2nd ed., pp. 228–253). Sudbury, MA: Jones & Bartlett.

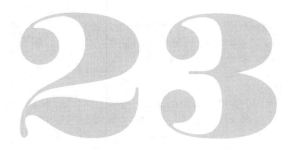

Fatigue and Weakness Evaluation and Management

Marianne Matzo
Patsy R. Smith
Deborah Witt Sherman

Key Points

- Fatigue in older adults may be underreported in patients who believe that fatigue is a normal part of aging.
- COPD-related fatigue is complicated by interactions with other symptoms and is manageable through planned rest periods and treatment of related symptoms and comorbid conditions.
- Patients may need to be evaluated and treated for symptoms of fatigue, including anxiety and depression before treatment begins.
- Participation in an exercise program that includes a class or short exercise sessions in the home can be effective in reducing symptoms of pain, depression, and fatigue associated with rheumatoid arthritis as has been found in other chronic conditions.
- Quality of life is an important goal of care and an outcome variable in palliative care; it is a priority of patients, families, and health professionals.
- Evaluation of fatigue at the end of life must be targeted to those causes which, if treated, have the best likelihood of improving the quality of life for the patient: anemia, polypharmacy, cognitive function, anxiety and depression, complications of therapies, nutrition, and infection.
- A daily fatigue journal is an important communication tool between the patient and the practitioner that supports counseling for symptom management.

Case Study: Ms. Seigal is a 72-year-old woman with a history of bilateral mastectomy and a four cycle course of chemotherapy followed by radiation secondary to metastatic breast cancer. Her most recent diagnosis of heart failure is a complication of cancer treatment though she is a 5-year survivor of the treatment. She realizes that cure is not the intent of her current treatment regimen, but rather to prevent further disease progression and promote her quality of life. Members of the palliative care team followed Ms. Seigal for 2 years after treatment by the Cancer Center. She is now being cared for by a hospice team who is concerned with her physical, emotional, social, and spiritual health. The hospice nurse assesses her symptoms, including fatigue. Ms. Seigal reports "feeling exhausted with little or no physical or emotional energy for self-care or housekeeping." She is a single woman who owns an advertising agency, has assigned the day-to-day operation to a business partner, but still feels the pressures of supervising and overseeing her business. She emphasizes the emotional investment she has in the business she built from scratch. Ms. Seigal indicates that she feels the same sense of overwhelming tiredness and fitful restlessness at night that she felt during and after her cancer treatment. Although she eventually regained her strength, she described this feeling as worse in that she "can't seem to get going in the morning, it takes the complete breath out of me just to get my clothes on." She also complained of "difficulty thinking straight and concentrating." She has no immediate family but does have "some help from the folks at the community church."

The hospice nurse requests the assistance of the palliative care nurse practitioner, who recognizes the cumulative effects of surviving cancer surgery, chemotherapy and radiation, and the emotional and existential burdens of diagnosis with another life-threatening illness. The hospice nurse and the palliative care nurse practitioner agree that a complete history, review of systems, physical examination, and laboratory data are warranted to discover the underlying, multidimensional aspects of the fatigue and weakness described by Ms. Seigal, and the changes that have occurred within the last 6 months. They also recognize that depression and fatigue can be correlated in patients with complex chronic medical conditions, specifically heart failure, and agree to an assessment of Ms. Seigal's emotional well-being.

Ms. Seigal has experienced the physical and emotional trauma of surgery, anesthesia, and anesthetics, as well as fatigue induced by chemotherapy. She became neutropenic and anemic during the chemotherapy regimen and was treated with Procrit and Neulasta. Her fatigue was exacerbated by radiation therapy 3 years ago, which nearly 100% of patients experience toward the end of the cycle and from which few, if any, experience full restoration of energy. Given the extensive history of Ms. Seigal, and the various etiologies of fatigue and weakness, the hospice nurse and the palliative care nurse practitioner form a team in accordance with Ms. Seigal's goals and preferences, the extent of her chronic heart failure, and co-existing symptoms, to develop a comprehensive plan of care that conforms to recommended competencies for end-of-life nursing care and guidelines for quality palliative care (National Consensus Project for Quality Palliative Care, 2009). The goals of care will be to focus on evaluation and management of symptoms that exacerbate fatigue, preventing fatigue by managing the activities that increase fatigue, and restoring energy with ultimate improvement in her overall quality of life.

Introduction

Fatigue is one of the most common symptoms experienced by persons with cancer, chronic pain (Jakobs son, Hallberg, & Westergren, 2007), multiple sclerosis (Tartaglia, Narayanan, & Arnold, 2008; Tellez et al., 2005), primary biliary cirrhosis (Biagini et al., 2008) and other incurable, progressive illnesses. Fatigue has a negative influence on quality of life when associated with medical conditions such as heart failure (Heo, Doering, Widener, & Moser, 2008; Stephen, 2008) and end stage renal disease with hemodialysis (O'Sullivan & McCarthy, 2007), and with inflammatory conditions such as rheumatoid arthritis (Repping-Wuts, Fransen, van Achterberg, Bleijenberg, & van Riel, 2007), ankylosing spondylitis (Turan et al., 2007). The ensuing fatigue affects how patients interact with others, their self-perception, ability to function, and sense of hopefulness. Its impact compounds the suffering associated with life-threatening illness.

Fatigue is not limited to muscular force or decline in function related to exercise tolerance across age and length of activity (Russ, Towse, Wigmore, Lanza, & Kent-Braun, 2008), or the emotional exhaustion experienced in relation to work (De Vries, Michielsen, & Van Heck, 2003; Leone, Huibers, Knottnerus, & Kant, 2007). Chronic fatigue is an invisible thief which can steal physical and mental abilities, deeply affecting the quality of life of the older adult and posing great challenges to care providers (Yennurajalingam & Bruera, 2007) including nurses in acute care, long-term care, and the palliative care team. Like pain, fatigue is what the patient says it is; it is a subjective experience that must be taken seriously by health-care practitioners. It is important to the delivery of competent palliative care to recognize the complexity of fatigue as it is related to various disease states, to understand the experience of fatigue of older adults, and to therapeutic intervention aimed at its management in chronic disease and at the end of life (Yennurajalingam & Bruera).

PREVALENCE OF FATIGUE

The overall prevalence of fatigue, generally defined as diminished physical and mental energy, is associated with numerous chronic medical conditions (Portenoy, 2003). Generalized muscle fatigue involves changes in muscle force, velocity, and power (Fitts, 2008), yet its etiology in chronic conditions at the end of life is not clearly understood. Chronic, unrelenting fatigue is a common symptom in patients with chronic disease at the end of life, with a complex array of complaints including variations in level of irritability, nighttime sleeplessness, and daytime sleepiness. The clinical definition of fatigue at this stage of life includes lacking physical or mental energy, especially in patients with multiple sclerosis where fatigue is reported to occur in "most" patients (Johansson, Ytterberg, Hillert, Holmqvist, & von Koch, 2008; Tartaglia et al., 2008). A study of older adults with heart failure (Stephen, 2008) revealed that the intensity of fatigue was related to a lower quality of life and that fatigue was persistent in patients where the condition was stable.

A National Institutes of Health (NIH) consensus statement identified a lack of consensus on the prevalence, definition, and treatment of fatigue (as well as depression and pain) as presented in cancer patients (National Institutes of Health, 2002, July 15–17). The consensus panel indicated that estimates of fatigue among patients with cancer ranged from 4% all the way to 91%, agreeing that fatigue is the most commonly reported complaint in this patient population. Cancer-related fatigue, though it remains poorly understood, is multi-dimensional and includes psychosocial factors, side effects of chemotherapy, radiation treatments, medical states that include anemia, malnutrition, and infections, and exacerbation of other symptoms such as depression, sleep disturbance, and chronic pain (Portenoy, 2003; Wagner & Cella, 2004). Fatigue is both physical and cognitive, and evaluation of symptoms is necessary for effective treatment.

People living with HIV/AIDS should be evaluated for the co-occurrence of fatigue and depression (Voss, Portillo, Holzemer, & Dodd, 2007). Fatigue is a common symptom burden for patients with HIV/AIDS. In a study of the correlates of fatigue in a sample of persons with HIV/AIDS, 58% of the participants reported moderate to severe fatigue using the revised signs and symptoms checklist for persons with HIV disease (SSC-HIV rev.),

a 74-item checklist with a 0–12 fatigue scoring range (Voss, 2005). Similar to previous reports in which fatigue affected a greater percentage of women with AIDS (69%) than men (49%) (Breitbart, McDonald, Monkman, & Passik, 1998), Voss (2005) reported greater intensity of fatigue among female (6.3 on 0–12 scale) participants than among males (5.4 on 0–12 scale). Additionally, Voss (2005) reported cultural and ethnic differences in the intensity of fatigue among participants who were African American, Caucasian, and Hispanic.

Palliative care nurses are encouraged to recognize that fatigue does not occur in a vacuum and should not be assessed as such. The frail older adult and patients at the end of life should be assessed for energy to perform daily living activities as well as co-occurring symptoms related to chronic medical conditions. The results of a retrospective study of the medical records of 100 consecutive cancer patients who had been referred to a palliative care consult team within a tertiary acute care hospital indicated, based on Edmonton symptom assessment scale (ESAS) that fatigue, appetite, and well-being were the most intense symptoms reported (Jenkins, Schulz, Hanson, et al, 2000). The authors concluded that the assessment and management of fatigue should be a priority of the palliative care team.

THE CONCEPT OF FATIGUE

The historical development of the concept of fatigue indicates specific identifying criteria of fatigue: 1) subjective perception; 2) alteration in neuromuscular and metabolic processes; 3) decrease in physical performance; and 4) deterioration in mental and physical activity (Dean & Anderson, 2001). There remains no clear consensus regarding the definition of fatigue or a description of the phenomenon. However, there is an appreciation of the differentiation between "normal" fatigue from which the majority of the population can recover after a period of rest, and pathologic fatigue associated with disease or its treatments that is common near the close of life and in patients receiving palliative care (Ream, 2007). The analysis of pathologic fatigue and weakness, its etiology, severity, duration, and impact are important aspects of the conceptual and operational definition fatigue.

Although there is no generally accepted standard definition of fatigue documented in the literature it is agreed that fatigue symptoms include a disabling and generalized weakness leaving the individual with feelings of significant distress or impairment (Lindqvist, Widmark, & Rasmussen, 2004; Portenoy, 2003; Ream, 2007). There is also agreement that fatigue is subjective, meaning it is described by the individual and, like pain, it is what the individual says it is. Fatigue is also generally accepted as unpleasant, with variation in duration and intensity. Since there are no clear criteria for differences in fatigue, chronic fatigue, and chronic fatigue syndrome the duration (6 months) of the condition helps to distinguish its chronicity (Ranjith, 2005). In a recent concept analysis of chronic fatigue, Jorgensen (2008) examined the use of the term in the disciplines of medicine, psychology, nursing, and medical sociology. Jorgensen reported that medicine associates the etiology of fatigue with physiological variables; psychology associates the condition with an overlap of coexisting psychopathology, and linking the condition to thoughts and behaviors; medical sociologists considered fatigue states in relation to underlying chronic illness with an impact on both the body and the living experience (sociomatic).

Nurse researchers were viewed as instrumental in laying the foundation of fatigue as a conceptual framework wherein the distinctive characteristics of the acute and chronic conditions were described (Aaronson et al., 1999; Jorgensen, 2008; Piper, 1989). In an ethno-scientific qualitative study of perceived differences among tiredness, fatigue, and exhaustion, participants in advanced cancer states, their family members and nurses, were interviewed regarding their experiences with each condition (Olson, Krawchuk, & Quddusi, 2007). The researchers reported findings to support these three conditions as separate and distinct, though similar, states on a progression model, which the researchers named the "fatigue adaptation model."

An early definition of fatigue included the influence of circadian rhythm on the feeling of tiredness, the variation in duration and intensity such that it encourages restorative rest or an aversion to activity ensues (Piper; Piper, Lindsey, & Dodd, 1989). The North American Nursing Diagnosis Association (NANDA) has defined fatigue as "an overwhelming, sustained sense of exhaustion and decreased capacity for physical or emotional work" (Tiesinga, Dassen, & Halfens, 1996). One of the most comprehensive definitions of fatigue, relevant to palliative care, is "the awareness of a decreased capacity for physical and/or mental activity due to an imbalance in the availability, utilization, and/or restoration of resources needed to perform activity" (Aaronson et al., 1999).

Neill (2005) conducted an analysis of the narratives of women with multiple sclerosis and rheumatoid arthritis in an attempt to learn about their life patterns in relation to the NANDA patterns. She found that the life pattern corollary of energy fatigue was meaningful as a primary pattern in the daily life of the women she studied. These chronic conditions are associated with low energy and fatigue, and thus have a great impact on the women's ability to work, take care of the home, or engage in social activities.

At various points in the course of illness, older adults may interpret fatigue differently. Older adults newly diagnosed with a life-threatening illness may have experienced fatigue as an early indication or warning symptom of the diagnosis. Over the course of treatment(s) for any number of conditions fatigue may be understood as the side effect of treatment, while for others with recurrence or exacerbation of illness, fatigue is interpreted as the end of a very long struggle (Dean & Anderson, 2001).

The concept of fatigue also encompasses emotional, cognitive, and behavioral dimensions. Psychosocial etiologic factors of fatigue in the medically ill include anxiety or depressive disorders, stress, and related environmental reinforcements (Portenoy, 2000). In healthy individuals, overexertion may produce ordinary fatigue, which is relieved relatively quickly by rest (Aaronson, Pallikkathayil, & Crighton, 2003); fatigue may also be interpreted as satisfaction given the accomplishment of hard work. However, fatigue associated with illness is perceived as more severe, comes on after a shorter period of time, and with less exertion than ordinary fatigue. It is often described as a general feeling of tiredness or "sapped" energy that occurs on a daily basis and is present intermittently throughout the day or during the evening after a day of normal activities.

Fatigue has been characterized by patients by such descriptors as "worn out, weary, exhausted, sleepiness, low energy, tired, worn down, bone-tired, and rubber knees." Patients have said they feel weakness, "a lack of physical strength . . . trapped in a failing body . . . struggling in vain . . . " (Lindqvist et al., 2004 p. 240), suggesting that palliative care nurses should talk with patients about their feelings to gain understanding of the physical and psychological impact of fatigue. A qualitative study of the experience of fatigue in cancer patients (Magnusson, Moller, Ekman, & Wallgren, 1999), fatigue is illustrated as a process with three major categories. These categories are 1) experiences of loss, need, psychological stress, emotional affection, malaise, abnormal weakness, and difficulty taking initiative; 2) the consequences of fatigue, specifically social limitation, affected self-esteem, and affected quality of life; and 3) the action taken for coping with fatigue. More recently, a study of cancer-related fatigue in patients with advanced disease states indicated signification relationships between fatigue and multiple psychological and physical characteristics including physical and psychological symptoms of well-being (Yennurajalingam, Palmer, Zhang, Poulter, & Bruera, 2008). They found primary associations among psychological and physical symptoms of cancer related fatigue including feelings of well-being, drowsiness, anorexia, and anxiety. These authors indicate that how fatigue is expressed is important in planning and delivering care for patients with cancer who experience fatigue.

Palliative care nurse practitioners, hospice nurses, and general care nurses use terms such as listless, lassitude, lethargy, and malaise to describe the fatigue observed in patients. Some practitioners differentiate fatigue from weakness, while others believe that they accompany each other and comprise a syndrome known as asthenia (Dean & Anderson, 2001). Fatigue that persists through resting and is present at awakening is termed asthenia, and may be considered within the context of clinically chronic and inflammatory conditions previously mentioned involving the nervous system or endocrine system (Kasatkin & Spirin, 2007; Saguil, 2005). Asthenia and chronic fatigue are clearly related and are also unpleasant sensations of whole-body tiredness experienced when an individual's physiologic resources are exceeded and coexists with muscular weakness.

MULTIDIMENSIONAL ASPECTS OF FATIGUE

Fatigue is like pain, a multidimensional symptom, a subjective experience associated with diverse etiologies (Portenoy, 2003). The complex phenomenon that is fatigue has physical, emotional, cognitive, and behavioral descriptors (Jorgensen, 2008) to which subgroups are not clearly measurable. For example, asthenia, fatigue, chronic fatigue, pathologic fatigue, and chronic fatigue syndrome imply varying levels of fatigue but existing criteria do not clearly distinguish subgroups from each other (Jorgensen; Portenoy; Ranjith, 2005). The consent among these authors is that physical etiologies of fatigue in the medically ill older adult include the underlying disease itself, associated treatment of disease (chemotherapy, radiation, surgery, biological response modifiers), co-occurring systemic disorders (anemia, infection, pulmonary disorders, hepatic failure, heart failure, renal failure, malnutrition, neuromuscular and neurogenic disorders), sleep disorders, chronic pain, use of centrally acting drugs, as well as lack of mobility and lack of exercise (Chochivov & Breitbart, 2000). From a physiological perspective, fatigue has been attributed to excessive energy consumption and the depletion of hormones, neurotransmitters or other essential substrates (Aaronson et al., 1999).

Independent categories of fatigue. Clinical fatigue, classified into independent categories, includes fatigue at rest (asthenia, chronic fatigue), fatigue on physical loading (pathological fatigue, acute fatigue), and fatigue as related to another condition (cancer-related fatigue, treatment-related fatigue) or exacerbation of a condition such as multiple sclerosis (Kasatkin & Spirin, 2007; Portenoy, 2003). Fatigue is also linked clinically to metabolic changes such as infection, fever, tissue injury, anemia, hypoxemia, malnutrition; or to conditions involving sleep or mood disorders including major depression (Portenoy).

In the case of cancer-related fatigue, asthenia, and weakness, three associated physiologic mechanisms may affect the CNS or muscles:

1) Direct tumor effects (mechanically by destruction, such as metastasis, or metabolically by lipolytic factors or tumor degradation products).
2) Tumor induced products (such as tumor necrosis factors [asthenin/cachectin], and other cytokines such as PEG2, Il-1, Ifn, or IL6).
3) Tumor accompanying factors (cachexia, infection, anemia, hypoxia, neurologic disorders, pharmacologic side effects, paraneoplastic, metabolic, or dehydration) (Neuenschwander & Bruera, 1998).

In cancer populations, there has been a documented relationship between asthenia and cachexia, although one may exist without the other. However, in patients with advanced cancer, both are usually present with asthenia as an epiphenomenon of the cachexia syndrome. In malignancy, changes is carbohydrate, fat, and protein metabolism, as well as direct tumor factors and cytokines previously mentioned, lead to cachexia and resultant loss of muscle mass. This partially explains cachexia-related asthenia.

Clinical classification of fatigue. Research indicates that the mechanisms or pathophysiology of fatigue, weakness, and asthenia differ from one clinical condition to another and are not consistent in the literature (Kasatkin & Spirin, 2007). The individual perception of fatigue is multidimensional and may include physical, psychological, and cognitive complaints, each contributing to the physiologic basis for the syndrome (Evans & Lambert, 2007). Fatigue has been classified as either acute physiologic, secondary to a medical condition, or chronic (Rosenthal et al., 2008). Physiologically, fatigue is classified according to two types: central or peripheral. Signal, Taylor, and McNair (2008) reviewed central and peripheral influences on neuromuscular fatigue in people after experiencing stroke, or cerebrovascular accident (CVA). They reported that patients experience a relatively decreased level of peripheral neuromuscular fatigue and an increased level of central fatigue after suffering a stroke. In central fatigue, the motor pathways in the central nervous system (CNS) fail to sustain recruitment and/or frequency of motor units or the generation of descending volleys in the motor cortex due to neurotransmitter modulation (Anish, 2005). Research data suggest that alterations in brain dopamine and 5-HT levels may influence arousal level, sleepiness, mood, and the perception of fatigue. These findings suggest that fatigue can contribute to functional impairment, therefore, the recognition and treatment of fatigue by a palliative care provider is an important consideration. Admittedly, the role of neurotransmitters in the development of central fatigue requires further study of correlates with chronic disease as well as extensive physical exercise (Anish).

In peripheral fatigue, there are metabolic changes in the muscle and a failure in the muscle fiber components' potential resulting in decreased postural stability (Dickin and Doan, 2008). This failure to exert effort results from a combined effect of failure in the neural drive, such as fatigue in the mind or central nervous system, and failure of neurotransmission in the muscles though continued research is in progress to understand the mechanisms (Anish, 2005). Peripheral fatigue has known association with chronic diseases related to muscle wasting, inflammation, or joint abnormalities including rheumatoid arthritis and systemic lupus erythematosus, (Swain, 2000), HIV-AIDS, and neurologic abnormalities including Parkinson's Disease.

Fatigue leads to a decline in mental or intellectual activities and a diminished motivation or capacity to attend (Tartaglia et al., 2008; van Kessel et al., 2008). Tartaglia et al. (2008) studied mental fatigue and its impact on motor task impulse activation in patients with MS. They found that MS patients with physical fatigue also experience fatigue for mentally challenging tasks, which can also affect unrelated motor activities, unrelated to age. Similarly, van Kessel et al. (2008) randomized patients with MS into groups for two study treatments: cognitive behavioral therapy (CBT) sessions to address contributory factors related to fatigue including behavioral, cognitive, emotional, and environmental issues; and relaxation training (RT) sessions during which relaxation techniques were taught and practiced without advice or strategies for maintaining the practices. van Kessel et al. reported that both methods result in significant improvements, with the CBT group showing more improvement in fatigue-related impairment, depression and anxiety, and stress level.

Acute (physiologic) fatigue. Acute or physiologic fatigue is a protective state that is identifiably linked to a single cause, in usually healthy individuals. Acute fatigue is a clinically significant state of tiredness and diminished ability to expend effort as in exercise-induced states (Anish, 2005) to which individuals may recover after a period of restoration. Antecedents to acute fatigue may be associated with physical exertion or lack of sleep that limits the usual activities of daily living (Evans & Lambert, 2007). Acute fatigue has a rapid onset and short direction, is viewed as normal in the usually healthy person, and can be alleviated by restorative techniques such as rest, diet, exercise, and stress management. Acute fatigue may have immediate effects on activities of daily living and minimal effects on quality of life.

Chronic fatigue. By contrast, chronic fatigue has no known physiologic purpose and can occur without any relationship to exertion or activity. Chronic fatigue is commonly associated with severe deconditioning or limited mobility as seen in patients with anemias and diminished aerobic capacity including those with heart failure, chronic lung conditions, and neurological disorders (Evans & Lambert, 2007). Chronic fatigue is frequently experienced by patients with life-threatening illness, is insidious in onset, and persists over time, typically longer than 6 months (Swain, 2000). Chronic fatigue is viewed as abnormal or pathological, is not effectively relieved by rest or sleep, and typically is not related to routine daily exertion. Therefore, chronic fatigue has a significant negative effect on independence, instrumental activities of living, and quality of life (Rosenthal et al., 2008).

Chronic fatigue syndrome (CFS) is an illness with symptoms of fatigue that are more intense than the feelings experienced by persons who have a difficult workday, or who have a stressful interaction. When unexplained fatigue occurs for more than 6 months, and is accompanied by an array of primary symptoms, the Centers for Disease Control and Prevention (CDC) recommends further evaluation and differentiation of CFS from illnesses that may mimic its symptoms (Centers for Disease Control and Prevention, 2006). For example, persons with CFS commonly complain of impaired cognitive function that lasts more than a day or two, and persons with co-occurring conditions or other illnesses may exhibit psychological problems including depression, irritability, mood swings, anxiety, and panic attacks (Centers for Disease Control and Prevention). Symptoms that occur with other disease conditions in which fatigue also occurs signal healthcare professionals to evaluate possible coexistence to determine the level of contribution to functional decline and impairment.

Secondary fatigue. When the body is experiencing the stress and pathology of chronic disease or cancer, the body reserves can become depleted and ultimately unable to counterbalance the physiologic insults (Evans & Lambert, 2007). The patient may experience fatigue in association with the advanced stage of chronic disease, and concurrent malnutrition, anemia and cachexia, and further deconditioning and weakness. The patient interview should include reviewing the effect of fatigue on lifestyle, the presence of other physical or mental conditions, and possible side effects of medicines or drugs (Rosenthal, Majeroni, Pretorius, Malik, 2008).

Cancer-related fatigue is reported by nearly 100% of patients undergoing radiation therapy and 95% of those receiving chemotherapy; it is also associated with anemia, cytokine activation, and mood changes including anxiety and depression (Lundberg & Rattanasuwan, 2007). A study of Thai Buddhist patients described consuming concerns about cancer treatment and outcomes that produced uncertainty, fear, weakness and difficulty sleeping leading to feelings of fatigue (Lundberg & Rattanasuwan). A 3-year longitudinal study of breast cancer patients treated with chemotherapy, radiation therapy, and tamoxifen revealed that depressed mood, muscle and joint pain, and hemoglobin level, as well as menopausal status were still related to fatigue at the 3-year follow-up evaluation (Nieboer et al., 2005). Coexisting symptoms such as nausea and vomiting, inadequate nutrient intake, pain, immobility, loss of muscle mass, infection, metabolic disturbances, shortness of breath, possible gastric obstruction, and anxiety or depression also are associated with the experience of fatigue in the older adult.

The treatment for cancer (surgery, radiation, chemotherapy, bio-therapeutic therapy) can cause feelings of fatigue. The anticipation of surgery generates anxiety resulting from preoperative regimens and contributes to the postoperative fatigue that can result from pain, direct tissue damage, anesthesia, sedatives, analgesics, and immobility (Paddison, Booth, Fuchs, and Hill, 2008). The study of women with breast cancer surgery revealed that postsurgical fatigue was predicted by level of preoperative distress and fatigue, level of education, and previous experience the person had with the same procedure (Paddison, Booth, Fuchs, and Hill, 2008). Paddison, Booth, Fuchs, and Hill (2008) studied patients of colorectal surgery and reported that locally occurring proinflammatory cytokines and neopterin may increase postsurgical fatigue; therefore, treating inflammation may reduce the fatigue experienced after major surgery. A secondary analysis of data on patients after coronary artery bypass graft surgery confirms the negative impact fatigue on postsurgical recovery (Barnason et al., 2008).

For patients treated with radiotherapy, nearly 100% experience dose-dependent fatigue, which tends to peak toward the end of the cycle. Approximately 95% of patients who receive chemotherapy report that fatigue is one of the worst symptoms they experience within the first 2 weeks after treatment. Bio-therapeutic agents (interferon, interleukins) are used as maintenance therapies in older adults, especially those in remission from acute myeloid leukemia (Melchert & Lancet, 2008). Interferon and interleukins can induce dose-related fatigue through side effects of flu-like symptoms including chills, fever, weakness, and dyspnea (Delglin & Vallerand, 2005).

Patients with chronic conditions, such as fibromyalgia, may manifest progressive symptoms of psychogenic fatigue, physiologic fatigue, and pain (Jain & Jain, 2008). Given the unknown etiology of fibromyalgia, there are limited treatment options for this disease, with relief primarily achieved by the palliation of symptoms. Recent studies provide positive results from appropriate treatment of causes and contributors to fatigue including sleep disorders, hormonal imbalances, infections, and malnutrition (Teitelbaum, 2008). Exercise is also recommended in levels that help sufferers to feel better without initially aiming at training or conditioning. Older adults who live with chronic conditions like fibromyalgia, rheumatoid arthritis, or chronic fatigue syndrome should be evaluated for co-morbid depression and the impact on overall quality of life and quality of health (Jakobsson et al., 2007). Interventions such as psychotherapy and medication management should be initiated to prevent suicidal ideation or attempt.

The causes of HIV-related fatigue are typically related to psychological and, or physiological factors (Barroso, 2002; Voss, Sukati et al., 2007) that influence symptoms associated with fatigue (Voss, Dodd, Portillo, & Holzemer, 2006). Fatigue is related to lack of restorative rest or exercise, anemia as manifested by low hemoglobin and hematocrit levels (Barroso, 2002), disturbances sleep or inadequate sleep, and activity patterns (Lee, Portillo, & Miramontes, 2001). The fatigue experience in patients with HIV/AIDS includes complaints of tiredness and exhaustion, with varying reports that women in some studies experience higher fatigue severity than men (Voss, 2005; Voss, Portillo et al., 2007).

Voss (2005) posits that the multi-tasking lifestyles generally attributed to women may account for reports of increased fatigue severity. Voss also found that women without family responsibilities who lived alone reported lower levels of fatigue severity. Barroso reported that fatigue severity was unrelated to individual viral load, and that fatigue occurred in patients at any stage of the infection (Barroso, 2002). Further, Voss found that a cluster of symptoms including fatigue, shortness of breath, lipodystrophy and depression contribute significantly to individual perceptions of quality of life, physical health, and mental or psychological well-being. Additional conditions that influence fatigue in the patient with HIV/AIDS include inadequate nutrition, infections and fever (Voss, Sukati et al., 2007), thyroid problems, and side-effects of medications (Delglin & Vallerand, 2005). Psychological distress such as depression, and physiological changes such as shortness of breath and lipodystrophy may compound the fatigue (Voss, 2005).

CORRELATES OF FATIGUE IN SPECIFIC PATIENT POPULATIONS

Fatigue has been associated with the use of centrally acting drugs, such as opioids and other narcotic agonist analgesics. Fatigue is also associated with advanced disease and combined therapies for life-threatening or chronic diseases, and with older age in connection with declining health (Rosenthal et al., 2008). Reporting on a study of patients with end-stage heart failure, Nordgren and Sorensen (2003) reported troublesome fatigue in 69%, and breathlessness in 88% of participants. Patients typically experience increasing fatigue as heart failure progresses to Stages C and D, characterized by symptoms of systolic dysfunction and refractory symptoms of dyspnea and fatigue while resting (Hunt et al., 2005). Breathlessness and dyspnea may be treated with opioids (narcotic agonist analgesics) which may contribute pharmacologically to the experience of fatigue (Hemani & Letizia, 2008). Given that fatigue is integral to the experience of heart failure, interventions are needed to assist patients to cope with the experience of fatigue, such as pacing of activities, relaxation, and restful sleep.

Fatigue—Pediatric Considerations

For children with advanced cancer, fatigue is the most common symptom reported in the last month of life (Ulrich & Mayer, 2007). The prevalence rate of this symptom is reported as 96% with 57% reporting as suffering significantly from it (Wolfe, Grier, & Klar, 2000). Jamsell and colleagues (2006) reported that in a study of 449 parents whose children had died of cancer, 86% reported that fatigue and significantly affected their child's well-being. In children, as in adults, fatigue typically results in decreased activity, loss of control, and a sense of loneliness and isolation (Ulrich & Mayer, 2007). Left untreated, fatigue can negatively impact quality of life, and interfere with opportunities for growth and closure at the end of life.

Assessment of fatigue is dependent on subjective reports of the patient. In children, clinicians may need to rely on the reports of the parents regarding the experience of fatigue. Hockenberry (Hockenberry, Hinds, & Barrera, 2003) developed a fatigue rating tool that took into consideration the perspective of the child, parent, and staff. Hinds (Hinds, Hockenberry-Eaton, & Gilger, 1999) documented that children conceptualize fatigue as a physical sensation while adolescents merge the concept with mental tiredness. Parents and staff share the view that the child's fatigue is manifested by physical, emotional, and mental changes that interfere with the child's ability to participate in activities (Hinds et al., 1999).

To date there is no evidence to support that interventions aimed at the management of fatigue are any different between children and adults, although there are no evidence-based studies documenting the efficacy of these interventions in children. One study assessing the effect of massage on fatigue in children with cancer was unable to document any effect on fatigue (Post-White, 2006). For children, studies are needed regarding assessment of fatigue in light of developmental stages. Education for children with life-threatening illnesses, their families, and clinicians is needed regarding recognition and treatment of this symptom in order to lessen this source of suffering.

Fatigue in the Older Adult

Fatigue is a common symptom among older adults and is particularly evident in the older adult in long-term care facilities. In a review of literature related to the unmet symptom needs of residents in long-term care, fatigue was named as one of the more common symptoms in persons with cancer who were not near the end of life (Duncan, Forbes-Thompson, & Bott, 2008).

The authors also reported that assessment and evaluation of fatigue was not specified in the minimum data set (MDS) required by each nursing home certified by Medicare or Medicaid (Centers for Medicare & Medicaid Services, 2002). In a study of resident-to-resident aggression among residents of long term care, researchers conducted 15 focus group interviews with 7 residents and 96 staff members in one facility (Rosen et al., 2008). The residents formed one focus group and staff of differing job levels and responsibilities formed the remaining groups. Although fatigue was named as a nonfrequent trigger or reason for aggression, the research report indicated that fatigue may occur during both public (group) and private (bathroom) activities involving residents, and may also be related to end-of-day fatigue of staff persons (Rosen et al., 2008). Policy recommendations for prevention of resident violence and aggression include specific staff training in geriatrics and long term care, and staff levels that allow staff members sufficient time to attend to the physical and emotional needs of residents (Robinson & Tappen, 2008). Each study suggests that fatigue may be poorly recognized and undertreated in older people in nursing home facilities.

Treatment of the older adult in palliative care must encompass the potential for confounding pathology secondary to aging. Clear associations between fatigue and depression (National Institute of Mental Health, 2002), cancer-related treatment modalities (National Institutes of Health, 2002, July 15–17; Portenoy, 2003), heart failure (Heo et al., 2008; Stephen, 2008), anemia (Balducci, Ershler, & Gaetano, 2008), malnutrition (Eliopoulos, 2005), end-stage renal disease (Bonner, Wellard, & Caltabiano, 2008; O'Sullivan & McCarthy, 2007), and fibromyalgia (Geisser et al., 2008) appear in the literature. A study by Karlsen, Larsen, Tandberg, & Jorgensen (1999), compared the prevalence of fatigue in patients with Parkinson's disease (PD) with healthy older adults to determine if fatigue was an independent symptom of PD. Forty-four percent of the elders with PD and 18% of the elder control subjects reported fatigue. Fatigue was associated in this study with depression, dementia, the use of sleeping pills, disease severity and duration, and levodopa dose. In a similar study patients with PD and a control group of age and gender matched non-individuals were evaluated for fatigue and depression (Zenzola et al., 2003). Both research teams concluded that fatigue was a multidimensional, independent symptom of PD that influenced, but was not causally related to, depressive symptoms.

Healthcare providers, in accordance with basic nursing competencies for end-of-life care (American Association of Colleges of Nursing, 2005) and guidelines for palliative care (National Consensus Project for Quality Palliative Care, 2009) should regularly and carefully assess symptoms of fatigue and weakness, and the symptoms that frequently accompany these, for all older adult patients and persons near the end-of-life. Nurses and palliative care nurse practitioners are expected to assess for and recognize the need to treat generally occurring symptoms that may include pain, breathlessness (dyspnea), constipation, anxiety, changes in appetite, nausea, vomiting, changes in sleep pattern, and alterations in cognition and function. Often the conventional wisdom is that because a person is of advanced age, fatigue is a normal consequence of the aging process. Many elders and their families erroneously consider fatigue to be inevitable, and therefore not a symptom to be treated. In fact, older adults may not even report symptoms of weakness and fatigue to their primary care provider. Even for the older adult in palliative care many causes of fatigue can be successfully treated by examining for and treating the underlying cause. The goal for the healthcare provider related to the symptom fatigue is to improve the patient's quality of life by treating the symptom and teaching the older adult coping mechanisms and lifestyle changes.

Fatigue is commonly included in characterizations of frailty. A 3-year prospective study of women aged 65 and over treated with ACE-inhibitors (angiotensin-converting enzyme inhibitors) in the Women's Health Initiative Observational Study (WHI-OS) revealed no association with frailty development (Gray et al., 2009). In a similar prospective study of frailty indicators, risk factors, and frailty outcome predictors among participants in the Women's Health Initiative Observational Study (WHI-OS), the terms poor endurance and exhaustion were used to describe a reduction in physical functioning, just one of the multiple components of frailty (Woods et al., 2005). The research report indicated that baseline frailty was a predictor of negative outcomes (death, hip fracture, disability in activities of daily living, and hospitalizations) among the participants. Unfortunately, exhaustion (fatigue) was measured as one of the multiple components of frailty, thus disallowing its independent examination as a contributor to the negative outcomes (Woods et al.).

Depressive symptoms were also associated with baseline frailty in the WHI-OS, and being underweight, overweight, or obese were described as risk factors for frailty (Woods et al., 2005), a component of which is poor physical functioning or exhaustion. The concept of fatigue in depression screening is often measured with criteria that reflect energy level (ability to get going), or effort required to conduct daily activities (American Psychiatric Association, 2000). Depression may be the primary contributor particularly if the fatigue is accompanied by poor appetite and unexplained weight loss. The American Psychiatric Association identifies fatigue as a symptom of depression (American Psychiatric Association, 2000), but often it is difficult to determine if chronic fatigue is etiologically unrelated to an affective disorder or if the symptoms of chronic fatigue precipitated the depression (Aaronson et al., 1999).

Fatigue is identified by researchers as occurring in patients with inflammatory conditions including biliary cirrhosis (Biagini et al., 2008; Bjornsson, Simren, Olsson, & Chapman, 2005), rheumatoid arthritis (Repping-Wuts et al., 2007), ankylosing spondylitis (Turan et al., 2007), and after an episode of infectious mononucleosis (Petersen, Thomas, Hamilton, & White, 2006). Biagini and colleagues studies a group of 49 patients with biliary cirrhosis and 30 health adults, and reported that fatigue scores were higher among patients with biliary cirrhosis, and scores were also higher when those patients had concurring illnesses including depression.

Björnsson, Simren, Olsson, and Chapman studied 96 patients with biliary cirrhosis and a group of matched persons from the general population, patients with functional gastrointestinal disorders, and patients with organic gastrointestinal disorders such as inflammatory bowel disease. They reported that patients with functional gastrointestinal disorders and organic gastrointestinal disorders had higher fatigue scores than the persons from the general population and those with biliary cirrhosis. Both these studies indicate the necessity to evaluate fatigue in patients with biliary cirrhosis, while present, may not be related to actual liver function, but related to the comorbidities including depression, alteration in sleep patterns and quality, or other psychological or psychiatric conditions.

In a study of 68 patients with ankylosing spondylitis, researchers reported an increase in fatigue that was associated with greater disease severity, functional disability, and disease activity (Turan et al., 2007). Repping-Wuts and colleagues (2007) studied a group of 150 patients with rheumatoid arthritis and found that the general health of the patient and the level of disability predicted high scores on measures of fatigue. Severe persistent fatigue was defined as a score of at least 35 at the beginning of the study and after 12 months using the fatigue subscale of the checklist individual strength questionnaire. These two studies underscore the relationships among fatigue, functional disability, and level of general health. It is therefore important to assess for fatigue and institute measures to reduce its severity in patients with inflammatory conditions such as ankylosing spondylitis and rheumatoid arthritis.

One study of 84 patients with heart failure indicated that fatigue was a common symptom in 95% of participants while engaged in daily activities (Heo et al., 2008). While fatigue was just one of several physical symptoms self-reported by participants, it was often associated with dyspnea; higher levels of symptoms were associated with poorer quality of life in relation to health. Significant measures of physical symptom status in these heart failure patients included employment status, patient perceived control over the management of the condition, anxiety, and depression. In another study of patients with heart failure, a group of 53 older adults completed the fatigue subscale of the profile of mood states (Stephen, 2008). Results indicated that, without regard to actual age, older adults who believed that fatigue was related to their aging scored higher on fatigue intensity than older adults who did not believe the relationship. Stephen found that the intensity of fatigue was predicted by the severity of the illness, negative affect (e.g., sadness and depression), perception of health status, satisfaction with life, severity of current co-occurring symptoms, and marital status).

A study of 19 women and 17 men with chronic obstructive pulmonary disease (COPD), not asthma or cancer, were compared with a control group of regional participants statistically matched for sex, marital status, and social support, to explore fatigue and its impact on the daily lives of participants (Theander & Unosson, 2004). Findings indicated that fatigue had a great impact on how participants with COPD felt each day, and on their ability to perform daily tasks. Nearly half (44%) of the participants reported that fatigue was experienced daily and was one of their worst symptoms. Participants in this study also reported higher fatigue scores as measured by the fatigue impact scale (FIS) (Theander & Unosson), developed for assessment of the perceived impact of fatigue on quality of life for persons with chronic illness (Fisk et al., 1994).

Fatigue and weakness were reported in 96% of patients with chronic obstructive pulmonary disease (COPD) near the end of life in a descriptive, retrospective study using informants of the deceased (Elkington, White, Addington-Hall, Higgs, & Edmonds, 2005). The researchers found that accompanying symptoms including low mood, sleep disturbances, anxiety, pain, and breathlessness were frequently among the patients' end-of-life experiences. In a study of persons with moderate to severe COPD researchers were able to demonstrate the between fatigue and the daily function and activities of persons with COPD (Kapella, Larson, Patel, Covey, & Berry, 2006). The sample of 130 participants reported situation-specific fatigue that was controllable and responsive to planned amounts of rest and sleep. They developed a model describing the direct influence of depressed mood on fatigue, and the indirect influence of anxiety and quality of sleep on fatigue, thereby contributing to diminished functional capacity. In a state of the science article examining over 75 articles related to anxiety and depression in patients with COPD, Putman-Casdorph and McCrone (2009) acknowledge the complexity of anxiety and depression and their negative impact on physical performance, compliance with prescribed regimen, symptom burden, and overall quality of life.

In a study of patients with Hodgkin's disease (aged 19–74 years, 56% male) (Loge, Abrahamsen, Ekeberg, & Kaasa, 2000), fatigue was also correlated with psychiatric morbidity, specifically depression and anxiety ($r = -0.41, 0.44$ respectively). Twenty-six percent had

fatigue for 6 months or longer. A multiple logistic regression analysis revealed that advanced age, anxiety and no self-reported psychiatric problems during treatment were predictors of fatigue.

Differences in fatigue by treatment methods in women with breast cancer has been studies by numerous researchers (Halkett, Kristjanson, & Lobb, 2008; Hwang et al., 2008; Minton & Stone, 2008). Minton and Stone conducted a literature review to address the issue of fatigue after treatment for breast cancer in survivors. Their findings indicate that fatigue may persist for five years following therapeutic intervention including surgery, radiotherapy, and chemotherapy. Halkett, Kristjanson, and Lobb conducted semi-structured interviews with 34 patients who discussed their experiences with radiotherapy treatments for breast cancer. They found that fear of fatigue, or "anticipating tiredness" (Halkett et al., p. 881), was often greater than the actual experiences of side effects. A randomized control study of 37 women with breast cancer in radiotherapy examined the effect of exercise on their quality of life, including levels of fatigue (Hwang et al., 2008). The study protocol included use of the Brief Fatigue Inventory (Korean version). Results indicated a significant difference ($p < .05$) between the two groups. Fatigue decreased after exercise and radiotherapy in the treatment, but increased after radiotherapy in the control group. Although these studies did not specifically address co-occurring illnesses, the findings in each suggest the need for anticipatory guidance regarding the side-effects, such as fatigue, of various treatment regimens, and methods for managing or decreasing the fatigue.

Severe fatigue is a complaint of cancer patients even before the start of therapeutic intervention which might add to the fatigue occurs (Goedendorp et al., 2008). In the study of 240 patients with varying forms of cancer, almost a fourth of participants with a diagnosis of cancer reported severe fatigue 1–3 years before starting treatment. For example, fatigue was categorized by disease process, and of the 23.5% of participants who complained of severe fatigue, the highest occurrence was in persons with 'other' tumors (33.3%), including gastrointestinal, urogenital, or gynecological. Of participants who complained of severe fatigue, 14.3% were persons with prostate cancer and 20.3% were persons with breast cancer. Participants with severe fatigue after diagnosis but before therapy also experienced more pain, less physical activity, more sleep disturbance, more depressive feelings and more anxiety than participants without severe fatigue. The researchers found that although anxiety might be a normal and expected response to a diagnosis of cancer, there was no significant association between the diagnosis of cancer and severe fatigue.

In a randomized control study of the effect of exercise on common symptoms in patients with rheumatoid arthritis, 220 patients participated in a guided exercise group, exercise at home with a videotape, or in a control group (Neuberger et al., 2007). All exercises were low impact during which one foot is always in contact with the floor. Findings indicated that fatigue, pain, and depression diminished among participants in the exercise class, whereas participants in the home exercise program experienced no changes (possibly related to less intensity and duration of exercise sessions in the nonguided home exercise participants). Participants who believed that exercise would be beneficial to their overall health tended to exercise more.

Numerous reviews of literature focused on fatigue, pain, and depression in patients with cancer confirm the complex etiology of fatigue (Barnes & Bruera, 2002; *National Institutes of Health State-of-the-Science Conference Statement: Symptom Management in Cancer: Pain, Depression, and Fatigue, July 15–17, 2002*, 2004; Rao & Cohen, 2004). Specified categories of cancer-related fatigue contributing factors include the cancer treatment and its complications, co-morbidities, nutritional status, medications, and psychological factors. Multiple instruments assist practitioners in the evaluation of fatigue and involve measurement of functional capacity and performance, and patient self-report using a visual analogue or numerical rating scale, or a survey. The researchers specify the need for targeted treatment of underlying contributors to fatigue such as anemia, sepsis, pain, nutrition and hydration, mood disorders and accompanying symptoms, sleep-rest disturbances, and endocrine or metabolic disorders.

FATIGUE AND QUALITY OF LIFE

Regardless of the age of the patient, fatigue has a profound effect on an older adult's quality of life. Researchers conducted a study of 526 older adults aged 75 and older in groups representing those who reported pain and those who did not report pain, and those who did or did not require in-home assistance with daily activities (Jakobsson et al., 2007). Decreased ability to carry out role performance tasks is associated with mobility, sleep quality, and mood, which were found to have an impact on overall quality of life for persons in pain. The findings indicated that fatigue was one factor that contributed to the health-related quality of life experienced by participants; the remaining contributors were associated with the need for special living accommodations, functional problems with walking or mobility (Jakobsson et al.). This study supports that in order to promote health-related quality of life, fatigue, as a symptom that often coexists with pain, must be appropriately assessed and effectively treated.

Assessment of Fatigue

As a subjective symptom, practitioners most often rely on the elder's self-report of fatigue to evaluate its severity. However, the assessment of fatigue does include observable characteristics and the impact of the symptom on quality of life. A comprehensive assessment of fatigue obtained through a health history, review of systems, including fatigue assessment, physical examination, and laboratory data, can assist the practitioner in discriminating between physiologic and psychogenic fatigue, depression, and the presence of correctable fatigue. Chapter 23 appendix, part A reviews the characteristics of the commonly used fatigue assessment tools.

Health History. The health history should include a medical, psychiatric, family, social, and medication history, which may reveal associated conditions, such as diabetes, hypothyroidism, sleep apnea, anxiety or depressive disorders, inherited metabolic disorders or a history of alcohol or illegal drug use, and the possibility of sexually transmitted infections often associated with fatigue, even in older populations.

Review of Systems. The review of systems regarding fatigue focuses on changes in other body systems that may indicate potential health problems associated with fatigue, such as respiratory disorders (e.g., dyspnea), cardiac problems, anemia, cancers, depression, or electrolyte disorders. In older adult populations, including those with chronic, incurable illness, fatigue may also be a side effect of medical treatments, including both prescription and over-the-counter medications. Furthermore, in speaking with the patient, it is important to determine their emotional status, particularly whether the person speaks of his/her own death or suicidal ideations.

The Fatigue Assessment. The fatigue assessment includes questions related to the six dimensions of fatigue (Piper, 1995) (Chapter 23 appendix, part B), specifically the:

1) Temporal dimension, which includes the assessment of the timing of fatigue (when it occurs), onset (from seconds to years), duration (chronic for more than 6 months), and the pattern (wake up fatigued, evening fatigue, transient etc), and changes in this dimension over time.
2) Sensory dimension, which focuses on how the fatigue feels. For example, is the fatigue localized? (e.g., tired eyes, arms, legs), or generalized? (e.g., whole body tiredness, weariness, weakness, lethargy), and what is the intensity or severity of fatigue (using 0–10 scale)? Additional assessment questions include what exacerbates the fatigue? (e.g., pain, nausea, vomiting, environmental heat, or noise). What helps the patient feel better or alleviates the symptoms (e.g., rest, food, listening to music etc.)?
3) Mental/cognitive dimension, which questions the patient's ability to concentrate and focus,

attention span, recall, and if they report being "mentally tired."

4) Affective/emotional dimension, which assesses the patient's irritability, impatience, mood changes, depression and the significance of the fatigue.

5) Behavioral dimension, which considers the effect that the fatigue has on the patient's ability to perform activities of daily living (bathing, dressing, cooking, socializing, sexual activity). Family and practitioner observations regarding the patient's posture, gait, appearance (e.g., drooping shoulders), or lack of energy should also be assessed. Acute behavioral manifestations can include a change in alertness, while chronic manifestations may not be obvious to the practitioner because of the ability of many patients to adapt to their fatigue. If the patient also has a dementing illness, the behavioral dimensions may be the only clue that the practitioner has regarding the presence of fatigue.

6) Physiologic dimension, which includes biological mechanisms such as laboratory tests, a complete physical examination and determining if co-morbid conditions such as diabetes, cardiac illness, or other disease factors are present.

Table 23.1 also provides questions related to the assessment of the pattern of sleep and rest, older persons' perceptions/expression of fatigue, and the impact on their quality of life (Cahill, 1999).

Physical Examination. The pyhsical examination includes the following assessment parameters:

- Vital signs, to determine if fever, low blood pressure, or weak pulse may be the cause of fatigue;
- General appearance, including affect (anxious, depressed, agitated, tearful, angry or flat), self-care behaviors, speech patterns, intonation, and general responsiveness;
- Assessment of cardiac, respiratory, renal, musculoskeletal, and skin status to identify physiologic conditions, including signs of infection or dehydration/nutrition that may be associated with fatigue; and
- Appropriate laboratory testing, such as complete blood count and other laboratory studies (electrolytes, blood gases, thyroid function tests), which may confirm diseases suspected.

Measuring Fatigue

Given its subjectivity and the general lack of consensus in the literature regarding a definition of fatigue, the measurement of fatigue remains a challenge. In a recent study of fatigue in participants with COPD, Theander, Cliffordson, Torstensson, Jakobsson, and Unosson (2007) examined the validity of the FIS and reported reliability coefficients of .98 Cronbach's alpha and .94 test-retest stability indicating statistically significant performance. Researchers reported a significant correlation between the level of fatigue and participant reports of fatigue greater than or less than 6 hours daily. The research group then reduced the number of items on the FIS to 25 from the original 40 and psychometric performance was maintained with Cronbach's alpha at .96 and test-retest stability at .94 for the total scale.

23.1 | Assessment of Patterns of Sleep/Rest, Perceptions/Expressions of Fatigue, and Impact on Quality of Life

SLEEP/REST PATTERNS	PERCEPTIONS/EXPRESSIONS OF FATIGUE	IMPACT ON QUALITY OF LIFE
Do you nap?	What do you believe is the cause of your fatigue?	Do you feel the quality of your life has changed because of fatigue?
Do you feel rested after a nap?	Are you distressed by fatigue?	Can you work?
Do you have difficulty falling asleep at night or staying asleep?	What do you think is the meaning of this symptom?	Do you socialize?
Has the quality of your sleep at night changed?	Do you feel hopeful?	Has fatigue affected your relationship with others?
How do you feel when you awaken?	Has your appetite changed?	Are you able to enjoy life?
Has your sleeping environment changed?	Do you have other symptoms, such as pain?	Has fatigue affected your outlook?

Construct validity is difficult to establish for an instrument since fatigue measure may examine various aspects of fatigue, such as its character, precursors, or causes, or the effects of fatigue, and each aspect can be addressed from a physiological, psychosocial, or behavioral perspective (See Chapter 23 appendix, part A). Significant aspects of fatigue to assess when measuring fatigue vary among scales, and may include combinations of symptoms that are physical, cognitive, affective, or behavioral Participants in a qualitative investigation of fatigue among working adults described fatigue in characteristic themes that included manifestations in the physical, emotional, and behavioral realms (Aaronson et al., 2003). For example, objective physical manifestations of fatigue included the signs of slumped shoulders or drawn and slackened face that others can readily see, whereas the subjective physical manifestations of fatigue included symptoms not readily seen by others such as lack of energy and endurance, or weakness (Aaronson et al., 2003). Study participants described emotional, mental and behavioral symptoms that might also represent depressive symptoms including sadness, inability to concentrate, and irritability.

As the first characteristic of fatigue, subjective quantification can be measured by the multidimensional assessment of fatigue (MAF) measure (Tack, 1991), which examines the experience of fatigue in the past week and its severity, perceived distress, the timing of fatigue, and interference with activities of daily living. The MAF provides a Global Fatigue Index (Chapter 23 appendix, part C) developed to capture the subjective experience of fatigue for patients with rheumatoid arthritis (Belza, Henke, Yelin, Epstein, & Gilliss, 1993) and has been used with multiple patient populations including persons with COPD (Belza et al., 2005; Belza et al., 2001) and older adults (Belza, 1995). The Global Fatigue Index has also been shown to be a valid and reliable measure of fatigue in community based patients with HIV (Bormann, Shivley, Smith, & Gifford, 2001).

As the second characteristic of fatigue, subjective distress can be measured by a single item on the MAF or by the Symptom Distress Scale (McCorkle & Young, 1978). The Symptom Distress Scale (SDS) was originally developed as to contain 10 items on symptoms which included a single item on fatigue, addressed as "tiredness" in which patients respond to a 5-point semantic differential:

| Could not feel more tired | 5 4 3 2 1 | I am not tired at all |

A more recent version of the SDS is a 13-item self-administered questionnaire that assesses the subjective distress of the patient and demonstrates satisfactory validity and reliability (Cooley et al., 2005). Additionally, significant ($p < .05$) correlation has been found between fatigue and other physical and psychological symptoms, and highlights the potentially confounding relationship between fatigue and these co-occurring symptoms experienced by different clinical populations (Yennurajalingam et al., 2008).

The effect of fatigue on activities (third characteristic of fatigue) of daily living can be measured by an 11-item subscale of the MAF which provides a Global Fatigue Index with scores 1–50 indicating *no fatigue* to *severe fatigue* (Belza et al., 2005). The GFI has been shown to be sensitive to changes in the level of fatigue and as such is useful as a monitoring tool for patient response to treatment and rehabilitation. The report of activity interference may provide a more sensitive measure for assessing changes in fatigue or evaluation of the success of an intervention.

As the fourth characteristic of fatigue, correlates of fatigue can be assessed by evaluation of comorbidities and primary conditions, exacerbations, side effects of treatment, and psychosocial factors (Wagner & Cella, 2004). Measurement of comorbidities and primary conditions require attention to anemias, nutritional status, thyroid function, and infection. Additional correlates that affect fatigue that should be measured include sleep disturbance and changes in function, depression and anxiety, chronic pain, and adjustment to chronic illness. The Profile of Mood States (POMS) (McNair, Lorr, & Droppleman, 1992) is also a well-established measure of mood disturbance and includes subscales that measure fatigue and vigor.

These fatigue rating scales are best used in research studies. A brief visual rating scale is recommended as the most efficient assessment tool for clinical practice (National Institutes of Health, 2002, July 15–17). The measure may include one or two items that ask the client to rate the severity of fatigue from 1 (no fatigue) to 10 (severe fatigue), and/or the degree to which fatigue prevents or interferes with desired daily activities (degree of impairment from fatigue), also from 1 (no interference) to 10 (severe interference). A cut score of about 5 has been suggested for 10-point scales, or 3 for 4–5-point scales, so that persons with at least moderate fatigue will be captured (Butt et al., 2008; Kirsh, Passik, Holtsclaw, Donaghy, & Theobald, 2001; Wagner & Cella, 2004). Clinicians should consistently use the same scale and give the same instructions each time. The patient should be asked to rate their fatigue at the time of assessment and in the last 24 h.

MANAGEMENT OF FATIGUE

The goal of the management of fatigue for the older adult palliative care patient is to achieve the best quality of life that is possible given their specific circumstances. Having the energy to do what is important to the older adult so that they may finalize specific tasks or interact in special relationships is a valuable outcome for treatment. Within the context of palliative care, the management of fatigue must be determined in relation to its ability to protect individuals from activities that may lead to suffering and subsequent detrimental consequences (Radbruch et al., 2008). Its major impact on the quality of life in patients at the end-of life must be considered by nurses delivering palliative care.

Interventions for fatigue may focus on treating symptoms that exacerbate fatigue, preventing fatigue from progressing to extreme exhaustion for which there may be no means of recovery (Olson et al., 2007). Nurses may assist patients and families to balance rest with activity and identify those activities that increase fatigue or that restore energy. Interventions for fatigue include nonpharmacologic and pharmacological management, and are selected in accordance with the underlying cause of the fatigue. A multi-stage approach is recommended in the National Comprehensive Cancer Network Cancer-related Fatigue Guidelines: a) screening of patients for the presence of fatigue; b) evaluation of fatigue to determine its intensity or severity and its relationship to the stage of underlying disease processes; c) management with nonpharmacologic and pharmacologic interventions; and d) re-evaluation of the patients for improvement, alleviation of symptoms, or worsening of condition followed by effective adjustment of management strategies (National Comprehensive Cancer Network, 2009).

Learning to cope with fatigue is important to promoting quality of life. Energy conserving strategies may be used to manage and alter the fatigue, specifically: avoid unnecessary or excessive use of energy by pacing yourself and taking extra rest periods; energy restoration to avoid further deconditioning and deterioration in physical functioning through keeping their muscles strong through exercising; continue to be self-reliant by only asking for help when necessary, while taking into account the possibility of escalating fatigue at the end of life (National Comprehensive Cancer Network, 2009). Encourage patients to rejuvenate their energy through relaxation strategies such as "sitting down and resting," "putting your feet up with a cup of tea," and resting before activities by reading, watching television or taking relaxing baths. In a case report of a retired nurse at the end of life, fatigue was described in association with a myriad of symptoms including anemia, weight loss, loss of interest, social isolation, dyspnea, chronic pain, deconditioning, and medications (Yennurajalingam & Bruera, 2007). This patient refused testing for additional medical information that was not directed at improving her quality of life: an important point that highlights the importance of patient autonomy. It was important to the patient and her palliative care team that her symptoms be evaluated for the purpose of determining which interventions might reduce fatigue, thereby improving her quality of life (Yennurajalingam & Bruera, 2007).

Nonpharmacological Interventions

Nonpharmacological interventions for fatigue include education/cognitive interventions, exercise, energy balance and conservation, and nutritional considerations. Education/cognitive interventions include preparatory information and anticipatory guidance regarding the likelihood of fatigue as a side-effect of many treatment options, the disease itself, or the emotional reaction to the disease. It should be a standard of care that older adults are educated about cancer related fatigue to empower them to anticipate fatigue patterns and apply early home interventions (Ream, 2007).

Older adults are often comforted to know that fatigue is often an expected outcome, and not a sign of disease progression. An analogy that can be helpful in conceptualizing fatigue is of fatigue as a depletion of a "bank account" of energy. Patients are encouraged to plan the pace of activities for conservation of energy so that there is sufficient energy for selected, though perhaps fewer, activities (Ream, 2007). There is also a recommendation for acupressure or acupuncture for the relief of fatigue as has been demonstrated in patients with end stage renal disease (Cho & Tsay, 2004; McDougall, 2005).

Patients may be encouraged to keep a daily journal to identify the factors and activities associated with fatigue, energy depletion, and its restoration (Radbruch et al., 2008). The journal could provide a daily entry regarding information learned about engagement in activities, level of energy or fatigue, and impact of treatment on energy or fatigue. Such a journal will also help the older adult communicate with the healthcare provider regarding various concerns which may be alleviated by effective symptom management. The journal provides the practitioner with objective evidence of how the patient is doing on a day-to-day basis and may then counsel the older adult to plan their schedule to optimize peak energy times for high priority tasks. The older adult is then encouraged to accept help from available support persons for remaining tasks.

Exercise is an effective intervention for older adults who are fatigued and has been shown to reduce fatigue and increase overall feelings of physical and psychological well-being in older adults (Puetz, O'Connor, & Dishman, 2006). Exercise can take place in a structured rehabilitation or physical therapy department, particularly for those who would benefit from rehabilitation therapy for neuro-musculoskeletal deficits and for those who are fatigued due to cardiac or respiratory problems (Anish, 2005; Cramp & Daniel, 2008; Przybylowski et al., 2007). For others, there may be simply a personal commitment to walk outdoors on a regular basis. Whichever is chosen, the exercise program should be individualized with consideration for the patient's physical condition and other medical problems.

Patients should be instructed not to exercise to exhaustion but the activity should be done for several days of the week to be beneficial. Movement can prevent loss of muscle tone that is difficult to regain, and helps reduce the incidence of falls. Endorphins are released with even the slightest activity, resulting in increased mood and well-being. Exercise that utilizes the entire body will help maintain tone, strength and flexibility. Walking, swimming, gardening, or golf are all good considerations; encourage the patient to exercise at least 6 hours before their typical bedtime so that they will not have difficulty falling asleep.

For patients with progressive illness, Potter (1998) suggests that more appropriate than admitting patients to rehabilitation centers (which have a daily exercise program of 4 hours a day), is admission of these patients to a palliative care unit. On the palliative care unit, the majority of time can be devoted to promoting quality of life and comfort, and the older adult does not have to watch others improve dramatically while they are just too tired to participate. This approach balances quality of life and the limited amount of therapy, which may be better tolerated.

Energy use and conservation involves finding a balance between rest and exercise that will give patients the most energy to do the things that they would like to do. Sleep disturbance, including insomnia, have been shown to be components of cancer-related fatigue and should be treated (Rao & Cohen, 2004). Although patients may believe that more rest and sleep will increase energy, sleep is not restorative of energy in chronic conditions associated with fatigue. Suggest that the older person sleep no longer than is necessary which establishes a more solid, less fragmented sleep pattern. Waking up and going to sleep at the same time each day strengthens the circadian cycles, the disruption of which can contribute to depression (Rao & Cohen, 2004). Since cancer patients have been shown to have worse sleep quality and more sleep disturbance (Fernandes, Stone, Andrews, Morgan, & Sharma, 2006), strategies for establishing rest and sleep patterns may assist in improving sleep quality Strategies noted by nursing home residents in a study in Taiwan included taking prescribed medicines, lying down, changing position in bed, or take a walk, and think pleasant thoughts (Tsai, Wong, & Ku, 2008).

In a review of nonpharmacological management of fatigue in patients with specific autoimmune conditions including multiple sclerosis, systemic lupus erythematosus, and rheumatoid arthritis, recommendations were in the categories of low to moderate impact exercise, behavioral therapies (self-help information, readings, life modifications), and physiological treatment of symptoms (Neill, Belan, & Ried, 2006). Additionally, a review of fatigue among health professionals offered several strategies that may also be applicable to older adults in palliative care: encourage individuals to have some exposure to outside light each day, avoiding bright light before bedtime, establish a specific bedtime (with routines to prepare for sleep) and wake time (Owens, 2007). In addition to an established bedtime, a light bedtime snack and something warm to drink promotes sleep.

Bedtime routines can help the reticular activating system in the brain shut down for about the last half-hour in readying for sleep. Strategies to promote a restful sleep also include the reduction of environmental stimuli (e.g. noise, light), diversional activities to encourage sleep (music, aromatherapy, massage), and the avoidance of alcohol and stimulants (e.g. caffeine, nicotine, steroids). Adjusting the room temperature and humidity, as well as using pillows may also be helpful in providing support and comfort. Neill, Belan, and Ried (2006) concluded that cooling activities should be tailored to the comfort of the individual and may include cool baths or placing the extremities in cool water. If the patient is unable to fall asleep in 20 min, suggest getting out of bed and going into another room to read with a dim light, and returning to bed when they get sleepy.

Acknowledge that fatigue is not a sequestered symptom but one that will affect all aspects of the older adult's life. As such, the patient will need to save their energy and plan for activities that are very important to them. They should be asked what activities they enjoy most and be encouraged to schedule those activities for the time of the day that they have the most energy. Breaks should be scheduled during activities to help restore energy levels; taking short therapeutic naps (15–20 minutes) between the hours of 3 PM and 5 PM tend to be more restoring than getting into a longer, deeper sleep (Owens, 2007). Energy conservation techniques should be reinforced with the older adult; e.g. do activities sitting down, use a power scooter for grocery shopping; store frequently used items at chest level to avoid bending and stretching; put a terry robe on after the shower instead of using energy to dry off; or wear slip-on shoes. Providing devices such as a raised toilet seat, a reaching device, and walker can also help conserve energy for elders with progressive fatigue.

Older adults should also be encouraged to ask for help with specific chores. Some elders will see this type of interdependence as very threatening; try to help them see their energy as something to be "budgeted" and used for something that they enjoy or that is very important for them to do. Jakobsson and colleagues (2007) studied factors related to quality of life among older adults who were dependent on others for help with daily living and who were in pain. Their findings underscored the importance of evaluating and treating the complexity of accompanying symptoms, including fatigue and depression. The elder should be encouraged to feel that they have the option to "spend" their energy on anything that they wish, yet being mindful of their energy as a limited resource. Often reframing their fatigue as one of their resources gives them the enfranchisement that they need to ask for help.

Spending time with family and friends is also very important in promoting a sense of well-being, which may lessen the perception of fatigue. Prioritizing who they would like to visit with can be helpful, as well as planning such visits at a time of day when the patient has most energy to avoid excessive fatigue. Health professionals may also assist in addressing the negative impact of psychologic and social stressors and how to avoid or modify them (Winninghan, Nail, Burke, 1994).

Nutritional status is also an important consideration; low fat foods and small meals might be metabolized easier resulting in less energy used for digestion. Given that nutrition and hydration are important in preventing fatigue, increasing fluids may be of benefit, unless contraindicated by other medical problems. Protein intake and supplements can also be encouraged if the elder is having trouble with regular food. Recent data suggest that for patients with chronic fatigue syndrome, equal benefit was experienced from a low sugar, low yeast dietary regimen or from a diet of healthy eating, with evidence of decreased fatigue and improved quality of life (Hobday, Thomas, O'Donovan, Murphy, & Pinching, 2008). The healthy eating control group and the low sugar low yeast group treatment group each demonstrated difficulty maintaining compliance with dietary recommendations. Food intake and appetite entries might be a helpful addition to a daily journal for some patients, though food journaling was not found helpful in the study by Hobday and colleagues (2008). Pharmacological intervention may be necessary to boost appetite and energy.

Pharmacologic Interventions

Palliative care for the fatigued elder is different from the management typically provided for other symptoms. Pharmacologic management of other symptoms in palliative care often involves medications that are available to treat the actual cause of the symptom. Yet with fatigue, the cause may not be treatable, and in many cases medications may not be the primary intervention for this symptom (Matzo & Sherman, 2001). Furthermore, each medication that the patient receives should be reviewed for its potential for producing sedation and fatigue. Symptoms, such as vomiting and pain, should be optimally treated as their relief often decreases associated fatigue, improving feelings of general well-being. Elders should be made aware that the fatigue experienced with opioid therapy may decrease as tolerance to opioids develops. Optimizing the use of non-opioid analgesics and adjuvant therapies may also reduce fatigue associated with pain management.

Treatment of proinflammatory cytokines (tumor necrosis factor) has been associated with improvements in symptoms of fatigue. Etanercept, studied in a randomized, double-blind placebo study of patients with psoriasis, was associated with improvements in fatigue and depression scores (Tyring et al., 2006).

In addition to treating symptoms, such as pain, vomiting or dyspnea, that induce fatigue, other medications, such as corticosteroids, stimulants, and antidepressants have been of benefit (refer to Table 23.2). There is empirical support for the use of low-dose corticosteroids for patients with fatigue and loss of general feelings of well being, with recommendations for withdrawal of the medication if improvement does not occur within 5–7 days (Ream, 2007; Ream & Stone, 2004). Corticosteroids can improve appetite and elevate mood, resulting in an improved sense of well-being although the duration of effect may be limited. It must be remembered, however, that corticosteroids may easily be overlooked as a contributor to fatigue (Cornuz, Guessous, & Favrat, 2006). Most commonly, dexamethasone 1–2 mg twice daily or prednisone 5–10 mg twice daily is prescribed.

In a review of the pharmacological treatment of cancer-related fatigue, the psychostimulant methylphenidate (ritalin) was found to reduce fatigue over a period of 5 weeks when compared to placebo (Minton, Richardson, Sharpe, Hotopf, & Stone, 2008). Dosing of 10–20 mg per day is recommended, based on patient improvement over a period of 2–5 weeks (Minton et al., 2008; Ream, 2007). The dose can be gradually increased until favorable effects occur or until toxicities, such as anorexia, insomnia, anxiety, confusion, tremor, or tachycardia, supervenes. A report of the National Comprehensive Cancer Network (2009) indicated that dextroamphetamine produced short-term reduction of fatigue in survivors of breast cancer, patients with advanced cancer, and persons with HIV. Benefits were short-lived, however, with no continuation of improvement noted after 8 days, the duration of the study by Cella, Davis, Breitbart, and Curt (2001). Mixed results have been reported on the use of carnitine as a micronutrient replacement, or on the use of modafinil as an agent to promote wakefulness in persons with advanced cancer; further studies were recommended (National Comprehensive Cancer Network, 2009). To limit toxicities in the medically ill population, dose escalation should be undertaken with caution, and over longer intervals (Portenoy, 2000).

When fatigue is associated with clinical depression, a trial of an antidepressant drug is appropriate. Depression and cancer-related fatigue may occur as separate conditions, and should be treated accordingly (Minton et al., 2008). Antidepressants such as serotonin-specific reuptake inhibitors (SSRIs) have fewer side effects than older antidepressants and are preferred in patients with such chronic conditions as ischemic heart disease, hypertrophic prostatic conditions, or glaucoma that is not controlled (Rao & Cohen, 2004). SSRIs are not associated with food and drug interaction restrictions. A sedating antidepressant can provide peaceful sleep as

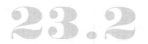

| Pharmacologic Therapies for the Treatment of Fatigue |

CLASS OF DRUG	EXAMPLES	MECHANISM OF ACTION	COMMENTS
Corticosteroids (glucocorticoids)	Dexamethasone (1–2 mg BID)	Mechanism of action is unclear, low dosing recommended.	May mask the signs of acute infections
	Prednisone/prednisolone (5–10 mg BID) Methyl-prednisolone Hydrocortisone	Duration and benefits limited to weeks, may boost appetite and energy; may improve activity levels and strength	Evidence is inconclusive regarding lessening of fatigue; effectiveness may be short-lived (Radbruch et al., 2008)
Stimulants	Methylphenidate (2.5–5 mg daily or BID)	Stimulates CNS and respiratory centers, increases appetite & energy levels, improves mood, reduces sedation (Bruera, Chadwick, & Brennis, 1985)	Titrate to effect, rapid onset of action, fewer side effects than many antidepressants, may cause agitation (Beers & Berkow, 2000). Risk of toxicity increases with dose
	Dextroamphetamine (2.5–5 mg daily or BID) and pemoline (18.75 mg daily or BID) have been used anecdotally.		No controlled comparisons between efficacies of each of these drugs. Response to one does not predict response to others. Sequential trials to determine the most useful drug are suggested (Breitbart, Esch, Porteny, 1997)
	Modafinil (200 mg daily with titration up to 400 mg daily)	Inhibits GABA; promotes release of neurotransmitters dopamine, norepinephrine, and serotonin (Radbruch et al., 2008)	Routine use of stimulants in palliative care is controversial as related to evaluation of evidence, and concerns that fatigue at the end of life may not be responsive (Radbruch et al., 2008).
	Amantadine	Centrally-acting: affects cholinergic, dopaminergic, adrenergic, glutamatergic neurotransmission	
Antidepressants	Trazodone (25–50 mg at bedtime, increase to 25–50 mg/day as tolerated to a maximum of 300 mg/day) (Beers & Berkow, 2000)	Reduces depressive symptoms associated with fatigue. Can improve sleep. Primary choice for treatment of depression in cancer patients	
■ Selective serotonin reuptake inhibitors (SSRIs)	Paroxetine (10 mg) Fluoxetine (10 mg) Sertraline (25 mg)	Inhibits serotonin reuptake	Give once daily in the morning. Some SSRIs have long half-lives and should be used cautiously in the terminally ill older adult
■ Tricyclic antidepressants	Amitriptyline (10–25 mg q hs) Nortriptyline (25 mg 3–4 times daily)	Block reuptake of various neurotransmitters at the neuronal membrane. Can improve sleep	Amitriptyline contraindicated in patients on MAOIs or post MI. Use with caution in elders with cardiovascular disease, adverse reaction includes arrhythmias
Erythropoietin	150 Units/kg SQ 3 times a week	Increases hemoglobin with effects on energy, activity & overall quality of life while decreasing transfusion requirements (Krammer et al., 1999)	Monitor hematocrit and reduce dose if HCT approaches 36% or increases by > 4 points in 2 weeks

well as mitigating the depression; potential neurologic and cardiac disadvantages may be of a lesser concern for the dying elder or for the palliative care patient at the end of life.

If the elder has had chemotherapy, the fatigue may be a result of anemia. Treatment with recombinant erythropoietin has been shown in randomized studies to increase hemoglobin level, which improves the patient with cancer-related fatigue energy levels and quality of life (Minton et al., 2008; Ream, 2007) although the impact on the intensity of fatigue may be limited in advanced cancer states (Yennurajalingam & Bruera, 2007). When the elder's hemoglobin level returns to 11 g/dL or 12 g/dL, many of the symptoms of anemia are assuaged. Treatment may also include addressing such nutrient deficiencies as iron, folate, or vitamin B-12. Anemia can also be treated with blood transfusions, but this intervention is not without substantial risks to the patient's health (Yennurajalingam & Bruera) and carries the potential of increasing health-care costs in the wake of transfusion complications. Risks associated with blood transfusions include systemic infections (e.g. HIV; hepatitis A, B, C) from inadequate screening of the blood supply, acute hemolytic reactions, bacterial contamination, subtle immune modulation, transfusion graft versus host disease, iron overload, and allergic reactions including urticaria, anaphylaxis (Yennurajalingam & Bruera).

It is important to evaluate the efficacy of both pharmacologic and nonpharmacologic fatigue interventions on a regular basis. Systematic documentation regarding the assessment, management, and evaluation of the success of the interventions in relieving fatigue is essential to quality care.

Fatigue in Family Caregivers

Family caregivers are often profoundly fatigued by the stressors inherent in care giving. Caregivers bear the physical and emotional burden of assisting elder patients with activities of daily living, as well as with treatments. They often must assume new roles and responsibilities and at times deal with additional financial distress (Abbey, 2000). As a result, family caregivers may also develop anxiety or depressive disorders associated with fatigue. Severe family fatigue is commonly experienced in four situations: 1) Inadequate relief of patient's pain and suffering; 2)Inadequate resources to cope with home care; 3) Unrealistic expectations of family caregivers of themselves or professional health-care supports; and 4) Emotional distress that persists even when there is adequate relief of patient suffering (Cherny, 2000).

Palliative care recognizes the patient and family as the unit of care, and therefore assessment and interventions to relieve caregiver burden are essential. Validating the needs and concerns of family caregivers

is important. Helping family caregivers to set priorities with regard to competing demands, optimizing stress and coping strategies, encouraging relaxation and rest, while assisting caregivers with respite care, are important interventions in preventing or alleviating caregiver fatigue (Abbey, 2000).

Case Study conclusion: Ms. Seigal's fatigue was managed through several therapeutic approaches. Laboratory data revealed a persistent anemia, which was treated with iron supplements. Discussion also focused on a well-balanced diet and daily multi-vitamin supplementation. Ms. Seigal agreed to make a personal commitment to regular exercise by walking outdoors for 20 min each day to promote muscle tone, increase endorphin levels, decrease fatigue, and improve mood and sense of well-being. The palliative care nurse helped Ms. Seigal to learn to balance rest with activity, shortening her work day, prioritizing activities, and carrying out activities when she had the greatest energy. Ms. Seigal was comforted by an understanding that fatigue is a common response to surgery, chemotherapy, and radiation for up to 5 years, versus considering her fatigue as indicative of disease progression.

Screening by the palliative care team also indicated that Ms. Seigal suffered from depressive symptoms, which exacerbated her perception of fatigue. To treat her depressive symptoms, Ms. Seigal continued meeting with the psychologist referred by the cancer center to discuss her feelings and fears (talk therapy). She was prescribed a selective serotonin reuptake inhibitor and vitamin B-12 by the palliative care nurse practitioner (pharmacologic therapy), and was encouraged to re-join the women's circle at her local senior center (social support). She refused a blood transfusion and erythropoietin therapy. Ms. Seigal was a participant in a breast cancer support group and recognized the value of providing support to those who were in the position where she had been, accepting help from willing friends (social support). She was counseled regarding strategies to promote a restful night sleep, including establishing regular bedtime routines, and establishing a quiet, relaxing environment. The plan of care involved continual evaluation of the efficacy of such interventions for fatigue. If necessary, a trial of dexamethasone would also be considered to decrease a sense of fatigue and promote maximal sense of well-being. During the follow-up evaluation, Ms. Seigal expressed a lessening of fatigue, greater sense of control, and improvement in health-related quality of life.

CONCLUSION

Healthcare professionals view fatigue as a clue to illness, a side effect of therapeutic intervention, progressive illness, the residual physical change of illness and treatment or the psychological and emotional strain of illness or caregiving. To the older adult and their family, fatigue is a symptom that keeps them from moving forward fully with life (Greenberg, 1998). Health professionals can be supportive by acknowledging fatigue as real and taking fatigue and its frustrations seriously. Understanding the possible etiology of fatigue and the meaning of the symptom to the patient are important in determining its management. Assisting older adults to live fully as they move along the illness trajectory may require consideration of nonpharmacologic, as well as pharmacologic therapies to comprehensively and effectively treat fatigue. Learning how to prevent fatigue and/or restore energy is important to improving the elder patient's function, their ability to socialize, and ultimately their adjustment to a "new normal" baseline as they live with a life-limiting or chronic illness (Harpham, 1999).

EVIDENCE-BASED PRACTICE

Olson, K., Turner, A. R., Courneya, K. S., Field, C., Man, G., Cree, M., et al. (2008). Possible links between behavioral and physiological indices of tiredness, fatigue, and exhaustion in advanced cancer. *Supportive Care in Cancer, 16*(3), 241–249.

Research question. The authors utilized an evidence-based model to develop an Edmonton fatigue framework (EFF), for the study of tiredness, fatigue, and exhaustion in advanced cancer.

Design and setting. Data were gathered from published studies pertaining to fatigue in depression, chronic fatigue syndrome, cancer, shift workers, and athletes published between 1995–2004 and further expanded in 2006.

Findings. The EFF provides new insights into possible links between behavioral and physiological indices of tiredness, fatigue, and exhaustion as they occur in both ill and non-ill states. Specific to people with advanced cancer, the authors documented that the cancer diagnosis and the subsequent treatment results in declines in cognitive function, sleep quality, nutrition, and muscle endurance. These declines, along with the interaction among these declines are the likely cause of fatigue in this population.

Conclusions. The authors suggest that effective interventions for patients with advanced cancer could benefit from a focus on the interactions among cognitive function, sleep quality, nutrition, and muscle endurance. Symptoms should be evaluated in clusters when interventions are being evaluated.

REFERENCES

Aaronson, L. S., Pallikkathayil, L., & Crighton, F. (2003). A qualitative investigation of fatigue among healthy working adults. *Western Journal of Nursing Research, 25*(4), 419–433.

Aaronson, L. S., Teel, C. S., Cassmeyer, V., Neuberger, G. B., Pallikkathayil, L., Pierce, J., et al. (1999). State of the science: Defining and measuring fatigue. *Image: Journal of Nursing Scholarship, 31*(1), 45–50.

American Association of Colleges of Nursing. (2005). *Peaceful death: Recommended competencies and curricular guidelines for end-of-life nursing care.* Retrieved from http://www.aacn.nche.edu/Education/deathfin.htm

American Psychiatric Association. (2000). *Diagnostic and statistical manual of mental disorders* [Text Revision] (4th ed.). Washington, DC: American Psychiatric Association.

Anish, E. J. (2005). Exercise and its effects on the central nervous system. *Current Sports Medicine Reports, 4*(1), 18–23.

Balducci, L., Ershler, W., & Gaetano, G. (Eds.). (2008). *Blood disorders in the elderly.* New York: Cambridge University Press.

Barnason, S., Zimmerman, L., Nieveen, J., Schulz, P., Miller, C., Hertzog, M., et al. (2008). Relationships between fatigue and early postoperative recovery outcomes over time in elderly patients undergoing coronary artery bypass graft surgery. *Heart and Lung: Journal of Acute and Critical Care, 37*(4), 245–256.

Barnes, E. A., & Bruera, E. (2002). Fatigue in patients with advanced cancer: A review. *International Journal of Gynecological Cancer, 12*(5), 424–428.

Barroso, J. (2002). HIV-related fatigue. *American Journal of Nursing, 102*(5).

Belza, B., Henke, C. J., Yelin, E. H., Epstain, W. V., & Gillis, C. L. (1993). Correlates of fatigue in older adults with rheumatoid arthritis *Nursing Research 42*, 93–99.

Belza, B., Steele, B. G., Cain, K., Coppersmith, J., Howard, J., & Lakshminarayan, S., et al. (2005). Seattle obstructive lung disease questionnaire: Sensitivity to outcomes in pulmonary rehabilitation in severe pulmonary illness. *Journal of Cardiopulmonary Rehabilitation, 25*(2), 107–114.

Belza, B., Steele, B. G., Hunziker, J., Lakshminaryan, S., Holt, L., & Buchner, D. M., et al. (2001). Correlates of physical activity in chronic obstructive pulmonary disease. *Nursing Research, 50*(4), 195–202.

Biagini, M. R., Tozzi, A., Milani, S., Grippo, A., Amantini, A., Capanni, M., et al. (2008). Fatigue in primary biliary cirrhosis: A possible role of comorbidities. *European Journal of Gastroenterology and Hepatology, 20*(2), 122–126.

Bjornsson, E., Simren, M., Olsson, R., & Chapman, R. W. (2005). Fatigue is not a specific symptom in patients with primary biliary cirrhosis. *European Journal of Gastroenterology and Hepatology, 17*(3), 351–357.

Bonner, A., Wellard, S., & Caltabiano, M. (2008). Levels of fatigue in people with ESRD living in far North Queensland [research]. *Journal of Clinical Nursing, 17*, 90–98.

Bormann, J., Shivley, M., Smith, T. L., & Gifford, A. L. (2001). Measurement of fatigue in HIV-positive adults: Reliability and validity of the global fatigue index. *Journal of the Association of Nurses in AIDS Care, 12*(3), 75–83.

Butt, Z., Wagner, L. I., Beaumont, J. L., Paice, J. A., Peterman, A. H., Shevrin, D., et al. (2008). Use of a single-item screening tool to detect clinically significant fatigue, pain, distress, and anorexia in ambulatory cancer practice. *Journal of Pain and Symptom Management, 35*(1), 20–30.

Cella, D., Davis, K., Breitbart, W., & Curt, G. (2001). Cancer-related fatigue: Prevalence of proposed diagnostic criteria in a

United States sample of cancer survivors. *Journal of Clinical Oncology, 19*(14), 3385–3391.

Centers for Disease Control and Prevention. (2006). *CFS: Diagnostic symptoms.* Retrieved October 2008 from http://www.cdc.gov/cfs/cfssymptomsHCP.htm

Centers for Medicare & Medicaid Services. (2002). *MDS 2.0 for nursing homes.* Retrieved February 6, 2009 from http://www.cms.hhs.gov/NursingHomeQualityInits/20_NHQIMDS20.asp

Cho, Y. C., & Tsay, S. L. (2004). The effect of acupressure with massage on fatigue and depression in patients with end-stage renal disease. *Journal of Nursing Research, 12*(1), 51–59.

Cooley, M. E., McCorkle, R., Knafl, G. J., Rimar, J., Barbieri, M. J., Davies, M., et al. (2005). Comparison of health-related quality of life questionnaires in ambulatory oncology. *Quality of Life Research, 14*(5), 1239–1249.

Cornuz, J., Guessous, I., & Favrat, B. (2006). Fatigue: A practical approach to diagnosis in primary care. *Canadian Medical Association Journal, 174*(6), 765–767.

Cramp, F., & Daniel, J. (2008). Exercise for the management of cancer-related fatigue in adults. *Cochrane Database of Systematic Reviews,* (2), CD006145.

Dagnelie, P. C., Pijls-Johannesma, M. C. G., Pijpe, A., Boumans, B. J. E., Skrabanja, A. T. P., Lambin, P., et al. (2006). Psychometric properties of the revised piper fatigue scale in Dutch cancer patients were satisfactory. *Journal of Clinical Epidemiology, 59*(6), 642–649.

De Vries, J., Michielsen, H. J., & Van Heck, G. L. (2003). Assessment of fatigue among working people: A comparison of six questionnaires. *Occupational and Environmental Medicine, 60*(90001), i10–15.

Dean, G. E., & Anderson, P. R. (2001). Fatigue. In B. R. Ferrell & N. Coyle (Eds.), *The textbook of palliative nursing* (pp. 91–100). New York: Oxford University Press.

Delglin, J. H., & Vallerand, A. H. (2005). *Davis's drug guide for nurses* (9th ed.). Philadelphia: F. A. Davis.

Duncan, J. G., Forbes-Thompson, S., & Bott, M. J. (2008). Unmet symptom management needs of nursing home residents with cancer. *Cancer Nursing 31*(4), 265–273.

Eliopoulos, C. (2005). *Gerontological nursing* (6th ed.). Philadelphia: Lippincott Williams & Williams.

Elkington, H., White, P., Addington-Hall, J., Higgs, R., & Edmonds, P. (2005). The healthcare needs of chronic obstructive pulmonary disease patients in the last year of life. *Palliative Medicine, 19*(6), 485–491.

Evans, W. J., & Lambert, C. P. (2007). Physiological basis of fatigue. *American Journal of Physical Medicine and Rehabilitation, 86*(1), S29–S46.

Fernandes, R., Stone, P., Andrews, P., Morgan, R., & Sharma, S. (2006). Comparison between fatigue, sleep disturbance, and circadian rhythm in cancer inpatients and healthy volunteers: Evaluation of diagnostic criteria for cancer-related fatigue. *Journal of Pain and Symptom Management, 32*(3), 245–254.

Fisk, J. D., Ritvo, P. G., Ross, L., Haase, D. A., Marrie, T. J., & Schlech, W. F., et al. (1994). Measuring the functional impact of fatigue: Initial validation of the fatigue impact scale. *Clinical Infectious Diseases, 18,* S79–S83.

Fitts, R. H. (2008). The cross-bridge cycle and skeletal muscle fatigue. *J Appl Physiol, 104*(2), 551–558.

Geisser, M. E., Strader Donnell, C., Petzke, F., Gracely, R. H., Clauw, D. J., & Williams, D. A., et al.(2008). Comorbid somatic symptoms and functional status in patients with fibromyalgia and chronic fatigue syndrome: Sensory amplification as a common mechanism. *Psychosomatics, 49*(3), 235–242.

Goedendorp, M. M., Gielissen, M. F., Verhagen, C. A., Peters, M. E., Bleijenberg, G., Gielissen, M. F. M., et al. (2008). Severe fatigue and related factors in cancer patients before the initiation of treatment. *British Journal of Cancer, 99*(9), 1408–1414.

Gray, S. L., LaCroix, A. Z., Aragaki, A. K., McDermott, M., Cochrane, B. B., Kooperberg, C. L., et al. (2009). Angiotensin-converting enzyme inhibitor use and incident frailty in women aged 65 and older: Prospective findings from the women's health initiative observational study. *Journal of the American Geriatrics Society, 57*(2), 297–303.

Halkett, G. K., Kristjanson, L. J., & Lobb, E. A. (2008). 'If we get too close to your bones they'll go brittle': Women's initial fears about radiotherapy for early breast cancer [Research Support, Non-U.S. Gov't]. *Psycho-Oncology, 17*(9), 877–884.

Hemani, S., & Letizia, M. (2008). Proving palliative care in end-stage heart failure. *Journal of Hospice and Palliative Nursing, 10*(2), 100–105.

Heo, S., Doering, L. V., Widener, J., & Moser, D. K. (2008). Predictors and effect of physical symptom status on health-related quality of life in patients with heart failure. *American Journal of Critical Care, 17*(2), 124–132.

Hinds, P. S., Hockenberry-Eaton, M. J., & Gilger, E. (1999). Comparing patient, parent, and staff descriptions of fatigue in pediatric oncology patients. *Cancer Nursing, 22*(4), 277–288.

Hobday, R. A., Thomas, S., O'Donovan, A., Murphy, M., & Pinching, A. J. (2008). Dietary intervention in chronic fatigue syndrome. *Journal of Human Nutrition and Dietetics, 21*(2), 141–149.

Hockenberry, M. J., Hinds, P. S., & Barrera, P. (2003). Three instruments to assess fatigue in children with cancer: The child, parent, and staff perspectives. *Journal of Pain and Symptom Management, 25*(4), 319–328.

Hunt, S. A., Abraham, W. T., Chin, M. H., Feldman, A. M., Francis, G. S., Ganiats, T. G., et al. (2005). ACC/AHA 2005 guideline update for the diagnosis and management of chronic heart failure in the adult: A report of the American college of cardiology/American heart association task force on practice guidelines (writing committee to update the 2001 guidelines for the evaluation and management of heart failure): Developed in collaboration with the American college of chest physicians and the international society for heart and lung transplantation: Endorsed by the heart rhythm society. *Circulation, 112*(12), e154–235.

Hwang, J. H., Chang, H. J., Shim, Y. H., Park, W. H., Park, W., Huh, S. J., et al. (2008). Effects of supervised exercise therapy in patients receiving radiotherapy for breast cancer. *Yonsei Medical Journal, 49*(3), 443–450.

Jain, R., & Jain, S. (2008). Fibromyalgia: A review of recent treatment guidelines and emerging therapies in the pipeline. *Psychiatric Times, 25,* 20–23.

Jakobsson, U., Hallberg, I. R., & Westergren, A. (2007). Exploring determinants for quality of life among older people in pain and in need of help for daily living. *Journal of Nursing and Healthcare of Chronic Illness in association with Journal of Clinical Nursing, 16*(3a), 95–104.

Jamsell, L., Kreicbergs, U., & Onelov, E. (2006). Symptoms affecting children with malignancies during the last month of life: A nationwide follow-up. *Pediatrics, 117*(4), 1314–1320.

Johansson, S., Ytterberg, C., Hillert, J., Holmqvist, L. W., & von Koch, L. (2008). A longitudinal study of variations in and predictors of fatigue in multiple sclerosis [short report]. *Journal of Neurological and Neurosurgical Psychiatry, 79,* 454–457.

Jorgensen, R. (2008). Chronic fatigue: An evolutionary concept analysis. *Journal of Advanced Nursing, 63*(2), 199–207.

Kapella, M. C., Larson, J. L., Patel, M. K., Covey, M. K., & Berry, J. K. (2006). Subjective fatigue, influencing variables, and consequences in chronic obstructive pulmonary disease. *Nursing Research, 55*(1), 10–17.

Kasatkin, D. S., & Spirin, N. N. (2007). Possible mechanisms of the formation of chronic fatigue syndrome in the clinical picture of multiple sclerosis [Review]. *Neuroscience and Behavioral Physiology, 37*(3), 215–219.

Kirsh, K. L., Passik, S., Holtsclaw, E., Donaghy, K., & Theobald, D. (2001). I get tired for no reason: A single item screening for cancer-related fatigue. *Journal of Pain and Symptom Management, 22*(5), 931–937.

Kukull, W. A., McCorkle, R., & Driever, M. (1986). Symptom distress, psychosocial variables and survival from lung cancer. *Journal of Psychosocial Oncology, 4,* 91–104.

Lee, K. A., Portillo, C. J., & Miramontes, H. (2001). The influence of sleep and activity patterns on fatigue in women with HIV/AIDS. *Journal of the Association of Nurses in AIDS Care, 12*(Suppl), 19–27.

Leone, S. S., Huibers, M. J. H., Knottnerus, J. A., & Kant, I. J. (2007). Similarities, overlap and differences between burnout and prolonged fatigue in the working population. *Q J Med, 100,* 616–627.

Lindqvist, O., Widmark, A., & Rasmussen, B. H. (2004). Meanings of the phenomenon of fatigue as narrated by 4 patients with cancer in palliative care. *Cancer Nursing 27*(3), 237–243.

Lundberg, P. C., & Rattanasuwan, O. (2007). Experiences of fatigue and self-management of thai buddhist cancer patients undergoing radiation therapy. *Cancer Nursing 30*(2), 146–155.

McCorkle, R., & Young, K. (1978). Development of a symptom distress scale. *Cancer Nursing, 1*(5), 373–378.

McDougall, G. J. (2005). Research review: The effect of acupressure with massage on fatigue and depression in patients with end-stage renal disease. *Geriatric Nursing, 26*(3), 164–165.

Melchert, M., & Lancet, J. (2008). Acute myeloid leukemia in the elderly. In L. Balducci, W. Ershler & G. Gaetano (Eds.), *Blood disorders in the elderly.* New York: Cambridge University Press.

Minton, O., Richardson, A., Sharpe, M., Hotopf, M., & Stone, P. (2008). A systematic review and meta-analysis of the pharmacological treatment of cancer-related fatigue. *Journal of the National Cancer Institute, 100*(16), 1155–1166.

Minton, O., & Stone, P. (2008). How common is fatigue in disease-free breast cancer survivors? A systematic review of the literature. *Breast Cancer Research and Treatment, 112*(1), 5–13.

National Comprehensive Cancer Network. (2009). *NCCN clinical practice guidelines in oncology: Cancer-related fatigue.* National Comprehensive Cancer Network.

National Consensus Project for Quality Palliative Care (Writer). (2009). *Clinical practice guidelines for quality palliative care.*

National Institute of Mental Health. (2002). *Depression.* Bethesda, MD: National Institute of Mental Health.

National Institutes of Health (2002, July 15–17). Symptom management in cancer: Pain, depression, and fatigue. *NIH Consensus and State-of-the-Science Statements*: National Institutes of Health (2004). *National Institutes of Health State-of-the-Science Conference Statement: Symptom Management in Cancer: Pain, Depression, and Fatigue.* Paper presented at the Journal of the National Cancer Institute Monographs. Retrieved *July 15–17, 2002.* from http://jncimono.oxfordjournals.org/cgi/content/abstract/jncimono;2004/32/9

Neill, J. (2005). Exploring underlying life patterns of women with multiple sclerosis or rheumatoid arthritis: Comparison with NANDA dimensions. *Nursing Science Quarterly, 18*(4), 344–352.

Neill, J., Belan, I., & Ried, K. (2006). Effectiveness of non-pharmacological interventions for fatigue in adults with multiple sclerosis, rheumatoid arthritis, or systemic lupus erythematosus: A systematic review. *Journal of Advanced Nursing, 56*(6), 617–635.

Neuberger, G. B., Aaronson, L. S., Gajewski, B., Embretson, S. E., Cagle, P. E., Loudon, J. K., et al. (2007). Predictors of exercise and effects of exercise on symptoms, function, aerobic fitness, and disease outcomes of rheumatoid arthritis. *Arthritis and Rheumatism, 57*(6), 943–952.

Nieboer, P., Buijs, C., Rodenhuis, S., Seynaeve, C., Beex, L. V. A. M., van der Wall, E., et al. (2005). Fatigue and relating factors in high-risk breast cancer patients treated with adjuvant standard or high-dose chemotherapy: A longitudinal study. *Journal of Clinical Oncology, 23*(33), 8296–8304.

Nordgren, L., & Sorensen, S. (2003). Symptoms experienced in the last six months of life in patients with end-stage heart failure. *European Journal of Cardiovascular Nursing, 2*(3), 213–217.

O'Sullivan, D., & McCarthy, G. (2007). An exploration of the relationship between fatigue and physical functioning in patients with end stage renal disease receiving haemodialysis [original research]. *Journal of Nursing and Healthcare of Chronic Illness in association with Journal of Clinical Nursing, 16*(11c), 276–284.

Olson, K., Krawchuk, A., & Quddusi, T. (2007). Fatigue in individuals with advanced cancer in active treatment and palliative settings. *Cancer Nursing, 30*(4), E1–10.

Owens, J. A. (2007). Sleep loss and fatigue in healthcare professionals. *Journal of Perinatal and Neonatal Nursing, 21*(2), 92–100.

Petersen, I., Thomas, J. M., Hamilton, W. T., & White, P. D. (2006). Risk and predictors of fatigue after infectious mononucleosis in a large primary-care cohort. *Qjm, 99*(1), 49–55.

Piper, B. F. (1989). Fatigue: Current basis of practice. In S. G. Funk, E. M. Funk & M. T. Champagne (Eds.), *Key aspects of comfort* (pp. 187–198). New York: Springer Publishers.

Piper, B. F., Dibble, S. L., Dodd, M. J., Weiss, M. C., Slaughter, R. E., & Paul, S. M., et al. (1998). The revised piper fatigue scale: Psychometric evaluation in women with breast cancer. *Oncology Nursing Forum, 25*(4), 677–684.

Piper, B. F., Lindsey, A. M., & Dodd, M. J. (1989). The development of an instrument to measure the subjective dimension of fatigue. In S. G. Funk, E. M. Funk & M. T. Champagne (Eds.), *Key aspects of comfort* (pp. 199–208). New York: Springer Publishers.

Portenoy, R. (2003). Fatigue. In M. B. Max & J. Lynn (Eds.), *Symptom research: Methods and opportunities.*: National Institutes of Health; Department of Health and Human Services.

Post-White, J. (2006). Complementary and alternative medicine in pediatric oncology. *Journal of Pediatric Oncology Nursing, 23,* 244–253.

Przybylowski, T., Bielicki, P., Kumor, M., Hildebrand, K., Maskey-Warzechowska, M., Korczynski, P., et al. (2007). Exercise capacity in patients with obstructive sleep apnea syndrome. *Journal of Physiology and Pharmacology, 58*(Suppl 5 (Pt 2)), 563–574.

Puetz, T. W., O'Connor, P. J., & Dishman, R. K. (2006). Effects of chronic exercise on feelings of energy and fatigue: A quantitative synthesis. *Psychological Bulletin, 132*(6), 866–876.

Putman-Casdorph, H., & McCrone, S. (2009). Chronic obstructive pulmonary disease, anxiety, and depression: State of the science. *Heart and Lung: Journal of Acute and Critical Care, 38*(1), 34–47.

Radbruch, L., Strasser, F., Elsner, F., Goncalves, J. F., Loge, J., Kaasa, S., et al. (2008). Fatigue in palliative care patients—an EAPC approach. *Palliative Medicine, 22*(1), 13–32.

Ranjith, G. (2005). Epidemiology of chronic fatigue syndrome [Review]. *Occupational Medicine (Oxford), 55*(1), 13–19.

Rao, A., & Cohen, H. J. (2004). Symptom management in the elderly cancer patient: fatigue, pain, and depression. *Journal of the National Cancer Institute Monographs, 2004*(32), 150–157.

Ream, E. (2007). Fatigue in patients receiving palliative care. *Nursing Standard, 21*(28), 49.

Ream, E., & Stone, P. (2004). Clinical interventions for fatigue. In J. Armes, M. Krishnasamy & I. Higginson (Eds.), *Fatigue in cancer* (pp. 255–277). New York: Oxford University Press.

Repping-Wuts, H., Fransen, J., van Achterberg, T., Bleijenberg, G., & van Riel, P. (2007). Persistent severe fatigue in patients with rheumatoid arthritis [original]. *Journal of Nursing and Healthcare of Chronic Illness; Journal of Clinical Nursing, 16*(11c), 377–383.

Robinson, K. M., & Tappen, R. M. (2008). Policy recommendations on the prevention of violence in long-term care facilities. *Journal of Gerontological Nursing, 34*(3), 10–14.

Rosen, T., Lachs, M. S., Bharucha, A. J., Stevens, S. M., Teresi, J. A., Nebres, F., et al. (2008). Resident-to-resident aggression in long-term care facilities: Insights from focus groups of nursing home residents and staff. *Journal of the American Geriatrics Society, 56*(8), 1398–1408.

Rosenthal, T. C., Majeroni, B. A., Pretorius, R., Malik, K., Rosenthal, T. C., Majeroni, B. A., et al. (2008). Fatigue: An overview. *American Family Physician, 78*(10), 1173–1179.

Russ, D. W., Towse, T. F., Wigmore, D. M., Lanza, I. R., & Kent-Braun, J. A. (2008). Contrasting influences of age and sex on muscle fatigue. *Medicine and Science in Sports and Exercise, 40*(2), 234–241.

Saguil, A. (2005). Evaluation of the patient with muscle weakness [Review]. *American Family Physician, 71*(7), 1327–1336.

Stephen, S. A. (2008). Fatigue in older adults with stable heart failure. *Heart and Lung, 37*(2), 122–131.

Tartaglia, M. C., Narayanan, S., & Arnold, D. L. (2008). Mental fatigue alters the pattern and increases the volume of cerebral activation for a motor task in multiple sclerosis patients with fatigue. *European Journal of Neurology, 15*, 413–419.

Teitelbaum, J. (2008). From fatigued to FANTASTIC! *Total Health, 30*(1), 22–26.

Tellez, N., Rio, J., Tintore, M., Nos, C., Galan, I., & Montalban, X., et al. (2005). Does the modified fatigue impact scale offer a more comprehensive assessment of fatigue in MS? *Multiple Sclerosis, 11*(2), 198–202.

Theander, K., Cliffordson, C., Torstensson, O., Jakobsson, P., & Unosson, M. (2007). Fatigue impact scale: Its validation in patients with chronic obstructive pulmonary disease. *Psychology, Health and Medicine, 12*(4), 470–484.

Theander, K., & Unosson, M. (2004). Fatigue in patients with chronic obstructive pulmonary disease. *Journal of Advanced Nursing, 45*(2), 172–177.

Tsai, Y. F., Wong, T. K., & Ku, Y. C. (2008). Self-care management of sleep disturbances and risk factors for poor sleep among older residents of Taiwanese nursing homes. *Journal of Clinical Nursing, 17*(9), 1219–1226.

Turan, Y., DuruM. T., Bal, S., Guvenc, A., Cerrahoglu, L., & Gurgan, A., et al. (2007). Assessment of fatigue in patients with ankylosing spondylitis. *Rheumatology International, 27*, 847–852.

Tyring, S., Gottlieb, A., Papp, K., Gordon, K., Leonardi, C., Wang, A., et al. (2006). Etanercept and clinical outcomes, fatigue, and depression in psoriasis: Double-blind placebo-controlled randomised phase III trial. *Lancet, 367*(9504), 29–35.

Ulrich, C. K., & Mayer, O. H. (2007). Assessment and management of fatigue and dyspnea in pediatric palliative care. *Pediatric Clinics of North America, 54*, 735–756.

van Kessel, K., Moss-Morris, R., Willoughby, E., Chalder, T., Johnson, M. H., & Robinson, E., et al. (2008). A randomized controlled trial of cognitive behavior therapy for multiple sclerosis fatigue. *Psychosomatic Medicine, 70*(2), 205–213.

Voss, J. (2005). Predictors and correlates of fatigue in HIV/AIDS. *Journal of Pain and Symptom Management, 29*(2), 173–184.

Voss, J., Dodd, M., Portillo, C., & Holzemer, W. (2006). Theories of fatigue: Application in HIV/AIDS. *Journal of the Association of Nurses in AIDS Care, 17*(1), 37–50.

Voss, J., Portillo, C. J., Holzemer, W. L., & Dodd, M. J. (2007). Symptom cluster of fatigue and depression in HIV/AIDS. *Journal of Prevention and Intervention in the Community, 33*(1–2), 19–34.

Voss, J., Sukati, N. A., Seboni, N. M., Makoae, L. N., Moleko, M., Human, S., et al. (2007). Symptom burden of fatigue in men and women living with HIV/AIDS in Southern Africa. *Journal of the Association of Nurses in AIDS Care, 18*(4), 22–31.

Wagner, L. I., & Cella, D. (2004). Fatigue and cancer: Causes, prevalence and treatment approaches. *British Journal of Cancer, 91*(5), 822–828.

Wolfe, J., Grier, H. E., & Klar, N. (2000). Symptoms and suffering at the end of life in children with cancer. *New England Journal of Medicine, 342*(5), 326–333.

Woods, N. F., LaCroix, A. Z., Gray, S. L., Aragaki, A., Cochrane, B. B., Brunner, R. L., et al. (2005). Frailty: Emergence and consequences in women aged 65 and older in the women's health initiative observational study. *Journal of the American Geriatrics Society, 53*(8), 1321–1330.

Yennurajalingam, S., & Bruera, E. (2007). Palliative management of fatigue at the close of life: "It feels like my body is just worn out". *JAMA, 297*(3), 295–304, E291.

Yennurajalingam, S., Palmer, J. L., Zhang, T., Poulter, V., & Bruera, E. (2008). Association between fatigue and other cancer-related symptoms in patients with advanced cancer. *Supportive Care in Cancer, 16*(10), 1125–1130.

Zenzola, A., Masi, G., Mari, M., Defazio, G., Livrea, P., & Lamberti, P., et al. (2003). Fatigue in Parkinson's disease. *Neurological Sciences, 24*(3), 225–226.

A. Cancer-Related Fatigue Instruments

INSTRUMENT	DESCRIPTION	ADMINISTRATION	VALIDITY	COMMENTS
Brief fatigue inventory (BFI)	9-item questionnaire, 11-point Likert scale, evaluation period: past week, current, past 24 h	Self-report, second party (interview), estimated time for completion: 5 min	Validated in men and women, internal reliability verified, test-retest reliability not evaluated, construct verified convergent: FACT (fatigue and anemia subscales) and POMS (fatigue and vigor subscales) divergent, not evaluated discriminators: albumin, hemoglobin, and ECOG-PSR	Able to capture physical and psychological aspects, useful for screening and outcome assessments, able to distinguish severe fatigue, but less reliable when differentiating mild-to-moderate symptoms
Cancer fatigue scale (CFS)	15-item questionnaire, 5-point Likert scale subscales: physical, affective, cognitive, evaluation period: current	Self-report, second party (interview), estimated time for completion: 2–3 min	Validated in men and women, internal reliability verified, test-retest reliability verified up to 8 days, construct: no healthy controls convergent: VAS-F and hospital anxiety and depression scale divergent: mini-mental state discriminators: ECOG-PSR (physical and affective subscales)	Able to capture physical and psychological aspects, validation performed in Japanese population, which may affect generalization, telephone test-retest: lower mean values but retained validity

(Continued)

INSTRUMENT	DESCRIPTION	ADMINISTRATION	VALIDITY	COMMENTS
Fatigue symptom inventory (FSI)	14-item questionnaire, 11-point Likert scale (12 questions), remaining questions pertain to number of days/week (0–7) fatigue is experienced and the pattern of daily fatigue (4-point Likert scale), evaluation period: past week, current	Self-report, second party (interview), estimated time for completion: 5 min	Validated in men and women, internal reliability: interference subscale test-retest reliability: low-to-moderate, correlations construct verified convergent: POMS-F, SF-36, SLDS-C, and CES-D divergent: MC-20 discriminators not evaluated	Similar questions as BFI, able to capture physical and psychological aspects, useful for screening and outcome assessments (single assessments only, not repeated, measures), identified a second version of this tool that used a 5-point Likert scale for the final question pertaining to daily pattern of fatigue
Functional assessment of cancer therapy (FACT-G)	27-item questionnaire, 5-point Likert scale, general cancer assessment tool derived from FACIT database, evaluates physical, functional, emotional, and social well-being (QOL); two questions regarding patient-physician relationships, evaluation period: past wk	Self-report, second party (interview), estimated time for completion: 5 min	Validated in men and women, internal reliability verified, test-retest reliability verified, construct: no healthy controls convergent: POMS, SF-36, SLDS-C, and CES-D, divergent: MC-20 discriminators: ECOG-PSR	General focus, useful for screening and outcome assessments
Functional assessment of cancer therapy fatigue subscale (FACT-F)	13-item questionnaire administered with FACT-G 5-point Likert scale, evaluation period, past week	Self-report, second party (interview), estimated time for completion: 5–10 min	Validated in men and women, internal reliability verified, test-retest reliability: 3–7 days, construct: no healthy controls convergent: PFS, POMS-F and -V (fatigue and vigor), divergent: MC-20, discriminators: hemoglobin and ECOG-PSR	Able to capture physical and psychological aspects, useful for screening and outcome assessments

INSTRUMENT	DESCRIPTION	ADMINISTRATION	VALIDITY	COMMENTS
Functional assessment of cancer, anemia subscale (FACT-An)	20-item questionnaire (13 of which are identical to FACT-F) administered with FACT-G, 5-point Likert scale assesses symptoms associated with anemia, evaluation period: past week	Self-report, second party (interview), estimated time for completion: 5–10 min	Validated in men and women, internal reliability verified, test-retest reliability: 3–7 days, construct: no healthy controls convergent: PFS, POMS-F and -V, divergent: MC-20, discriminators: hemoglobin and ECOG-PSR	Able to capture physical and psychological aspects, useful for screening and outcome assessments
Lee fatigue scale (LFS or VAS-F)	18-item visual analog scale, fatigue subscale: 13 items, energy subscale: 5 items, evaluation period: current	Self-report, second party (interview), estimated time for completion: < 5 min	Validated in men and women, internal reliability verified, test-retest reliability: limited data construct verified convergent: POMS (F and V) and Stanford sleepiness scale divergent not evaluated, discriminators not evaluated	Able to capture physical and psychological aspects useful for screening and outcome assessments, although this tool has been used to assess cancer fatigue, original validation performed in patients with sleep disorders
Multidimensional assessment of fatigue (MAF) scale (Belza, Henke, Yelin, Epstain, & Gillis, 1993), provides a global fatigue index (Belza, 2001)	16-item questionnaire, 10-point scale for items 1–14; 5-point scale for item 15, 5 dimensions: degree, severity, distress, impact, timing	Self-report, item 16 is not included in the scoring, estimated completion time: 10 min, scores range 1 (no fatigue) – 50 (severe fatigue)		
Multidimensional fatigue inventory (MFI-20)	20-item questionnaire, 5-point Likert scale scales: general, physical, mental, reduced motivation, reduced activity, evaluation period: past 24 h	Self-report, second party (interview), estimated time for completion: 5–10 min	Validated in men and women, internal reliability verified, test-retest reliability not evaluated, construct verified convergent: VAS (single item), BDS and Rhoten fatigue scale divergent not evaluated, discriminators not evaluated	Able to capture physical and psychological aspects, useful for screening and outcome assessments

(Continued)

INSTRUMENT	DESCRIPTION	ADMINISTRATION	VALIDITY	COMMENTS
Multidimensional fatigue symptom inventory (MFSI)	Same authors as FSI, 83-item questionnaire, 5-point Likert scale, rational subscale: global, somatic, affective, cognitive, and behavioral aspects, empirical subscale: general, physical, emotional, mental, aspects; also evaluates vigor, short form (MFSI-SF): developed to evaluate only empiric information, evaluation period: past wk	Self-report, second party (interview), estimated time for completion: 10 min	Validated in women, internal reliability: both subscales, test-retest reliability: significant and equivalent, correlations noted for both subscales, construct verified convergent: POMS-F and SF-36 (vitality), STAI, and CES-D, divergent: MC-20, discriminators: ECOG-PSR	Able to capture physical and psychological aspects, validation performed in women only, which may affect generalization, useful for screening, however, may be too long or cumbersome for outcome assessments
Piper fatigue scale (PFS)	27-Item questionnaire, 22 items: 11-point Likert scale, used to estimate fatigue scores, 5 items: open-ended, subscales: behavioral-severity, affective meaning, sensory, and cognitive-mood, evaluation period: current	Self-report, second party (interview), estimated time for completion: 5 min	Validated in women, internal reliability verified, test-retest reliability not evaluated, construct, no healthy controls, convergent: demographic profile (investigator-developed), POMS, and fatigue symptom checklist, divergent: POMS-Vigor, discriminators not evaluated	Able to capture physical and psychological aspects, useful for screening and outcome assessments, used clinically to assess CRF in men; however, formal validation efforts have not yet been published
Revised Piper fatigue scale (Dagnelie et al., 2006)	22-items with 10-point numerical rating in four subscales: behavioral/severity; affective meaning; sensory; and cognitive/mood	Self-report questionnaire	Psychometric properties validated in Dutch cancer patients: 16 males, 13 females with lung cancer; 35 women with breast cancer, construct validity was established with the MFI, criterion related validity was moderate with the MFI and the Rotterdam symptom checklist (RSCL)	Significantly lower ($p < 0.01$) scores were found in sensory and cognitive/mood subscales among Dutch breast cancer patients when compared to the original study population (Piper et al., 1998); no significant differences in behavioral/severity or affective meaning subscales

INSTRUMENT	DESCRIPTION	ADMINISTRATION	VALIDITY	COMMENTS
Profile of mood states (POMS)	65-item questionnaire, 5-point Likert scale, subscales: tension-anxiety, anger-hostility, vigor-activity, fatigue-inertia, and confusion-bewilderment, short form: 30 items (derived from the six subscales); developed for the elderly and individuals with medical disorders or disabilities, evaluation period: past wk	Self-report, second party (interview), estimated time for completion: 5–7 min (some individuals may require more time)	Validated in men and women, internal reliability: all subscales, test-retest reliability: all subscales construct verified, convergent: Hopkins symptom distress scale, manifest anxiety scale, BDS, and interpersonal behavior inventory, divergent: MC-20, discriminators not evaluated	Only able to capture psychological aspects, useful for screening, however may be too long or cumbersome for outcome assessments, flexible scoring: entire document or individual subscales
Schwartz cancer fatigue scale (SCFS) [original version]	28-item questionnaire, 5-point Likert scale, subscales (factors): physical, emotional, cognitive, and temporal, evaluation period: past 2–3 days	Self-report, second party (interview), estimated time for completion: 5 min	Validated in men and women, internal reliability verified, test-retest reliability not evaluated, construct: limited evaluation convergent: VAS-F, divergent not evaluated, discriminators not evaluated	Able to capture physical and psychological aspects, described validation under experimental conditions, but validation was not maintained when used in a clinical setting
Schwartz cancer fatigue scale (SCFS-6) [revised version]	6-item questionnaire, 5-point Likert scale, subscales (factors): physical and perceptual developed because further testing was unable to confirm validation of original version, evaluation period: past 2–3 days	Self-report, second party (interview), estimated time for completion: 1–2 min	Validated in men and women, internal reliability verified, test-retest reliability not evaluated, construct verified convergent not evaluated, divergent not evaluated, discriminators: limited evaluation	Able to capture physical and psychological aspects, requires further validation (in the clinical setting), items are identical to those in POMS, computerized version has been developed

(Continued)

INSTRUMENT	DESCRIPTION	ADMINISTRATION	VALIDITY	COMMENTS
Symptom distress scale (SDS) (Cooley et al., 2005)	13-items, 5-point Likert scale, assessment of 11 symptoms (nausea, appetite, insomnia, pain, fatigue, bowel pattern, concentration, cough, appearance, outlook, breathing); and a frequency report for two symptoms (pain, nausea); evaluates feelings on day of administration	Self-report, estimated completion time: 5 min., scores range 13 (little distress) – 65 (severe symptom distress)	Validity: reported accurately, used and completed by over 98% of participants; preferred by participants with lower education when compared with other questionnaires; internal reliability demonstrated by repeated measure (Kukull, McCorkle, & Driever, 1986)	Developed for symptom assessment in adults diagnosed with cancer

BDS = Beck depression scale; CES-D = Center for epidemiological studies-depression scale; ECOG-PSR = Eastern collaborative oncology group performance status rating; FACIT = Functional assessment of chronic illness therapy; MC-20 = Marlowe-Crowne social desirability scale; QOL = quality of life; SF-36 = Health outcomes study short form; SLDS-C = Satisfaction with life domains scale-cancer; STAI = State-trait anxiety inventory; VAS-F = Visual analog scale-fatigue.

Adapted from *Pharmacotherapy* 22(11):1433–1441, 2002.

B. Piper Fatigue Scale

Directions: Many individuals can experience a sense of unusual or excessive tiredness whenever they become ill, receive treatment, or recover from their illness/treatment. This unusual sense of tiredness is not usually relieved either by a good night's sleep or by rest. Some call this symptom "fatigue" to distinguish it from the usual sense of tiredness.

For each of the following questions, please fill in the space provided for that response that best describes the fatigue you are experiencing now or for today. Please make every effort to answer each question to the best of your ability. If you are not experiencing fatigue now or for today, fill in the circle indicating "0" for your response. Thank you very much!

1. How long have you been feeling fatigue? (Check one response only.)

   ☐ 1. Not feeling fatigue

   ☐ 2. Minutes

   ☐ 3. Hours

   ☐ 4. Days

   ☐ 5. Weeks

   ☐ 6. Months

   ☐ 7. Other (please describe)

2. To what degree is the fatigue you are feeling now causing you distress?

   No distress   A great deal

☐	☐	☐	☐	☐	☐	☐	☐	☐	☐
1	2	3	4	5	6	7	8	9	10

3. To what degree is the fatigue you are feeling now interfering with your ability to complete your work or school activities?

   None   A great deal

☐	☐	☐	☐	☐	☐	☐	☐	☐	☐
1	2	3	4	5	6	7	8	9	10

4. To what degree is the fatigue you are feeling now interfering with your ability to socialize with your friends?

   None   A great deal

☐	☐	☐	☐	☐	☐	☐	☐	☐	☐
1	2	3	4	5	6	7	8	9	10

5. To what degree is the fatigue you are feeling now interfering with your ability to engage in sexual activity?

   None   A great deal

☐	☐	☐	☐	☐	☐	☐	☐	☐	☐
1	2	3	4	5	6	7	8	9	10

6. Overall, how much is the fatigue, which you are now experiencing, interfering with your ability to engage in the kind of activities you enjoy doing?

None   A great deal

☐   ☐   ☐   ☐   ☐   ☐   ☐   ☐   ☐   ☐

1   2   3   4   5   6   7   8   9   10

7. How would you describe the degree of intensity or severity of the fatigue that you are experiencing now?

Mild   Severe

☐   ☐   ☐   ☐   ☐   ☐   ☐   ☐   ☐   ☐

1   2   3   4   5   6   7   8   9   10

8. To what degree would you describe the fatigue that you are experiencing now as being?

Pleasant   Unpleasant

☐   ☐   ☐   ☐   ☐   ☐   ☐   ☐   ☐   ☐

1   2   3   4   5   6   7   8   9   10

9. To what degree would you describe the fatigue that you are experiencing now as being?

Agreeable   Disagreeable

☐   ☐   ☐   ☐   ☐   ☐   ☐   ☐   ☐   ☐

1   2   3   4   5   6   7   8   9   10

10. To what degree would you describe the fatigue that you are experiencing now as being?

Protective   Destructive

☐   ☐   ☐   ☐   ☐   ☐   ☐   ☐   ☐   ☐

1   2   3   4   5   6   7   8   9   10

11. To what degree would you describe the fatigue that you are experiencing now as being?

Positive   Negative

☐   ☐   ☐   ☐   ☐   ☐   ☐   ☐   ☐   ☐

1   2   3   4   5   6   7   8   9   10

12. To what degree would you describe the fatigue which you are experiencing now as being:

Normal   Abnormal

☐   ☐   ☐   ☐   ☐   ☐   ☐   ☐   ☐   ☐

1   2   3   4   5   6   7   8   9   10

13. To what degree are you now feeling:

Strong   Weak

☐   ☐   ☐   ☐   ☐   ☐   ☐   ☐   ☐   ☐

1   2   3   4   5   6   7   8   9   10

14. To what degree are you now feeling:

Awake   Sleepy

☐   ☐   ☐   ☐   ☐   ☐   ☐   ☐   ☐   ☐

1   2   3   4   5   6   7   8   9   10

15. To what degree are you now feeling:

Lively   Listless

☐   ☐   ☐   ☐   ☐   ☐   ☐   ☐   ☐   ☐
1   2   3   4   5   6   7   8   9   10

16. To what degree are you now feeling:

Refreshed   Tired

☐   ☐   ☐   ☐   ☐   ☐   ☐   ☐   ☐   ☐
1   2   3   4   5   6   7   8   9   10

17. To what degree are you now feeling:

Energetic   Unenergetic

☐   ☐   ☐   ☐   ☐   ☐   ☐   ☐   ☐   ☐
1   2   3   4   5   6   7   8   9   10

18. To what degree are you now feeling:

Patient   Impatient

☐   ☐   ☐   ☐   ☐   ☐   ☐   ☐   ☐   ☐
1   2   3   4   5   6   7   8   9   10

19. To what degree are you now feeling:

Relaxed   A great deal

☐   ☐   ☐   ☐   ☐   ☐   ☐   ☐   ☐   ☐
1   2   3   4   5   6   7   8   9   10

20. To what degree are you now feeling:

Exhilarated   Depressed

☐   ☐   ☐   ☐   ☐   ☐   ☐   ☐   ☐   ☐
1   2   3   4   5   6   7   8   9   10

21. To what degree are you now feeling:

Able to concentrate   Unable to concentrate

☐   ☐   ☐   ☐   ☐   ☐   ☐   ☐   ☐   ☐
1   2   3   4   5   6   7   8   9   10

22. To what degree are you now feeling:

Able to remember   Unable to remember

☐   ☐   ☐   ☐   ☐   ☐   ☐   ☐   ☐   ☐
1   2   3   4   5   6   7   8   9   10

23. To what degree are you now feeling:

Able to think clearly   Unable to think clearly

☐   ☐   ☐   ☐   ☐   ☐   ☐   ☐   ☐   ☐
1   2   3   4   5   6   7   8   9   10

24. Overall, what do you believe is *most* directly contributing to or causing your fatigue?

_____

_____

_____

25. Overall, the *best* thing you have found to relieve your fatigue is:

_____

_____

_____

26. Is there anything else you would like to add that would describe your fatigue better to us?

_____

_____

_____

27. Are you experiencing any other symptoms right now?

_____

_____

_____

Scoring Piper Fatigue Scale (PFS) Survey Results:

PFS current format and scoring instructions:

1. The PFS in its current form is composed of 22 numerically scaled, "0"–"10" items that measure four dimensions of subjective fatigue: behavioral/severity (6 items; # 2–7); affective meaning (5 items: # 8–12); sensory (5 items: # 13–17); and cognitive/mood (6 items: # 18–23). These 22 items are used to calculate the four sub-scale/dimensional scores and the total fatigue scores.
2. Five additional items (# 1 and # 24–27) are not used to calculate subscale or total fatigue scores but are recommended to be kept on the scale as these items furnish rich, qualitative data. Item # 1, in particular gives a categorical way in which to assess the duration of the respondent's fatigue.
3. To score the PFS, add the items contained on each specific subscale together and divide by the number of items on that subscale. This will give you a subscale score that remains on the same "0"–"10" numeric scale. Should you have missing item data, and the respondent has answered at least 75%–80% of the remaining items on that particular subscale, calculate the subscale mean score based on the number of items answered, and substitute that mean value for the missing item score (mean item substitution).
4. Recalculate the subscale score. To calculate the total fatigue score, add the 22 item scores together and divide by 22 in order to keep the score on the same numeric "0"–"10" scale!

Severity Codes:
0	NONE
1–3	MILD
4–6	MODERATE
7–10	SEVERE

Source: Piper, B. F., Dibble, S. L., Dodd, M. J., Weiss, M. C., Slaughter, R. E., & Paul, S. M. (1998). The revised Piper Fatigue Scale: Psychometric evaluation in women with breast cancer. *Oncology Nursing Forum, 25*(4), 677–684.

C. Global Fatigue Index

Multidimensional Assessment of Fatigue (MAF) Scale

Fatigue Dimension	Questions	Scoring
Degree	1. To what degree have you experienced fatigue?	1 (not at all) – 10 (a great deal)
Severity	2. How severe is the fatigue which you have been experiencing?	1 (not at all) – 10 (a great deal)
Distress	3. To what degree has fatigue caused you distress?	1 (not at all) – 10 (a great deal)
Impact on activities of daily living (11 items)	4. Household chores?	1 (not at all) – 10 (a great deal)
	5. Cook?	1 (not at all) – 10 (a great deal)
	6. Bathe or wash?	1 (not at all) – 10 (a great deal)
	7. Dress?	1 (not at all) – 10 (a great deal)
	8. Work?	1 (not at all) – 10 (a great deal)
	9. Visit or socialize with friends or family?	1 (not at all) – 10 (a great deal)
	10. Engage in sexual activity?	1 (not at all) – 10 (a great deal)
	11. Engage in leisure and recreational activities?	1 (not at all) – 10 (a great deal)
	12. Shop and do errands?	1 (not at all) – 10 (a great deal)
	13. Walk?	1 (not at all) – 10 (a great deal)
	14. Exercise, other than walking?	1 (not at all) – 10 (a great deal)
Timing	15. Over the past week, including today, how often have you been fatigued?	0 (hardly any days) – 4 (every day)
	16. To what degree has your fatigue changed during the past week?	1 (decreased) – 4 (increased)

Scoring: Total score for items 1,2, and 3. Average items 4–14 (ADLs). Item #15 multiply the score by 2.5. Item 16 is not included in the score. Score range 1–50; the higher the score the greater impairment from fatigue.

Source: Reprinted from Belza, B., Steele, B. G., Hunziker, J., Lakshminaryan, S., Holt, L., & Buchner, D. M. (2001). Correlates of physical activity in chronic obstructive pulmonary disease. *Nursing Research, 50*(4), 195-202.

24

Skin Care Needs of Palliative Patients

Elizabeth A. Ayello
R. Gary Sibbald
Kevin Y. Woo

Key Points

- Prevention of skin injury may need to be balanced against the overall goals of care.
- Pressure ulcers are common occurrences during the dying process.
- Wound care should be aimed at providing comfort; relieving pain, odor, and containing exudates; and improving patient's quality of life.

Case Study: Ms. DL is a 57-year-old female with metastatic ovarian cancer to the lower neck and breast areas that has gradually expanded over the last 3 years (See Figure 24.1). Some of the lesions have become elevated above the skin surface with central ulceration. There is a heavy exudate, surface bleeding from tiny telangiectatic vessels, and an odor that is very disturbing to the patient. She has had previous radiotherapy and chemotherapy but reached the maximal dose of radiation and is now unresponsive to currently available chemotherapy. She is embarrassed to go out in public because of the visibility of the lesions on the neck and the associated odor. The pain was partially controlled with a combination of methadone and a fentanyl patch supplemented with oxycodone for breakthrough. She has become lethargic and confused at times.

As part of the interprofessional team looking after this patient:

1) How would you approach the control of the exudate and odor?

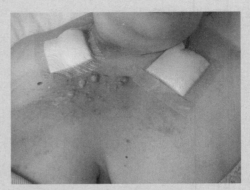

Figure 24.1   Lesions for Case Study

2) Do you have any suggestions for the management of her pain?

Introduction

Cancer can arise from any organ in the body. Because the skin is the largest external organ, the visible changes in the skin are typically very apparent to the patient and their family because it is the largest external organ. The physical appearance of skin wounds and/or damage to the skin from drainage as well as the odor, can be physically and emotionally upsetting. Skin injuries not only cause pain, but also may require changes in other aspects of the patient's overall management and treatment plan.

Skin assessment is an important part of care of the older adult or any person who is at the end of their life. Prevention of skin injury may need to be balanced against the overall goals of care. Actual observation of the skin and of the total patient is needed to identify patients at risk for skin injury and to begin prevention protocols. There is however, no consensus in the literature as to what constitutes a minimum skin assessment. Baranoski and Ayello (2008) have suggested five elements to include in a basic skin assessment. They are skin temperature, color, moisture, turgor, and if the skin is intact or has areas of injury such as open areas. Once areas of skin injury are identified, it is imperative to document the changes and have an appropriate healthcare professional determine the correct wound etiology. In palliative care, the goal may not be wound healing, but rather wound maintenence, control of wound odor, exudate, infection and bleeding, as well as alleviation of wound pain. This knowledge will guide the clinician in developing the proper treatment plan.

In this chapter, several common skin problems (skin tears, pressure ulcers, tumor and treatment-related skin injuries, ostomy skin, and fistulas) will be discussed.

Skin Damage from Radiation Therapy

Radiation therapy damages cellular DNA resulting in cell death. This is why rapidly dividing cells such as skin, hair, or mucosa cells die after being irradiated (Turnbull, 2007). Skin reactions may include erythema, desquamation, either dry (dry, flaky, scaly skin when sweat and sebaceous glands are damaged) or moist (blistering, peeling sloughing skin), or even ulceration (Oncology Nursing Society, 2008).

While the patient is undergoing radiation therapy, care should be taken not to remove any of the treatment field markers on the skin. Avoid activities that could cause mechanical skin damage such as vigorous rubbing, heat, or shaving of the skin in the treatment area. Use of any topical products such as lotions, creams, deodorants, is generally discouraged. Any product with metal components or ingredients (for example silver or zinc oxide) should not be used during radiation treatment. (Turnbull, 2007) Patient care goals include keeping the skin intact as well as in correct moisture balance. The Oncology Nursing Society recommends products with vitamin A and E, or Aloe Vera gels for treating erythema although topical steroids should also be considered with the presence of a topical contact irritant dermatitis. Talcum, corn starch, or baby powder use is controversial as they often contain heavy metals but if they are applied, an even layer can be obtained with a cotton ball dabbed on the affected area rather than sprinkling the powder from a container that often leads to local clumping.

Skin Changes at Life's End (SCALE)

Despite optimal nursing care, not all pressure ulcers at life's end are preventable (Sibbald et al., 2008). An expert group of panelists have been assembled to make recommendations for the documentation and treatment of pressure ulcers at life's end. The recommendations are summarized in Table 24.1

PRESSURE ULCERS

Pressure ulcers are common occurrences during the dying process. Eckman (1989) reported the results of a randomized study of 130 funeral homes across the United States. Of the 1,378 deceased persons, 1 out of 4 (23.6%) had a pressure ulcer. The number of ulcers ranged from 1–14. 31% had one ulcer while 68.6% had more than one ulcer. Table 24.2 demonstrates the number of cases by location when location of death was known.

Kennedy (1989) reported that 56% of patients who died in an intermediate care facility developed a pressure ulcer within the 6 weeks prior to their death.

24.1 | Pressure Ulcer Treatment

FEB 2009	SCALE RECOMMENDATIONS
A)	Skin Changes at Life's End (SCALE) and related physiologic changes occur as a result of the dying process and may be manifest as subjective symptoms or observable signs. These changes may occur in spite of appropriate interventions and are therefore unavoidable.
B)	SCALE reflects tissue damage from decreased tissue oxygenation and removal of metabolic wastes. The skin becomes dysfunctional thereby resulting in decreased tolerance to pressure and other external forces/ insults.
C)	SCALE stakeholder discussions (patients, policy makers, payers, and healthcare professionals) can act as a stimulus for evidence-based research and education.
1)	Obtain patient history and describe and document the skin or wound abnormality exactly as assessed.
2)	Address patient-centered concerns including pain and activities of daily living.
3)	Changes associated with SCALE may include: ■ *Symptoms:* Progressive limitation of mobility, increasing weakness, loss of appetite (suboptimal nutrition), weight loss, cachexia, incontinence, impaired immune function. ■ *Signs:* Wasting, decreased blood perfusion (decreased local skin temperature, mottled discoloration, tissue death), loss of skin integrity. ■ *Investigations:* Low serum albumin/ prealbumin, low hemoglobin, impaired tissue oxygenation.
4)	If the underlying etiology or cause of skin changes cannot be determined, obtain a differential diagnosis from a qualified healthcare professional.
5)	Consider the 4 P's for determining goals of care and the appropriate strategies: prevention, prescription (treatable), preservation (maintenance without deterioration), palliation (usually nonhealable, not likely to improve).
6)	Expectations around the patient's end of life issues should be communicated among the members of the interprofessional team and the patient unit. The discussion should include the potential for SCALE: skin breakdown, pressure ulcers, and other skin changes.
7)	Regularly perform a total skin assessment and document all areas of concern. Pay special attention to bony prominences (e.g. sacrum, sacral-coccygeal, ischium, hips, & heels), tips of digits.
8)	Care of the patient should be documented. The plan of care is reflected in the entire patient record. Charting by exception is an appropriate method of documentation in certain healthcare settings.

24.2 | Guidelines for Reassessment for Pressure Ulcer Risk by Setting

LOCATION	% OF CASES	% OF ULCERS
HOSPITAL	44.3%	44.6%
NURSING HOME	37.8%	40.2%
FAMILY HOME	14.2%	12%

EXHIBIT 24.1: NPUAP RESEARCH IMPLICATIONS AND RECOMMENDATIONS

RECOMMENDATIONS:
- Significant gaps in knowledge.
- Large multi-site studies of hospice patients needed.
- Extent and nature of ulcers need clarification.
- Pressure ulcer prevention at end of life.

QUESTIONS:
- To what extend can pressure ulcer be attributed to "dying condition"
- What are "best practices" for pressure ulcer prevention at "end-of-life"?
- What is palliative pressure ulcer care?
- When does palliative care replace goal of healing the wound?

Furthermore, Kennedy has described the following characteristics of the Kennedy terminal ulcer: Pear shaped, coccyx or sacrum, red, yellow or black, sudden onset, and death was imminent. The presence of a pressure ulcer "complicates care, increases costs, and threatens quality of life" for hospice patients as proposed by Colburn (1987). The incidence of pressure ulcers may be higher in hospice patients (Hansen et al, 1991). "Time in bed increases as their condition deteriorates, which occurs concomitantly as multi-system failure and growing weakness predispose them to risk factors including decreased activity and mobility, depleted nutrition and hydration, incontinence, and changes in sensory perception and consciousness" (Langemo, Bates-Jensen, Hanson, 2001, p. 143). "Strategies used to prevent pressure ulcers in other populations may seem to be in direct conflict with palliative care strategies" (Langemo, Bates-Jensen, Hanson, 2001, p. 143). It is unclear exactly what protocols are best to use when the goals of care are comfort rather than cure or healing, preventing extension of wound, and limiting impact of the wound demise on the elder's quality of life.

The National Pressure Ulcer Advisory Panel (NPUAP) (2001) reviewed studies over a 10-year period to determine the prevalence and incidence of pressure ulcers in the palliative care/hospice patient population. This report (see Exhibit 24.1 for the summary of implications and recommendations) reviewed the existing evidence base of 7 studies on hospice or palliative care. Incidence rates ranged from a low of 8% (Olson, Tkachuk & Hanson, 1998) to 85% (Waltman, Bergstrom, Armstrong, Norvell, & Braden, 1991). The majority of patients in these studies had cancer. Hanson and colleagues (1992) reported an incidence of 13% stages I and II pressure ulcers. Locations of these pressure ulcers were the sacrum (38.4%), elbows (30.7%), and heels (15.4%). Pressure ulcers often occurred within 2 weeks of death. Waltman and colleagues (1991) found a higher incidence of pressure ulcers in elder patients with cancer (85%) compared to a matched group without cancer (70%). In this prospective study, average time to death after developing a pressure ulcer was 3 weeks.

Preventing Pressure Ulcers: Risk Assessment

New joint international guidelines for the prevention and treatment of pressure ulcers are slated to be released in 2009 by the European Pressure Ulcer Advisory Panel and the National Pressure Ulcer Advisory Panel in the USA. (Watch the organization websites for the release of this information). The current use of risk assessment scales to identify patients at risk for pressure ulcers are recommended by the AHCPR Clinical Practice Guidelines (Panel for the prediction and prevention of pressure ulcers in adults, AHCPR, 1992). Most studies that have used the risk assessment scales have been in long-term care, hospital, or home care settings. Unfortunately, these studies do not always report if the older adults in these settings are palliative care patients. A widely used scale in the United States is the Braden Scale. This scale has six factor subscales — sensory perception, moisture, activity, mobility, nutrition, and friction/shear, which are ranked to provide a total risk score. The Braden scale is considered to have good reliability and specificity (AHCPR, 1992). One study by Hanson, Langemo, Olson, Hunter, and Burd (1994) reported data from the Braden Scale used to identify pressure ulcer risk in hospitalized cancer patients. Incidence was 8%, sensitivity 82%, and specificity 84% (Hanson et al., 1994). Based on patients on a palliative care unit in England, Chaplin (2000) developed a pressure ulcer risk assessment tool. This scale referred to as the Hunters Hill Marie Curie Centre pressure ulcer risk assessment tool, has two more subscales than the Braden scale as it has eight, rather than six, Braden subscales. While both have a subscale for sensory/perception, moisture, mobility, activity, and friction/shear, the Hunters Hill Marie Curie Center Pressure Ulcer Risk Assessment Tool has a subscale for skin condition which is graded on a scale of 1 (skin condition good) to the number 4 (skin integrity broken) and includes weight change pattern in the nutrition subscale. Perhaps one of the biggest difference between this scale and the Braden scale (low scores are at risk, with 18 being onset of pressure ulcer risk) is that no impairments have low subscale numbers while area of high impairment have the highest numbers, therefore, total scores of 12 or lower are at low risk, while scores 13 or higher are at medium risk.

The AHCPR (1992) pressure ulcer guidelines recommend that patients be evaluated on admission to a care setting and at periodic intervals. Guidelines for reassessment for pressure ulcer risk by specific settings have been suggested (Ayello & Braden, 2001). While Exhibit 24.3 gives these recommendations, just how applicable these are to palliative care patients is not known.

Prevention Interventions

Pressure ulcers are suggestive of deterioration and part of the disease trajectory Brink, Fries-Smith, and Linkewich (2006). Sometimes the primary treatment and prevention goal of care id displaced by a greater need for comfort (Brink et al., 2006). A study of 546 palliative home care patients found risk factors included male gender, inability to lay flat, catheter or ostomy care, and a reduced ability to perform activities of daily living were associated with an increased risk of pressure ulcers (Brink et al., 2006)

The purpose of doing a risk assessment is to identify which older adults need prevention interventions. The goal of reducing risk factors is the prevention of pressure ulcers; the utilization of prevention strategies for at-risk older adults is to spare them painful and sometimes tiresome treatments. Older adults are considered to be 'at risk' when their Braden scale reaches 18, intervention protocols have been linked to levels of risk (Ayello & Braden, 2001; Braden Scale Website, 2009).

EXHIBIT 24.2: INTERVALS FOR PRESSURE ULCER RISK ASSESSMENT

ACUTE CARE
Initial assessment on admission
Reassessment every 24–48 h or whenever the patient's condition changes

LONG TERM CARE
Initial assessment on admission
Reassessment weekly for first 4 weeks, then monthly to quarterly or whenever the patient's condition changes

HOME HEALTHCARE
Initial assessment on admission
Reassessment with every RN visit

Attention to an elder's score on subscales can also help to target prevention interventions to that specific factor that is most placing the patient at risk. Based on the AHCPR (1992) guidelines, Exhibit 24.3 gives pressure ulcer prevention guidelines.

The AHCPR (1992) guidelines may need to be modified based on the overall goals of the older adult's care. For palliative care patients, following the recommended every 2-hour repositioning schedule may cause the patient undue pain, and nursing staff may decide not to follow this usual practice. The patient and the family need to clearly understand the implications for skin injury. This variation in the patient's treatment plan also need to be documented in the patient's record.

Teaching the patient and their family about pressure ulcer prevention is very important (Ayello, Mezey, & Amella, 1997). Consider using the booklet developed by the New Jersey Hospital Association and their collaborator; Patient teaching booklets developed by AHCPR may not be appropriate for all patients as the reading level is higher than the usual recommended 5–6 grade reading level (Ayello, 1992).

Pressure Ulcer Location

The sacrum is the number one location for pressure ulcer occurrence, heels are second (Baldwin, 2001; Cuddigan, Hollinger, Brown, & Horslen, 2001). In specific palliative care patients, other sites may be at risk for pressure ulcer breakdown. For example, elders with

EXHIBIT 24.3: AHCPR (1992) PRESSURE ULCER PREVENTION PROTOCOL

INSPECTION AND CARE OF SKIN
Frequency of inspection—daily & document
- Bathing—avoid hot water, soaps
- Use moisturizers to treat dry skin
- Avoid low humidity environment
- Do not massage reddened bony prominences
- Manage incontinence (see AHCPR incontinence guidelines)

MECHANICAL LOADING AND SUPPORT SURFACES
1) Turning and positioning schedules—reposition q 2h—use a written schedule
2) Full position changes, use positioning devices
3) 30 lateral positions
4) "Pillow bridging"
5) Small shift changes
6) No donuts
7) Use lifting devices
8) Use protective devices and support surfaces
9) Do range of motion exercises
10) Keep head of bed at < 30°
11) Use of support surfaces?

COPD who are on long-term oxygen therapy, the part of the ears underneath the oxygen tubing must be checked for pressure ulcers.

Pressure Ulcer Staging

Pressure ulcers are staged based on the visible assessment of the depth of tissue that has been damaged in the wound bed. Bennett (1995) has urged clinicians to use appropriate lighting sources such as natural or halogen lighting as well as evaluating skin temperature and consistency to detect stage I pressure ulcers in clients with darkly pigmented skin. The National Pressure Ulcer Advisory Panel (NPUAP) increased the original 1988 four staging definitions by adding two additional categories of unstagable (ulcers covered with eschar) and suspected deep tissue injury (sDTI) (purple or maroon discolored localized areas of intact skin or blood filled blister (www.npuap.org). The NPUAP and the EPUAP will be premiering new international staging definitions on their websites sometime in 2009. The EPUAP and the centers for Medicare and Medicaid services (CMS) have not adopted the unstagable and sDTI categories. Some key points from the staging system are listed below:

Stage I: A stage I pressure ulcer is an observable pressure related alteration of intact skin whose indicators as compared to an adjacent or opposite area on the body may include changes in one or more of the following:

- skin temperature (warmth or coolness)
- tissue consistency (firm or boggy feel) and /or
- sensation (pain, itching)

The ulcer appears as a defined area of persistent redness in a lightly pigmented skin whereas in darker skin tones, the ulcer may appear with persistent red, blue, or purple hues.

Stage II: Partial thickness skin loss involving epidermis and/or dermis. The ulcer is superficial and presents clinically as an abrasion, blister, or shallow crater. It may also appear as a serum filled blister. There is no slough in a stage II pressure ulcer.

Stage III: If there is any slough on the wound bed, then the ulcer is at least a stage III. Full-thickness skin loss involving damage or necrosis of subcutaneous tissue that may extend down to, but not through, underlying fascia. Clinically the ulcer presents as a deep crater with or without undermining of adjacent tissue.

Stage IV: Full-thickness skin loss with extensive destruction, tissue necrosis ordamage to muscle, bone, or supporting structures (e.g., tendon, joint capsules, etc.).

Pressure Ulcer Treatment

The AHCPR (Bergstrom et al., 1994) pressure ulcer treatment guidelines recommend using normal saline and some commercially available wound cleaners to cleanse the ulcer. These solutions do not kill cells like cytotoxic agents such as Dakin's solution (sodium hypochlorite solution) and acetic acid. Cytotoxic agents are typically not recommended for cleaning of pressure ulcers. For palliative care patients, the use of these solutions may be warranted, because the goal is *no longer healing*. The benefits of odor control from these solutions may make them an appropriate choice for older adults who are at the end of their lives. Use gentle irrigation of 4–15 psi to irrigate pressure ulcers; this can be achieved by using a 19-gauge needle with a 35 cc syringe. The psi from a bulb syringe is below 4, so it may provide adequate pressure to clean the pressure ulcers.

Pressure ulcers may need ongoing debridement of necrotic tissue. Autolytic debridement can be achieved by using film, hydrocolloid, hydrogel, or other dressings (Ayello, Cuddigan, Kerstein, 2002). Debridement using enzymes is another method that is effective in the palliative care setting because there is little pain associated with this intervention. Surgical debridement may be best for infected wounds with advancing cellulitis with appropriate systemic antibiotic coverage (Kirshen, Woo, Ayello, & Sibbald, 2006). Mechanical debridement accomplished by wet-to-dry dressings is painful and can cause additional damage as well as bleeding of the tissue, so it is not generally recommended for use with palliative care patients, when comfort is the goal.

Beginning with the discovery of moist wound healing by Winter (1962), many new types of dressings have become available. With the hundreds of different types of dressings available, selecting the right dressing can be confusing for the clinician. A good way to approach this decision is by assessing the pressure ulcer wound characteristics and then matching the dressing to meet those needs. For many clinicians, the key determining factor is the amount of exudate in the pressure ulcer wound. For example, wounds with low amounts of exudate can be managed by a dressing with low absorbent capabilities. If the wound bed were dry, then using dressings that adds moisture to the wound would be indicated. See Exhibit 24.4 for a brief summary of selected dressings.

Quality of Life Issues, Including Pressure Ulcer Associated Pain

Pain is common for people with pressure ulcers, yet pain management is often inadequate (Dallam et al., 1995). Although they are few in number, some studies have provided clinicians with insights into quality of life issues for patients with pressure ulcers (Langemo, Melland, Hanson, Olson, & Hunter, 2000) and their

EXHIBIT 24.4: SELECTED DRESSINGS

LOW EXUDATES ABSORPTION

Film dressings
- Easily applied
- Can see the wound site
- Waterproof, good for incontinent patients
- Adhesive may cause skin injury during removal
- Generally not recommended for use with infected wounds

Hydrogel dressings
- Available as sheets or gels
- Effective for painful wounds
- High water content, so effective for to use for wounds that are dry
- Require a secondary dressing to keep in place

Hydrocolloid dressings
- Available in many shapes and sizes
- Very moldable
- Some are adhesive, some are not
- Can remain in place for many days

MODERATE TO HIGH EXUDATES ABSORPTION

Calcium alginate dressings
- Made from seaweed
- Available in sheet and rope forms
- Effective for packing wounds
- Not effective on wounds without enough exudate to convert the fiber to a hydrogel (do not use on dry wounds)
- Be aware that the wound may have the odor of "low tide"
- Switch to another dressing if exudate diminish, as it can dry out a wound with low exudate
- Requires a secondary dressing to hold in place

Foam dressings
- Very useful for wet, weepy wounds
- Effective for packing deep wounds
- Requires a secondary dressing
- Can be used underneath compression stockings, and multiple layer bandaging systems

Negative pressure wound therapy
- Great for wounds with large amounts of exudate
- Requires learning the technique for placing the specialized foam / dressings into the wound,
- Positioning the tubing, applying the specialized drape, and attaching to the vacuum source.

Antimicrobial dressings
- Effective for infected wounds
- Requires a secondary dressings
- No MRI if silver dressings used

caregivers (Baharestani, 1994). Themes common to both of these studies were: pain, lack of knowledge, the meaning of the pressure ulcer, and life style changes

imposed by the pressure ulcer. A recent article by Pieper, Langemo, and Cuddigan (2009) provides extensive tables of pressure ulcer pain studies.

Acute pain in a person with a pressure ulcer often indicates extension of the injury or secondary complications such as infection, periwound maceration or friction and shear injury. Treatment must consider both the nociceptive (gnawing, aching, tender, or throbbing) or neuropathic components (burning, stinging, shooting, and stabbing) that need to be treated with a combination of appropriate long and short acting agents.

Total management also requires attention to nutritional needs. Adequate nutrition may be difficult for elders experiencing anorexia from cancer or other chronic disease. It also may be inconsistent with the elder's wishes, directives, and the goals of management.

Pressure ulcers are a result of unrelieved pressure. Providing an adequate pressure relieving support cushion, mattress, or bed, may greatly decrease the older adult's pain, prevent skin breakdown, or prevent further tissue destruction in an existing pressure ulcer. Use static support surfaces should be initiated if the patient can turn (AHCPR, 1992). Always check to see if the support surface is "bottoming out" by placing a hand under the support surface. If the patient's bottom can be felt, then the support surface is not adequate. If this is the case then deep foam pressure redistribution static or dynamic support surfaces should be obtained.

SKIN TEARS

Scope of the Problem

Unlike chronic wounds such as pressure ulcers, skin tears are acute wounds. Malone, Rozario, Gavinski, and Goodwin (1991) have defined skin tears as "traumatic wound resulting from separation of the epidermis from the dermis". Although the exact number of skin tears is unknown, Thomas, Goode, LaMaster, Tennyson, and Parnell (1999) have reported that 1.5 million skin tears occur each year in institutionalized adults.

The Aging Skin

Aging skin predisposes a patient to skin tears due to many changes that are normal aspects of the aging process. As skin ages, there is a decrease in the dermal thickness leading to a thinning of the skin, especially over the legs and forearms. With the decrease in fatty layers and subcutaneous tissues, the bony prominences are less protected. The skin's elastin fibers lose their ability to recoil. Sensation, metabolism, and sweat gland production are also diminished resulting in dry skin that lacks some of the protection mechanisms. An important change that translates into skin tear injury risk is the decrease in the size of the rete ridges in the basement membrane of the skin. As these ridges become flatter with aging, it becomes easier to accidentally separate the epidermis from dermis (Kaminer & Gilchrest, 1994; Mason, 1997).

Location and Cause

Most skin tears (80%) occur in the upper extremities on the arms and hands over areas of senile purpura that are most prominent on sun damaged regions of the extensor aspect of the hands and forearms. (Malone et al., 1991; McGough-Csarny & Kopac, 1998; Payne & Martin, 1990). Skin tears on the back and buttocks can be mistaken for stage II pressure ulcers. For about half of skin tears, there is no apparent cause. When the cause is known, 1/4 are from wheelchair injuries, 1/4 caused by accidentally bumping into objects, 18% from transfers, and 12.4% from falls (Malone et al., 1991). Long-term steroid use and decreased hormone levels in older females may also be risk factors for skin tears (O'Regan, 2002).

A retrospective study by White, Karam, and Cowell (1994) identified dependent patients who required total care for all ADLs as being most at risk for skin tears. The skin tears occurred during routine activities of dressing, bathing, positioning, and transferring. The next most common at risk areas in independent ambulatory residents were the lower extremities. Last, were those slightly impaired residents whose skin tear injuries resulted from hitting furniture or equipment such as wheelchairs (White, Karam, & Cowell, 1994).

The method of skin cleansing in routine bathing practices may affect the occurrence of skin tears. Soap increases skin pH to an alkaline level rather than the normal "acid mantel" of the skin (Mason, 1997). Mason (1997) found a lower rate of skin tears in long-term residents (34%) who were bathed every other day with emollient soap. Use of the newer no-rinse bathing products (responsible bathing) may also be advantageous. (LeBlanc, Christensen, Orsted, & Keast, 2008) Birch and Coggins (2003) have reported a decline of skin tears from 23%–3% in a long-term care facility when a no-rinse, one-step bed bath protocol rather than the traditional soap and water was used.

White, Karam, and Cowell (1994) developed a skin integrity risk assessment tool to identify persons at risk for skin tears. The tool utilizes three groups (I, II, or III) for leveling the risk of skin tear occurrence. Implementation of a skin tear risk prevention plan of care depends on the number of criteria that a patient meets in a group or a combination of criteria in groups II or III. Additional research with this assessment tool would be valuable in establishing its reliability and validity.

In their 6-month study of residents in a Veteran's Administration (VA) nursing home care unit and nine community nursing homes, McGough-Csarny and Kopac (1998) identified ten risk factors for skin tears; six of these accounted for skin tears in 65% of their sample. They were advanced age, sensory loss, and compromised nutrition, history of previous skin tear, cognitive impairment, and dependency. Fifty-percent of the sample had bruising and poor locomotion as contributing factors. Two other factors present in 40% of the sample were polypharmacy and assistive device. Using these 10 identified risk factors, they report a plan to develop an instrument to assess skin tear risk.

Classifying Skin Tears

The Payne-Martin Classification system for assessing skin tears (Payne & Martin, 1990, 1993) is used to identify the type of skin tear. It has three categories. Category I are skin tears without any tissue loss. Category II skin tears have a partial tissue loss of the epidermal flap. Skin tears with complete tissue loss where the epidermal flap is absent are designated as category III (Payne & Martin, 1993).

The Payne-Martin Classification system has been used in subsequent studies. McGough-Csarny and Kopac (1998) used this system in their 6-month study of residents in a VA nursing home unit, and nine community nursing homes. These authors reported that category I and category III were the easiest tears for staff to identify. Thomas and colleagues (1999) utilized this system in their study comparing the healing of skin tears with foam versus transparent film dressings. Although the Payne-Martin Classification system has been used in some studies (McGough-Csarny & Kopac, 1998; Thomas et al., 1999), further research to determine the tools efficacy in documentation is warranted.

Plan of Care to Prevent or Treat Skin Tears

Once a patient has been identified as being at risk for developing skin tears, a protocol to prevent skin injury should be implemented. There is no universal agreement as to the best practice to prevent or treat skin tears in the literature; one example can be found in the Chapter 24 appendix. The following suggested protocols are based on the literature (Baranoski, 2000, 2001a, 2001b; Camp-Sorrell, 1991; Krasner, 1991; LeBlanc et al. 2008, LeBlanc & Baranoski, 2009; Malone et al., 1991; Mason, 1997; McGough-Csarny & Kopac, 1998; O'Regan, 2002; Payne & Martin, 1990; Thomas et al, 1999; White, Karem, & Cowell, 1994) and expert clinical opinion:

Skin Tears Prevention Protocol

- Use proper position, turning, lifting, and transferring techniques.
- Use a lift sheet to move and turn patients.
- Have the patient wear long sleeves and pants to add a layer of protection.

- Pad bed rails, wheelchair arm, leg supports, and any other equipment that the patient may use.
- Use non--adherent dressings on frail skin. Be gentle when removing these products to prevent skin injury.
- Use stockinettes, gauge wrap, or some of the commercially available drain holders to secure dressings and drains. If you use tape, use only paper tape.
- Support dangling arms and legs with pillows or blankets.
- Consider use of waterless, no rinse cleansers. Use emollient soaps. Avoid using alcohol on the skin as it is drying.
- Pat dry skin instead of rubbing while bathing patients.
- Use moisturizing agents on dry skin.
- Keep the environment well lit to prevent falls.
- Educate staff and caregivers to practice gentle care. This includes being careful that their nails do not scratch an elders vulnerable skin nor should they slide and watches or jewelry over the arm of an at risk person.

Skin Tears Treatment Protocol

- Continue using the skin tear prevention protocol.
- Gently clean the skin tear with normal saline.
- Let the area air dry or pat dry carefully.
- Approximate the skin tear flap.
- Apply petroleum-based ointment, steri-strips or a moist non-adherent wound dressing.
- Calcium Alginate dressings facilitated closing in 7–10 days (Nazarko, 2005).
- Two studies reported healing with octylcyanoacrylate skin glue (LeBlanc et al., 2008; Milne & Corbett, 2005).
- Use caution if using film dressings as skin damage can occur when removing this dressing.
- Consider putting an arrow to indicate the direction of the skin tear on the dressing to minimize any further skin injury during dressing removal.
- Always assess the size of the skin tear, consider doing a wound tracing.
- Document assessment and treatment findings.

PERISTOMAL (OSTOMY) SKIN

Secondary to the original surgery or because of complications (obstruction from recurrent tumor) some patients may require urinary or fecal diversions. This is most commonly seen in patients with colon, rectal, cervical, bladder, or other pelvic malignancies (Turnbull, 2007). Once a patient develops an incontinent ostomy, protecting the skin around the stoma—the peristomal skin, and preventing its breakdown, becomes an important nursing goal. A wound, ostomy, continence nurse (CWOCN, formerly ET) is an excellent resource in planning and implementing care for these elders.

The Wound, Ostomy, and Continence Nurses Society (WOCN) have a website and maintain a directory of nurses by geographic area who are available for clinical consults (see their website – www.wocn.org)

Assessing Peristomal Skin

Peristomal skin must be assessed with each pouching system change. Recently, a new tool to bring consistency to describing peristomal skin complications was published in English and three other languages. The tool contains three criteria; discoloration, erosion, and hyperplasia or raised lesions that can be measured with size and severity for a maximum score of 5 points for each criteria. (Claessens, Serrano, English, & Martins, 2008). Normal peristomal skin should be intact without discoloration and no difference between the peristomal skin and adjacent skin surfaces. Peristomal skin damage may be evidenced by erthyema, maceration, denudation, skin rash, ulceration, or blister formation. In darkly pigmented patients, the damaged skin may appear lighter or darker than the surrounding skin (Erwin-Toth, 2001).

Protecting the peristomal skin from the damaging effects of urinary or fecal effluent is paramount. The proteolytic enzymes found in the effluent from small bowel stomas can rapidly erode the skin. If the urine from a urinary diversion becomes alkaline, it is more damaging to the skin than normally acidic urine. Large amounts of liquid effluent can result in maceration, if allowed to pool on the skin.

Maintaining Peristomal Skin Integrity

Maintaining the integrity of peristomal skin can be accomplished, in part, by observing correct pouching principles. Similarly, peristomal skin must be protected from mechanical trauma, which can occur from inappropriate cleaning. To avoid skin stripping, use adhesive removers to remove skin barriers and pouching systems. Gently peel the adhesive barriers off the skin by supporting with one hand, and using the adhesive remover as the edge of the barrier that is attached to the skin. Application of skin sealants prior to application of skin barriers of the pouching system can provide protection for the peristomal skin. Avoid too frequent or unnecessary changing of the pouch/skin barrier.

The nurse should be sure to use the correct products on peristomal skin. Alcohol based products should never be used, especially if the peristomal skin is denuded. If solvents are used, the skin should be cleaned, and the solvent is removed before applying the ostomy pouch. The older adult should be assessed for sensitivity to the ostomy products PRIOR to using the product; this includes assessing for latex sensitivity.

Skin sealants come in a variety of forms—wipes, gels, and sprays. These products, when dried, provided a thin film to the skin surface, and thus decrease the chance of skin stripping. Some skin sealants contain alcohol, so care should be taken not to use them on denuded skin because they can cause the elder additional pain or burning on application.

A variety of skin barriers can be used to protect the peristomal skin from effluent. These are available as rings, wafers, pastes, and powders. In addition to protecting the skin, they also create a level pouching surface, which can prevent leakage of effluent underneath the pouch seal in "difficult to fit" stomas. A properly sized and applied skin barrier can protect the skin from the damaging effects of ostomy effluent. Skin barriers vary in their resistance to breakdown by urine or feces. Karaya dissolves with urine, so avoid its use with urinary diversions.

Skin barriers that are powders can be "dusted" onto the denuded skin. Using a skin sealant product over this product can help provide an absorptive protective layer for the peristomal skin. Some skin barriers can cause pain when used on denuded skin. Check that the skin sealant product does not have alcohol in it, as this can be painful when applied to denuded and irritated skin. Some companies make "no sting" skin barriers that do not cause pain or "burning" when applied to irritated denuded skin.

Selecting the right ostomy pouching system for your patient may require the assistance of the CWOCN (ET) nurse. Pouching systems are provided as one or two pieces. A one-piece system has the skin barrier permanently attached to the ostomy pouch. A two-piece ostomy pouching system has the advantage of the skin barrier remaining on the skin for several days with the ease of snapping the pouch off the skin barrier for emptying of contents. Pouches can be drainable or closed end. There are also pouches specially designed for pediatric patients.

Pouches should be selected that are correct for the type of drainage coming from the ostomy. For example, fecal pouches will not work for urinary diversions. Urinary ostomy pouches have a spout on the bottom for proper emptying of the urine. For fecal pouches, the opening is wide and closed, and, in most cases, with a special ostomy clamp. Most modern day ostomy pouching systems are odor proof when correctly closed and the seal is intact. If the elder has an unusually large amount of drainage, one of the high-output pouches should be used. Treatments such as chemotherapy or radiation may affect the patient's stool consistency and amount of output. Adjustments in the size of the pouch, more frequent emptying of the pouch and changes in ostomy irrigations may need to be implemented. It is imperative when selecting the appropriate pouch, that it is the correct size for the ostomy stoma. A too large or too small, a pouch opening size can cause leakage and/or trauma to the stoma (Bryant and Fleischer, 2000).

Total Ostomy Care Management

Care of the older adult patient with an ostomy involves more than just assessing the peristomal skin and pouching system. The elder's emotional and psychosocial acceptance of the stoma is important; for some people, the creation of a diverting ostomy may bring relief from the symptoms of obstruction, but may also serve as a permanent reminder of the progression of their disease. Supporting the patient to adjust to this change in body image, over coming concerns about odor, learning new psychomotor self care skills, and dietary adjustments are just some of the comprehensive care elements that the nurse may need to obtain the consultation of a WOCN (ET) nurse to meet the patient's needs.

FISTULAS

Fistulas are abnormal openings between two organs or an organ and the skin. An internal fistula is inside the body while an external fistula tracts outside the body to the skin, most commonly through the GI tract or bladder but sometimes through the vagina or rectum. Fistulas can occur with certain diseases (e.g. malignancies including obstructions, Crohn's disease, or diverticulitis,) or from treatment modalities such as radiation or surgery including postoperative adhesions. A high-output fistula has more than 200ml/24 h (Rolstead & Bryant, 2000). Assessment of the perifistula skin is critical because irrigation from the effluent can be caustic to the skin and result in irritation and erosion. The perifistula skin should be assessed for signs of fungal infections as well as for redness, popular rash, and satellite lesions.

Identification of the fistula to determine its origin is important for developing the plan for closure, which can be spontaneous (about 50%), or surgical. Goals of management for an older adult with a fistula should include: maintaining fluid and electrolyte balance (assess for dehydration and metabolic acidosis), protection of the perifistula skin, odor control, effluent containment and measurement, nutritional management, and patient comfort. Holistic care of an elder with a fistula might include total parenteral nutrition to meet the nutritional needs, therapeutic communication to respond to the patient's emotional needs from having a foul smelling fistula, protecting the skin from injury from the effluent, and eliminating odor.

Women who have had pelvic radiation can then develop vaginal fistulas, which are often distressing to the patient and challenging to the nurse. Containment of the feces and odor are difficult and require frequent dressing changes. For nonambulatory patients, urinary incontinence pouches, commercially available vaginal drain devices, or a breast shield or vaginal diaphragm attached to a malecot catheter may be used (Rolstead & Bryant, 2000).

Management Options

Pouching

A pouching system may be the primary choice for management for older adults with odorous fistulas. Using a clear pouch will enable the caregiver or nurse to easily see the type and amount of effluent. Pouching is superior to dressings because it provides better protection for the skin. A pouch with a spout on the bottom works well for fistulas with thin effluent drainage, for thicker drainage, a fecal pouch that can be closed with a clamp is a better choice. Wound management pouches come in a variety of sizes and are useful for treating abdominal fistulas (Schaffner, Hocevar, Erwin-Toth, 1994). For patients with odorless fistulas and output (100cc/24 h), dressings may be used. A dressing that is absorbent such as foams, calcium alginates, or hydrocolloids should be used. In these cases, use a petroleum or zinc based ointment to protect the perifistula skin from maceration or breakdown. Some patients have such large wounds with enterocutaneous fistulae that the usual commercially available pouches are too small and will not fit. O'Brien, Landis-Erdman, and Erwin-Toth (1998) have described the management of one such fistulae and large wound using a surgical isolation bag with skin barrier while packing the wound with moistened gauze.

The more enzymes and liquidly of the fistula output, the greater the need to place additional skin barrier seals around the fistula opening prior to placing a high output pouch. For older adults who have abdominal fistulas with irregular skin surfaces, skin barrier pastes or strips may need to be placed around the fistula opening in order to "build it up" so the abdominal plane can be "filled in" and then a pouch placed over it. Sometimes, a patient has two fistula openings; if they are close together, one pouch may fit over both fistula orifices. If not, "saddle bagging" two pouches may be the best option.

Tubes and Suction

Another way to manage fistulas is to use drainage tubes, with or without suction. Beitz and Caldwell (1998) have described the management of a high output enterocutaneous fistula using a drain tube (JP) connected to low wall suction (60 mm of pressure) that was covered with saline soaked gauze and a large surgical plastic drape. When using this technique, be careful in placing the catheter tube so it does not inadvertently cause injury to the tissue. Harris and Komray (1993) have also used a similar system to manage a pharyngocutaneous fistula. This system should not be confused with the negative pressure wound therapy (NPWT) previously discussed under the pressure ulcer section. According to the manufacturers, NPWAT. should not be used for fistulas.

Trough

Another method of managing enterocutaneous fistula is by using the trough procedure. This technique is used for fistulas that are deep within wounds (Wiltshire, 1996). It is made up of several layers of transparent dressing with an ostomy pouch on the bottom of the wound (Rolstead & Bryant, 2000).

Patient Comfort

Promoting patient comfort is a major priority in caring for a patient with a fistula. The amount of pain or discomfort that a particular management option may cause a patient should influence the decision regarding which management option to select. The goal is to choose the method that will cause the least discomfort and disruption to the patient and caregiver. Medicating the patient prior to removal and application of fistula containment measurements is essential.

TUMOR NECROSIS AND SKIN INJURY FROM FECAL INCONTINENCE

Tumor Necrosis and Skin Care

In some older adults with advanced cancer, the tumor can invade the skin, which results in ulcerated fungating wounds. For example, in patients with breast cancer, the tumor can grow outward onto to the skin in a blackened cauliflower-like appearance (see Exhibit 24.5, Giving Voice to Patient-Centered Concerns). This results in maceration of the surrounding skin as well as extensive odor from bacterial infection from organisms such

---

EXHIBIT 24.5: GIVING VOICE TO PATIENT-CENTERED CONCERNS

Here are some of the comments from a patient in our case study about important aspects of her care.

Initial approach—"From the very beginning, the wound care team treated me with respect. You asked me if I was ok. You called me by my name. It was not just about my boops, my illnesses or my wounds."

What made the difference—"You acknowledged that my feelings about my body image were an important component to me. I always put on my jewelry, did my hair and dressed up nice to come to the wound clinic. Even though I have several wounds on my chest, you always remarked about my pretty necklace."

Pain— "When my wounds were painful, you understood that I had to work through the pain. I was addicted to the feeling of feeling better. Even something as simple as lifting the laundry can be very heavy with the pain and these wounds on my chest.

as *Pseudomonas aeruginosa*, staphylococcus, proteus, and klebsiella (Haisfield-Wolfe & Baxendale-Cox, 1999; Haisfield-Wolfe & Rund, 1997). Nodules may enlarge and erupt spontaneously through the abdominal skin in patients with carcinomatosis. While the majority of metastatic skin lesions are found on the anterior trunk, they may also be found on the pelvis, flank, head and neck, and posterior trunk (Bauer, Gerlach, & Doughty, 2000). Haisfield-Wolfe and Baxendale-Cox (1999) have suggested the use of a staging classification for assessment of malignant cutaneous wounds. Parameters to include are wound depth, color of the wound, drainage, pain, odor, and presence of tunneling or undermining.

Management Strategies

In an effort to palliate symptoms, radiation or chemotherapy may be used to shrink the tumors that have grown onto the skin. Maida, Ennis, Kuziemsky, and Trozzolo (2009) identified 8 key symptoms associated with malignant wounds from a prospective series of 472 cancer patients. Approximately two-thirds of the malignant wounds were associated with at least one of these symptoms: pain, mass effect, aesthetic distress, exudate, odor, pruritus, bleeding and crusting. Management strategies suggested by Alvarez et al. (2007) include the mnemonic SPECIAL (stabilizing the wounds, preventing new wounds, eliminating odor, control pain, infection prophylaxis, advanced, absorbent wound dressings, lessen dressing changes).

Wound Cleansing

Although the evidence base for management of such extensive wounds is limited, options for addressing the patient care needs are anecdotally reported. Frequent irrigation of the wound with large amounts of fluid may be important to reduce the bacterial burden on the wound surface (Bauer et al., 2000). For patients who can get into the shower, cleansing these fungating wounds may provide physical as well as psychological benefits. Instruct the patient not to aim the shower water directly at the wound, but rather above the ulcerated area so the water can trickle down over the wound without undue force. Use of a hand held shower device might be preferred by some patients (Bauer et al., 2000). For patients who cannot tolerate being showered or where the tissue is very friable, gentle cleaning with saline or commercially available wound cleansers may be substituted.

Exudate Management

Management of these wounds can be challenging and they generally have large amounts of exudate because of the tumor's hyperpermeability to fibrinogen and colloids, but primarily due to the secretion of vascular permeability factor secreted by the tumor (Bauer et al., 2000). There may also be drainage of fecal material in the case of patients with abdominal carcinomatosis. Dressings should be used that are absorbent (foam, calcium alginate, or cotton absorbent dressing pads). Often there is much necrotic tissue in these wounds and debridement is required. Autolytic debridement techniques such as the use of calcium alginate dressings, hydrogel dressings, or other non-adherent modern dressings are advocated. Others (Bauer et al., 2000) recommend using a petroleum-impregnated gauze dressing. Picture frame the skin area around the fungating wound with protective skin barriers such as hydrocolloid dressing strips. Use of Montgomery straps to hold the secondary dressing in place will also reduce damage to skin that can be caused by the frequent removal of tape. Cutting the crotch off mesh underpanties and putting this around the chest wall like a tube top can also be used to hold the bulky dressings in place (Bauer et al., 2000). Mechanical debridement, such as wet-to-dry dressings, should be avoided due to the obvious risk of causing more bleeding and increasing pain. The safety of using enzymatic debriding agents in cancer wounds is not yet known.

Controlling Bleeding in Friable Areas

Bleeding commonly occurs in these types of wounds because tumor cells take over the function of platelets, and the growth and clotting factors that they secrete damage normal tissue (Bauer et al., 2000). Preventing the dressings from drying out can minimize tissue trauma from the removal of soiled dressings. Calcium alginate dressings (Haisfield-Wolf & Rund, 1997) have a hemostatic effect and are a good choice for bleeding wounds. Silver nitrate sticks can be used to control small amounts of blood.

Pain management

Pain also results from the tumor growing on the skin and from treatment procedures. Seaman (1995) suggests using ice packs or topical anesthetic aerosol spray (Hurricane) to alleviate wound pain. Some clinicians have reported using the negative pressure wound therapy dressing system (NPWT) solely for pain management and comfort for elders with these types of extensive wounds. Topical extemporaneously compounded opioids or preparations containing amide local anesthetics (lidocaine & prilocaine including EMLA{Eutectic Mixture of Local Anesthetics}, pramoxine)have also been used to relieve wound pain.(Alvarez et al., 2007).

Odor management

Odor may be one of the most distressing problems for the patient and their caregivers. Seaman (1995) suggests first using one of the commercially available wound gel deodorizers; some patients may experience burning with application of these products. The use of metrogel (0.8% topical antibiotic wound deodorizing gel) (Newman, Allwood, & Oakes, 1989; Rice, 1990; Seaman, 1995) to control even the most horrific odors has been reported. Metronidazole tablets can be dissolved into normal saline and used to irritate the wound (McMullen, 1995). Metronidazole tablets (250 mg or 500 mg) can be crushed and sprinkled directly onto the wound bed (Bauer et al., 2000). Healthcare professionals should wear a mask to avoid inhaling the particles. Taking metronidazole systemically or using the IV solution as an irrigation solution has also been recommended.

Topical application of yogurt or buttermilk has been used to combat the extensive odors from tumor necrosis (Welch, 1981; Schulte, 1993). The newer antimicrobial cadexomer iodine or silver dressings are also excellent at reducing odor with the added plus of also controlling the bacterial burden in the surface compartment wound. Another advantage is that some of these dressings can stay in place for up to 7 days, which reduces the pain from dressing change. Odor control within patient's environment may be achieved by utilizing aromatherapy products, such as peppermint oils/sprays, or charcoal under the bed (Cormier, McCann, & McKeithan, 1995).

QUALITY OF LIFE ISSUES

The clinician should be aware of his or her nonverbal and verbal communication to patients during dressing changes. Patients and/or family members may have difficulty coping with wound odor or appearance, and will look to the clinician to see his or her reaction. Seeing the extensive deterioration of one's own body, coupled with overpowering smells, and weeping feces may be extremely overwhelming to patients. The clinician's resolve to problem-solve and provide the patient with the appropriate wound management is vital in helping these patients overcome their (sometimes self-imposed) isolation and hiding.

Skin care needs from fecal incontinence. Changes in bowel habits may occur in older adults undergoing cancer treatments such as radiation or chemotherapy. Bliss, Larson, Burr, and Savik (2001) tested the reliability of a four-category stool consistency classification system, and found it to be a valid tool for use by nurses and lay caregivers. Precision in describing the characteristics of the stool is important for clinicians. By understanding if a patient truly is having diarrhea or loose stools, the clinician can then develop an appropriate plan to protect the skin. For example, Grogan and Kramer (2002) have described the use of the rectal trumpet (nasopharyngeal airway) to contain fecal incontinence in critically ill and geriatric patients. This technique proved to be less traumatic than other methods of fecal containment (diapers, perineal incontinence pouches, and balloon catheters).

Educating elders about skin care is an important part of nursing interventions. Ideally, this type of teaching will occur prior to any skin injury. For example, Haisfield-Wolfe and Rund (2002) created a booklet for cancer patients with guidelines for skin care. The 30 female oncology patients who were receiving chemotherapy found the booklet helpful in doing their own self-assessment for perineal skin changes.

Case Study conclusion: Ms. DL required treatment systemically for the secondary infection, due to gram negative and anaerobic organisms, that was leading to the increased pain, exudate, and odor. A combination antibiotic of clavulinic acid and amoxicillin was administered with improvement in the symptoms. For cleansing of the wounds, a dilute acetic acid compress was used for 10 min prior to dressing changes. The wounds contained slough that was autolytically debrided with hypertonic saline ribbon gauze alternating with a calcium alginate and silver combination product (see Figure 24.2). With the treatment program, the dressing changes (with moist saline gauze and an antibiotic ointment) occurring 3 to 4 times a day were reduced to daily, with an improvement in pain, odor, and the amount of the exudate.

Psychologically the improved management of the cutaneous lesions lead to an increased self confidence and the ability to resume social relationships and to consent to an interview for an advanced wound care program to highlight the importance of palliative wound care centered around patient concerns.

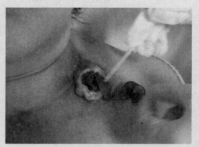

Figure 24.2   Hypertonic Saline Ribbon Gauze Debridement

CONCLUSION

The nurse and the health-care team can be faced with a multiple of skin problems when caring for patients receiving palliative care. Focusing on the wound etiology and classifying wounds as healable, maintenance, or palliative (nonhealing) can provide realistic expectations for patients, their family unit and care givers as well as the healthcare professional team. Local wound care should be aimed at providing comfort, relieving pain, odor, containing exudate and improving patient's quality of life permitting them to resume as many activities of daily living as possible. Local wound care may be aimed at moisture reduction rather than moisture balance with antibacterial activity of agents such as povidone iodine or chlorhexidine and its derivatives more important than tissue toxicity. Debridement is often conservative to remove slough or devitalized tissue but not to create active bleeding of an acute wound within a chronic wound. The focus should be patient and symptom centered and not curative.

EVIDENCE-BASED PRACTICE

Wallace, M., Fulmer, T. (2002). Fulmer SPICES: An Overall Assessment Tool of Older Adults. *Dermatology Nursing,14*(2), 142.

Purpose. Normal aging brings about inevitable and irreversible changes. These normal aging changes are partially responsible for the increased risk of developing health-related problems within the elderly population. Prevalent problems experienced by older adults include sleep disorders, problems with eating or feeding, incontinence, confusion, evidence of falls and skin breakdown. Familiarity with these commonly occurring disorders helps the nurse prevent unnecessary iatrogenesis and promote optimal function of the aging patient. Flagging conditions for further assessment will allow the nurse to implement preventative and therapeutic interventions.

Best tool. The most appropriate instrument for obtaining the information necessary to prevent health alterations in SPICES developed by Terry Fulmer, PhD, RN, FAAN at New York University, Division of Nursing. SPICES are an acronym for the common syndromes of the elderly requiring nursing intervention:

S is for Sleep Disorders

P is for Problems with eating or feeding

I is for Incontinence

C is for Confusion

E is for Evidence of Falls

S is for Skin Breakdown

Target population. The problems assessed through SPICES occur commonly among the entire elderly population. Therefore, the instrument may be used for both healthy and frail older adults.

Validity/Reliability. The instrument has been used extensively to assess the elderly population. Notably, members of the Geriatric Nurse Resource Project at Yale University Medical Center use the tool to assess and prevent the most frequent health problems of older adults. It is also being used at New York University Medical Center. Psychometric testing has not been done.

Strengths and limitations. The SPICES acronym is easily remembered and may be used to recall the common problems of the elderly population in all clinical settings. It provides a simple system for flagging areas in need of further assessment and provides a basis for standardizing quality of care around certain parameters. SPICES are an alert system and refer to only the most frequently occurring health problems of older adults. Through this initial screen, assessments that are more complete are triggered. It should not be used as a replacement for a complete nursing assessment.

EVIDENCE-BASED PRACTICE

Lentz, L. (2003). Daily Baths: Torment or Comfort at End of Life? *Journal of Hospice & Palliative Nursing, 5*(1) 34–39.

Abstract Review. As far back as the Middle Ages, bathing has been a ritualistic pleasure. In more recent times, bathing improves an individual's hygiene and social acceptance. Since Florence Nightingale, nurses and their assistants have considered the traditional bath a daily professional responsibility. In 1994, Skewes introduced an alternative to the traditional bath called a bag bath. This article challenges those who care for bed-bound or demented patients to change their traditional bathing practices and incorporate the bag bath process to improve quality of life. Bathing the bed-bound elder patient poses risks to skin integrity because of skin dryness and fragility. Bathing the demented patient poses behavior problems associated with fear of the process. The bag bath concept offers relief to these individuals, thereby improving skin integrity, comfort, self-esteem, and quality of life. The use of warm washcloths soaked in a mixture of water, an emollient concentrate to cleanse the skin has been shown to improve patient satisfaction while reducing staff time and savings in labor, and supply costs. It is time to consider this alternate daily bathing approach for the bed-bound and demented patient populations, and to replace the torment with comfort at the end of life.

REFERENCES

Alvarez, O. M., Kalinski, C., Nusbaum, J., Hernandez, L., Pappous, E., Kyriannis, C., et al. (2007). Incorporating wound healing strategies to improve palliation (Symptom Management) in patients with chronic wounds. *Journal of Palliative Medicine,* 10(5),1161–1189.

Ayello, E. A. (1992). Teaching the assessment of patients with pressure ulcers. *Decubitus, 5,* 53–54.

Ayello, E. A. (1993). A critique of the AHCPR's "Preventing pressure ulcers: A patient's guide" as a written instructional tool. *Decubitus, 6*(3), 44–50.

Ayello, E. A., Braden, B. (2001). Why is pressure ulcer risk assessment so important? *Nursing 2001, 31*(11), 75–79.

Ayello, E. A., Cuddigan, J., Kerstein, M. (2002). Skip the knife: Debriding wounds without surgery. *Nursing, 32*(9), 58–63.

Ayello, E. A., Mezey. M., & Amella, E. J. (1997). Educational assessment and teaching of older clients with pressure ulcers. *Clinics in Geriatric Medicine, 13* (3), 483–496.

Bales, S., Finlay, I., Harding, K. G. (1995). Pressure sore prevention in a hospice. *Journal of Wound Care, 4*(10), 465–468.

Baranoski, S. (2000). Skin tears: The enemy of frail skin. *Advances in Skin and Wound Care, 13*(3), 123–126.

Baranoski, S. (2001a). Skin tears: Guard against this enemy of frail skin. *Nursing Management,32*(8), 25–31.

Baranoski, S. (2001b). Skin: the forgotten organ. *16th Annual Clinical Symposium of Advances in Skin and Wound Care,* Lake Buena Vista, Florida, September 2001.

Baranoski, S., & Ayello, E. A. (2008).*Wound care essentials: Practice principles* (2nd ed.). Springhouse, PA: Lippincott.

Baldwin, K. (2001). Incidence and prevalence of pressure ulcers in children. *Advances in Skin and Wound Care, 15*(3), 121– 124.

Baharestani, M. M. (1994). The lived experience of wives caring for their frail, home bound, elderly husbands with pressure ulcers. *Advances in Wound Care, 7*(3), 40–52.

Bauer, C., Gerlach, M. A., Doughty, D. (2000). Care of metastatic skin lesions. *JWOCN, 27*(4), 247–251.

Beitz, J. M., Caldwell, D. (1998). Abdominal wound with enterocutaneous fistula: A case study. *Journal of Wound Ostomy Continence Nursing, 25*(2), 102–106.

Bennett, M. A. (1995). Characteristics of intact dark skin. *Advances in Wound Care, 8*(6), 34–35.

Bergstrom N., Bennett M. A., Carlson C. E., et al. (December 1994). *Treatment of pressure ulcers.Clinical practice guideline, No. 15.* Rockville, MD: U.S. Department of Health and Human Services. Public Health Service, Agency of Health Care Policy and Research. *AHCPR Publication No. 95-0652.*

Bliss, D. Z., Larson, S. J., Burr, J. K., Savik, K. (2001). Reliability of a stool consistency classification system. *JWOCN, 28*(6), 305–13.

Braden Scale. (2009). Accessed on May 1, www.bradenscale.com

Brink, P., Fries-Smith, T., Linkewich, B. (2006). Factors associated with pressure ulcers in palliative home care. *Journal of Palliative Medicine, 9*(6), 1369–1375.

Bryant, D., & Fleischer, I. (2000). Changing an ostomy appliance. *Nursing, 30*(11), 51–53.

Camp-Sorrell, D. (1991). Skin tears: What can you do? *Oncology Nursing Forum, 18*(1), 135.

Chaplin, J. (2000). Pressure sore risk assessment in palliative care. *Journal of Tissue Viability, 10*(1), 27–31.

Claessens, I., Serrano, J. L. C., English, E., Martins, L. (2008). Peristomal skin disorders and the ostomy skin tool. *JWCET, 28*(2),26–27.

Colburn, L. (1987). Pressure ulcer prevention for the hospice patient. Strategies for care to increase comfort. *American Journal of Hospital Care, 4*(2), 22–26.

Cormier, A. C., McCann, E., McKeithan, L. (1995). Reducing odor caused by metastatic breast cancer skin lesions. *Oncology Nursing Forum, 22,* 988–999.

Cuddigan, J., Hollinger, K., Brown, C., Horslen, S. P. (2001). Pressure ulcers in infants and children. In J. Cuddigan, E. A. Ayello,

& C. Sussman (Eds.),. *Pressure ulcers in America: Prevalence, incidence, and implications for the future* (pp. 163–166). Reston, VA: National Pressure Ulcer Advisory Panel (NPUAP).

Dallam, L., et al. (1995). Pressure ulcer pain: Assessment and quantification. *JWOCN, 22* (5), 211–218.

Eckman, K. (1989). The prevalence of pressure ulcers among persons in the U.S. who have died. *Decubitus, 2*(2), 36–41.

Erwin-Toth, P. (2001). Caring for a stoma is more than skin deep. *Nursing, 31*(5), 36–40.

Grogan, T. A., Kramer, D. J. (2002). The rectal trumpet: Use of a nasopharyngeal airway to contain fecal incontinence in critically ill patients. *J WOCN, 29*(4), 193–201.

Haisfield-Wolfe, M. E., Rund, C. (2002). The development and pilot testing of a teaching booklet for oncology patients' self assessment and perineal skin care .*JWOCN, 29*(2), 88–92.

Haisfield-Wolfe, M. E., Rund, C. (1997). Malignant coetaneous wounds: A management protocol. *Ostomy Wound Management 42*(1), 56–66.

Haisfield-Wolfe, M. E., Baxendale-Cox, L. M. (1999). Staging of malignant cutaneous wounds: A pilot study. *Oncology Nursing Forum 26,* 1055–1064.

Hanson, D., Langemo, D. K., Olson, B., Hunter, S, Burd, C. (1994). Evaluation of pressure ulcer prevalence rates for hospice patient's post-implementation of pressure ulcer protocols. *American Journal of Hospital and Palliative Care, 11*(6), 14–9.

Hanson, D., Langemo, D. K., Olson, B., Hunter, S., Sauvage, T. R., Burd, C., et al. (1991). The prevalence and incidence of pressure ulcers in the hospice setting: Analysis of two methodologies. *American Journal of Hospice and Palliative Care, 8*(5), 18–22.

Harris, A. Komray, R. R. (1993). Cost-effective management of pharyngocutaneous fistulas following laryngectomy. *Ostomy/Wound Managemen, 39,* 36–44.

Hatcliffe, S., & Dawe, R. (1996). Clinical Audit: Monitoring pressure sores in a palliative care setting. *Intern Jo of Palliative Care Nursing, 2*(4), 182, 184–186.

Henderson, C. T., Ayello, E. A., Sussman, C., Leiby, D. M., Bennett, M. A., Dungog, E. F., et al. (1997). Draft definition of stage 1-pressure ulcers: Inclusion of persons with darkly pigmented skin. *Advances in Wound Care, 10* (5), 16–19.

Kaminer, M., Gilchrest, B. (1994). Aging of the skin. In W. Hazzard (Ed.), *Principles of geriatric medicine and gerontology* (pp. 411–415). New York: McGraw-Hill.

Kennedy, K. L. (1989). The prevalence of pressure ulcers in an intermediate care facility. *Decubitus 2*(2), 44–45.

Kirshen, C., Woo, K., Ayello, E. A.,Sibbald, R. G. (2006). Debridement, A vital component of wound bed preparation. *Advances in Skin and Wound Care, 19*(9), 506–17, quiz, 518–19.

Krasner, D. (1991). An approach to treating skin tears. *Ostomy/Wound Management. 32*(1), 56–58.

Langemo, D., Bates-Jensen, B., Hanson, D. (2001). Pressure ulcers in individuals at the end of life: Palliative care and hospice. (pp. 143–151). In J. Cuddigan, E. A. Ayello, & C. Sussman (Eds.), *Pressure ulcers in America: Prevalence, incidence, and implications for the future.* Reston, VA: National Pressure Ulcer Advisory Panel (NPUAP).

Langemo, D., Melland, H., Hanson, D., Olson, B., Hunter, S. (2000). The lived experience of having a pressure ulcer: a qualitative analysis. *Advances in Skin and Wound Care 13*(5), 225–235.

LeBlanc, K., Baranoski, S. (2009 in press). Prevention and management of skin tears. *Advances in Skin and Wound Care.*

LeBlanc, K., Christensen, D., Orsted, H. L., Keast, D. H., (2008). Best practice recommendations for the prevention and treatment of skin tears. *Wound Care Canada, 6*(1),14–32.

Maida, V., Corbo, M., Dolzhykov, M., Ennis, M., Irani, S., Trozzolo, L., et al. (2008). Wounds in advanced illness: A prevalence and incidence study based on a prospective case series. *Int Wound J, 5*(2), 3–5–14.

Maida, V., Ennis, M., Kuziemsky, C., Trozzolo, L. (2009). Symptoms associated with malignant wounds: a prospective case series.*Journal of Pain and Symptom Management, Feb 37*(2), 206–222.

Malone, M. L., Rozario, N., Gavinski, M., Goodwin, J. (1991). The epidemiology of skin tears in the institutionalized elderly. *Journal of the American Geriatric Society, 39*(6), 591–595.

Mason, S. (1997). Types of soap and the incidence of skin tears among residents of a long-term care facility. *Ostomy/Wound Management, 43*(8), 26–41.

McGough-Csarny, J., Kopac, C. A. (1998). Skin tears in institutionalized elderly: An epidemiological study. *Ostomy/Wound Management, 44*(3A), 14S–24S.

McMullen, D. (1992). Topical metronidazole, part II. *Ostomy/Wound Management 38*, 42–47.

Milne, C. T., Corbett, L. Q. (2005). A new option in the treatment of skin tears for the institutionalized resident: formulated 2-octycyanacrylate topical bandage. *Geriatric Nurs 26*, 321–325.

National Pressure Ulcer Advisory Panel. (NPUAP). (2001). J. Cuddigan, E. A. Ayello, & C. Sussman (Eds.). *Pressure ulcers in America: Prevalence, incidence, and implications for the future.* Reston, VA: NPUAP.

Nazarko, L. (2005). Preventing and treating skin tears. *Nursing and Residential Care, 7*(12), L549–L550.

Newman, V., Allwood, M., Oakes, R. A. (1989). The use of metonidazole gel to control the smell of malodorous lesions. *Palliative Medicine, 3*, 303–305.

Olson, B., Tkachuk, L., Hanson, J. (1998). Preventing pressure sores in oncology patients.*Clinical Nursing Research, 7*(2), 207–224.

Oncology Nursing Society. (ONS). (2008). Radiation oncology nursing practice and education. Available at www.guidelines. gov. Accessed September 13.

O'Brien, B., Landis-Erdman, J., & Erwin-Toth, P. (1998). Nursing management of multiple enterocutaneous fistulae located in the center of a large open abdominal wound: A case study. *Ostomy/Wound Management, 44*(1), 20–24.

O'Regan, A. (2002). Skin tears: A review of the literature. *WCET Journal, 22*(2), 26–31.

Panel for the Prediction and Prevention of Pressure Ulcers in Adults. (AHCPR). (May, 1992). *Pressure ulcers in adults: Prediction and prevention. Clinical practice guideline, Number 3.AHCPR Publication No. 92–0047.* Rockville, MD: Agency for Health Care Policy and Research, Public Health Service, U.S. Department of Health and Human Services.

Payne, R. L., Martin, M. L. (1993). Defining and classifying skin tears: Need for a common language. *Ostomy/Wound Managemen,. 39*(5), 16–24.

Payne, R. L., Martin, M. L. (1990). The epidemiology and management of skin tears in older adults. *Ostomy/Wound Management, 26*(1), 26–37.

Pieper, B., Langemo, D., Cuddigan, J. (2009). Pressure ulcer pain: A systematic literature review and the national pressure ulcer advisory panel white paper. *Ostomy/Wound Management, 55*(2), 16–31.

Rice, T. (1990). Metronidazole use in malodorous skin lesions. *Rehabilitation Nursing, 17*, 244–245.

Rolstead, B. S., Bryant, R. (2000). Management of drain sites and fistulas. In R. Bryant, (Ed.), *Acute and chronic wounds—Nursing management* (2nd ed., pp. 317–341). St. Louis: Mosby.

Schaffner, A., Hocevar, B. J., & Erwin-Toth, P. (1994). Small bowel fistulas complicating midline surgical wounds. *Journal of Wound Ostomy Continence Nursing, 21*, 161–165.

Schulte, M. J. (1993).*Oncology Nursing Forum, 20*, 1262.

Seaman, S. (1995). Home care for pain, odor, and drainage in tumor-associated wounds. *Oncology Nursing Forum, 22*, 987.

Sibbald, R. G., Krasner, D. L., Lutz, J., Alvarex, O., Ayello, E. A., Baranoski, S. (2008). Skin changes at life's end (SCALE): A preliminary consensus statement. *JWCET, 28*(4),15–22.

Thomas, D., Goode, P., LaMaster, K, Tennyson, T., Parnell, L. K. S. (1999). A comparison of an opaque foam dressing versus a transparent film dressing in the management of skin tears in institutionalized subjects. *Ostomy/Wound Management, 45*(6), 22–28

Turnbull, G.B. (2007). Ostomy care and radiation therapy. *Ostomy/Wound Management, 53*(11), 24–26.

Waltman, N. L., Bergstrom, N., Armstrong, N., Norvell, K., Braden, B. (1991). Nutritional status, pressure sores, and mortality in elderly patients with cancer. *Oncology Nursing, Forum, 18*(5), 867–873.

Welch, L. B. (1981). Simple new remedy for the odor of open lesions.*RN 44*, 42–43.

White, M., Karam, S., Cowell, B., (1994). Skin tears in frail elders. A practical approach to prevention. *Geriatric Nursing, 15*(2), 95–99.

Wiltshire, B. L. (1996). Challenging enterocutaneous fistula: A case presentation. *Journal of WOCN, 23*(6), 297– 301.

Winter, G. D. (1962). Formation of scab and the rate of epithelialization of superficial wounds in the skin of domestic pig. *Nature, 193*, 293–294.

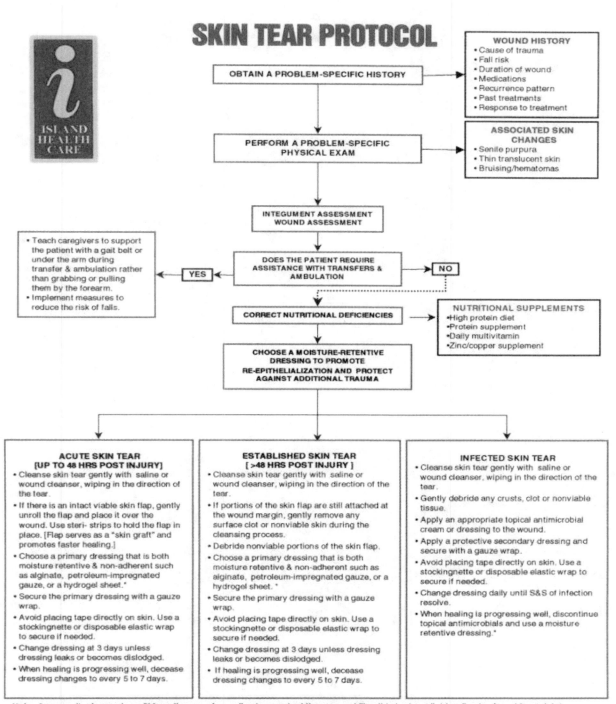

SKIN TEAR PROTOCOL

ISLAND HEALTH CARE

OBTAIN A PROBLEM-SPECIFIC HISTORY

WOUND HISTORY
- Cause of trauma
- Fall risk
- Duration of wound
- Medications
- Recurrence pattern
- Past treatments
- Response to treatment

PERFORM A PROBLEM-SPECIFIC PHYSICAL EXAM

ASSOCIATED SKIN CHANGES
- Senile purpura
- Thin translucent skin
- Bruising/hematomas

INTEGUMENT ASSESSMENT
WOUND ASSESSMENT

DOES THE PATIENT REQUIRE ASSISTANCE WITH TRANSFERS & AMBULATION

YES

NO

- Teach caregivers to support the patient with a gait belt or under the arm during transfer & ambulation rather than grabbing or pulling them by the forearm.
- Implement measures to reduce the risk of falls.

CORRECT NUTRITIONAL DEFICIENCIES

NUTRITIONAL SUPPLEMENTS
- High protein diet
- Protein supplement
- Daily multivitamin
- Zinc/copper supplement

CHOOSE A MOISTURE-RETENTIVE DRESSING TO PROMOTE RE-EPITHELIALIZATION AND PROTECT AGAINST ADDITIONAL TRAUMA

**ACUTE SKIN TEAR
[UP TO 48 HRS POST INJURY]**
- Cleanse skin tear gently with saline or wound cleanser, wiping in the direction of the tear.
- If there is an intact viable skin flap, gently unroll the flap and place it over the wound. Use steri- strips to hold the flap in place. [Flap serves as a "skin graft" and promotes faster healing.]
- Choose a primary dressing that is both moisture retentive & non-adherent such as alginate, petroleum-impregnated gauze, or a hydrogel sheet.*
- Secure the primary dressing with a gauze wrap.
- Avoid placing tape directly on skin. Use a stockingnette or disposable elastic wrap to secure if needed.
- Change dressing at 3 days unless dressing leaks or becomes dislodged.
- When healing is progressing well, decease dressing changes to every 5 to 7 days.

**ESTABLISHED SKIN TEAR
[>48 HRS POST INJURY]**
- Cleanse skin tear gently with saline or wound cleanser, wiping in the direction of the tear.
- If portions of the skin flap are still attached at the wound margin, gently remove any surface clot or nonviable skin during the cleansing process.
- Debride nonviable portions of the skin flap.
- Choose a primary dressing that is both moisture retentive & non-adherent such as alginate, petroleum-impregnated gauze, or a hydrogel sheet. *
- Secure the primary dressing with a gauze wrap.
- Avoid placing tape directly on skin. Use a stockingnette or disposable elastic wrap to secure if needed.
- Change dressing at 3 days unless dressing leaks or becomes dislodged.
- If healing is progressing well, decease dressing changes to every 5 to 7 days.

INFECTED SKIN TEAR
- Cleanse skin tear gently with saline or wound cleanser, wiping in the direction of the tear.
- Gently debride any crusts, clot or nonviable tissue.
- Apply an appropriate topical antimicrobial cream or dressing to the wound.
- Apply a protective secondary dressing and secure with a gauze wrap.
- Avoid placing tape directly on skin. Use a stockingnette or disposable elastic wrap to secure if needed.
- Change dressing daily until S&S of infection resolve.
- When healing is progressing well, discontinue topical antimicrobials and use a moisture retentive dressing.*

Note: Some patients may benefit from the use of an adhesive product [transparent film, thin hydrocolloid, adhesive foam] to maintain dressing integrity. Adhesive dressings can cause reinjury and should be used with caution.

Cuzzell, J. (2002). Wound Assessment and Evaluation: Skin Tear Protocol. *Dermatology Nursing, 14*(6), 405.

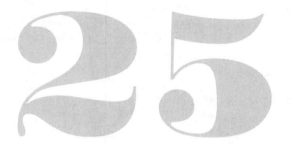

Peri-Death Nursing Care

Marianne Matzo
Jane A. Hill

- Nurses caring for patients who are near death should be aware of the patient's and family's physical and emotional experiences during the dying experience.
- Special considerations for children and elderly patients who cannot make their own decisions should be addressed with the family.
- Families should be informed of the physical processes that occur during the dying process and the nursing interventions and activities that occur after death.
- Nurses should engage in a discussion with families about the options for organ donation, autopsy, and various postmortem responsibilities, rights, and rituals appropriate to the culture, and assist them with accessing resources.
- Nursing interventions do not terminate with a patient's death and should include bereavement care and assistance with accessing appropriate resources.

Case Study: When I pulled up to the house, there was hardly any place to park my car because every available spot was taken by her family members' cars. I walked up to the house, and there were children playing on the porch, their parents and aunts and uncles talking together. Mrs. Jerion was in a hospital bed in the living room, surrounded by bustling activity. The Benny Goodman Orchestra played on the radio and dinner was being cooked in the kitchen. Mr. Jerion was at his wife's side, the woman he had met more than 50 years ago. Mrs. Jerion was actively dying from liver cancer, and it was clear to everyone that she would likely die within the next day. Her skin was darkly jaundiced, and her Foley catheter was draining a small amount of amber-colored urine. She lay with her eyes open and watched the activity around her, but had stopped talking except to answer direct questions. She denied pain or discomfort and looked to be at peace.

At this point, the family was primarily concerned about Mr. Jerion. He had yet to talk about the fact that his wife was dying and would just wander around among his children as though he were lost in his own house. Dealing with their own grief at losing their mother, they had no idea how to help their father with his pain over the impending death of his wife.

Introduction

As an experiential process, dying and death for the individual, his or her family, and the health care practitioner can be one of the most profound and significant events experienced in one's lifetime. The last hours of life are conceptualized as the peri-death period, which specifically encompasses the symptoms and experiences right before death occurs, the actual death, and the care of the body after death. This time requires intensive holistic nursing care.

The purpose of this chapter is to relate the role of the nurse during the peri-death period and convey the core knowledge necessary for nurses to help facilitate a "good" death. The information in this chapter should be considered a requirement for nurses educated at a basic level. The role of the advanced practice nurse regarding peri-death nursing includes mentoring and modeling appropriate behaviors for the novice nurse, as well as directing symptom management. Additionally, the role includes supporting the novice nurse through the dying experience, and support of the family during the decision-making process regarding autopsy and funeral arrangements.

PERI-DEATH 1: SYMPTOMS AND EXPERIENCES BEFORE DEATH

The peri-death period begins with a preparation phase, the hallmark of which is the realization or acknowledgment that death is inevitable and temporally near. The patient and family members begin to prepare for the death. Similarly, the preparation phase for the terminally ill person is also a time when patients and families have many decisions to make regarding home or hospital care, hospice referral, advance directives, and Do-Not-Resuscitate orders.

The patient may be so uncomfortable with the physical (e.g., pain, dyspnea, fatigue) and emotional (e.g., depression, dependency) aspects of dying that he or she may feel ready for life to end. This sense of readiness may be in tension with a reluctance to die based upon fear of the unknown and concern for how the family will cope after the death. Family members are confronted with their role in the dying process, the prospect of losing their loved one, and the conflicts that arise from these and other issues. The patient's role within the family may change as the family learns how to provide care.

Any, all, or none of the following symptoms may occur during the final stages of the dying process. In-depth nursing interventions for the person with advanced disease can be found in the previous chapters of this book. The focus here is on the physiological changes that occur as death is imminent and the nursing interventions that are appropriate at this time.

Pain

As the body begins to shut down and die, the need for pain medication may change or decrease. Drugs most often used to manage pain at the end of life are MS Contin, Morphine Sulfate Instant Release (MSIR), Oxy-Contin, and Oxycodone, and administration should be individualized to achieve optimum pain control with minimal side effects (Lynch & Dahlin, 2007). The liver conjugates these drugs and active metabolites remain in the body, exerting a pharmacological effect until they are cleared by the kidneys. As the body is dying, renal and hepatic function is compromised and the drugs are cleared from the system very slowly. This results in an increase in serum opioid concentrations, which results in increased drowsiness or mild confusion. A nursing priority should be to keep the patient pain free and comfortable but with the understanding that the dosage to accomplish this may be considerably less than what had been previously needed for effective pain management.

Patients, health care providers, and family need an understanding of the importance and value of pain management during the dying process. The patient may seek pain relief or may view pain as a way to atone for sins and refuse to be medicated. Healthcare professionals may worry about determining the appropriate dose which will either offer relief of pain and suffering or hasten death (Rushton, 2008). Like the nurse, the family may fear being the person to give the "last dose" of morphine before the patient dies. Not adequately medicating for pain, though, can interfere with the memories that the family will carry with them for the rest of their lives. They will remember the death of their loved one as a time of agony and pain rather than a time that could have been used for conversations that are more meaningful and memorable.

The role of the nurse in management of pain and other distressing symptoms is to assess the level of pain the patient is having and the patient and family's attitudes toward pain. The assessment must be based on an informed understanding of the patient's values and goals, and assure patients and families that comfort and alleviation of pain is a priority. Encouraging patients to report their pain before it becomes intense will prevent unbearable suffering. Determining the adequacy of the pain control and its duration is important assessment data so that those dosages can be appropriately adjusted. Pain relief is an attainable goal, but may require sedation in order to achieve adequate control (Bruce, Hendrix, & Gentry, 2006).

Given that pain medications frequently cause constipation, nurses must be vigilant in assessing for constipation. Caregivers should be encouraged to continue prophylaxis bowel regimens to prevent or alleviate its associated discomfort. Other nonpharmacological interventions that alleviate pain are a calm environment, soothing music, and aromatherapy. Simple human touch or therapeutically intended touch, such as Reiki or therapeutic touch, can relieve stress, be a source of comfort or support, and overcome fear of abandonment.

Anorexia/Dehydration

As patients approach the end of life, they may say they are not hungry, which is a normal predeath finding. Decreased eating results in a metabolic imbalance whereby the energy a patient takes in does not cover the energy they expend, resulting in a state of dehydration. Although healthy people who are experiencing dehydration will report pain, abdominal cramps, nausea, vomiting, and dry mouth, patients who are terminally ill do not report such symptoms. At the end of life, patients typically only complain of having a dry mouth, which is often unrelated to hydration status and most often is the result of medication side effects, increased respiration, or mouth breathing.

Food represents more than nutrition to many families and can have a vital role in helping them to maintain hope and providing comfort to the patient. It is regrettable that attempts to feed the dying patient are not only frustrating for everyone involved but can also add to the patient's suffering (Cimino, 2003). In many cases, artificial hydration and nutrition provide an opportunity to "do something" at a time when the mistaken perception is that there is little else the nurse can do for them. The family's choice to provide food should be respected (Zerwekh, 2006) and balanced with the patient's wishes.

Intravenous fluids are sometimes given to reverse delirium for a person who is actively dying (Emanuel, Farris, von Gutten, & von Roenn, 2008). This increases urinary output, which may result in the necessity for a Foley catheter. It may increase respiratory secretions and increase cough as well as increasing gastrointestinal fluids, leading to abdominal distention, nausea, or vomiting. Increasing the intravascular volume in the presence of decreasing renal function can further result in peripheral edema and increase the incidence of decubitus ulcers. Pain can result from the IV site and restraints may become necessary to prevent the patient from removing the tubing. The presence of the IV may act as a physical barrier to the family and may be a cause of anxiety to them. In essence, artificial nutrition and hydration at this stage may lead to symptoms of congestive heart failure, increased tracheal and bronchial secretions, nausea and vomiting, painful edema, and diarrhea rather than improving symptoms or prolonging life (Bavin, 2007).

In contrast, there are many benefits to the patient in withholding food and fluids as death nears. With calorie deprivation comes an increased production of ketones, which results in an elevation of naturally occurring opioid peptides or endorphins that provide analgesia. An electrolyte imbalance, if present, will also result in increased analgesia. Decreased fluid intake will result in fewer pulmonary fluids, which ease respiration, lessens coughing, and reduces drowning sensations. If a tumor is present, dehydration may make it smaller in size by reducing the edematous layer around the tumor resulting in less pressure and pain. Discontinuing total parenteral nutrition can reduce the burden of sepsis, while stopping tube feedings can reduce diarrhea (AAHPM, 2006). Whatever the decision, nurses should discuss end-of-life choices related to patient goals and values (Suter, Rogers, & Strack, 2008).

Nursing interventions focus on meticulous mouth, nasal, and conjuctival care to alleviate mouth dryness and prevent sores, dental problems, infections, and discomfort. Scrupulous cleaning and moistening of the mouth can be one of the most important interventions to prevent suffering in a patient nearing death (Emanuel et al., 2008; Field & Cassel, 1997). The mouth and teeth can be cleaned with a soft-bristled toothbrush or sponge-covered oral swabs. To maintain moisture in mucosal membranes, the mouth should be rinsed frequently with water. A spray bottle can be used to mist the mouth often; a room humidifier is also very helpful. Commercial salivary substitutes or supplements such as Salivart, Oral Balance, Salagen, and MoiStir, or a baking soda mouthwash (1 teaspoon salt, 1 teaspoon baking soda, and 1 quart tepid water) can also help keep the patient comfortable. Chamomile tea is also very soothing and can be used to clean the mouth or offered to the patient to sip on. End-of-life halitosis is a frequent phenomenon. Two drops of essential peppermint oil in one ounce of purified drinking water can be used on a toothette when providing oral care. It is not an immediate cure for halitosis, but with multiple uses can refresh breath and leave a pleasant taste and aroma for the patient (K.T. Young, personal communication, September 8, 2008). Generously applying lip lubricant can prevent dry, chapped lips and alleviate associated discomfort. Avoid petroleum-based products if the patient is on oxygen. Ophthalmic lubricating gel or artificial tears can be used to hydrate conjunctiva. Family members should be shown how to give good mouth, nasal, and conjunctival care and be supported by the nurse in their efforts. It is essential for everyone involved in the care of the patient to realize that not providing food and fluids is not the same as not caring for the patient, only that the concentration of care is on meeting the needs of the dying person and providing comprehensive symptom management (Emanuel et al., 2008).

If the patient is experiencing oral pain, morphine or morphine elixir can be used if the pain is severe or during mouth care and meals. Topical agents for mouth pain include Viscous Xylocaine 2% solution, 5–15 ml, swish and spit every 2 to 4 hours as needed. KBX solution (Kaopectate, Benadryl, Xylocaine viscous in equal parts), 5–15 ml, swish for 1 minute, then spit or swallow every 2 to 4 hours as needed may also be ordered. Xylocaine provides topical anesthesia; the Benadryl is a short-acting anesthetic; and the Kaopectate (Mylanta may be substituted) serves as an alkalizing agent (Schaefer, 2008; Gates & Fink, 1997).

If the patient is still sipping fluids, encourage those fluids that contain salt to help prevent electrolyte imbalance. Fluids such as bullion soup, tomato juice, or sport drinks like Gatorade may be well tolerated. Avoid citrus juices or foods that may irritate the mouth, as well as temperature extremes of foods. It is important not to force food or fluids at this point and to support the family who may have a difficult time accepting the patient's refusal to eat or drink. Families can be reminded that even in the case of acute illness, such as the flu, food and fluids can create additional distress.

As death approaches, patients often lose their ability to swallow because of weakness or a decrease in neurological function. The gag reflex may diminish and secretions will tend to accumulate in the tracheobronchial tree. Positioning is important to prevent the accumulation of secretions in the back of the throat and upper airways (Ferrell, Virani, & Grant, 1999). This phenomenon, known as a death rattle, occurs in 31–92% of dying patients, and is present in 76% of patients within 48 hours before death (Owens, 2006). Scopolamine transdermal patches can be used to decrease secretion production and decrease the occurrence of the "death rattle," which although not distressing to the patient can be very upsetting to the family (Hoyal, Grant, Chamberlain, Cox, & Campbell, 2002). Oropharyngeal suctioning is not recommended, as it is frequently ineffective and may stimulate the patient and distress the family even more (Emanuel et al., 2008).

Weakness and Fatigue

Fatigue is a primary complaint of patients in the last hours and days of life. The tiredness may be a result of both the disease and the treatment for the disease, as well as malnutrition and disrupted sleep patterns. Fatigue may interfere with a person's ability to move, bathe, or toilet (Emanuel et al., 2008; Field & Cassel, 1997).

The nurse should be aware that while the patient is at high risk for a pressure ulcer, turning and positioning should be done as frequently as possible but only as often as comfort permits. Bony prominences should be padded and supported if this is comfortable for the patient. If any of these interventions result in increased pain or suffering, they should not be implemented. Initially, this may be difficult for the novice nurse to support, as it is contrary to the basic nursing skills they have been taught. When a patient is actively dying, intervention goals should focus on comfort; any intervention that compromises this goal should be discontinued.

Dyspnea

Dyspnea is a common symptom experienced at the end of life and results from the lungs' inability to function in proportion to the metabolic demands of the body and may be indicative of significant neurologic compromise (Field & Cassel, 1997). When a person has trouble breathing, there must be either an increase in ventilation or a decrease in activity. Terminal dyspnea occurs in as many as 75% of patients in the peri-death period (LaDuke, 2001). Changes in respiration are normal and should be anticipated prior to death. Physiologically increased carbon dioxide in the blood stimulates respiration. During the peri-death period, increased pulmonary congestion and poor gas exchange result in a rise in carbon dioxide levels, but the brain is less responsive to this signal (Pitorak, 2003). The breathing pattern can become irregular and include shallow breathing altered with apnea lasting 5–60 seconds (Cheyne-Stokes breathing) (Emanuel et al., 2008).

Families should be warned that dyspnea and loud respirations are a possibility during the peri-death period. Patients may fear they will suffocate while they are dying, and families fear they will have to watch their loved one struggle to breathe. Nurses should educate the patient and family regarding what they can expect and give assurances that medications will be used to effectively palliate these symptoms (Emanuel et al., 2008; Tarzian, 2000).

Nursing interventions include positioning the patient with the head of the bed raised and/or turning the person on one side. For opioid-naive patients, low-dose opiates, such as morphine 5 mg PO every 4 hours, can alleviate the sensation of breathlessness. If morphine is already being used for pain, an increase of 2.5 mg times their regular dose is generally effective. Oxygen is typically only effective if the dyspnea is secondary to hypoxia (e.g., COPD, pulmonary fibrosis), although it may provide a placebo effect (Horn, 1992). A fan blowing a gentle breeze toward the patient's face can also be very effective. Suctioning is usually not recommended, as it may incidentally increase secretion production. Emotion-focused interventions such as relaxation techniques, prayer and meditation, and distraction may alleviate the anxiety often associated with dyspnea (Spector, Connolly, & Carlson, 2007; Horn, 1992).

Multisystem Failure

As the body is shutting down, there is a decrease in blood perfusion and a resulting shutdown of the major organs (e.g., renal and hepatic). Decreased cardiac output and intravascular volume results in tachycardia and hypotension. Additionally, the body will conserve blood volume for vital organs, which results in peripheral cooling (as the body conserves heat) and peripheral and central cyanosis. The skin may therefore become mottled and discolored, which is normal before death and a sign that it is imminent. Mottling is typically seen on the earlobes and the soles of the feet before other areas.

Urine output is greatly diminished, and there can be a loss of sphincter control resulting in urinary or fecal incontinence. It may be a good idea to insert a urinary catheter to reduce the need for frequent bedding changes and to prevent skin breakdown. The catheter also helps the continent patient conserve energy by removing the need to use a bedpan or urinal.

Neurological dysfunction is a result of multiple, concurrent, and nonreversible organ failure. Consequently, the patient may experience reduced cerebral perfusion, hypoxemia, metabolic imbalances, acidosis, accumulation of toxins from renal and hepatic failure, and sepsis (Zerwekh, 2006; Ferrell et al., 1999). The net effect of these changes may be a decreased level of consciousness or terminal delirium.

Terminal Delirium

Terminal delirium can be manifested as confusion, anxiety, agitation, or restlessness; restlessness and delirium are typical symptoms that are indicative that the patient is close to death. These can be distressing symptoms for patients and their families and are estimated to occur in up to 88% of patients who develop delirium in the last 24–48 hours of life (Macleod, 2006). Confusion is a mental state in which a person reacts inappropriately to their environment because they are confounded or disoriented. It may be the side effect of medications or caused by the dying process itself (Field & Cassel, 1997). Anxiety is the biological and emotional reaction to stressful situations, including the approach of death.

The patient may experience dread, danger, or tension with somatic complaints that includes shortness of breath, nausea, or diarrhea (Field & Cassel, 1997). Moaning and grimacing can accompany agitation and restlessness and may be misinterpreted by the nurse as pain (Ferrell et al., 1999). Uncontrollable pain is not likely to develop during the last hours of life if not previously present (Emanuel et al., 2008). The patient may be restless and make repetitive motions (e.g., pulling on clothing or the sheets). The underlying cause of the restlessness may be opioid toxicity, metabolic disorders, and lowered seizure threshold, or full bladder or bowel (Zerwekh, 2006; Heming & Colmer, 2003).

Nursing interventions to manage terminal delirium should focus on the treatment of the underlying physical cause if it is practical and possible. Antianxiety agents like benzodiazepines (lorazepam, diazepam, alprazolam) and neuroleptics (Haldol) for drug toxicity can help to quiet distressing symptoms. Methotrimeprazine can be effective if the patient's jerking movements are secondary to renal failure and it possesses antiemetic characteristics (Kaye, 2003). Barbiturates or propofol has been suggested, as have other antiepileptics such as IV phenytoin, phenobarbital, or carbamazepine (Emanuel et al., 2008).

The family is in need of education and support regarding the cause and the irreversible nature of the behavior. Maintaining a calm environment, spiritual comfort, and emotional support are vital at this time. The family can be advised to continue to talk to the patient and calm the patient with their words. Light massage of the arms, back, or forehead can be very soothing. Soft music and low lights can also be effective. It may be suggested that the number of people in the room be decreased if there is a lot of activity. Refraining from asking the patient many questions can diminish agitation.

Eventually the patient's level of consciousness will decrease and they may even become unable to be aroused. This is a very upsetting time for families because the patient may seem unresponsive and withdrawn, but it is a normal aspect of the dying process.

At this time, the patient is starting to "let go" in preparation for death and is detaching from relationships and the physical environment. A patient may ask to be with only one person toward the end or seem distracted from the family. Reassure the family that this is not a personal rejection, only another aspect of the dying process. A dying person may talk about seeing people who have already died or talk about taking a trip with a long-deceased relative. Patients may describe feeling separate from their body. This is a normal experience and is not considered a hallucination.

Even if the patient is unresponsive, encourage family members to talk with him or her. Assume that the patient hears everything; this is the time for loved ones to say "Good-bye," "I'm sorry," "I love you," or "Thank you." The patient may have difficulty letting go, and the nurse may need to encourage the family to give the patient permission to die. Encourage the family to show affection to the patient, touch them, and let them know they will be missed.

Affirming Life and Maintaining Hope

Two very important goals of palliative care nursing are to help patients live until they die, and to encourage hope. First, the nurse can help patients live until they die by encouraging socialization, listening, being honest, and helping them finish any unfinished business. Dialogues about death with healthcare professionals, families and friends can benefit all involved (Wasserman, 2008). By offering patients choices regarding routines, food, and activities, nurses promote continued independence and the ability to help maintain control over their lives. Of course, the degree of independence depends on patients' energy level and ability (Zerwekh, 2006; Birchenall & Streight, 1997). Furthermore, patients' wishes should be respected even if those wishes are inconsistent with the family's or healthcare provider's values.

Second, hope is an important component of the emotional stages of dying and death. It has been a factor in helping the patient and family continue through the difficult months and years leading up to the death. Hope is what maintains a person's spirit and helps the person to go on; as the person is dying, *what* he or she hopes for may change, but it does not go away. There may be hope for the "miracle" of a complete cure; it is not acceptable for the nurse to take this hope away or to tell the patient and family to be "realistic."

Their hopes may change from that of cure to the hope for a full night's sleep, a visit from an important person, or for less pain. Persons with hope have been found to live longer and have a greater quality of life than those who are hopeless (Birchenall & Streight, 1997). Benzein & Savemen (2008) posit that patients who told their story were able to relieve an unrecognized burden. What is important for the nurse is to be present for the patient and family wherever they are in this process and support the feelings that are experienced. The rights of the dying can be found in Exhibit 25.1. Listening and caring for their needs are important nursing functions at this time of life.

Palliative Care for the Aged and Individuals with Dementia

In the 21st century, the needs of healthcare will continue to change. It is predicted that by 2030 the Medicare population will almost double from the current 40 million to 77 million (CMS, 2002). This will create a significant challenge for current hospice, palliative care, and end-of-life care practices and providers.

Although the body of research regarding end-of-life care continues to grow, information about the very old or individuals with dementia is more in its infancy. These individuals have unique issues in that they may

---

EXHIBIT 25.1: THE DYING PERSON'S BILL OF RIGHTS

- I have the right to be treated as a living human being until I die.
- I have the right to maintain a sense of hopefulness, however changing its focus may be.
- I have the right to be cared for by those who can maintain a sense of hopefulness, however challenging this might be.
- I have the right to express my feelings and emotions about my approaching death, in my own way.
- I have the right to participate in decisions concerning my care.
- I have the right to expect continuing medical and nursing attention even though "cure" goals must be changed to "comfort" goals.
- I have the right not to die alone.
- I have the right to be free from pain.
- I have the right to have my questions answered honestly.
- I have the right not to be deceived.
- I have the right to have help from and for my family in accepting my death.
- I have the right to die in peace and dignity.
- I have the right to retain my individuality and not be judged for my decisions, which may be contrary to the beliefs of others.
- I have the right to discuss and enlarge my religious and/or spiritual experiences, regardless of what they may mean to others.
- I have the right to expect that the sanctity of the human body will be respected after death.
- I have the right to be cared for by caring, sensitive, knowledgeable people who will attempt to understand my needs and will be able to gain some satisfaction in helping me face my death.

Note: This Bill of Rights was created at a workshop on "the terminally ill patient and the helping person" in Lansing, Michigan, sponsored by the Southwestern Michigan In-service Education Council and conducted by Amelia J. Barbus, Associate Professor of Nursing, Wayne State University, in 1975.

From S. A. Sorrentino, *Assisting with Patient Care* (p. 843). St. Louis, MO: Mosby, 1999. Used with permission.

lose some of their capacity to make decisions or choose to designate surrogates to make those decisions for them. Research indicates surrogate decision making encourages the surrogate to "exercise considerable discretion in the decision making" (Berger, DeRenzo, & Schwartz, 2008, p. 48).

Individuals with dementia often enter an end-of-life stage without acknowledgement by the family or caregivers, which may lead to inappropriate care during the end stages of dementia (Peacock, 2008). A patient with progressive dementia has the potential for an extended life unless complicating conditions develop (Zerwekh, 2006). One effort to enhance end-of life practices for individuals with dementia includes *The Palliative Excellence in Alzheimer Care Efforts* (PEACE) program offered by the University of Chicago (promotingexcellence.org).

Decision making for family members can be compounded by ambivalence, struggles with opposing beliefs, and moral issues. Family members may require additional conversations, and interventions by healthcare workers to help resolve those conflicts (Peacock, 2008). Advance directives and living wills may create as many problems as they solve, as the patient priorities in the context of aging rather than a specific illness may be more tenuous (Berger et al., 2008).

Special Considerations Related to the Dying Child

Palliative care for the child encompasses a holistic approach to physical, psychological, and spiritual care. Consideration for both the dying child and their family supporting optimal functioning until the time of death is a vital role for the nurse (Ethier, 2007; Drake, Frost, & Collins, 2003). Ethical considerations have a significant role in decisions related to a dying child. Identifying if, when, and how much to tell a child about their impending death is an important decision for the family. Talking with children about impending death demands an understanding of the child's perception of death based on previous experiences and developmental stage (Lynch & Dahlin, 2007).

Children are often very perceptive and may know far more than adults assume. Offering time for discussion related to death and the dying process helps the child recognize that he or she will not be alone in the process and will be loved and remembered (Ethier, 2007). End-of-life communication will not typically send a dying child into a deep depression. Attempts to protect children from knowledge about their impending death place barriers between them and the people who can best help them understand and deal with their experience. Honest and accurate information about a child's impending death can address separation issues in young children; fears, phobias, and regression in school-age children; emotional lability in pre-adolescents; and anger, insecurity, and body image in older adolescents (Beale, Baile, & Aaron, 2005).

Children experience a variety of symptoms in the dying process which may be similar or different from those of adults, but discomfort, seizure management, pain in nonverbal patients, and feeding issues are most common (Sumner, 2006). These symptoms may be a result of the disease process, previous treatment history, or side effects of palliative medication. It is important to assess the onset of those symptoms, severity, duration, and the impact those symptoms have on the child's comfort. This requires extensive investigation and developmentally appropriate interventions and strategies to identify and manage those symptoms (IOM, 2003). Physical signs and symptoms that occur for children as death approaches include sleeping more, decreased appetite, and less fluid intake. The urine frequency and output will diminish, and breathing may become slow and shallow, with occasional deep sighs. There may be some gasping and periods of apnea. The skin may be cool to the touch, and appear pale, grayish-blue (Ethier, 2007).

Nurses should help families understand that what they see may be different from what the child experiences. If the families are given the opportunity to care for the child, utilizing what they feel is best for the child, a gift of confidence is given to the family. Basic caring-bathing, holding, dressing—becomes significantly important during the peri-death period (Emanuel et al., 2008). Caring for the child does not stop at the time of death. Families may choose to engage in the same activities as if the child were alive, and they should be encouraged if cultural and religious values allow it (IOM, 2003).

Family Support During the Last Hours of Life

Supporting the family during the last hours of the patient's life is an important nursing role. When possible, one nurse should be assigned to be with the family through the last phase of life. Enough time with the dying person should be given to the family so that they have the opportunity to resolve any final interpersonal issues. If the death is occurring at home the family should have access to a Symptom Relief Kit with detailed, easy to understand instructions for its use (Chapter 25 appendix). Depending on cultural and religious considerations, the family should be afforded privacy and clergy support. The primary nurse should communicate with the family regarding what they can expect the dying process to be like and how they will know when the person has died.

Many people have not been with someone who is actively dying and do not know what to expect. Even though no two deaths are alike, it helps to give significant others an idea of what the final stage of life may be like and the symptoms they may see during this period. Exhibit 25.2, which shows the final stages of dying, is an information sheet written for the general population regarding the dying process and is a good handout for students.

EXHIBIT 25.2: VNS GUIDELINES FOR CARE DURING THE DYING PROCESS

When a person enters the final stage of the dying process, two different dynamics are at work. On the physical plane, the body begins the final process of shutting down, which will end when all the physical systems cease to function. Usually this is an orderly, progressive series of physical changes that are not medical emergencies. These physical changes are the natural way in which the body prepares itself to stop. The most appropriate kinds of responses are comfort-enhancing measures.

The other dynamic of the dying process is emotional and spiritual in nature. The "spirit" of the dying person begins the final process of release from the body, its immediate environment, and all attachments. This release also tends to follow its own priorities, which may include the resolution of whatever is *unfinished* of a practical nature and exercising permission from family members to "let go." The most appropriate kinds of responses to the emotional/spiritual changes are those that support and encourage this release and transition.

When a person's body is ready and wanting to stop, but the person is still unresolved or is not reconciled about some important issue or relationship, the person may tend to linger in order to finish whatever needs finishing. On the other hand, when a person is emotionally/spiritually resolved and ready for this release, but his/her body has not completed its final physical process, the person will continue to live until the physical shutdown is completed.

The experience we call "death" occurs when the body and the spirit complete the natural process of shutting down, reconciling, and finishing. These processes need to happen in a way appropriate and unique to the values, beliefs, and lifestyle of the dying person. The physical and emotional/spiritual signs and symptoms of impending death that follow are offered to help you understand the natural kinds of things that may happen and how you can respond appropriately. Not all these signs and symptoms will occur with every person, nor will they occur in this particular sequence. Each person is unique and needs your full acceptance, support, and comfort.

The following signs and symptoms are indicative of how the body prepares itself for the final stage of life:

Coolness: The person's hands, arms, feet and legs may be increasingly cool. At the same time, the color of the skin may change. The underside of the body may become darker and the skin mottled or discolored. This is a normal indication that the circulation of blood is decreasing to the body's extremities and being reserved for the most vital organs. Keep the person warm with a nonelectric blanket.

Sleeping: The person may spend an increasing amount of time sleeping and appear to be uncommunicative or unresponsive, at times difficult to arouse. This normal change is due in part to changes in the metabolism of the body. Sit with your loved one, speak softly and naturally. Plan to spend time when the person seems most alert and awake. Try not to talk as if the person were not there. Speak directly as you normally would, even though there may be no response. Never assume the person cannot hear; hearing is the last of the senses to be lost.

Fluid and Food Decrease: The person may have a decrease in appetite and thirst, wanting little or no food or fluid. The body will naturally begin to conserve energy that would be expended on these tasks. Do not try to force food or drink into the person. To use guilt or manipulation only makes the person more uncomfortable. Small chips of ice, frozen Gatorade or juice may be refreshing in the mouth. If the person is able to swallow, fluids may be given in small amounts by syringe (ask the hospice nurse for guidance). Glycerin swabs may help keep the mouth and lips moist and comfortable. A cool, moist washcloth on the forehead may also increase physical comfort.

Incontinence: Control of urine and/or bowels may be lost as the muscles in that area begin to relax. Discuss with your hospice nurse what can be done to protect the bed and keep your loved one clean and comfortable. If it would make the person more comfortable, the nurse may suggest a catheter to drain the bladder into a collection bag. The person's normal urine output may decrease and become dark due to the decrease in circulation through the kidneys.

Congestion: The person may have gurgling sounds coming from the chest as though marbles were rolling around inside. These sounds may become very loud. This normal change is due to the decrease of fluid intake and the inability to cough up normal secretions. The sound of the congestion does not indicate the onset of severe or new pain. Suctioning usually increases the secretions. The nurse or home health aide can show you how to keep the mouth clean with "touthettes."

Breathing Pattern Change: The person's regular breathing pattern may change and become irregular, e.g., shallow breaths with periods of no breathing for 5 to 30 seconds and up to a full minute. This is called Cheyne-Stokes breathing. The person may also experience periods of rapid shallow panting. Elevating the head and/or turning the person on one side may bring comfort. Use your hands to touch and soothe. Speak gently.

Disorientation: The person may seem to be confused about the time, place, and identity of people, including those close and familiar. This is due in part to metabolism changes. Identify yourself by name before you speak rather than asking the person to guess who you are. Speak softly, clearly, and truthfully when you need to communicate something important, such as, "It's time to take your medication," and explain the reason for the communication, such as, "So you won't begin to hurt." Never use this method to try to manipulate the person to meet your own needs or values. It may be difficult to make this distinction.

Restlessness: The person may make restless and repetitive motions, such as pulling at bed linen or clothing. This often happens and is due to the decrease in oxygen circulation to the brain and to metabolism changes. Do not interfere with or try to restrain such motions. Occasionally the person may twitch or make jerking motions. This may have to do with medication or the disease itself. Sometimes other medication helps decrease this twitching. To have a calming effect, speak in a quiet, natural way; lightly massage the forehead, back, or arms; read to the person, or play some soothing music. Try to decrease the number of people around the person. Asking a lot of questions may increase the person's agitation.

EMOTIONAL SYMPTOMS AND RESPONSES

Withdrawal: The person may seem unresponsive, withdrawn, or in a comatose-like state. This indicates preparation for release, a detaching from surroundings and relationships, and a beginning of letting go. Because hearing remains almost all the way to the end, now is the time to say whatever you need to say that will help the person let go. The person may only want to be with a very few or even just one person. This is another sign of preparation for release. If you are not part of this inner circle at the end, it does not mean you are not loved or are unimportant. It means you have already fulfilled your tasks, and it is time for you to say good-bye.

Vision-like experiences: The person may speak or claim to have spoken to persons who have already died, or to see places not presently accessible or visible to you. This does not indicate hallucinations or a drug reaction. The person is beginning to detach from this life and is preparing for the transition. Do not contradict, explain, belittle, or argue about what the person claims to have seen or heard. Affirm the experiences. They are normal and natural.

Letting Go: The person may continue to perform repetitive and restless tasks. This may indicate that something is still unresolved or unfinished and preventing the letting go. The hospice team can assist you in identifying what may be happening and help the person find release from tension or fear. As hard as it might be, you need to give the person permission to let go.

Saying Good-Bye: When the person is ready to die, and you are able to let go, saying goodbye is your final gift of love. It achieves closure and makes the final release possible. It may be helpful to hold or touch and say the things you want to say. It may be as simple (or as complicated) as saying "I love you." It may include recounting favorite memories, places, and activities you shared. It may include saying "I'm sorry for whatever I've done to cause any tensions or difficulty." You may also want to say "Thank you." Tears are a normal and natural part of saying good-bye. You don't need to apologize for them or try to hide them. They are a natural expression of your sadness and loss. It is all right to say "I will miss you so much."

HOW WILL YOU KNOW WHEN DEATH HAS OCCURRED?

Although you may be prepared for the dying process, you may not be prepared for the actual moment. It may be helpful for you and your family to think about and discuss what you would do if you were alone when the death occurs. The death of a hospice patient is expected and is not an emergency. Nothing must be done immediately. The signs of death include such things as:

- No heartbeat
- Release of bowel and bladder
- No response
- Eyelids slightly open
- Pupils enlarged
- Eyes fixed on a certain spot
- No blinking
- Jaw relaxed and mouth slightly open

You may now notify a hospice nurse or the on-call nurse as you have been instructed. The nurse will make the pronouncement and notify your physician. The body does not have to be moved until you are ready. The nurse can call the funeral home, but you or a member of your family will probably need to speak with the funeral director.

LATER ON

Hospice staff and volunteers continue to be available to support you and your family through the Bereavement Program. We will contact you a week or so after the death has occurred, after all the "busyness" is over and the visitors have gone. If you need or want to communicate with us before then, please do not hesitate to call. Even if you just need a place to go for comfort and support, call or stop in.

We salute you for all you have done during this difficult time. We know it has been an enormous commitment and a true act of love. We feel honored to have shared this experience with you in spite of your pain. You accompanied someone you love as far as you could on life's final journey. We hope you feel good about what you've done. We hope this feeling will sustain you, give you courage, and allow you eventually to go on with your life.

Source: The Visiting Nurses Association of Manchester and Southern NH. Manchester, NH. Used with permission.

Terminal Sedation

Sedation for the imminently dying is an intervention to relieve intractable symptoms of patients who are suffering at the end of their life. It involves the definitive decision to make the dying elder "unconscious to prevent or respond to otherwise unrelievable physical distress" (Quill & Byock, 2000, p. 409), but not to intentionally end their life. This intervention should only occur when the symptoms or suffering cannot be relieved in any other way.

Jansen and Sulmasy (2002) differentiate sedation of the imminently dying from sedation toward death and see these two practices as morally distinct from each other. Sedation of the imminently dying is a practice in which "1) the patient is close to death (hours, days, or at most a few weeks); 2) the patient has one or more severe symptoms that are refractory to standard palliative care; 3) the patient's physician vigorously treats these symptoms with therapy known to be efficacious; 4) this therapy has a dose-dependent side effect of sedation that is a foreseen but unintended consequence of trying to relieve the patients symptoms; and 5) this therapy may be coupled with the withholding or withdrawing of life-sustaining treatments that are ineffective or disproportionately burdensome" (p. 845). This type of sedation fulfills the conditions set forth in the rule of double effect (see chapter 7) and is considered to be morally justifiable. These authors define sedation toward death as "a practice in which 1) the patient need not be imminently dying; 2) the symptoms believed to be refractory to treatment are simply the consciousness that one is not yet dead; 3) the patient's physician selects therapy intended to render the patient unconscious as a means of treating the refractory symptoms; and 4) other life-sustaining treatments are withdrawn to hasten death" (p. 845). The aim of the healthcare practitioner in this case is to cause the patient to be unconscious and to shorten life.

Indications for terminal sedation are uncontrolled physical suffering such as intractable pain, dyspnea, seizures, or delirium. Exhibit 25.3 offers general guidelines for terminal sedation and Exhibit 25.4 lists medications and guidelines for their use in sedating an imminently dying patient. The level of sedation that eliminates objective signs of discomfort is maintained until the elder dies; death will typically occurs within hours or days of the initiation of sedation (Quill & Byock, 2000). There is no literature to support the belief that imminently dying patients die more quickly when sedated to control intractable symptoms. Panke (2003) suggests that patients with unrelieved symptoms may die sooner secondary to "increased physiologic stress, diminished immunocompetence, decreased mobility, increased risk of thromboembolism and pneumonia, increased difficulty breathing, and greater myocardial oxygen requirements" (p. 31).

Terminal sedation requires participation of the entire healthcare team for monitoring the elder and support of their family. The sedation is maintained by continuous subcutaneous or intravenous infusion. Opioids that have already been initiated for pain and other symptoms should be continued to prevent unobservable pain or opioid withdrawal, but opioids should not be used to maintain the sedation itself (Quill & Byock, 2000).

PERI-DEATH 2: DEATH

Signs of Death

Signs of death include cessation of a heartbeat and respiration, release of bowel and bladder, slightly open and not blinking eyelids, glazed eyes, and fixed and dilated pupils. There is a drop in body temperature, and as the blood settles the body color turns to a waxen pallor, the jaw is relaxed and slightly open, and there is no response from the patient. These signs do not occur in sequence, and it may take a few minutes for the body to completely stop (Green & Green, 2006; Ferrell et al., 1999). If the death occurs at home, the family should be told that it is not considered an emergency, but be given a number to call to inform hospice staff or their physician of the death. The body does not have to be moved immediately, so the family should not feel rushed or pressured to act.

When Death Has Occurred

Post-death nursing care involves preparing the body for the morgue or funeral home and helping the family

EXHIBIT 25.3: GENERAL GUIDELINES FOR TERMINAL SEDATION

GUIDELINE DOMAIN	TERMINAL SEDATION
Palliative care	Must be available, in place, and unable to adequately relieve current suffering
Usual patient characteristics	Severe, immediate, or otherwise un-relievable symptoms (for example, pain, shortness of breath, nausea, vomiting, seizures, delirium) or to prevent severe suffering (for example, suffocation sensation when mechanical ventilation is discontinued)
Terminal prognosis	Usually days to weeks
Patient informed consent	Patient should be competent and fully informed or noncompetent with severe, otherwise irreversible suffering (clinician should use advance directive or consensus about patient wishes and best interests)
Family participation in decision	Clinician should strongly encourage input from and consensus of immediate family members
Incompetent patient	Can be used for severe, persistent suffering with the informed consent of the patient's designated proxy and family members. If no surrogate is available, team members and consultants should agree that no other acceptable palliative therapies are available.
Second opinion(s)	Should be obtained from an expert in palliative care and a mental health expert (if uncertainty exists about patient's mental capacity)
Healthcare practitioner participation in decision	Input from staff involved in immediate patient care activities is encouraged; physician and staff consent is required for their own participation

Adapted from: Quill, T. E., & Byock, I. R. (2000). Responding to intractable terminal suffering: The role of terminal sedation and voluntary refusal of food and fluids. *Annals of Internal Medicine, 132*(5), 408–414.

EXHIBIT 25.4: MEDICATIONS USED IN TERMINAL SEDATION

MEDICATION	TYPE	USUAL STARTING DOSAGE	USUAL MAINTENANCE DOSAGE	ROUTE
Midazolam	Rapid, short-acting benzodiazepine	0.5–1.5 mg/hr after bolus of 0.5 mg	30–100 mg/d	Intravenous or subcutaneous
Lorazepam	Benzodiazepine	1–4 mg every 4–6 hr orally or dissolved buccally; infusion of 0.5–1.0 mg/hr intravenously	4–40 mg/d	Oral, buccal, subcutaneous, or intravenous
Propofol	General anesthetic; ultrarapid onset and elimination	5–10 mg/hr; bolus doses of 20–50 mg may be administered for urgent sedation, but continuous infusion is required	10–200 mg/d	Intravenous
Thiopental	Ultrashort-acting barbiturate	5–7 mg/kg of body weight to induce unconsciousness	Initial rate may range from 20 to 80 mg/h; average maintenance rates range between 70 and 180 mg/h	Intravenous
Pentobarbital	Long-acting barbiturate	2–3 mg/kg, slow infusion, to induce unconsciousness	1 mg/h, increasing as needed to maintain sedation	Intravenous
Phenobarbital	Long-acting barbiturate	200 mg loading dose, repeated every 10–15 minutes until patient is comfortable	Approximately 50 mg/h	Intravenous or subcutaneous

Note: Goal of treatment is to relieve suffering by inducing sedation. Dosage should be increased by approximately 30% every hour until sedation is achieved. Once desired level of sedation is achieved, infusion is usually maintained at that level as long as the patient seems comfortable. If symptoms return, dosages should be increased in 30% increments until sedation is achieved. The ranges above are representative. Individual patients may require lower or higher doses to achieve the desired goal. Previous doses of opioids and other symptom-relieving medications should be continued.

Adapted from: Quill, T.E., & Byock, I.R. (2000). Responding to intractable terminal suffering: The role of terminal sedation and voluntary refusal of food and fluids. *Annals of Internal Medicine, 132*(5), 40.

through decisions regarding autopsy and burial. When death has occurred, the blood will begin to pool in the areas of the body closest to the ground; if the corpse was supine this would be the back and buttocks. A purple-red discoloration of the skin is evident, which results from the blood accumulating in the dependent vessels; this is called *livor mortis.* The body begins to cool, and this fall in body temperature after death is called *algor mortis* (Pattison, 2008; Kastenbaum & Kastenbaum, 1989). Initially, at the time of death, the muscles in the body relax, but within 2–6 hours *rigor mortis* begins. Rigor mortis is the stiffening of all muscle groups beginning with the eyelids, neck, and jaw. During the next 4–6 hours, it will spread to the other muscles including the internal organs. Rigor mortis will usually last between 24 and 48 hours depending on the ambient temperature; after this time the muscles relax and secondary flaccidity develops (Beattie, 2006; Iserson, 2001).

Care of the body by the nurse should include closing the eyes, inserting dentures and closing the mouth, and elevating the head of the bed so that the blood does not drain into the face and discolor it. Any IV or catheter can be removed at this time, and the physical environment should be straightened. Removal of tubes and equipment is dependent on institutional protocol. Follow the agency protocol regarding jewelry; if there is a wedding ring, secure it on the finger with tape. The body should be bathed in plain water and dried; a bed protector should be placed under the body. If there are dressings on wounds, they should be replaced with clean ones. The hair should be combed, the extremities straightened, and the right great toe tied with an identification tag (Pattison, 2008; Sorrentino, 1999).

If the family wants to participate in the preparation of the deceased for the funeral home, they should be encouraged to do so. The family should also be offered the opportunity to bathe and dress the body if they wish. Some people find comfort in giving the last bath and it helps them to believe that no one else will touch the body in this way again.

When the body and the room have been prepared, family and those close to the patient can be encouraged to say a final goodbye. Within the confines of cultural, personal, and religious practices, the family can be invited to touch or hold the person's body and to take the time they need. This time spent with the deceased can help to promote the transition from acute grief to a new stage of the grieving process (Pattison, 2008; Ferrell et al., 1999). Accepting the reality of the death is considered one of the first tasks of mourning necessary for working through the grief (Worden, 1992). Seeing the dead body helps the bereaved see the reality of the death and to say good-bye. The body should not be transported to the morgue or mortuary until the family is prepared and they have given their permission. The family's wishes should be respected regarding their presence during the removal of the body (Beattie, 2006).

When the family has given permission for the body to be moved, the nurse should follow the institutional protocol regarding shrouding the body. If a person has died at home and it is an expected death, the undertaker is called and they remove the body as it is. In a hospital or nursing home setting, the body is wrapped in a shroud or body bag. The shroud should be secured with safety pins or ties and a second identification tag attached to the shroud or body bag. The body is then taken to the morgue (Beattie, 2006; Sorrentino, 1999).

The nurse can offer help with making personal phone calls to give the family time to become accustomed to the immediate loss. The physician should be notified of the death and the nurse should be certain to follow agency protocol regarding the removal of medications and equipment. If the family wishes, support from their clergy or bereavement professionals can be offered.

In many states, the nurse can sign the death certificate if the death occurs in the hospital or nursing home or at the family home if hospice is involved. Once the death certificate is signed, the family can contact the mortuary and the body can be transported to the funeral home or crematorium. If the nurse or physician is unwilling to sign the death certificate because of a suspicious nature of the death, the medical examiner is called, who assumes responsibility for the body (Iserson, 2001). If the death is sudden and unexpected or if it occurs at home, the medical examiner must be notified and he or she will decide if an autopsy is required. The family has no authority to stop an officially mandated autopsy (Lynn & Harrold, 2006).

The next of kin may request an autopsy even if the medical examiner declines to do one. The nurse should be available to educate the family about the autopsy and assist them in their decision-making process. An autopsy will help determine the cause of death but the family may be charged a fee for this service (as much as $2,000). Autopsies also serve other purposes, as shown in Exhibit 25.5.

The word autopsy comes from the Greek *autopsia,* which means seeing with one's own eyes. Pathologists, who are physicians who have specialized in human anatomy, perform them. Organs are removed and inspected, and body fluids are analyzed. There are three degrees of autopsy: complete, limited, and selective. A complete autopsy exposes all body cavities (including the head) for examination; limited autopsy usually excludes the head; and selective autopsy involves examination of only one or more organs specific to the nature of the illness (Iserson, 2001).

If the deceased has requested that his or her organs be donated, the nurse is often the person responsible for notifying the proper agencies for organ and tissue harvesting. Organ donation is the practice of giving a part of the deceased body for transplantation into another person. Persons designate this wish to donate organs by signing the back of their driver's license, indicating their preferences; by specifying organ donation in an advance directive; or by filling out an organ donor card. Organ donor cards can be ordered from the United Network for Organ Sharing (UNOS) (804–782–4800 or http://www.unos.org). Persons younger than 18 years of age generally must have the consent of parents

EXHIBIT 25.5: THE BENEFITS OF AUTOPSIES

TO MEDICAL PRACTICE AND SCIENCE
Discover or elucidate new diseases
Explain unknown or unanticipated medical complications
Confirm, refute, or modify clinical diagnosis
Assist in the development/quality assurance of new technology, procedures, and therapy
Educate medical students, residents, other health practitioners
Continue physician education

TO THE JUDICIAL SYSTEM
Classify and explain sudden, unexpected and/or unnatural deaths

TO PUBLIC WELFARE
Identify infectious and contagious diseases
Provide data for vital health, death, and disease statistics
Identify and monitor occupational and environmental health hazards
Quality control and risk assessment in hospital practices
Provide a source of organs and tissues for medical and scientific purposes
Provide materials and hypotheses for research
Improve accuracy, and therefore usefulness, of vital statistics

TO THE DECEASED'S FAMILY
Assist grief process
Provide a means for tissue donation
Discover contagious diseases within the family
Assist in genetic counseling and identification of family health risks
Provide information for insurance/death benefits
Confirm, refute, or modify clinical diagnosis

From Iserson, K. V.: *Death to Dust: What Happens to Dead Bodies?,* 2nd ed., Table 4.1, page 143, COPYRIGHT 1994, 2001 by Kenneth V. Iserson. Reprinted by permission of Kenneth V. Iserson and Galen Press, Ltd., Tucson, AZ.

or guardians to sign an organ donor card. The Anatomical Gift Act of 2006 has been adopted by many states. Specifics of the act can be found at http://www.anatomicalgiftact.org. Some states will record the intent to donate an organ in a donor registry, which is a central repository of information regarding the intent to donate. When a potential donor is identified, the donor registry is contacted to determine the person's intent (Office of the Inspector General, 2002). Complete information on organ donation and times required for specific organ removal can be found at *The Organ Procurement and Transplantation Network* web page, http://www.optn.org or at Donate Life http://www.donatelife.net (OPTN, 2008).

Even with the proper documentation, the family may refuse to allow a relative's organs to be donated. In the United States, an estimated 12,000 individuals eligible for organ donation die each year, but less than half of those donate (www.kidney.org). Based on data retrieved in November 2008, the OPTN indicates there are more than 100,000 individuals registered for transplants in the United States, but unless the deceased has specified that he or she does not want his or her organs donated, the senior next of kin may donate all or part of a relative's body (Iserson, 2001).

Depending on what organ is being donated, the time for organ removal varies (Exhibit 25.6). Eyes must be removed within 24 hours of the death, but once they are in a preservative they can wait 10 to 14 days to be transplanted. Tissue (e.g., bone, skin, and tendons) can wait 24 hours to be removed from the deceased and can be preserved (depending on the method of preservation) for 3 to 5 years. If the body has been refrigerated within 4 hours of the death, saphenous veins can be harvested in the following 10 hours and heart valves within 24 hours (OPTN, 2008; Iserson, 2001).

Once the organs are removed from the body, it is ready for embalming or cremation. Embalming is the process by which the corpse is preserved and prepared for viewing; it is common for health reasons and protects mourners from being in the presence of a decaying body, but is not legally required (Shannon, 2006; Quested, 2003). "Basically, the embalmer is a creator of illusions—of pleasant illusions which banish the traces of suffering and death and present the deceased in an attitude of normal, restful sleep. In the practice of embalming this illusion is called a 'memory picture'" (Strub & Frederick, 1967, p. 133). There is no legal requirement that the body be embalmed, even if it is going to be viewed. The average cost for embalming is about $500 (Shannon, 2006; Iserson, 2001).

There are four embalming methods which all involve the injection of chemicals to preserve the body. Arterial embalming injects the chemicals into the blood vessels; cavity embalming injects the chest and abdomen; hypodermic embalming injects under the skin; and surface embalming is the application of chemicals

EXHIBIT 25.6: GUIDELINES FOR ORGAN AND TISSUE DONATION

ALL TISSUE AND ORGAN DONORS

- Death by brain or heart criteria (many centers only accept organ donation from those dead by brain criteria).
  - ☐ No malignancy other than a primary brain tumor without a shunt
  - ☐ No body-wide infection or injury to tissue
  - ☐ No known neurologic disease or AIDS risk factors
  - ☐ Resuscitated cardiac arrest (does not preclude donation)

TISSUE SPECIFIC (CAN BE RECOVERED UP TO 24 HOURS AFTER DEATH)

- Heart Valves
  - ☐ Age 3 months to 55 years with no prior heart surgery
  - ☐ No disease of heart valves
  - ☐ No injections into the heart
- Bone
  - ☐ Age 16–65 years
  - ☐ No steroid or insulin use
  - ☐ No collagen-vascular disease (e.g. lupus, rheumatoid arthritis)
  - ☐ No neurological disease.
- Corneas
  - ☐ Any age with no eye disease
  - ☐ No leukemia or retinoblastoma

ORGAN SPECIFIC

- Kidney
  - ☐ No kidney malfunction or infection
  - ☐ Generally younger than age 75 years
  - ☐ Allowable time from donor to recipient, 15–18 hours
- Heart
  - ☐ Generally younger than 65 years
  - ☐ No enlargement of the heart
  - ☐ Allowable time from donor to recipient, 4–5 hours
- Liver
  - ☐ No liver malfunction or cirrhosis
  - ☐ Generally younger than 65 years
  - ☐ Allowable time from donor to recipient, 12–18 hours
- Lung
  - ☐ Age 10–65 years
  - ☐ No lung disease
  - ☐ No fluid or infection in the lungs
  - ☐ Allowable time from donor to recipient, 5–6 hours
- Pancreas
  - ☐ Younger than 60 years
  - ☐ No pancreatic malfunction
  - ☐ Allowable time from donor to recipient, 12–15 hours

Adapted from Iserson, K. V.: *Death to Dust: What Happens to Dead Bodies?*, 2nd ed. Tucson, AZ: Galen Press, Ltd., 2001: 76 (Table 3.4).

in gel or liquid form to the body surface (Mayer & Taylor, 2005; Iserson, 2001). The size of the body, age, water content, temperature, decomposition, condition of the body's blood vessels, and premortem medication regime (e.g., gentamycin inactivates embalming fluid) will dictate the types, solution strengths, and injection rates of the embalming chemicals.

Primarily, formaldehyde and methyl alcohol are used as preservative chemicals because they change the cell proteins to prevent putrefaction. Embalmers inject these chemicals into the body using a centrifugal pump that pushes the fluids into the body with 5–10 psi of pressure. At the same time, blood and fluid are drained from the body by gravity or electrical aspirators. The embalmer will look for evidence that the chemicals have reached the hands and face and facilitate this process by massaging and repositioning the corpse. When the embalming fluid reaches the hands, they are placed in their final position over the chest or abdomen and the fingers are held together by using cyanoacrylate (e.g., Superglue). The muscles will gradually harden over the 8- to 12-hour period following the embalming; once they are set, the body's position will not be able to be moved.

If there is going to be a viewing at the funeral home, the body is prepared with the use of cosmetics. The hair is styled and the deceased is dressed. The body is then "casketed" in the coffin; typically, the right shoulder is lower than the left so the body does not look like it is flat on its back.

Cremation is an increasingly popular alternative to embalming and burial. Cremation is a process to reduce the "corpse and its container to ashes and small bone fragments" (Iserson, 2001, p. 236). Temperatures of between 1400 and 1800 degrees are used to burn the body, which evaporates water (70–80% of non-bone tissue), burns soft tissue, and reduces the average-sized adult to 4–8 pounds of ash (cremains). It takes about 2–3 hours to cremate a body, and what is left is grey ash and bone fragments. The cremains are then processed through an electric grinder to pulverize the bone fragments into an even consistency. The costs for this service ranges between $1,000 and $2,500 (Harris, 2007).

Prosthetic devices do not burn (e.g., dental gold, metal plates, and screws) and are removed with a magnet from the ashes. Pacemakers with lithium batteries will explode when burned and are removed before cremation. The body does not have to be embalmed before cremation nor does the family need to purchase a coffin. The only requirement is that the body be burned in a combustible container (e.g., cardboard or particleboard). Typically, there is a 24- to 48-hour waiting period after the death before cremation can legally take place.

Crematories are the facilities that contain the oven or retorts where the cremation will take place. It is becoming increasingly common for funeral homes to build crematories on the site and to offer a wide range of disposal options. There are no local, state, or federal laws that require a body to be cremated in a casket, but some facilities may require a container of some sort (Harris, 2007). Some cemeteries will have a columbarium for the interment of the urn containing the cremains. Memorial gardens are also available for scattering or burying the ashes and giving visitors a place to visit or place a marker. Some people will divide the cremains to bury, scatter, keep in an urn, share among family members, or even wear in specially designed jewelry. The cremains can be made into a diamond or sent up in a rocket.

Burning the body as a way of disposal dates back to prehistoric times. Our primitive ancestors believed they could return to their bodies and harm the living and therefore feared the dead; destroying the corpse removed that danger. Ancient civilizations believed that cremation would provide the dead with heat and warmth in the next world and protected the body from mutilation by animals or other humans. Native Americans believe that souls are conveyed to paradise by means of fire.

Peri-Death Religious and Cultural Rituals

Nursing care does not stop when a patient dies. There is tremendous variability around the world regarding the care of dead bodies and funeral practices. In India, there are funeral pyres; there are second burial rites by Indonesian hill tribes; and there is pervasiveness of embalming practices in the United States (Quested, 2003). Throughout the dying process, and particularly at the very end of life, the nurse must be aware of cultural and religious values, practices, and traditions of the patient and the family. Customs and rituals have tremendous significance in the healing process following death, and the grief response is often structured by these rituals. The nurse's role is to help the family carry out the rites and practices that provide solace and support. The nurse should be open-minded and understanding of the physical, psychosocial, and spiritual needs of the dying patient and his or her family and offer them respect and privacy (Purnell & Paulanka, 2008).

Rituals and customs vary based on a person's faith background or culture. For those of the Roman Catholic faith, priests will offer the Sacrament of the Anointing of the Sick, which in the past was called Extreme Unction or the Last Rites. The sacrament is for those who are seriously ill; the family, friends, and priest gather at the bedside to pray for healing. If it is God's will that the person not recover from his/her illness, then the prayer is that God will accompany the dying person toward the rewards of heaven (Miller, 1993; Green & Green, 2006). The nurse can ask the family if they would like the priest to be called. The priest would hear the patient's confession of sins, absolve the individual, and offer the Sacrament of the Sick. The comfort this ritual can bring to the dying Catholic and his or her family cannot be underestimated.

The preference of the Catholic Church is that the body of the deceased be present for the funeral rites; Masses with cremated remains present can be performed. When cremated remains are present, they must be contained in a "worthy vessel," placed on a table, or in the place normally occupied by the casket, and must be covered with a pall, that is, a heavy drape or cloth. The prayer of committal would read "earthly remains" in place of "body" (Archdiocese of San Antonio, 2002; Green & Green, 2006).

Out of respect for the human body, the cremains should to be treated with regard and buried in a grave or entombed in a mausoleum or columbarium. Scattering at sea, from the air or ground, or keeping the cremains at home are not considered reverent disposition. The Church still recommends burial or inurnment (placing the cremains in an urn) in a Catholic cemetery. Throughout the history of the Church, the Catholic cemetery has served as a visible sign of the faith community: a statement of continued belief in that everlasting life, even in death (Archdiocese of Chicago, 2008). Mourning traditionally has been expected to be kept to a minimum, with the view that people should "get on with their lives" (Bhungalia & Kemp, 2002).

In the Church of Jesus Christ of Latter-Day Saints (Mormons), church members of the same gender who have permission to be admitted into the temple are the ones who dress deceased members. The body is dressed in white undergarments that are covered by a robe, cap, and apron. Prior to burial, a white cap is placed on a deceased man, and a deceased woman's face is veiled (Iserson, 2001; Green & Green, 2006).

A Hindu who is dying may also request holy rites before death; readings and hymns from holy books are also comforting. Some may wish to lie on the floor to symbolize their closeness to the earth. A Hindu priest would administer the holy rites, which may include tying a thread around the wrists or neck of the dying person, sprinkling blessed water from the Ganges, of placing a sacred tulsi leaf in the dying person's mouth. Some Hindus may wish to return to India to die, especially to the holy city of Banaras. Many believe that to die in Banaras ensures a rebirth in heaven or even a release from continued rebirth. At a minimum, a Hindu will request to die at home because death in the hospital is very distressing. Only another Hindu should touch the dead body; if it is necessary for a non-Hindu to touch it, disposable gloves should be worn. Sacred threads, jewelry, and other religious objects should not be removed. The body should not be washed but only wrapped in a plain sheet. Washing of the body is a part of the funeral rite and is typically carried out only by family members; a mixture of milk and yogurt is used to cleanse the body. In India, a funeral would take place within 24 hours; adult Hindus are cremated although young children and infants may be buried (Green, 1989a, 1989b, 1989c; Green & Green, 2006).

The dying person of the Muslim faith may wish to lie or sit facing Mecca. If it is possible, the bed should be positioned to accommodate this wish. Those of Islamic faith believe the body belongs to God, so reasons for autopsies must be clear and legitimate. Likewise, organ donation and cremation are not acceptable. In Iran, embalming is not practiced, and a person is immediately placed in a casket if he or she has died during the day. If death occurs at night, a copy of the Qur'an should be placed on the chest of the deceased and a lighted candle at the head (Iserson, 2001; Purnell & Paulanka, 2008); the body is watched during the night by a person reading the Qur'an.

Following the death, non-Muslims should wear gloves when touching the body. If there is no family available to carry out postmortem care, the nurse should wear gloves in administering care of the body. However, the body is not washed and hair and nails are not cut; the eyes are closed. According to Green and Green (2006), the normal Muslim procedure is that the body is straightened immediately after death. This is done by flexing the elbows, shoulders, knees and hips first, before straightening them. This is thought to ensure that the body does not stiffen, thus facilitating its washing and shrouding. Turn the head towards the right shoulder. This is so the body can be buried with the face towards Mecca.

The body is then covered with a sheet that cloaks the whole body until a Muslim is available to perform the ritual bath. The ritual bath includes washing the body three times, first with lotus water, and then camphor water, and last with plain water (Iserson, 2001). This bathing is done from head to toe and front to back. All body orifices are closed and packed with cotton (to prevent body-fluid leakage that is considered unclean). Prayers from the Qur'an are read (especially verses of hope and acceptance) and the body is wrapped in a special cotton shroud. This shroud is made from three pieces of white unsewn cloth, 9 yards long, which are wrapped above, below, and around the midsection. Muslims are buried in a brick- or cement-lined grave with the head facing east toward Mecca. In Iran, the body is buried directly in the earth with the shroud removed from the face and one side of the face turned to be in contact with the earth (Purnell & Paulanka, 2008).

When those of the Jewish faith are dying, they may want to hear or recite special prayers, such as the Shema, which confirms one's belief in one God; or psalms, in particular Psalm 23 ("The Lord is my Shepherd"). Jews also have a personal confession prayer called *Viddui*, which is said by the dying person or by another individual when death is imminent (Purnell & Paulanka, 2008). Observant Jews are often buried in shrouds called *takhrikhim*. These are plain white cotton garments that are generally hand-sewn and made without buttons, zippers, or fasteners of any kind and cover the entire body (Hill & Daniels, 2007).

The person may also wish to hold the written prayer in his or her hand (Green, 1989d). A relative remains with the dying person to ensure the soul does not leave the body when she or he is alone; it is a sign of disrespect to leave the body alone. Even after death, the body is not left alone until the funeral, so that the body is not left defenseless (Purnell & Paulanka, 2008). The eyes should be closed after death, preferably by a child of the deceased; the body should be covered and left untouched (Green, 1989e). Autopsies are not permitted, although organ transplants are. The body should be handled as little as possible by non-Jews, and burial should take place within 24 hours. Burial is usually only delayed for the Sabbath. Embalming and cosmetics are not part of traditional practice. Orthodox Jews are always buried, although Jews who are more liberal may select cremation. The body is wrapped in a shroud and a prayer shawl. The casket is made of wood, so that the body and the casket decay at the same rate. There is no wake or viewing of the body. At the funeral, the *Kaddish,* the *prayer* for the dead, is said, which praises God and reaffirms faith (Purnell & Paulanka, 2008).

For those who are Buddhist, an important consideration is the state of mind at the time of death; dying thoughts and desires are crucial in determining the next rebirth of the deceased. A Buddhist monk or minister should be notified at the time of death to chant verses to the dead and the family. Buddhists may be cremated because Buddha was cremated (Purnell & Paulanka, 2008). The length of time between death and burial can vary between 3 and 7 days depending on the Buddhist tradition. Family members plan the burial; the tradition is to wear white to the funeral.

In terms of differences based on cultural backgrounds, Cuban Americans who are dying are usually attended by large groups of family and friends. Depending on their religious affiliation, a Catholic priest, Protestant minister, rabbi, or *santero* may be called to perform death rites. For followers of *santero,* these rites may include animal sacrifice, ceremonial displays, and chants (Purnell & Paulanka, 2008). After the death, candles are lit to light the path of the spirit to the afterlife. Burial is the common custom although there is no restriction to cremation.

African Americans generally prefer to have people with terminal illness cared for in the home, but prefer death to occur in the hospital for fear of bad luck being brought to the home. Family members and extended family stay by the bedside of the dying patient, as they believe God is ultimately in control of outcomes. Grief is expressed openly and publicly. Autopsy is acceptable, although organ donation is not typical. Death does not end the connection to the family (Purnell & Paulanka, 2008; American Geriatrics Society [AGS], 2004).

Mexican Americans may take turns sitting vigil over the dying person; dying in a hospital is not desirable because the spirit may become lost. Spiritual amulets, rosary beads, or other religious artifacts are kept near the patient. Typically, organ donation or autopsy is not allowed. When death occurs, family and friends will often come long distances for the funeral. A *velorio* is a festive watch of the deceased body before burial. Traditional families may exhibit hyperkinetic shaking and seizure-like activity called *ataque de nervios,* which is a way to release emotions related to grieving. The family may erect altars in their homes in honor of the anniversary of their relative's death and may include candles, decorations, and having the deceased's favorite meal at a graveside picnic (Purnell & Paulanka, 1998).

Native Americans have different traditions in each tribe. There is a belief that the spirit of the deceased remains where the person has died; therefore family may not want the person to die at home. At the same time, it is considered inappropriate for the person to die alone. If the person dies at home, the house must be abandoned or a ceremony is held to cleanse it. Families gather together at the time of death and material possessions are dispersed. When a person dies, a cleansing ceremony is performed or else the spirit of the deceased may try to take over someone else's spirit. Those who work with the dead also must have a ceremonial cleansing to protect themselves from the dead person's spirit. No embalming is done; the deceased are buried in sacred ground with their shoes on the wrong feet, rings on their index fingers, and with many gifts surrounding them; or the body is cremated (Purnell & Paulanka, 2008).

For Appalachians, a death is an important event, even for extended family. The funeral is a significant social occasion and family and friends will come great distances to attend. The body is displayed for long periods of time so that all can see the body who wish to. The deceased is buried in his or her best clothes and some people have custom-made clothes for burial. At the funeral home, personal possessions are displayed and it is common to bury these items with the person. Gravesites are typically on hillsides because of the fear they will be flooded out in low-lying areas (Purnell & Paulanka, 2008).

Subgroups from China, Vietnam, Laos, Thailand, and Burma together are called the Hmong. The Hmong believe that proper burial and worship of the dead and other ancestors directly affects the safety, health, and prosperity of the family. The belief is that the spiritual world coexists with the physical world and that the spirits are able to influence human life. The preference is to die at home because they believe their soul will wander for all of eternity without a resting place if they were to die elsewhere. Some groups believe that death should take place in the hospital so as not to bring bad luck into the home. Autopsy and cremation are acceptable practices to some families. For these groups, burial occurs in the afternoon.

The Chinese will place a coin in the deceased's mouth so that the deceased has money to pay anyone who interferes in the journey. Additionally, symbolic money may be burned to signify the transmission of wealth to the celestial bank, and has recently translated to burning symbolic paper items which includes houses, cell phones, and cars (Chung & Wegars, 2005). In northern China, the body is placed in burial clothes, and an unpadded quilt is used as a shroud. The face is covered with cloth or paper and the feet are tied with colored string. The wife or oldest son wipes the eyes of the deceased with cotton floss before the coffin is closed. Instead of being buried immediately after the funeral, the body may be stored so that a husband and wife can be buried together (Iserson, 2001).

The Japanese bathe their dead, shave some of the hair, and dress the person in white. The deceased wears a ceremonial hat or triangular piece of white paper tied to the forehead and may also include white socks and white gloves. Special favorite items may be placed in the coffin (Green & Green, 2006). Koreans use perfume to wash the body and dress the body in silk or hemp clothes tied in seven places that correlate with the seven stars in the Ursa Major constellation (Iserson, 2001).

Literature is extremely limited related to Wiccans, Pagans, and Nature Spiritualists (WPNS) and end-of-life preferences. The passage from this life is generally referred to as "into the Summerland." It is important to include priests, priestesses, and death midwives in the dying process to provide herbal therapies and complementary care. In preparation for death, Pagans may perform rituals or prayers in a circle surrounding the patient. Individuals may sing, pray, or chant, focusing energy on the patient. Alternative healing methods include the use of crystals and stones, Reiki, sound healing, massage, music, and color therapy. Generally, the patient's coven, priest, priestess, or chosen family member will administer last rites. The death midwife may help the family with cleansing, anointing, and dressing the body (Smith-Stoner & Young, 2007).

PERI-DEATH 3: THE FUNERAL AS A CEREMONY OF DEATH

Across cultures, people accept a responsibility to care for, respect, and honor their dead. The funeral can serve to dispose of the dead body, transmit the body to the afterlife, and enable the bereaved community and family to adjust to their new role in society (Brooks-Gordon, Ebetehaj, Herring, Johnson, & Richards, 2007). For most ethnic groups and religious groups, the process of physically preparing the body for the funeral and burial is handled by persons outside the family, but includes some form of preparation for the afterlife. The undertaker—a person who "undertook" the responsibility to keep the body safe and make the funeral arrangements—has been a part of society since ancient times. The general public interchangeably refers to the person who prepares the body for burial and conducts all aspects of the funeral service as the undertaker,

mortician, embalmer, or funeral director (Iserson, 2001; Green & Green, 2006).

In modern society, funeral directors may coordinate all the details of the funeral for the family, but are also expected to manage the survivor's distress. They supervise preparation of the body for viewing or burial, oversee embalming procedures if embalming is desired, coordinate cremation planning, instruct and support the pallbearers, arrange the transportation of the family and the deceased to the cemetery, place death notices in the newspaper, and otherwise facilitate the family's burial decisions. Most funeral directors in the United States have at least a bachelor's degree, and 51% of current mortuary science graduates are women. Though funeral direction was historically a family business, this is no longer true (Iserson, 2001; NFDA, 2008; Habenstein & Lamers, 2007). Funeral homes employ embalmers, cosmetologists, hairdressers, and hearse and limousine drivers.

The funeral director may orchestrate all aspects of the funeral, but it is not mandated (NFDA, 2008). Those who work in the funeral industry know that the funeral must be perfectly organized and executed because they will not get a second chance to make things right. It was originally believed that the funeral held merely theological value, but for many people the funeral is one of the first steps of successful grieving. The funeral is *"of* the person who has died. . . . It is *for* those who survive" (Raether, 1993, p. 211).

For families that have a wake, this is the first component of postdeath ritual. It may be one of the few times the entire family will reassemble for an event. It is a time for family and friends to view the dead body and to pay their final respects. Seeing the dead body emphasizes the fact that the person is dead; declining to see the body may delay grieving. "I was recently again reminded of how valuable and legitimate a funeral service can be. I accompanied a friend to the funeral of his mother. She had died of a chronic and wasting illness and I had been present at her deathbed. My friend experienced a deep and profound consolation seeing his mother with the lines of suffering erased from her face and lying at peace" (Raether, 1993, p. 211).

The second component of postdeath rituals is the funeral. It is a ceremonial service typically consisting of music, prayers, poetry, eulogies, and it may be part of a funeral Mass where Communion is celebrated. Some people will plan their funerals before they die, which can be comforting to those who are dying as well as their families (Raether, 1993; Shannon, 2006).

The committal service is the concluding funeral rite. It is the final act of caring for the deceased and is celebrated at the grave, tomb, or crematorium, and has seen little change during the past century. Those changes that have occurred reflect compassion for the bereaved (Habenstein & Lamers, 2007). This service is a "symbolic demonstration that the kind of relationship which has existed between the mourner and the deceased is now at an end" (Raether, 1993, p. 212).

Eight specific therapeutic values have been assigned to the funeral process as delineated by Raether (1993, p. 209). First, the "therapy of direct expression" denotes that the funeral furnishes the setting and opportunity for the bereaved to express their grief physically. Funerals offer "therapy of language" by providing the bereaved an opportunity to talk about what has happened, voice their feelings, and begin to feel relief in the telling.

The "therapy of sharing" is the coming together of the family and significant others to provide emotional and physical support to each other. Time spent with the bereaved is an important aspect of burying the dead. Immersion in the many aspects of the funeral process also encompasses the "therapy of activity." The routine of greeting mourners at the funeral home or interacting with those who offer their sympathy prevents the bereaved from withdrawing and allowing their energy to be focused in the immediate postdeath period. The funeral also provides the "therapy of ceremony" that is both glorifying and ennobling. The liturgical aspect of the funeral ceremony encompasses the views of the meaning of life and the nature of life hereafter. Given that accepting the reality of the death is difficult for many people, the "therapy of viewing" establishes a final and amended view of the deceased. This revised image replaces those composed during the illness or at the time of death and may bring comfort to the mourner. Finally, the "therapy of suffering" addresses the guilt that mourners may be experiencing and provides the occasion to verbalize what had been left unsaid previously.

Another important aspect of the postdeath experience for the bereaved is the formation of a new identity within their community. The role of widow, of no longer having a child, or of one who has lost a parent brings with it a change in how the bereaved interact and correspond to society at large. Social groups may shrink, volunteer opportunities may be lost, and favorite activities may be forfeited due to the loss of the deceased. Nurses need to be aware of the difficulties inherent in these role shifts and offer alternatives and community-support referrals during this transitional stage.

ANALYSES OF THE PERI-DEATH EXPERIENCE

As with any application of the nursing process, the nurse should evaluate the effectiveness of the interventions that have been utilized. In the case of peri-death nursing, there is no way to obtain objective data from the older adult who has just died to determine the efficacy of care. Although family members can be surveyed regarding their experiences, they can truly only report their perceptions as viewed through their own lens. In

reality, guilt, remorse, or grief may cloud this lens.

Ternestedt, Andershed, Eriksson, and Johansson (2002) propose seven questions that the nurse can use to perform a retrospective analysis of the quality of patient care given at the end of life. These questions are as follows:

1) Did the patient receive adequate symptom relief and was the care adequate?
2) Could the patient make his or her own decisions during the final phase of his or her life?
3) Could the patient maintain important social relationships to the end of his or her life?
4) Could the patient maintain an acceptable self-image and feeling of personal worth during the final phase of his or her life?
5) Were there signs of conflict resolution and did the patient sum up his or her life?
6) Did the patient accept the fact that death was near, or did he or she struggle against death?
7) Did the patient have a very good death? A good death? A bad death? (Ternestedt et al., 2002, p. 157).

These questions should be asked by the healthcare practitioners after each person has died to attain knowledge about the care of dying older adults and determine areas where improvement can be made.

> **Case Study conclusion:** After having assessed Mrs. Jerion, I sat next to her husband, who was at the bedside holding her hand. I said, "You have been married for a long time." "Yes," he said, "50 years last June." "How did you meet?" I asked. And he began to talk . . . he told me funny stories about their courtship, how her father did not want her to date him . . . about their life together and raising their children. As their children and their children's spouses sat and listened to him reminisce, Mrs. Jerion would occasionally smile. When he stopped talking, I said that it sounded to me like they had had a wonderful time together and a good life. He agreed, and hugged his wife. As I left, his daughter thanked me for taking care of her father, that this was more talking than he had done in a quite a while. She felt that they could continue the conversation with him and help him to process the loss of the bride he loved so much.
>
> Mrs. Jerion died that night, surrounded by her loving family and the man for whose sake she had defied her father. It was a peaceful death for everyone involved.

CONCLUSION

When the nurse is providing end-of-life care, the focus of care is the dying older adult and their family. When the death occurs, the work of the nurse is not over because the family is still in need of nursing care and interventions. The goal of postdeath nursing care is to promote optimal adjustment and to help the family and significant others with the tasks of bereavement (see chapter 11). Bereavement is an important developmental stage; the nurse should provide interventions that offer the opportunity for healing and growth, a redefinition of self, and opportunities to make new plans. Follow-up with the family is important during the bereavement period. The nurse should encourage memorial rituals commemorating the deceased's life and death. Unique opportunities exist in peri-death nursing to support the dying patient and the patient's family in making what is a painful and difficult process one that is also priceless.

EVIDENCE-BASED PRACTICE

Walling, A. M., Brown-Saltzman, K., Barry, T., Jue Quan, R., & Wenger, N.S. (2008). Assessment of implementation of an order protocol for end-of-life symptom management. *Journal of Palliative Medicine (11)*6, pp. 857–865.

Objectives. Use of end-of-life management protocols have been shown to improve symptoms at the end of life. End-of-life symptoms have not typically been managed well due to knowledge deficits and concerns related to double effect. The study was designed to institute a protocol that integrated palliative care principles, models, pharmacologic principles, and ancillary interventions to determine benefits and limitations of palliative care order sets.

Design. Feasibility assessment interviews with physicians and nurses using an "end-of-life symptom management order (ESMO)" (p. 858).

Setting. Physicians and nurses in a quaternary care medical center were asked to complete a brief self-administered instrument or were interviewed to answer questions relating to implementation of the ESMO protocol.

Participants. Eighty-nine physicians and 91 nurses who cared for 127 patients during a 342-day study were surveyed.

Measurements. The survey instrument asked questions that included items related to symptom management, opiate dosing, time spent discussing end-of-life issues, and appropriateness of the EMSO protocol. Open-ended responses were also encouraged to determine timeliness of the implementation of the protocol. Pilot questions were given to residents to ensure 10-minute survey completion.

Results. EMSO protocols are identified as important to clinicians providing end-of-life care. One of the most common concerns of nurses is opiate use at the end of life, and hospital protocols for unrestricted opiate use are feasible. Timely implementation of the protocols were hindered, and it is recommended that advance care planning efforts be initiated sooner to be able to implement protocols to assist patients with symptom management.

Conclusions. Protocols for end-of-life care are useful but are only one means of improving care. Advanced care planning and clinician training related to increased confidence in opiate administration are still crucial. Evaluation of the EMSO protocol outcomes has not occurred.

EVIDENCE-BASED PRACTICE

Bailey, F. A., Ferguson, L., Williams, B. R., Woodby, L. L., Redden, D. T., Durham, R. M., et al. (2008). Palliative care intervention for choice and use of opioids in the last hours of life. *Journals of Gerontology Series A-Biological Sciences and Medical Sciences, 63*(9), 974–978.

Objectives. Pain and dyspnea are the most common symptoms that a patient who is at the end of his or her life will experience; the most effective drug to manage these symptoms are opioid medications. This study sought to document the effectiveness of a physician-led Inpatient Comfort Care Program in the management of pain and dyspnea for dying patients in an acute care setting of a VA hospital.

Design. This pre-intervention/post-intervention trial followed actively dying patients in the last 72 hours of life. Data (derived from the Computerized Patient Record System) from patients who had died in the 6-months prior to the start of the Comfort Care Program were compared to those in a 6-month period after the program was fully functional.

Setting. Acute care setting of a VA hospital.

Intervention. The intervention included staff education to better identify actively dying patients and a Comfort Care Order Set to guide care in the last hours of life.

Participants. Data abstracted from computerized medical records of 191 veterans who died during a 6-month period before ($N = 98$) and after ($N = 93$) the intervention were used to examine changes in choice and amount of medication administered in the last 3 days of life.

Measurements. Data collected included orders for opioid medications (type and amount), and medication administration records to determine if the medications were given. Medication administration was determined by totaling the doses of all opioids given and converting the doses to oral morphine equivalents using a standard equianalgesic conversion table.

Results. Findings show a significant increase in orders, specifically for morphine, from 47.4% to 81.7% ($p < .001$). Orders for hydromorphone or oxycodone did not increase significantly, and no patients had orders for meperidine or codeine. There was an increase in the administration of opioids from 16.7% to 73.0% ($p < .001$). The amount of opioid administered (in oral morphine equivalents) increased from 31.9 mg/72 hours pre-intervention to 52.9 mg/72 hours post-intervention ($p = .12$).

Conclusions. The results indicate that the availability of morphine as a preferred opioid and the number of patients who received opioid medication during the last 3 days of life increased after introduction of the inpatient palliative care program.

REFERENCES

American Academy of Hospice and Palliative Medicine. (AAHPM) (2006). *Statement on artificial nutrition and hydration near the end of life.* Retrieved August 7, 2008, from http://www.aahpm.org/positions/nutrition.html

American Geriatrics Society. (2004). *Older African–Americans.* In *Doorway thoughts: Cross-cultural health care for older adults* (Vol. 1, pp. 43–53). Sudbury, MA: Jones and Bartlett.

Archdiocese of Chicago. (2008). *Catholic cemeteries.* Retrieved November 11, 2008, from http://www.catholiccemeterieschicago.org/sacredplaces.php

Archdiocese of San Antonio. (2002). *Cremation for catholics? Catholic cemeteries and mausoleums.* Retrieved July 15, 2004, from http://www.catholiccemeteriesofsa.org/index.htm

Bailey, F. A., Ferguson, L., Williams, B. R., Woodby, L. L., Redden, D. T., Durham, R. M., et al. (2008). Palliative care intervention for choice and use of opioids in the last hours of life. *Journal of Gerontology Series A-Biological Sciences and Medical Sciences, 63*(9), 974–978.

Bavin, L. (2007). Artificial rehydration in the last days of life: Is it beneficial? *International Journal of Palliative Nursing, 13*(9), 445–449.

Beale, E., Baile, W. F., & Aaron, J. (2005). Silence is not golden: Communicating with children dying from cancer. *Journal of Clinical Oncology, 23*(15), 3629–3631.

Beattie, S. (2006). Hands on help: Post-mortem care. *RN, 69*(10), 24ac1–4.

Berger, J. T., DeRenzo, E. G., & Schwarz, J. (2008). Surrogate decision making: Reconciling ethical theory and clinical practice. *Annals of Internal Medicine, 149,* 48–53.

Birchenall, J., & Streight, E. (1997). *Home care aide.* St. Louis, MO: Mosby.

Bruce, S. D., Hendrix, C. C., & Gentry, J. H. (2006). Palliative sedation in end-of-life care. *Journal of Hospice and Palliative Nursing, 8*(6), 320–327.

Craig, G. (2000). On withholding nutrition and hydration in the terminally ill. In D. Dickenson (Ed.). *Death, dying and bereavement.* London: Open University Press/Sage.

Benzein, E. G., & Saveman, B. I. (2008). Health-promoting conversations about hope and suffering with couples in palliative care. *International Journal of Palliative Nursing, 14*(9), 439–445.

Bhungalia, S., & Kemp, C. (2002). (Asian) Indian health beliefs and practices related to end of life. *Journal of Hospice and Palliative Nursing, 4*(1), 54–58.

Brooks-Gordon, B., Ebetehaj, F., Herring, J., Johnson, M., & Richards, M., (2007). *Death rites and rights.* London: Hart

Center for Medicare and Medicaid Services. (CMS) (2002). *Healthcare industry and market update.* Retrieved November 13, 2008, from http://www.cms.hhs.gov/CapMarketUpdates/Downloads/hcimu101002.pdf

Chung, S. F. & Wegars, P. (2005). *Chinese–American death rituals; Respecting the ancestors.* Lanham, MD: AltaMira Press:

Cimino, J. (2003). The role of nutrition in hospice and palliative care of the cancer patient. *Topics in Clinical Nutrition, 18,*154–161.

Drake, R., Frost, J., & Collins, J. J. (2003). The symptoms of dying children. *Journal of Pain and Symptom Management, 26*(1), 594–603.

Emanuel, L., Ferris, F. D., von Gunten, C. F., & Von Roenn, J. H. (2008). The last hours of living: Practical advice for clinicians [Electronic Version]. *EPEC™-O: Education in Palliative and End-of-life Care for Oncology. (Module 6: Last Hours of Living © The EPEC Project™, Chicago, IL, 2005,* 18. Retrieved August 11, 2008 from http://www.medscape.com/viewprogram/5808

Ethier, A. M. (2007). Palliative care in childhood terminal illness. In M. J. Hockenberry (Ed.). *Wong's nursing care of infants and children* (8th ed., pp. 958–988). St. Louis: Mosby.

Ferrell, B. R., Virani, R., & Grant, M. (1999). Analysis of end of life content in nursing textbooks. *Oncology Nursing Forum, 26,* 869–876.

Field, M., & Cassel, C. (1997). *Approaching death: Improving care at the end of life.* Washington, DC: National Academy Press.

Gates, R. A., & Fink, R. M. (1997). *Oncology nursing secrets.* St. Louis, MO: Mosby.

Green, J. (1989a). Death with dignity: Baha'i Faith. *Nursing Times, 85*(10), 50–51.

Green, J. (1989b). Death with dignity: Buddhism. *Nursing Times, 85*(9), 40–41.

Green, J. (1989c). Death with dignity: Hinduism. *Nursing Times, 85*(6), 50–51.

Green, J. (1989d). Death with dignity: Islam. *Nursing Times, 85*(5), 56–57.

Green, J. (1989e). Death with dignity: Judaism. *Nursing Times, 85*(8), 65–65.

Green, J. & Green, M. (2006) Dealing *with death* (2nd ed.). London & Philadelphia: Jessica Kingsley.

Habenstein, R. W., & Lamers, W. M. (2007). *The history of American funeral directing.* (6th ed.). Brookfield, WI: National Funeral Directors Association.

Harris, M. (2007). *Grave matters: A journey through the modern funeral industry to a natural way of burial.* New York: Scribner.

Heming, D., & Colmer, A. (2003). Care of dying patients. *Nursing Standard, 8*(10), 47–56.

Hill, J., & Daniels, P. (2007). *Life events and rites of passage.* Detroit: Omnigraphics.

Horn, L. W. (1992, March/April). Terminal dyspnea: A hospice approach. *American Journal of Hospice and Palliative Care,* 24–32.

Hoyal, C., Grant, J., Chamberlain, F., Cox, R., & Campbell, T. (2002). Improving the management of breathlessness using a clinical effectiveness programme. *International Journal of Palliative Nursing, 8*(2), 78–87.

Iserson, K. V. (2001). *Death to dust: What happens to dead bodies?* Tucson, AZ: Galen Press.

Kastenbaum, R., & Kastenbaum, B., (Eds.). (1989). *Encyclopedia of death.* Phoenix, AZ: Oryx Press.

Kaye, P. (2003). *A–Z pocket book of symptom control.* Northampton, MA: EBL.

LaDuke, S. (2001). Terminal dyspnea and palliative care. *American Journal of Nursing, 101*(11), 26–31.

Lynch, M., & Dahlin, C.M. (2007). The national consensus project and national quality forum preferred practices in care of the imminently dying: Implications for nursing. *Journal of Hospice and Palliative Nursing, 9*(6), 316–322.

Lynn, J., & Harrold, J. (2006). *Handbook for mortals: Guidance for people facing serious illness.* [Electronic version] New York: Oxford University Press.

Macleod, A., & Whitehead, L. (1997) Dysgraphia and terminal delirium. *Palliative Medicine, 11*(2), 127–132.

Macleod, A. D. (2006). The management of terminal delirium. *Indian Journal of Palliative Care, 12*(1), 22–28.

Mayer, R. G., & Taylor, J. (2005). *Embalming: History, theory and practice*(4th ed.). New York: McGraw-Hill.

Miller, E. J. (1993). A Roman Catholic view of death. In K. Doka & J. D. Morgan (Eds.), *Death and spirituality*(pp. 33–50). Amityville, NY: Baywood.

National Funeral Directors Association. (NFDA). (2008). Retrieved November 8, 2008 from http://www.nfda.org/

Office of the Inspector General. (2002). *Organ donor registries executive report # OEI-01-01-00350.* Retrieved July 15, 2004, from http://oig.hhs.gov/oei

OPTN (2008). *The organ procurement and transplantation network.* Retrieved December 6, 2008 from http://www.optn.org.

Owens, D. P. (2006). Management of upper airway secretions at the end of life. *Journal of Hospice and Palliative Nursing, 8*(1), 12–14.

Panke, J. (2003). Difficulties in managing pain at the end of life. *Journal of Hospice and Palliative Nursing, 5*(2), 83–90.

Pattison, N. (2008). Care of patients who have died. *Nursing Standard, 22*(28), 42–48.

Pitorak, E. F. (2003). Care at the time of death: How nurses can make the last hours of life a richer, more comfortable experience. *American Journal of Nursing, 103*(7), 42–52.

Purnell, L. D., & Paulanka, B. J. (1998). *Transcultural health care: A culturally competent approach* (2nd ed.), Philadelphia: Davis.

Purnell, L. D. & Paulanka, B. J. (2008). *Transcultural health care: A culturally competent approach* (3rd ed.). Philadelphia: Davis.

Quested, B. (2003). Nursing care of dead bodies: A discursive analysis of last offices. *Journal of Advanced Nursing, 41,* 553–560.

Raether, H. C. (1993). Rituals, beliefs, and grief. In K. Doka & J. D. Morgan (Eds.). *Death and spirituality*(pp. 207–216). Amityville, NY: Baywood.

Rushton, C. H. (2008). Treating distress at the end of life: The principle of double effect. *AACN Advanced Critical Care, 19*(3), 340–344.

Mitra, J. K., Mishra, S., & Bhatnagar, S. (2006). Advanced head and neck cancer: Care beyond cure. *Internet Journal of Pain Symptom Control and Palliative Care, 4*(2). Retrieved from OVID database November 12, 2008.

Shannon, J. B. (2006). *Death and dying sourcebook* (2nd ed.). Detroit: Omnigraphics

Smith-Stoner, M. R., & Young, N. C. (2007). Spiritual needs of Wiccan, Pagan, and Nature Spiritualists at end of life. *Journal of Hospice and Palliative Nursing 9*(5), 279–286.

Soden, K., Hoy, A., Hoy, W., & Clelland, S. (2002). Artificial hydration during the last week of life in patients dying in a district general hospital. *Palliative Medicine, 16,* 542–543.

Sorrentino, S. A. (1999). *Assisting with patient care.* St. Louis, MO: Mosby.

Spector, N., Connolly, M. A., & Carlson, K. K., (2007). Dyspnea: Applying research to bedside practice. *AACN Advanced Critical Care, 18*(1), 45–60.

Strub, C. G., & Frederick, L. G. (1967). *The principles and practice of embalming.* Dallas, TX: Frederick.

Sumner, L. H. (2006). Pediatric care: The hospice perspective. In B. R. Ferrell & N. Coyle (Eds.), *Textbook of palliative nursing* (2nd ed.). New York: Oxford University Press.

Suter, P. M., Rogers, J. A. & Strack, C. (2008). Artificial nutrition and hydration for the terminally ill: A reasoned approach. *Home Healthcare Nurse, 26*(1), 23–29.

Tarzian, A. J. (2000). Caring for dying patients who have air hunger. *Journal of Nursing Scholarship, 32,* 137–143.

Ternestedt, B., Andershed, B., Eriksson, M., & Johansson, I. (2002). A good death. *Journal of Hospice and Palliative Nursing, 4*(3), 153–160.

Transition rituals: A faith-by-faith guide to rites for the deceased. Retrieved August 16 , 2009, from http://www.beliefnet.com/Health/Health-Support/Grief-and-Loss/2001/05/Transition-Rituals.aspx

Uniform Anatomical Gift Act. (2007). Retrieved November 9, 2008 from http://www.anatomicalgiftact.org

Walling, A. M., Brown-Saltzman, K., Barry, T., Jue Quan, R., & Wenger, N. S. (2008). Assessment of implementation of an order protocol for end-of-life symptom management. *Journal of Palliative Medicine, 11*(6), 857–865.

Wasserman, L. (2008). Respectful death: A model for end-of-life care. *Clinical Journal of Oncology Nursing, 12*(4), 621–626.

Worden, W. (1992). *Grief counseling and grief therapy* (2nd ed.). London: Rutledge.

Zerwekh, J.V. (2006). *Nursing care at the end of life: Palliative care for patients and families.* Philadelphia: Davis.

Health-Care Provider Information Sheet

SYMPTOM RELIEF KIT

Pain or dyspnea:*

- Morphine solution 0.25–0.5 ml (20 mg/ml solution) PO/SL q 2 PRN, may increase up to 1–2 ml q 1–2 h PRN
- Titration:
  □ May increase current opioid dose by 25–50% every 24 hrs PRN moderate pain
  □ May increase current opioid dose by 50–100% every 24 hrs PRN severe pain
  □ If pain still not adequately controlled w/current opiate and/or patient requiring 3 or more rescue doses per day, may equianalgesically adjust the dose of the current opiate pain medication every 24 hrs using the following calculation:
  Add the 24 hrs total rescue dose + total 24 hr = new 24 hr dose
  Adjust the "rescue dose" or "breakthrough dose" using the new 24 hr dose

Loud, wet respirations, or excessive secretions:

- Hyoscyamine (Levsin) 0.125 mg (1–2 tablets) PO/SL q 6 hr PRN.
- OR Scopolamine 0.5mg gel apply 1 syringe to neck below ear q 4 hrs PRN TOPICAL – apply to neck/below ear
- OR Scopolamine patch 1.5 mg (start with one patch, can increase up to three every 72 hrs TOPICAL)

Unrelieved respiratory fluid accumulation:

Furosemide (Lasix) 40 mg IV/ IM/PO/SC. May repeat.

Nausea or vomiting:

- Prochlorperazine 25 mg suppository PR q 8 h PRN. Compazine Spansule 10–15 mg q 12 hrs or Compazine 10mg q 6 hrs PO
- Compazine 25 mg suppository q 6 hrs PR
- Phenergan 12.5–25 mg q 4–6 hrs PRN PO

- Zofran 4 mg q 6–8 hrs PRN PO
- Tigan suppository 200 mg q 6 hrs PR
- Scopolamine 0.5 mg gel q 8 hrs TOPICAL to decrease nausea – apply to neck/below ear

Severe agitation or restlessness:

- Determine if client is in pain and treat accordingly;
- Determine if client is constipated or having urinary retention, take appropriate action;
- If agitation persists, administer Pentobarbital suppository PR q 6 h PRN
- Ativan 0.25–1 mg q 4 hrs PRN PO
- Xanax 0.25–0.5 mg q 6–8 hrs PRN PO

Temperature elevation

- Tylenol 325 mg 1 or 2 q 4–6 hrs PO PRN temperature elevation 101
- Ibuprofen 200–800 mg q 4 hours PRN PO

Candidiasis

- Nystatin oral suspension 5 cc swish and swallow qid PO
- Diflucan 100 mg bid PO x 3 days then qd x 10–14 days PRN candidiasis or Diflucan (Fluconazole) 100 mg troche qd x 3–5 days PO

Mouth care

- Artificial Saliva QS PRN PO; BVM (Benadryl, Viscous Lidocaine, Maalox 1:1:1) 1 tsp swish and swallow q 4 hrs PRN oral scores PO
- Hydrogen peroxide 1.5%, Deoxyl-D-Glucose (DDG) 1%, Dexamethazone 1% swish and spit 3–4 x qd PRN oral scores
- Lemon glycerine swabs PRN
- Pilocarpine 2 mg lollipop may suck on 1–2 qd PRN dry mouth PO

*Clients taking opioids for pain will need to increase their usual morphine dose (for breakthrough pain) for effective treatment of dyspnea.